Parkinson's Disease and Movement Disorders

Under the Banner of
Parkinson's Disease and Movement Disorder Society

Parkinson's Disease and Movement Disorders

Under the Banner of
Parkinson's Disease and Movement Disorder Society

Second Edition

Editor

Kalyan B Bhattacharyya MD DM MAMS FIAN FRCP (Edin)
Editor-in-Chief (IAN Yearbook Neurology)
Former Professor and Head
Department of Neurology, RG Kar Medical College and Hospital
Kolkata, West Bengal, India

Co-Editors

Jimmy A Lalkaka MD DM (Neuro)
Consultant Neurologist, Associate Professor
Department of Neurology
Bombay Hospital Institute of Medical Sciences
Mumbai, Maharashtra, India

Charulata Savant Sankhla MD DNB
Faculty, Department of Neurology
PD Hinduja National Hospital
Mumbai, Maharashtra, India

Pettarusp Murzban Wadia MD DNB (Med) DM DNB (Neuro)
Clinical Fellowship Movement Disorders University of Toronto
Consultant Neurologist and Movement Disorder Specialist
Department of Neurology, Jaslok Hospital and Research Centre
Mumbai, Maharashtra, India

Foreword

Niall Patrick Quinn

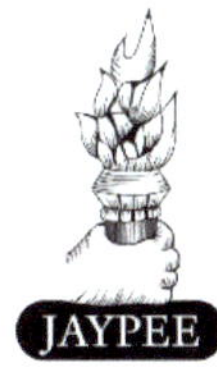

JAYPEE BROTHERS MEDICAL PUBLISHERS
The Health Sciences Publisher
New Delhi | London

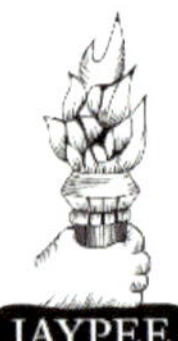

Jaypee Brothers Medical Publishers (P) Ltd

Headquarters
EMCA House
23/23-B, Ansari Road, Daryaganj
New Delhi 110 002, India
Landline: +91-11-23272143, +91-11-23272703
+91-11-23282021, +91-11-23245672
E-mail: jaypee@jaypeebrothers.com

Corporate Office
Jaypee Brothers Medical Publishers (P) Ltd.
4838/24, Ansari Road, Daryaganj
New Delhi 110 002, India
Phone: +91-11-43574357
Fax: +91-11-43574314
E-mail: jaypee@jaypeebrothers.com

Overseas Office
JP Medical Ltd.
83, Victoria Street, London
SW1H 0HW (UK)
Phone: +44-20 3170 8910
E-mail: info@jpmedpub.com

EU GPSR Authorised Representative
Logos Europe, 9 rue Nicolas Poussin
17000, La Rochelle, France
Phone: +33 (0) 6 67 93 73 78
E-mail: Contact@logoseurope.eu

Website: www.jaypeebrothers.com
Website: www.jaypeedigital.com

Inquiries for bulk sales may be solicited at: jaypee@jaypeebrothers.com

Parkinson's Disease and Movement Disorders* / *Kalyan B Bhattacharyya

First Edition: 2005

Second Edition: 2022, Reprint: **2025**

ISBN: 978-93-5465-035-2

Printed in India

DEDICATION

This book is dedicated to
the memory of Professor C David Marsden (1938–1998),
the MASTER OF MOVEMENT DISORDERS

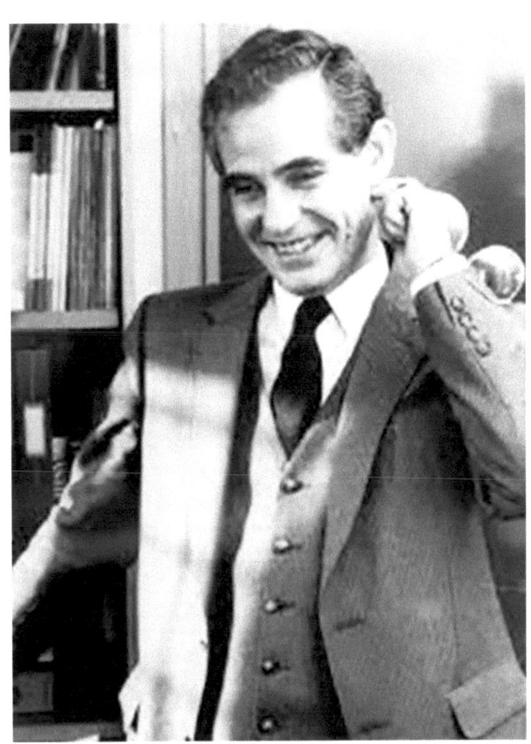

Contributors

EDITOR

Kalyan B Bhattacharyya MD DM MAMS FIAN FRCP (Edin)
Editor-in-Chief (IAN Yearbook Neurology)
Former Professor and Head
Department of Neurology
RG Kar Medical College and Hospital
Kolkata, West Bengal, India

CO-EDITORS

Jimmy A Lalkaka MD DM (Neuro)
Consultant Neurologist
Associate Professor
Department of Neurology
Bombay Hospital Institute of Medical Sciences
Mumbai, Maharashtra, India

Charulata Savant Sankhla MD DNB
Faculty
Department of Neurology
PD Hinduja National Hospital
Mumbai, Maharashtra, India

Pettarusp Murzban Wadia MD DNB (Med) DM DNB (Neuro) Clinical Fellowship Movement Disorders University of Toronto
Consultant Neurologist and Movement Disorder Specialist
Department of Neurology
Jaslok Hospital and Research Centre
Mumbai, Maharashtra, India

CONTRIBUTING AUTHORS

Abhilekh Srivastava MBBS MD DM
Consultant, Fortis Flt. Lt. Rajan Dhall
Vasant Kunj, New Delhi, India

Achal Kumar Srivastava MD DM
Professor, Department of Neurology
All India Institute of Medical Sciences
New Delhi, India

Aditya Ashok Murgai MD DM
Consulting Neurologist and Movement Disorders Specialist
Fortis Memorial Research Institute
Gurugram, Haryana, India

Alexander Storch MD
Director and Professor of Neurology
Department of Neurology
University of Rostock, Rostock, Germany

Anil Venkatichalam DM Neurology
Fellowship in Movement Disorders (Canada)
Consultant Neurologist
Nanavati Hospital
Mumbai, Maharashtra, India

Anthony E Lang OC MD FRCPC
Professor
Edmond J. Safra Program in Parkinson's Disease
Toronto Western Hospital
Toronto, Ontario, Canada

Arpit Agrawal MBBS MD
Senior Resident
Department of Neurology
All India Institute of Medical Sciences
New Delhi, India

Arun B Taly MBBS MD DM
ICMR Emeritus Medical Scientist
Formerly Senior Professor of Neurology
NIMHANS
Bengaluru, Karnataka, India

Arup Kumar Dutta MD DM
Associate Professor
Department of Neurology
RG Kar Medical College and Hospital
Kolkata, West Bengal, India

Asha Kishore MD DM
Senior Consultant and Movement Disorders Specialist
Centre of Excellence for Neuroscience
Aster Medcity
Kochi, Kerala, India

AV Srinivasan MD (Med) DM (Neuro) PhD FAAN FIAN DSc (Hons) FRCP (London)
Emeritus Professor of Neurology
The Tamil Nadu Dr MGR Medical University Chennai, Tamil Nadu, India
Consultant Neurophysician AVS Clinic
Raja Annamalai Puram
Chennai, Tamil Nadu, India

Azad M Irani DNB (Int Med) DNB (Neuro)
Consultant Neurologist
Department of Neurology
Jaslok Hospital and Research Centre
Mumbai, Maharashtra, India

Beomseok Jeon PhD MD
Medical Director
Movement Disorder Center
Seoul National University Hospital
Seoul, South Korea
Professor
Department of Neurology
College of Medicine
Seoul National University
Seoul, South Korea

Bhagyadhan Patel DM DNB
Neuromuscular Disorder Specialist
Consultant Neurophysician
Brain and Nerve Clinic
Ahmedabad, Gujarat, India

Bhaskar Ghosh Dip Card MD DNB DM (Neurology) MNAMS FICP Fellowship in Movement Disorders
Former Additional Chief Health Director
Neurology, BR Singh Hospital, Kolkata, West Bengal, India

Bhimsen Singhal MD DSc FRCP FAMS
Director of Neurology
Bombay Hospital Institute of Medical Sciences
Mumbai, Maharashtra, India

Charulata Savant Sankhla MD DNB
Faculty, Department of Neurology
PD Hinduja National Hospital
Mumbai, Maharashtra, India

Daniel J van Wamlen MD PhD
Neurologist; Postdoctoral Clinical Research Fellow
King's College London
Department of Basic and Clinical Neurosciences, Institute of Psychiatry, Psychology and Neuroscience
London, United Kingdom
Parkinson Foundation Centre of Excellence, King's College Hospital, Denmark Hill, London, United Kingdom

Debjani Roy Chowdhury MD DM
Consultant Neurologist
AMRI Hospitals, Salt Lake
Kolkata, West Bengal, India

Deepa Dash MD DM
Clinical Fellow
The Ottawa Hospital
Ottawa, Canada

Dhiman Das MD DM
Associate Professor
Department of Neurology
RG Kar Medical College and Hospital
Kolkata, West Bengal, India

Dipali Nemade MD MPH
PGY4 Resident
Department of Neurology
Marshall University School of Medicine
Huntington, United States

Divya KP MD DM
Assistant Professor
Department of Neurology
Sree Chitra Tirunal Institute for Medical Sciences and Technology
Thiruvananthapuram, Kerala, India

Gautam Wali PhD
Research Scientist
Kolling Institute
University of Sydney
Australia

Govind Madhaw MD DM
Senior Resident
Department of Neurology
All India Institute of Medical Sciences
Rishikesh, Uttarakhand, India

Greg Daniel Kuhlman MD MBA
Assistant Professor
James J and Joan A Gardner Family Center for Parkinson's Disease and Movement Disorders
Department of Neurology
University of Cincinnati
Cincinnati, Ohio, United States

Gurusidheshwar Wali MBBS MD DM
Chief Consultant and Director
Neurospecialities Centre
Belgaum, Karnataka, India

Hee Jin Kim MD
Associate Professor
Department of Neurology
Konkuk University School of Medicine
Seoul, South Korea

Heli S Shah MD DM
Consultant Neurologist
Sterling Hospital
Jivraj Mehta Hospital
Ahmedabad, Gujarat, India

Hrishikesh Kumar MD DM
HOD, Neurology
In-Charge, Movement Disorders Program
Director of Research
Vice Chairman
Institute of Neurosciences Kolkata
Kolkata, West Bengal, India

Indu Ghanshyam Bhana MBBS MD General Medicine DM Neurology
Consultant Neurologist
Jupiter Hospital
Indore, Madhya Pradesh, India

Jimmy A Lalkaka MD DM (Neuro)
Consultant Neurologist
Associate Professor
Department of Neurology
Bombay Hospital Institute of Medical Sciences
Mumbai, Maharashtra, India

JS Katpal MBBS MD Medicine
Consultant Neurologist
Choithram Hospital and Research Center
Indore, Madhya Pradesh, India

K Ray Chaudhuri MD FRCP DSc
Professor of Movement Disorders and Neurology
King's College London, Department of Basic and Clinical Neurosciences
Institute of Psychiatry, Psychology and Neuroscience
London, United Kingdom
Parkinson Foundation Centre of Excellence, King's College Hospital
Denmark Hill, London, United Kingdom

Kalyan B Bhattacharyya MD DM MAMS FIAN FRCP (Edin)
Professor and Head
Department of Neurology
RG Kar Medical College and Hospital
Kolkata, West Bengal, India

Swetha Tandra MD DM (Neurology)
Assistant Professor
Department of Neurology
Nizam's Institute of Medical Sciences
Hyderabad, Telangana, India

Kamakshi Dhamija MD DM
Postdoctoral Fellow in
CNS Demyelinating Disorders
Department of Neurology
NIMHANS Bengaluru
Kolkata, West Bengal, India

Kaushik Sen MBBS MD DM
Head of the Department
Medica Superspecialty Hospital
Kolkata, West Bengal, India

Khushnuma Mansukhani MD
Head
Department of Electrophysiology
Bombay Hospital Institute of
Medical Sciences
Mumbai, Maharashtra, India

Madhuri Behari MBBS MD DM
Director, Neurology
Fortis Flt. Lt. Rajan Dhall
Vasant Kunj, New Delhi, India

Mahendra Thakre MD DNB
Senior Resident
PD Hinduja National Hospital and
Medical Research Centre
Mumbai, Maharashtra, India

Manan Mayur Mehta MD (Medicine)
DM (Neurology)
Consultant Neurologist
Mehta Neurology Center and
Tricolour Hospitals
Vadodara, Gujarat, India

Mandar Jog MD FAAN
Professor, Department of Clinical
Neurological Sciences, Neurosciences
Physiology and Pharmacology
Neurology, Western University
London, Ontario, Canada
Director, Movement Disorders Centre
and NPF Centre of Excellence
Division of Neurology
London Health Sciences Centre
London, Ontario, Canada

Manish Mahajan MD DNB Neurology
Senior Consultant
Department of Neurology and Head of
Neuroimmunology
Artemis Hospital Gurgaon
Gurugram, Haryana, India

Maria Amelia Barretto MA PhD CEO
Parkinson's Disease and Movement
Disorder Society, Bombay Hospital and
Medical Research Centre
Mumbai, Maharashtra, India

Mark Hallett MD
Chief
Human Motor Control Section
NINDS
NIH, Building 10, Room 7D37
10 Center Dr MSC 1428
Bethesda, Maryland, United States

Meenakshisundaram Umaiorubahan MD, DM, FAAN, FIAN,
FRCP (Edinburgh) FRCP (Glasgow)
Director of Neurosciences
SRM Institutes for Medical Science
Chennai, Tamil Nadu, India

Meher Ursekar MD
Head of Neuroradiology
Sir HN Reliance Foundation Hospital and
Research Centre
Mumbai, Maharashtra, India
Teacher
Theory of Knowledge (IB Diploma
Program) at Bombay International School
Mumbai, Maharashtra, India

Mohammed Faruq MBBS
Senior Scientist
Genomics and Molecular Medicine
Institute of Genomics and Integrative
Biology (CSIR)
New Delhi, India

Monika Porwal (BAGUL) MBBS MD
Medicine DNB Neurology
Consultant Neurologist
Mahatma Gandhi Memorial Medical
College
Indore, Madhya Pradesh, India

Natasha Tipnis MD (Medicine) DNB
(Neurology)
Senior Resident in Neurology
Department of Neurology
Jaslok Hospital and Research Centre
Mumbai, Maharashtra, India

Navaz Irani MA
Programme Manager
Parkinson's Disease and Movement
Disorder Society
Bombay Hospital and Medical Research
Centre
Mumbai, Maharashtra, India

Nicole D'Souza BPT MPT
Head of Therapy and Research
Parkinson's Disease and Movement
Disorder Society
Bombay Hospital and Medical Research
Centre
Mumbai, Maharashtra, India

Nikita Changlani BA Psy
Research Assistant
Paul L Foster School of Medicine
Texas Tech University Health Sciences
Center
El Paso, Texas, United States

Niraj Kumar MD DM PDF
Additional Professor
Department of Neurology
All India Institute of Medical Sciences
Rishikesh, Uttarakhand, India

Nirmal Surya MD DNB (Neuro) FIAN
MNAMS FRCP
Founder Trustee and Chairman
Epilepsy Foundation India
Doctor of Medicine
Surya Neuro Center
Mumbai, Maharashtra, India

Nishan Mol MD
Senior Resident
Department of Neurology
National Institute of Mental Health and
Neurosciences
Bengaluru, Karnataka, India

Padma MV Srivastava MD DM
FRCP (Edin) FAMS FNASc FIAN
Professor and Head
Department of Neurology
All India Institute of Medical Sciences
New Delhi, India

Pankaj A Agarwal MD DNB DM
Senior Consultant
Department of Neurology
Head, Movement Disorders Clinic
and In-Charge
Deep Brain Stimulation (DBS) Program
Global Hospitals, Mumbai
Honorary Teaching Faculty
Department of Neurology
Seth GS Medical College and
KEM Hospital
Mumbai, Maharashtra, India

Paresh K Doshi MS MCh (Neurosurgery)
Director of Neurosurgery and Functional
Neurosurgery
Department of Neurosurgery
Jaslok Hospital and Research Centre
Mumbai, Maharashtra, India

Payal Shah MD (Pediatrics) Fellowship
Pediatric Neurology (MUHS)
Assistant Professor
Departments of Pediatrics and Neurology
Bai Jerbai Wadia Hospital for Children
Mumbai, Maharashtra, India

PD Thompson AM MB PhD FRACP
Emeritus Professor of Neurology
University of Adelaide
Adelaide, Australia

Pettarusp Murzban Wadia MD DNB (Med) DM DNB (Neuro) Clinical Fellowship Movement Disorders, University of Toronto
Consultant Neurologist and Movement Disorder Specialist
Movement Disorder Clinic
Department of Neurology
Jaslok Hospital and Research Centre
Mumbai, Maharashtra, India

Poorna J Visa MBBS PG Diploma in Pharmacology (University of Auckland)
Clinical Assistant
AVS Clinic, Raja Annamalai Puram,
Chennai, Tamil Nadu, India

Porrselvi Ammaiappan Palanisamy PhD Cpsychol
Cognitive Neuropsychologist
Unified Brain Health Care
Chennai, Tamil Nadu, India

Pramod Kumar Pal MD DNB DM FIAN FRCP
Professor, Department of Neurology
National Institute of Mental Health and Neurosciences
Bengaluru, Karnataka, India

Prashanth LK DM
Consultant Neurologist
Specialist: Parkinson's Disease and Other Movement Disorders
Parkinson's Disease and Movement Disorders Clinic, and Vikram Hospitals
Bengaluru, Karnataka, India

Preeti Devnani MD ABPN FAASM
Clinical Director
Cleveland Clinic Abu Dhabi
Abu Dhabi, United Arab Emirates

Priyanka Korepu DNB
Nuclear Medicine Consultant
Newmedd Diagnostics
Bengaluru, Karnataka, India

Rachael Fernandes MSc
Research Assistant
Sleep Disorders Clinic
Mumbai, Maharashtra, India

Ravi Yadav MD DM MNAMS
Professor of Neurology
National Institute of Mental Health and Neurosciences
Bengaluru, Karnataka, India

Rebecca Banerjee PhD
Senior Post-doctoral Research Fellow
Movement Disorders Program
Institute of Neurosciences Kolkata
Kolkata, West Bengal, India

Rima Ramesh Sansi MBBS DNB EDiNR
Consultant Radiologist
Sevenhills Healthcare Pvt Ltd
Mumbai, Maharashtra, India

Rinsha Rafeeqe MBBS
Junior Resident
Kannur Medical College Anjarakandy
Kannur, Kerala, India

Robert Chen MA MBBChir MSc FRCPC
Professor
Division of Neurology
Department of Medicine
University of Toronto and Krembil Research Institute
Toronto, Ontario, Canada

Rohan Mahale DM
Associate Professor of Neurology
Department of Neurology
National Institute of Mental Health and Neurosciences
Bengaluru, Karnataka, India

Roopa Rajan MBBS MD DM
Associate Professor
Department of Neurology
All India Institute of Medical Sciences
New Delhi, India

Rukmini Kandadai Mridula DNB DM (Neurogy)
Associate Professor
Department of Neurology
Nizam's Institute of Medical Sciences
Hyderabad, Telangana, India

Rupam Borgohain DM (Neuro)
Professor and Head
Department of Neurology
Nizam's Institute of Medical Sciences
Hyderabad, Telangana, India

Rukmini Mridula Kandadai DNB (Gen Med) DM (Neuro)
Associate Professor
Department of Neurology
Nizam's Institute of Medical Sciences
Hyderabad, Telangana, India

Sangeeta H Ravat MD DM
Professor and Head
Department of Neurology
King Edward Memorial (KEM) Hospital and Seth GS Medical College
Mumbai, Maharashtra, India

Sanjay Pandey MD DM
Director Professor, Neurology
Govind Ballabh Pant Institute of Postgraduate Medical Education and Research
New Delhi, India

Sanjib Sinha MD DM
Professor and Head
Department of Neurology
NIMHANS
Bengluru, Karnataka, India

Sarbani Sengupta DCH MRCP (General Medicine) MRCPS FRCP
Head, Department of Medicine
Additional Chief Health Director
BR Singh Hospital and Center for Medical Education and Research
Kolkata, West Bengal, India

Sarosh M Katrak MD DM FRCPE
Emeritus Director
Department of Neurology
Jaslok Hospital and Research Centre
Mumbai, Maharashtra, India

Satish V Khadilkar MD DM DNBE FIAN FICP FAMS FRCP (London)
Dean and Professor and Head
Department of Neurology
Bombay Hospital Institute of Medical Sciences, Mumbai
Professor Emeritus
Sir J.J. Group of Hospitals
Mumbai, Maharashtra, India

Seetha Lekshmi B MBBS MD
Senior Resident in Neurology
Department of Neurology
All India Institute of Medical Sciences
New Delhi, India

Shabbir Merchant MD
Assistant Professor of Neurology
Division of Movement Disorders
Medical University of South Carolina
Charleston, United States

Shivam Om Mittal MD
Consultant Neurologist
Parkinson's and Movement Disorders
Center, Cleveland Clinic Abu Dhabi
Abu Dhabi, United Arab Emirates

Shruti Agrawal MD DM
Fellow In Epilepsy
Department of Neurology
King Edward Memorial (KEM) Hospital
Seth GS Medical College
Mumbai, Maharashtra, India

Shweta Prasad MBBS
PhD Scholar
Department of Clinical Neurosciences
Department of Neurology
National Institute of Mental Health and
Neurosciences
Bengaluru, Karnataka, India

Shyamal Kumar Das MD DM
Professor Neuromedicine
In-Charge, Movement Disorders Clinic
Bangur Institute of Neurology
Kolkata, West Bengal, India

Soaham Dilip Desai MBBS MD DM
Senior Consultant Neurologist
Professor and Head, Neurology
Department of Neurology,
Shree Krishna Hospital and
Pramukhswami Medical College
Bhaikaka University
Karamsad, Anand, Gujarat, India

Sonali Bhattad MD DM
Senior Resident, Neurology
Govind Ballabh Pant Institute of
Postgraduate Medical Education and
Research, New Delhi, India

Srinivas Raju MBBS MD DMO
Consultant Neurologist
Columbia Asia Hebbal and Bangalore
Baptist Hospital
Bengaluru, Karnataka, India

Subhash Kaul MD DM
Senior Consultant Neurologist
Krishna Institute of Medical Sciences
Hyderabad, Telangana, India

Sudhir V Shah MD DM
Professor and HOD
Smt NHL Muncipal Medical College
and SVPIMSR
Ahmedabad, Gujarat, India
Director of Neurosciences
Sterling Hospital
Ahmedabad, Gujarat, India

Sujith Ovallath MD DM DNB
Consultant Neurologist and Movement
Disorder Specialist
Professor and Head of Neurology
Director
James Parkinson's Movement Disorder
Research Centre
Kannur Medical College Anjarakandy
Kannur, Kerala, India

Sumit Singh MBBS MD DM Neurology
Chief of Neurology
Artemis Hospital Gurgaon
Gurugram, Haryana, India

Supriyo Choudhury MD
Consultant Clinical Pharmacologist
Senior Research Fellow (Neurology)
Assistant Director of Research
Institute of Neurosciences Kolkata
Kolkata, West Bengal, India

Suryaprabha Turaga MD (Gen Med)
DM (Neuro)
Additional Professor
Department of Neurology
Nizam's Institute of Medical
Sciences
Hyderabad, Telangana, India

Swetha Reddy Tandra MD (Gen Med)
DM (Neuro)
Assistant Professor
Department of Neurology
Nizam's Institute of Medical Sciences
Hyderabad, Telangana, India

Urvashi Shah PhD
Consultant Neuropsychologist
Department of Neurology
KEM Hospital and Global Hospitals
Mumbai, Maharashtra, India

Utkarsh Patel MD DNB
Consultant Neurophysician
Arvita Neurology Superspeciality Clinic
Ahemdabad, Gujarat, India

Valentina Leta MD
Neurologist; Clinical Reaserach Fellow
King's College London, Department
of Basic and Clinical Neurosciences
Institute of Psychiatry, Psychology and
Neuroscience, London, United Kingdom
Parkinson Foundation Centre of
Excellence, King's College Hospital
Denmark Hill, London, United Kingdom

Varhsa A Patil MD DNB DM
Consultant Neurologist
Bombay Hospital Institute of
Medical Sciences
Mumbai, Maharashtra, India

Vikram R Lele MD DNB
Director, Department of Nuclear
Medicine and PET-CT, Jaslok Hospital
and Research Centre
Mumbai, Maharashtra, India

Vikram Shivkumar MD
Assistant Professor of Neurology
Marshall University School of Medicine
Huntington, United States

Vinay Goyal MD DM FIAN
Director Neurology
Medanta - The Medicity
Gurugram, Haryana, India

Viraj Sanghi MD DNB (Neurology)
Fellowship Paed Neurology (Toronto, Canada)
Senior Consultant, Paediatrics
Neurologist
SRCC Children's Hospital, Mumbai
Honorary Consultant
KEM Hospital and Seth GS Medical College
Mumbai, Maharashtra, India

Viral Ashvinbhai Barfiwala MBBS MD
DNB
Consultant Neurologist
Jaslok Hospital and Research Centre
Mumbai, Maharashtra
Advanced Neuro Clinic
Surat, Gujarat, India

Vrajesh Udani MD
Consultant, Child Neurology and Epilepsy
PD Hinduja National Hospital and
Medical Research Center
Mumbai, Maharashtra, India

Yatin Sagvekar DNB Neurology
Associate Consultant
Reliance Hospital
Navi Mumbai, Maharashtra, India

Foreword

I am delighted to commend this comprehensive textbook, published Under the Aegis of the Parkinson's Disease and Movement Disorders Society of India, founded in 2003 on the initiative of Professor Bhimsen Singhal.

This project was conceived by Professors Bhimsen Singhal and Kalyan Bhattacharyya, who was also Editor-in-Chief, with Drs Pettarusp Murzban Wadia, Jimmy A Lalkaka, and Charulata Savant Sankhla as coeditors.

When I qualified as a doctor in 1973, levodopa, the first effective treatment for a progressive neurodegenerative disorder, had only recently appeared on the scene. Three years later I did my first neurology post under the late Professor David Marsden, to whose memory this book is dedicated, and got "hooked" on Movement Disorders.

I vividly recall my very first neurology conference at the WFN Parkinson's Disease Conference in the Airport Hotel in Frankfurt in 1982, attended by 200 souls. Having read the papers of many experts in the field, I was fortunate to see and hear for the first time many of our great pioneers, since deceased, including Peggy Hoehn, Melvin Yahr, Roger Duvoisin, Hiro Narabayashi, Rolf Hassler, Oleh Hornykiewicz, and Andre Barbeau.

It took a number of years before the discipline of movement disorders became more widely recognized. However, things began to change in the mid-80s, when David Marsden in London, and Stanley Fahn in New York, founded the Movement Disorder Society and the Movement Disorders Journal.

At that time, Indian Neurology had not yet introduced Movement Disorder clinics and meetings. However, with the increasing number of neurologists in India, the Indian Academy of Neurology established a subsection. This was followed by the founding in 2011 of the Movement Disorder Society of India (MDSI), and later its affiliation with the MDS Asian and Oceanic Section of the International Parkinson and Movement Disorder Society.

Indian Movement Disorder Neurology has developed and flourished brilliantly in recent years, and this thorough, comprehensive and detailed textbook marks a crowning achievement for the 113 authors and coauthors who have contributed 55 chapters to this monumental piece of work. This impressive and up-to-date volume of over 514 pages is the authoritative movement disorder reference in India, and a showcase for the breadth and depth of Indian Neurology. It is also a definitive and eminently affordable source for neurologists worldwide, ranking alongside Marsden's Book of Movement Disorders, finally completed posthumously 9 years ago, fittingly by an Indian, Kailash Bhatia.

Niall Patrick Quinn MA MD FRCP
Emeritus Professor of Clinical Neurology
University College London

Preface to the Second Edition

The pharmacological management of Parkinson's disease (PD) has improved significantly over the years since the introduction of levodopa in 1967. Newer molecules and delivery systems along with surgical interventions—lesioning and deep brain stimulation—are now available for use when the situation arises. The recognition and management of nonmotor symptoms have also had a positive impact on the quality of life of persons with PD. We hope that some day we shall have neuroprotective agents to prevent the progression of the disease.

However, despite all the advances in medical therapy, persons with PD and their caregivers continued to feel isolated and lonely. We realized that they needed more than just medicines to help them on their long journey. We were keen to set up an infrastructure with a multidisciplinary approach to help them and their families and also increase public awareness of this disease. This led to the foundation of the Parkinson's Disease and Movement Disorder Society (PDMDS), an all India nonprofit charitable society, in 2001. In 2003, an International symposium of Parkinson's disease with more than 40 international experts and a large audience of neurologists from all over India was organized in Mumbai. A special parallel session for persons with PD and their carers was conducted at the same time. In this meeting, the "Global declaration for Parkinson's disease was launched for the first time by Mrs Mary Baker—former chairperson of the working group of Parkinson's disease of the World Health Organization". Over the ensuing years, it has been gratifying to see the significant strides that the PDMDS has made under the able stewardship of Dr Maria Barretto and her team. From two initial support care centers in Mumbai, the PDMDS now has 64 community-based support centers in urban, rural, and tribal areas, spread over 24 states across the country. The PDMDS has, so far, impacted the lives of more than 50,000 people with PD and their carers.

India has a vast population of more than 136 crore people. There are very few (around 2,000) neurologists and still fewer "movement disorder" specialists for Parkinson's disease to cater to this large section of the society. They are also mainly located in urban areas. So, the burden of treatment falls on general physicians and local healthcare workers. With increase in longevity, we are also witnessing a significant increase in people with age-related neurological illnesses such as stroke, dementia, and Parkinson's disease.

The management of Parkinson's disease is complex, requiring knowledge and skill. Realizing the great need to educate the medical personnel on the optimal management of this disease, the first edition of the book "Parkinson's Disease and Movement Disorders" with Drs TN Mehrotra and Kalyan B Bhattacharyya was published under the aegis of the PDMDS in 2005. After a lapse of several years, it was decided to bring out the second edition under the able leadership of Dr Kalyan B Bhattacharyya assisted by his editorial team of movement disorder experts—Drs Pettarusp Murzban Wadia, Charulata Savant Sankhla, and Jimmy A Lalkaka (all members of the PDMDS governing council). This book covers nearly all aspects of the diagnosis and management of PD and other movement disorders and will serve as a reference book for physicians, neurologists, and all those involved in the care of PD patients and other movement disorders.

We are very grateful to all the distinguished neurologists and movement disorder specialists from India and abroad who have spent their precious time to contribute chapters for this book.

Bhimsen Singhal
Founder—PDMDS
and the PDMDS Family

Preface to the First Edition

Parkinson's disease is a common disorder. Most physicians as well as neurologists have patients of parkinsonism in their practice. The care of patients with parkinsonism is complex.

In the early stages as well as the diagnosis is made many patients may only need education about the disease and reassurance. However, over the ensuing years the clinicians may be orchestrating pharmacologic interventions and a variety of community and medical services to cope with a diversity of problems that may be associated with parkinsonism.

There are number of monographs on parkinsonism and movement disorders. However, there is none published by experts in this field from our country. In this book we have attempted to gather experiences of our colleagues engaged in handling these patients.

Optimal care of parkinsonian patients requires more than just intelligent use of antiparkinsonian drugs and hence we have also discussed often less appreciated aspects of management. I hope that this publication will help our fellow colleagues, physicians and neurologists alike to offer better care to the people suffering from Parkinson's disease.

TN Mehrotra
Kalyan B Bhattacharyya

Acknowledgement

We express our deep sense of gratitude to Professor BS Singhal for guiding us all along during the preparation of this book.

Contents

SECTION 6: ATYPICAL PARKINSONSIM

SECTION 7: HYPERKINETIC MOVEMENT DISORDERS

SECTION 8: SECONDARY MOVEMENT DISORDERS

PLATE 1

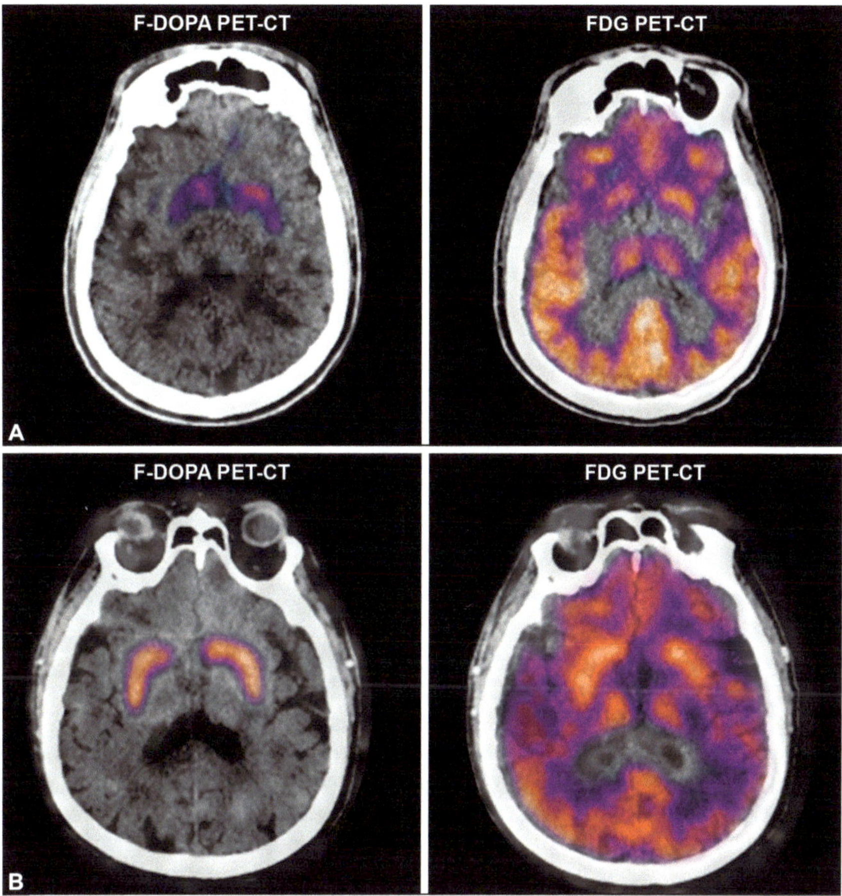

(^{18}F-DOPA-PET: 18F-fluoro-L-DOPA positron emission tomography; CT: computed tomography; ET: essential tremor; PD: Parkinson's disease)

FIGS. 3A AND B: Positive ^{18}F-DOPA-PET scan demonstrating decreased ^{18}F-DOPA uptake within the bilateral posterior greater than anterior putamen consistent with PD (3a, left panel) and uniform uptake within the bilateral caudate and putamen in a case of ET (3b, left panel). The right panel shows FDG-PET showing decreased metabolism in the striatum bilaterally in PD (3a) c.f. ET (3b). Both the patients had mildly asymmetrical (L>R) postural tremor of 3 years duration. ***(Chapter 31)***

Courtesy: Dr Noaline Sinha, Consultant Nuclear Medicine, Artemis Hospital, Gurugram, India.

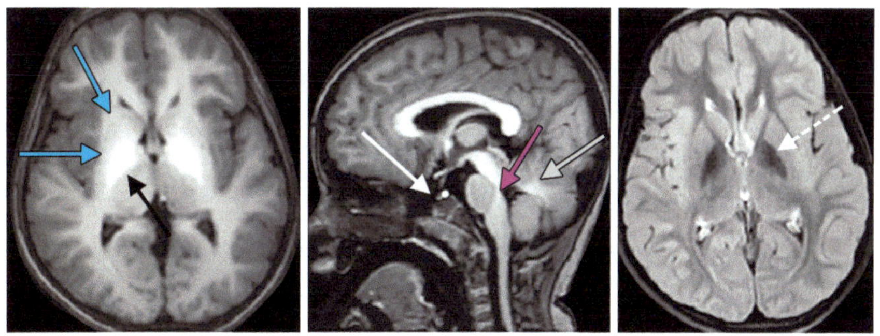

(GP: globus pallidus; HMNDYT2: hypermanganesemia with dystonia type 2)

FIG. 4: HMNDYT2: Typical T-1 hyperintensity predominantly in the globus pallidus (black arrows), brainstem (pink arrow), and dentate nucleus (gray arrow) note absence of significant change in corpus striatum (blue arrow). T2 shows GP hypointensity. ***(Chapter 40)***

Source: Modified from Tuscl 2016.

PLATE 2

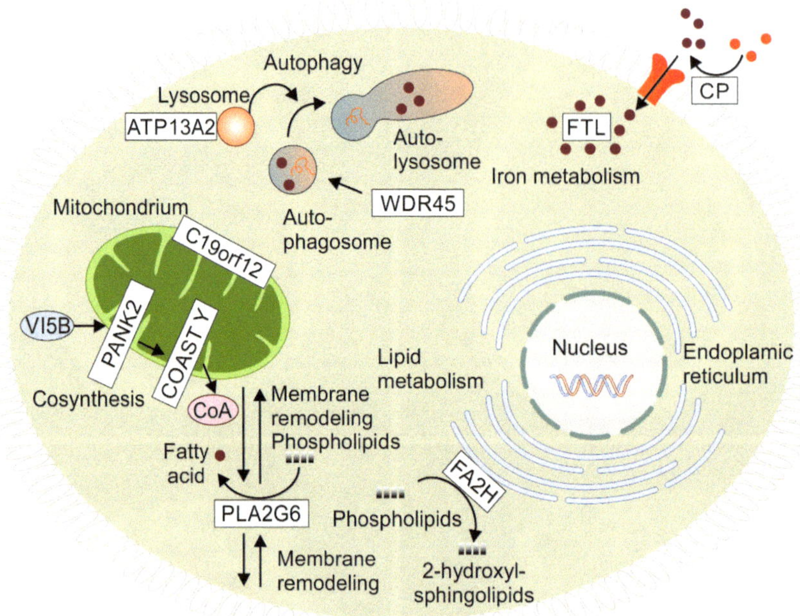

FIG. 6: NBIA: Overview of genes and pathways involved in neurodegeneration with brain iron accumulation (NBIA). Schematic representation of a cell indicating the pathophysiologic mechanisms postulated for NBIA. Nine reported NBIA genes (white box, black outline) and their associated cellular processes are shown. Ceruloplasmin (CP) and ferritin light polypeptide (FTL) are important regulators of cellular iron homeostasis. Phospholipase A2 (PLA2G6) and fatty acid 2-hydroxylase (FA2H) are involved in lipid metabolism and membrane remodeling. Pantothenate kinase 2 (PANK2) and CoA synthase (COASY) are key enzymes in the biosynthesis of coenzyme A (CoA) utilized in a multitude of cellular processes, including the synthesis of fatty acids. WD repeat domain 45 (WDR45) and ATPase type13A2 (ATP13A2) play a role in the degradation process of autophagy. The function of the mitochondrial membrane protein C19orf12 is still unknown, but it is postulated to be associated with fatty acid biogenesis. ***(Chapter 40)***

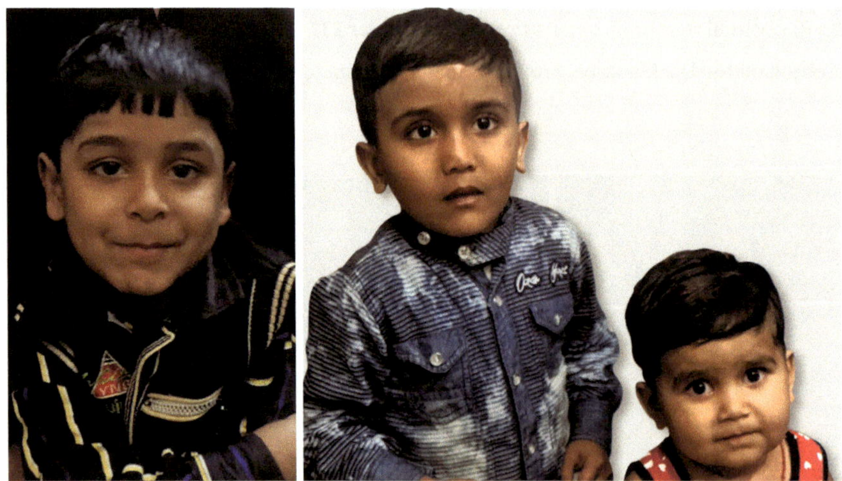

FIG. 8: One unrelated (top) and brother/sister with confirmed PKAN—both with characteristic facies (personal observation). ***(Chapter 40)***

PLATE 3

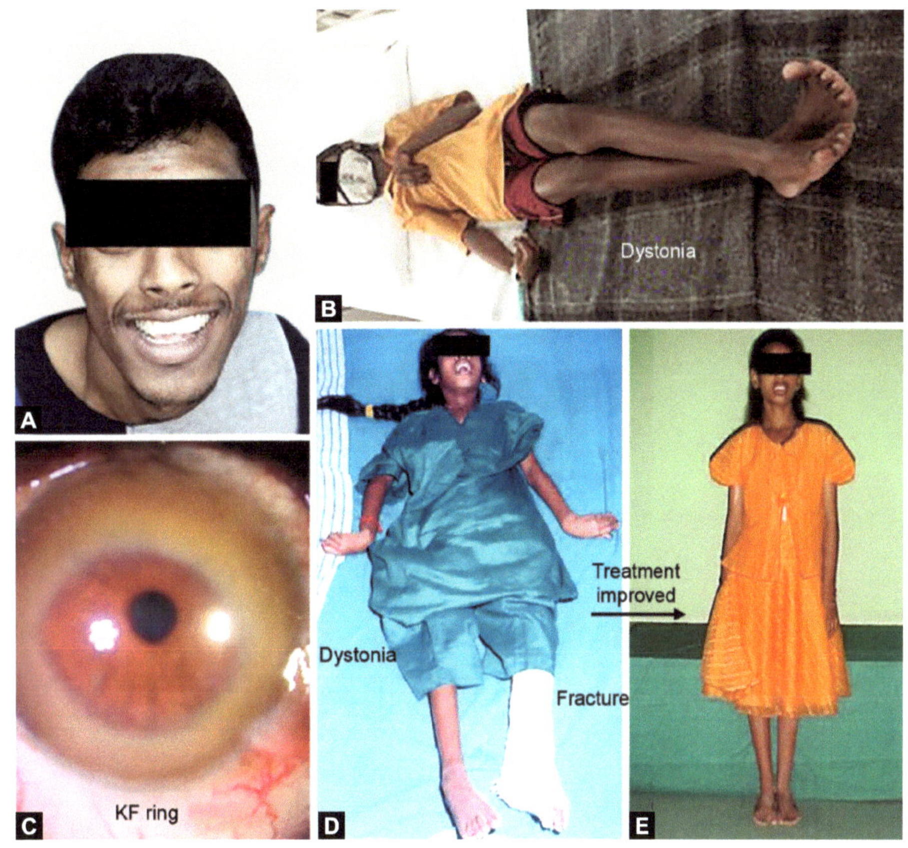

(KF: Kayser–Fleischer)

FIGS. 1A TO E: It shows various clinical features in patients with Wilson's disease. ***(Chapter 41)***

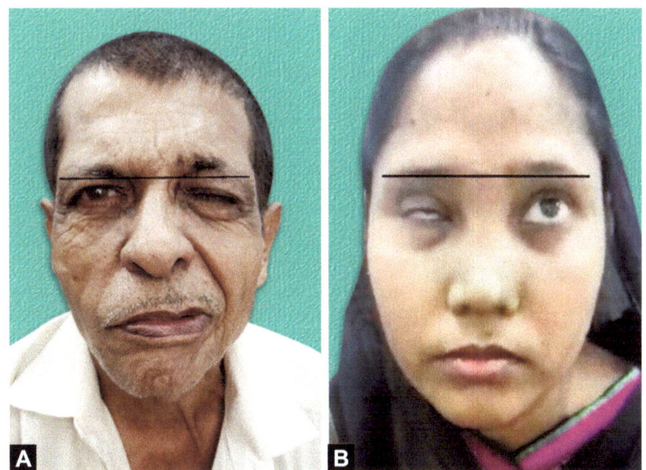

FIGS. 1A AND B: (A) Organic left hemifacial spasm (HFS)—the "other Babinski" sign. Elevation of left eyebrow at the same time as left eye closure due to concurrent contraction of frontalis and orbicularis oculi muscles in HFS; and (B) Functional (psychogenic) right eye closure. The right eyebrow is *relatively* depressed compared to the unaffected left eyebrow. The "other Babinski" sign is, therefore, absent. ***(Chapter 51)***

SECTION

1

INTRODUCTION TO MOVEMENT DISORDERS

CHAPTER 1

The Masters of Movement Disorders

Kalyan B Bhattacharyya

INTRODUCTION

Movement disorder is an established subspecialty in the field of neurology and it encompasses within its ambit, the study of several disorders, such as Parkinson's disease, dystonias, chorea, athetosis, tremors, tics, and other related conditions. Although, many physicians and neurologists contributed enormously to enrich the subject, a detailed account of every work is beyond the scope of this review. We shall, therefore, concentrate on some of the important and pathbreaking works carried out by the masters of neurology.

THOMAS SYDENHAM (1624–1689)

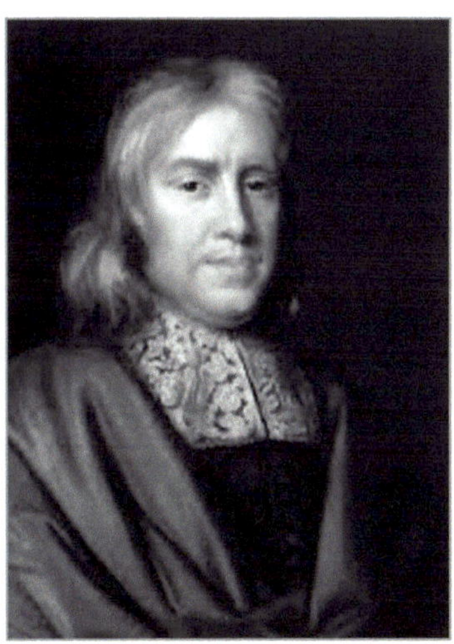

In 1886, Thomas Sydenham, an English physician, wrote an account of "*chorea minor*", a frequent complication of rheumatic fever in those days in the Western world. This is in all likelihood, the first documented evidence of the description of movement disorders in the United Kingdom.[1,2]

Sydenham enrolled in Magdalen College, Oxford in 1642 when the discontent against the ruling of King Charles I had been raging in England and there was every attempt to introduce the system of democracy by the Puritans under the leadership of Oliver Cromwell. Sydenham was highly influenced by Cromwell, was drawn toward the civil war, and left academic pursuits in helping in the overthrow of the monarchy of King Charles Stuart in the 1640s.[1] The revolt led to the execution of the King on the 30th of January 1649. Thereafter, he returned to Oxford in 1645, completed his medical education at the Wadham College in 1848, and was elected as Fellow of All Souls College. Almost 30 years later, he completed his MD from Pembroke College, Cambridge in 1676, where his son was an undergraduate student at that time.[1,2]

Sydenham wrote his account in Latin but a verbatim English translation was appended at the end of the paper, written by Pechy in 1906, which appeared in the celebrated textbook, *Neurology*, by Kinnier Wilson, published posthumously in 1940. It reads:[3]

> *"Chorea Saint Viti is a sort of convulsion, which chiefly invades boys and girls from 10 years of age to puberty; firstly, it shows itself by a certain Lameness, or rather instability of one of the legs which the patient drags after him like a fool; afterward, it appears in the hand of the same side, which is affected with the disease, can by no means keep in the same posture for one moment... If a drink be put into his hand, he represents a thousand gestures, like jugglers, before he brings it to his mouth for whereas he cannot carry it to his mouth in a right*

line, his hand being drawn hither and thither by the convulsions, he turns it suddenly into his mouth and drinks greedily as if the poor wretch was designed to make sport."

This brilliant clinical account was, however, not readily agreed upon by one and all and in 1785, William Cullen, one of the most premier physician from Edinburgh thought that though the convulsive disease of Sydenham encompassed both "*diverse states mimicking the gesticulations of ludicrous antics of a stage clown*" and the "*convulsive agitations of the body with the retention of consciousness, as described by Limmaeus*", were in essence, identical.[1,2]

Incidentally, the term, Chorea Sancti Viti, was originally used for dancing mania, a form of hysteria, which was common in Europe in the 15th and 16th century since the affected persons were brought to the chapels of St Vitus.[1,4] Subsequently, it was known as *Chorea Magna*, and Sydenham's disease as *Chorea Minor* and, later, the eponym was assigned to him. The old entity, "*Dancing Mania*", had largely disappeared by the time Sydenham arrived, and it is most unlikely that he ever encountered such a condition. His description was based on the complications of rheumatic fever only, which he might have had confused with *Chorea Sancti Viti*.[1,2]

Sydenham's interest centered around clinical medicine. A famous painting depicts him examining a patient in a tender manner and John Locke, the renowned philosopher and his close friend, observing him from a distance. During his time, most of the physicians were *systematists* who believed that all physical phenomena could be explained by a single chemical cause. On the contrary, Sydenham directed his attention toward the patient's symptoms and developed a general chemical description of individual diseases. John Arbuthnot, a leading Scottish physician called him "*aemulus Hippocratis*", literally meaning the "*rival of Hippocrates*",[5] and he is universally known as the *Father of Clinical Medicine,* and Hermann Boerhaave, the Dutch physician and botanist, described him as "*Angliae lumen, artis phoebum, veram Hippocratici viri speciem*", meaning "*The light of England, the skill of Apollo, the true face of Hippocrates.*"[1] Bedside examination was all that mattered to him and he had little regard for the anatomical and physiological basis of maladies. It is on record that once he said, "*This is all very fine, but it won't do. Anatomy, Botany, Nonsense! Sir, I know an old woman in Covent Garden who understands Botany better, and as for anatomy, my butcher can dissect a joint full and well; no, young man, all that is stuff; you must go to the bedside, it is there alone you can learn disease.*"[1]

JAMES PARKINSON (1755–1824)

In all probability, James Parkinson is the most talked-about personality in the world literature on movement disorders. Eponyms are nowadays generally discouraged and expunged, since they do not tell us anything about the disease entity and may actually obfuscate its clarity. Yet if any eponym, in all likelihood, shall survive the ruthless grind of time, surely it is the disease described by James Parkinson in 1817. The clinical picture described >200 years ago has been acknowledged as the most classical account which could hardly be improved upon, barring an occasional omission and aberration here and there.

In 1817, James Parkinson wrote an account of the disease, entitled, "*An essay on the Shaking Palsy*", and published by Sherwood, Neely, and Jones, London. The book ran into 66 pages and five chapters namely, (1) *Definition, history, illustrative cases, (2) Pathognomonic symptoms examined, tremor coactus, scleroderma festinans, (3) Shaking palsy distinguished from other diseases with which it may be confounded, (4) Proximate cases, remote cases,* and *(5) Considerations respecting the means of cure.*[1,6] His description of the condition has entered into the classics of the medical literature. Jefferson, his biographer, wrote:

> *"It sharply illumined a clinical entity which had been only dimly apprehended before that date...Even now the essay can be read with profit, not only because it is a superb model of lucid clinical description, but because it is written with such lucid mastery of style that it must give pleasure to anyone with a taste for English prose. It is also a model of logical use of clinical experience...Considering the limited scope of neurological knowledge in his day, it is astonishing that his deductions were so close to the target zone of the substantia nigra..."*[7]

In the beginning, he summarized as follows:[1,6]

> *"Involuntary tremulous motion, with lessened muscular power, in parts not in action and even when supported; with a propensity to bend the trunk forward, and to pass from a walking to a running pace, the senses and intellect being uninjured."*

Here are some excerpts from the actual text.[1,6]

> *"So slight and imperceptible are the first inroads of this malady, and so extremely slow its progress, that it rarely happens that the patient can form any recollection of the precise period of its commencement. The first symptoms perceived are a slight sense of weakness, with a proneness to trembling... most commonly in one of the hands and arms... in <12 months or more, the morbid influence is felt in some other part. After a few more months the patient is found to be less strict than usual in preserving an upright posture...*
>
> *While at meals the fork is not being duly directed, frequently fails to raise the morsel from the plate, which, when seized, is with much difficulty conveyed*

to the mouth the disease proceeds, ...the hands fail to answer the dictates of the will. Walking becomes a task which cannot be performed without considerable attention.... The legs are not raised to that height, ... so that utmost care is `necessary to prevent frequent falls... writing can now be hardly accomplished; ...propensity to lean forward becomes invincible,...being at the same time, irresistibly impelled to take much quicker and shorter steps, and thereby to adopt unwillingly a running pace... the bowels...had all along been torpid, the expulsion of feces requiring mechanical aid. ...His words are now scarcely intelligible...no longer able to feed himself... saliva is constantly draining from the mouth, mixed with particles of food he is no longer able to clear from inside of the mouth.

...The power of conveying the food to the mouth is at length so much impeded that he is obliged to consent to be fed by others. As the disease proceeds toward its last stage, the trunk is almost permanently bowed ... and the tremulous agitation becomes violent... The chin is now almost immovably bent down upon the sternum... The power of articulation is lost. The urine and feces are passed involuntarily; and at the last, constant sleepiness, with slight delirium and other marks of extreme exhaustion, announce the wished-for release."

Parkinson drew his conclusions from observing only six patients. He treated one to the terminal stage of the illness, casually encountered two others in the streets of London, followed up one more for 2 weeks while he was treating him for abscess, saw one at a distance who had been walking at a running pace accompanied by a helper, and the last case was of considerable interest, since tremor disappeared following an attack of apoplexy.[1,2,4] Medical historians feel that the first case he described was in all probability one of multiple system atrophy.[4]

During his life and even later, Parkinson received little recognition in his own country or in Europe for his brilliant observation. German Sée, a contemporary of Jean Martin Charcot in Paris and an examiner for Joseph Babinski at the time of his MD examination in 1892, where incidentally, he failed, addressed him as *"Patterson"* in 1850. However, in 1888, the peerless Jean-Martin Charcot from Salpétrière, Paris, immortalized him, conferring the eponym, *"la Maladie de Parkinson"*, or *"Parkinson's disease"*,[4] though it is on record that Sanders called it *"Paralysis Agitans"* in 1855 and even a giant like William Gowers too, retained the same name in his famous *"Manual"*, published as late as in 1886.[1]

If "Parkinson" was incomplete anywhere in his clinical description, it is to be seen in the summary itself. He wrote that the intellect was unimpaired, though it is now proved incontrovertibly that the senses and the intellect are certainly impaired, designated nowadays, as the nonmotor symptoms of the disease.[1,2] This apart, he ignored rigidity in his patients and that was for the simple reason that examination of the muscle tone as a clinical sign was not yet described and he mentioned that the tremor was more prominent during sleep.[4] He also felt that the seat of the lesion was in the upper cervical cord, extending up to the medulla, a view that was rectified ages later by the work of Konstantin Tretiakoff from Soviet Russia in 1919, who described the nigral lesions.[1,2]

It is interesting to know that Wilhelm von Humboldt, an education reformer, statesman, and prolific writer from Germany, published in 1824, an account of his own motor illness that supplemented Parkinson's classic treatise. His intellect remained undisturbed and additionally, he described many new features of the disease. At the age of 61 years, he felt that he had been trembling in the hands and had difficulty in buttoning his shirt. He also recognized that his handwriting was becoming smaller and smaller with the passage of time and 2 years later, he wrote to Johann Wolfgang Goethe, the great German litterateur and his friend, that his movements were getting slow. Three years later, he said that he was having difficulty in turning in bed and the tremor worsened in stressful situations. However, two curious features were observed in him namely, his tremor improved with age and his handwriting was worse while writing in German than while writing in Latin.[1]

Parkinson breathed his last in 1824, and it is of considerable interest that the leading British journals at that time, such as, *The Medico-Chirurgical Review*, *The London Medical and Physical Journal*, and the *London Medical Repository* did not publish any obituary of this outstanding clinician.[1,2,4] However, there was renewed interest in his life in more recent times. The articles by AD Morris in *The Lancet*, entitled *"James Parkinson. Born April 11, 1755"*, published in 1955, and that of M Jefferson in *British Medical Journal* in 1973, entitled, *"M James Parkinson (1755–1824)"* report that there is no verified portrait of James Parkinson even in the National Art Gallery.[7-9] Photography was invented decades after his death by Henry Fox Talbot (1800–1877) in England in the 1840s. Three photographs bearing his name can be traced from various sources. The bearded man is in all likelihood, James Cumine Parkinson, a midshipman, who lost his interest in his vocation and later settled in the colonies of New Zealand and Tasmania. The one dressed in garish apparel with a cane stick in hand was a dentist who died in 1889. However, Simon RW Scott wrote that the *"Elusive Parkinson"*, represented in a painting in a book, *"The Villager's Friend and Physician"*, written and sketched by Parkinson himself, is the true James Parkinson, and he is seen lecturing before the gathering, though the evidence is scanty.[10,11]

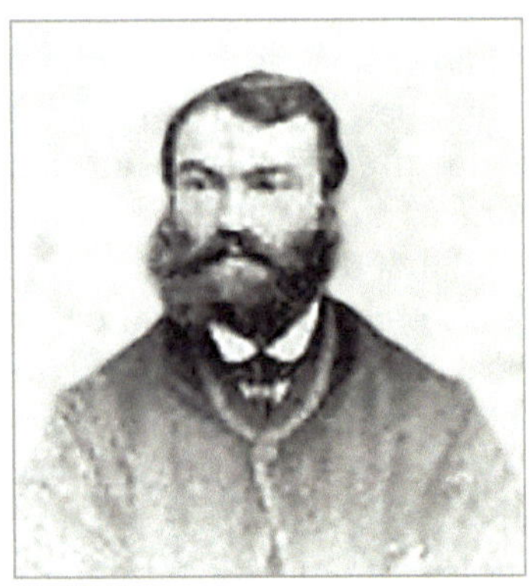

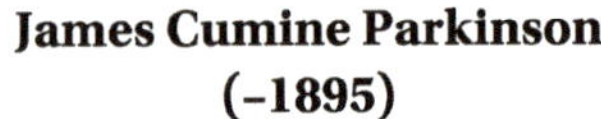

James Cumine Parkinson (-1895)

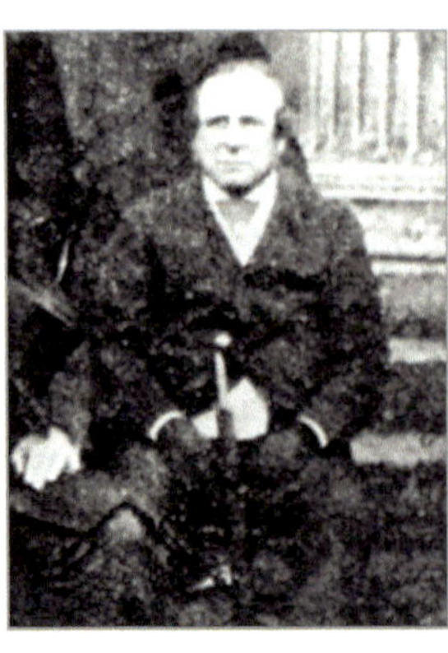

James Parkinson (1832–1887)

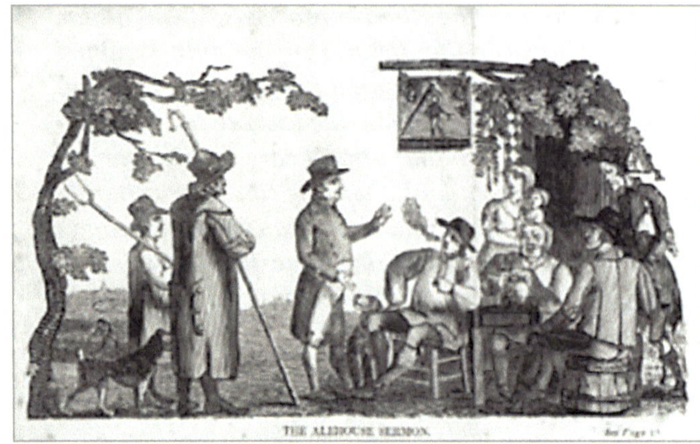

James Parkinson, the Village Physician (1755–1824)

The only written description provided by his friend and a fellow paleontologist, Gideon Mantell, reads,

> *"Mr Parkinson was rather below middle stature, with an energetic, intelligent, and pleasing expression of countenance, and of mild and courteous manners; readily imparting information either on his favorite science or on professional subjects."*[7]

Indeed, James Parkinson was a colorful and multifaceted personality, with much of a muchness of a genius, not recognized in his lifetime, and who left the world, unwept, unhonored, and unsung. As a matter of fact, JG Rowntree, one of the earliest biographers of Parkinson, wrote in 1912, in *Johns Hopkins Hospital Bulletin*, that, *"English born, English bred, forgotten by the English and the world at large, such was the fate of James Parkinson"*.[11,12]

GEORGE HUNTINGTON (1850–1916)

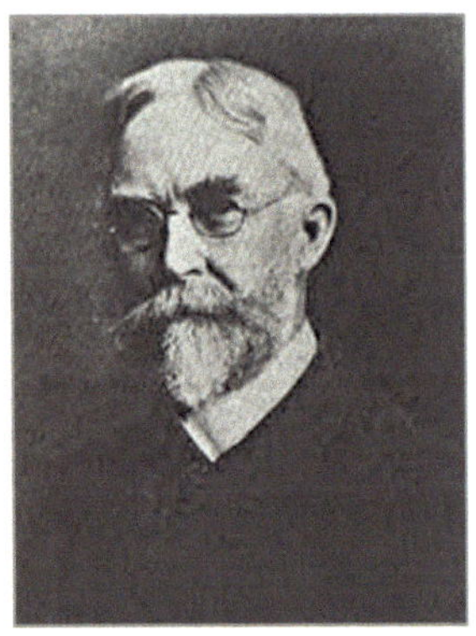

George Huntington was born into a family of general practitioners in East Hampton, USA. He practiced in his native place and soon he reported cases of dementia and chorea in middle-aged persons which ran into families, conforming to the autosomal dominant mode of transmission. He also referred to a series of such cases examined by his father and grandfather in the past, worked on these cases, and studied their families in great detail and his father's correctional notes are evident in his original manuscript. He moved to Pomeroy, Ohio in 1871 and when he was only 20 years of age, he presented his observations entitled, *"On chorea"* in 1872, before the Meigs and Mason Academy of Medicine. He wrote:

> *"The movements gradually increase when muscles hitherto unaffected take on the spasmodic action, until every muscle in the body becomes affected... As the disease progresses the mind becomes more or less impaired, in many accounting to insanity, while in others mind and body gradually fail until death relieves them of their suffering. When either or both the parents have shown manifestations of the disease, one or more of the offspring invariably suffer from the condition. It never skips a generation to again manifest itself in another..."*

However, it is on record that in 1860 Johan Christian Lund, a Norwegian physician, noted a high prevalence of dementia along with jerky movements in subjects in the remote areas in Setesdalen, Norway, and for that reason the disease is often referred to as *"Setesdalsrykkja"* in that country. Even though previous workers had reported this condition, it was the lucidity and the clarity of expression which marked Huntington's description and that earned him the eponym *"Huntington's disease"*, previously known as *"Huntington's Chorea"*. The name was modified since chorea was not the sole feature of the condition.

Though Huntington described the entity in great detail, the condition has been described in the past. It is noteworthy that a disease presenting similarly had been known to many generations in the families in colonial New England and was called *"magrums"* or *"megrims"* by the local inhabitants. The victims of the disease were treated as despicable witches and they were burnt to death publicly.

Physicians of earlier days like Thelenius, reported one such subject in 1816, while Ruspf brought to light one more patient in 1834. Walters followed close on the heels and published his observations in Dunglison's *Practice of Medicine* in 1842. This was later to be the subject for the thesis of Charles Gorman of Pennsylvania in 1848 and was reported again by Groving Lyon in *American Medical Times* in 1863. The German literature reported cases described by Adolf Kussmaul and Carl Hermann Nothnagel in 1872, and thus the eponym was more or less firmly established.[1,13]

The disease was imported to United States of America form Bures, Suffolk in the United Kingdom by the wife of a young Englishman in 1630, the match being, however, disapproved by the boy's family, as the girl's father was choreic. Undaunted, this brave young man married the girl and they emigrated to USA, and most unwittingly, transmitted the disease through their children. It is further on record that some of the Puritans who emigrated to the USA in the ship named "Mayflower", were put to death on the charge of witchcraft after the trial of Salem, Massachusetts. Their grotesque posture and curious grimaces prompted people to treat them with utter disdain.

In 1902, SE Jelliffe began studying the history of Huntington's disease in New England and it was left to Vassie in 1932 documented that almost all these patients could be traced to only six individuals who had migrated from the Anglican village of Bures in Suffolk and one remarkably curious family could be traced for 300 years through twelve generations, where all the patients had fully expressed the disease. Many others could be tracked down to a family in Somerset in UK who later settled in Tasmania, Australia. Alois Alzheimer, Pierre Marie, Jean Lhermitte, and Oskar Vogt among others, performed intensive autopsy studies on the brains of these patients.[1,14-16]

The Maracaibo Story

In the mid-1950s, Americo Negrette, a young Venezuelan physician, arrived at San Luis near the city and lake of Maracaibo, where he was to spend 1 year in the national service. This percipient young physician observed some people behaving curiously with shakes as if they were uncontrollably inebriated. The neighbors were good enough to suggest that these strange people would soon be invalid to the extent that voluntary activities could not be performed easily and they would eventually die. The condition was known as *"el mal de San Vito"*, meaning *"the inauspicious dance"* among the local inhabitants.[1,14-16]

Negrette in his enthusiasm took a detailed history, examined the subjects, and concluded that the problem was one of dementia and choreiform movements. He further observed that the transmission of the disease conformed to an autosomal dominant pattern and concluded that he was dealing with cases of Huntington's chorea. He left for posterity his remarkable treatise, *"Chorea de Huntington. Maracaibo, Venezuela: University of Zulia 1958"*, that has firmly found its pride of place in the history of medicine.[1,15,17]

In 1972, Ramon Avilla Giron, who worked along with Negrette, carried with him the video recordings of these patients in order to present them in Huntington's disease Centenary Celebration which was organized in New York at that time. There was unanimous agreement about the disease entity among the experts. The study further showed that these Venezuelans were all descendants from one woman, Maria Concepcion Soto, who lived in the early 18th century and who perhaps inherited the gene from a European sailor.[1,15,17]

Nancy Wexler, a psychoanalyst, from the National Institute of Neurological and Communicative Disorders and Stroke, whose mother was a victim of Huntington's disease, attended the meeting and she was inspired to get to the core of the problem. She organized a trip to Lake Maracaibo in July 1979 and in collaboration with Thomas Chase of the National Institute of Health, Bethesda, USA, formed The Venezuelan Collaborative Huntington's Disease Society and Nancy Wexler was appointed its executive director. The principal investigators were Sir Ernesto Bonilla from Zulia and Nancy Wexler herself and they were aided by other neurologists, geneticists, anthropologists, and historians. The team of geneticists led by James Gusella, discovered that the genetic locus for the disease was in the short arm of chromosome 4 and a landmark paper was published in *Nature* in 1983.[15] In 1992, Anita Harding, from Queen Square, London, identified that the number of trinucleotide repeats had a direct relationship with the severity of the disease and in 1993 the Huntington's Disease Collaborative Research Group could isolate the gene at the precise location at 4p 16.3 position.[15] In 1996, a transgenic mouse model *(the R6 line)* was created that could be made to exhibit the clinical features of Huntington's disease.[15]

In 1908, William Osler, the peerless physician, wrote, *"In the history of medicine, there are few instances in which a disease has been more accurately, more graphically, or more briefly described."*[15] Huntington wrote in his personal memoirs:

> *"Over 50 years ago, in riding with my father on his professional rounds, I saw my first case of "that disorder", which was the way in which the natives always referred to the dreaded disease. It made a most enduring impression upon my boyish mind, an impression every detail of which I recall today, and an impression which was the very first impulse to my choosing chorea as my virgin contribution to medical lore. We suddenly came upon two women, mother and daughter, both tall, thin, almost cadaverous, both bowing, twisting, grimacing. I stared in wonderment... Then my medical instruction had its inception. From this point on, my interest in the disease has never wholly ceased."*[15,18]

George Huntington died of pneumonia in 1916.

SAMUEL ALEXANDER KINNIER WILSON (1878–1939)

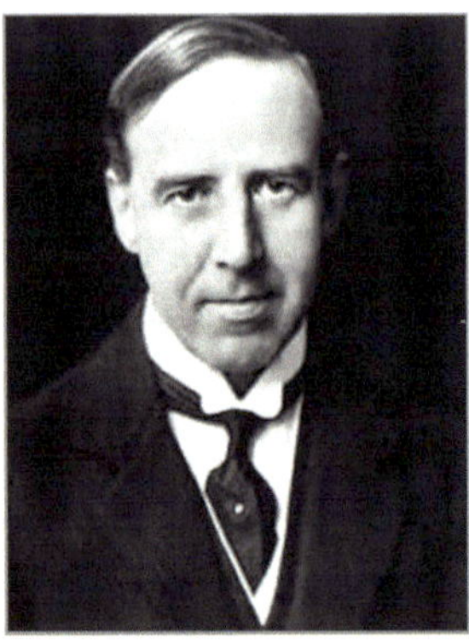

Wilson was born in New Jersey, United States of America in 1878. He studied at the University of Edinburgh and graduated to MA in 1897 and MB Ch B in 1902. Thereafter, he moved to France and worked with Joseph Babinski and Pierre Marie at Bicêtre. On his return to London, he was appointed as the last House Physician to Hughlings Jackson, and then to William Gowers at the National Hospital, Queen Square. He became a full Physician in 1925. Along with Gordon Holmes, he constituted the core of *"Queen Square Neurology"* that was almost synonymous with British neurology in the first half of the last century. He was also in charge of the neurological department at King's College from 1919 and to acknowledge his contributions, one ward was named after him. He was the first British physician to have practiced neurology exclusively.[1,13]

The entity which bears the eponym Wilson's disease constituted his thesis for his MD degree, and it earned him a gold medal. It was entitled, *"Progressive lenticular degeneration: A familial nervous disease associated with cirrhosis of the liver."* Later, in 1912, he published his work in the celebrated journal, *Brain,* which ran for 214 pages and it was the only article in that volume.[1,19] The original description of the entity was as follows:

> *"It is characterized by a definite symptom complex, whose chief features are: generalized tremor, dysarthria, and dysphagia, muscular rigidity and hypertonicity, emaciation, spasmodic contractions, contracture, emotionalisms. There are also certain mental symptoms, either transient... or more chronic... The mental symptoms may be very slight and are sometimes absent."*[1,3]

And further,

> *"Progressive lenticular degeneration is, I believe, the first definitely established morbid entity whose most striking characteristic is a specific association between the disease of one of the viscera and disease of a particular part of the gray matter of the central nervous system-viz., the lenticular nucleus."*[1,3]

Wilson initially called it *"progressive lenticular degeneration"* and coined the term in 1911. He alluded to some cases described by his predecessors and acknowledged the works of William Gowers. He felt that Gowers in 1888 described two cases of *"brother and sister under the title "Tetanoid Chorea", associated with Cirrhosis of the Liver."* He further wrote that Ormerod in 1890 described *"Cirrhosis of Liver in a Boy with Obscure and Fatal Nervous Symptoms"*, and wrote:

> *"In Ormerod's case, the putamen were softened on both sides where in Gower's... no very definite nervous lesion could be found. All had hepatic cirrhosis."*[1,3]

On the other hand, Wilson found no reason to accept the entity, *pseudosclerosis*, described by Westphal in 1883 and Strümpell in 1898, as cases belonging to this category, since hepatic cirrhosis could not be documented. He felt that those cases had,

> *"... little in common, except tremor. So doubtful was he himself of their nature that he attributed them to "a neurosis" which may perhaps, though not very suitably, be described as "pseudosclerosis" because in some way they recalled the picture of cerebrospinal gray degeneration, "i.e., multiple sclerosis."*[1,3]

Strümpell tried to revive the entity but Wilson critical of Strümpell's observations. He wrote,

> *"Plainly, these cases of Westphal and Strümpell are so heterogeneous as to be useless for the extraction of any specific clinicopathological entity therefrom... In not one of these cases (except a syphilitic case of Strümpell's) and of a number more published later...was allusion made to cirrhosis of the liver, for the simple reason that it did not occur."*[1,3]

Incidentally, Wilson was so rigid on the presence of hepatic cirrhosis as a necessary component of the condition, that some clinicians even referred to cases with hepatic lesions and without any cerebral stigmata as, *"Abdominal Wilson's disease"*![1]

Such was the impact of Kinnier Wilson in neurology that David Marsden and Stanley Fahn, two contemporary giants in the field of movement disorders, wrote in the Editorial of the journal, *Movement Disorders* in 1987:

> *"Kinnier Wilson was the father of basal ganglia research. We stand on his shoulders, and it is a pleasure to do tribute to his memory."*

Kinnier Wilson died of the complications of malignancy in 1939, though there is an element of controversy regarding his year of expiry. His book *Neurology* was published posthumously in 1940.

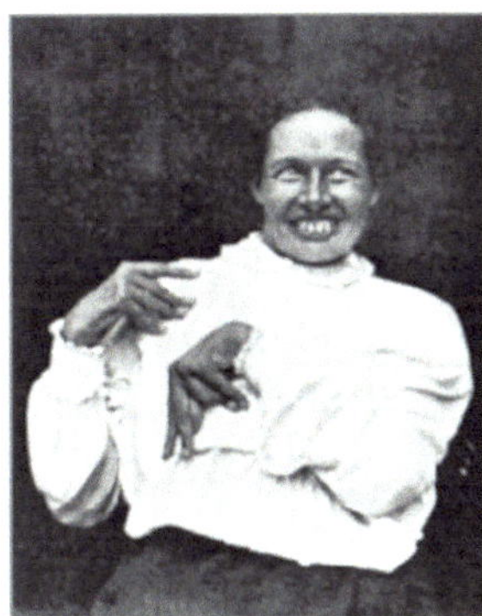
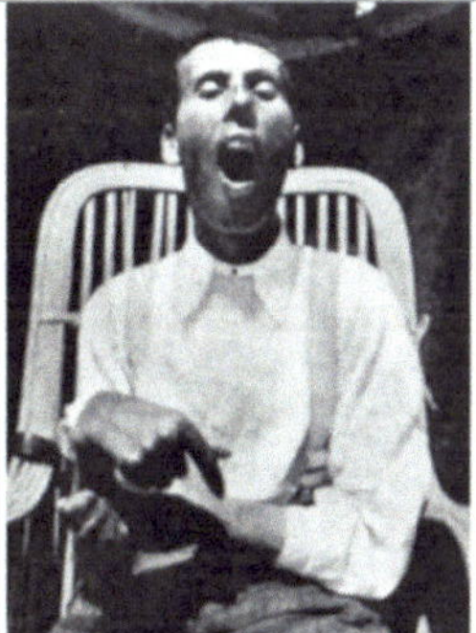
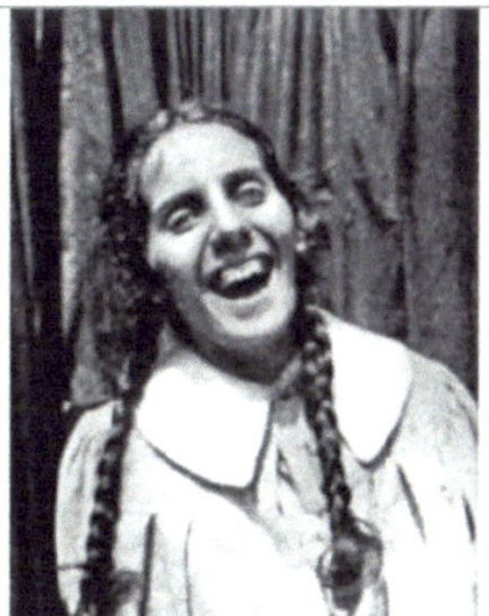
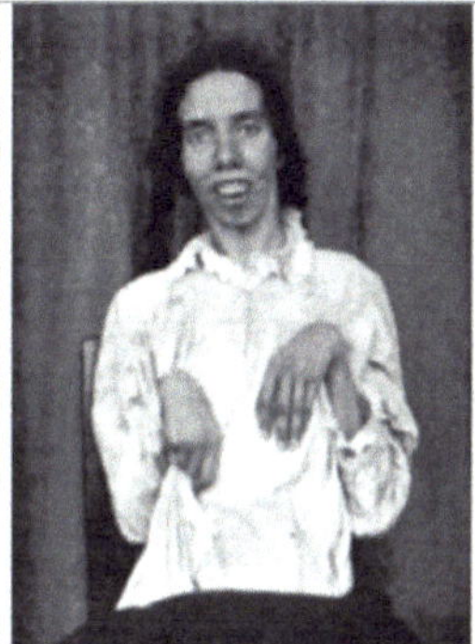
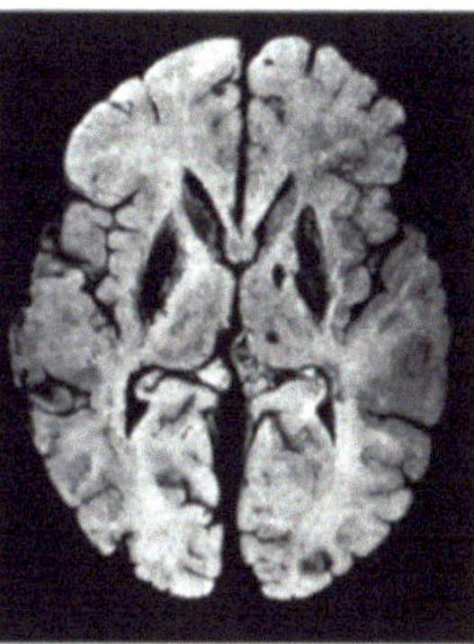

Four cases of Kinnier Wilson and the autopsy findings in one of them.

CHARLES DAVID MARSDEN (1938–1998)

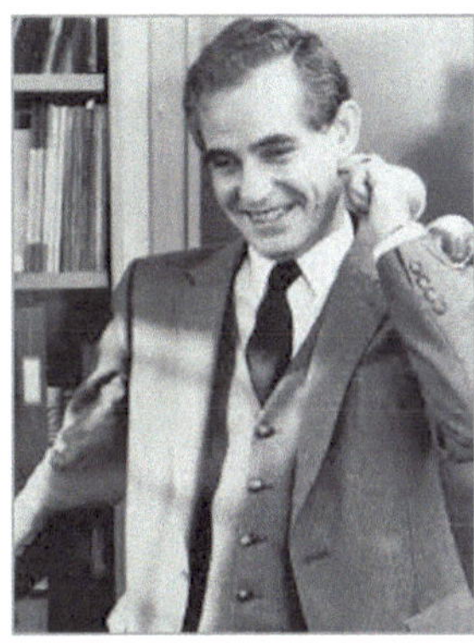

David Marsden was the supreme master in the field of movement disorders in the last century. Indeed, he was one of the greatest figures in the study of movement disorders.

He was born in 1938 and studied at St Thomas Medical School. Even at that preparatory period, he likened the substantia nigra to the basement of a house and wondered why it was dark. He even started speculating that the key to the mysteries of the basal ganglia lay in the understanding of neuromelanin.[20,21] While he was in his early 20s, he was in communication with Oleh Hornykiewicz from Austria, who had just demonstrated a severe deficiency of dopamine in the substantia nigra in Parkinson's disease. In the middle of his medical study, he shifted from clinical neurology to the study of physiology and wrote a thesis on the pigmentation of the substantia nigra. He was appointed as Honorary Lecturer at Queen Square in 1970 and 2 years later, took up the position of the first-ever Professor of neurology[4] at the Maudsley and King's College Hospital, London.[1]

Marsden collaborated with a number of young neuroscientists and loads of papers of outstanding scientific quality started flowing from his center. He attracted Fellows from all over the world and they came to be known as the Denmark Hill fellows, named after the street that runs between the King's College and the Maudsley Hospital. They include Roger Duvoisin, Paul Bedard, Mark Hallett, Dan Tarsy, Eldad Melamed, Wolfgang Oertel, Alberto Albanese, Giovanni Abbruzzese, Fabrizio Stocchi, Tony Lang, Jose Obeso, Niall Quinn, Philip Thompson, Kailash Bhatia, and others.[20] In 1983 he was elected a Fellow of the Royal Society at the age of 45 years. The following year, the London University conferred the Doctor of Science degree on him and in 1987, he moved to National Hospital, Queen Square as the Professor of Clinical Neurology, the premier chair in the United Kingdom. He worked in that capacity till 1995, when he was appointed the Dean of the Institute of Neurology. He went to Bethesda, the USA in 1998 as Fogerty Fellow to work on apraxia.[1,20]

Marsden's gamut of research in movement disorders had been staggering and his output overwhelming. His opinion was the gold standard and the last word in any international meeting anywhere. The following is just a glimpse of the vastness of his scientific output.

- Conducted epoch-making works on dystonia, a complicated mishmash for a long time. He brought order into the whole conundrum of disorders such as blepharospasm, writer's cramp, and torticollis among others, and proved incontrovertibly that these were organic diseases and not hysterical manifestations of psychiatric disorders.
- Defined myoclonus in electrophysiological terms and in collaboration with Mark Hallett and classified it as cortical, subcortical, and other varieties.[22]
- Along with David Parkes worked on the pharmacodynamics of levodopa and the long-term complications associated with its use.[23]
- Along with Pat Merton, an outstanding neurophysiologist and Bert Morton, a technical wizard, popularly known as the "3Ms", carried out seminal works on the servo action of the human thumb, the importance of the long latency reflexes and adduced evidence for the evidence of a transcortical component in stretch reflexes. This was a significant departure from the classical Sherringtonian concept that stretch reflexes are monosynaptic and spinal in nature.[24-26]

- Worked on evoked potentials and transcranial electrical and magnetic stimulation that helped to develop novel and pioneering surgical techniques for the management of Parkinson's disease and other movement disorders.[1]
- Along with Peter Jenner, the neuropharmacologist from King's College, London, developed the MPTP marmoset model of Parkinson's disease.[1]

One great contribution of Marsden is the foundation of the Parkinson's Disease Society Brain Bank of the United Kingdom in collaboration with Andrew Lees during a flight in an aircraft.[27,28] This apart, he founded the Movement Disorders Society in 1985 along with his comrade-in-arms, Stanley Fahn from Columbia, and they also coedited the journal *Movement Disorders* for its first 10 years. He was appointed as the editor of the *Journal of Neurology, Neurosurgery, and Psychiatry* for 10 years and gave it a new shape and direction, and a commemorative volume was published in his honor in 1989 when he stepped down from that assignment. He was on the editorial boards of >20 journals, held >40 visiting fellowships, received numerous awards, and was on the councils of the Royal Society, Medical Research Council, and the Royal College of Physicians.[20]

The essential quality which Marsden possessed was his unique capability to see the truth in a medley of conflicting data. Peter Jenner wrote *"where no one could see meaning and, with one sweep of his hand, he would remove the dross and clear a path with absolute brilliance that captured the key findings and explained all."* Niall Quinn wrote, *"One secret of his success was his attention to detail whilst at the same time, clearly seeing the bigger picture. He did best particularly in his clinics and ward rounds, and especially in his "book rounds". The SHO or the Registrar would begin the history and after several sentences, David would say, "Stop!", and ask one of his Fellows what he or she thought of the story so far, and by iterating this process, gave insight into the way he would approach the question of differential diagnosis."*[20] In his obituary in *Journal of Neurology Neurosurgery and Psychiatry* David Brooks, Professor of Neurology, Hammersmith Hospital, London, wrote that such was his clinical acumen that in future while confronted with a difficult and mixed movement disorders problem, he would almost hear Marsden's baritone voice in the background in an oracular fashion *"and what did we think this patient had the last time we saw him?"*[29] In 1998, he received the prestigious Fogarty-in-Residence Fellowship for a year to work at the National Institute of Health, Bethesda, USA. However, within a month, he died of a hitherto undiagnosed congenital heart problem and with that, the world of neurology lost a genius untimely. Indeed, Marsden was the role model for generations of experts on movement disorders.

ARVID CARLSSON (1923–2018)

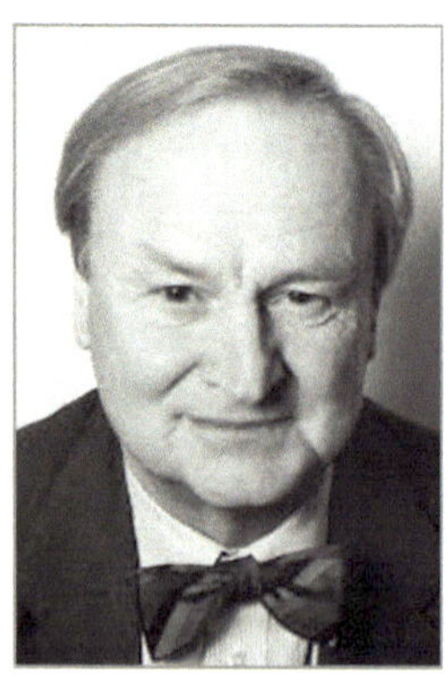

Levodopa (L-DOPA) was first synthesized in the western world in 1911 by the Polish biochemist Casimir Funk (1884–1967) though the credit for isolating it from the seeds of Vicia faba, a leguminous plant which grows abundantly in India and the neighbouring counties goes to Markus Guggenheim (1885–1970), a biochemist from Sweden in 1913.[30] Guggenheim himself consumed it and vomited violently. He shelved his idea and later, in his celebrated treatise, *Die Biogenen Amine*, he devoted only two pages to his own discovery. Sir Henry Dale, the peerless neuropharmacologist and the Nobel Laureate for the year 1936, suggested the name, *dopamine*. It was already documented that a dose of injection of reserpine lowered the level of serotonin in the brain and it was speculated that its antihypertensive action was hyposerotoninergic in effect.

Carlsson was born in Uppsala, Sweden, and studied Medicine at the University of Lund. Later, he spent some time at Bethesda, USA. While working in the cardiac laboratory of Herman Blaschko in Oxford, he felt that the action was brought about by catecholamines and it was observed that L-DOPA was present in high concentration in the basal ganglia. Following his return to Sweden he set up his own laboratory at the University of Lund and in 1957 he showed that following the administration of reserpine in rabbits there was complete disappearance of norepinephrine from the adrenal medulla and the brain. Additionally, the akinetic effect of reserpine resembled the clinical picture of parkinsonism which was quickly reversed by L-DOPA. Incidentally, the precursor of serotonin, 5-hydroxytryptophan, had no such effect.

He devised a sensitive fluorescent assay device to measure dopamine in the brain, observed its high concentration in the striatum, and showed that a dose of reserpine, a dopamine-depleting agent, when injected into rabbits, leads to features that closely resemble those of Parkinson's disease. Levodopa reversed the clinical state.[31-33] This was the first experiment that proved the efficacy of levodopa in the management of Parkinson's disease, and it earned him the Nobel Prize in the year 2000.

This is the set of the famous photographs of the pair of rabbits, reserpinized, and rendered lethargic and immobile, while the one below shows the rejuvenated and alert ones with the use of levodopa.[33]

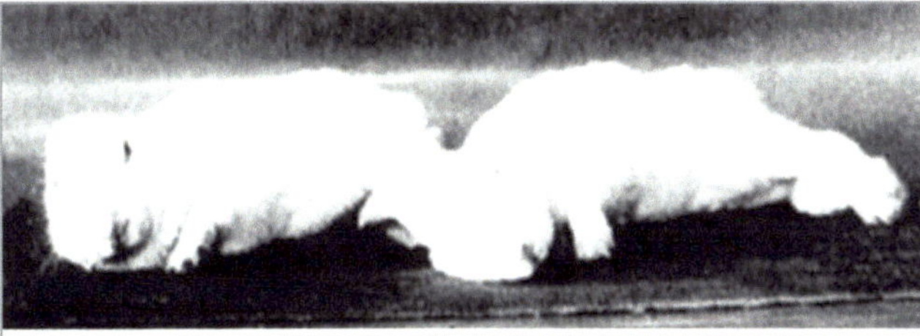

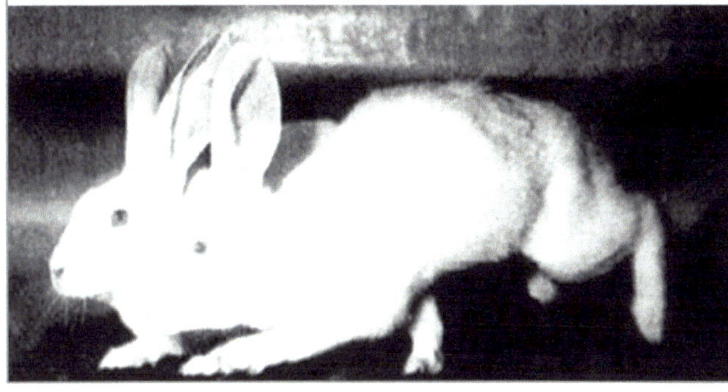

In his Nobel Lecture in 2000, Carlsson said:

> *"...This work had resulted in my doctoral thesis in 1951 and a series of subsequent papers,... I came to work under Dr. Brodie for about 5 months,... Brodie and his colleagues had made a breakthrough discovery, namely that the administration of reserpine, a recently introduced antipsychotic and antihypertensive drug, caused the virtually complete disappearance of serotonin from the brain and other tissues...*
>
> *... I proposed to Brodie that we investigate the effect of reserpine on the catecholamines in view of their similarity to serotonin. But Brodie thought that this would be a waste of time... But I felt that a look at the catecholamines would be worthwhile... I wrote to him (Professor Nils Åke Hillarp) and proposed collaboration and he agreed... We demonstrated the depletion of catecholamines from the adrenal medulla of rabbits following treatment with reserpine...depletion of catecholamines could be the cause of the behavioral inhibition induced by reserpine... We gave DOPA...and discovered the dramatic reversal of the reserpine-induced syndrome...*
>
> *...Later we found the unique distribution of dopamine in the brain.... This, taken together with the fact that a characteristic side-effect of reserpine is to mimic very faithfully the syndrome of Parkinsonism...led us to conclude that depletion of dopamine will induce the Parkinson syndrome and that treatment with L-DOPA will alleviate the syndrome by restoring the dopamine level..."*[34]
>
> *... All this I presented at the First International Catecholamine Symposium in October 1958... the debate...revealed a profound and nearly unanimous skepticism... Dale expressed the view that L-DOPA was a poison... Marthe Vogt concluded that...the action of serotonin and catecholamines, respectively, in the brain would not have a long life... John Gaddum, an outstanding pharmacologist from Cambridge...stated that nobody has ventured to speculate on the relationship between catecholamines and the functions of the brain...'*[35]

Unfortunately, Carlsson's work was not taken seriously and he had to face vitriolic criticisms from many authorities including Sir Henry Dale and John Gaddum. That a chemical substance released from the brain was the panacea for such a devastating malady was beyond the imagination and the limits of the credibility of his detractors. Dale was not convinced about Carlsson's observations and commented that DA had not yet fulfilled the criterion for a neurotransmitter. He felt that the actions were possibly attributable to L-DOPA being a '*mysterious brain toxin and when combined with a monoamine oxidase inhibitor led to excitation and could be lethal*'.[36]

The indifferent reception left Carlsson a disillusioned scientist. However, his steely nerve did not allow him to harbor any sense of resignation, and his passion for catecholamines, Parkinson's disease and the brain, went on unabated, and finally, he got his reward when he was awarded the coveted Nobel Prize.

OLEH HORNYKIEWICZ (1926–2020)

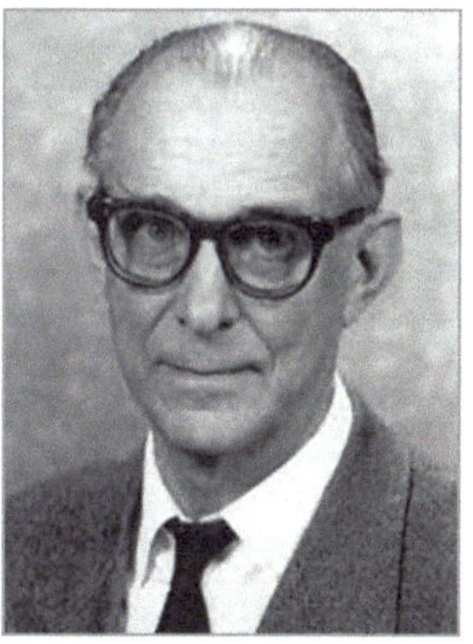

Oleh Hornykiewicz (1926–2020), a young neuroscientist from Austria, returned to Vienna from Oxford in 1958. He worked on DA and observed its high concentration in the striatum.[34,36] With his assistant Herbert Ehringer (1932–), he decided to study the DA content in the brain in patients with PD, post-encephalitic parkinsonism, and Huntington's disease (HD). They reported DA deficiency in the range of 90% in PD and post-encephalitic parkinsonism, while it was normal in HD.[36] He postulated that most of the major motor symptoms of PD were related to the deficiency of DA and the symptoms appeared after 80% reduction of DA in the nigral cells.[36]

In 1961, Hornykiewicz collected L-DOPA and urged upon his associate, Walther Birkmayer (1910–1996), to carry out trials on 20 patients with PD and **postencephalitic** parkinsonism. They injected it in gradually incremental dosage in strengths of 50 mg, 100 mg, and 150 mg.[28] In the third group, there was a marked improvement in hypokinesia. They treated more than 200 patients along with isocarboxazid, a MAO-inhibitor, and by 1964 the results showed that in about 20% of patients there was lasting relief for about 3 hours.[29] In an interview with B Sommer, a geriatric psychiatrist, he said,

> *'... Bedridden patients who were unable to sit up, patients who could not stand up when seated, who when standing could not start walking, performed these activities with ease... The drug worked from the first dose, and its beneficial action from bradykinesia was reported to last from 3 to 24 hours... Pretreatment with the monoamine oxidase inhibitor isocarboxazid, considerably prolonged the anti-akinetic effect.'*[34]

The response to Hornykiewicz's works was tepid and many international authorities repudiated his ideas. Denny-Brown commented, *'You have presented reasons against the common assumption that lesions in the substantia nigra are responsible for parkinsonism'*, while Rolf Hassler, an anatomist from Frankfurt said, *'The interpretation of your observations does not agree with many known facts about the direction of the nigrostriatal connections...'* Mettler wrote, *'The attribution of such a complex clinical syndrome to a rather small and homogeneous structure has not appeared logical'*, while Bertler and Rosengren said, *'The effect of L-DOPA is too complex to permit a conclusion about disturbances of the striatal system in Parkinson's disease.'*[37] Jasper's comments were acerbic and he wrote that *'L-DOPA is the right therapy for the wrong reason'*, and even Arvid Carlsson was not far behind in snide remark and said, *'...not possible to draw any conclusion about the relative importance of dopamine... for the central effects.'*[37] Roger Duvoisin stated, *'Despite enthusiastic claims of therapeutic benefit, no evidence has been presented that DOPA effects are in any way specific....'*[37] The issue was getting so convoluted with growing controversies, that in 1965 even Hornykiewicz had to concede that possibly L-DOPA did not have a potential future.[37]

Much later in 2010, when L-DOPA was firmly established as the drug of choice in PD long ago, Hornykiewicz wrote,

> *'...one would have expected unanimous support ... This was indeed the case with the vast majority of clinical neurologists, but not the rule among the basic brain scientists... Among those strongly critical of DA and levodopa were the best minds of the contemporary neuroscience...'*[37]

Later, when DA was found to be useful for the management of PD, the world of neurology found it hard to accept the fact that when the Nobel Prize in 2000 was awarded to Carlsson, Hornykiewicz was overlooked. More than 250 eminent neurologists wrote to the Nobel Committee, expressing their disappointment. However, Hornykiewicz stated politely that scientists take to investigative studies not in order to win prizes and receive universal recognition though he regretted that the Nobel Committee was amiss in their assessment that Carlsson was the chief architect in discovering low DA content in the brain in PD. True to what he said, Hornykiewicz and his team were the scientists behind this fundamental discovery.[36]

GEORGE COTZIAS (1918–1977)

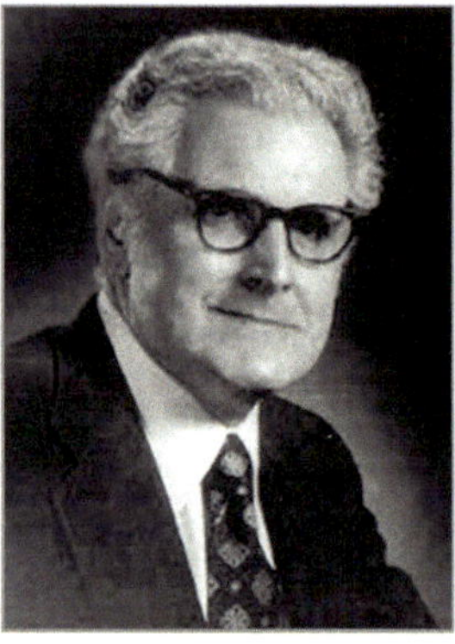

Cotzias proved undeniably the efficacy of L-DOPA in clinical practice. He used L-DOPA in a small dosage, increased it slowly, and carried on the treatment for a long duration, ultimately attaining the dose of 12 g per day. He published his observations in the *New England Journal of Medicine* in 1967, and thereafter, an exhaustive report titled, *'Modification of parkinsonism: Chronic treatment with L-DOPA'*, appeared in 1969 in the same journal, where he described the appearance of some involuntary movements. He wrote that of the 28 patients studied, there were various grades of improvement which was sustained for two years.[34]

It is pertinent to question why Cotzias' method of using the low and slowly incremental dosage of L-DOPA was a success. A cogent argument was that he did not use it in order to dramatically increase the level of dopamine in the striatum; rather, his hope was to replenish the lost melanin in the substantia nigra, which he felt, was the cause of PD.[34] In his seminal paper in 1969, he wrote that one of the biochemical abnormalities in PD was the decrease in melanin in the substantia nigra and this might be interrelated since tyrosine is hydroxylated to dihydroxyphenylalanine, a precursor for the synthesis of melanin and catecholamines in the melanocytes. He surmised that the interrelation between melanogenesis and PD was of fundamental importance.[36] This view was endorsed by David Marsden of (1938–1998), one of the most influential experts in movement disorders of the latter half in the last century. In his *Robert Wartenberg Lecture* delivered before the American Academy of Neurology in 1982, he said, *'... I stepped sideways from the mainstream of medical education into the research laboratory to try to discover why the substantia nigra was black! In my naiveté, I thought that this must constitute some key to the function of this region of the brain and I even believed..., that neuromelanin holds the key to the cause of Parkinson's disease.'*[38] However, in spite of the improvement in the symptoms of PD, the works of Cotzias were also not immediately recognized, as had been the case with the previous investigators. In fact, Melvin Yahr and Roger Duvoisin, unquestionable experts in PD, wrote in 1968,

> *'Cotzias et al, (1967) have reported oral administration of L-DOPA in dosages of up to 16 gper day... However, there has also been an appreciable incidence of undesirable side effects... Though undoubtedly at this dosage...a sustained effect ...can be obtained, the role of dopa...is far from established.'*[36]

Fahn made an interesting remark that when Cotzias presented his observations at a symposium in Montreal in 1967, Carlsson and he himself were present there and were impressed. Thereafter, Roger Duvoisin visited Cotzias' laboratory to witness the patients under trial and returned to Columbia, content with the work.[36] Such was the impact of Cotzias' work on the effect of L-DOPA that Irving Cooper, the celebrated American neurosurgeon, who demonstrated the amelioration of PD following accidental ligation of the anterior choroidal artery in 1953 declared that surgical procedures be postponed for at least for 1 year.[36]

On the slow and incremental dose of L-DOPA, Cotzias wrote,

> *'We recognized that the oral route of administration must be used... We defined our needs as follows: to saturate...either or both the enzymes, dopa decarboxylase...and the melanin-forming enzymes, i.e., tyrosinase, within the brain. This simplistic notion confirmed...with the method used by biochemists wishing to saturate an enzyme with substrate. They do this by gradually increasing the amounts of the substrate presented to the enzyme.'*[36]

MELVIN YAHR (1917–2004)

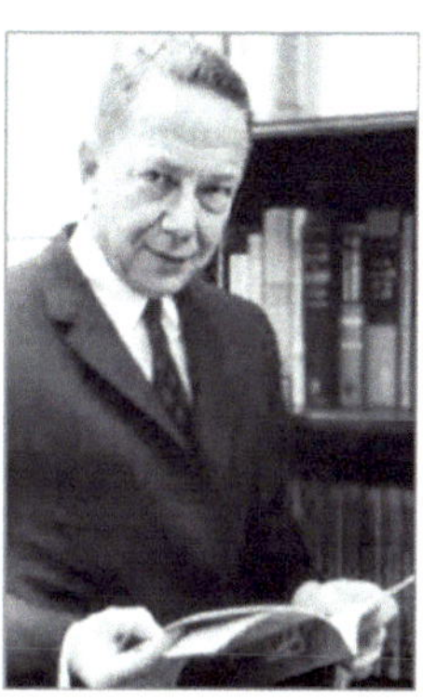

Melvin Yahr from Mount Sinai decided to carry out a double-blind study of L-DOPA on PD patients. He recruited 60 patients, (56 had PD, 3 of postencephalitic parkinsonism, and 1 suffering from progressive supranuclear palsy). They were hospitalized for a period of 4–12 weeks and were on 5–10 tablets per day. The placebo group received 1 tablet in a daily dosage of 750 mg to 1 g. Placebo tablets were gradually replaced by 0.5 g of L-DOPA every 28–48 hours until an optimal therapeutic response was observed, and a total dose of 8 g per day was administered, or till side effects appeared. L-DOPA was rapidly withdrawn in 9 patients, replaced by placebo, and the patients were clinically examined by two independent observers every day. The patients were followed up for 4–12 months and 49 subjects showed considerable improvement. Yahr et al, concluded that L-DOPA was an effective drug and was superior to all other modalities prevalent at that time.[36]

Close on the heels of Cotzias many other workers performed open-label trials met with success to a varying extent, and it was finally approved by the USA Food and Drug Administration in 1970. In 1973, Bernheimer et al, noted morphological and neurochemical correlations in the dopamine level in PD treated with L-DOPA and two years later, Lloyd and his colleagues from Canada analyzed the brain tissue in postmortem studies in PD subjects treated with L-DOPA and controls. There was a 9- to 15-fold increase in L-DOPA concentration in the substantia nigra in the former group.[36]

Thus, a short account of the fundamental works of the stalwarts in the field of movement disorders is presented here. However, one shall be amiss if some notable names like Gilles de la Tourette, André Barbeau, Herbert Ehringer, Walther Birkmayer, Roger Duvoisin, Margaret Hoehn, and others are not paid obeisance and remembered, at least in passing.

Note: This article deals only with those experts in Movement Disorders who are no longer with us. There are a number of giants in the field who are presently working and churning out works of extraordinary quality in order to unravel the mysteries of these disorders with unabated zeal and enthusiasm.

REFERENCES

1. Bhattacharyya KB. Eminent Neuroscientists: Their lives and works. Kolkata, India: Academic Publishers; 2011.
2. Bhattacharyya KB. Movement Disorders. Twentieth Century Neurology: The British Contribution (Ed.) FC Rose. London: Imperial College Press; 2001. pp. 129-51.
3. Wilson SAK. *Sydenham's Chorea in "Neurology"*. Edward Arnold & Co, London. 1940;1:605-6.
4. Rose FC. History of British Neurology. London: Imperial College Press; 2012. pp. 47-9.
5. Bhattacharyya KB. Pioneers in Movement Disorders. J Assoc Phys Ind. 2016;64:75-6.
6. Parkinson J. An Essay on the Shaking Palsy. London: Sherwood; 1817.
7. Jefferson M. James Parkinson (1755-1824): Aspects of the history of Parkinson's disease. Br Med J. 1973;2:601-4.
8. Morris AD. James Parkinson: A Biographical Overview. In: Rose FC (Ed). James Parkinson: His Life and Times. Binkhauser, Boston. 1989.
9. Pearce JMS. A brief history of Parkinson's disease. J Assoc Neurol East Ind. 1996;2:94-9.
10. Scott SRW. The wrong James Parkinson. Practical Neurol. 2015;1:1136.
11. Bhattacharyya KB. Hallmarks of clinical aspects of Parkinson's disease through centuries. Int Rev Neurobiol. 2017;132:1-23.
12. Rowntree LG. James Parkinson: Bulletin of the Johns Hopkins Hospital. 1912;23:33.
13. Foster JB. Companion to Clinical Neurology. Brain. 1995;118(5): 1357-8.
14. Bhattacharyya KB. The History of Huntington's disease. J Assoc Neurol East Ind. 1996;100-6.
15. Bhattacharyya KB. The story of George Huntington and his disease. Ann Ind Acad Neurol. 2016;19:25-8.
16. Haymaker W, Schiller F. Founders of Neurology. Springfield, Illinois: Charles C Thomas; 1970. pp.305-7.
17. Negrette A. Corea de Huntington, 2nd edition. Maracaibo: Talleres Graficos de la Universidad del Zulia; 1963.
18. Huntington G. On Chorea. Medical and Surgical Reporter. Philadelphia: SW Butler; 1872.
19. Compston A. From the Archives. Brain. 2009;132(2):1997-2001.
20. Quinn N, Rothwell J, Jenner P. Charles David Marsden, 15 April 1938–29 September 1998. Biogr Mems Fell R Soc. 2012;58:203-28.
21. Marsden CD. The mysterious motor functions of the basal ganglia: The Robert Wartenberg Lecture. Neurology. 1982; 32(5):514-39.
22. Hallett M, Chadwick D, Marsden CD. Ballistic movement overflow myoclonus a form of essential myoclonus. Brain. 1977;100(2):299-312.
23. Marsden CD, Parkes JD, Rees JE. A year's comparison of treatment of patients with Parkinson's disease with levodopa combined with carbidopa versus treatment with levodopa alone. Lancet. 1973;2(7844):1459-62.
24. Marsden CD, Merton PA, Morton HB. Is the human stretch reflex cortical rather than spinal? Lancet. 1973;1(7806): 759-61.
25. Marsden CD, Merton PA, Morton HB. Servo action in human voluntary movement. Nature. 1972;238(5360):140-3.
26. Marsden CD, Merton PA, Morton HB. Stretch reflex and servo action in a variety of human muscles. J Physiol. 1976;259(2): 531-60.
27. Zubko LEBM, Franco MKP, Meira AT, Germiniani FMB, Camargo CHF, Teive HAG. The legacy of Charles David Marsden: A role model in the field of movement disorders. Eur Neurol. 2019;81(5-6):319-22.
28. Lees AJ. C David Marsden (April 15, 1938–September 29,1998). In Memoriam. Mov Disord. 1999;14:3-5.
29. Brooks D. Professor C David Marsden 1938–98. J Neurol Neurosurg Psychiatry. 1999;66(1):2.
30. Ovallath S, Sulthana B. Levodopa: History and therapeutic applications. Ann Ind Acad Neurol 2017;20:185-189.
31. Yeragani VK, Tancer M, Chokka P, Baker GB. Arvid Carlsson, and the story of dopamine. Ind J Psychiatry. 2010;52(1):87-8.
32. Carlsson A, Lindqvist M, Magnusson T. 3, 4-Dihydroxyphenylalanine and 5-hydroxytryptophan as reserpine antagonists. Nature. 1957;180(4596):1200.
33. Carlsson A. Basic concepts underlying recent developments in the field of Parkinson's disease. Contemp Neurol Ser. 1971; 8:1-31.
34. Fahn S. The medical treatment of Parkinson's disease from James Parkinson to George Cotzias. Mov Disord. 2015;30(1): 4-18.
35. Carlsson A. A half century of neurotransmitter research: Impact on neurology and psychiatry. Nobel Lecture. 2000: 303-22.
36. Lees AJ, Tolosa E, Olanow CW. Four pioneers of L-dopa treatment: Arvid Carlsson, Oleh Hornykiewicz, George Cotzias, and Melvin Yahr. Mov Disord. 2015;30(1):19-36.
37. Hornykiewicz O. A brief history of levodopa. J Neurol 2010; 257(suppl 2):249-52.

CHAPTER 2

Basal Ganglia Anatomy and Functions

Aditya Ashok Murgai, Mandar Jog

INTRODUCTION

Basal ganglia (BG) are a group of large subcortical nuclei important for motor learning, action selection, motor control, motivation, and reward. BG circuits are organized in a way to facilitate desired voluntary movement and inhibit competing movements. They form the extrapyramidal system which is involved in various movement disorders such as Parkinson's disease, Huntington's disease, and Tourette's syndrome. Over the years many anatomical, functional neuroimaging, and neurophysiology studies have tried to understand the functions of BG and its circuits. Another approach of understanding BG functions has been to study the deficits that occur in patients with BG disorders. In the following sections we would discuss in detail about BG microstructure, circuits, and their role in motor control, behavior, and cognition.

BASAL GANGLIA STRUCTURE

The principal components of the BG are the striatum, subthalamic nucleus (STN), pallidum, and substantia nigra. The striatum can be functionally and anatomically divided into a dorsal and ventral portion. The dorsal striatum is composed of the putamen and caudate nucleus (CN) and the ventral striatum includes the nucleus accumbens (NA). For such a large nucleus, the striatum is unique as it lacks glutamatergic neurons and most of the output cells are gamma-aminobutyric acid-ergic (GABAergic). The STN is a biconvex-shaped nucleus, approximately 9 × 7 × 4 mm (length, height, weight). Subthalamic nuclei lies just below the thalamus and can also be considered an input nucleus as it receives input from the cerebral cortex. It also receives input from the globus pallidus external (GPe) and gives excitatory output to globus pallidus interna (GPi) nucleus. The STN is divided into dorsolateral, ventromedial, and medial portions, which differ in their connectivity and functions. Dorsolateral STN, which is the sensorimotor region receiving direct projections from the primary motor cortex (M1) and supplementary motor area (SMA). The ventromedial STN contains the associative region, receiving projections from the premotor cortex (PMC), prefrontal cortex (PFC), SMA, frontal eye field (FEF), and supplementary eye field. Lastly, the medial portion which represents the limbic region and receives projections from the caudal cingulate motor cortex.[1] The GP is separated into two nuclei: The more laterally positioned nucleus is called the GPe, whereas the medial nucleus is called the GPi, both receiving GABAergic input from the striatal neurons.[2]

The putamen and caudate are the main input nuclei while the GPi along with substantia nigra pars reticulata (SNr) form the main output nuclei of BG. The BG provide output to the thalamus, the superior colliculus (SC), and the pedunculopontine nucleus (PPN). BG influence motor, sensory, and cognitive information processing through their innervation of the thalamus, eye movements through innervation of SC, and locomotion and postural control through innervation of the PPN.[2]

Striatum receives dopaminergic input from the ventral midbrain, which consists of three main groups of neurons. Ventral tegmental area (A10) projects to NA and ventral pallidum and is involved in addiction and motivation, substantia nigra compacta (SNc) (A9) and retro-rubral field (A8), both project to the striatum.[3] Substantia nigra can be separated into two regions, SNc and SNr. SNr cells are involved in saccadic eye movements and there is some evidence showing their role in cognitive processing.[4] In the following sections we will discuss the microanatomy of the striatum, STN, and GP in greater.

Striatal Compartments: Striosomes and Matrix

Striatum comprising of putamen and caudate is composed of two distinct compartments, the striosomes (patches) and matrix.[5] Acetylcholine esterase (AChE) staining of striatum shows weak AChE activity in striosomes in a background of more intense AChE staining of matrix. Also, striosomes shows strong immunoreactivity for enkephalin, substance P, GABA, and neurotensin, whereas the matrix compartment shows immunoreactivity for parvalbumin.[3] Both the compartments have medium spiny neurons (MSNs) and the dendrites of MSNs in striosomes and matrix remain restricted to their respective compartment with minimal interaction.

Each cortical area projects to both the patches and the matrix of the striatum. Deep layer V and layer VI corticostriate neurons project principally to the patches, whereas, superficial layer V and layer II and III corticostriatal neurons project mainly to the matrix. However, allocortical areas provide a greater input to the patches and neocortical areas to the matrix.[5]

Striatal Neurons: Projection Neurons and Interneurons

There are two populations of neurons in the striatum, projection neurons (striatofugal) and interneurons. Striatofugal neurons are MSNs (medium as they are about 20 μm in diameter and spiny as their dendrites have numerous spines) which constitute about 90% of striatal neurons and interneurons constitute the remaining 10%. The soma of MSN gives rise to 5–10 smooth primary dendrites that become densely invested with spines about 20 μm from the soma.[6] These dendrites branch moderately to about 30–35 dendritic tips and form a roughly spherical arbor unless distorted by the presence of a boundary between the striosome and matrix compartments which they do not cross (**Fig. 1**).[7]

Medium spiny neuronal membrane potential fluctuates between a relatively hyperpolarized "Down" state (–80 mV) and a relatively depolarized "Up" state (–50 mV). These neurons usually fire while in the Up state exhibiting a phasic burst pattern with a low firing rate. The occurrence of Up and Down states in striatal neurons requires phasic changes in the cortical and thalamic inputs to striatal neurons.[8] Excitatory cortical inputs on MSN end on the head of spines and dopaminergic terminals from the SNc terminate in close association with the corticostriate inputs on the spine necks or dendritic shafts (**Fig. 1**).[9]

The sources of the striatofugal direct and indirect pathways are also GABAergic neurons that can be segregated into two populations based on their peptide content, and by the preferential expression of dopamine receptors. Direct pathway neurons contain substance P/dynorphin and preferentially express D1-receptors whereas, indirect pathway neurons contain enkephalin and preferentially express D2-receptors. Striatal MSNs synapse with GPi/SNr, which gives output to the thalamus and then to cortex forming the direct pathway. Indirect pathway involves striatal MSNs, GPe, STN, GPi/SNr, thalamus, and cortex (**Fig. 2**). The input into GPi/SNr from the striatum and STN is such that the striatum provides a focused, context-dependent inhibition, while the STN provides a less specific and divergent excitation. Because the output from the GPi/SNr is inhibitory, this results

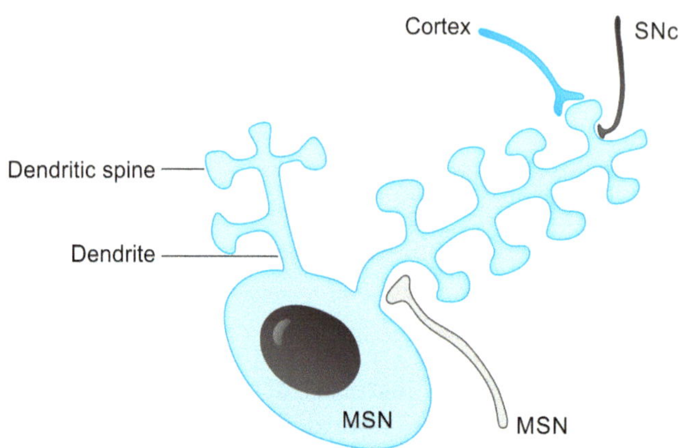

FIG. 1: Schematic image of a medium spiny neuron (MSN) structure. The glutaminergic input from cortex goes to the head of the dendritic spine, whereas the modulatory dopaminergic input from substantia nigra pars compacta (SNc) goes to the shaft of the dendritic spine.

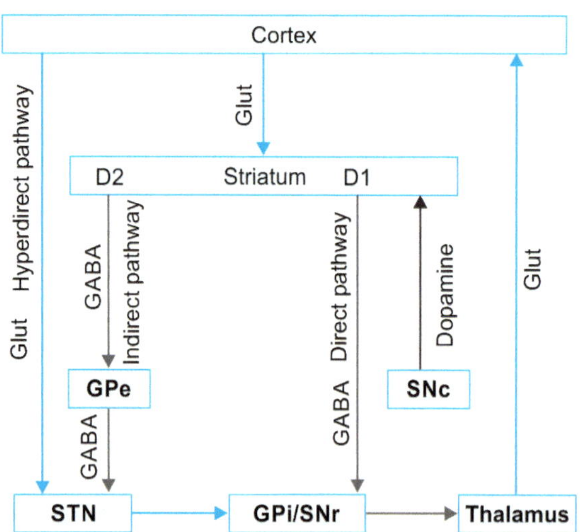

(GABA: gamma-aminobutyric acid; GPe: globus pallidus external; GPi: globus pallidus interna; SNc: substantia nigra compacta; SNr: substantia nigra reticulata; STN: subthalamic nucleus)

FIG. 2: Direct, indirect, and hyperdirect pathways in basal ganglia. The excitatory output is shown in blue and inhibitory output in gray color.

in a focused facilitation associated with a surround inhibition of motor phenomenon. This organization results in selective facilitation of desired movements and inhibition of competing movements.[10] Dopamine acts on D1 receptors increasing the production of cyclic adenosine monophosphate (cAMP) resulting in facilitation of the pathway through long-term potentiation whereas dopamine acting on D2 receptors causes reduction of cAMP resulting in long-term depression in the indirect pathway. Hence, dopamine has a facilitatory effect on the motor output from BG.

Striatal interneurons are inhibitory and use GABA as a neurotransmitter. These neurons are classified into four groups. The most abundant group of interneurons consist of large aspiny cholinergic neurons, comprising 0.3–2% of the neurons in the rodent striatum. They show a continuous and constant firing pattern and hence are also known as tonically active neurons (TANs). Aspiny cholinergic neurons can fire spontaneously unlike MSNs and have synaptic connections with MSNs and other interneurons. These neurons exhibit a relatively depolarized resting membrane potential between -55 and -60 mV and do not display the discrete "Up" and "Down" states like MSNs. The remaining interneurons are GABAergic, distinguishable on electrophysiological, morphological, and neurochemical bases. Parvalbumin (calcium binding protein) positive GABAergic interneuron, also known as fast-spiking interneurons (FSI) can fire at a high frequency of up to 300 Hz. The second type of GABAergic interneurons are medium size, calretinin (calcium binding protein) positive interneurons. The third type of GABAergic interneurons use nitric oxide as the neurotransmitter. TAN and FSI interneurons modulate the activity of striatofugal neurons and are under dopaminergic control whereas, calretinin and nitrergic GABAergic interneurons innervate TAN and FSI interneurons.[3]

ULTRASTRUCTURE OF GLOBUS PALLIDUS AND SUBTHALAMIC NUCLEUS

The STN is a lens-shaped densely populated structure. It is predominantly made up of glutamatergic projection neurons with 7.5% of GABAergic interneuron cells.[11] The STN consisted of tightly packed neurons distributed within a neuropil filled with large numbers of blood vessels and thinly myelinated fibers. STN neurons, dendrites, and initial axon segments are tightly apposed without any intervening glial membranes.[12]

The GP is divided by a thin lamina into an inner and outer segment. The entopeduncular nucleus in rodent is considered homologous to the GPi in primates. Unlike STN and striatum, the neurons are sparsely distributed across GP. Most of the cell bodies in GP are large (35–70 μ) in size.[13,14] These large pallidal neurons are characterized by sparsely branched dendritic arborizations with thick, smooth, and long dendrites.[15] Ultrastructural of GP shows highly prevalent synaptic interaction between glutamic acid decarboxylase (GAD) immune-reactive axon terminals and GAD positive pallidal neurons.[16]

BASAL GANGLIA CIRCUITS

Basal ganglia receive cortical input from multiple cortical areas including primary motor cortex, somatosensory cortex, PMC, supplementary motor cortex, dorsolateral PFC, orbitofrontal cortex, and anterior cingulate cortex. Alexander, DeLong, and Strick in 1986 proposed five cortico-BG circuits involved in motor, oculomotor, cognition, emotion, and motivation.[17] They proposed that each circuit receives multiple, partially overlapping corticostriate inputs, which are progressively integrated and projected to a restricted cortical area. The thalamocortical projections of the motor circuit terminate largely within the SMA while the corticostriate inputs to this circuit include projections from the SMA, motor, premotor, and sensory cortex. Oculomotor circuit consists of fibers from FEFs (Brodmann's area 8) along with projections from dorsolateral prefrontal cortex (DLPFC) and posterior parietal cortex (area 7), projecting to the body of the CN. The caudate projects to the GPi/SNr, which then projects to the ventro-anterior (VA)/dorso-medial (DM) nuclei of thalamus and back to FEF. Oculomotor circuit is involved in generation of saccadic eye movement. SNr neurons show pause in activity just before the onset of saccadic eye movement and this is associated with a burst activity in SC neurons producing a saccade. DLPFC also known as association circuit consists of projections from DLPFC to the CN to GPi/SNr, which then projects to VA nucleus of thalamus and back to DLFPC. The cortical connections to caudate suggest a role of this circuit in forward planning of complex motor tasks. It is believed that when a motor task becomes automatic, the motor circuit takes over that task from the dorsolateral prefrontal circuit. There is some evidence to suggest that this circuit also participates in processes subserving spatial memory. Lateral orbitofrontal circuit consists of fibers projecting from orbitofrontal cortex to CN to GPi/SNr, which then projects to VA/DM thalamic nuclei and back to orbitofrontal cortex. Bilateral lesions of this circuit have shown to interfere with appropriate switches in behavioral set. Anterior cingulate or limbic circuit consists of fibers from the anterior cingulate cortex, hippocampus, and entorhinal cortex projecting to ventral striatum (NA) to ventral pallidum, which projects to DM nucleus of thalamus and then back to anterior cingulate cortex. This circuit is believed to be involved in motivation.[17]

Basal Ganglia and Cerebellum

The cerebellar circuits and BG circuits were believed to be anatomically and functionally distinct and interact at the level of cortex. Recent animal studies have shown bidirectional disynaptic connection between cerebellar cortex and striatum through the dentate nucleus. Also, anatomical connection has been found between cerebellar cortex and STN through the pontine nuclei. These connections suggest that BG and cerebellum exchange information in real time to provide appropriate input to the frontal cortex.[18] A recent model proposes that cerebellar, BG, and motor cortex are interlinked and their abnormal interactions results in abnormal movements in Parkinsonism and levodopa-induced dyskinesias.[19]

Basal Ganglia and Motor Control

Over last few decades various functions of BG have been proposed including selection of action and suppression of potentially competing actions, regulation of speed and size of the movement, online correction of motor error, motor learning, and production of overlearned motor skills.[20] There are two basic theories for the motor control, learning, and action selection by striatum. The oldest and the most long-standing theory is of lateral inhibition by MSNs which works on the principle of winner takes it all. Lateral inhibition is important in the selection of competing motor programs. It is based on the fact that each MSN has numerous inhibitor GABAergic connections with the neighboring MSNs, which causes their inhibition in order to increase the signal to noise ratio of the striatal output. Another theory is based upon feed-forward model of inhibition by the FSI in the striatum, which are GABAergic. These neurons get their input directly from the cortex and not from within the striatum and hence the name feed forward. Computational modeling of BG has shown the importance of both the models in proper BG functioning. Lateral inhibition is required for motor learning, action initiation and control, and the impairment may result in chorea and bradykinesia. Feedforward inhibition is expected to be involved in selection of appropriate actions and its impairment has been observed in Tourette's disease and obsessive-compulsive disorder.[21]

A study by Crutcher et al. published in 1990 showed that SMA neurons discharge significantly earlier than those in motor cortex, which in turn were earlier than those in putamen.[22] Late onset of movement-related activity argues against a role of the putamen in the initiation of movement but some putamen neurons do have activity several hundred milliseconds in advance of movement. This early putamen neuronal activity is thought to be related to instruction cue, which conveys information regarding the correct direction of movement, how far to move, or whether to move at all. This is followed by the "go" signal which provides information on when to move. Thus, BG are responsible for the quality and correctness of a movement and may not play an important role in initiation of movement.[23]

Medium spiny neurons are difficult to excite and need strong convergent input from cortex to become active. Corticostriatal system fibers from different functionally related cortical areas converge on the same neuron or groups of MSNs (ensemble). These neurons are activated only when a sufficient number of their excitatory corticostriatal afferents are active.[9] Dopamine release has a focusing or attentional effect facilitating the output of a particular ensemble of striatal neurons at the expense of others thus having a gating role. Dopamine effect on MSNs also leads to synaptic plasticity, building and shaping striatal output modules, and a role in the process of reward-based motor and behavioral learning.[9,24] Hence BG are involved in forming reward-based associations, which over the course of practice train show Hebbian learning in thalamocortical circuits.[20] It is believed that BG circuits are necessary for new skill learning, but become less important in retention and recall of well-learned motor skills. Another hypothesis to explain BG function is of movement gain. It is based on a simple concept that BG regulate the speed and size of movement (movement gain). Gain hypothesis is supported by the neurophysiological findings showing that movement-related activity in the pallidum is correlated with the amplitude or velocity of the limb movements.[20]

Basal Ganglia Role in Reward and Language Processing

Ventral striatum (NA) projections to the ventral pallidum translates limbic motivation signals into motor output and this accounts for the limbic-motor integration. Lesional studies have shown the ventral pallidum may be crucial for learning or performing learned responses related to rewards. Growing evidence suggests role of ventral pallidum in food reward, sex, social affiliation, drug abuse, winning money, and other rewards. Hence, ventral pallidum might be viewed as a convergent point for hedonic and motivational signaling pathways in the brain and hence a final pathway for reward.[25] Striatum also plays an important role in language processing including lexical processing (e.g., word retrieval) and grammatical rule application (syntax). A positron emission tomography (PET) study in Huntington disease patients showed that the left striatum encompasses linguistic (lexical processing and rule application) and arithmetic circuits. Ventrally located regions in striatum are dedicated to rule computations and dorsal regions to lexical processing.[26]

CONCLUSION

Basal ganglia network is a complex structure consisting of multiple subcortical nuclei and parallel circuits. The most important function of the BG is in motor control including selection of action, suppression of competing actions, regulation of speed and size of the movement, and motor learning. BG also play a crucial role in behavior, reward, and language processing.

REFERENCES

1. Tewari A, Jog R, Jog MS. The Striatum and Subthalamic Nucleus as Independent and Collaborative Structures in Motor Control. Front Syst Neurosci. 2016;10:17.
2. Utter AA, Basso MA. The basal ganglia: an overview of circuits and function. Neurosci Biobehav Rev. 2008;32(3):333-42.
3. Lanciego JL, Luquin N, Obeso JA. Functional neuroanatomy of the basal ganglia. Cold Spring Harb Perspect Med. 2012;2(12): a009621.
4. Basso MA, Sommer MA. Exploring the role of the substantia nigra pars reticulata in eye movements. Neuroscience. 2011;198:205-12.
5. Gerfen CR. The Neostriatal Mosaic: Striatal patch-matrix organization is related to cortical lamination. Science. 1989; 246(4928):385-8.
6. Gerfen CR, Wilson CJ. Chapter II The basal ganglia. Handbook Chem Neuroanat. 1996;12:371-468.
7. Tepper JM, Sharpe NA, Koós TZ, Trent F. Postnatal development of the rat neostriatum: electrophysiological, light- and electron-microscopic studies. Dev Neurosci. 1998;20(2-3): 125-45.
8. Wilson C. Up and down states. Scholarpedia J. 2008;3(6):1410.
9. Groenewegen HJ. The basal ganglia and motor control. Neural Plast. 2003;10(1-2):107-20.
10. Mink JW. The Basal Ganglia and involuntary movements: impaired inhibition of competing motor patterns. Arch Neurol. 2003;60(10):1365-8.
11. Hamani C, Florence G, Heinsen H, Plantinga BR, Temel Y, Uludag K, et al. Subthalamic Nucleus Deep Brain Stimulation: Basic Concepts and Novel Perspectives. eNeuro. 2017;4(5).
12. Chang HT, Kita H, Kitai ST. The fine structure of the rat subthalamic nucleus: an electron microscopic study. J Comp Neurol. 1983;221(1):113-23.
13. Fox CA, Andrade AN, Lu Qui IJ, Rafols JA. The primate globus pallidus: a Golgi and electron microscopic study. J Hirnforsch. 1974;15(1):75-93.
14. Difiglia M, Rafols JA. Synaptic organization of the globus pallidus. J Electron Microsc Tech. 1988;10(3):247-63.
15. Yelnik J, Percheron G, François C. A Golgi analysis of the primate globus pallidus. II. Quantitative morphology and spatial orientation of dendritic arborizations. J Comp Neurol. 1984;227(2):200-13.
16. Oertel WH, Nitsch C, Mugnaini E. Immunocytochemical demonstration of the GABA-ergic neurons in rat globus pallidus and nucleus entopeduncularis and their GABA-ergic innervation. Adv Neurol. 1984;40:91-8.
17. Alexander GE, DeLong MR, Strick PL. Parallel organization of functionally segregated circuits linking basal ganglia and cortex. Annu Rev Neurosci. 1986;9:357-81.
18. Caligiore D, Pezzulo G, Baldassarre G, Bostan AC, Strick PL, Doya K, et al. Consensus Paper: Towards a Systems-Level View of Cerebellar Function: the Interplay Between Cerebellum, Basal Ganglia, and Cortex. Cerebellum. 2017;16(1):203-29.
19. Kishore A, Popa T. Cerebellum in levodopa-induced dyskinesias: the unusual suspect in the motor network. Front Neurol. 2014;5:157.
20. Turner RS, Desmurget M. Basal Ganglia Contributions to Motor Control: A Vigorous Tutor. Curr Opin Neurobiol. 2010;20(6): 704-16.
21. Moyer JT, Halterman BL, Finkel LH, Wolf JA. Lateral and feedforward inhibition suppress asynchronous activity in a large, biophysically-detailed computational model of the striatal network. Front Comput Neurosci. 2014;8:152.
22. Crutcher MD, Alexander GE. Movement-related neuronal activity selectively coding either direction or muscle pattern in three motor areas of the monkey. J Neurophysiol. 1990;64(1): 151-63.
23. Mink JW. The basal ganglia: focused selection and inhibition of competing motor programs. Prog Neurobiol. 1996;50(4): 381-425.
24. Schultz W. Getting formal with dopamine and reward. Neuron. 2002;36(2):241-63.
25. Smith KS, Tindell AJ, Aldridge JW, Berridge KC. Ventral pallidum roles in reward and motivation. Behav Brain Res. 2009;196(2):155-67.
26. Teichmann M, Gaura V, Démonet J-F, Supiot F, Delliaux M, Verny C, et al. Language processing within the striatum: evidence from a PET correlation study in Huntington's disease. Brain. 2008;131(Pt 4):1046-56.

CHAPTER 3

Epidemiology of Movement Disorders in India and in Other Countries

Bhaskar Ghosh, Shyamal Kumar Das

INTRODUCTION

Epidemiology is a powerful tool in medical science to estimate the magnitude of a disease in the community and also to find out the association of causative factors. Epidemiology is also a key to proper health care planning and to resource mobilization. Essentially, it has three arms: (1) Descriptive or observational study, (2) Analytical study, and (3) Interventional study. Descriptive study consists of determining the prevalence rate (presence of total number of cases at any specified time period) and incidence rate (number of new cases added to each year). Prevalence is a function of both disease incidence and duration. Improved diagnostic capabilities can produce an apparent increase in prevalence. Ideally incidence and prevalence are determined by screening entire populations defined by specific geographic or political boundaries: Community or population-based studies.[1] Estimates of prevalence based on populations identified by other methods, such as participants in a hospital clinic, do not reflect accurately the general population of an area as cultural, economic, or other factors may influence case selection (selection bias). Analytical studies include prospective cohort study or follow-up study and case-control study to find out the association of risk factors or etiologies. In prospective cohort study individuals are observed over time and frequency of new disease in exposed and unexposed person is determined.

Movement disorders are relatively a younger branch of neurosciences and emphasis has been placed over the last two decades in the last century. There are a number of epidemiological studies from Western countries, but there are only few studies from third world countries. In India there are few community-based studies, which have recorded the frequency of different movement disorders. In this communication, we have tried to give in brief the report of different epidemiological studies from different countries and as well as community and clinic based information from India.

DIFFICULTIES IN EPIDEMIOLOGICAL STUDIES OF MOVEMENT DISORDERS

There is no antemortem diagnostic test for Parkinson disease (PD) and most of the other movement disorders excepting some genetic diseases such as Huntington disease (HD) and Wilson disease (WD). Consequently, diagnostic accuracy is a challenge in epidemiological studies in movement disorders. Expertise is the most important asset, which determines the diagnostic accuracy dramatically. In some communities, essential tremor (ET) accounted for 10–40% of the false-positive diagnosis of PD.[2] Conversely, true PD patients may be misdiagnosed as depression or, in the very elderly as, normal aging. Neurodegenerative disorders, such as progressive supranuclear palsy (PSP) and multisystem atrophy, may not be distinguished easily from PD in the early course of illness.[3]

Temporal differences in diagnostic practices also can limit comparability across studies. Many of the neuro-degenerative disorders with multiple system involvement and Parkinsonism generally were recognized only in the last several decades. These may have been included in earlier studies of movement disorders. Some cases of arteriosclerotic Parkinsonism might be later considered to be typical PD.[4-6] In other reports, Parkinsonism of known cause (drug-induced Parkinsonism and postencephalitic Parkinsonism) were grouped along with PD in determining incidence or prevalence rates.[4,5,7] Since these three types of Parkinsonism are distinct, such grouping could result in erroneous conclusions about disease patterns or risk factors.

OVERVIEW OF MOVEMENT DISORDERS IN INDIA

There are very few epidemiological studies showing the data of movement disorders either in the community or in the clinic. One study from South India by Gourie Devi et al. has provided a prevalence rate of 254 per 100,000 (urban 39 and rural 221) of cases with movement disorders.[8] In a clinic based study of 1,354 patients seen over 10 years in the Bangur Institute of Neurology (BIN), Kolkata, following disorders were recorded as follows: Dystonia (37%), Parkinsonism (22%), tremor (15%), choreoathetosis (4%), tics (4%), metabolic (3%), and miscellaneous (15%) (unpublished data).

EPIDEMIOLOGY OF PARKINSON DISEASE

Parkinson disease is an uncommon disorder beginning in late life. The latency from onset of neurodegeneration to appearance of clinical signs is unknown. In such a situation, prospective cohort studies are problematic, because a large number of unaffected individuals must be followed for decades. But cross-sectional methods, such as case-control studies, are faster and more economical. In case-control studies, individuals already affected with the disease of interest are compared to individuals without the illness, and exposures proposed to relate to the illness are compared. In some cases (such as toxin-induced Parkinsonism) identification and intensive investigation of an unusually high incidence of a disease, either in space or in time (a cluster), may provide important clues to disease etiology.

DESCRIPTIVE EPIDEMIOLOGY

Prevalence Rate (Table 1)

The prevalence rate of PD varies between 18 and 418 per 100,000 worldwide,[9] although the variations are much less marked when the differences between the study methodologies are considered. Age adjustment and restriction to studies using similar methodology reduce the variation between prevalence rates to between 102 and 190 per 100,000 population, at least in Western countries.

Clusters of high prevalence of PD have been reported, e.g., in Iceland or on the Faroe Islands, where prevalence of PD was considerably higher.[9] Conversely low prevalence rates were observed in other populations, such as Bulgarian Gypsies[10] and in Northern Africa.[11]

In India, the prevalence of PD varied markedly from one study to other. The prevalence rate is 8 per 100,000 from Bangalore (Southern India),[12] 328.3 per 100,000 in Urban Parsi community of Mumbai (Western India),[13] 14.1 per 100,000 in Kashmir (Northern India),[14] 16 per 100,000 (Rural) and 80 per 100,000 (Urban) in Malda district of West Bengal (Eastern India),[15,16] 68 per 100,000 in Baruipur area of West Bengal.[17]

A study from National Institute of Mental Health and Neurosciences (NIMHANS), Bangalore, involving both urban and rural population presented in an abstract form by Gourie Devi et al., had recorded a crude prevalence rate of 27/100,000 and rates for urban and rural were 14 and 41, respectively. Men had slightly higher rate (31/100,000) than female (24/100,000). The age specific rates showed a dramatic increase from 28 in the fourth decade to 573/100,000 in ninth decade. The differences in prevalence rates reflect in large part marked differences in methodology and ascertainment criteria, they may also indicate actual differences in occurrence of PD, which may be due to differences in genetic background or, alternatively, in environmental exposure.

Incidence (Table 1)

A better indicator for the frequency of a chronic disease in the population than prevalence is the incidence rate, as it is independent of survival, which may vary in temporally or geographically separated population. However such studies require larger study populations and/or longer observation times and are therefore much rare and not many studies in PD have been reported (**Table 1**). The incidence rates in these studies range from 1.5 to 21/100,000-population per year.

The wide variability in incidence rates is also due to same reasons as in case of prevalence rates.

Age

Both the incidence and the prevalence of PD increase with increasing age of the population. PD is rare before the age of 50 and its incidence increases with increasing age.[7] This is true in all community-based studies, regardless of the absolute prevalence of the disease in the population including one recently concluded study from West Bengal.[17] Some examples of age-specific prevalence in different communities are shown in **Table 2**. Possible explanations for the near exponential correlation between increasing age and PD prevalence include age-related neuronal vulnerability or a causal mechanism dependent on the passage of time.

TABLE 1: Estimated crude incidence and crude prevalence of Parkinson's disease in some studies.

Reference age on day of prevalence	*Type of study*	*No. of cases*	*Location*	*Crude incidence/ 100,000/year*	*Crude prevalence/ 100,000/year*	*Age at onset*	
Gourie-Devi et al.[12] 1987	D		Bangalore, South India		8		
Bharucha et al.[13] 1988	D	46	Parsi community, Mumbai, India		328		
Razdan et al.[14] 1994	D		Anantnag district of South Kashmir, India		14		
Das et al.[15] 1996	D	4	Malda district of West Bengal, India (Rural)		16		
Das et al.[16] 1998	D		Malda district of West Bengal, India (Urban)		80		
Saha et al.[17] 2003	D	11	Baruipur area of West Bengal, India		68		
Li et al.[18] 1985	D	28	Six cities of China	44	63.3		
Melcon et al.[19] 1997	D	51	Junin, Buenos Aires, Argentina*	399–669*	64		
Morgante et al.[20] 1992	D	63	Sicily, Italy	257			
Schoenberg et al.[21] 1985	D	31	Copiah County, Mississippi, USA	347			
Wang et al.[22] 1991	D	566	29 provinces of China	1.5	15		
Milanov et al.[10] 2000	D	1 and 119	Gypsies and Caucasians in Bulgaria		16 and 137		
Ashok et al.[11] 1986	C	163	Benghazi, Libya	4.5	31		
Fall et al.[23] 1996	C	170	Ostergotland, Sweden	11	115	65.6	73.7
Gudmunsson et al.[24] 1967	C	453	Iceland	16	162	61.1	68
Kurland[5] 1958	C	56	Rochester, New York, USA	20	187		
Marttila et al.[2] 1976	C	484	Turku, Finland	15	120		
Rajput et al.[25] 1984	C	138	Rochester, New York, USA	21			
Sutcliffe et al.[26] 1995	C	383	Northampton, UK	12	121		
Tandberg et al.[27] 1995	C	245	Rogaland, Norway		111	64.4	73.5
Wermuth et al.[28] 1997	C	82	Faroe Islands		187.6	64.2	73.4

*Different prevalence with eight different criteria-sets for the diagnosis.

Note:
C: Community based study.
D: Door to door surveys.

Because of the strength and consistency of the risk factor, comparisons of disease frequency among populations must be adjusted for their differing age distributions.[9] One would expect crude (unadjusted) PD incidence and prevalence to be higher in a community with a greater proportion of elderly individuals. Similarly, evaluation of any putative risk factor requires concomitant adjustment for the distribution of that risk factor with respect to age. This may be one of the reasons for lower rate of PD in our country as Indian population is younger than Western population. Proper age standardization with a standard population is absolutely necessary.

In personally observed cases of PD at the Movement Disorders Clinic at BIN and also at B R Singh Hospital and Center for Medical Education and Research, Headquarter Hospital of Eastern Railway, Kolkata about 20% patients are below the age of 40 years. The reason for this may be due to genetic predisposition.

Gender

There are also conflicting result of sexwise prevalence of PD. Although marginal male predominance of PD is reported by many record and clinic-based studies, few door to door studies could confirm this. Saha et al.[17] showed increased prevalence in females in a rural population of Bengal, that too increasing with age being in the order of 214.2 per 100,000 in female and 164.2 per 100,000 in male in the age group of 51–60 years increasing to 1666.7 per 100,000 in female and 552.5 per 100,000 male in the age group of 70+ years. Other studies have shown conflicting results (**Table 3**).[2,11,18-38] Overall, the increased prevalence in male is probably due to a biological function (increased X-linked genetic disposition or influence of sex hormones on disease risk) or alternatively, greater exposure to a causative environmental factor in men or male-related lifestyle factor.

TABLE 2: Age-specific prevalence of Parkinson's disease.

		Prevalence (per 100,000) by age groups in years					
Reference	**Location**	**0–39**	**40–49**	**50–59**	**60–69**	**70–79**	**80–89**
Saha et al.[17]	Baruipur, West Bengal, India			189.2	844.2	1,109.6 >70 years	1,109.6
Fall et al.[23] 1996	Östergötland, Sweden		19.1	53.4	210.0	614.3	971
Harada, Nishikawa, and Takahashi[29] 1983	Yonago, Japan	4.7	39.9	85.5	245.1	698.4	752.7
Li et al.[16] 1985	Six cities of the People's Republic of China			92.0	145.0	615 >70 years	
Marttila and Rinne[2] 1976	Turku, Finland	0.8	27.8	136.2	503.5	736.1	468.8 >79 years
Mayeux et al.[30] 1992	New York, USA		23	45.7	234.8	525.6	1,145 >80 years
Morgante et al.[20] 1992	Sicily, Italy		0.0	115.6	621.4	1,978.3	3,055
Mutch et al.[31] 1986	Aberdeen, Scotland		46.6	77.9	54.0	839.6	1,925 >79 years
Okada et al.[32] 1990	Izumo, Japan	23.2	19.6	63.6	338.6	478.7	335.7
Rosati et al.[33] 1980	Sardinia, Italy	3.3	38.6	204.5	342.1	311.3	82.6
Sutcliffe and Meara[26] 1995	Northampton, UK*		6.8	93.3	251	760	1,222 >80 years
Svenson[34] 1991	Alberta, Canada		46.6	77.9	254.0	839.6	1,925 79 years
Wang et al.[35] 1994	Kin-Hu, People's Republic of China		0.0	780.0	1,750		2,500 >80 years

*Mean values are calculated from 5-year groups.

TABLE 3: Parkinson's disease: Gender ratio of age-adjusted prevalence.

Reference	Location	Male-to-female ratio
D'Alessandro et al.[36]	San Marino	1.24
Harada et al.[29]	Yonago, Japan	0.86
Li et al.[18]	Chinese cities	3.70
Rosati et al.[33]	Sardinia, Italy	1.38
Sutcliffe and Meara[26]	Northampton, UK	1.3
Marttila and Rinne[2]	Turku, Finland	0.98
Ashok et al.[11]	Benghazi, Libya	1.04
Rajput et al.[25]	Rochester, New York, USA	1.48
Mayeux et al.[30]	New York, USA	1.73
Imaizumi and Kaneko[37]	Japan	1.29*

*Mortality data.

Race

Parkinson disease prevalence generally appears to be highest in Europe and North America, whereas rates in Japan, China, India, and Africa are markedly lower. These observations suggest that there is a greater risk of PD among whites. There are two interesting observations regarding the Indians with risk of PD. In the Parsi community in Mumbai,[13] prevalence was stated to be similar to that found in Europe and North America. The Persians are descendants from Iran, who migrated to India between the seventh and tenth centuries and formed a close community. These facts may also account for the high prevalence observed, despite their Asian residence. The prevalence of PD in Bulgarian Gypsies was found to be much less as compared to Caucasians.[10] The origin of the Gypsies is thought to be in North India,[39] who later moved to Balkans in the 14th and 15th century. Around 800,000 Gypsies living in Bulgaria have the characteristics of true genetic isolates. No difference exists between the Caucasians and Gypsies in regard to environment, type of work, food, medical care, and habits such as smoking. It is interesting to note that all marriages of Gypsies are only to other Gypsies, so they exist as genetic isolates. Since the Gypsies originated in India, the prevalence of PD is comparable to other Indian or Asian population.

Time Trends

With regard to time trends for the incidence of PD, a population-based study evaluating the incidence of PD in Olmsted County, Minnesota from 1935 through 1988 showed that the annual incidence of PD increased from 9.2 per 100,000 for the interval between 1935 and 1944 to 16.3 per 100,000 for the interval between 1975 and 1984.[39] On the other hand, Zhang et al., performed a meta-analytical study by adjusting reported data with a single standard population and concluded that the prevalence and incidence of PD appear to have remained unchanged over the past 40 years.[9] As there are very few longitudinal data for PD incidence and the data might lack consistency for diagnostic criteria and study methods over time, at present it is difficult to reliably evaluate the changes in time trends of PD.

ANALYTICAL EPIDEMIOLOGY

Genetic Factors

Family history has consistently been reported to be associated with increased risk of PD compared with controls, suggesting that genetic factors play a role in the etiology of PD.[40-42] However, it is uncertain whether this reflects an increased genetic susceptibility, pure genetic inheritance, shared familial exposure, or biased recall in families of patients with PD. Twin studies are of particular value to address this question. If genetic factors play an important role in the etiology of a disorder, the concordance rates in monozygotic twins should be higher than in dizygotic twins. However, most twin studies have not confirmed an overall increased risk of PD in monozygotic twins as compared to dizygotic twins,[43,44] though in twins with age of onset of PD below 50 years the concordance rates in monozygotic twins were significantly higher than in dizygotic twins.[45] These results suggest that genetic factors contribute significantly to the development of PD in those with young onset but do not play a major role in causing typical PD.

Last few years in PD research have shown that there are families in whom PD is genetically determined. However, mutations in the α-synuclein gene inherited as autosomal dominant pattern account for only small number of cases.[46] The autosomal recessively (AR) inherited Parkin gene, on the other hand, appears to account for a substantial minority of cases of sporadic PD.[47]

Environmental Factors

Although the cause or causes of PD remain obscure, a number of factors have been associated with an increased or decreased risk of PD (**Box 1** and **2**).

Box 1 Putative factors reported with increased risk for Parkinson's disease.

Demographic factors:
- Age—elderly
- Gender—men
- Race—white

Genetic factors:
- Family history of PD or essential tremor
- Onset of PD before 50 years of age in twin study
- Families with a number of kindreds with PD and Parkinsonism

Life experience:
- Head injury and trauma
- Emotional stress
- Personality (shyness and depressed mood)

Dietary factors:
- Dairy products in men
- Animal fat consumption

Infectious agents or diseases:
- HIV, Japanese B encephalitis, coxsackie B, influenza A, herpes simplex, measles, mumps, diphtheria, croup, and rheumatic fever

Environmental exposures:
- Rural living
- Farming activity
- Well-water drinking
- Neurotoxin—MPTP and MPTP-like compounds
- Pesticide exposure—insecticides, herbicides, fungicides, rodenticides, fumigants, and wood preservatives
- Metal exposure—lead, manganese, mercury, iron, copper, and amalgam

Occupational factors:
- Teachers, healthcare services, social science (law, library), and oil/gas field

(HIV: human immunodeficiency virus; MPTP: 1-methyl-4-phenyl-1,2,3,6-tetrahydropyridine; PD: Parkinson's disease)

Box 2 Putative factors reported with reduced risk for Parkinson's disease.

Antioxidants:
- Beta-carotene, vitamin A, vitamin C, and vitamin E (α-tocopherol)

Dietary factors:
- Niacin-containing food
- Coffee
- Tea

Life experience:
- Cigarette smoking
- Alcohol drinking

Infectious disease:
- Measles in childhood

While head injury, emotional stress, and premorbid personality have been linked to PD in numerous reports, the associations between these factors and PD are controversial because of the difficulties of recall bias, accuracy of diagnosis, and long duration of time between injury and onset of PD. A number of studies reported that different lifestyle elements such as rural living, farming activity, or well-water drinking may act as risk factors for PD. So far reports on pesticide exposure show either no convincing correlation or an increased risk of developing PD. Reports on heavy metals have been conflicting. Further studies are required in these areas.

Interestingly, a recent prospective longitudinal study involving 8,004 subjects over 30 years of follow-up found a significant inverse relation between the incidence of PD and higher coffee and caffeine consumption with a dose-response relationship.[48] Those who did not drink coffee had a 5-fold greater risk when compared with those who drank 28 ounces or more coffee a day. The effect persisted even after the results were adjusted for cigarette smoking. This study revealed that other nutrients in coffee, including niacin, were unrelated to PD incidence, and it suggests that the mechanism is related to caffeine intake and not to other nutrients contained in coffee.

Infectious agents were considered as a possible cause for PD because encephalitis lethargica often preceded Parkinsonism during the influenza pandemic of the early 1920s. A number of studies reported that some infectious agents or diseases, such as HIV, Japanese B encephalitis, coxsackie B, influenza B, herpes simplex, measles, mumps, diphtheria, or rheumatic fever might be linked to post-infectious Parkinsonism either acutely or as a long-term complication. Some researchers suggest that exposure to an influenza virus in the fetus or childhood might predispose one to PD in adulthood.[49]

Various studies have documented the beneficial effects of smoking and PD though other views are also prevailing. In animal model, the beneficial role of nicotine has been demonstrated on age, and MPTP induced dopaminergic neuronal loss.[50] The proposed protective effect of cigarette smoking could be confounded by many factors including a greater propensity to quit smoking, because they turn ill before being diagnosed and the possibility that the patients with PD who smoke have greater mortality than those who do not smoke. Recently, a study of occupational risk factors for PD in British Columbia found school teachers and those in healthcare service occupations with significantly increased risk for PD and suggested that this observation might reflect higher exposure to viral respiratory tract infections circulating in school and healthcare facilities.[51] However, referral bias and recall bias could not be ruled out entirely in this study since the sample was based on population attending a specialty referral clinic. Further studies with more extensive and more direct measures of exposure to respiratory tract illness are being undertaken to substantiate the findings. A recent study has suggested that higher intake of dairy products may increase the risk of PD in men.[52] However, this finding needs further evaluation and the underlying active components need to be identified.

THE INDIAN DATA

In the previous paragraphs, the results of community-based prevalence studies from India have already been discussed. In a clinic-based analysis of 150 cases of PD seen over 5 years, Sengupta et al. have recorded male dominance (M:F-2.85:1), younger age of onset in 21.3% of case (below 40 years), and the peak of disease onset was in the fifth decade in the majority group (28.6%).[53] Tremor was the common single presenting symptom noticed in 41% and on examination it was observed in 97% of cases. Disease-associated limb dystonia was noted in 4% of cases. Drug-induced dyskinesia was present in 9% and family history in 2% of cases. Thus, from these studies, it was evident that PD in India was mostly tremor dominant, having an earlier age of onset with a somewhat lower frequency of dyskinesia. Incidentally, requirement of levodopa in these groups of patients was also low. In another study, Behari et al., from All India Institute of Medical Sciences (AIIMS), New Delhi, recorded positive family history in 21% of cases among consecutive 104 cases of PD.[54,55]

Behari et al., further, studied epidemiological data on risk factors of PD from India.[56] In a case-control study, they investigated environmental and genetic risk factors in the etiology of idiopathic PD. They found positive correlation with the male gender, family history of PD, past history of depression of up to 10-year duration and well water drinking of >10-year duration. However, tobacco smoking of up to 20-year duration and exposure to pets had protective effect. Vegetarian diet, occupational physical stress, rural living, farming, exposure to insecticides, herbicides, rodenticides, alcohol intake, and family history of neurodegenerative diseases had no significant correlation with occurrence of PD. Results of their study supported the hypothesis of multifactorial etiology of PD with environmental factors acting on a genetically susceptible host.[55]

Mortality

Although the mortality rate represents a unique population-based statistics and has been used to examine both the time trends and the geographical distribution of PD. Phillips et al. found that only 37% of patients had PD coded as the underlying cause of death in all diagnosed cases.[56] The reason is that PD is not a primary or direct cause of death. Overall, in the United States, the average annual age-adjusted PD mortality between 1962 and 1984 was estimated as 2 deaths per 100,000 for white men and 1 death per 100,000 for nonwhite men, 1 death per 100,000 for white women, and <1 death per 100,000 for nonwhite women. Mortality increased in persons above 75 years of age but declined for those younger than age of 70 years.[57] Generally, mortality rates for PD increased in the older age groups but decreased for younger ages.

Survival

Although the life expectancy of PD patients has been prolonged, the life span of PD patients is still somewhat less than that of the general population. Improved survival as the result of introducing effective symptomatic therapy and decreased or delayed mortality from other disorders may partly account for the decreased mortality in younger people. Tanner et al. reported that relative survival for people with PD diagnosed before the age of 60 years is similar to that for the general population though the relative survival is less than expected for those who are older at diagnosis.[58] A study examining prognosis of PD patients in Japan showed that the most common cause of death for all patients regardless of age, was pneumonia.[59] This suggests that in addition to providing improved antiparkinsonian therapy to patients, PD-related conditions such as pneumonia should also be treated more aggressively.

ATYPICAL PARKINSONISM

According to PD data brain bank data, 15–20% of cases that are treated clinically antemortem as PD, have atypical features in autopsy. Pathologically, these are similar to PSP, multiple system atrophy (MSA), corticobasal ganglionic degeneration, vascular Parkinsonism, and Alzheimer disease. Prevalence and incidence studies on these disorders are lacking.

To find out the causative factors, Caparros-Lefebvre et al. recorded a high percentage of PSP from a group of Parkinsonian patients in French-West Indies.[60] This has been thought to be due to the intake of herbal tea and fruits of the *Annonae* species. Bhattacharyya and Chaudhuri (unpublished observations) have reported *sporadic atypical Parkinsonism* among migrant ethnic minority population in the UK from Africa and Indian subcontinents and from Eastern India. Afro-Caribbean patients have bradykinetic dominant disease with marked axial and peripheral rigidity, early postural instability, and neuropsychiatry manifestations particularly complex visual hallucination. Subjects of Indian subcontinent origin appear to have a mixed pattern, that is, bradykinesia with rest and postural tremor, relative intolerance to levodopa, and early onset of axial dystonias. On the other hand, patients recruited from Eastern India were often found to be less responsive to levodopa and levodopa induced dyskinesias appeared early. They have postulated that the both genetic and environmental factors might be the possible causative factors.[61]

EPIDEMIOLOGY OF DYSTONIA

Prevalence

Since dystonia is commonly underdiagnosed or under-reported, it is difficult to get its true prevalence. It has been recognized that dystonia is relatively common in Jewish population, particularly in Jews of Eastern European ancestry.[62-65] In them the prevalence rate is 4.3 per 100,000 for generalized dystonia.[65] In other ethnic groups the prevalence rate varied. In Mayo Clinic in Rochester, Minnesota, over three decades yielded prevalence rates of 3.4 per 100,000 for generalized dystonia and 29.5 per 100,000 for focal dystonia.[66] In Spain, the prevalence of focal dystonia was 27.9 per 100,000 population.[67] In Northern England, the prevalence for generalized dystonia was 1.42 per 100,000 and for focal dystonia 13 per 100,000.[68] In a recent multinational European study, the overall prevalence rate of focal dystonia based on diagnosed cases was 11.7 per 100,000.[69,70] All the above reports were based on hospital-based studies. Population-based studies showed reduced prevalence from China[18] (3 per 100,000), Egypt[71] (10/100,000 all focal dystonias), and also from Japan[72] (generalized 0.2 and focal 6.1 per 100,000).

Among the different types of focal dystonia, the most common type in one study was cervical dystonia followed by blepharospasm. Writer's cramp and spasmodic dysphonia were relatively uncommon.[68] European collaborative study has also recorded cervical dystonia in 38%, blepharospasm in 20%, and writer's cramp in 9% of cases with primary dystonias.[70]

Incidence

Age-adjusted annual incidence in the early epidemiological study in Israel population was 0.43 per million in the total Jewish population, 0.98 in European Jews, and 0.11 in Afro-Asians Jews.[66] In Rochester, Minnesota, in the years 1950–1982, annual incidence rate of all focal dystonias was reported as 2.4 per 100,000 and of generalized dystonia with 0.2 per 100,000.[66]

Age

Age of onset is generally older in patients with blepharospasm and oromandibular dystonia than in patients with other focal dystonias and younger for generalized dystonia.[66,68]

Gender

With the exception of writer's cramp, focal and segmental dystonia has mostly been reported to be more common in females than in males.[68,70] Epidemiological study of dystonia by Europe Collaborative Group studied 957 cases of primary (idiopathic) dystonia and found a significant excess of female patients for segmental and focal dystonia.[70] A novel observation was a significantly earlier age at onset in males as opposed to females for primary segmental (mean age: 44.6 vs. 53.3) and focal dystonia (43.8 vs. 47.8). This was also apparent in cervical dystonia, blepharospasm, and laryngeal dystonia. For writer's cramp and focal limb dystonia, this trend was reversed with an earlier age at onset in females. These results suggest that focal dystonia should not be treated as a homogenous group and sex-linked factors may play a role.[73,74]

Genetic Factors

A gene for generalized primary torsion dystonia (PTD) with childhood onset, which contains a three-nucleotide (GAG) deletion and codes for the previously unknown protein torsin A, has been identified on chromosome 9q34 (*DYT-1*).[75] It is responsible for most of the cases of early limb-onset PTD in both Jewish and non-Jewish kindreds.[75,76] Transmission mostly follows autosomal dominant pattern of inheritance with low penetrance. In a minority of cases, late onset dystonia is associated with a positive family history but it is not usually associated with *DYT-1* gene. Other loci causing PTD have recently been mapped on chromosome 18p (*DYT-7*), chromosome 8 (*DYT-6*), chromosome 1p (*DYT-13*), and other loci are likely to be identified in adult onset focal dystonia. The D5 receptor gene has also been implicated in cervical dystonia.[75] These findings provide evidence of genetic heterogeneity of dystonia.

Fletcher et al. observed that family history of tremor or stuttering was significantly more common among patients with PTD than control subjects in a case-control study.[77,78]

Environmental Factors

Environmental factors have a role in the expression of genetic predisposition to develop adult-onset PTD. Patients often report trauma or significant viral infection preceding the onset of symptoms,[63,77] but epidemiological evidence regarding the role of such factors is controversial. Defazio et al. reported that head or face trauma with loss of consciousness and family history of tremor or dystonia were associated with an increased risk of adult-onset dystonia, whereas hypertension and cigarette smoking exerted a protective effect.[79]

Prognosis

Progression of dystonia is likely in cases of early-onset dystonia, whereas in most cases of adult-onset primary dystonia there is no or minimal spread to contiguous body parts.[66,68] Early onset dystonia starts in the lower limbs, but in 20% of those with onset before the age of 22 years, symptoms begin with torticollis and in 66% of them, they do not spread.[69] Remission of dystonia occurs in a minority of patients.[65,77]

Indian Scenario

There was no community-based prevalence and incidence data in India on dystonia. Two clinic-based data from tertiary care centers from Southern India (Trivandram, Kerala) and Eastern India (Kolkata, West Bengal) have recorded the various types of dystonia, age of onset, and underlying etiology in an abstract form. The study from Southern India has analyzed 114 cases of dystonias seen over 10 years and showed that 70% had adult onset, 15% childhood onset, and the rest was of adolescent onset [80] The male and female ratio is 2.4:1. Among the various types of dystonia, generalized dystonia constitutes 22% followed by focal dystonia (59%), segmental dystonia (13%), and hemidystonia (0.5%). Primary dystonia was noted in 62% of cases and familial cases were noted in about 10% of situations.

Data from BIN, Eastern India is also clinic based on 300 cases of dystonias seen over 5 years.[81] Male to female ratio was 3:1. Out of the total cases, adult onset dystonia constitutes the majority (71%), followed by childhood onset (17%), and the rest (12%) are of adolescent onset. The various types of dystonia include focal dystonia (66%), generalized (13%), segmental (11.33%), and hemidystonia (9.33%). Out of the cases of focal dystonias, the distribution is as follows: Limb dystonia in 25.3% (writer's cramp 17.3%, leg dystonia 3.6%, and other occupational cramps 4.3%), cranial dystonias in 16% (blepharospasm 10%, and oromandibular 6%), cervical dystonia in 10%, and trunkal dystonias in 4%. Primary dystonias constitute about 82%. Thus, there is a difference in the pattern of focal dystonias characterized by higher frequency of blepharospasm and cervical dystonias in the Western study. This discrepancy in the pattern of dystonias may be due to referral bias or may be true related to genetic predisposition and environmental interaction.

In a case-control study on dystonias, Behari et al. from AIIMS, New Delhi, have shown traditional chewing of betel leaves may be responsible for frequent occurrence of orofacial dystonias.[82]

EPIDEMIOLOGY OF ESSENTIAL TREMOR

Essential tremor is probably the most common movement disorder. However, prevalence rates vary widely as epidemiologic studies are hampered by the lack of a marker or a clearly delineated clinical phenotype. It is likely that ET is clinically, pathophysiologically, and genetically a heterogeneous condition,[83,84] and phenotypic overlap in the phenotype with other conditions exist. Till date, a reliable clinical differentiation of individual patients with tremor is currently not possible.

Prevalence

Taking into account the limitations of comparability of studies using different ascertainment and diagnostic methods, the prevalence rates range from 0.01 to 22%.[85] One study defined ET as an action tremor and used community-based rather than service-based designs. Louis et al. reported a wider range of prevalence rates from 0.4 to 3.9% in the overall population and from 1.3 to 5% in those over the age of 60 years.[85,86]

Incidence

Incidence data are far fewer than prevalence rates, ranging from 8 per 100,000 per year[87] to 23.7 per 100,000 in a longitudinal study in Rochester, Minnesota.[88] This study also showed an increase in annual age- and sex-adjusted incidence rate from 5.8 in 1935–1949 to 23.7 in 1964–1979, most likely resulting from under diagnosis of ET in earlier years.

Age

Despite the differences in diagnosis, it is clear that the prevalence of ET increases with age. Age at onset showed bimodal distribution with peak in second and sixth decade. A study from Minnesota has shown that the incidence rates continuously increased up to the oldest age group with a sharp increase after the age of 49.[88]

Gender

Apart from a few studies that found a higher prevalence in women or men,[89,90] ET is largely found to be equally common in women and men.

Race

Although few comparative data are available, two studies have reported a slightly higher prevalence rate of ET in white than in black Americans.[89,90]

Genetic Factors

Essential tremor is generally thought to be an autosomal and dominantly inherited condition with high but age-dependant penetrance.[91,92] However, the reported percentage of patients with ET with a family history ranges from 17.4 to 100%. This wide range may be due to error in reporting or heterogeneity of the condition. Isolated families of ET with linkage to different chromosomes have been established (chromosome 3q13—*FET-1* and chromosome 2p22-25—*ETM* or *ET 2*).[93-95] Some studies have reported anticipation in successive generations of families, though others could not confirm it.

A relation has been observed in some patients with ET who subsequently developed PD compared to general population, though no genetic confirmation has been found.[96]

Environmental Factors

Exposure to agricultural chemicals and domestic animals has been suggested as a potential risk factor for the occurrence of ET in one study, but it was a small study and statistically insignificant.[97]

Prognosis

Tremor severity and disability increases with advancing age and tremor duration. Life expectancy of patients with ET is similar to that of general population although ET has also been claimed to increase longevity.[98] In a recently concluded study, it has been reported that, increase in tremor severity may be related to the inherent worsening of the disease with increasing duration that this is independent of age and age-related processes such as neuronal attrition and change in tremor frequency.[99]

Indian Scenario

The prevalence rate of ET available from India varies from 8 to 1,663 per 100,000 from various community-based studies.[12,13,15,88] A door-to-door survey for neurological diseases was conducted in the Parsi community of 14,010 people (Parsis living in the colonies in Mumbai).[88] Neurologists used defined diagnostic criteria to evaluate persons with positive results on the screening survey. Total of 233 people (104 men and 129 women) were identified as having ET. The overall prevalence ratio was 1,663.1 (corrected) per 100,000 population. Age-specific prevalence ratios increased with age. Age-adjusted prevalence ratios were similar for men and women.[76] Devi et al., NIMHANS, Bangalore, have recorded a crude prevalence of 23/100,000 (rural 25, semiurban 17).[12]

In two clinic-based study from India, various types of tremor have been reported. Shukla et al., from AIIMS, reported 106 patients of non-Parkinsonian and non-cerebellar tremor. Male to female ratio was 4:1 with mean age 44.4 years.[100] Essential (60%) and dystonic tremor (22%) were the most common and family history was positive in 52.4% of cases. Ganguly et al. from BIN, Kolkata, have reported a total of 168 cases who primarily presented with tremor.[101] Out of them rest tremor was in 70 cases (41.6%), dystonic tremor in 16 cases (9.5%), ET in 42 cases (25%), enhanced physiological tremor in 23%, cerebellar and rubral tremor in 6%, WD in 3.65%, psychogenic in 4.5%, and following exposure to toxins in 2.3% of cases.

EPIDEMIOLOGY OF CHOREA-INDIAN PICTURE

Gourie Devi et al. from NIMHANS, Bangalore, reported a prevalence rate of 9 per 100,000 of cases with chorea in a community based study on combined rural and urban population in Southern India.[12] The underlying break-up of the different etiologies has not been mentioned. In a clinic-based study from Eastern India, Sen et al. reported 56 patients of chorea-athetosis out of which only 6 patients had predominantly athetosis.[102] Drug-induced causes have been excluded.

Underlying causes could be found in 35 cases and these include neurogenetic conditions in 19 cases, immunologic in 4 cases (rheumatic), structural in 6 cases (cerebrovascular accidents and trauma), infective in 2 cases(tuberculosis), and hypoxia in 4 cases.[102] Genetically confirmed HD has been observed in 7 cases only. It is interesting that as contrary to the expectation, the number of rheumatic chorea is less, possibly due to referral bias or the typical nature of the illness characterized by spontaneous remission.

EPIDEMIOLOGY OF HUNTINGTON'S DISEASE

Huntington's disease is an autosomal dominantly inherited disorder with complete penetrance. It is caused by an expanded trinucleotide repeat (CAG) in a gene on chromosome 4p16.3, which codes for huntingtin protein.[103] Recently, in transgenic mouse, it has been shown that environmental factors can also influence the age of onset. This is a significant observation as environmental manipulation may have the potentiality of modifying disease expression.[104]

Prevalence

Huntington disease occurs worldwide with prevalence rates between 2 and 12 per 100,000.[105] It is observed that most European populations, both Northern and Southern, show a relatively high prevalence (4–8 per 100,000),[106] but lower prevalence rates have been reported in black populations, as well as in Finland, Japan, and China. Lower frequency of HD has been associated with smaller CAG repeat lengths and different distribution of CCG alleles in these populations compared with Western European populations, suggesting that in addition to European emigration, new mutations could make a contribution to the geographic variation of prevalence rates.[107,108,]

In India, there is conflicting results of prevalence of HD. Harper from population surveys and death rate analysis in the light of genetic studies concluded that the disorder may also be frequent in India and parts of Central Asia.[109] But using the records of Churchill Hospital, Oxford, and those of genetics centers, and other national institutions, Shiwach[109] reported that the minimum prevalence of HD among immigrants from the Indian subcontinent was almost half of that found in the indigenous UK population. However, according to him, this observed prevalence was probably depressed, and therefore, may not differ greatly from that estimated for European populations. All the identified cases were immigrants from Pakistan and in India from Punjab and Gujarat and none were from Bangladesh. Pramanik et al. based on genetic studies concluded that the overall prevalence of HD in Indian population may not be as high as in the Western population.[110]

Age at Onset

The age at onset is usually in the mid-40s, but it ranges from 2 to >80 years. A study from NIMHANS, Bangalore, on 26 genetically confirmed HD patients from 19 Indian families, predominantly from South India, showed that adult onset HD was the most common while Juvenile HD (onset <20 years) was observed in approximately 15% of patients.[111]

Survival

Median survival has been reported to be as long as 16.2 years,[112] and many patients survive >20 years, probably depending on the quality of care during advanced stages. The main causes of death are pneumonia and cardiovascular disease,[113] but the risk of suicide is also increased in patients with HD as well as unaffected siblings at risk for HD.[114]

EPIDEMIOLOGY OF WILSON'S DISEASE

Wilson's disease is an inherited AR disorder of copper metabolism transmitted by a mutant gene on chromosome 13q14–21 and results in abnormal accumulation of copper giving rise to protean manifestations.

Prevalence and Incidence

The prevalence of WD is estimated at one in 30,000 in most populations, with a corresponding carrier frequency in the general population of one in 90. The prevalence is as high as one in 10,000 in Japan, China, and Sardinia. The higher prevalence rate in Japan is presumably due to a higher consanguinity rate. In the Chinese population, there is a tight linkage between WD and two gene loci for esterase D and retinoblastoma in the long arm of chromosome 13. The high proportion of patients with hepatic presentation accounts for early onset of WD in the Japanese and Chinese series. Skeletal involvement, leg hyperpigmentation, dark complexion, amenorrhea, epileptic seizures, and cerebral white matter degeneration are relatively more common among WD patients in Asia. Excessive copper in the liver appears to have a protective effect against hepatocellular carcinoma and type B hepatitis.[115] The incidence of WD is 1:40,000–1:100,000[116] in the homozygous form.

Age of Onset

Age of onset of WD in India was reported to be earlier. A study from AIIMS, New Delhi, revealed that the age of onset of initial symptomatology ranged from 3 to 11 years with a mean of 7.2 years (for the hepatic presentation 6.8 years VS. 8 years for the neurologic patients).[117] Another study from Eastern India reported the mean age of onset 11.13 years.[117,118] Other studies from India have also reported early age of onset.[119-121] In the Western series, it was noted at a later age (mean age 11–18 years)[122] where hepatic presentation was mostly between 14 and 15 years and neurological presentation was between 18 and 21 years.[123] Presentation with psychiatric manifestations occurred at a further later age (25.3 ± 2.4 years).[123] Indian study revealed the earliest hepatic presentation at the age of 3 years.[117] However, initial neurologic presentation have been described before the age of 5 years and after the age of 50 years.[117, 124-129]

Thus, it is possible that the disease manifests at a younger age in Indian children. The average intake of copper in India ranges from 5.7 to 7.1 mg/day and is higher than the reported 0.34–1.1 mg/day in the Western countries.[130] The practice of cooking food in copper pots might be contributory.[120,121] An analogous situation was reported by one of the authors for Indian Childhood Cirrhosis, a condition with heavy hepatic copper deposition.[131]

Gender

In most of the studies, it was observed that males were more affected than the females.

EPIDEMIOLOGY OF TIC DISORDERS

Variability of symptoms, ignorance, absence of biologic marker, and controversies in diagnostic criteria pose problems for conducting epidemiological studies. There is extreme paucity of data on this disorders in India. Tic disorders, as we see in the clinic-based study, may be the tip of the iceberg and grossly under-reported because of the nature of disorders.

Prevalence Study

Most epidemiological studies in adults have yielded prevalence of 30–50 per 100,000. Surveys in school children have yielded higher rates, which stand between 0.1 and 3%.[132] Attention deficit hyperactivity disorder, obsessive compulsive disorder, depression, or self-injurious behavior are common comorbid disorders. The prevalence relationship of these to Tourette syndrome (TS) is unknown. These conditions may be the variable expressions of a single disorder, a shared underlying etiology, selection bias, or consequence of social and personal impact.

The prevalence of TS in children with special educational need is higher and ranges between 7.5 and 8.6%.[132] Tics are frequent in children with emotional and behavioral difficulties (65%), with learning difficulties (24%), problem children (6%), and with autism (6.3%). There has been increase in the prevalence of TS in the last decade, because of greater recognition and higher referral to hospitals.

Incidence Study

A study from Rochester, Minnesota has recorded annual incidence rate of 0.46 per 100,000. This may be an underestimate because of the reasons cited above.[133,134]

Natural History[135]

The average onset of age of motor tics is 7 years, but it ranges from 2 to 21 years. Progressive worsening of tics occur up to the age of 10 years, followed by gradual decline in late adolescence or early adulthood. By the age of 18, half of the cohorts is virtually free from tics. Phonic tics usually occur at the age of 11 years.

Risk Factors

- *Genetic*: The inheritance is autosomal dominant with variable expression and penetrance. The candidate gene has still not been cloned.[136] There is also growing evidence for bilineal transmission with the father typically having motor tics and mother suffering from obsessive-compulsive syndrome.
- *Environmental factors*: Infection and birth injury in addition to genetic vulnerability may determine the phenotypic manifestation of TS. Recent description of PANDAS (*P*ediatric *A*utoimmune *N*europsychiatric *D*isorders *A*ssociated with *S*treptococcal infection) links the recurrence of obsessive compulsive disorder and tic disorder with prepubertal symptom onset to streptococcal infection.[137]

Tics in India

The only community-based study from NIMHANS, Bangalore, where Gourie Devi et al. have reported prevalence rate of 2 per 100,000 for tics disorder.[12] In a clinic based study from Eastern India, Sengupta et al. reported 28 well-documented cases of tic disorders (4.3% of all cases) with good follow up. Males were sufferers in 89.3% of cases and 78.5% of the cases presented in first two decades. TS was noted in 9 cases (32%) and 5 of them had positive family history. Comorbid disorders such as attention deficit hyperactivity disorder and obsessive-compulsive disorders were noted in 35.7% and 28.5% of cases, respectively.

CONCLUSION

We have attempted to provide an overview of the current status of epidemiology of movement disorders globally as well as in India. The pattern of the diseases is similar to that in the Western countries in general, but markedly different in frequency. However, to obtain a reasonable figure about the prevalence and incidence studies on movement disorders in India, epidemiological studies from different parts with age standardization need to be carried out in view of heterogeneity of the population. Due to increasing of longevity of the population, it is expected that there will be an increasing burden of adult-onset movement disorders such as PD, tremor, dystonia, and chorea, which will put burden on the individual, family, and community. However newer investigative methods such as neuroimaging and genetic studies will lead to precise diagnosis and these will be supplementary to neuroepidemiological studies.

ACKNOWLEDGMENT

We are grateful to Prof AK Maity, Director Bangur Institute of Neurology, Prof D Sen (Ex-Director), Prof Trishit Roy, Head of the department of Neuromedicine, Prof B Maity (Ex-Head), my colleagues—Prof PK Ganguly, Dr A Senapati, Dr G Ganguly, and Dr SP Saha, our Post-doctoral residents and staff of BIN, particularly Mr Ramswarup for their whole hearted support for continuation of epidemiology and movement disorders program in this institute.

REFERENCES

1. Schlesselman JJ. Case-Control Studies: Design, Conduct, Analysis. New York: Oxford University Press; 1982.
2. Marttila RJ, Rinne UK. Epidemiology of Parkinson's disease in Finland. Acta Neurol Scand. 1976;53(2):81-102.
3. Koller WC. Classification of Parkinsonism. In: Koller WC (Ed). Handbook of Parkinson's disease. New York: Marcel Dekker; 1987. pp. 51-80.
4. Brewis M, Poskanzer DC, Rolland C, Miller H. Neurological disease in an English city. Acta Neurol Scand. 1966;42(suppl 24): 9-89.
5. Kurland LT. Epidemiology: Incidence, geographic distribution and genetic considerations. In Field W (Ed). Springfield: Pathogenesis and treatment of Parkinsonism; 1958. pp. 5-49.
6. Martin WE, Young WI, Anderson VE. Parkinson's disease: A genetic study. Brain. 1973;96(3):495-506.
7. Rajput AH, Offord KP, Beard CM, Kurland LT. A case control study of smoking habits, dementia and the other illnesses in Idiopathic Parkinson's disease. Neurol. 1987;37(2):226-32.
8. Gourie-Devi M, Gururaj G, Satischandra P, Subbakrishna DK. Prevalence of Parkinson's disease in Bangalore: A door-to door survey of urban and rural population. Neurol India. 1999;47(S1):73.
9. Zhang ZX, Roman GC. Worldwide occurrence of Parkinson's disease: an updated review. Neuroepidemiology. 1993;12(4): 195-208.
10. Milanov I, Kmetski TS, Lyons KE, Koller WC. Prevalence of Parkinson's disease in Bulgarian gypsies. Neuroepidemiology. 2000;19(4):206-9.
11. Ashok PP, Radhakrishnan K, Sridharan R, Mousa ME. Epidemiology of Parkinson's disease in Benghazi, North-East Libya. Clin Neurol Neurosurg. 1986;88(2):109-13.
12. Gourie Devi M, Rao VN, Prakashi R. Neuroepidemiological study in semi-urban and rural areas in South India: Pattern of neurological disorders including motor neurone disease. In: Gourie-Devi M (Ed). New Delhi: Oxford and IBH; 1987. pp. 10-21.
13. Bharucha NE, Bharucha EP, Bharucha AE, Bhise AV, Schoenberg BS. Prevalence of Parkinson's disease in the Parsi community of Bombay, India. Arch Neurol. 1988;45(12):1321-3.
14. Razdan S, Kaul RL, Motta A, Kaul S, Bhatt RK. Prevalence and pattern of major neurological disorders in rural Kashmir (India) in 1986. Neuroepidemiology. 1994;13(3):113-9.
15. Das SK, Sanyal K. Neuroepidemiology of major neurological disorders in rural Bengal. Neurol India. 1996;44(2):47-58.
16. Das S, Sanyal K, Moitra A. A pilot study on neuroepidemiology in urban Bengal. Indian J Public Health. 1998;42(2):34-6.
17. Saha SP, Bhattacharya S, Das SK, Maity B, Roy T, Raut DK. Epidemiology study of Neurological disorder in a rural population of Eastern India. J Indian Med Assoc. 2003;101(5): 299-304.
18. Li SC, Schoenberg BS, Wang CC, Cheng XM, Rui DY, Bolis CL, et al. A prevalence survey of Parkinson's disease and other movement disorders in the People's Republic of China. Arch Neurol. 1985;42(7):655-7.
19. Melcon MO, Anderson DW, Vergara RH, Rocca WA. Prevalence of Parkinson's disease in Junin, Buenos Aires Province, Argentina. Mov Disord. 1997;12(2):197-205.
20. Morgante L, Rocca WA, Di Rosa AE, De Domenico P, Grigoletto F, Meneghini F, et al. Prevalence of Parkinson's disease and other types of parkinsonism: a door-to- door survey in three Sicilian municipalities. The Sicilian Neuro-Epidemiologic Study (SNES) Group. Neurology. 1992;42(10):1901-7.
21. Schoenberg BS, Anderson DW, Haerer AF. Prevalence of Parkinson's disease in the biracial population of Copiah County, Mississippi. Neurology. 1985;35(6):841-5.
22. Wang YS, Shi YM, Wu ZY, He YX, Zhang BZ. Parkinson's disease in China. Coordinational Group of Neuroepidemiology, PLA. Chin Med J. 1991;104(11):960-4.
23. Fall PA, Axelson O, Fredriksson M, Hansson G, Lindvall B, Olsson JE, et al. Age-standardized incidence and prevalence of Parkinson's disease in a Swedish community. J Clin Epidemiol. 1996;49(6):637-41.

24. Gudmundsson KR. A clinical survey of Parkinsonism in Iceland. Acta Neurol Scand. 1967;43(S33):9-61.
25. Rajput AH, Offord KP, Beard CM, Kurland LT. Epidemiology of Parkinsonism: Incidence, classification, and mortality. Ann Neurol. 1984;16(3):278-82.
26. Sutcliffe RL, Meara JR. Parkinson's disease epidemiology in the Northampton District, England, 1992. Acta Neurol Scand. 1995;92(6):443-50.
27. Tandberg E, Larsen JP, Nessler EG, Riise T, Aarli JA. The epidemiology of Parkinson's disease in the county of Rogaland, Norway. Mov Disord. 1995;10(5):541-9.
28. Wermuth L, Joensen P, Bunger N, Jeune B. High prevalence of Parkinson's disease in the Faroe Islands. Neurology. 1997;49(2):426-32.
29. Harada H, Nishikawa S, Takahashi K. Epidemiology of Parkinson's disease in a Japanese city. Arch Neurol. 1983;40(3): 151-4.
30. Mayeux R, Denaro J, Hemenegildo N, Marder K, Tang MX, Cote LJ, et al. A population-based investigation of Parkinson's disease with and without dementia. Relationship to age and gender. Arch Neurol. 1992;49(5):492-7.
31. Mutch WJ, Dingwall-Fordyce I, Downie AW, Paterson JG, Roy SK. Parkinson's disease in a Scottish city. Br Med J (Clin Res Ed). 1986:292(6519):534-6.
32. Okada K, Kobayashi S, Tsunematsu T. Prevalence of Parkinson's disease in Izumo City, Japan. Gerontology. 1990;36(5-6):340-4.
33. Rosati G, Granieri E, Pinna L, Aiello I, Tola R, De Bastiani P, et al. The risk of Parkinson's disease in Mediterranean people. Neurology. 1980;30(3):250-5.
34. Svenson LW. Regional disparities in the annual prevalence rates of Parkinson's disease in Canada. Neuroepidemiology. 1991;10(4):205-10.
35. Wang SJ, Fuh JL, Liu CY, Lin KP, Chang R, Yih JS, et al. Parkinson's disease in Kin-Hu, Kinmen: a community survey by neurologists. Neuroepidemiology. 1994;13(1–2):69-74.
36. D'Alessandro R, Gamberini G, Granieri E, Benassi G, Naccarato S, Manzaroli D. Prevalence of Parkinson's disease in the republic of San Marino. Neurology. 1987:37(10):1679-82.
37. Imaizumi Y, Kaneko R. Rising mortality from Parkinson's disease in Japan, 1950–1992. Acta Neurol Scand. 1995;91(3):169-76.
38. Vekerdi J. On the social prehistory of the gypsies. Orient Hung. 1981;25:243-54.
39. Tanner CM, Thelen JA, Offord KP. Parkinson's disease incidence in Olmsted County, MN: 1935–1988. Neurology. 1992;42 (Suppl 3):194.
40. Tanner CM, Goldman SM. Epidemiology of Parkinson's disease. Neurol Clin. 1996;14(2):317-35.
41. Taylor CA, Saint-Hilaire MH, Cupples LA, Thomas CA, Burchard AE, Feldman RG, et al. Environmental, medical, and family history risk factors for Parkinson's disease: a New England-based case control study. Am J Med Genet. 1999;88(6):742-9.
42. Rybicki BA, Johnson CC, Peterson EL, Kortsha GX, Gorell JM. A family history of Parkinson's disease and its effect on other PD risk factors. Neuroepidemiology. 1999;18(5):270-8.
43. Duvoisin RC, Eldridge R, Williams A, Nutt J, Calne D. Twin study of Parkinson disease. Neurology. 1981;31(1):77-80.
44. Marttila RJ, Kaprio J, Koskenvuo M, Rinne UK. Parkinson's disease in a nationwide twin cohort. Neurology. 1988;38(8):1217-9.
45. Tanner CM, Ottman R, Goldman SM, Ellenberg J, Chan P, Mayeux R, et al. Parkinson disease in twins: an etiologic study. JAMA.1999;281(4):341-6.
46. Chan DK, Mellick G, Cai H, Wang XL, Ng PW, Pang CP, et al. The alpha-synuclein gene and Parkinson disease in a Chinese population. Arch Neurol. 2000;57(4):501-3.
47. Lucking CB, Durr A, Bonifati V, Vaughan J, De Michele G, Gasser T, et al. Association between early onset Parkinson's disease and mutations in the parkin gene. N Engl J Med. 2000;342(21):1560-7.
48. Ross GW, Abbott RD, Petrovitel H, Morens DM, Grandinetti A, Tung KH, et al. Association of coffee and caffeine intake with the risk of Parkinson disease. JAMA. 2000;283(20):2674-9.
49. Martyn CN, Osmond C. Parkinson's disease and the environment in early life. J Neurol Sci. 1995;132(2):201-6.
50. Prasad C, Ikegami H, Shimizu I, Onaivi ES. Chronic nicotine intake decelerates aging of nigrostriatal dopaminergic neurons. Life Sci. 1994;54(16):1169-84.
51. Tsui JK, Calne DB, Wang Y, Schulzer M, Marion SA. Occupational risk factors in Parkinson's disease. Can J Public Health. 1999;90(5):334-7.
52. Chen H, Zhang SM, Hernan MA, Willett WC, Ascherio A. Diet and Parkinson's disease: a potential role of dairy products in men. Ann Neurol. 2002;52(6):793-801.
53. Sengupta P, Sen A, Kundu TN. Study of clinical pattern and response to treatment in patients of Parkinson Disease attending movement disorders clinic at BIN, Kolkata. Annals of Indian academy of Neurology. 2001; 4:150.
54. Behari M, Wani MA. Clinical and genetic study of Parkinson's disease. Ann Indian Acad Neurol. 2000;3:129.
55. Behari M, Srivastava AK, Das RR, Pandey RM. Risk factors of Parkinson's disease in Indian patients. J Neurol Sci. 2001;190: 49-55.
56. Phillips NJ, Reay J, Martyn CN. Validity of mortality data for Parkinson's disease. J Epidemiol Community Health. 1999;53(9):587-8.
57. Lilienfeld DE, Chan E, Ehland J, Godbold J, Landrigan PJ, Marsh G, et al. Two decades of increasing mortality from Parkinson's disease among the US elderly. Arch Neurol. 1990;47(7):731-4.
58. Tanner CM, Thelen JA, Offord KP, et al. Relationship of age at diagnosis to survival in Parkinson's disease. Mov Disord. 1992;7:104.
59. Nakashima K, Maeda M, Tabata M, Adachi Y, Kusumi M, Ohshiro H. Prognosis of Parkinson's disease in Japan. Eur Neurol. 1997;38(Suppl 2):60-3.
60. Caparros-Lefebvre D. Elbaz A. Possible relation of atypical Parkinsonism in the French West Indies with consumption of tropical plants: a case control study. Lancet. 1999;354(9175): 281-6.
61. Chaudhuri KR, Hu MT, Brooks DJ. Atypical Parkinsonism in Afro-Caribbean and Indian origin immigrants to the UK. Mov Disord. 2000;15(1):18-23.
62. Alter M, Kahana E, Feldman S. Differences in torsion dystonia among Israeli ethnic groups. Adv Neurol. 1976;14:115-20.
63. Cooper IS, Cullinan T, Riklan M. The natural history of dystonia. Adv Neurol. 1976;14:157-69.
64. Korczyn AD, Kahana E, Zilber N, Streifler M, Carasso R, Alter M. Torsion dystonia in Israel. Ann Neurol. 1980;8(4):387-91
65. Zilber N, Korczyn AD, Kahana E, Fried K, Alter M. Inheritance of Idiopathic torsion dystonia among Jews. J Med Genet. 1984;21(1):13-20.
66. Nutt JG, Muenter MD, Aronson A, Kurland LT, Melton LJ. Epidemiology of focal and generalized dystonia in Rochester, Minnesota. Mov Disord. 1998;3(3):188-94.

67. Sempere AP, Duarte J, Coria F, Cabezas C, Claveria LE. Prevalence of idiopathic focal dystonia in the province of Segovia, Spain. J Neurol. 1994;241:S124.
68. Duffey PO, Butler AG, Hawthorne MR, Barnes MP. The epidemiology of the primary dystonias in the north of England. Adv Neurol. 1998;78:121-5.
69. Greene P, Kang UJ, Fahn S. Spread of symptoms in idiopathic torsion dystonia. Mov Disord. 1995;10:143-52.
70. The Epidemiological Study of Dystonia in Europe (ESDE) Collaborative Group. A prevalence study of primary dystonia in eight European countries. J Neurol. 2000;247(10):787-92.
71 Kandil MR, Tohamy SA, Fattah MA, Ahmed HN, Farwiez HM. Prevalence of chorea, dystonia and athetosis in Assiut, Egypt: a clinical and epidemiological study. Neuroepidemiology. 1994;13(5):202-10.
72. Nakashima K, Kusumi M, Inoue Y, Takahashi K. Prevalence of focal dystonias in the western area of Tottori Prefecture in Japan. Mov Disord. 1995;10(4):440-3.
73. Soland VL, Bhatia KP, Marsden CD. Sex prevalence of focal dystonias. J Neurol Neurosurg Psychiatry. 1996;60(2):204-5.
74. Sex-related influences on the frequency and age of onset of primary dystonia. Epidemiologic Study of Dystonia in Europe (ESDE) Collaborative Group. Neurology. 1999;53(8):1871-3.
75. Ozelius LJ, Page CE, Klein C, Hewett JW, Mineta M, Leung J, et al. The *TOR1A (DYT1)* gene family and its role in early onset torsion dystonia. Genomics. 1999;62(3):377-84.
76. Klein C, Brin MF, de Leon D, Limborska SA, Ivanova-Smolenskaya IA, Bressman SB, et al. De novo mutations (GAG deletion) in the DYT1 gene in two non-Jewish patients with early onset dystonia. Hum Mol Genet. 1998;7(7):1133-6.
77. Claypool DW, Duane DD, Ilstrup DM, Melton LJ. Epidemiology and outcome of cervical dystonia (spasmodic torticollis) in Rochester, Minnesota. Mov Disord. 1995;10(5):608-14.
78. Fletcher NA, Harding AE, Marsden CD. A case-control study of idiopathic torsion dystonia. Mov Disord. 1991;6(4):304-9.
79. Defazio G, Berardelli A, Abbruzzese G, Lepore V, Coviello V, Acquistapace D, et al. Possible risk factors for primary adult onset dystonia: a case-control investigation by the Italian Movement Disorders Study Group. J Neurol Neurosurg Psychiatry. 1998;64(1):25-32.
80. George J, Kishore A, Radhakrishnana KR. Retrospective study of the etiological profile and clinico-anatomical correlation of dystonic disorders. Neurol India. 1999;47:74.
81. Sen A, Sengupta P, Ganguly G. Clinical pattern of dystonia in a tertiary care center in West Bengal. Annals Indian Acad Neurol. 2000;3:146.
82. Behari M, Sharma AK, Changkakoti M, Sharma N, Pandey RM. Case-control study of Meige's syndrome. Result of a Pilot Study. Neuroepidemiology. 2000;19:275-80.
83. Munchau A, Schrag A, Chuang C, MacKinnon CD, Bhatia KP, Quinn NP, et al. Arm tremor in cervical dystonia differs from essential tremor and can be classified by onset age and spread of symptoms. Brain. 2001;124(9):1765-76.
84. Louis ED, Ford B, Barnes LF. Clinical subtypes of essential tremor. Arch Neurol. 2000;57(8):1194-8.
85. Louis ED, Ottman R, Hauser WA. How common is the most common adult movement disorder? Estimates of the prevalence of essential tremor throughout the world. Mov Disord. 1998;13(1):5-10.
86. Bharucha NE, Bharucha EP, Bharucha AE, Bhise AV, Schoenberg BS. Prevalence of essential tremor in the Parsi community of Bombay, India. Arch Neurol. 1988;45(8):907-8.
87. MacDonald BK, Cockerell OC, Sander JW, ShorvonSD. The incidence and lifetime prevalence of neurological disorders in a prospective community-based study in the UK. Brain. 2000;123(4):665-76.
88. Rajput AH, Offord KP, Beard CM, Kurland LT. Essential tremor in Rochester, Minnesota: a 45-year study. J Neurol Neurosurg Psychiatry. 1984;47(5):466-70.
89. Haerer AF, Anderson DW, Schoenberg BS. Prevalence of essential tremor: results from the Copiah County study. Arch Neurol. 1982;39(12):750-1.
90. Louis ED, Marder K, Cote L, Pullman S, Ford B, Wilder D, et al. Differences in the prevalence of essential tremor among elderly African Americans, whites, and Hispanics in northern Manhattan, NY. Arch Neurol. 1995;52(12):1201-5.
91. Herskovits E, Figueroa E, Mangone C. Hereditary essential tremor in Buenos Aires (Argentina). Arq Neuropsiquiatr. 1988;46(3):238-47.
92. Bain PG, Findley LJ, Thompson PD, Gresty MA, Rothwell JC, Harding AE, et al. A study of hereditary essential tremor. Brain. 1994;117(4):805-24.
93. Gulcher JR, Jonsson P, Kong A, Kristjánsson K, Frigge ML, Kárason A, et al. Mapping of a familial essential tremor gene, FET1, to chromosome 3q13. Nat Genet. 1997;17(1):84-7.
94. Higgins JJ, Pho LT, Nee LE. A gene (ETM) for essential tremor maps to chromosome 2p22-p25. Mov Disord. 1997;12(6): 859-64.
95. Higgins JJ, Loveless JM, Jankovic J, Patel PI. Evidence that a gene for essential tremor maps to chromosome 2p in four families. Mov Disord. 1998;13(6):972-7.
96. Pahwa R, Koller WC. Is there a relationship between Parkinson's disease and essential tremor? Clin Neuropharmacol. 1993;16(1): 30-5.
97. Salemi G, Aridon P, Calagna G, Monte M, Savettieri G. Population-based case control study of essential tremor. Ital J Neurol Sci. 1998;19(5):301-5.
98. Jankovic J, Beach J, Schwartz K, Contant C. Tremor and longevity in relatives of patients with Parkinson's disease, essential tremor, and control subjects. Neurology. 1995;45(4): 645-8.
99. Louis ED, Jurewicz EC, Watner D. Community-based data on associations of disease duration and age with severity of essential tremor: implications for disease pathophysiology. Mov Disord. 2003;18(1):90-3.
100. Shukla G, Behari M. A clinical study of non-parkinsonian and non-cerebellar tremor attending a specialty movement disorders clinic. Neurol India. 2004;52(2):200-2.
101. Ganguly G, Das S, Ganguly PK. Evaluation of tremor cases at the movement disorders clinic. Ann Indian Acad Neurol. 2000;3:120.
102. Sen A, Sengupta P, Mitra K. A clinical pattern of choreo-athetosis in patients attending Movement Disorders clinic, Bangur institute of neurology, Kolkata. J Association East Ind. 2001;6:25-32.
103. A novel gene containing a trinucleotide repeat that is expanded and unstable on Huntington's disease chromosomes. The Huntington's Disease Collaborative Research Group. Cell. 1993;72(6):971-83.

104. Di Maio I, Squitieri F, Napolitano G, Campanella G, Trofatter JA, Conneally PM, et al. Onset symptoms in 510 patients with Huntington's disease. J Med Genet. 1993;30(4):289-92.
105. Tanner CM, Goldman SM. Epidemiology of movement disorders. Curr Opin Neurol. 1994;7(4):340-5.
106. Harper PS. The epidemiology of Huntington's disease. Hum Genet. 1992;89(4):365-76.
107. Squitieri F, Andrew SE, Goldberg YP, Kremer B, Spence N, Zeisler J, et al. DNA haplotype analysis of Huntington disease reveals clues to the origins and mechanisms of CAG expansion and reasons for geographic variations of prevalence. Hum Mol Genet. 1994;3:2103-14.
108. Andrew SE, Hayden MR. Origins and evolution of Huntington disease chromosomes. Neurodegeneration. 1995;4(3):239-44.
109. Shiwach RS, Lindenbaum RH. Prevalence of Huntington's disease among UK immigrants from the Indian subcontinent. Br J Psychiatry. 1990;157:598-9.
110. Pramanik S, Basu P, Gangopadhaya PK, Sinha KK, Jha DK, Sinha S, et al. Analysis of CAG and CCG repeats in Huntingtin gene among HD patients and normal populations of India. Eur J Hum Genet. 2000;8(9):678-82.
111. Murgod UA, Saleem Q, Anand A, Brahmachari SK, Jain S, Muthane UB. A clinical study of patients with genetically confirmed Huntington's disease from India. J Neurol Sci. 2001;190(1-2):73-8.
112. Roos RA, Hermans J, Vegter-van der Vlis M, van Ommen GJ, Bruyn GW. Duration of illness of Huntington's disease is not related to age at onset. J Neurol Neurosurg Psychiatry. 1993;56(1):98-100.
113. Sorensen SA, Fenger K. Causes of death in patients with Huntington's disease and in unaffected first-degree relatives. J Med Genet. 1992;29(12):911-4.
114. Di Maio L, Squitieri F, Napolitano G, Campanella G, Trofatter JA, Conneally PM. Suicide risk in Huntington's disease. J Med Genet. 1993;30(4):293-5.
115. Chu NS, Hung TP. Geographic variations in Wilson's disease. J Neurol Sci. 1993;117(1–2):1-7
116. Haslam RHA. Movement disorders. In: Textbook of Pediatrics. Behrman RE, Kliegman RM, Arvin AM (Eds). Philadelphia: WB Saunders Company; 1996. pp. 1709-12.
117. Kalra V, Khurana D, Mittal R. Wilson's disease--early onset and lessons from a pediatric cohort in India. Indian Pediatr. 2000;37(6):595-601.
118. Sinha S, Jha DK, Sinha KK. Wilson's disease in Eastern India. J Assoc Physicians India. 2001;49:881-4.
119. Singh S, Dilawari JB, Chawla Y, Walia BN. Wilson's disease in young children from Northern India. Trop Gastroenterol. 1989;10(1):46-50.
120. Bhave SA, Purohit GM, Pradhan AV, Pandit AN. Hepatic presentation of Wilson's disease. Indian Pediatr. 1987;24(5):385-93.
121. Bhave SA. Pediatric Wilson's disease in India. Med J West India. 1990;8:14-7.
122. Park RH, McCabe P, Fell GS, Russell RI. Wilson's disease in Scotland. Gut. 1991;32(12):1541-5.
123. Huang CC, Chu NS. Wilson's disease: clinical analysis of 71 cases and comparison with previous Chinese series. J Formos Med Assoc. 1992;91(5):502-7.
124. Walshe JM, Yealland M. Wilson's disease: the problem of delayed diagnosis. J Neurol Neurosurg Psychiatry. 1992;55(8): 692-6.
125. Walshe JM. Wilson's disease presenting with features of hepatic dysfunction: a clinical analysis of eighty-seven patients. Q J Med. 1989;70(263):253-63.
126. Fitzgerald MA, Gross JB, Goldstein NP, Wahner HW, McCall JT. Wilson's disease of late adult onset: report of case. Mayo Clinic Proc. 1975;50(8):438-42.
127. Czlonkowska A, Rodo M. Late onset Wilson's disease. Report of a family. Arch Neurol. 1981;38(11):729-30.
128. Ross ME, Jacobson IM, Dienstag JL, Martin JB. Late-onset Wilson's disease with neurological involvement in the absence of Kayser-Fleischer rings. Ann Neurol. 1985;17(4):411-3.
129. Madden JW, Ironside JW, Triger DR, Bradshaw JP. An unusual case of Wilson's disease. Q J Med. 1985;55(216):63-73.
130. Soman SD, Panday VK, Joseph KT, Raut SJ. Daily intake of some major and trace elements. Health Phys. 1969;17(1):35-40.
131. Kalra V, Ghai OP, Shapcott D. Biochemical profile of copper in patients and siblings of Indian Childhood Cirrhosis. Indian Pediatr. 1982;19(11):901-4.
132. Apter A, Pauls DL, Bleich A, Zohar AH, Kron S, Ratzoni G, et al. An epidemiologic study of Gilles de la Tourette's syndrome in Israel. Arch Gen Psychiatry. 1993:50(9):734-8.
133. Kurlan R, McDermott MP, Deeley C, Como PG, Brower C, Eapen S, et al. Prevalence of tics in school children and association with placement in special education. Neurology. 2001;57(8): 1383-8.
134. Lucas AR, Beard CM, Rajput AH, Kurland LT, et al. Tourette syndrome in Rochester, Minnesota, 1968–1979. Adv Neurol. 1982;35:267-9.
135. Erenberg G, Cruse RP, Rothner AD. The natural history of Tourette syndrome: a follow-up study. Ann Neurol. 1987;22: 383-5.
136. Kurlan R, Eapev V, Stern J, McDermott MP, Robertson MM. Bilineal transmission in Tourette's syndrome families. Neurology. 1994;44(12):2336-42.
137. Swedo SE, Leonard HL, Mittleman BB, Allen AJ, Rapoport JL, Dow SP, et al. Identification of children with Pediatric autoimmune neuropsychiatric disorders associated with streptococcal infections by a marker associated with rheumatic fever. Am J Psychiatry. 1997;154(1):110-2.

CHAPTER 4

Approach to Higher Level Gait Disorders

PD Thompson

INTRODUCTION

The concept of a higher level gait disorder was derived from Hughling's-Jackson's division of the nervous system into an organizational hierarchy from the lowest, simplest, most-organized automatic actions to the highest, least organized, modifiable, and complex sensorimotor functions.[1] Walking is a complex process in which the movements involved in maintaining equilibrium, an upright posture, and stepping are mediated by middle (basal ganglia, cerebellar, corticospinal, and reticulospinal) and lower (peripheral motor, proprioceptive sensory, and vestibular) levels of the nervous system under the direction of higher cortical control. Higher cortical levels link cognitive executive control with visuospatial information enabling flexibility and adaptability in walking taking into account the intended goal, spatial environment, and other circumstances. Higher cortical centers also supervise the inter-relation between the fundamentals of gait, equilibrium and stepping, adjusting truncal position to allow stepping to begin and monitoring body sway during walking. With learning and experience walking becomes "automatic" or "habitual" in that conscious monitoring is not necessary to remain upright and continue stepping. Yet conscious voluntary control can intervene, switching the stepping strategy to a goal directed mode if balance is threatened, a change in terrain occurs, or when learning new locomotor tasks.

Disease can interfere with walking at lower (arthritic, neuropathic, myopathic, vestibulopathic, and sensory ataxia) and middle (spasticity, cerebellar ataxia, dystonia, chorea, or Parkinsonism) levels each presenting with characteristic clinical neurological signs.[1] Many gait disorders, particularly in the elderly do not conform to these patterns and there is a long history of descriptions of poorly understood patterns emphasizing the clinical signs, the anatomical sites of identified lesions, and various or unknown pathologies (**Box 1**). In most of these descriptions pathology when identified involved the frontal lobes and it is now recognized that higher level gait disorders interrupt a locomotor network encompassing the frontal lobes and connections with other cortical areas, the basal ganglia and brainstem locomotor centers including the cerebellum.[2] The concept of higher level gait disorders provided a framework for the analysis of these poorly understood gait disorders according to disruption of higher level control of the fundamentals of gait, equilibrium and stepping.[1] Disease can disturb each of these functions

Box 1 Earlier descriptions of higher level gait disorders used the following terms.

- Frontal ataxia, frontal gait disorder
- Gait apraxia
- Trepidant abasia
- Astasia-abasia
- Marche a petits pas
- Arteriosclerotic Parkinsonism
- Magnetic apraxia
- Slipping clutch syndrome
- Senile paraplegia
- Senile gait disorder
- Lower body (half) Parkinsonism
- Parkinsonian ataxia

in isolation, interfering with maintenance of an upright standing posture (dysequilibrium, postural instability, poor truncal mobility, and falls), difficulty starting to walk (failure of gait ignition and start hesitation), shuffling, failure to maintain stepping (freezing), or in any number of combinations. Accordingly, the clinical features of a higher level gait disorder vary considerably, depending on whether the predominant deficit relates to dysequilibrium or difficulty stepping. This may change as the disease progresses.

CAUTIOUS GAIT PATTERNS

A cautious gait pattern is often the presenting feature of a higher level gait disorder. If balance is impaired, standing and stepping will be affected. This is apparent in normal individuals attempting to walk on a slippery surface. Similarly, any neurological disease that interferes with sensorimotor function can alter balance, equilibrium, and walking. The compensatory response to perceived instability, particularly if there have been falls, is a cautious gait in which a slightly stooped posture on a widened stance base is adopted, stride length is shortened, walking speed is slower, and turning occurs en bloc. Improvement in stepping with minor external support is an important clue to a cautious gait where shuffling steps are compensatory for subtle dysequilibrium.

STEPPING PATTERNS IN HIGHER LEVEL GAIT DISORDERS

The typical gait pattern consists of short, shallow, shuffling steps, on a slightly widened stance with an upright trunkal posture and preserved or exaggerated arm swing.[3,4] Shuffling steps are most noticeable when starting to walk (start hesitation) and on turning, especially in narrow spaces or when passing through doorways. Multitasking and distraction also precipitate shuffling steps. The shuffling stepping pattern overlaps with freezing (see below). The normal fluid interplay between trunkal motion and associated arm swing during walking is lacking and in combination with an upright trunkal posture create the appearance of a "military two step" gait. As the gait disorder evolves, steps become shorter and the shuffling more pronounced to the extent the feet appear stuck to the ground ("magnetic feet"). The stance base also widens further indicating compensation for increasing unsteadiness due to dysequilibrium (see below). Dysequilibrium and the risk of falls in turn affect the capacity to step. Accordingly, shuffling steps can be considered a primary locomotor deficit, exemplified by freezing, but also may be compensatory for dysequilibrium.

DYSEQUILIBRIUM IN HIGHER LEVEL GAIT DISORDERS

Relatively little has been written about the neurological assessment of dysequilibrium even though equilibrium is of crucial importance in maintaining the upright trunkal posture necessary for bipedal walking. Dysequilibrium is often overlooked in the examination of gait when there are obvious and dramatic stepping changes. The initial deleterious effects of dysequilibrium on walking encountered in higher level gait disorders are subtle but can be distinguished from the imbalance of cerebellar ataxia (see below). Higher level gait disorders due to dysequilibrium initially manifest as a cautious, shuffling gait or present with apparently unexplained falls due to inadequate postural responses including the failure of rescue and protective reactions to correct trunkal perturbations, control truncal motion and maintain an upright posture.[5] Dysequilibrium is also accompanied by deteriorating trunkal mobility. Trunkal mobility is examined by the ability to position the trunk appropriately and safely when sitting down and standing up, and turning or rolling over while lying in bed. The initial encounter with the patient with dysequilibrium, before the formal examination, is often revealing (as is the characteristic of frontal cognitive deficits). On entering the consulting room, the patient with impaired trunkal movement staggers, leaning to one side with lurching steps, moving too quickly and attempting to sit without properly aligning themselves with the chair. When sitting down, trunkal positioning is inappropriate without due care in placing the trunk safely over the seat of the chair. On standing up, the legs are not placed squarely beneath the trunk but scissored, with flexed posturing and other movements and postures that hinder balance and stability. Formal examination of trunkal movements reveals difficulty sitting down, standing up, lying down, an inability to roll over or sit up without assistance. The trunkal posture and the extent and direction of body sway during quiet standing should be noted. A wide stance base indicates instability and is often accompanied by increased body sway. A flexed trunkal posture with arm movements searching for support may be compensatory for dysequilibrium. Extension of the trunk may also be seen in dysequilibrium along with a tendency to tilt backwards or take a few spontaneous steps of retropulsion. The pull test, conducted with the examiner standing behind the patient, placing their hands on the patient's shoulders and gently pulling backwards, examines postural righting reflexes and corrective rescue reactions. The tendency to sway, tilt and fall backwards is further demonstrated by an impaired pull test in which minor displacement of the upper body precipitates falls backwards or uncontrolled retropulsion without compensatory movements to arrest the trunkal motion, a step backwards to stabilise the trunk or windmill rescue movements of the arms. Inadequate or absent postural righting reflexes and corrective rescue responses are important signs of dysequilibrium. As dysequilibrium progresses, toppling falls and increasing shuffling steps on a wide stance base lead to loss of mobility and independence.

NEUROLOGICAL CLINICAL SIGNS IN HIGHER LEVEL GAIT DISORDERS

Several clinical signs are useful in distinguishing higher level gait disorders from Parkinson's disease especially in the early stages when this distinction may be difficult. Facial expression is normal, voluntary upper limb and hand movements are preserved. Standing is unstable on a wide base when caused by dysequilibrium but heel shin ataxia when supine is not present (distinguishing cerebellar gait ataxia from dysequilibrium). There is a tendency to fall with impaired postural responses on the pull test, tilting or falling backwards. A degree of cognitive impairment, upper motor neurone signs of hyperreflexia, extensor plantar responses, frontal signs such as slow responses, grasp reflexes, gegenhalten or paratonic rigidity, motor perseveration, hypokinesia and pseudobulbar palsy (dysarthria, emotional lability) are commonly present. These signs typically accompany subcortical small vessel disease.[3,4] However, in some cases higher level gait disorders can progress without deterioration in cognition or other pyramidal and "extrapyramidal" signs.[6]

FALLS

A history of "sudden", "spontaneous", or "unexplained" falls without loss of consciousness, tripping, or stumbling over an obstacle is a common presenting symptom of dysequilibrium. Such falls in the elderly are often attributed to "mechanical" or musculoskeletal factors, but the presence of head injury or leg fracture should raise the possibility of inadequate postural responses or rescue reactions and dysequilibrium. In this situation, the patient usually cannot describe how or explain why they fall. However, a careful history will reveal the fall occurred during a postural adjustment when standing from a seated position, turning, leaning, bending over, or following a minor perturbation. Postural adjustments when performing multiple tasks at once such as carrying an object while walking, reaching into a cupboard, the fridge or bookshelf, turning while carrying a dinner plate, etc., are common precipitants of falls in dysequilibrium. Further inquiry will reveal the gradual evolution over many months of declining gait with subtle imbalance, loss of confidence, a fear of falling, dislike of open or crowded spaces, shiny floors, moving walkways or crossing roads. Examination will demonstrate a compensatory cautious gait. If attention is diverted during multitasking, attentional resources become inadequate, voluntary conscious compensation fails and a fall, often backward, results. The wide extent of central cerebral networks involved in equilibrium and locomotion confers considerable compensatory reserve for dysequilibrium but the pathologies that disrupt equilibrium by interfering with postural responses also affect voluntary compensatory control of trunkal motion. When there are diminished resources (cognitive, attentional, executive, and visuospatial) maintaining locomotion and equilibrium, the competing demands of environmental distraction (walking through doorways and turning corners) or the performance of multiple tasks simultaneously or sequentially divert attention from walking and falls occur. This is especially the case when locomotion is under the high attentional demand of voluntary goal directed control. Ultimately, voluntary compensation becomes inadequate rendering locomotion increasingly difficult.

FREEZING OF GAIT

Stepping failure on starting to walk, start hesitation, or during walking, freezing, is characterized by the appearance of short shallow ineffective steps lasting a few seconds. Freezing is often accompanied by trembling movements of the legs and a body posture leaning forward with hip, knee and foot plantar flexion, standing on the toes. Episodic freezing is typically precipitated by turning in confined spaces, walking through doorways, encountering unexpected obstacles, entering crowded environments, crossing streets, or any external distracting stimulus. Freezing of gait is most commonly encountered in advanced Parkinson's disease and the majority of studies of the mechanisms of freezing concern Parkinson's disease.[7-10] Freezing in Parkinson's disease does not correlate with severity of rigidity or bradykinesia, consistent with the notion that freezing is a higher order stepping defect and one aspect of a higher level gait disorder. Pathophysiological mechanisms invoked to explain freezing of gait include a central locomotor deficit with altered patterns of leg muscle activation,[7,8] faulty coupling of postural and stepping components of locomotion,[7,8] impaired shifting of trunkal posture when starting to walk or turning,[4] disruption of basal ganglia—supplementary motor area loops controlling self-initiated movement and reliance on external cues driving motor activity,[7,8] executive dysfunction impairing appropriate selection of trunkal and limb movements-related to postural control.[9] Right cerebral hemisphere locomotor circuitry is more affected than the left in freezing, potentially resulting in an imbalance between hemispheric executive control of movement initiation, decreasing left hemisphere initiation of movement and increasing right hemisphere inhibition of action.[8] Reduced connectivity in the locomotor network between right pedunculopontine nucleus and medial right frontal cortex has also been demonstrated.[10] Freezing and impaired postural control in higher level gait disorders appears related to frontal and basal ganglia pathology,[4] while lesions causing freezing are located in a network encompassing the cerebellar locomotor region.[11]

PURE AKINESIA WITH GAIT FREEZING

Freezing may be the initial feature of higher level gait disorders due to frontal white matter disease such as vasculopathy or hydrocephalus. It is increasingly recognized that freezing can present as a relatively-isolated gait disturbance, described variously as pure akinesia, gait ignition failure, frozen gait, primary progressive freezing gait, and pure akinesia with gait freezing.[12-19] This syndrome manifests as start hesitation with short shuffling steps, an inability to initiate the first step to start walking, with ineffective shuffling on the spot ("slipping clutch phenomenon") or the feet appearing to stick to the floor ("magnetic feet"). The first step may be triggered by the use of an external cue such as stepping over the handle of an upturned walking stick, walking up stairs, or in response to an auditory signal. Once walking is underway, stepping appears relatively normal with good sized paces, a steady rhythm or cadence, and preserved arm swing. Primary progressive freezing gait or pure akinesia with gait freezing may be accompanied by "akinesia" of handwriting (micrographia) and speech (hypophonia), rigidity, postural tremor, hyper-reflexia, and the emergence of retroplusion, postural instability, and falls resulting in progressive loss of mobility over 5 years.[17,18] Progressive supranuclear palsy tauopathy is the most common pathology identified[16,19] but others have included pallidonigroluysian degeneration, diffuse Lewy body disease, and corticobasal degeneration.[20,21] Apraxia of eyelid opening may occur but a supranuclear ophthalmoplegia does not appear and dementia is infrequent in this presentation of progressive supranuclear palsy.[12,16,19]

STEPPING FAILURE OR DYSEQUILIBRIUM?

Stepping difficulty is readily evident on history and examination but short steps are a nonspecific feature in many elderly gait disorders and compensatory for postural instability with subtle dysequilibrium.[22] This is an important consideration when deciding whether start hesitation or shuffling is "primary" in the sense of a locomotor network failure to deliver stepping commands or "secondary" to profound dysequilibrium causing imbalance, loss of postural control, and an inability to step without the risk of falling. In lower half Parkinsonism due to frontal white matter vascular disease, the initial anterolateral postural shifts toward the support limb before gait initiation are preserved, but abnormally variable in amplitude and direction, and accompanied by one or more aborted hesitant steps before the first step is completed.[4] These errant postural adjustments are potentially destabilizing and interfere with gait initiation.[4] Similarly, reduced stride length and shallow steps are considered secondary to the broad-based dysequilibrium in normal pressure hydrocephalus.[23] Walking in subcortical arteriosclerotic encephalopathy exhibits elements of Parkinsonism and ataxia but the speed is slower than cerebellar or Parkinsonian gait, stride length is reduced and steps are variable in length and timing on a wide stance base compensating for instability.[24] Postural sway is increased during induced instability indicating dysequilibrium.[25]

IMAGING AND PATHOLOGY

Higher level gaid disorders are most commonly associated with frontal pathology, notably small vessel ischemic change in deep periventricular white matter of the frontal lobes[26] and hydrocephalus, but a number of pathologies have been described (**Box 2**). Motor fibers from motor cortex leg area, connecting the frontal motor cortex, supplementary motor area, basal ganglia, cerebellum, thalamus, and midbrain locomotor region, within the locomotor network, are located in the deep periventricular frontal white matter perhaps explaining the lower half predominance of higher level gait disorders.[3] Periventricular white matter signal change is associated with dysequilibrium, falls, and declining cognitive performance.[27,28] Sophisticated imaging in higher level gait disorders[29,30] and hydrocephalus[31] demonstrate disruption of frontal and callosal white matter integrity in areas that appeared normal on standard imaging. These and other studies reinforce the notion that higher level gait disorders are due to frontal white matter pathologies-related to cerebrovascular disease or aging. However, a reduction in gray matter volume in the mesencephalic locomotor region, consistent with atrophy was reported in patients with higher

Box 2 Pathologies interrupting the locomotor network from the frontal lobes to basal ganglia, cerebellum, and midbrain locomotor region that present with a higher level gait disorder.

- Subcortical arteriosclerotic encephalopathy (vascular Parkinsonism)
- Progressive supranuclear palsy
- Pallidonigroluysian atrophy
- Normal pressure hydrocephalus
- Diffuse Lewy body disease
- Parkinson's disease (late stages)
- Corticobasal degeneration

level gait disorders manifesting as impaired step execution and postural control.[32]

DIFFERENTIAL DIAGNOSIS

A shuffling stepping pattern that dominates the initial clinical picture of a higher level gait disorder frequently creates the impression that locomotor hypokinesia is the primary deficit. As a result, Parkinson's disease is often suspected. The shuffling gait of a higher level gait disorder is distinguished from Parkinson's disease by the normal facial expression, normal upper limb motor function, preserved arm swing during walking, an upright trunkal posture, a wide-based stance, and the absence of a resting or dependant tremor. This clinical picture is the basis of "lower half Parkinsonism".[3,33]

Instability and unsteadiness suggest cerebellar ataxia. However, frequent falls, especially when turning, multitasking, leaning forward or backward, poor control of trunkal motion with increased multidirectional body sway, tilting backward when standing, impairment of postural righting reflexes and corrective rescue reactions distinguish the dysequilibrium of a higher level gait disorder from cerebellar gait ataxia. Unprovoked spontaneous falls are unusual in most cerebellar diseases. Heel shin ataxia and the rhythmic trunkal oscillation of an anterior lobe trunkal ataxia are not features of dysequilibrium in higher level gait disorders.

Difficulty standing from a sitting or squatting position, sitting down, or turning in bed indicate impaired trunkal mobility and a higher level gait disorder. Impulsive initiation of gait or directional change without apparent appreciation of the risk of falling (a "reckless" gait) is another clue to the presence of frontal cognitive gait dysfunction particularly in progressive supranuclear palsy. In such patients, the pull test will reveal poor righting reflexes and absent or imperfect corrective rescue reactions that are not features of cerebellar gait ataxia.

CONCLUSION

Higher level gait disorders are common, particularly in the elderly. These gait disorders are variable, complex, and the initial presentation can be misleading. The precise basis of the breakdown of gait in the elderly is poorly understood as is the physiological basis for bipedal locomotion. A model for examining gait according to the fundamentals of walking is suggested as a starting point to classify gait disorders. It is evident the striking clinical signs of shuffling steps, magnetic feet, and propensity to fall in these cases contrasts with the relative ease of leg and foot movements when sitting or lying. This observation gave rise to the popular concept of "gait apraxia".[34] The disorganized linkage between trunkal and limb movements in patients with frontal motor syndromes and higher level gait disorders were also construed as an apraxia of gait and trunk movements,[35] and recently modified to an "apraxia of postural transitions" to explain the inappropriate limb positioning, postural synergies, and rescue reactions.[36] The presence of other frontal and corticospinal signs along with the possibility that the stepping difficulty may in part be voluntary compensation for a fear of falling secondary to dysequilibrium, challenge the validity of the term "apraxia" in this situation. Moreover, abnormal trunkal movement and postural control appears central to higher level gait disorders in contrast to the original concept of apraxia being related to skilled limb movement.[37,38] Finally, in discussing the term gait apraxia, Elble[39] stressed the importance of describing the clinical phenomena of higher level gait disorders, recognizing four key features: (1) Inappropriate limb movement, postural synergies, and interaction with the environment, (2) Variable performance, influenced by the environment, and emotion, (3) Hesitation and freezing, and (4) Absent or inappropriate rescue reactions. These clinical descriptions summarize the features of higher level gait disorders discussed in this review.

REFERENCES

1. Nutt JG, Marsden CD, Thompson PD. Human walking and higher-level gait disorders, particularly in the elderly. Neurology. 1993;43(2):268-79.
2. Takakusaki K, Chiba R, Nozu T, Okumura T. Brainstem control of locomotion and muscle tone with special reference to the role of the mesopontine tegmentum and medullary reticulospinal systems. J Neural Transm (Vienna). 2016; 123(7):695-729.
3. Thompson PD, Marsden CD. Gait disorder of subcortical arteriosclerotic encephalopathy: Binswanger's disease. Move Disord. 1987;2(1):1-8.
4. Elble RJ, Cousins R, Leffler K, Hughes L. Gait initiation by patients with lower-half parkinsonism. Brain. 1996;119(5):1705-16.
5. Weiner WJ, Nora LM, Glantz RH. Elderly in patients: postural reflex impairment. Neurology. 1984;34(7):945-7.
6. Huber-Mahlin V, Giladi N, Herman T, Perez C, Gurevich T, Hausdorff JM. Progressive nature of a higher level gait disorder: A 3-year prospective study. J Neurol. 2010;257(8): 1279-86.
7. Nutt JG, Bloem BR, Giladi N, Hallett M, Horak FB, Nieuwboer A. Freezing of gait: moving forward on a mysterious clinical phenomenon. Lancet Neurol. 2011;10(8):734-44.

8. Snijders AH, Takakusaki K, Debu B, Lozano AM, Krishna V, Fasano A. Physiology of freezing of gait. Ann Neurol. 2016;80(5): 644-59.
9. Giladi N, Hubler-Martin V, Herman T, Hausdorff JM. Freezing of gait in older adults with high level gait disorders: association with impaired executive function. J Neural Transm (Vienna). 2007;114(10):1349-53.
10. Fling BW, Cohen RG, Mancini M, Nutt JG, Fair DA, Horak FB. Asymmetric pedunculopontine network connectivity in parkinsonian patients with freezing of gait. Brain. 2013;136(8):2405-18.
11. Fasano A, Laganiere SE, Lam S, Fox MD. Lesions causing freezing of gait localize to a cerebellar functional network. Ann Neurol. 2017;81(1):129-41.
12. Matsuo H, Takashima H, Kishikawa M, Kinoshita I, Mori M, Tsujihata M, et al. Pure akinesia: An atypical manifestation of progressive supranuclear palsy. J Neurol Neurosurg Psychiatry. 1991;54(5):397-400.
13. Imai H, Nakamura T, Kondo T, Narabayashi H. Dopa-unresponsive pure akinesia or freezing. A condition within a wide spectrum of PSP? Adv Neurol. 1993;60:622-5.
14. Atchison PR, Thompson PD, Frackowiak RSJ, Marsden CD. The syndrome of gait ignition failure: A report of six cases. Move Disord. 1993;8(3):285-92.
15. Achiron A, Ziv I, Goren M, Goldberg H, Zoldan Y, Sroka H, et al. Primary progressive freezing gait. Move Disord. 1993;8(3): 293-7.
16. Riley DE, Fogt N, Leigh RJ: The syndrome of "pure akinesia" and its relationship to progressive supranuclear palsy. Neurology. 1994;44(6):1025-9.
17. Factor SA, Higgins DS, Qian J. Primary progressive freezing gait: a syndrome with many causes. Neurology. 2006;66(3): 411-4.
18. Factor SA, Jennings DL, Molho ES, Marek KL. The natural history of the syndrome of primary progressive freezing gait. Arch Neurol. 2002;59(11):1778-83.
19. Williams DR, Holton JL, Strand K, Revesz T, Lees AJ. Pure akinesia with gait freezing: a third clinical phenotype of progressive supranuclear palsy. Mov Disord. 2007;22(15):2235-41.
20. Giladi N, Kao R, Fahn S. Freezing phenomenon in patients with parkinsonian syndromes. Mov Disord. 1997;12(3):302-5.
21. Elkouzi A, Bit-Ivan EN, Elble RJ. Pure akinesia with gait freezing: A clinicopathologic study. J Clin Mov Disord. 2017;4:15.
22. Elble RJ, Hughes L, Higgins C. The syndrome of senile gait. J Neurol. 1992;239(2):71-5.
23. Stolze H, Kuhtz-Buschbeck JP, Drucke H, Jöhnk K, Diercks C, Palmié S, et al. Gait analysis in idiopathic normal pressure hydrocephalus-which parameters respond to the CSF tap test? Clin Neurophysiol. 2000;111(9):1678-86.
24. Ebersbach G, Sojer M, Valldeoriola F, Wissel J, Müller J, Tolosa E, et al. Comparative analysis of gait in Parkinson's disease, cerebellar ataxia and subcortical arteriosclerotic encephalopathy. Brain. 1999;122(7):1349-55.
25. Trenkwalder C, Paulus W, Krafczyk S, Hawken M, Oertel WH, Brandt T. Postural stability differentiates "lower body" from idiopathic parkinsonism. Acta Neurol Scand. 1995;91(6): 444-52.
26. Ishii N, Nishihara Y, Imamura T. Why do frontal lobe symptoms predominate in vascular dementia with lacunes? Neurology. 1986;36(3):340-45.
27. Whitman GT, Tang Y, Lin A, Baloh RW. A prospective study of cerebral white matter abnormalities in older people with gait dysfunction. Neurology. 2001;57(6):990-4.
28. Masdeu JC, Wolfson L, Lantos G, Tobin JN, Grober E, Whipple R, et al: Brain white-matter changes in the elderly prone to falling. Arch Neurol. 1989;46(12):1292-6.
29. de Laat KF, Tuladhar AM, van Norden AG, Norris DG, Zwiers MP, de Leeuw FE. Loss of white matter integrity is associated with gait disorders in cerebral small vessel disease. Brain. 2011;134(1):73-83.
30. Kafri M, Sasson E, Assaf Y, Balash Y, Aiznstein O, Hausdorff JM, et al. High level gait disorder: associations with specific white matter changes observed on advanced diffusion imaging. J Neuroimaging. 2013;23(1):39-46.
31. Hattingen F, Jurcoane A, Melber J, Blasel S, Zanella FE, Neumann-Haefelin T, et al. Diffusion tensor imaging in patients with adult chronic idiopathic hydrocephalus. Neurosurgery. 2010;66(5):917-24.
32. Demain A, Westby GWM, Fernandez-Vidal S, Karachi C, Bonneville F, Do MC, et al. High-level gait and balance disorders in the elderly: a midbrain disease? J Neurol. 2014;261(1): 196-206.
33. Glass PG, Lees AJ, Bacellar A, Zijlmans J, Katzenschlager R, Silveira-Moriyama L. The clinical features of pathologically confirmed vascular parkinsonism. J Neurol Neurosurg Psychiatry. 2012;83(10):1027-9.
34. Meyer JS, Barron DW. Apraxia of gait: A clinico-physiological study. Brain 1960;83(2):261-84.
35. Petrovici I: Apraxia of gait and of trunk movements. J Neurol Sci. 1968;7(2):229-43.
36. Dale ML, Curtze C, Nutt JG. Apraxia of gait- or apraxia of postural transitions. Parkinsonism Relat Disord. 2018;50:19-22.
37. Thompson PD. Higher level gait disorders. Curr Neurol Neurosci Rep. 2007;7(4):290-4.
38. Nutt JG. Higher-Level Gait Disorders: An open frontier. Mov Disord. 2013;28(11):1560-5.
39. Elble RJ. Gait and dementia: Moving beyond the notion of gait apraxia. J Neural Transm (Vienna). 2007;114(10):1253-8.

SECTION

2

PARKINSON'S DISEASE

CHAPTER 5

Genetics of Parkinson's Disease

Asha Kishore, Divya KP

INTRODUCTION

Parkinson's disease (PD) is a debilitating neurodegenerative disorder with worldwide incidence rates of 8–18 per 100,000 person-years.[1] PD increases with age affecting >1% of the population over the age of 60 years, making it the most prevalent movement disorder and the second most common neurodegenerative disorder after Alzheimer's dementia.[2] The defining characteristics of PD include bradykinesia, tremor, rigidity, and postural instability. PD is associated with a myriad of nonmotor symptoms including disorders of mood and affect such as apathy, anhedonia, and depression, cognitive dysfunction in the form of working memory deficits and complex behavioral disorders. Sensory dysfunction with hyposmia or pain is quite common, as are disturbances of sleep-wake cycle. Autonomic dysfunction such as orthostatic hypotension, urogenital dysfunction, and constipation is also present in a majority of patients. Many of the nonmotor symptoms can antedate the occurrence of motor signs or become increasingly prevalent with advancing disease. Symptoms such as loss of smell, constipation, anxiety/depression, and rapid eye movement (REM) sleep behavioral disorders (RBD) have been described up to 10 years or more prior to the onset of the typical disease.[3]

Parkinson's disease occurs more in men (prevalence = 2.865/1,000; incidence = 0.490/1,000 person-years) than in women (prevalence = 1.934/1,000; incidence = 0.328/1,000 person-years). The overall male:female (M:F) ratio was 1.48 for prevalence and 1.49 for incidence. Prevalence and incidence M:F ratios increases by 0.05 and 0.14, respectively, per 10 years of age. Incidence was similar in both genders aged below 50 years (M:F ratio <1.2) and over 1.6 times higher in men than women above 80 years.[4]

Since the description about PD in 1817 by James Parkinson, success in elucidating an etiological factor has been elusive. Majority of PD cases are sporadic without a family history of the disease. Neuropathologically, PD is defined by loss of dopaminergic neurons in the substantia nigra pars compacta (SNc) of the midbrain and the presence of cytoplasmic and axonal accumulation of an aggregated protein, alpha-synuclein (encoded by the gene *SNCA*) which is globular and called as Lewy bodies (LBs) in the perikarya and spindle or thread-like and known as Lewy neurites (LNs) in axons of the remaining neurons.[5] Clinical diagnosis of PD is made when the motor symptoms and signs appear and by this time >50% of dopaminergic neurons would have been lost in the SNc.[6] The neurodegenerative process in PD is a combination of both cell-autonomous mechanisms including dysregulation of calcium homeostasis, impaired turnover of mitochondria, and alterations in mitochondrial bioenergetics and non-cell-autonomous mechanisms involving neuroinflammation and prion-like behavior of misfolded proteins.[7]

GENETIC FORMS OF PARKINSON'S DISEASE

Twin study is a good tool for assessing the influence of hereditary factors in diseases. [^{18}F]-DOPA PET was used to study dopaminergic function in twin pairs who were at baseline clinically discordant for PD. The concordance for subclinical striatal dopaminergic dysfunction at baseline was found to be significantly higher in 18 monozygotic (MZ) than in 16 dizygotic (DZ) twin pairs (55% vs. 18%, respectively). All asymptomatic MZ twins showed progressive loss of dopaminergic function over

7 years and four developed clinical PD while none of the DZ twin pairs became clinically concordant. On follow-up, the combined concordance levels for subclinical dopaminergic dysfunction and clinical PD were 75% in the 12 MZ and 22% in the 9 DZ twin pairs. These findings suggested a substantial role for inheritance in "sporadic" PD.[8] Conclusion from the population-based Swedish Twin Registry (STR) was that concordance rates for PD were somewhat higher (4% for MZ and same-sexed DZ twin pairs) but the heritability estimate was nonsignificant. Their longitudinal analyses demonstrated that PD and Parkinsonism were modestly heritable.[9]

Approximately 5–10% of all PD is caused by highly penetrant monogenic but rare mutations segregating with the disease in families. The spectrum of genetic variants underlying PD etiology ranges from rare variants with very large effects (i.e., fully or highly penetrant mutations in single genes) to genetic variants exerting only modest effects but that are relatively common in the general population. **Figure 1** shows the penetrance of various genes associated with PD.

GENE DISCOVERY RESEARCH STRATEGIES

- *Linkage mapping* is a useful tool for the identification of highly-penetrant pathogenic mutations when DNA samples from large families segregating the disease are available. This strategy is easier in a disease with a recessive pattern of inheritance, because the analysis of only 2–3 affected siblings born from consanguineous parents might be informative enough to find a causative gene using homozygosity mapping.
- *Candidate gene studies*: Investigates the association between genetic variants in genes with a plausible role in disease pathophysiology and a phenotype of interest. Candidate genes are most often selected for study based on a prior knowledge of the gene's biological functional impact on disease. The reason for focusing on allelic variation in specific biologically relevant regions of the genome is that certain mutations will directly impact the function of the gene and lead to the phenotype or disease state being investigated.[10]
- *Genome-wide association studies (GWAS)*: Assesses the association between a large number (typically several hundred thousands to millions) of polymorphisms across genome and a phenotype of interest. This technique is to identify genetic variants that are common in the population which individually have very small effect sizes (odds ratios <1.5), but "modulate the risk of" (rather than cause) disease. GWAS require large number of cases and well-matched population controls.[11]
- *Next-generation sequencing (NGS)*: Next-generation sequencing technologies enable much higher sequencing capacity at lower cost.[12] It is now possible to rapidly sequence the entire chromosomal region delimited by a linkage mapping or a GWAS strategy and sequence only the exons contained therein.[13]

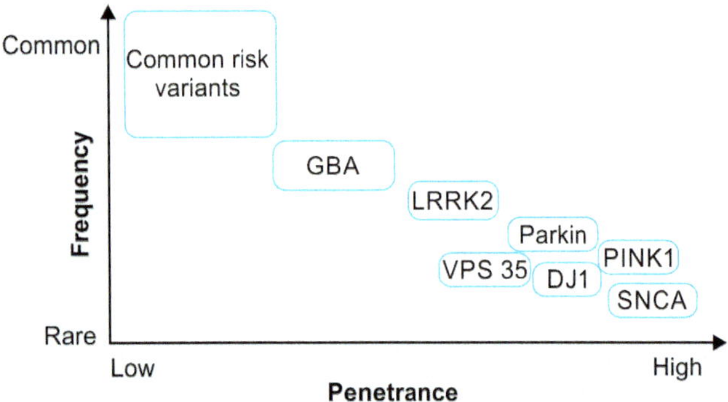

(GBA: glucocerebrosidase; LRRK2: leucine-rich repeat kinase 2; PINK1: PTEN induced putative kinase 1; PTEN: phosphatase and tensin homolog; SNCA: alpha-synuclein; VPS35: vacuolar protein sorting 35 retromer complex component)

FIG. 1: Showing penetrance of various genes in Parkinson's disease.

Monogenic Forms of Parkinson's Disease (Table 1)

Refer to Table 1 for confirmed genes implicated in monogenic PD.

THE AUTOSOMAL DOMINANT FORMS OF PARKINSON'S DISEASE

Mutations in three genes (*SNCA, LRRK2,* and *VPS35*) are conclusively established as a cause of autosomal dominant (AD) forms of PD. The evidence for a fourth gene, eukaryotic translation initiation factor 4 gamma 1 (*EIF4G1*), remains incomplete. Heterozygous mutations in the glucocerebrosidase (*GBA*) gene are important and strong risk factors for PD and diffuse Lewy-body disease (DLB).

Alpha-synuclein

Alpha-synuclein was the first genetic mutation reported to cause AD PD. Patients with *SNCA* mutations usually have early-onset PD (EOPD) (age of onset <50 years) with a good response to levodopa treatment, initially. The disease progresses rapidly and often develops dementia, atypical features such as central hypoventilation and myoclonus. LBs are present and spread through the substantia nigra, locus ceruleus, hypothalamus, and cerebral cortex.[14]

The *SNCA* gene is located on human chromosome 4 and encodes the protein *SNCA*. The physiological function of *SNCA* is in the regulation of neurotransmitter release, synaptic function, and plasticity of dopaminergic neurons. Misfolding and aggregation of the SNCA protein into neurotoxic species are at the center of the current pathogenetic theories for PD.[15] Missense mutations in

TABLE 1: Confirmed genes implicated in monogenic Parkinson's disease (PD).

Nomenclature	*Gene loci*	*Gene*	*Inheritance*	*Clinical presentation*	*Status*
PARK1	4q21–22	*SNCA*	AD	YOPD	Confirmed
PARK2	6q25.2–q27	*Parkin*	AR	YOPD	Confirmed
PARK3	2p13	Unknown	AD	Classical PD	Unconfirmed
PARK4	4q21–q23	*SNCA*	AD	YOPD	Same as PARK 1
PARK5	4p13	*UCHL1*	AD	Classical PD	Unconfirmed
PARK6	1p35–p36	*PINK1*	AR	YOPD	Confirmed
PARK7	1p36	*DJ1*	AR	YOPD	Confirmed
PARK8	12q12	*LRRK2*	AD	Classical PD	Confirmed
PARK9	1p36	*ATP13A2*	AR	Kufor–Rakeb disease	Confirmed
PARK10	1p32	Unknown	Risk factor	Classical PD	Confirmed
PARK11	2q36.27	Unknown	AD	Late onset PD	Not independently confirmed
PARK12	Xq21–q25	Unknown	Risk factor	Classical PD	Confirmed susceptibility locus
PARK13	2p12	*HTRA1*	AD or risk factor	Classical PD	Unconfirmed
PARK14	22q13.1	*PLA2G6*	AD	Early onset dystonia parkinsonism	Confirmed
PARK15	22q12–q13	*FBXO7*	AD	Pallidopyramidal syndrome	Confirmed
PARK16	1q32	Unknown	Risk factor	Classical PD	Confirmed susceptibility locus
PARK17	16q11.2	*VPS35*	AD	Classical PD	Confirmed
PARK18	3q27.1	*EIF4G1*	AD	Classical PD	Unconfirmed

(AD: autosomal dominant; AR: autosomal recessive; PD: Parkinson's disease; YOPD: young-onset Parkinson's disease)

SNCA locus were identified in familial forms of PD (A53T, A30P, E46K, and H50Q)[16] as well as in sporadic PD patients (A18T and A29S).[17] Duplications and triplications of the *SNCA* locus cause familial Parkinsonism and correlate with disease severity.[18]

Mutations in the *SNCA* gene are rare and include point mutations and whole-locus multiplications (duplications or triplications) of the wild gene. Ala53Thr mutation are reported in few families of Greek ancestry and occasionally in Asia;[19] Ala30Pro and Glu46Lys have been found in single families of German and Spanish origin, respectively. Duplications are detected in approximately 1-2% of the PD families. Point mutations and triplications are extremely rare. The brain pathology is characterized by an abundance of *SNCA*-positive neuronal inclusions [LBs and LNs], the phenotype ranges from typical features of PD to more atypical and aggressive phenotypes (including myoclonus, severe autonomic dysfunction, and dementia in addition to Parkinsonism), and resembling dementia with LBs [(DLB) or multiple system atrophy (MSA)].

Two novel missense mutations were recently identified in this gene in PD patients. The first mutation, c.150T>G, leads to the p.His50Gln (H50Q) missense change in the SNCA protein. Further data, is needed, to clarify whether His50Gln is a PD-causing mutation or a benign neutral rare variant. The second mutation, c.152G>A, occurs two nucleotides downstream in the SNCA open reading frame, leading to the p.Gly51Asp (G51D) missense change in the protein.[20] Parkinsonian symptoms in the carriers of Gly51Asp occurred often before the age of 40 years and before 20 years in one (juvenile Parkinsonism). Levodopa response is moderate, and the disease progression is very rapid, with death in <10 years from onset in some. Atypical features, such as pyramidal signs, cognitive deterioration, psychiatric disturbances, myoclonus, and seizures, were present. The pathology in the carriers of Gly51Asp is characterized by brain atrophy, more severe in the frontotemporal lobes, severe neuronal loss in sites typical for PD, but also in the striatum, hippocampus, and cerebral cortex, with abundant and pleomorphic SNCA positive inclusions, some resembling LBs and LNs but other similar to the glial and neuronal cytoplasmic inclusions of the MSA. The patients with SNCA duplications often display a classical PD phenotype, whereas the more rare cases carrying triplications display more severe phenotypes.[21]

Leucine-rich Repeat Kinase 2

Mutations in the gene encoding leucine-rich repeat kinase 2 (*LRRK2)* was first identified in 2004 and have since been shown to be the single most common cause of inherited PD. *LRRK2* belongs to the ROCO protein family. This class of multidomain proteins is characterized by the presence of a 200–250 amino acid Ras of complex protein (Roc) domain, followed by a 300–400 amino acid domain termed COR (C-terminal of Roc).[22]

Mutations in the gene encoding *LRRK2* cause AD, late-onset PD that is clinically similar to idiopathic disease. *LRRK2* is a multidomain protein containing several protein interaction motifs as well as dual enzymatic domains of GTPase and protein kinase activities. The PARK8 locus (*LRRK2*) was originally mapped in a large Japanese family, the Sagamihara family, presenting with AD Parkinsonism. Brain autopsy in four members of the Sagamihara family revealed pure nigral neuronal degeneration without coexisting pathology.[23] In contrast, nigral neuronal loss, tauopathy, and LB synucleinopathy have been described elsewhere for other families with *LRRK2* mutations.[24]

Mutations in *LRRK2* is the most frequent cause of familial PD, particularly in certain populations in north African Arab region.[25] A minimum of six highly penetrant, pathogenic mutations have been described in *LRRK2* (Asn1437His, Arg1441Cys/Gly/His, Tyr1699Cys, Gly2019Ser, and Ile2020Thr),[26] among which the most common mutation Gly2019Ser (rs34637584) has an estimated carrier frequency of 4% in familial and 1% in "sporadic" PD patients.[27]

The *LRRK2* gene product, also called dardarin, is a large and complex protein (285 kD). Recent biochemical studies have demonstrated that *LRRK2* has kinase activity in vitro and that the *LRRK2* G2019S and I2020T mutations have elevated kinase activity as tested for autophosphorylation.[28] These results are consistent with the notion that *LRRK2* mutations cause PD by way of a "gain-of-function" or hyperactivity of *LRRK2*.

LRRK2 is unique among the PD-causing genes, because a missense mutation, G2019S, is a frequent determinant of not only familial but also sporadic PD. Thus, *LRRK2* has emerged as a promising therapeutic target for combating PD. Inhibitors of *LRRK2* kinase are protective in vitro and in vivo models of *LRRK2*-induced neurodegeneration.[29]

Vacuolar Protein Sorting 35 Retromer Complex Component

Latest PD gene, *VPS35* (encoding vacuolar protein sorting 35 retromer complex component), was identified by whole-exome NGS.[30] The same mutation p.Asp620Asn (c.1858G>A) was independently identified in an Austrian.[31] and Swiss[30] kindred, respectively. *VPS35* p.Asp620Asn has since been confirmed to represent a causative, AD PD mutation in independent datasets. The *VPS35* protein is involved in the retrograde transport of proteins from endosomes to the trans-Golgi network.[32]

Eukaryotic Translation Initiation Factor 4 Gamma 1

Variants in the *EIF4G1* have been identified to be responsible for AD PD (PARK18). *EIF4G1* is associated with LB pathology.[33] Mutations in the *EIF4G1* gene was initially detected by a genome-wide linkage approach in a large French family, where the missense p.Arg1502 His mutation was initially identified.[34] However, subsequent studies have failed to replicate those initial findings.

Glucocerebrosidase

Dominantly-inherited heterozygous mutations in the *GBA* gene are a frequent and strong risk factor for PD.[35] Patients with *GBA* pathogenic mutations have typical PD with possibly a slightly earlier onset age. Evidence linking *GBA* mutations to the clinical characteristics of PD, including disease phenotype, progression, and prognosis, has been extensively documented. The most commonly presenting feature is an asymmetric resting tremor, although postural instability and gait difficulties are also relatively frequent. *GBA* carrier status has a significant impact on the natural history of PD with patients reporting an earlier age of symptom onset and severe motor impairment.[36,37] There is a higher prevalence of dementia and a distinct pattern of cognitive deficits, characterized by greater impairment in memory, executive function, and visuospatial abilities.[38] Other nonmotor clinical features are also highly prevalent, with the most common being anosmia and dysautonomia, as well as REM sleep disorder, depression, anxiety, and psychotic features presenting as hallucinations.[39]

Other Autosomal Dominant Forms of Parkinson's Disease with Incomplete Evidence of Pathogenicity

A heterozygous mutation c.169C>A, p.P57T in *RIC3* acetylcholine receptor chaperone (11p15) segregated with disease in two affected cousins (with some nonmotor phenotypes) from a 14-member Indian PD family with an AD mode of inheritance. A different heterozygous mutation c.502G>C, p.V168L was detected in an unrelated PD patient. Both mutations were absent in 144 healthy control and in 74 non-PD whole exome sequencing (WES) data available in-house and in 186 age and sex-matched controls screened by polymerase chain reaction (PCR) sequencing. *RIC3* is a chaperone of neuronal nicotinic acetylcholine receptor subunit α-7 (CHRNA7). The novel demonstration provides strong evidence for the role of cholinergic pathway for the first time in PD etiology.[40]

AUTOSOMAL-RECESSIVE PARKINSON'S DISEASE GENES

Autosomal recessive (AR) homozygous or compound heterozygous loss-of-function mutations have been identified in three genes using traditional gene mapping approaches: *PARK2* (RBR E3ubiquitin protein ligase, commonly known as Parkin),[41] *PINK1* (phosphatase and tensin homolog (PTEN) induced putative kinase 1),[42] and *PARK7* (Parkinson protein 7, commonly known as DJ-1).[43] While mutations in these genes are all relatively rare in the general PD population, they appear to be responsible for a substantial proportion of EOPD (mean age at onset of homozygous mutation carriers for *Parkin*, *PINK1*, and DJ-1~39 years).[43] The most commonly mutated AR PD gene is *Parkin*, which accounts for 8.6% of EOPD (<50 years) cases, followed by *PINK1* (3.7%) and DJ-1(0.4%).[44]

Parkin

Parkin was the second identified PD gene and the first gene irrefutably causing an AR form of the disorder. The disease usually starts in the third or fourth decade of the patients' life and is usually slowly progressive with an excellent response to dopaminergic treatment. However, some of the Parkin-mutation carriers have an onset even in childhood and homozygous mutations in Parkin are the most frequent cause of juvenile PD (age of onset < 21 years). Parkin mutations are the most common known cause of EOPD, accounting for up to 77% of the familial cases with an age of onset <30 years[45] and for 10–20% of EOPD patients in general.[46]

Parkin is the second largest gene in human genome and codes for a 465-amino acid protein with a modular architecture. The Parkin protein functions as an E3 ubiquitin ligase in the process of ubiquitination, a form of post-translational modification that conjugates ubiquitin protein(s) to lysine residue(s) of target proteins, which in turn determines their cellular fate.

PINK1

The majority of *PINK1* mutations reported are either missense or nonsense mutations, and, only few families with whole-exon deletions (exons 4–8, 6–8, and 7 and one with a heterozygous whole-gene deletion have been reported).[47-50]

More than 60 different missense and nonsense mutations have been found, affecting all 8 *PINK1* exons at nearly equal frequencies. *PINK1* is a 581 amino acid ubiquitously expressed protein kinase. It consists of an amino terminal 34 amino acid mitochondrial targeting motif, a conserved serine-threonine kinase domain (amino acids 156–509; exons 2–8), and a carboxy-terminal autoregulatory domain. Two-thirds of the reported mutations in *PINK1* are loss-of-function mutations affecting the kinase domain, demonstrating the importance of *PINK1*'s enzymatic activity in the pathogenesis of PD. Interestingly, recent studies provided evidence that *PINK1* and Parkin function in a common pathway for sensing and selectively eliminating damaged mitochondria from the mitochondrial network.[51] Psychiatric signs and symptoms have repeatedly been described for *PINK1*-related PD.

DJ-1

DJ-1 is mutated in about 1–2% of EOPD cases.[52,53] *DJ-1* was first identified as a causative PD gene in two consanguineous families of Dutch and Italian origin[47] and mutation analyses have revealed both point and structural mutations (Glu163Lys, Leu166Pro, exon 1e5 deletion, g.168-185dup).[36] Clinical characteristics *DJ-1* mutation carriers are comparable with typical signs and symptoms of classical levodopa-responsive PD.

The seven coding exons of the *DJ-1* gene code for a 189-amino acid-long protein that is ubiquitously expressed and functions as a cellular sensor of oxidative stress. Pathophysiologically, *DJ-1* has been involved in the protection of neurons from oxidative stress and may also play a role in mitochondrial function.[54,55]

DNAJC6

Whole exome sequencing has also led to the successful identification of AR mutations in *DNAJC6* [encoding DNAJ heat shock protein family (Hsp40) member C6, a.k.a. auxilin] as a cause of EOPD, predominately with a typical signs and symptoms. Initially, a homozygous splicing mutation (c.801-2A>G) in *DNAJC6* was identified using homozygosity mapping followed by WES in two affected brothers of a small consanguineous family from Palestine. Clinically, the brothers presented with signs of parkinsonism, missing response to levodopa, and very rapid progression of motor symptom.[55] Age at onset of *DNAJC6*-linked Parkinsonism with prominent atypical signs and symptoms appears to be very early with an average of 10 years (range 7–11) across the seven reported cases from three families.[56] The reported carriers of AR *DNAJC6* mutations who showed signs and symptoms of typical PD had a mean age of onset of 31 years.[55]

Auxilin (encoded by *DNAJC6*) is a clathrin-associated protein expressed predominately in neurons and enriched in nerve terminals suggesting again that vesicle trafficking is an important feature in PD pathogenesis.[57]

Autosomal Recessive Juvenile Atypical Parkinsonism

PARK9 (also termed Kufor-Rakeb syndrome) is characterized by juvenile, levodopa-responsive Parkinsonism, pyramidal signs, dementia, and supranuclear gaze palsy, and is caused by recessive mutations in the ATPase type 13A2 (*ATP13A2*) gene. The *ATP13A2* gene encodes a lysosomal membrane transporter.[58]

Recessive mutations in the phospholipase A2, group VI (*PLA2G6*) gene, described initially as the cause of infantile neuroaxonal dystrophy and neurodegeneration associated with brain iron accumulation, were later identified in patients with levodopa-responsive dystonia-Parkinsonism, pyramidal signs, and cognitive/psychiatric features, with onset in early adulthood. Magnetic resonance imaging (MRI) shows brain atrophy with or without iron accumulation.[58]

Mutations in the F-box only protein 7 gene (*FBXO7*) cause PARK15, a recessive form of juvenile Parkinsonism with pyramidal disturbances. The brain pathology in patients with PARK15 remains unknown. *FBXO7* immunoreactivity in the LBs of typical PD and in glial cytoplasmic inclusions of multiple system atrophy has been recently reported suggesting an involvement of this protein in the pathogenesis of the common forms of synucleinopathies.[59]

Recently, mutations in another gene *SYNJ1* were identified as the cause of AR juvenile Parkinsonism.[60,61] *SYNJ1* encodes synaptojanin 1, playing a very close role in the postendocytic recycling of synaptic vesicles.

Major Risk Loci

The investigation of *MAPT*, which encodes the microtubule-associated protein tau, as a candidate gene in PD (100–103) has been motivated by shared neuropathological characteristics (and overlapping clinical features of Parkinsonism) across several neurodegenerative diseases. Specifically, brain tissues in Alzheimer's disease, tauopathies [supranuclear palsy and "frontotemporal dementia and Parkinsonism linked to chromosome 17" (FTLD-17)], and PD all show an aggregation of intraneuronal hyperphosphorylated tau. *MAPT* is located in an interval on chromosome 17 that is characterized by a large inversion with two haplotypes, H1 and H2, in Caucasian populations.[62] Of these, H1 has been identified to confer risk for PD.[63] Notably, individuals from East Asia are homozygous for the H1 haplotype;[64] accordingly, due to absence of the "allele contrast" (i.e., H1 vs. H2), no association between *MAPT* and PD has been reported in Asian populations.[65]

Gene-environment Interactions in Parkinson's Disease

The establishment of gene-environment (GxE) interaction effects has proven to be difficult in most complex diseases, PD representing no exception. The first genome wide interaction analyses reported for this sample highlighted a potential genome-wide significant interaction of coffee consumption and SNP rs4998386 in GRIN2A.[66] This finding, however, could not be validated in several independent population-based datasets.[67] The other set of genome-wide GxE analyses in the same dataset reported a suggestive result for smoking history.[68] However, this latter finding currently lacks any independent support. Thus, in order to result in robust and replicable results, this field of genetic research in PD requires the compilation of carefully ascertained population-based datasets of sufficient size to detect or refute GxE effects on a genome-wide scale.

Parkinson's Disease in Indian Patients

Indian data show a skewed female to male ratio of 1:3 among PD patients in hospital-based studies. It may partly be due to the fact that more men than women seek medical care for comparably severe medical illness in Indian context.[69] Most commonly reported six mutations in *LRRK2* gene were screened among Indian PD patients, using PCR-restriction fragment length polymorphism (PCR-RFLP) method. Mutations G2019S, R1441C, R1441G, and R1441H were screened in 1,012 individuals (PD, 800; controls, 212) while mutations I2012T and I2020T were screened in 748 PD patients. None of these six mutations were seen except in a single female young-onset PD patient who showed a heterozygous G2019S mutation. The absence of mutations was reconfirmed by sequencing of probands from several AD PD families. These observations suggest that these mutations may be a rare cause of PD among Indians.[70]

CONCLUSION

The past 20 years have seen the identification of numerous causative genes and genetic risk variants in PD. These discoveries have substantially improved our understanding of PD pathophysiology. It can be expected that additional causative genes for Parkinsonian phenotypes will be discovered upon a more wide spread employment of high-throughput genomic technologies. Though we are far from understanding the exact sequence of molecular events leading to SNCA aggregation and cell death, the hitherto identified PD genes may serve as novel targets for disease prevention and early therapeutic strategies.

REFERENCES

1. Dorsey ER, Constantinescu R, Thompson JP, Biglan KM, Holloway RG, Kieburtz K, et al. Projected number of people with Parkinson disease in the most populous nations, 2005 through 2030. Neurology. 2007;68(5):384-6.
2. de Lau LML, Breteler MMB. Epidemiology of Parkinson's disease. Lancet Neurol. 2006;5(6):525-35.
3. Schrag A, Horsfall L, Walters K, Noyce A, Petersen I. Prediagnostic presentations of Parkinson's disease in primary care: a case-control study. Lancet Neurol. 2015;14(1):57-64.
4. Moisan F, Kab S, Mohamed F, Canonico M, Le Guern M, Quintin C, et al. Parkinson disease male-to-female ratios increase with age: French nationwide study and meta-analysis. J Neurol Neurosurg Psychiatry. 2016;87(9):952-7.
5. Spillantini MG, Schmidt ML, Lee VM, Trojanowski JQ, Jakes R, Goedert M. Alpha-synuclein in Lewy bodies. Nature. 1997;388(6645):839-40.
6. Cheng HC, Ulane CM, Burke RE. Clinical progression in Parkinson disease and the neurobiology of axons. Ann Neurol. 2010;67(6):715-25.
7. Hirsch EC, Jenner P, Przedborski S. Pathogenesis of Parkinson's disease. Mov Disord. 2013;28(1):24-30.
8. Piccini P, Burn DJ, Ceravolo R, Maraganore D, Brooks DJ. The role of inheritance in sporadic Parkinson's disease: evidence from a longitudinal study of dopaminergic function in twins. Ann Neurol. 1999;45(5):577-82.
9. Wirdefeldt K, Gatz M, Reynolds CA, Prescott CA, Pedersen NL. Heritability of Parkinson disease in Swedish twins: a longitudinal study. Neurobiol Aging. 2011;32(10):1923.e1-8.
10. Zhu M, Zhao S. Candidate gene identification approach: progress and challenges. Int J Biol Sci. 2007;3(7):420-7.
11. Keller MF, Saad M, Bras J, Bettella F, Nicolaou N, Simon-Sanchez J, et al. Using genome-wide complex trait analysis to quantify 'missing heritability' in Parkinson's disease. Hum Mol Genet. 2012;21(22):4996-5009.
12. Metzker ML. Sequencing technologies—the next generation. Nat Rev Genet. 2010;11(1):31-46.
13. Gilissen C, Hoischen A, Brunner HG, Veltman JA. Disease gene identification strategies for exome sequencing. Eur J Hum Genet. 2012;20(5):490-7.
14. Polymeropoulos MH, Higgins JJ, Golbe LI, Johnson WG, Ide SE, Di Iorio G, et al. Mapping of a gene for Parkinson's disease to chromosome 4q21-q23. Science. 1996;274(5290):1197-9.
15. Olanow CW, Brundin P. Parkinson's disease and alpha synuclein: is Parkinson's disease a prion-like disorder? Mov Disord. 2013;28(1):31-40.
16. Polymeropoulos MH, Lavedan C, Leroy E, Ide SE, Dehejia A, Dutra A, et al. Mutation in the α-synuclein gene identified in families with Parkinson's disease. Science. 1997;276(5321):2045-7.
17. Hoffman-Zacharska D, Koziorowski D, Ross OA, Milewski M, Poznanski JA, Jurek M, et al. Novel A18T and pA29S substitutions in α-synuclein may be associated with sporadic Parkinson's disease. Parkinsonism Relat Disord. 2013;19(11):1057-60.
18. Chartier-Harlin MC, Kachergus J, Roumier C, Mouroux V, Douay X, Lincoln S, et al. α-synuclein locus duplication as a cause of familial Parkinson's disease. Lancet. 2004;364(9440):1167-9.
19. Tan EK, Tan C, Shen H, Chai A, Lum SY, Teoh ML, et al. Alpha synuclein promoter and risk of Parkinson's disease: microsatellite and allelic size variability. Neurosci Lett. 2003;336(1):70-2.
20. Kiely AP, Asi YT, Kara E, Limousin P, Ling H, Lewis P, et al. Alpha-Synucleinopathy associated with G51D SNCA mutation: a link between Parkinson's disease and multiple system atrophy? Acta Neuropathol. 2013;125(5):753-69.
21. Sironi F, Trotta L, Antonini A, Zini M, Ciccone R, Della Mina E, et al. Alpha-Synuclein multiplication analysis in Italian familial Parkinson disease. Parkinsonism Relat Disord. 2010;16(3): 228-31.
22. Bosgraaf L, Van Haastert PJ. Roc, a Ras/GTPase domain in complex proteins. Biochim Biophys Acta. 2003;1643(1–3):5-10.
23. Funayama M, Hasegawa K, Kowa H, Saito M, Tsuji S, Obata F. A new locus for Parkinson's disease (PARK8) maps to chromosome 12p11.2-q13.1. Ann Neurol. 2002;51(3):296-301.
24. Wszolek ZK, Pfeiffer RF, Tsuboi Y, Uitti RJ, McComb RD, Stoessl AJ, et al. Autosomal dominant parkinsonism associated with variable synuclein and tau pathology. Neurology. 2004;62(9):1619-22.
25. Zimprich A, Biskup S, Leitner P, Lichtner P, Farrer M, Lincoln S, et al. Mutations in LRRK2 cause autosomal-dominant parkinsonism with pleomorphic pathology. Neuron. 2004;44(4):601-7.
26. Ross OA, Soto-Ortolaza AI, Heckman MG, Aasly JO, Abahuni N, Annesi G, et al. Association of LRRK2 exonic variants with susceptibility to Parkinson's disease: a case-control study. Lancet Neurol. 2011;10(10):898-908.
27. Healy DG, Falchi M, O'Sullivan SS, Bonifati V, Durr A, Bressman S, et al. Phenotype, genotype, and worldwide genetic penetrance of LRRK2-associated Parkinson's disease: a case-control study. Lancet Neurol. 2008;7(7):583-90.
28. Smith WW, Pei Z, Jiang H, Dawson VL, Dawson TM, Ross CA. Kinase activity of mutant LRRK2 mediates neuronal toxicity. Nat Neurosci. 2006;9(10):1231-3.
29. Lee BD, Shin JH, VanKampen J, Petrucelli L, West AB, Ko HS, et al. Inhibitors of leucine-rich repeat kinase-2 protect against models of Parkinson's disease. Nat Med. 2010;16(9):998-1000.
30. Vilarino-Güell C, Wider C, Ross OA, Dachsel JC, Kachergus JM, Lincoln SJ, et al. VPS35 mutations in Parkinson disease. Am J Hum Genet. 2011;89(1):162-7.
31. Zimprich A, Benet-Pages A, Struhal W, Graf E, Eck SH, Offman MN, et al. A mutation in VPS35, encoding a subunit of the retromer complex, causes late-onset Parkinson disease. Am J Hum Genet. 2011;89(1):168-75.
32. Trinh J, Farrer M. Advances in the genetics of Parkinson disease. Nat Rev Neurol. 2013;9(8):445-54.
33. Deng H, Wu Y, Jankovic J. The EIF4G1 gene and Parkinson's disease. Acta Neurol Scand. 2015;132(2):73-8.
34. Chartier-Harlin MC, Dachsel JC, Vilarino-Guell C, Lincoln SJ, Lepretre F, Hulihan MM, et al. Translation initiator EIF4G1 mutations in familial Parkinson disease. Am J Hum Genet. 2011;89:398-406.
35. Sidransky E, Nalls MA, Aasly JO, Aharon-Peretz J, Annesi G, Barbosa ER, et al. Multicenter analysis of glucocerebrosidase mutations in Parkinson's disease. N Engl J Med. 2009;361(17):1651-61.
36. Winder-Rhodes SE, Evans JR, Ban M, Mason SL, Williams-Gray CH, Foltynie T, et al. Glucocerebrosidase mutations influence the natural history of Parkinson's disease in a community-based incident cohort. Brain. 2013;136(Pt 2):392-9.

37. Lopez G, Kim J, Wiggs E, Cintron D, Groden C, Tayebi N, et al. Clinical course and prognosis in patients with Gaucher disease and parkinsonism. Neurol Genet. 2016;2(2):e57.
38. Mata IF, Leverenz JB, Weintraub D, Trojanowski JQ, Chen-Plotkin A, Van Deerlin VM, et al. GBA variants are associated with a distinct pattern of cognitive deficits in Parkinson's disease. Mov Disord. 2016;31(1):95-102.
39. Cilia R, Tunesi S, Marotta G, Cereda E, Siri C, Tesei S, et al. Survival and dementia in GBA-associated Parkinson's disease: the mutation matters. Ann Neurol. 2016;80(5):662-73.
40. Sudhaman S, Muthane UB, Behari M, Govindappa ST, Juyal RC, Thelma BK. Evidence of mutations in RIC3 acetylcholine receptor chaperone as a novel cause of autosomal-dominant Parkinson's disease with non-motor phenotypes. J Med Genet. 2016;53(8):559-66.
41. Kitada T, Asakawa S, Hattori N, Matsumine H, Yamamura Y, Minoshima S, et al. Mutations in the parkin gene cause autosomal recessive juvenile parkinsonism. Nature. 1998;392(6676):605-8.
42. Valente EM, Abou-Sleiman PM, Caputo V, Muqit MMK, Harvey K, Gispert S, et al. Hereditary early-onset Parkinson's disease caused by mutations in PINK1. Science. 2004;304(5674):1158-60.
43. Bonifati V, Rizzu P, van Baren MJ, Schaap O, Breedveld GJ, Krieger E, et al. Mutations in the DJ-1 gene associated with autosomal recessive early-onset parkinsonism. Science. 2003;299(5604):256-9.
44. Kilarski LL, Pearson JP, Newsway V, Majounie E, Knipe MDW, Misbahuddin A, et al. Systematic review and UK-based study of PARK2 (parkin), PINK1, PARK7 (DJ-1) and LRRK2 in early-onset Parkinson's disease. Mov Disord. 2012;27(12):1522-9.
45. Lucking CB, Durr A, Bonifati V, Vaughan J, De Michele G, Gasser T, et al. Association between early-onset Parkinson's disease and mutations in the parkin gene. N Engl J Med. 2000;342(21):1560-7.
46. Klein C, Lohmann-Hedrich K. Impact of recent genetic findings in Parkinson's disease. Curr Opin Neurol. 2007;20(4):453-64.
47. Cazeneuve C, San C, Ibrahim SA, Mukhtar MM, Kheir MM, Leguern E, et al. A new complex homozygous large rearrangement of the PINK1 gene in a Sudanese family with early onset Parkinson's disease. Neurogenetics. 2009;10(3):265-70.
48. Camargos ST, Dornas LO, Momeni P, Lees A, Hardy J, Singleton A, et al. Familial Parkinsonism and early onset Parkinson's disease in a Brazilian movement disorders clinic: Phenotypic characterization and frequency of *SNCA, PRKN, PINK1*, and *LRRK2* mutations. Mov Disord. 2009;24(5):662-6.
49. Marongiu R, Brancati F, Antonini A, Ialongo T, Ceccarini C, Scarciolla O, et al. Whole gene deletion and splicing mutations expand the PINK1 genotypic spectrum. Hum Mutat. 2007;28(1):98.
50. Youle RJ, Narendra DP. Mechanisms of mitophagy. Nat Rev Mol Cell Biol. 2011;12(1):9-14.
51. Pankratz N, Pauciulo MW, Elsaesser VE, Marek DK, Halter CA, Wojcieszek J, et al. Mutations in DJ-1 are rare in familial Parkinson disease. Neurosci Lett. 2006;408(3):209-13.
52. Junn E, Taniguchi H, Jeong BS, Zhao X, Ichijo H, Mouradian MM. Interaction of DJ-1 with Daxx inhibits apoptosis signal-regulating kinase 1 activity and cell death. Proc Natl Acad Sci USA. 2005;102(27):9691-6.
53. Kim RH, Smith PD, Aleyasin H, Hayley S, Mount MP, Pownall S, et al. Hypersensitivity of DJ-1-deficient mice to 1-methyl-4-phenyl-1,2,3,6-tetrahydropyrindine (MPTP) and oxidative stress. Proc Natl Acad Sci USA. 2005;102(14);5215-20.
54. Olgiati S, Quadri M, Fang M, Rood JPMA, Saute JA, Chien HF, et al. DNAJC6 mutations associated with early-onset Parkinson's disease. Ann Neurol. 2016;79(2):244-56.
55. Elsayed LEO, Drouet V, Usenko T, Mohammed IN, Hamed AAA, Elseed MA, et al. A novel nonsense mutation in DNAJC6 expands the phenotype of autosomal-recessive juvenile-onset Parkinson's disease. Ann Neurol. 2016;79(2):335-7.
56. Eisenberg E, Greene LE. Multiple roles of auxilin and hsc70 in clathrin-mediated endocytosis. Traffic. 2007;8(6):640-6.
57. Bras J, Verloes A, Schneider SA, Mole SE, Guerreiro RJ. Mutation of the parkinsonism gene ATP13A2 causes neuronal ceroid-lipofuscinosis. Hum Mol Genet. 2012;21(12):2646-50.
58. Paisan-Ruiz C, Li A, Schneider SA, Holton JL, Johnson R, Kidd D, et al. Widespread Lewy body and tau accumulation in childhood and adult onset dystonia-parkinsonism cases with PLA2G6 mutations. Neurobiol Aging. 2012;33(4):814-23.
59. Zhao T, Severijnen LA, van der Weiden M, Zheng PP, Oostra BA, Hukema RK, et al. FBXO7 immunoreactivity in alpha-synuclein-containing inclusions in Parkinson disease and multiple system atrophy. J Neuropathol Exp Neurol. 2013;72(6):482-8.
60. Krebs CE, Karkheiran S, Powell JC, Cao M, Makarov V, Darvish H, et al. The Sac1 domain of SYNJ1 identified mutated in a family with early-onset progressive parkinsonism with generalized seizures. Hum Mutat. 2013;34(9):1200-7.
61. Quadri M, Fang M, Picillo M, Olgiati S, Breedveld GJ, Graafland J, et al. Mutation in the SYNJ1 gene associated with autosomal recessive, early-onset parkinsonism. Hum Mutat. 2013;34(9):1208-15.
62. Stefansson H, Helgason A, Thorleifsson G, Steinthorsdottir V, Masson G, Barnard J, et al. A common inversion under selection in Europeans. Nat Genet. 2005;37(2):129-37.
63. Martin ER, Scott WK, Nance MA, Watts RL, Hubble JP, Koller WC, et al. Association of single-nucleotide polymorphisms of the tau gene with late-onset Parkinson disease. JAMA. 2001;286(18):2245-50.
64. Lill CM, Roehr JT, McQueen MB, Kavvoura FK, Bagade S, Schjeide BMM, et al. Comprehensive research synopsis and systematic meta-analyses in Parkinson's disease genetics: the PD Gene database. PLoS Genet. 2012;8(3):e1002548.
65. Satake W, Nakabayashi Y, Mizuta I, Hirota Y, Ito C, Kubo M, et al. Genome-wide association study identifies common variants at four loci as genetic risk factors for Parkinson's disease. Nat Genet. 2009;41(12):1303-7.
66. Hamza TH, Chen H, Hill-Burns EM, Rhodes SL, Montimurro J, Kay DM, et al. Genome-wide gene-environment study identifies glutamate receptor gene GRIN2A as a Parkinson's disease modifier gene via interaction with coffee. PLoS Genet. 2011;7(8):e1002237.
67. Ahmed I, Lee PC, Lill CM, Nielsen SS, Artaud F, Gallagher LG, et al. Lack of replication of the GRIN2A-by-coffee interaction in Parkinson disease. PLoS Genet. 2014;10(11):e1004788.
68. Hill-Burns EM, Singh N, Ganguly P, Hamza TM, Montimurro J, Kay DM, et al. A genetic basis for the variable effect of smoking/nicotine on Parkinson's disease. Pharmacogenomics J. 2013;13(6):530-7.
69. Behari M, Srivastava AK, Das RR, Pandey RM. Risk factors of Parkinson's disease in Indian patients. J Neurol Sci. 2001;190(1-2):49-55.
70. Punia S, Behari M, Govindappa ST, Swaminath PV, Jayaram S, Goyal V, et al. Absence/rarity of commonly reported LRRK2 mutations in Indian Parkinson's disease patients. Neurosci Lett. 2006;409(2):83-8.

CHAPTER 6

Signs and Symptoms of Parkinson's Disease

JS Katpal, Monika Porwal (Bagul)

INTRODUCTION

Parkinsonism is a syndrome manifested by a combination of six cardinal features: Tremor-at-rest, rigidity, bradykinesia, loss of postural reflexes, flexed posture, and freezing (motor blocks).[1] Combination of these signs is used to define definite, probable, and possible Parkinsonism. Most common form is idiopathic Parkinson disease (PD), first recognized by James Parkinson in 1817, previously referred to as "paralysis agitans", Charcot later in 19th century referred it as "maladie de Parkinson".[2] It was not until 100 years after Parkinson's landmark paper that the loss of dopamine-containing cells in the substantia nigra (SN) was recognized.[2,3]

CLINICAL FEATURES

Clinically, PD is heterogeneous and its phenomenology is well recognized, consisting of prodromal phase which is characterized by nonspecific findings such as mood disorder, frequent medical consultations, increased frequency of various pains, shoulder pain, generalized body ache, and stiffness or limb paresthesias, fibromyalgia, constipation, sleeplessness, and reduction in volume of voice.[4] More specific complaints included problems with fine motor skills, decreased sense of smell, loss of appetite, tremor occurring with anxiety, and reduced arm swing on the affected side, decreased emotional expression, and personality changes including introversion and inflexibility.[5] Up to 46% PD patients had characteristic asymmetric presentation that correlated with handedness.[6] In some cases, Parkinsonism may remain confined to one side and may be associated with hemiatrophy. Mean age at onset for hemiparkinsonism-hemiatrophy was 44.2 (15–63) years with mean duration 9.7 (2–20) years with dystonia present in 21 (70%) PD patients.[7]

Further clinical subtypes of PD include: (1) Younger age of onset with slow progression of disease, (2) Older age of onset with rapid progression of disease, (3) Tremor-predominant, and (4) Postural instability and gait difficulty (PIGD) dominated by rigidity and bradykinesia.[2] Patients presenting with axial predominant symptoms such as dysphagia, dysarthria, freezing of gait, and loss of equilibrium carry poor prognosis and also lack response to dopaminergic drugs (**Fig. 1**).[8] The "ten steps" test (abnormal tandem gait) has 82% sensitivity and 92% specificity for patients with atypical Parkinsonism than in typical PD patients.[9]

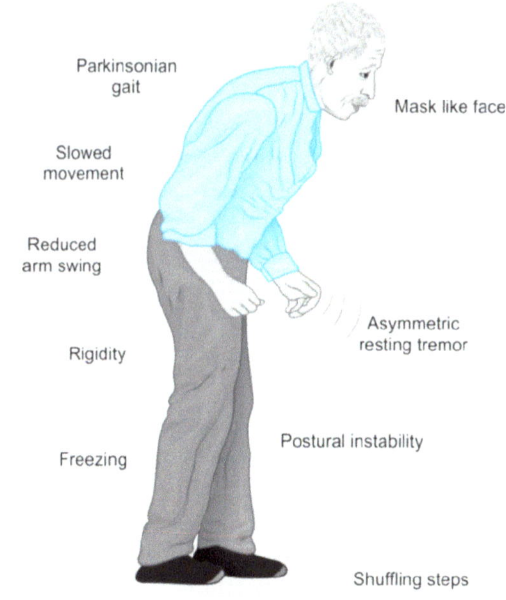

FIG. 1: Clinical features of Parkinson disease.

BRADYKINESIA

It is the most characteristic clinical hallmark of PD, manifested by slowness in activities of daily living, slow rapid alternating and fine motor movements, and slow reaction times.[2] Other manifestations include drooling due to failure to swallow saliva, monotonic, and hypophonic dysarthria, loss of facial expression (hypomimia), and reduced arm swing when walking (loss of automatic movement).[2] Micrographia due to reduced motor output or weakness of agonist force coupled with distortions in visual feedback. Bradyphrenia refers to slowness of thought.[10] Pathophysiology of bradykinesia is unclear, but it is thought to result from failure of basal ganglia output circuits to reinforce cortical mechanisms that execute and prepare commands to move.[11] With sudden emotional surge, immobile patient may make fast movements or even catch a ball, this phenomenon is known as kinesia paradoxa which indicates that PD patients have difficulty in accessing intact motor programs without using any external trigger.[12] The Bereitschafts potential [premovement electroencephalographic (EEG) potential] is reduced in PD patients which indirectly reflects inadequate activation of supplementary motor area by basal ganglia.[13] Positron emission tomography (PET) scans demonstrated decreased 18F-fluorodeoxyglucose uptake in striatum and accumbens-caudate complex which is proportional to the degree of bradykinesia in PD patients.[14]

TREMOR

Rest tremor is the most typical sign of PD with frequency between 4–6 Hz, almost always most prominent in distal part of an extremity, such hand tremors called as "pill-rolling tremors", often exacerbated during walking and counting backward.[15] Head tremors involving lips, chin, and jaw are a common manifestation of essential tremors (ETs) and is rare in PD.[16] Some PD patients complain of "inner tremor", which is internal and nonvisible tremor. Tremors as initial presenting symptom of PD confer a favorable prognosis with slow disease progression and therefore termed as "benign tremulous Parkinsonism", having family history of tremor and poor response to levodopa.[15]

Second type of tremor is postural tremor, which may be the initial presentation of PD and is more prominent and disabling than rest tremor.[16] Postural tremors without Parkinsonism or other etiologies are known as ET and both can be differentiated when arms assume an outstretched horizontal position, postural tremor of ET usually appears immediately while in PD there is delay in onset of tremor with latency of few seconds to minute, and re-emerges during postural holding termed as re-emergent tremor.[17]

Third type of tremor is kinetic tremor, an enhanced physiologic tremor that impairs normal reach-to-grasp movement.[18] Pallidum plays a fundamental role in generation of rest tremor of PD. It has a complicated pathophysiology which results from dysfunction of both circuits that is striato-pallidal-thalamo-cortical and cerebello-dentato-thalamo-cortical.

Another form of PD-associated tremor occurs due to abnormal neuronal activity at globus pallidus internus (GPi) leads to muscle discharges that can be auscultated with a stethoscope.[19]

RIGIDITY AND FLEXED POSTURE

Rigidity, tested by passively flexing, extending, and rotating the body part, is manifested by increased resistance throughout the range of movement.[1,20] Cog wheeling is often encountered, if there is associated tremor.[20] Rigidity may be present proximally (e.g., neck, shoulders, and hips) and distally (e.g., wrists and ankles). Painful shoulder, due to rigidity, is one of the frequent initial manifestations of PD often misdiagnosed as arthritis, bursitis, or rotator cuff injury.[20] Increased resistance to passive movement of a limb about a joint during voluntary movement of a contralateral limb is termed as "Froment's maneuver".[1,20]

Flexed neck and trunk with flexed elbows and knees occur later in the disease are commonly seen in PD patients. "Striatal hand" deformity is characterized by ulnar deviation of hands, flexion at metacarpophalangeal joints, and extension at interphalangeal joints, and there may be extension of the big toe (striatal toe) or flexion of the other toes, seen in some of the PD patients.[21] Other abnormalities include extreme neck flexion (dropped head/head ptosis/anterocollis/bent spine), scoliosis, and trunk tilting, referred to as "Pisa syndrome" and truncal flexion (camptocormia).[21] Extreme flexion of thoracolumbar spine that increases during walking and resolves in supine position termed as camptocormia is more common with severe PD.[22]

LOSS OF POSTURAL REFLEXES

Loss of postural reflexes, a characteristic feature in PD patients, usually occurs in more advanced stages of the disease along with freezing of gait and worsens with worsening disease severity.[23] Festination is seen in many PD patients is manifested by faster walking as if chasing their center of gravity and tends to collapse into the chair when attempt to sit.[24] When performing complex motor and cognitive tasks concurrently, PD patients tend to sacrifice motor performance to complete tasks and therefore, make more errors. Measures contributing to falls in PD patients include frontal impairment, poor balance, and leg weakness.[24] Female gender, symmetrical onset, postural, and autonomic instability appear to be the most frequent predictors of falls in PD.[2] Measures for predicting falls with best sensitivity (78%) and specificity (84%) are: Unified

Parkinson's Disease Rating Scale (UPDRS) score,[25] freezing of gait score,[23] symptomatic postural orthostasis, Tinetti score,[26] and extent of postural sway in anterior-posterior direction.

Cholinergic hypofunction related to pedunculopontine nucleus (PPN) degeneration rather than dopaminergic degeneration have been implicated in disturbed balance and falls associated with PD. Subcortical cholinergic activity was significantly more decreased in multiple system atrophy-Parkinsonian (MSA-P) and progressive supranuclear palsy (PSP) than in PD.[24]

FREEZING

Freezing, also referred as motor blocks, one of the most disabling symptom of PD patients, consists of start hesitation when they initiate to walk and sudden transient inability to move feet (as if glued to the ground), sometimes considered as akinesia (loss of movement).[24] Mostly, it affects legs but can also involve upper limbs and eyelids (apraxia of eyelid opening or closure).[27] It is the most common cause of falls in PD patients that can result in injuries. Mostly, it is noticed when they turn or walk through narrow passages (such as doors or elevator) or while street crossing with heavy traffic, or when approaching a destination (target hesitation).[28] Patients adopt various cues or tricks to overcome these freezing attacks: Marching on to commands (left, right, left, right), stepping over objects like a pavement stone, cracks on the floor, end of a walking stick, etc., walk to music, shift body weight, rocking movements, etc.[24] It may occur during "off" phenomenon but may also occur during "on" time termed as "on freezing", independent of bradykinesia, and tremor.[29] Freezing occurs frequently in men and less frequent in patients presenting with tremor.[24] If freezing occurs early in the disease course, alternative diagnosis should be considered as in PSP, MSA, and vascular (lower body) Parkinsonism.[30,31] Pathophysiology of freezing involves noradrenergic deficiency due to locus coeruleus degeneration. Moreover, treatment whether medical or surgical, generally do not provide satisfactory control of freezing (**Table 1**).[28]

OTHER MOTOR ABNORMALITIES

Re-emergence of primitive reflexes is attributed to breakdown of frontal lobe inhibitory mechanisms normally presents in infancy and early childhood, hence, termed release signs.[32] Glabellar tap reflex or Myerson sign, elicited through repeated stimuli to glabellar region of forehead, inducing concomitant blinking with each tap.[33] Other "frontal" and "cortical disinhibition" signs such as applause sign is not specific for PD.[33] Bulbar symptoms (dysarthria, hypophonia, dysphagia, and sialorrhea) result from orofacial-laryngeal bradykinesia and rigidity.[34] Respiratory difficulties occur d/t rigid respiratory muscles and levodopa-induced respiratory dyskinesias. Hypokinetic dysarthria seen in PD patients

TABLE 1: Stages of Parkinson disease.

	Early PD		*Mild-stage PD*	*Advanced PD*	
Stages of Parkinson's disease (PD)	*1*	*2*	*3*	*4*	*5*
Severity of symptoms	**Mild**	**Mild**	**Moderate**	**Severe**	**Severe**
	Symptoms of PD are mild and only seen on one side of the body (unilateral involvement)	Symptoms of PD on both sides of the body (bilateral involvement) or at the midline	Symptoms of PD are characterized by loss of balance and slowness of movement	Symptoms of PD are severely disabling	Symptoms of PD are severe and are characterized by an inability to rise
	Symptoms	**Symptoms**	**Symptoms**	**Symptoms**	**Symptoms**
	• Tremor of one hand • Rigidity • Clumsy leg • One side of the face may be affected, impacting the expression	• Loss of facial expression on both sides • Decreased blinking • Speech abnormalities • Rigidity of the muscles in the trunk	• Balance is compromised • Inability to make the rapid, automatic, and involuntary adjustments • All other symptoms of PD are present	• Patients may be able to walk and stand unassisted, but they are noticeably incapacitated • Patient is unable to live an independent life and needs assistance	• Patients fall when standing or turning • May freeze or stumble when walking • Hallucinations or delusions

is characterized by low volume (hypophonia), uniform pitch (aprosody) and loudness (monotonicity), short speech rush (tachyphemia), imprecise consonants, and hesitation.[4] Childhood stuttering that had remitted can recur with onset of PD.[4] Patients with parkin mutations (*PARK2*) tend to develop levodopa-induced dyskinesias, hallucinations, dopa-responsive dystonia, dystonic gait, cervical dystonia, hemiparkinsonism-hemiatrophy, festination, freezing, retropulsion, rest leg tremor, orthostatic tremor on standing, marked sleep benefit, ataxia, peripheral neuropathy, hyper-reflexia, and dysautonomia.[35]

NONMOTOR MANIFESTATIONS

Nonmotor nondopaminergic symptoms of PD occur in 88% of all patients, seriously impact quality of life, particularly in advanced stages of disease.[36] Other problems included excessive daytime sleepiness, falls, freezing, fractures, postural hypotension, urinary incontinence, dysarthria, choking, and hallucinations.[37] Clinical-pathologic correlations suggested three groups of patients: (1) Younger-onset typical PD; brainstem Lewy bodies predominate; (2) Older-onset PD with shorter survival and higher Lewy body loads; and (3) Early malignant, dementia-dominant with severe neocortical disease, consistent with dementia with Lewy bodies (DLB).[38]

AUTONOMIC DYSFUNCTION

Autonomic dysfunction such as orthostatic hypotension, sphincter dysfunction, sweating dysfunction, and sexual impotence occurs frequently in PD but is typically presenting feature of MSA.[39] Dysautonomia is predominantly peripheral (ganglionic and postganglionic) in PD, while in MSA lesion is primarily preganglionic.[39] Axial hyperhidrosis occurs as a compensatory phenomenon for reduced sympathetic function of extremities. Such symptoms occurred frequently during "off" periods and during "on with dyskinesia" periods. Presence of α-synuclein deposits in dermis is associated with autonomic failure usually viewed as variant synucleinopathies.[1,4] Bladder symptoms are frequent in PD patients and require constant medical attention. Hypersexuality is also related to dopaminergic drugs. Aging, female gender, lower education, and depression were significantly associated with decreased sexual desire.[40] Drooling (sialorrhea), the most embarrassing symptom of PD, is due to a difficulty with swallowing. Dysphagia along with delayed gastric emptying and constipation represents the most frequent gastrointestinal manifestations of PD. Impaired coordination of breathing and swallowing may contribute to aspiration pneumonia in PD. Seborrhea, hair loss, and leg edema represent peripheral involvement in PD.[41]

COGNITIVE AND NEUROBEHAVIORAL ABNORMALITIES

Cognitive deficits affecting attention, episodic memory, fluency, psychomotor function, executive, and visuospatial functions have been found in 30% early PD patients.[42] Neurobehavioral abnormalities such as depression, dementia, word-finding difficulties, and tip-of-the-tongue phenomenon are usually late features of PD.[43] Thinking, verbal functions, and reasoning are relatively spared in PD patients.[43] Death, suicidal ideation, and anhedonia are other frequent symptoms of PD.[43] Abulia, catatonia, waxy flexibility, akinetic mutism, refusal to eat or drink, staring, grimacing, echo phenomenon, stereotypy, rigidity, posturing, and severe apathy have been recognized in PD.[42]

SCOPA-COG (Scales for Outcomes of Parkinson's Disease-Cognition) Scale is used to assess "frontal-subcortical" cognitive defects in PD patients while PD-Cognitive Rating Scale (PD-CRS) assesses "instrumental-cortical" functions.[44] PD patients have limited perception of large spatial configurations that is seeing trees for the forest.[1] Because of ceiling effect, Mini-Mental State Examination (MMSE) fails to detect early cognitive decline, therefore, Montreal Cognitive Assessment (MoCA) has been developed to detect it.[45]

Psychosis in PD is characterized by paranoid delusions, visual hallucination, illusions, and false sense of presence in contrast to auditory hallucinations and thought disorder typically seen in patients with schizophrenia.[46] It is frequently associated with depression, anxiety, apathy, and dementia.[42] Risk factors for hallucinations include older age, duration of illness, depression, cognitive disorder, daytime somnolence, poor visual acuity, family history of dementia, and dopaminergic drugs.[47]

About "premorbid Parkinsonian personality", suggests that since childhood, PD patients tend to be more introverted, cautious, socially alert, tense, nervous, and rigid. Since, dopamine is involved in reward system, slight deficiency may predispose some individuals to exhibit a "nonsmoking personality", and a tendency to be "honest".[48]

Types of obsessive-compulsive disorder in PD include: (1) Order and symmetry; (2) washing and cleaning; (3) repeated checking, religious, sexual obsessions, and (4) punding.[49] Punding is characterized by intense fascination with repetitive handling, examining, sorting, and arranging of objects, inordinate writing, doodling, painting, collecting things, shuffling through personal papers, journaling/blogging, and internet play, excessive cleaning or gardening or sorting household objects, humming or singing, and reciting long, meaningless soliloquies without an audience.[50] Hedonistic homeostatic dysregulation is seen in males with young-onset or early-onset PD (YOPD) presenting as cyclic mood disorder with hypomania or manic psychosis.[51] Dopamine dysregulation syndrome includes compulsive dopaminergic replacement, compulsive foraging, euphoria, dysphoria, phobias, hypersexuality, pathologic gambling, compulsive shopping, aggression, craving, binge eating, insulting gestures, paranoia, jealousy, impulsivity, and other behaviors.[52] Dopaminergic drugs have been demonstrated to precipitate or exacerbate behavioral symptoms which improves with reduction of dose of dopamine agonists.[53]

SLEEP DISORDERS

Sleep disorders are being increasingly recognized as a feature of PD.[54] A 15 questionnaire instrument for assessing sleep and nocturnal disability has been described while most studies attribute excessive daytime drowsiness and irresistible sleep attacks to anti-PD medications while some authors believe that sleep disturbances are an integral part of PD.[55] Increasing the night-time sleep with antidepressants or benzodiazepines may not alleviate daytime drowsiness.[56] Mechanism of restless legs syndrome in PD patients involves degeneration of diencephalospinal dopaminergic pathway.[57] Rapid eye movement (REM) sleep behavior disorder (RBD) is considered as a preparkinsonian state and predictor of dysautonomia mainly orthostatic hypotension.[58] RBD Screening Questionnaire (RBDSQ) is a sensitive instrument to capture most characteristics of RBD. It is often exacerbated by dopaminergic therapy. PD patients with RBD are less likely to have tremors, higher frequency of falls, and are less responsive to medications.[59]

In PD patients with RBD, sleep walking has also been demonstrated, vice versa individuals with RBD have increased risk of developing Parkinsonism. Since, loss of dopamine in PD generally progresses from putamen to caudate and eventually to limbic areas which is responsible for excessive daytime sleepiness and sleep-onset REM in PD.[60]

SENSORY ABNORMALITIES

Sensory complaints such as paresthesias, akathisia, and orogenital pains are frequently observed in PD patient. Impaired olfaction occurs typically in 90% of PD and Alzheimer disease patients.[61] Hyposmia, dysautonomia, and sleep disorder may predate other clinical symptoms of PD by at least 4 years and associated with 10% increased risk of developing PD.[62] All hyposmic individuals developing PD had an abnormal reduced baseline 2 betacarboxymethoxy-3-beta-(4[^{123}I] iodophenyl) tropane (β-CIT) single-photon emission computed tomography (SPECT) scan.[63] Two-step approach using olfactory testing followed by dopamine transporter (DAT) SPECT scanning in hyposmic individuals appears to have a high sensitivity and specificity in detecting PD. Hyposmia is usually not present in ET, PSP, corticobasal degeneration, vascular Parkinsonism, or Parkinsonism due to *parkin* and *DJ1* mutation.[63] Some PD patients experience impaired color discrimination, contrast sensitivity, visual speed, visual construction, and visual memory while sparing visual acuity.[60,61] Other features include: Decreased blink rate, visual hallucinations, blepharospasm, and decreased convergence. Many PD patients also experience dyspnea, facial flushing, hunger (sweet cravings), and weight loss.[1]

CLINICAL RATING SCALES AND OTHER ASSESSMENTS

Most commonly used clinical rating scales are UPDRS, Hoehn-Yahr Staging Scale, and Schwab-England Scale of activities of daily living.[64] Two short, and reliable scales that can be used for research and practice are: The Short (0–3) Parkinson's Evaluation Scale (SPES) and the SCOPA.[65] New MDS-UPDRS has been modified to integrate nonmotor and motor elements that is—(1) nonmotor experiences of daily living; (2) motor experiences of daily living; (3) motor examination; (4) motor complications, along with the original UPDRS structure of four parts with a total summed score. All items have five responses with uniform anchors of 0 = normal, 1 = slight, 2 = mild, 3 = moderate, 4 = severe.[66]

In standard pull test, a sudden, quick, and firm shoulder pull is done from back without warning but with prior explanation (executed only once) and if patient takes >2 steps backward, it is considered abnormal.[67] In push and release test, patients are instructed to stand and keep their eyes open and examiner stands behind them. Now, patient is instructed to push backward against palms of examiner's hands placed on patient's scapulae while examiner flexes his elbows so as to allow slight backward movement of trunk and then examiner suddenly removes his hands, so that patient can take a backward step to regain balance.[67]

CONCLUSION

To conclude Parkinson disease is a neurodegenerative disorder and as the condition progresses, the symptoms get worse and it can affect activities of daily living. Having detailed knowledge about signs and symptoms of disease can help in early diagnosis which can lead to slow progression and reduce mortality and morbidity,

Thus patients can have a normal or near-normal life expectancy.

REFERENCES

1. Jankovic J, Lang AE. Movement disorders: Diagnosis and assessment. In Bradley WG, Daroff RB, Fenichel GM, Jankovic J (eds). Neurology in clinical practice, 5th edition. Philadelphia: Butterworth-Heinemann (Elsevier); 2008. pp. 293-322.
2. Parkinson J. An Essay on the Shaking Palsy. London: Sherwood, Neely and Jones; 1817.
3. Parkinson Study Group: Mortality in DATATOP: A multicenter trial in early Parkinson's disease. Ann Neurol 1998;43(3):318-25.
4. Jankovic J. Pathophysiology and clinical assessment of parkinsonian symptoms and signs. In Pahwa R, Lyons K, Koller WC (eds). Handbook of Parkinson's Disease. New York: Marcel Dekker; 2003. pp. 71-107.
5. Jankovic J, Rajput AH, McDermott MP, Perl DP. The evolution of diagnosis in early Parkinson disease. Arch Neurol. 2000;57: 369-72.
6. Uitti RJ, Baba Y, Whaley NR, Wszolek ZK, Putzke JD. Parkinson disease: Handedness predicts asymmetry. Neurology. 2005;64:1925-30.
7. Jankovic J, Tintner R. Dystonia and parkinsonism. Parkinsonism Relat Disord. 2001;8:109-21.
8. Suchowersky O, Reich S, Perlmutter J, Zesiewicz T, Gronseth G, Weiner WJ. Practice Parameter: Diagnosis and prognosis of new onset Parkinson disease (an evidence-based review): Report of the Quality Standards Subcommittee of the American Academy of Neurology. Neurology. 2006;66(7):968-75.
9. Abdo WF, Borm GF, Munneke M, Verbeek MM, Esselink RA, Bloem BR. Ten steps to identify atypical parkinsonism. J Neurol Neurosurg Psychiatry. 2006;77(12):1367-9.
10. Giovannoni G, Van Schalkwyk J, Fritz VU, Lees A. Bradykinesia akinesia incoordination test (BRAIN TEST): An objective computerized assessment of upper limb motor function. J Neurol Neurosurg Psychiatry. 1999;67:624-9.
11. Berardelli A, Rothwell JC, Thompson PD, Hallett M. Pathophysiology of bradykinesia in Parkinson's disease. Brain. 2001;124:2131-46.
12. Williams DR, Watt HC, Lees AJ. Predictors of falls and fractures in bradykinetic rigid syndromes: A retrospective study. J Neurol Neurosurg Psychiatry. 2006;77:468-73.
13. Dick JP, Rothwell JC, Day BL, Cantello R, Buruma O, Gioux M, et al. The Bereitschaftspotential is abnormal in Parkinson's disease. Brain. 1989;112(1):233-44.
14. Whone AL, Brefel-Courbon C, Moore RY, Rascol O, Brooks DJ. Tremor at diagnosis is predictive of slower disease progression in Parkinson's disease: An ^{18}F dopa PET study. Mov Disord. 2002;17(suppl 5):S140-1.
15. Antonini A, Moeller JR, Nakamura T, Spetsieris P, Dhawan V, Eidelberg D. The metabolic anatomy of tremor in Parkinson's disease. Neurology. 1998;51:803-10.
16. Jankovic J. Essential tremor: A heterogenous disorder. Mov Disord. 2002;17:638-44.
17. Jankovic J, Schwartz, KS, Ondo W. Re-emergent tremor of Parkinson's disease. J Neurol Neurosurg Psychiatry. 1999;67:646-50.
18. Hirsch EC, Mouatt A, Faucheux B, Bonnet AM, Javoy-Agid F, Graybiel AM, et al. Dopamine, tremor, and Parkinson's disease. Lancet. 1992;340(8811):125-6.
19. Brooks DJ, Playford ED, Ibanez V, Sawle GV, Thompson PD, Findley LJ, et al. Isolated tremor and disruption of the nigrostriatal dopaminergic system: An 18F-dopa PET study. Neurology. 1992;42(8):1554-60.
20. Hunker CJ, Abbs JH, Barlow SM. The relationship between parkinsonian rigidity and hypokinesia in the orofacial system: A quantitative analysis. Neurology. 1982;32:749-54.
21. Oerlemans WGH, de Visser M. Dropped head syndrome and bent spine syndrome: Two separate clinical entities or different manifestations of axial myopathy. J Neurol Neurosurg Psychiatry. 1998;65:258-9.
22. Djaldetti R, Mosberg-Galili R, Sroka H, Merims D, Melamed E. Camptocormia (bent spine) in patients with Parkinson's disease: Characterization and possible pathogenesis of an unusual phenomenon. Mov Disord. 1999;14(3):443-7.
23. Bartels AL, Balash Y, Gurevich T, Schaafsma JD, Hausdorff JM, Giladi N. Relationship between freezing of gait (FOG) and other features of Parkinson's: FOG is not correlated with bradykinesia. J Clin Neurosci. 2003;10(5):584-8.
24. Jankovic J, Nutt JG, Sudarsky L. Classification, diagnosis and etiology of gait disorders. In Ruzicka E, Hallett M, Jankovic J (eds). Gait disorders: Advances in Neurology. Philadelphia: Lippincott Williams & Wilkins; 2001. pp. 119-34.
25. Movement Disorder Society Task Force on Rating Scales for Parkinson's Disease: The Unified Parkinson's Disease Rating Scale (UPDRS): Status and recommendations. Mov Disord. 2003;18:738-50.
26. Tinetti ME, Williams TF, Mayewski R. Fall Risk Index for elderly patients based on number of chronic disabilities. Am J Med. 1986:80:429-34.
27. Boghen D. Apraxia of lid opening: A review. Neurology. 1997;48:1481-503.
28. Elble RJ, Cousins R, Leffler K, Hughes L. Gait initiation by patients with lower-half parkinsonism. Brain. 1996;119: 1705-16.
29. Lee MS, Kim HS, Lyoo CH. "Off" gait freezing and temporal discrimination threshold in patients with Parkinson disease. Neurology. 2005;64(4):670-4.
30. FitzGerald PM, Jankovic J. Lower body parkinsonism: Evidence for vascular etiology. Mov Disord. 1989;4:249-60.
31. Brooks DJ, Ibanez V, Sawle GV, Playford ED, Quinn N, Mathias CJ, et al. Striatal D2 receptor status in patients with Parkinson's disease, striatonigral degeneration, and progressive supranuclear palsy, measured with 11C-Raclopride and positron emission tomography. Ann Neurol. 1992;31(2):184-92.
32. Vreeling FW, Jollens J, Verhey FRJ, Houx PJ. Primitive reflexes in healthy, adult volunteers and neurological patients: Methodological issues. J Neurol. 1993;240:495-504.
33. Brodsky H, Dat Vuong K, Thomas M, Jankovic J. Glabellar and palmomental reflexes in parkinsonian disorders. Neurology. 2004;63:1096-8.
34. Hunter PC, Crameri J, Austin S, Woodward MC, Hughes AJ. Response of parkinsonian swallowing dysfunction to dopaminergic stimulation. J Neurol Neurosurg Psychiatry. 1997;63(5):579-83.

35. Schrag A, Schott JM. Epidemiological, clinical, and genetic characteristics of early-onset parkinsonism. Lancet Neurol. 2006;5:355-63.
36. Hillen ME, Sage JI. Nonmotor fluctuations in patients with Parkinson's disease. Neurology. 1996;47:1180-3.
37. Chaudhuri KR, Healy DG, Schapira AH; National Institute for Clinical Excellence. Non-motor symptoms of Parkinson's disease: Diagnosis and management. Lancet Neurol. 2006;5(3): 235-45.
38. Braak H, Ghebremedhin E, Rub U, Bratzke H, Del Tredici K. Stages in the development of Parkinson's disease-related pathology. Cell Tissue Res. 2004;318(1):121-34.
39. Bonuccelli U, Lucetti C, Del Dott P, Ceravolo R, Gambaccini G, Bernardini S, et al. Orthostatic hypotension in de novo Parkinson disease. Arch Neurol. 2003;60:1400-04.
40. Kaufmann H, Nahm K, Purohit D, Wolfe D. Autonomic failure as the initial presentation of Parkinson disease and dementia with Lewy bodies. Neurology. 2004;63:1093-5.
41. Winge K, Rasmussen D, Werdelin LM. Constipation in neurological diseases. J Neurol Neurosurg Psychiatry. 2003;74:13-9.
42. Aarsland D, Larsen JP, Lim NG, Janvin C, Karlsen K, Tandberg E, et al. Range of neuropsychiatric disturbances in patients with Parkinson's disease. J Neurol Neurosurg Psychiatry. 1999;67(4):492-6.
43. Starkstein SE, Petracca G, Chemerinski E, Merello M. Prevalence and correlates of parkinsonism in patients with primary depression. Neurology. 2001;57(3):553-5.
44. Marinus J, Visser M, Verwey NA, Verhey FRJ, Middelkoop HAM, Stiggelbout AM, et al. Assessment of cognition in Parkinson's disease. Neurology. 2003;61:1222-8.
45. Nasreddine ZS, Phillips NA, Bédirian V, Charbonneau S, Whitehead V, Collin I, et al. "The Montreal Cognitive Assessment, MoCA: a brief screening tool for mild cognitive impairment". J Am Geriatr Soc. 2005;53(4):695-9.
46. Emre W. What causes mental dysfunction in Parkinson's disease? Mov Disord. 2003;18(suppl 6):S63-71.
47. Fénelon G, Mahieux F, Huon R, Ziégler M. Hallucinations in Parkinson's disease: Prevalence, phenomenology and risk factors. Brain. 2000;123:733-45.
48. Marsh L, Williams JR, Rocco M, Grill S, Munro C, Dawson TM. Psychiatric comorbidities in patients with Parkinson disease and psychosis. Neurology. 2004;63(2):293-300.
49. Alegret M, Junque C, Valldeoriola F, Vendrell P, Martí MJ, Tolosa E. Obsessive-compulsive symptoms in Parkinson's disease. J Neurol Neurosurg Psychiatry. 2001;70(3):394-6.
50. Evans AH, Katzenschlager R, Paviour D, O'Sullivan JD, Appel S, Lawrence AD, et al: Punding in Parkinson's disease: Its relation to the dopamine dysregulation syndrome. Mov Disord. 2004;19(4):397-405.
51. Giovannoni G, O'Sullivan JD, Turner K, Manson AJ, Lees AJ. Hedonistic homeostatic dysregulation in patients with Parkinson's disease on dopamine replacement therapies. J Neurol Neurosurg Psychiatry. 2000;68(4):423-8.
52. Dodd ML, Klos KJ, Bower JH, Geda YE, Josephs KA, Ahlskog JE. Pathological gambling caused by drugs used to treat Parkinson disease. Arch Neurol. 2005;62(9):1377-81.
53. Evans AH, Lees AJ. Dopamine dysregulation syndrome in Parkinson's disease. Curr Opin Neurol. 2004;17:393-39.
54. Adler CH, Thorpy MJ. Sleep issues in Parkinson's disease. Neurology. 2005;64(suppl 3):S12-20.
55. Chaudhuri KR, Pal S, DiMarco A, Whately-Smith C, Bridgman K, Mathew R, et al: The Parkinson's disease sleep scale: A new instrument for assessing sleep and nocturnal disability in Parkinson's disease. J Neurol Neurosurg Psychiatry. 2002;73(6):629-35.
56. Pal PK, Calne S, Samii A, Fleming JAE. A review of normal sleep and its disturbances in Parkinson's disease. Parkinsonism Relat Disords. 1999;5:1-17.
57. Wetter TC, Collado-Seidel V, Pollmacher T, Yassouridis A, Trenkwalder C. Sleep and periodic leg movement patterns in drug-free patients with Parkinson's disease and multiple system atrophy. Sleep. 2000;23(3):361-7.
58. Albin RL, Koeppe RA, Chervin RD, Consens FB, Wernette K, Frey KA, et al. Decreased striatal dopaminergic innervation in REM sleep behavior disorder. Neurology. 2000;55(9): 1410-2.
59. Gagnon JF, Bedard MA, Fantini ML, Petit D, Panisset M, Rompré S, et al. REM sleep behavior disorder and REM sleep without atonia in Parkinson's disease. Neurology. 2002;59(4): 585-9.
60. Arnulf I, Bonnet AM, Damier P, Bejjani BP, Seilhean D, Derenne JP, et al. Hallucinations, REM sleep, and Parkinson's disease: A medical hypothesis. Neurology. 2000;55(2):281-8.
61. Hawkes C. Olfaction in neurodegenerative disorder. Mov Disord. 2003;18:364-72.
62. Double KL, Rowe DB, Hayes M, Chan DK, Blackie J, Corbett A, et al. Identifying the pattern of olfactory deficits in Parkinson disease using the brief smell identification test. Arch Neurol. 2003;60(4):545-9.
63. Booij J, Tissingh G, Boer GJ, Speelman JD, Stoof JC, Janssen AG, et al: [123I]FP-CIT SPECT shows a pronounced decline of striatal dopamine transporter labeling in early and advanced Parkinson's disease. J Neurol Neurosurg Psychiatry. 1997;62(2):133-40.
64. Goetz CG, Poewe W, Rascol O, Sampaio C, Stebbins GT, Counsell C, et al. Movement Disorder Society Task Force report on the Hoehn and Yahr staging scale: Status and recommendations. Mov Disord. 2004;19(9):1020-8.
65. Marinus J, Visser M, Stiggelbout AM, Rabey JM, Martínez-Martín P, Bonuccelli U, et al: A short scale for the assessment of motor impairments and disabilities in Parkinson's disease: The SPES/SCOPA. J Neurol Neurosurg Psychiatry. 2004;75(3): 388-95.
66. Bennett DA, Shannon KM, Beckett LA, Goetz CG, Wilson RS. Metric properties of nurses' ratings of parkinsonian signs with a modified Unified Parkinson's Disease Rating Scale. Neurology. 1997;49(6):1580-7.
67. Munhoz RP, Li JY, Kurtinecz M, Piboolnurak P, Constantino A, Fahn S, et al: Evaluation of the pull test technique in assessing postural instability in Parkinson's disease. Neurology. 2004; 62(1):125-7.

CHAPTER 7

Parkinson's Disease Pathogenesis: Key Players and Potential Therapeutic Targets

Rebecca Banerjee, Supriyo Choudhury, Hrishikesh Kumar

INTRODUCTION

Parkinson's disease (PD), the second most prevalent neurodegenerative disorder, afflicts 1% of the population above the age of 65 years.[1] The prevalence of PD in the United States is projected to steadily increase, reaching 2 million by 2030.[2,3] A similar trend could be expected in India with increasing number of evidence-based epidemiological studies of PD.[4] Pioneering works on PD from India are extremely valuable.[5]

The motor symptoms—resting tremor, muscle rigidity, bradykinesia, and postural instability occur due to nigrostriatal dysregulations and loss of neuromelanin-rich dopaminergic neurons of the substantia nigra pars compacta (SNpc).[6] An array of nonmotor symptoms manifested is attributed to the degeneration of nondopaminergic neuronal loci-autonomic nuclei, locus coeruleus, and glutamatergic neurons of the cerebral cortex.[7] Dementia commonly sets in late and in advanced PD. The cytologic pathological hallmarks of PD are inclusions known as Lewy bodies and Lewy neurites that were revealed from autopsied PD brains.[8] The true relationship between accumulation of inclusion bodies, neuronal death, and neurological deficits is unknown.

Ever since the first description of PD in 1817 by James Parkinson, disease-modifying therapy remains an unmet need. Extensive research has given several clues to PD complexity, intermingling of molecular factors, as well as the impact of environment, and genes. An early differential diagnosis and effective intervention of PD might materialize with a better grasp of core disease mechanisms and advanced neuroimaging methods like such as positron emission tomography (PET), single photon emission computed tomography (SPECT), and magnetic resonance imaging (MRI). This review provides an overview of key pathogenic factors in PD deduced from human, in vitro, and animal experiments. Current therapeutic modalities in PD with clinical applications have been highlighted here.

DISEASE ASSOCIATIVE FACTORS

Concept of PD as a singular entity is getting obsolete as therapeutically targeting single molecular pathway has not proved viable. This disease better fits in as a cluster of clinical, epidemiological, molecular, neuropathological, and genetic subtypes.[9] The disease associative factors—triggers, facilitators, and aggravators can be categorized within three temporal phases. Triggers remain hidden for early prodromal premotor phases of PD, except in genetic cases. Triggers could be multiple in the form of protein aggregation due to misfolding or impaired degradation, free radicals causing oxidative stress, mitochondrial dysfunction, neurotrophic factor deficits, and chronic neuroinflammation. The exact cascade of molecular events in PD is not deciphered.

Gene mutations have been directly linked to PD or linked to an increased risk for developing PD. Environmental factors such as toxins, pesticides, and head trauma have also been linked to PD.[6] The vast majority of PD cases, however, do not reveal a known genetic component or identifiable environmental exposure and the direct cause of idiopathic PD is puzzling. Valuable tools like recently developed patient-derived-induced pluripotent stem cells could potentially address the molecular basis for disease-relevant phenotypes in PD and its etiology (**Fig. 1**).[10] Moreover, sensitive modern day proteomic techniques

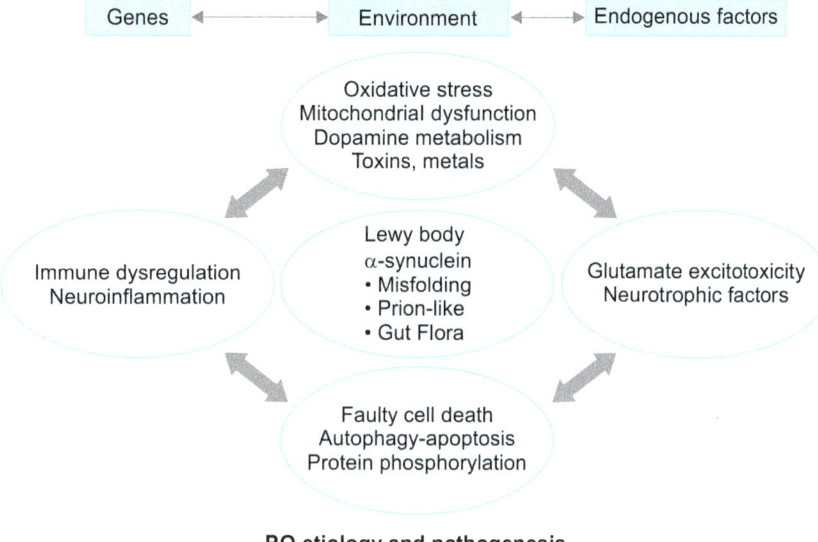

FIG. 1: Diagrammatic illustration of inter-related key pathogenic mechanisms in Parkinson's disease.

detecting alterations of the brain proteome in PD could aid in novel protein identification and biomarker discovery.[11] Furthermore, midbrain organoid culture, could make breakthrough in unveiling intraneuronal mechanisms of PD.[12]

PROPOSED MECHANISMS

Ample neuropathological evidence on human and experimental PD suggests existence of interacting complex signaling pathways in PD pathogenesis (**Fig. 1**). In terms of the mechanism of dopaminergic neuronal death in PD, no unanimous conclusion has been drawn. Several theories have been proposed for PD, but each one is steeped in controversies.[13] In this review, we have discussed in brief, few currently popular therapeutically targeted mechanisms in PD.

ALPHA-SYNUCLEIN AND LEWY BODY PATHOLOGY

Alpha-synuclein discovered as the first causative gene product for PD is enriched within Lewy bodies and Lewy neurites.[8,14] A causal connection might exist between Lewy body inclusions and the stages in the development of PD-related pathology, as described by Braak and colleagues.[15] Braak's hypothesis was postulated based on topographic distribution of Lewy bodies and neurites in autopsied PD patients and the most of the typical PD cases matched the Braak staging scheme. Despite promising fluid biomarkers in PD and in vivo neuroimaging tools, neuropathological staging, and postmortem confirmation of PD is still the gold standard and signifies the usefulness of Braak staging. Research implicates α-synuclein's pathogenic role in sporadic and familial PD.[16] Missense mutations in α-synuclein, copy number variants, and upregulation are each associated with PD. Altered α-synuclein homeostasis and misfolding are additional contributing factors in PD.[17] α-synuclein misfolding might be an early event, and its intervention at this stage of PD seems critical. Multitude of α-synuclein-directed therapeutics for reducing α-synuclein levels or propagation are in clinical research.[16,18]

Prion-like Spread of α-Synuclein

Hypothetically, in PD, pathogenic α-synuclein originating in the gut and then spreading in a prion-like fashion is gaining popularity.[18] Appearance of constipation before the onset of motor symptoms, gut dysbiosis, and peripheral synucleinopathy in PD patients are important clues to support this hypothesis. Several cell culture and animal experimental findings favored the prion-like seeding of synucleinopathy and conformed to the sequential progression of Braak stages in PD. It remains unexplained how α-synuclein shuttles in the physiological system and cross talks between peripheral organs and brain. Prion-like cell-to-cell transmissibility of α-synuclein was further bolstered up from postmortem observations, whereby pathological α-synuclein inclusions appeared in healthy grafted neurons in PD patients. Accumulation of α-synuclein within the peripheral autonomic nervous system, including the enteric nervous system, and the dorsal motor nucleus of the vagus support the concept that α-synuclein can spread from the enteric nervous system to the brain via the vagus nerve. This notion is supported by the decreased risk of PD following truncal vagotomy that also strengthens Braak's hypothesis.[19] Recently, phosphorylated α-synuclein deposits has been tracked in the enteric nervous system from biopsies of subjects collected several years before the actual onset of PD motor symptoms.[20] Besides the gut, abnormal α-synuclein deposits have been demonstrated even in the pancreas, heart, salivary glands, and skin. The proposed scheme of Braak staging in PD is highly debated and further mechanistic basis are warranted. Although the reliability of the Braak staging system has recently been challenged, it appears to be valid for PD patients with young-onset and long duration of motor symptoms.[21] Clinical immunotherapy trials in PD are currently targeting the "prion-like" cell-to-cell transfer process of α-synuclein.[18] Presently, it is unresolved which molecular species of α-synuclein is toxic and should be a biomarker and a therapeutic target in PD.

NEUROINFLAMMATION AND IMMUNE DYSREGULATION

Numerous evidences testify for the principal role of neuroinflammation in the progression of PD.[13] Targeting the immune system with immunotherapy are promising strategies for PD treatment. Investigations based upon postmortem PD brains not only confirm robust neuroinflammatory changes but reveal infiltration of T lymphocytes from the peripheral system.[22] Several autoimmune features present in PD along with major inflammatory pathology in the brain as well as in the periphery, even suggest PD to be an immunological disorder.[23] Peripheral markers of T cell response show changes in PD patients relative to controls and potentially applicable as diagnostic and therapeutic biomarkers.[22] Dopamine, the major neurotransmitter involved in PD also exerts an immunoregulatory role during neuroinflammation.[24] Further, the role of inflammasomes which are intracellular proinflammatory pattern-recognition receptors capable of initiating and propagating inflammation have recently cropped up in PD. Histopathologic studies revealed elevated nod-like receptor 3 protein (NLRP3)-inflammasome expression in mesencephalic neurons of PD patients.[25] This study also characterized a rare *NLRP3* gene polymorphism that possibly is associated with a decreased risk of PD. Intense research in the inflammasome PD field including our own research efforts has explicitly brought forth the importance of α-synuclein and NLRP3 inflammasome inflammatory activation in PD patients.[26-28]

Epidemiological studies on the use of anti-inflammatory drugs with reduced risk of developing PD though exciting has not yet been established.[29] New therapeutic strategies such as vaccination, optimal regulation of neuroinflammatory processes, and peripheral intervention to prevent the deleterious role of the immune system in the brain parenchyma could be beneficial.

MITOCHONDRIAL DYSFUNCTION AND OXIDATIVE STRESS

Substantial evidence gathered from investigation of human tissues, genetic and toxin-induced animal and cellular models indicate that mitochondrial dysfunction plays a central role in the pathophysiology of PD in both sporadic and familial forms of PD.[30] Deficits in mitochondrial functions due to defective bioenergetics, alterations in mitochondrial deoxyribonucleic acid (mtDNA), generation of reactive oxygen species (ROS), aberrant calcium homeostasis, and anomalies in mitochondrial dynamics and quality control are some of the key mechanisms that contribute to neuronal demise in PD.[31] Multiple therapeutic strategies targeting mitochondrial function and homeostasis have been tested in preclinical studies and clinical trials.

Antioxidant Therapies

Various preclinical studies have shown that antioxidants can ameliorate mitochondrial pathology in PD and thereby strongly suggest that antioxidants might protect in human PD.

Key Clinical Trials

The Deprenyl and Tocopherol Antioxidative Therapy of Parkinsonism (DATATOP) trial suggested that deprenyl, but not tocopherol, delayed the onset of disability in early and untreated PD (The Parkinson Study Group, 1993). However, whether this was a symptomatic effect, or a slowing of the underlying disease process was not clear. A trial of a newer monoamine oxidase-B inhibitor, rasagiline, though showed a benefit consistent with a disease modifying effect with a dose of 1 mg, with a higher dose of 2 mg the benefit was not seen.[31]

Effect of mitoquinone (MitoQ), a mitochondrial targeted antioxidant, was assessed for disease modification in PD patients.[32] Unfortunately, no benefit of MitoQ for disease progression in the double-blind and placebo-controlled study was found.

Coenzyme Q10 (CoQ10), a potent antioxidant supporting the function of mitochondria, was investigated on disease progression in a large phase 3 randomized, placebo-controlled, and double-blind clinical trial (Parkinson Study Group QE3 Investigators, 2014). While CoQ10 was safe and well-tolerated, the study failed to show any clinical benefit.

The drug EPI-589, which modifies cellular reduced glutathione (GSH) levels and has an antioxidant effect, is currently the subject of a phase 2 study.

Another promising antioxidant is N-acetylcysteine (NAC), a precursor to GSH. In a preliminary clinical study, NAC caused significant increase of dopamine transporter (DAT) binding in the caudate and putamen on DAT scan as well as Unified Parkinson's Disease Rating Scale (UPDRS) score improvement.[33]

Reactive Oxygen Species and Parkinson's Disease-associated Factors

Mitochondrial dysfunction, dopamine, neuroinflammation, iron, and genetic mutations solely or synergistically induce ROS generation which could induce dopaminergic neurons death via protein, lipid, and DNA oxidation.[34] Novel targets enhancing antioxidant status, anti-inflammatory pathways, and induction of cytoprotective genes could mitigate the oxidative stress buildup in PD.

Exogenous Toxins and Heavy Metals

Epidemiological as well as experimental data support the role of metals such as manganese, iron, aluminum, copper, lead, mercury, bismuth, thallium, and zinc in the pathogenesis of PD.[35] Chronic metal exposure, with manganese, being one of the major offender elements occurs through industrial toxicants, occupational exposure, contaminated seafood, dental amalgams, etc. Neurotoxicity likely results from elevated levels of heavy metals that promote oxidative stress, lipid peroxidation, and cellular stress in selectively vulnerable dopaminergic neurons. While lead actually diminishes dopamine synthesis, increased free iron generates highly toxic hydroxyl radicals via Fenton reaction. Besides, rural-living, well-water drinking, widespread use of pesticides, and fungicides like rotenone, paraquat, maneb, organophosphates, and organochlorine compounds are possible risk factors for PD. Epidemiological data on toxin exposure and development of PD are sparse although animal and in vitro pesticide models closely mimic PD pathways. While rotenone, a common pesticide, is an extremely potent mitochondrial complex I inhibitor; direct, or indirect neurotoxic effects are impacted upon by many other pesticides, inorganic manganese, and mercury containing fungicides.[36] On the other hand, exposure to algal bloom-infested aquatic ecosystem and aquatic organism consumption seems to play a role in PD due to the triggering of excitotoxicity by the cyanobacteria-producing beta-N-methylamino-L-alanine (BMAA).[37] Overall, possible detoxification of neurotoxins and chelation therapy of metals are future strategies to halt the progression of neurodegeneration in PD.

GENE MUTATIONS AND GENETIC RISK FACTORS

There has been immense progress in our understanding of genetics in PD.[38] Highly-penetrant mutations in different genes (*SNCA, LRRK2, VPS35, PARKIN, PINK1,* and *DJ-1*) are known to cause autosomal dominant or recessive monogenic PD. Furthermore, different variants with incomplete penetrance in the *LRRK2* and the *GBA* gene are strong-risk factors for PD and are especially prevalent in certain populations. The monogenic cases account for <5% of all PD, the majority being apparently sporadic cases. PD might be a complex genetic disorder as it fits within the wide-range of complex polygenic disorders influenced by both genetic and environmental factors. Large-scale genome-wide association studies (GWAS) have identified over 40 loci that are at risk for PD. Monogenic and idiopathic PD possibly have shared pathogenic mechanisms as evident from the overlap between monogenic and sporadic PD genes, particularly for the loci that contain the genes *SNCA* and *LRRK2*. Idiopathic PD cases with heterozygous variants in autosomal recessive genes suggest that these mutations might increase the risk of PD. Genetic studies from Indian population reveals novel variants for *LRRK2* and 5% of early-onset PD account for DJ-1 mutations.[39,40] Next generation DNA sequencing technologies would assist in unveiling the genetic landscape of PD. This would lead to a better understanding of pathological mechanisms, genetic counseling, prognosis, and identification of novel therapeutic targets.

FAULTY CELL DEATH MECHANISMS

Perturbation of cell death signaling is critical for long-lived cells such as neurons. Various cell death mechanisms—namely apoptosis, autophagy, and necrosis are implicated in PD. Restoring the interaction amongst molecules involved in cell death might protect against neurodegeneration. Alterations in the autophagy-lysosome pathway have been suggested as a contributory pathophysiological factor for PD. Evidence obtained from PD brain suggests for a dysregulation of autophagy to be associated with α-synuclein aggregation. The potential of autophagy enhancement as a disease-modifying therapy in PD are based on preclinical evidences.[41] Autophagy-related proteins in cerebrospinal fluid may be utilized as potential diagnostic and prognostic biomarkers of early-stage PD. The benefit of antiapoptotic agents in PD is yet to be seen.

IMPROPER PROTEIN PHOSPHORYLATION

Defective phosphorylation of various proteins as a consequence to dysfunction of specific kinases and phosphatases has been revealed through mainly genetic cases of PD. Increased phosphorylation of c-Abl, a nonreceptor protein kinase, regulates various cellular processes linked to PD and c-Abl inhibitors might be helpful in PD therapy.[42]

GUT MICROBIOME AND SKIN

Recently, gut microbiome seems to be a hot research topic in PD. There are substantial clinical and pathological findings supporting the link between intestinal microflora changes and compositional differences of gut microbiota in PD.[43] Moreover, antibiotic exposure and ingested toxins could adversely impact the enteric microbiome resulting in low-grade systemic inflammation thus, leading to damage of neurons in both enteric- and central nervous systems. Despite evidence for gut dysbiosis in PD, the microbiome field is still nascent and further mechanistic studies are warranted. It is possible that PD patients might benefit from microbial therapy and rectify the dysfunctional bidirectional gut-brain axis in PD. The gut microflora could even be dynamically modulated by nutritional status, diet, exercise, and stress. Involvement of oral and nasal microbiome cavities, two other important ports of pathogen entry has also been hinted upon in PD pathogenesis. Rather interesting, skin is also implicated in the pathogenesis of PD.[44] Skin disorders generally overlooked in PD, could be a mixed manifestation for nonmotor symptoms and side effects of medication. Chronic relapsing inflammatory skin disorders, seborrheic dermatitis, bulloid pemphigoid, and rosacea are common in PD. Autonomic dysfunction of sweating patterns reflects pathological changes in skin nerves. Apart from skin being a possible route for neuroinvasion, a positive association of PD and malignant melanoma has been recently reported. The nervous system, gastrointestinal tract, and skin are analogous in their embryological development but the causal link for the comorbid skin problems in PD is yet to be established. Skin biopsy from patients and manipulation of skin fibroblast-derived induced pluripotent stem cells offers new hope of therapeutic betterment in PD. Skin cells could perhaps become useful peripheral biomarkers in PD in future.

ROLE OF MICRORIBONUCLEIC ACID

Microribonucleic acids (miRNAs) are recently implicated in PD etiology and their expressions associated with pathophysiological processes.[45] MicroRNAs circulating in body fluids are one of the major promising biomarker candidates for PD. Recent findings indicate a regulatory role of different miRNAs on PD-related genes, and neuroinflammation. MicroRNAs involved in PD might be tailored into high-clinical-impact therapeutic molecular agents in PD.

ASSOCIATION OF INHERITED METABOLIC DISORDERS

The clinical convergence between PD and certain inherited metabolic disorders like lysosomal storage diseases as seen in type 1 Gaucher disease (GD); Niemann-Pick disease, copper, and iron dyshomeostasis—Wilson's disease and hemochromatosis; disorders of amino acid metabolism as in phenylketonuria, maple syrup urine disease, and finally a spectrum of mitochondrial degenerative disorders has instigated research into their overlapping genetic and biochemical dysregulatory status.[46] The discovery of shared pathways of an imbalanced homeostasis continues to expand our understanding of the clinical implications of oxidative stress, reduction in neurotransmitters, and aberrant protein accumulation in the process of neurodegeneration. Probable connections between metabolic syndrome—hypertension, hyperglycemia, hyperlipidemia, and higher risk for PD need further investigation.[47]

DOPAMINE METABOLISM

Dopamine homeostasis is critical in PD as the metabolism of dopamine sets dopaminergic neurons under constant oxidative stress and its oxidation can lead to endogenous neurotoxins.[48] A pilot study indicated that treatment with dopamine precursor "levodopa" increased oxidative stress levels in PD patients.[49] However, in a recent multicentric clinical trial study the effect of early initiation of levodopa on PD progression was not observed.[50]

GLUTAMATE-MEDIATED EXCITOTOXICITY

Glutamate-mediated neurotoxicity in PD arises secondary to the death of dopaminergic neurons that leads to altered neurotransmission due to an imbalance between excitatory and inhibitory neurotransmitters and calcium-dependent synaptic plasticity.[51] Many of the glutamate receptors antagonists have been adopted in clinical trials on PD patients.

NEUROTROPHIC FACTORS

Neuroprotective and neurorestorative actions of trophic factors are documented in experimental PD.[52] This has led to clinical trials with glial cell line-derived neurotrophic factor (GDNF), neurturin (NRTN), platelet-derived growth factor, and cerebral dopaminergic neurotrophic factor. Open-label studies with GDNF as well as a study with NRTN showed clinical improvement, particularly in patients with early-stage PD. Variants of fibroblast growth factor-20 (*FGF-20*), a susceptibility gene for PD, were recently studied among eastern Indians.[53]

SELECTIVE VULNERABILITY OF DOPAMINE NEURONS

There are several arguments over explaining why only a small population of dopaminergic neurons in the SNpc selectively degenerate in PD, despite the fact that the adjacent ventral tegmental area (VTA) dopaminergic neurons are relatively spared.[54] Various studies indicate that SNpc and VTA dopaminergic neurons have considerable heterogeneity in their molecular and electrophysiologic constitution.[55] Neurons within the SNpc intrinsically bear a unique anatomical, physiological, and biochemical phenotype that predisposes them to mitochondrial dysfunction or α-synuclein pathology.

CURRENT TREATMENT AND FUTURE THERAPY

Except for symptomatic treatment in PD, no success has been met that can stop or slow the disease. Levodopa, the gold standard of PD treatment today remains, based on discoveries made in 1950s but is not devoid of adverse long-term levodopa-induced motor complications.[56] In addition to this, the diagnosis of PD relies primarily on the clinical assessment of motor symptoms that become detectable only when a large part of the nigral dopaminergic neurons are already degenerated. Other treatment options include catechol-O-methyltransferase inhibitors to prevent peripheral metabolism of dopamine, monoamine oxidase-B inhibitors to prevent oxidative stress in glial cells, and deep brain stimulation using high-frequency (100–200 Hz) electrical signals to stimulate the subthalamic nucleus (STN) to reduce STN overactivity and mitigate the motor symptoms.[57,58] Gene therapy is emerging as a promising approach to treat PD whereby, some STN neurons are converted to an inhibitory phenotype through local transfer of glutamic acid decarboxylase (GAD). A phase 2 clinical trial delivering GAD into the STN of PD patients-demonstrated therapeutic effects.[59]

PD symptomatology, disease course, and neuropathology vary between patients, and therefore, a combinatorial therapeutic approach in PD could be more rewarding. Late detection of PD is a major impediment in the treatment of PD. The distressing nonmotor symptoms are resistant to the motor symptom-directed therapies in PD. Neural mechanisms underlying the dementing process and its associated cognitive deficits are also still poorly understood. Novel biomarker discovery could lead us to alternative pathogenic pathways in PD and new therapeutic targets. Molecular collates to brain pathology and symptoms should provide greater insight into the systemic nature of PD.

Immunomodulatory techniques and stem cell therapy have shown promise in experimental models. Targeted brain delivery of therapeutically potential molecules with the help of advanced nanomedicine strategy, molecular, and clinical tools brings hope for a better therapeutic design. A new neurotheranostics approach offering individualized personalized medicine might be beneficial to the PD patient more than conventional therapy.[60]

CONCLUSION

Conceptual and technical hurdles in discovering a cure for PD continue to baffle clinicians and scientists. While progress has been made in knowing the genetic contribution of PD, there is still a vast lacuna in understanding PD pathogenesis and molecular mechanisms. Lack of biomarkers and dependence on clinical evidence is a major obstacle for early diagnosis of PD. Clinical trial failures could be guideposts for future therapeutic designs. Epidemiological and therapeutic studies on the diverse, heterogeneous population, and ethnic gene pools from India could shed light on unknown pathomechanisms of PD. Bold research initiatives and innovation would eventually steer toward a cure for PD.

REFERENCES

1. de Lau LM, Breteler MMB. Epidemiology of Parkinson's disease. Lancet Neurol. 2006;5(6):525-35.
2. Bach JP, Riedel O, Klotsche J, Spottke A, Dodel R, Wittchen HU. Impact of complications and comorbidities on treatment costs and health-related quality of life of patients with Parkinson's disease. J Neurol Sci. 2012;314(1-2):41-7.
3. Dorsey ER, Constantinescu R, Thompson JP, Biglan KM, Holloway RG, Kieburtz K, et al. Projected number of people with Parkinson disease in the most populous nations, 2005 through 2030. Neurology. 2007;68(5):384-6.
4. Surathi P, Jhunjhunwala K, Yadav R, Pal PK. Research in Parkinson's disease in India: A review. Ann Indian Acad Neurol. 2016;19(1):9-20.
5. Das SK, Misra AK, Ray BK, Hazra A, Ghosal MK, Chaudhuri A, et al. Epidemiology of Parkinson disease in the city of Kolkata, India: a community-based study. Neurology. 2010;75(15):1362-9.

6. Kalia LV, Lang AE. Parkinson's disease. Lancet. 2015;386(9996): 896-912.
7. Schapira AHV, Chaudhuri KR, Jenner P. Non-motor features of Parkinson disease. Nat Rev Neurosci. 2017;18(7):435-50.
8. Spillantini MG, Schmidt ML, Lee VM, Trojanowski JQ, Jakes R, Goedert M. α-Synuclein in Lewy bodies. Nature. 1997;388 (6645):839-40.
9. Johnson ME, Stecher B, Labrie V, Brundin L, Brundin P. Triggers, facilitators, and aggravators: Redefining Parkinson's disease pathogenesis. Trends Neurosci. 2019;42(1):4-13.
10. Sison SL, Vermilyea SC, Emborg ME, Ebert AD. Using patient-derived induced pluripotent stem cells to identify Parkinson's disease-relevant phenotypes. Curr Neurol Neurosci Rep. 2018;18(12):84.
11. Pal R, Larsen JP, Moller SG. The potential of proteomics in understanding neurodegeneration. Int Rev Neurobiol. 2015;121:25-58.
12. Monzel AS, Smits LM, Hemmer K, Hachi S, Moreno EL, van Wuellen T, et al. Derivation of human midbrain-specific organoids from neuroepithelial stem cells. Stem Cell Reports. 2017;8(5):1144-54.
13. Hirsch EC, Jenner P, Przedborski S. Pathogenesis of Parkinson's disease. Mov Disord. 2013;28(1):24-30.
14. Polymeropoulos MH, Lavedan C, Leroy E, Ide SE, Dehejia A, Dutra A, et al. Mutation in the α-synuclein gene identified in families with Parkinson's disease. Science. 1997;276(5321):2045-7.
15. Braak H, Del Tredici K. Neuroanatomy and pathology of sporadic Parkinson's disease. Adv Anat Embryol Cell Biol. 2009;201:1-119.
16. Brundin P, Dave KD, Kordower JH. Therapeutic approaches to target alpha-synuclein pathology. Exp Neurol. 2017;298: 225-35.
17. Dettmer U. Rationally designed variants of α-synuclein illuminate its in vivo structural properties in health and disease. Front Neurosci. 2018;12:623.
18. George S, Brundin P. Immunotherapy in Parkinson's disease: micromanaging alpha-synuclein aggregation. J Parkinsons Dis. 2015;5(3):413-24.
19. Breen DP, Halliday GM, Lang AE. Gut-brain axis and the spread of α-synuclein pathology: Vagal highway or dead end? Mov Disord. 2019;34(3):307-16.
20. Stokholm MG, Danielsen EH, Hamilton-Dutoit SJ, Borghammer P. Pathological α-synuclein in gastrointestinal tissues from prodromal Parkinson disease patients. Ann Neurol. 2016;79(6): 940-9.
21. Jellinger KA. Is Braak staging valid for all types of Parkinson's disease? J Neural Transm (Vienna). 2019;126(4):423-31.
22. Baird JK, Bourdette D, Meshul CK, Quinn JF. The key role of T cells in Parkinson's disease pathogenesis and therapy. Parkinsonism Relat Disord. 2019;60:25-31.
23. Jiang T, Li G, Xu J, Gao S, Chen X. The Challenge of the Pathogenesis of Parkinson's Disease: Is Autoimmunity the Culprit? Front Immunol. 2018;9:2047.
24. Yan Y, Jiang W, Liu L, Wang X, Ding C, Tian Z, et al. Dopamine controls systemic inflammation through inhibition of NLRP3 inflammasome. Cell. 2015;160(1-2):62-73.
25. von Herrmann KM, Salas LA, Martinez EM, Young AL, Howard JM, Feldman MS, et al. NLRP3 expression in mesencephalic neurons and characterization of a rare NLRP3 polymorphism associated with decreased risk of Parkinson's disease. NPJ Parkinson's Dis. 2018;4(1):24.
26. Chatterjee K, Roy A, Banerjee R, Choudhury S, Mondal B, Halder S, et al. Inflammasome and α-synuclein in Parkinson's disease: A cross-sectional study. J Neuroimmunol. 2020;338:577089.
27. Han X, Sun S, Sun Y, Song Q, Zhu J, Song N, et al. Small molecule-driven NLRP3 inflammation inhibition via interplay between ubiquitination and autophagy: implications for Parkinson disease. Autophagy. 2019;15(11):1860-81.
28. Haque ME, Akther M, Jakaria M, Kim IS, Azam S, Choi DK. Targeting the microglial NLRP3 inflammasome and its role in Parkinson's disease. Mov Disord. 2020;35(1):20-33.
29. Hirsch EC, Vyas S, Hunot S. Neuroinflammation in Parkinson's disease. Parkinsonism Relat Disord. 2012;18(1):S210-2.
30. Grünewald A, Kumar KR, Sue CM. New insights into the complex role of mitochondria in Parkinson's disease. Prog Neurobiol. 2019;177:73-93.
31. Olanow CW, Rascol O, Hauser R, Feigin PD, Jankovic J, Lang A, et al. A double-blind, delayed-start trial of rasagiline in Parkinson's disease. N Engl J Med. 2009;361(13):1268-78.
32. Snow BJ, Rolfe FL, Lockhart MM, Frampton CM, O'Sullivan JD, Fung V, et al. A double-blind, placebo-controlled study to assess the mitochondria-targeted antioxidant MitoQ as a disease-modifying therapy in Parkinson's disease. Mov Disord. 2010;25(11):1670-4.
33. Monti DA, Zabrecky G, Kremens D, Liang T-W, Wintering NA, Cai J, et al. N-acetyl cysteine may support dopamine neurons in Parkinson's disease: preliminary clinical and cell line data. PLoS One. 2016;11(6):e0157602.
34. Banerjee R, Beal MF, Thomas B. Autophagy in neurodegenerative disorders: pathogenic roles and therapeutic implications. Trends Neurosci. 2010;33(12):541-9.
35. Bjørklund G, Hofer T, Nurchi VM, Aaseth J. Iron and other metals in the pathogenesis of Parkinson's disease: Toxic effects and possible detoxification. J Inorg Biochem. 2019;199: 110717.
36. Goldman SM. Environmental toxins and Parkinson's disease. Annu Rev Pharmacol Toxicol. 2014;54:141-64.
37. Nunes-Costa D, Magalhães JD, G-Fernandes M, Cardoso SM, Empadinhas N. Microbial BMAA and the Pathway for Parkinson's Disease Neurodegeneration. Front Aging Neurosci. 2020;7;12:26.
38. Bonifati V. Genetics of Parkinson's disease–state of the art, 2013. Parkinsonism Relat Disord. 2014;20(1):S23-8.
39. Kishore A, Ashok Kumar Sreelatha A, Sturm M, von-Zweydorf F, Pihlstrøm L, Raimondi F, et al. Understanding the role of genetic variability in LRRK2 in Indian population. Mov Disord. 2019;34(4):496-505.
40. Abbas MM, Govindappa ST, Sudhaman S, Thelma BK, Juyal RC, Behari M, et al. Early Onset Parkinson's disease due to DJ1 mutations: An Indian study. Parkinsonism Relat Disord. 2016;32:20-4.
41. Moors TE, Hoozemans JJ, Ingrassia A, Beccari T, Parnetti L, Chartier-Harlin M-C, et al. Therapeutic potential of autophagy-enhancing agents in Parkinson's disease. Mol Neurodegener. 2017;12(1):11.
42. Brahmachari S, Karuppagounder SS, Ge P, Lee S, Dawson VL, Dawson TM, et al. c-Abl and Parkinson's disease: mechanisms and therapeutic potential. J Parkinsons Dis. 2017;7(4): 589-601.
43. Lubomski M, Tan AH, Lim SY, Holmes AJ, Davis RL, Sue CM. Parkinson's disease and the gastrointestinal microbiome. J Neurol. 2020;267(9):2507-23.

44. Skorvanek M, Bhatia KP. The Skin and Parkinson's Disease: Review of Clinical, Diagnostic, and Therapeutic Issues. Mov Disord Clin Pract. 2016;4(1):21-31.
45. Leggio L, Vivarelli S, L'Episcopo F, Tirolo C, Caniglia S, Testa N, et al. microRNAs in Parkinson's disease: from pathogenesis to novel diagnostic and therapeutic approaches. Int J Mol Sci. 2017;18(12):2698.
46. Limphaibool N, Iwanowski P, Holstad MJV, Perkowska K. Parkinsonism in inherited metabolic disorders: key considerations and major features. Front Neurol. 2018;9:857.
47. Leehey M, Luo S, Sharma S, Wills AA, Bainbridge JL, Wong PS, et al. Association of metabolic syndrome and change in Unified Parkinson's Disease Rating Scale scores. Neurology. 2017;89(17):1789-94.
48. Banerjee R, Kaidery NA, Thomas B. (2015). Oxidative stress in Parkinson's disease: Role in neurodegeneration and targets for therapeutics. In S. Andreescu, & M. Hepel (Eds.), Oxidative Stress: Diagnostics, Prevention, and Therapy Volume 2 (pp. 147-176). (ACS Symposium Series; Vol. 1200). American Chemical Society. https://doi.org/10.1021/bk-2015-1200.ch005
49. Müller T, Trommer I, Muhlack S, Mueller BK. Levodopa increases oxidative stress and repulsive guidance molecule A levels: a pilot study in patients with Parkinson's disease. J Neural Transm. 2016;123(4):401-6.
50. Verschuur CVM, Suwijn SR, Boel JA, Post B, Bloem BR, van Hilten JJ, et al. Randomized delayed-start trial of levodopa in Parkinson's disease. N Engl J Med. 2019;380(4):315-24.
51. Ambrosi G, Cerri S, Blandini F. A further update on the role of excitotoxicity in the pathogenesis of Parkinson's disease. J Neural Transm. 2014;121(8):849-59.
52. Domanskyi A, Saarma M, Airavaara M. Prospects of neurotrophic factors for Parkinson's disease: comparison of protein and gene therapy. Hum Gene Ther. 2015;26(8):550-9.
53. Sadhukhan D, Das G, Biswas A, Ghosh S, Das SK, Ray K, et al. Evaluation of FGF 20 variants for susceptibility to Parkinson's disease in Eastern Indians. Neurosci Lett. 2018;675:68-73.
54. Dauer W, Przedborski S. Parkinson's disease: mechanisms and models. Neuron. 2003;39(6):889-909.
55. Brichta L, Greengard P. Molecular determinants of selective dopaminergic vulnerability in Parkinson's disease: an update. Front Neuroanat. 2014;8:152.
56. Espay AJ, Morgante F, Merola A, Fasano A, Marsili L, Fox SH, et al. Levodopa-induced dyskinesia in Parkinson disease: Current and evolving concepts. Ann Neurol. 2018;84(6): 797-811.
57. Bronstein JM, Tagliati M, Alterman RL, Lozano AM, Volkmann J, Stefani A, et al. Deep brain stimulation for Parkinson disease: an expert consensus and review of key issues. Arch Neurol. 2011;68(2):165.
58. Müller T. Catechol-O-methyltransferase inhibitors in Parkinson's disease. Drugs. 2015;75(2):157-74.
59. Niethammer M, Tang CC, LeWitt PA, Rezai AR, Leehey MA, Ojemann SG, et al. Long-term follow-up of a randomized AAV2-GAD gene therapy trial for Parkinson's disease. JCI Insight. 2017;2(7):e90133.
60. Kevadiya BD, Ottemann BM, Thomas MB, Mukadam I, Nigam S, McMillan J, et al. Neurotheranostics as personalized medicines. Adv Drug Deliv Rev. 2019;148:252-89.

CHAPTER 8

Young-onset Parkinson's Disease

Nishan Mol, Rohan Mahale, Ravi Yadav

INTRODUCTION

The term *movement disorders* came into existence in 1968. They are neurologic syndromes in which there is either an excess of movement (*hyperkinesia*) or a paucity of voluntary and automatic movements (*hypokinesia/bradykinesia/akinesia*), unrelated to weakness or spasticity. The slowness of movement is termed as *bradykinesia* and paucity or absence of movement (*akinesias*) and *hypokinesia* to describe a reduction in amplitude of movement.[1] Parkinson's disease (PD) is an α-synucleinopathy characterized by early prominent death of dopaminergic neurons in the substantia nigra (SN) pars compacta (SNpc) and wide spread presence of Lewy bodies in the brain including SN. PD is associated with motor symptoms that include bradykinesia, rigidity, rest tremors, and postural instability (advanced stage) and have levodopa response. Mild Parkinsonian syndromes can occur in up to 25% of elderly persons without PD.[2] Young-onset PD (YOPD) or also referred as early-onset PD commonly defined as onset of motor symptoms occurring in those aged 21–40 years and is clinically similar to older-onset PD (OOPD). Juvenile PD is defined as onset of motor symptoms of PD at or before age 20 years.[3] It is commonly familial. By contrast, YOPD is less commonly familial and both the clinical picture and the pathology, except some of the genetic forms, usually resemble that of OOPD. Secondary Parkinsonism is much less common in young-onset age group and becomes increasingly rare with increasing age at onset. Nevertheless, Wilson's disease, dopa-responsive dystonia, drug-induced Parkinsonism, and structural causes must be excluded in any young patient presenting with Parkinsonism even in the absence of other neurological feature and various other diagnoses might need consideration depending on the clinical phenotype.[4]

Young-onset PD affects people when they are in the prime of their productivity. The estimated prevalence of YOPD in Europe is 12–20 per 100,000, constituting 5–7% of PD patients in the western hemisphere and up to 45 per 100,000 among those living in Asian countries constituting 10–14% in Japan.[5] However, population-based epidemiological data and data on nonwhites with YOPD are limited. Patients with YOPD show increased genetic predisposition, have slower progression, frequently associated with psychiatric disorders such as depression, anxiety, and psychosis, and increased risk of levodopa-related complications as compared to OOPD. They have longer disease duration and suffer from more physical, economic, and psychological consequences.[6,7] Dementia in PD is more strongly associated with older age at onset than the duration of illness. Patients with OOPD have an increased risk of dementia as compared to those without PD. The risk of dementia in YOPD is less clear. The survival for PD patients was 32 years in YOPD [age at onset (AAO) ≤49 years], 18.5 years in PD with AAO = 50–69 years, and 9.3 years in PD with AAO ≥ 70 years.[8] The presence of positive family history of PD is about 20% in YOPD patients as compared to 6.9% of OOPD patients. The age-specific risk of PD is 7.8-fold higher in the relatives of patients with YOPD compared to 2.9-fold among the relatives of patients with OOPD.[9]

The diagnosis of YOPD is a challenge to neurologists even though YOPD have a clinical presentation similar to OOPD. Neurologists seem to give preference to diagnoses other than PD in patients with symptoms presenting at young-onset. YOPD patients more likely receive a functional (psychogenic) diagnosis.[10] There is also an element of decreased acceptance of the diagnosis of PD by younger patients resulting in delayed initiation of the appropriate therapy and further increasing the negative impact of the disease on all aspects of the patient's life.

The predominant initial motor symptoms in YOPD patients are the rigidity and painful cramps while gait instability as the predominant initial symptom was more frequent in older-onset patients. The frequency of tremors and bradykinesia is similar in both groups. Dystonia as a presenting motor symptom was reported in 20% of YOPD (AAO < 45) but only 3% of late-onset PD (LOPD) (AAO > 64).[11] The motor symptoms have slower progression in YOPD patients as compared to those with OOPD.[12] Levodopa-related motor fluctuations and dyskinesia with a shorter latency from treatment onset are more common in patients with YOPD compared to those with OOPD. There is increase in dopamine turnover as compared with the decrease in dopamine synthesis and storage rate in patients of YOPD. These greater alterations of dopamine turn over in YOPD lead to larger swings in synaptic dopamine levels, which may contribute to a greater risk of motor fluctuations in YOPD.[13] YOPD patients have longer presymptomatic phase and more damage to the dopaminergic system before motor symptoms develop. The greater extent of neuronal loss in YOPD patients with similar severity of motor symptoms as compared to OOPD patients contributes to increased frequency of dyskinesia in YOPD patients.[14] Hence delaying initiation of levodopa therapy in YOPD patients does not necessarily prevent levodopa-related complications. There is a common practice to avoid the use of levodopa as long as possible, especially in YOPD, and to consider alternatives such as dopamine agonists. This leads in the delay in initiation of effective treatment in individuals who need it the most, the productive patients with YOPD.[15] Dopamine agonists are associated with sudden sleep attacks and side effects such as edema and impulse control disorder such as hypersexuality, compulsive shopping, and gambling.[16] Levodopa should be started as soon as it is required to reduce motor disability and its impact on professional and family life, with fewer potentially serious side effects than dopamine agonists.

Nonmotor symptoms such as depression, loss of libido, sexual dysfunction, restless legs syndrome, and also occur in YOPD patients along with motor symptoms contributing to occupational and social disability. PD patients are at higher risk for addictive behaviors due to the disease itself, but also due to dopaminergic medications used to treat the motor symptoms of PD. Impulse control disorders, such as gambling, compulsive shopping, and sexual addiction were nearly three-fold more in patients taking dopamine agonists and a 50% increase associated with levodopa treatment.[16] Dopamine dysregulation syndrome (DDRS) has also been seen with YOPD patients, especially in males.[17] DDRS manifests in younger male patients with minimal motor symptoms but have dyskinesia and take dopaminergic medications despite being in a pronounced dyskinetic state. It is a manifestation of hyperdopaminergic state leading to compulsive symptoms with impulsivity secondary to hypersensitivity to reward in PD. In DDRS, patient self-medicate with high doses of dopaminergic medications, particularly the short-acting dopamine agonist apomorphine and levodopa. Dopamine transporter (DAT) scans in patients with YOPD have shown sparing of caudate as compared with the putamen. However, in OOPD patients, there is uniform involvement of caudate and putamen. Caudate is involved in psychomotor and complex cognitive functions. The relative sparing of caudate in YOPD patients may explain the lower prevalence of nonmotor symptoms in YOPD compared to OOPD.[18] The clinical symptomatology which are less frequent in YOPD is summarized in **Box 1**.

Box 1 Findings that are less frequent, less severe or delayed in YOPD compared to LOPD.[40]

- Disease progression
- Gait disturbances including freezing of gait
- Falls
- Dementia
- Anxiety
- Psychosis
- Double vision
- Gastrointestinal complaints (constipation and gastroparesis)
- Urinary complaints
- Impairment of taste and smell
- Daytime sleepiness
- REM sleep behavior disorders
- Insomnia
- Nightmares

(LOPD: late-onset Parkinson's disease; REM: rapid-eye-movement; YOPD: young-onset Parkinson's disease)

Young-onset PD patients are at risk of exhibiting anger and self-destructive patterns of behavior due to poorly developed coping skills. They are more vulnerable to the lure of "miracle cures" and unproven therapies such as supplements and stem cells. A multidisciplinary team approach is needed to educate them about their disease and providing adequate coping strategies and support system.[19]

GENETICS

Genetics contribute to the etiology of YOPD more commonly than PD with later-onset. Mutations (deletions, multiplications, and point mutations) in the *parkin* gene are the most common cause of autosomal recessive YOPD. The *parkin* gene (*PRKN*) in the PARK2 locus on the long-arm of chromosome 6 is an E3-type ubiquitin protein ligase that is involved in the proteosomal degradation of α-synuclein. It also protects mitochondrial deoxyribonucleic acid (DNA) from oxidative damage and stimulates its repair. Hence, loss of function mutation of *parkin* gene causes oxidative damage to mitochondrial DNA. Dystonia is a common feature, making it difficult to distinguish from dopa-responsive dystonia.[20] However, majority of patients with *parkin* mutation develop early and marked levodopa-induced motor fluctuations and dyskinesias. Patients show good response to anticholinergics and are very sensitive to small doses of levodopa; small doses can cause severe dyskinesia and occasional psychosis.[20] The disease progression is slow with low prevalence of dementia. Early postural instability, freezing, festination, autonomic dysfunction, brisk reflexes, and sleep benefit can also occur. The occurrence of psychiatric disturbance, including anxiety, psychosis, obsessive-compulsive disorder, and early behavioral disturbances is common.[21] Olfaction is relatively preserved in *parkin* mutation-related PD.[22] Histopathological studies have shown severe neuronal degeneration and gliosis in the SN, moderate decrease in locus coeruleus. Lewy bodies have not been found in PD patients with *parkin* mutation.

The second most common cause of autosomal recessive YOPD is *PINK1* (PTEN-induced putative kinase) gene mutation at PARK6 locus on chromosome 1p36–p35. The *PINK1* gene mutation suggests the involvement of kinase signaling pathway in the pathogenesis of dopaminergic nigral cell death. *PINK1* is localized to mitochondria in the intermembrane space.[23] It phosphorylates tumor necrosis factor (TNF) receptor-associated protein 1 (TRAP1) and protects against oxidative stress-induced cell death. It also phosphorylates cytoplasmic *parkin* attached to damaged mitochondria and helps in elimination of damaged mitochondria through mitophagy. Patients with *PINK1* mutation presents with asymmetric onset rest tremors, bradykinesia, and rigidity with good levodopa response and slow progression. The clinical phenotype is similar to *parkin*-related PD; however, dystonia and sleep benefit are less common. Dementia has also been reported in cases with deletions in *PINK1* gene.[24] Another gene-associated with YOPD is *DJ-1* at PARK7 locus in chromosome 1p36. It constitutes about 1% of YOPD. The clinical features are similar to *parkin* and *PINK1* mutation with high rate of dystonia and psychiatric disturbances. It is involved in protection from oxidative stress.[25]

Mutations of *ATP13A2* gene (*PARK*9) located on chromosome 1 (1p36.13) causes autosomal recessive young-onset atypical Parkinsonism (Kufor–Rakeb syndrome). The *ATP13A2* gene encodes a lysosomal P5-type transport ATPase protein. It protects against α-synuclein induced neurodegeneration. Kufor–Rakeb syndrome has signs of pyramidal degeneration, dementia, levodopa-responsive Parkinsonism, facial-faucial-finger mini-myoclonus, slow saccades, and supranuclear gaze paresis. Generalized brain atrophy and iron accumulation in the basal ganglia are also found in imaging studies. The levodopa-responsive Parkinsonism is associated with early levodopa-induced motor fluctuations and dyskinesias. Hallucinations and dystonia are also usually seen.[26] The *PLA2G6* gene encodes an enzyme, phospholipase A2, which hydrolysis glycerophospholipids and maintains cell membrane homeostasis. *PLA2G6* recessive mutations cause early-onset dystonia-Parkinsonism with the presence of Lewy bodies (PARK14). Patients with PARK14 mutations present with rapid cognitive decline, Parkinsonism, ataxia and/or dystonia, pyramidal features, eye movement abnormalities, psychiatric features such as depression, aggressive behavior, and irritability, dysautonomic signs such as urinary urgency or incontinence, a good response to levodopa, but with rapid-onset of treatment-induced dyskinesias.[27] The gene *FBXO7* encodes F-box protein 7, which is involved in mitochondrial maintenance in interaction with *PINK1* and *Parkin*. The mutations in the gene cause juvenile or young-onset Parkinsonism with pyramidal signs and less frequent tremors (PARK15). Cognitive decline, upgaze paresis, or dysautonomic features are less common. Patients usually had a good response to levodopa with treatment-induced psychiatric features and dyskinesias.[28] Mutations in the gene *DNAJC6* cause an impairment of synaptic vesicle recycling and could perturb endocytosis. This results in early-onset Parkinsonism with postural instability and good levodopa response (PARK19). Seizures, cognitive decline, and hallucinations can occur. Gaze paresis, autonomic dysfunction, and cerebellar signs are not seen. The disease progression is rapid with wheel-chair bound state within 2–10 years of onset.[29] Mutation of the gene *SYNJ1* that encodes a protein synaptojanin 1, a phosphoinositide phosphatase alter the endolysosomal pathway, resulting in a defect of synaptic vesicle recycling. This leads to early-onset autosomal recessive Parkinsonism (PARK20). The age at onset is between 20 and 40 years. Patients present with Parkinsonism with poor response to levodopa or early-onset of treated-induced dyskinesias. Most patients also have epilepsy and cognitive decline whereas, supranuclear upward vertical gaze limitation, dysarthria, and dysphagia are less frequent.[30] Mutations in *VPS13C* gene cause early-onset PD with good response to dopaminergic treatment (PARK23). This may be associated with dystonia and pyramidal signs progressing to spastic tetraplegia as the disease progress. Rapid cognitive decline can also occurs.[31]

Mutations (duplication, triplication, and point mutations) in *α-synuclein* gene (*SNCA*) at the chromosome 4q21–q23, although rare, cause PD to occur at a younger age (PARK4). The inheritance is autosomal dominant. Apart from the typical features of motor Parkinsonism, patient may have prominent dementia, psychiatric disturbances, myoclonus, and autonomic dysfunction. Histopathological studies have shown loss of dopaminergic neurons with extensive Lewy pathology in SN, brainstem nuclei, limbic system, hippocampus, and neocortex.[32] Mutations in the leucine-rich repeat kinase 2 (*LRRK2*) gene coding for the protein dardarin cause autosomal dominant PD. The usual age of onset is above 50 years with clinical features similar to idiopathic PD; however YOPD can occur with this gene mutation. The histopathology is highly variable. This includes typical Lewy-body pathology in the brainstem or more widespread Lewy-body deposition as seen in diffuse Lewy-body disease, neurofibrillary tangles similar to progressive supranuclear palsy, or pure nigrostriatal cell loss.[33] Mutation of the *VPS35* gene (PARK17) cause occurrence of PD in the fourth or fifth decade. It encodes a protein that regulates synaptic endocytosis and synaptic vesicle regeneration through the Rab-mediated endocytic pathway. Tremor is the predominant symptom, with good response to levodopa and no atypical signs. Disease progression is slow and cognitive impairment or neuropsychiatric signs are rare.[34] The gene *GCH1* encodes GTP cyclohydrolase 1 involved in the synthesis of tetrahydrobiopterin, a cofactor of tyrosine hydroxylase, and the synthesis of monoamines, including dopamine. Mutations in *GCH1* are the most common cause of dopa-responsive dystonia. However, the mutation can also present as early-onset PD with prominent nonmotor signs, such as cognitive impairment, hyposmia, dysautonomic features, and sleep disorders.[35] Mutation in *ATXN2* gene that causes spinocerebellar ataxia type 2 can also cause YOPD with clinical features similar to idiopathic PD. There was no cognitive decline or ophthalmoplegia or cerebellar symptoms.[36] The genetic forms of YOPD with mode of inheritance is summarized in **Box 2**. Lastly, heterozygous mutations in the *glucocerebrosidase* gene (GBA) cause PD to occur at a younger age. They frequently manifest with nonmotor symptoms of cognitive impairment, neuropsychiatric disturbances, and autonomic dysfunction with rapid disease progression and reduced survival rates. It is one of the strongest genetic risk factors for occurrence of sporadic PD.[37]

Box 2 Genetic forms of YOPD.[40]

Genetic forms:

- PARK-SNCA (PARK1 and 4, 4q21–23); autosomal dominant
- PARK-*Parkin* (PARK2, 6q25.2–27); autosomal recessive
- PARK-*PINK1* (PARK6, 1p36); autosomal recessive
- PARK-*DJ-1* (PARK7, 1p36); autosomal recessive
- PARK-*LRRK2* (PARK8, 12q12); autosomal dominant
- PARK-*ATP13A2* (PARK9, 1p36); Kufor–Rakeb syndrome; autosomal recessive
- PARK-*PLA2G6* (PARK14, 22q13.1); PLAN; autosomal recessive
- PARK-*FBXO7* (PARK15, 22q12–q13); early-onset Parkinsonian-pyramidal disease
- PARK-*VPS35* (PARK17, 12q11.2); autosomal dominant
- PARK-*DNAJC6* (PARK19, 1p31.3); autosomal recessive
- PARK-*SYNJ1* (PARK20, 21q22.11); autosomal recessive
- PARK-*VPS13C* (PARK23, 15q22.2); autosomal recessive
- *ATXN2* (12q24.12); autosomal dominant
- *GCH1* (14q22.2); autosomal dominant

(YOPD: young-onset Parkinson's disease)

About 50% of patients with YOPD and positive family history have *parkin* gene mutations. In isolated cases of early-onset PD, about 80% of those with onset before age 20 years will harbor a *parkin* gene mutation, but in patients with onset over age 30 years this figure is reduced to around 3%. Some cases of idiopathic YOPD may also be due to either very rare and atypical genetic abnormalities, or as yet unidentified genetic defects. However, most patients with YOPD will not have an identifiable genetic cause.[38]

Apart from genetic factors, environmental factors may also play a role in YOPD etiology. Aguiar et al. (2008) observed higher exposure to well-water drinking in the YOPD patient group. Most of the patients were exposed during the first or second decades of life, for an average period of 14.3 years.[39] The other potential environmental risk factors included pesticides, herbicides, and organic solvents exposure.

HOW TO DIAGNOSE?

The clinical presentation and presence or absence of family history should guide investigations in YOPD. Patients presenting with atypical features along with Parkinsonism requires detailed investigation to exclude secondary causes of Parkinsonism. The differential diagnoses for YOPD are illustrated in **Box 3**.[40] Wilson's disease, neurodegeneration with brain iron accumulation (NBIA), dopa-responsive dystonia, structural brain lesions, and drug-induced Parkinsonism should be considered and excluded. History of neuroleptic or antiemetic drug use should be sought, and measurement of serum copper, ceruloplasmin, urinary 24 hours copper excretion, assessment for Kayser–Fleischer rings, and brain magnetic resonance imaging (MRI) should be considered. Genetic testing is available for the detection of mutations in the GTP cyclohydrolase I (*GTP-CH1*) gene in suspected cases of dopa-responsive dystonia. In patients with pure Parkinsonism and juvenile to young-onset, *parkin* gene mutations are the most probable diagnosis.

MANAGEMENT

Pharmacological Treatment

To date, the most effective treatment for PD has been shown to be levodopa. It is effective in treating symptoms such as bradykinesia and rigidity. The effects of levodopa on postural stability, speech, and gait disturbance are less pronounced. The initiation of pharmacotherapy (timing and choice of medications) in YOPD is a complex

Box 3 Differential diagnosis of YOPD.[40]

- Wilson's disease
- NBIA-PKAN (PANK2, 20p13)
- MPAN (C19orf12, 19q12)—neurodegeneration with brain iron accumulation 4
- BPAN (WDR45, Xp11.23)—beta-propeller protein-associated neurodegeneration
- Huntington disease (Westphal variant) (HTT, 4p16.3)
- DYT3 (TAF1, Xq13.1)—Lubag disease
- DYT5 (GCH1, 14q22.1–q22.2)—dopa responsive dystonia
- DYT12 (ATP1A3, 19q13.2)—rapid-onset dystonia Parkinsonism
- DYT16 (PRKRA, 2q31.2)—young-onset dystonia Parkinsonism
- GBA, 1q21—Gaucher's disease
- Spinocerebellar ataxia 2 (ATXN2, 12q24)
- Spinocerebellar ataxia 3 (ATXN3, 14q32.12)
- Chorea-acanthocytosis (VPS13A, 9q21.2)
- Niemann-Pick type C (NPC1, 18q11.2 or NPC2, 14q24.3)
- Autosomal recessive hereditary spastic paraplegia (SPG-11; 15q21.1) and (SPG7, 16q24.3)
- Frontotemporal dementia and Parkinsonism linked to chromosome 17 (MAPT, 17q21.31)
- Cerebrotendinous xanthomatosis (CYP27A1, 2q35)
- Dentatorubral-pallidoluysian atrophy (ATN1, 12p13.31)
- Juvenile neuronal ceroid lipofuscinoses (multiple genes and disorders)
- Neuronal intranuclear (hyaline) inclusion body disease (NIID)
- Mitochondrial diseases
- 22q11.2 deletion syndrome
- Chediak–Higashi syndrome (LYST, 1q42.3)
- *Paraneoplastic:*
  - Anti-Ma2-paraneoplastic limbic encephalitis
  - Anti-N-methyl-D-aspartate receptor (anti-NMDAR) encephalitis
- *Central nervous system infections:*
  - Encephalitis lethargica
  - Japanese encephalitis
  - HIV/AIDS encephalitis
  - Mycoplasma
  - Neurosyphilis
  - Prion diseases
  - Progressive multifocal leukoencephalopathy
  - Toxoplasmosis
  - Subacute sclerosing panencephalitis
- *Miscellaneous*
  - Drug-induced Parkinsonism
  - Structural lesion (vascular, tumoral, and demyelinating)
  - Hydrocephalus
  - Hypoparathyroidism
  - Pseudohypoparathyroidism
  - Chronic liver failure
  - Extrapontine myelinolysis
  - Systemic lupus erythematosus
  - Carbon monoxide, cyanide, and methanol poisoning

treatment decision that depends on disease severity, functional disability, and psychosocial handicap. The treatment with levodopa is associated with the early and prominent occurrence of motor complications, namely dyskinesia which can occur as early as within the first week of treatment with levodopa. A quarter of patients developed after 5 years of levodopa treatment, and after 12 years, all patients had motor fluctuations with dyskinesias.[3] Therefore, the treatment with levodopa needs to be delayed in YOPD. However, the independent risk factor for the development of motor fluctuations and dyskinesias is the age of disease onset, younger the age of onset shorter is the latency to develop motor fluctuations.[41] The initiation of levodopa early at the disease onset may not solely contribute to early development of motor fluctuations and dyskinesias. Thus, delaying the initiation of levodopa in patients with YOPD is not appropriate as they need it the most, the otherwise productive patients with YOPD, with greater cumulative disability.[15]

Other medications include dopamine agonists, inhibitors of monoamine oxidase-B (MAO-B) (selegiline hydrochloride or rasagiline mesilate), and amantadine hydrochloride. They can be used alone or in combination with levodopa. The use of dopamine agonists rather than levodopa is associated with a decreased risk of developing motor complications. However, dopamine agonists have its own side effects as stated earlier, which are more prominent in YOPD. MAO-B inhibitors and amantadine are used as an adjunct to levodopa.

In the advanced stage of PD in YOPD, motor complications such as wearing-off, unpredictable offs, and dyskinesias predominate. Therefore addition and manipulation of doses of levodopa, dopamine agonists, MAO-B inhibitors, and inhibitors of catechol-O-methyl transferase (COMT) can all be helpful in improving these complications. COMT inhibitors in combination with levodopa enhance the efficacy of levodopa on motor symptoms of PD due to prolongation of its effect.

Young-onset PD patients face a lifetime of progressive disease and several years of therapy. They may be good candidates for continuous apomorphine infusions, stereotactic surgery, or continuous levodopa treatment once dose adjustment of oral antiparkinsonian drugs is exhausted.

Surgery

Deep Brain Stimulation

Stimulation of the subthalamic nucleus (STN) can ameliorate the on-off motor fluctuations and levodopa-induced dyskinesia.[42] The effects of STN stimulation on the cardinal motor symptoms of PD are comparable to a response from maximal dose of levodopa but without fluctuations and dyskinesia. A good presurgical levodopa-reactivity of motor symptoms is a predictive factor for good postsurgical improvement of motor function.[43] YOPD patients are better candidates for STN-deep brain stimulation (STN-DBS). Early introduction of STN stimulation appears to preserve a better motor function and quality of life during the prime of YOPD patient's life.[44] In YOPD patients, STN-DBS remains effective to improve motor disabilities over 7 years and is a safe procedure concerning cognitive outcome and morbidity.[45]

Novel Therapies

These therapies are currently in experimental stages of development and have not been Food and Drug Administration (FDA) approved. These therapies focus very little on the YOPD subgroup of patients. Further research is required to test their efficacy on YOPD patients specifically.

Gene Therapy

In-vivo gene therapy is a new approach. Gene transfer of glutamic acid decarboxylase (GAD), rate-limiting enzyme in gamma-aminobutyric acid (GABA) production modulate the production of GABA in the STN, and improve basal ganglia function in Parkinsonism in animal models. The effect of bilateral delivery of adeno-associated viral vector (AAV2)-GAD in the STN compared with sham surgery in patients with advanced PD showed significant improvement from baseline in Unified PD Rating Scale (UPDRS) scores compared with sham group over the course of 6 months.[46] However, usage of neurturin, a naturally occurring analog of glial cell-line-derived neurotrophic factor, by bilateral delivery of AAV2-neurturin into the putamen and SN showed no motor score improvement even after 12 months of follow-up.[47] YOPD patients could be the best candidates for gene therapy, because they have a slower disease progression and more competent compensatory mechanisms, and this could be beneficial for effects of transplantations.

Cell-based Therapy

The transplantation of fetal ventral mesencephalic (VM) tissue into the striatum of young PD patients showed marked motor improvement and increased fluorodopa uptake in the striatum on positron emission tomography (PET) imaging. The transplanted fetal VM tissue can survive up to a decade and provide sustained motor benefits in PD.[48]

Adjuvant Therapies

Along with the pharmacological treatment, physical and occupational therapy in YOPD patients should be used which assist in the rehabilitation process. The initiation of an exercise program from the earliest stages of PD might benefit secondary motor problems involving arm swing, gait, and posture. Exercise has been shown to improve physical function, health-related quality of life, leg strength, balance, and gait speed in PD. YOPD patients with speech difficulties might benefit from intensive voice therapy to maintain employment and social activity.

CONCLUSION

Young-onset PD is very similar to OOPD in many ways. However, the treatment approach is slightly different for YOPD patients as they have slower disease progression, an increased rate of dystonia at the onset, a lower rate of dementia, and an increased rate of levodopa-induced dyskinesias. YOPD patients are also ideal candidates for DBS therapy with medium to long-term lower incidence of stimulation and medication resistant symptoms. Regular physical exercise and physical therapy must be encouraged. Apart from the motor complications, YOPD patients also have psychological disability which is often overlooked and results in decrease in the quality of life. A comprehensive treatment plan that includes motor symptoms and nonmotor symptoms is necessary for YOPD patients to improve quality of life and occupational capabilities.

REFERENCES

1. Fahn S. Classification of movement disorders. Mov Disord. 2011;26(6):947-57.
2. Postuma RB, Berg D, Stern M, Poewe W, Olanow CW, Oertel W, et al. MDS clinical diagnostic criteria for Parkinson's disease. Mov Disord. 2015;30(12):1591-601.
3. Quinn N, Critchley P, Marsden CD. Young onset Parkinson's disease. Mov Disord. 1987;2(2):73-91.
4. Klepac N, Habek M, Adamec I, Barušić AK, Bach I, Margetić E, et al. An update on the management of young-onset Parkinson's disease. Degener Neurol Neuromuscul Dis. 2013; 2:53-62.
5. Golbe LI. Young-onset Parkinson's disease: a clinical review. Neurology. 1991;41:168-73.
6. Schrag A, Ben-Shlomo Y, Brown R, Marsden CD, Quinn N. Young-onset Parkinson's disease revisited-clinical features, natural history, and mortality. Mov Disord. 1998;13(6): 885-94.
7. Calne SM, Kumar A. Young onset Parkinson's disease. Practical management of medical issues. Parkinsonism Relat Disord. 2008;14(2):133-42.
8. Mehanna R, Moore S, Hou JG, Sarwar AI, Lai EC. Comparing clinical features of young onset, middle onset and late onset

Parkinson's disease. Parkinsonism Relat Disord. 2014;20(5): 530-4.
9. Payami H, Zareparsi S, James D, Nutt J. Familial aggregation of Parkinson's disease: a comparative study of early-onset and late-onset disease. Arch Neurol. 2002;59(5):848-50.
10. Thenganatt MA, Jancovic J. Functional (Psychogenic) Parkinsonism. In: Hallett M, Stone J, Carson A (Eds). Functional Neurologic Disorders, Handbook of Clinical Neurology. Amsterdam, Netherlands: Elsevier; 2017;139:259-62.
11. Wickremaratchi MM, Knipe MD, Sastry BS, Morgan E, Jones A, Salmon R, et al. The motor phenotype of Parkinson's disease in relation to age at onset. Mov Disord. 2011;26(3):457-63.
12. Kempster PA, O'Sullivan SS, Holton JL, Revesz T, Lees AJ. Relationships between age and late progression of Parkinson's disease: a clinico-pathological study. Brain 2010;133(Pt 6): 1755-62.
13. Sossi V, de la Fuente-Fernandez R, Schulzer M, Adams J, Stoessl J. Age-related differences in levodopa dynamics in Parkinson's: implications for motor complications. Brain. 2006;129(Pt 4): 1050-8.
14. de la Fuente-Fernandez R, Schulzer M, Kuramoto L, Cragg J, Ramachandiran N, Au WL, et al. Age-specific progression of nigrostriatal dysfunction inParkinson's disease, Ann Neurol. 2011;69(5):803-10.
15. Espay AJ, Lang AE. Levodopa and Parkinson disease-myths revisited-reply. JAMA Neurol. 2017;74(10):1270-1.
16. Vela L, Martinez Castrillo JC, Garcia Ruiz P, Gasca-Salas C, Macias Macias Y, Perez Fernandez E, et al. The high prevalence of impulse control behaviors in patients with early-onset Parkinson disease: a cross-sectional multicenter study. J Neurol Sci. 2016;368:150-4.
17. Barbosa P, Djamshidian A, Lees AJ, Warner TT. The outcome of dopamine dysregulation syndrome in Parkinson's disease: a retrospective postmortem study. Mov Disord Clin Pract. 2018; 5(5):519-22.
18. Liu SY, Wu JJ, Zhao J, Huang SF, Wang YX, Ge JJ, et al. Onset-related subtypes of Parkinson's disease differ in the patterns of striatal dopaminergic dysfunction: a positron emission tomography study. Parkinsonism Relat Disord. 2015;21(12):1448-53.
19. Robledo I, Jankovic J. Media hype: Patient and scientific perspectives on misleading medical news. Mov Disord. 2017;32(9):1319-23.
20. Khan NL, Graham E, Critchley P, Schrag AE, Wood NW, Lees AJ, et al. Parkin disease: a phenotypic study of a large case series. Brain. 2003;126(Pt 6):1279-92.
21. Lohmann E, Periquet M, Bonifati V, Wood NW, De Michele G, Bonnet AM, et al. How much phenotypic variation can be attributed to parkin genotype? Ann Neurol. 2003;54(2): 176-85.
22. Khan NL, Katzenschlager R, Watt H, Bhatia KP, Wood NW, Quinn N, et al. Olfaction differentiates parkin disease from early-onset parkinsonism and Parkinson disease. Neurology. 2004;62(7):1224-6.
23. Valente EM, Abou-Sleiman PM, Caputo V, Muqit MMK, Harvey K, Gispert S, et al. Hereditary early-onset Parkinson's disease caused by mutations in PINK1. Science. 2004:304(5674): 1158-60.
24. Li Y, Tomiyama H, Sato K, Hatano Y, Yoshino H, Atsumi M, et al. Clinicogenetic study of PINK1 mutations in autosomal recessive early-onset parkinsonism. Neurology. 2005;64(11):1955-7.
25. Dekker M, Bonifati V, van Swieten J, Leenders N, Galjaard RJ, Snijders P, et al. Clinical features and neuroimaging of PARK7-linked parkinsonism. Mov Disord. 2003;18(7):751-7.
26. Fonzo AD, Chien HF, Socal M, Giraudo S, Tassorelli C, Iliceto G, et al. ATP13A2 missense mutations in juvenile parkinsonism and young onset Parkinson disease. Neurology. 2007;68(19):1557-62.
27. Paisan-Ruiz C, Bhatia KP, Li A, Hernandez D, Davis M, Wood NW, et al. Characterization of PLA2G6 as a locus for dystonia-parkinsonism. Ann Neurol. 2009;65(1):19-23.
28. Fonzo AD, Dekker MCJ, Montagna P, Baruzzi A, Yonova EH, Guedes LC, et al. FBXO7 mutations cause autosomal recessive, early-onset parkinsonian-pyramidal syndrome. Neurology. 2009;72(3):240-5.
29. Olgiati S, Quadri M, Fang M, Rood JPMA, Saute JA, Chien HF, et al. DNAJC6 mutations associated with early-onset Parkinson's disease. Ann Neurol. 2016;79(2):244-56.
30. Quadri M, Fang M, Picillo M, Olgiati S, Breedveld GJ, Graafland J, et al. Mutation in the SYNJ1 gene associated with autosomal recessive, early-onset Parkinsonism. Hum Mutat. 2013;34(9):1208-15.
31. Lesage S, Drouet V, Majounie E, Deramecourt V, Jacoupy M, Nicolas A, et al. Loss of VPS13C function in autosomal-recessive Parkinsonism causes mitochondrial dysfunction and increases PINK1/Parkin-dependent mitophagy. Am J Hum Genet. 2016;98(3):500-13.
32. Kasten M, Klein C. The many faces of alpha-synuclein mutations. Mov Disord. 2013;28(6):697-701.
33. Zabetian CP, Samii A, Mosley AD, Roberts JW, Leis BC, et al. A clinic-based study of the LRRK2 gene in Parkinson disease yields new mutations. Neurology. 2005;65(5):741-4.
34. Vilarino-Guell C, Wider C, Ross OA, Dachsel JC, Kachergus JM, Lincoln SJ, et al. VPS35 mutations in Parkinson disease. Am J Hum Genet. 2011;89(1):162-7.
35. Mencacci NE, Isaias IU, Reich MM, Ganos C, Plagnol V, Polke JM, et al. Parkinson's disease in GTP cyclohydrolase 1 mutation carriers. Brain. 2014;137(Pt 9):2480-92.
36. Kim YE, Jeon B, Farrer MJ, Scott E, Guella I, Park SS, et al. SCA2 family presenting as typical Parkinson's disease: 34 year follow up. Parkinsonism Relat Disord. 2017;40:69-72.
37. Neumann J, Bras J, Deas E, O'Sullivan SS, Parkkinen L, Lachmann RH, et al. Glucocerebrosidase mutations in clinical and pathologically proven Parkinson's disease. Brain. 2009;132(7):1783-94.
38. Lucking CB, Durr A, Bonifati V, Vaughan J, De Michele G, Gasser T, et al. Association between early-onset Parkinson's disease and mutations in the parkin gene. N Engl J Med. 2000;342(21):1560-7.
39. Aguiar Pde C, Lessa PS, Godeiro C Jr, Barsottini O, Felício AC, Borges V, et al. Genetic and environmental findings in early-onset Parkinson's disease Brazilian patients. Mov Disord. 2008;23(9):1228-33.
40. Mehanna R, Jankovic J. Young-onset Parkinson's disease: Its unique features and their impact on quality of life. Parkinsonism Relat Disord. 2019;65:39-48.
41. Spica V, Pekmezovic T, Svetel M, Kostic VS. Prevalence of non-motor symptoms in young-onset versus late-onset Parkinson's disease. J Neurol. 2013;260(1):131-7.
42. Kumar R, Lozano AM, Kim YJ, Hutchison WD, Sime E, Halket E, et al. Double-blind evaluation of subthalamic nucleus deep brain stimulation in advanced Parkinson's disease. Neurology. 1998;51(3):850-5.

43. Welter ML, Houeto JL, Tezenas du Montcel S, Mesnage V, Bonnet AM, Pillon B, et al. Clinical predictive factors of subthalamic stimulation in Parkinson's disease. Brain. 2002;125(3):575-83.
44. Otaka T, Oshima H, Katayama Y, Kano T, Kobayashi K, Suzuki Y, et al. Impact of subthalamic nucleus stimulation on young-onset Parkinson's disease. Neuromodulation. 2010;13(1): 10-6.
45. Tsai ST, Hung HY, Hsieh TC, Lin SH, Lin SZ, Chen SY. Long-term outcome of young-onset Parkinson's disease after subthalamic stimulation—a cross-sectional study. Clin Neurol Neurosurg. 2013;115(10):2082-7.
46. LeWitt PA, Rezai AR, Leehey MA, Ojemann SG, Flaherty AW, Eskandar EN, et al. AAV2-GAD gene therapy for advanced Parkinson's disease: a double-blind, sham-surgery controlled, randomised trial. Lancet Neurol. 2011;10(4):309-19.
47. Olanow CW, Bartus RT, Baumann TL, Factor S, Boulis N, Stacy M, et al. Gene delivery of neurturin to putamen and substantia nigra in Parkinson's disease: A double-blind, randomized, controlled trial. Ann Neurol. 2015;78(2):248-57.
48. Piccini P, Brooks DJ, Björklund A, Gunn RN, Grasby PM, Rimoldi O, et al. Dopamine release from nigral transplants visualized in vivo in a Parkinson's patient. Nat Neurosci. 1999;2(12):1137-40.

SECTION

3

NON-MOTOR SYMPTOMS OF MOVEMENT DISORDERS

CHAPTER 9

Psychosis and Mood Disorders in Parkinson's Disease

Jimmy A Lalkaka, Varhsa A Patil, Bhimsen Singhal

INTRODUCTION

Of all the nonmotor symptoms (NMS) of Parkinson's disease (PD), neuropsychiatric manifestations are arguably the most disabling. They are associated with poor long-term outcomes and increased caregiver distress.[1] Dementia, depression, and psychosis are most common. Other clinically significant psychiatric complications include anxiety, disturbances of sleep, and wakefulness, impulse control disorders, apathy, and fatigue. This chapter gives an overview of psychosis and mood disorders (depression, anxiety, and apathy) in PD.

PSYCHOSIS

Psychosis generally occurs during the advanced stage of the disease. It has a lifetime cumulative prevalence of 60% in PD.[2] It is associated with a poor quality of life and is the single greatest risk factor for nursing home placement.[3] PD psychosis (PD-P) is an independent predictor of increased mortality[4] and also the most important factor responsible for caregiver distress.[5]

Clinical Features

Psychosis is a clinical syndrome of hallucinations and delusions. In hallucinations, stimuli in one of the five special senses are perceived, that have no basis in reality. Visual hallucinations (VH) are most common in PD-P, while auditory hallucinations (AH) are half as common.[6] Tactile and olfactory hallucinations are also known to occur.[7] The VH are typically vivid and well-formed, mostly of people or animals. They occur more in the evenings in a low stimulus environment. They disappear when the patient tries to approach them, but reappear in the same stereotyped form with variable frequency. Sometimes, AH accompany VH. They are heard as indistinct voices without the words being understood. Although hallucinations in PD are usually benign, they can sometimes be frightening. A person standing near the bed at night can make the patient shout for help. Insight into these hallucinations is retained initially, but is lost at a later stage.

Besides these major hallucinations, minor ones in the form of presence hallucinations, passage hallucinations and illusions also occur in PD-P. They have a high prevalence (42%) in newly diagnosed untreated patients.[8] In passage hallucinations, the patient sees a fleeting image of a shadow or small animal in the peripheral field of vision, but when he turns to look, he sees nothing. In presence hallucinations, the patient feels there is something behind him or to the side that is not seen or heard. It is not a true hallucination because none of the special senses is involved. Illusions are distorted interpretations of real images. They are almost always visual. A clock on the wall looks like a tree or a flower may appear like a face.

Delusions are irrational fixed beliefs that are not based on facts and are maintained despite evidence to the contrary. In PD-P, they are usually paranoid, and often lead to agitation.[6] Common examples are belief of infidelity of spouse (jealous delusions) and suspicion that the maid or a family member is stealing money. They are the most disabling of all psychotic symptoms with a prevalence of 1–7%.

DIFFERENTIAL DIAGNOSIS

The symptoms of PD-P must be differentiated from those of primary psychosis like schizophrenia. In the latter, hallucinations are mainly auditory with emotional content. People hear distinct voices saying nasty things about them. Whereas in PD-P, the VH predominate. If AH occurs, the voices are distant and indistinct, with no emotional content. Delusions are also different. In schizophrenia, grandiose, persecutory, and religious delusions are far more common.

Dementia with Lewy bodies (DLB) can sometimes be mistaken for PD-P due to presence of major VH. The contrasting features in DLB are that VH occur early in the disease, unrelated to drug use.

Delirium is marked by decreased attention, variable level of consciousness, and disorientation. It occurs more acutely and is usually related to a secondary treatable cause like infection.

RISK FACTORS

Risk factors for PD-P include older age, PD medication use, greater severity and longer duration of illness, rapid eye movement (REM) sleep behavior disorder (RBD), affective disorders, visual disturbances, and cognitive impairment including dementia.[9]

The majority of PD-P patients have sleep disturbances including RBD. In fact, some hallucinations are thought to represent a narcolepsy-like REM sleep disorder during daytime hours.[10] Cognitive impairment is one of the most important independent risk factors for psychosis, being more prevalent in PD-dementia (up to 75%) than in those without dementia.[11] There is also a strong correlation between visual perceptive disorders and VH. Poor vision due to cataract and dim lighting at night can cause VH in susceptible individuals.[9]

PATHOPHYSIOLOGY

A complex interplay between exogenous (drugs and intercurrent illness) and endogenous (PD pathology) factors is likely responsible for PD-P. Some postulated pathophysiological mechanisms are:

- Hypersensitivity of mesocorticolimbic D2/D3 receptors caused by chronic dopaminergic therapy.
- Cholinergic deficits and serotonergic/dopaminergic imbalance occurring in primary visual and visual association pathways.[12]
- Neurodegeneration of widespread limbic, paralimbic, and neocortical gray matter including prefrontal cortex is seen.[13]

ASSESSMENT SCALES

No widely used, validated, PD-P specific rating scale is available. Scales from non-PD conditions like schizophrenia that are recommended are: Neuropsychiatric inventory (NPI), Schedule for Assessment of Positive Symptoms (SAPS), the Positive and Negative Syndrome Scale and Brief Psychiatric Rating Scale. In the recent pimavanserin trial, a PD-modified scale called SAPS-PD was used.[14]

MANAGEMENT

A systematic and stepwise approach should be adopted for the management of PD-P.

The first step is to assess the severity of symptoms to decide on the need for intervention. If minor VH occurs infrequently and are not bothersome, they do not need to be treated immediately. Patients are often willing to tolerate them. However, they need close monitoring. Treatment must be started when symptoms become more frequent and disturbing.

The next step is to look for and treat any secondary cause such as infection, dehydration, electrolyte imbalance, or a subdural hematoma. They can trigger acute delirium and psychosis or worsen existing symptoms. A respiratory or urinary tract infection may sometimes present with psychosis even before the onset of fever.

The next approach is to review the drug history. First, all nonessential, non-PD medications such as tricyclic antidepressants (TCAs), bladder antispasmodics, muscle relaxants, and narcotic analgesics should be reduced or withdrawn, if possible. The recent addition of a new drug or increased dosage of an existing one may be the incriminating factor.

After this is done, the focus is shifted to PD medications. The aim is to withdraw or reduce them to a level that resolves psychosis without significant worsening of motor control. This process of withdrawal should be done gradually and sequentially, one drug at a time. Generally, one can start with anticholinergics, followed by amantadine, monoamine oxidase type B (MAO-B) inhibitor, catechol-O-methyltransferase (COMT) inhibitor, then dopamine agonist, and finally levodopa. There is no universal consensus on this sequential order of withdrawal. The above measures suffice to resolve psychosis in many patients, at least in the short-term. If psychotic symptoms still persist, an antipsychotic drug should be started.

Antipsychotic Drugs

The antipsychotic drug must be effective, well-tolerated, and safe. All conventional and most atypical antipsychotics (risperidone, olanzapine, and aripiprazole) should not be given because they worsen the Parkinsonian motor state and increase the risk of tardive syndromes. In addition, olanzapine did not show clinical benefit in PD-P.[15]

The three recommended drugs in PD-P are clozapine, quetiapine, and pimavanserin. Cognitive enhancing drugs (rivastigmine and donepezil) are used in patients with associated cognitive impairment. All antipsychotic drugs carry a black box warning of increased risk of death, especially in elderly patients with dementia.[16] For all of them, a baseline electrocardiogram must be taken to ensure a normal QTc interval.

Clozapine is a second generation atypical antipsychotic drug. It is a weak striatal D2 receptor blocker, but it has prominent activity at the dopamine D4 and serotonin $5HT_{2A}$ receptors. A good efficacy of this drug in PD-P has been established without deterioration of motor function. In fact, this drug improves PD tremor.[17] The average effective dose is 25–50 mg/day, significantly lower than the high dose of 300–900 mg/day required for schizophrenia. A rapid therapeutic response is usually seen within a week and with a dose as low as 6.25 mg/day. The main disadvantage of clozapine is that it causes agranulocytosis and neutropenia. Nondose-related agranulocytosis is rare (prevalence of 0.38%). It can be fatal, but it is reversible if stopped immediately. Transient neutropenia (8.3%) also resolves on discontinuation of the drug.[18] It is therefore mandatory to check blood count once a week for the first 6 months and thereafter at less frequent intervals. Clozapine also causes sedation and orthostatic hypotension. Increased sedation may worsen confusion in demented patients. Hence, it should be used with caution in this patient group.

Quetiapine has moderate affinity for dopamine D2 and $5HT_{2A}$ receptors. The quetiapine story makes interesting reading. Despite lack of efficacy in multiple trials, this drug has been widely prescribed by physicians who find it clinically useful.[19] Its improved safety profile and ease of administration have made it a pragmatic first choice drug in PD-P. It is started in a dose of 12.5 mg or 25 mg at night. Maintenance daily dose is 25–75 mg, much lower than that used for primary psychosis. Like clozapine, it can cause sedation and orthostatic hypotension.

Pimavanserin is a selective serotonin $5HT_{2A}$ inverse agonist without any dopaminergic, adrenergic, histaminergic, or muscarinic effects. It is the only drug approved by the Food and Drug Administration (FDA) for the treatment of PD-P. A double-blind, placebo-controlled trial showed a more than 2-folds benefit of pimavanserin over placebo.[20] Secondary measures of sleep and caregiver burden also improved. At the daily dose of 34 mg, improvement occurred after 4 weeks, and increased further by the end point of 6 weeks.[19] It is well-tolerated with no sedation or orthostatic hypotension. This makes it a safe drug to use in PD-P patients with cognitive impairment. There is no Parkinsonian worsening. A recent FDA analysis found no long-term side-effects or increased mortality with it.[21]

Rivastigmine and donepezil, the cholinesterase inhibitors, are useful in improving psychotic symptoms in PD patients with dementia.[22] They are generally well-tolerated, but can cause diarrhea, loss of appetite, and worsening of tremor.[23]

Electroconvulsive Therapy

Electroconvulsive therapy (ECT) has been used in the rare cases of PD-P which are refractory to all the above treatments. Improvement in motor symptoms has also been reported following ECT.[24]

CHOICE OF ANTIPSYCHOTIC DRUG

The selection of the appropriate antipsychotic drug depends on severity of symptoms, efficacy and safety profile of the drug, presence of cognitive impairment, experience of the physician, and patient preference.

Most physicians use quetiapine as first-line drug despite its lack of efficacy in clinical trials, for the reasons mentioned earlier. Clozapine is usually prescribed only if quetiapine or pimavanserin fail. Although it is very efficacious, the risk of agranulocytosis and the need for weekly blood monitoring have significantly restricted its use. It can still be the first option for those who do not mind regular blood monitoring.

When psychosis is severe and rapid control of symptoms is required, quetiapine or clozapine is chosen because of their rapid onset of action. When symptoms are reasonably tolerated and a 4 week delay in efficacy is acceptable, pimavanserin is selected. It is also the drug of choice in PD-P patients with dementia because it does not cause sedation or orthostatic hypotension. Pimavanserin is currently recommended for short-term use of up to 6 weeks.

Cholinesterase inhibitors are considered when minor psychotic symptoms are associated with mild to moderate dementia. Demented PD-P patients who are treated with a combination of pimavanserin and cholinesterase inhibitor have shown a greater benefit than those treated with pimavanserin alone.[25]

DEPRESSION

Depression affects up to 45% of PD patients. Major depression accounts for 5–20%, while nonmajor forms (minor or subsyndromic depression) make up an additional 10–30% of patients.[26,27]

Depression in PD has a profound impact on quality of life, sometimes more than the motor symptoms. Yet it remains under-recognized and under-treated, even in speciality care centers.

PATHOPHYSIOLOGY

There is a complex interaction of psychological factors arising from the stress of a chronic illness and neurobiological mechanisms. In support of the latter is the observation that depression sometimes precedes the onset of motor symptoms, when there is no physical disability.[28] Dopaminergic, serotonergic, and noradrenergic pathways in the limbic system have been implicated. In vivo radioactive ligand imaging has shown decreased binding in the locus coeruleus and limbic system in depressed versus nondepressed PD patients.[29] There is also widespread brainstem and cortical (mainly prefrontal cortex) pathology in depressed PD (dPD) patients.

CLINICAL FEATURES

Depression occurs at all stages of PD and can even precede the motor onset by months to years, making it a potential prodromal marker. Risk factors for depression in PD include female sex, a past or family history of depression, early-onset PD, cognitive impairment, psychosis, anxiety, and apathy.[30,31]

Depressed PD patients exhibit a low mood, pessimism, somatic symptoms, and mild intellectual impairment. As compared to their non-PD depressed counterparts, dPD patients have higher rates of anxiety, pessimism, suicidal ideation without suicidal behavior, and less guilt and self-blame. One of the reasons for under-diagnosis of depression in PD is that PD motor symptoms often overlap and mask underlying depression. A sad face, hunched posture, slow movement, fatigue, and sleep disturbance of depression can all mimic the signs of PD. Hence, a high index of suspicion is required to recognize depression in PD.

Depression, along with anxiety and pain, also occurs as a nonmotor fluctuation (NMF) in PD. Depressive symptoms are observed in the off-state and subside during the on-state. These NMF have been reported in 19–40% of PD patients and can even occur in the absence of motor fluctuations.[32]

ASSESSMENT SCALES

The Hamilton Depression Rating Scale (HAM-D), Beck's Depression Inventory (BDI), and Montgomery–Asberg Depression Rating Scale (MADRS) are recommended in dPD for screening purpose and for measurement of severity.[33]

PHARMACOTHERAPY

A survey of antidepressant drug use in PD showed that 20–25% of PD patients were taking an antidepressant at any given time, including de novo patients.[34] The common antidepressant drugs used in PD are the selective serotonin reuptake inhibitors (SSRIs), TCAs, and selective serotonin and norepinephrine reuptake inhibitors (SSNRIs). Relatively few double-blind placebo-controlled trials of antidepressant drugs in PD are available.

Tricyclic Antidepressants

Amitriptyline, nortriptyline, and desipramine are the commonly used TCAs in practice. Nortriptyline is, so far, the only TCA with proven efficacy from a randomized and placebo-controlled trial.[35] Adverse effects of TCAs are dry mouth, constipation, cardiac arrhythmias, sedation, and confusion. They are best avoided in elderly people with cognitive impairment.

Selective Serotonin Reuptake Inhibitors

The SSRIs are the most commonly used antidepressants in PD.[34] They include fluoxetine, sertraline, escitalopram, citalopram, and paroxetine. Paroxetine demonstrated efficacy in a placebo-controlled trial.[34] The SSRIs are often preferred over TCAs because of lower incidence of anticholinergic side-effects and arrhythmias. However, they may occasionally worsen Parkinsonism. Citalopram, >20 mg/day, may cause prolonged QTc interval.

Selective Serotonin and Norepinephrine Reuptake Inhibitors

Venlafaxine, an SSNRI, is being increasingly used in dPD patients. Its efficacy has been proven in a double-blind controlled trial[36] and it has a favorable safety profile.

Dopaminergic Drugs

The dopamine receptor agonist pramipexole has shown good antidepressant benefit in PD patients.[37] Ropinirole is also beneficial.[38] Rasagiline, an MAO-B inhibitor, had a negative outcome in a randomized controlled trial.[39] Levodopa is useful only in the subset of PD patients who exhibit depression and anxiety as a NMF in the off-phase. Adjusting levodopa dose improves depression in them.[40]

NONPHARMACOLOGICAL THERAPY

Cognitive-behavioral therapy (CBT) by a trained psychologist or counselor benefits dPD patients and their caregivers.[41] Many of them prefer psychotherapy to drugs. They must also be encouraged to participate in support groups and community self-help programs.

Repetitive transcranial magnetic stimulation (rTMS) has shown antidepressant benefit in the general population. It is also likely to help dPD patients.[42] The duration of benefit is usually short and has to be repeated at regular intervals.

Electroconvulsive therapy is used as a last resort for severe treatment-refractory dPD patients. An added benefit of ECT is temporary improvement in Parkinsonism.[43]

ANXIETY DISORDER

Up to 40% of PD patients experience anxiety.[44] It occurs in three forms: (1) Generalized anxiety disorder (GAD); (2) Panic attack; and (3) Social phobia. Anxiety often coexists with depression. In many patients, it is a NMF with episodic panic attacks or exacerbations during the off-period.[45] Other patients experience it as a constant and underlying mood disorder.

The etiology of anxiety is not known. Like depression, it can appear as a prodromal symptom, predating the onset of disease by up to 20 years.[46] Loss of dopaminergic and noradrenergic innervation in locus coeruleus and limbic system may be the causative neurobiological factor. Anxious PD patients have a poor quality of life with increased caregiver burden. Tremor and dyskinesia are often worsened by anxiety. A PD-specific validated anxiety rating scale called Parkinson Anxiety Scale is now available.[47]

TREATMENT

Like in depression, counseling and CBT help to alleviate anxiety in patients and their caregivers. There are no randomized controlled drug trials for treatment of anxiety in PD.

Levodopa

If anxiety presents as a NMF, then adjustment of levodopa dose will improve the off-period anxiety state and prevent a panic attack.

Antidepressant Drugs

Some antidepressant treatment trials have reported secondary benefit for anxiety symptoms also.[35] The SSRIs with their favorable side-effect profile are often used as first line treatment. The onset of anxiolytic effect is usually in 2–4 weeks.

Benzodiazepines

Benzodiazepines are used to relieve disabling anxiety symptoms and abort an acute panic attack. Alprazolam, lorazepam, and clonazepam are the commonly used drugs. They have a rapid onset of action and are effective in the short-term.[48] Prolonged use may cause dependence. They must be used with caution as they cause sedation, gait imbalance, and cognitive impairment.

Buspirone

It is an anxiolytic drug with partial 5HT1A agonism and low sedative potential. It has proven efficacy in PD-related anxiety.[49] The advantage of this drug over benzodiazepines is that it does not produce dependence. However, it has a slow onset of action over 3–4 weeks.

APATHY

Apathy occurs in about 40% of PD patients. It can overlap with depression and anxiety, but also occurs as an independent NMS.[50] It is a general sense of indifference with loss of motivation, diminished goal-directed behavior, and a reduced interest in interacting with people. Dopaminergic and cholinergic denervation in limbic areas play a role in PD-related apathy. There is also prefrontal lobe dysfunction with executive deficits, verbal memory deficits, and bradyphrenia.[51]

PHARMACOTHERAPY

Piribedil, a dopamine agonist, has been shown to improve apathy in PD.[52] Stimulants such as methylphenidate and amphetamine have also been used to treat PD-related apathy. Rivastigmine, a cholinesterase inhibitor, has also benefitted apathetic PD patients without depression or dementia.[53]

CONCLUSION

Our understanding of PD-related psychosis and mood disorders has increased in the last couple of decades. Few well-designed clinical trials have helped the physician to better manage these disorders. However, several lacunae and unresolved issues still remain. In the near future, we should make a concerted effort to improve research, education, training, and clinical care, so as to optimize the care of PD patients with neuropsychiatric manifestations.

REFERENCES

1. Chaudhuri KR, Healy DG, Schapira AHV. Non-motor symptoms of Parkinson's disease: Diagnosis and management. Lancet Neurol. 2006;5(3):235-45.
2. Forsaa EB, Larsen JP, Wentzel-Larsen T, Goetz CG, Stebbins GT, Aarsland D, et al. A 12 year population-based study of psychosis in Parkinson's disease. Arch Neurol. 2010;67(8):996-1001.
3. Goetz CG, Stebbins GT. Risk factors for nursing home placement in advanced Parkinson's disease. Neurology. 1993;43(11):2227-9.
4. Forsaa EB, Larsen JP, Wentzel-Larsen T, Alves G. What predicts mortality in Parkinson's disease? A prospective population-based long-term study. Neurology. 2010;75(14):1270-6.

5. Schrag A, Hovris A, Morley D, Quinn N, Jahanshahi M. Caregiver-burden in Parkinson's disease is closely associated with psychiatric systems, falls, and disability. Parkinsonism Relat Disord. 2006;12(1):35-41.
6. Chou KL, Messing S, Oakes D, Feldman PD, Breier A, Friedman JH. Drug-induced psychosis in Parkinson's disease: phenomenology and correlations among psychosis rating instruments. Clin Neuropharmacol. 2005;28(5):215-9.
7. Fénelon G, Soulas T, Zenasni F, de Langavant LC. The changing face of Parkinson's disease-associated psychosis: a cross-sectional study based on the new NINDS-NIMH criteria. Mov Disord. 2010;25(6):763-6.
8. Pagonabarraga J, Martinez-Horta S, Fernandez de Bobadilla R, Pérez J, Ribosa-Nogué R, Marín J, et al. Minor hallucinations occur in drug-naïve Parkinson's disease patients even from the premotor phase. Mov Disord. 2016;31(1):45-52.
9. Ffytche DH, Creese B, Politis M, Chaudhuri KR, Weintraub D, Ballard C, et al. The psychosis spectrum in Parkinson's disease. Nat Rev Neurol. 2017;13(2):81-95.
10. Arnulf I, Bonnet AM, Damier P, Bejjani BP, Seilhean D, Derenne JP, et al. Hallucinations, REM sleep, and Parkinson's disease: a medical hypothesis. Neurology. 2000;55(2):281-8.
11. Aarsland D, Ballard C, Larsen JP, McKeith I. A comparative study of psychiatric symptoms in dementia with Lewy bodies and Parkinson's disease with and without dementia. Int J Geriatr Psychiatry. 2001;16(5):528-36.
12. Ballanger B, Strafella AP, van Eimeren T, Zurowski M, Rusjan PM, Houle S, et al. Serotonin 2A receptors and visual hallucinations in Parkinson's disease. Arch Neurol. 2010;67(4):416-21.
13. Goldman JG, Stebbins GT, Dinh V, Bernard B, Merkitch D, deToledo-Morrell L, et al. Visuoperceptive region atrophy independent of cognitive status in patients with Parkinson's disease with hallucinations. Brain. 2014;137(3):849-59.
14. Voss T, Bahr D, Cummings J, Mills R, Ravina B, Williams H. Performance of a shortened scale for Assessment of Positive Symptoms for Parkinson's disease psychosis. Parkinsonism Relat Disord. 2013;19(3):295-9.
15. Ondo WG, Levy JK, Vuong KD, Hunter C, Jankovic J. Olanzapine treatment for dopaminergic-induced hallucinations. Mov Disord. 2002;17(5):1031-5.
16. Trifiro G, Verhamme KMC, Ziere G, Caputi AP, Ch Stricker BH, Sturkenboom MC. All-cause mortality associated with atypical and typical antipsychotics in demented outpatients. Pharmacoepidemiol Drug Saf. 2007;16:538-44.
17. Parkinson Study Group. Low dose clozapine for the treatment of drug-induced psychosis in Parkinson's disease. N Eng J Med. 1999;340(10):757-63.
18. Honigfeld G, Arellano F, Sethi J, Bianchini A, Schein J. Reducing clozapine-related morbidity and mortality: 5 years of experience with the Clozaril National Registry. J Clin Psychiatry. 1998;59(3):3-7.
19. Ondo WG, Tintner R, Voung KD, Lai D, Ringholz G. Double-blind, placebo-controlled, unforced titration parallel trial of quetiapine for dopaminergic-induced hallucinations in Parkinson's disease. Mov Disord. 2005;20(8):958-63.
20. Cummings J, Isaacson S, Mills R, Williams H, Chi-Burris K, Corbett A. Pimavanserin for patients with Parkinson's disease psychosis: a randomized placebo-controlled phase 3 trial. Lancet. 2014;383(9916):533-40.
21. Webster P. Pimavanserin evaluated by the FDA. Lancet. 2018;391(10132):1762.
22. Bullock R, Cameron A. Rivastigmine for the treatment of dementia and visual hallucinations associated with Parkinson's disease: a case series. Curr Med Res Opin. 2002;18(5):258-64.
23. Dubois B, Tolosa E, Katzenschlager R, Emre M, Lees AJ, Schumann G, et al. Donepezil in Parkinson's disease dementia: a randomized, double-blind efficacy and safety study. Mov Disord. 2012;27(10):1230-8.
24. Ueda S, Koyama K, Okubo Y. Marked improvement of psychotic symptoms after electroconvulsive therapy in Parkinson's disease. J ECT. 2010;26(2):111-5.
25. Espay AJ, Guskey MT, Norton JC, Coate B, Vizcarra JA, Ballard C, et al. Pimavanserin for Parkinson's disease psychosis: Effects stratified by baseline cognition and use of cognitive-enhancing medications. Mov Disord. 2018;33(11):1769-76.
26. Reijnders JS, Ehrt U, Weber WE, Aarsland D, Leentjens AF. A systematic review of prevalence studies of depression in Parkinson's disease. Mov Disord. 2008;23(2):183-9.
27. Chaudhury KR, Schapira AHV. Non-motor symptoms of Parkinson's disease: dopaminergic pathophysiology and treatment. Lancet Neurol. 2009;8(5):464-74.
28. Alonso A, Rodriguez LAG, Logroscino G, Hernan MA. Use of antidepressants and the risk of Parkinson's disease: a prospective study. J. Neurol Neurosurg Psychiatry. 2009; 80(6):671-5.
29. Remy P, Doder M, Lees A, Turjanski N, Brooks D. Depression in Parkinson's disease: Loss of dopamine and noradrenaline innervations in the limbic system. Brain. 2005;128(6):1314-22.
30. Tandberg E, Larsen JP, Aarsland D, Laake K, Cummings JL. Risk factors for depression in Parkinson's disease. Arch Neurol. 1997;54(5):625-30.
31. Leentjens AFG, Lousberg R, Verhey FRJ. Markers for depression in Parkinson's disease. Acta Psychiatr Scand. 2002;106(3): 196-201.
32. Seki M, Takahashi K, Uematsu D, Mihara B, Morita Y, Isozumi K, et al. Clinical features and varieties of non-motor fluctuations in Parkinson's disease: a Japanese multicenter study. Parkinsonism Relat Disord. 2013;19(1):104-8.
33. Schrag A, Barone P, Brown RG, Leentjens AF, McDonald WM, Starkstein G, et al. Depression rating scales in Parkinson's disease: critique and recommendations. Mov Disord. 2007;22(8):1077-92.
34. Richard IH, Kurlan R. A survey of antidepressant drug use in Parkinson's disease. Parkinson Study Group. Neurology. 1997;49(4):1168-70.
35. Menza M, Dobkin RD, Marin H, Mark MH, Gara M, Buyske S, et al. A controlled trial of antidepressants in patients with Parkinson disease and depression. Neurology. 2009;72(10):886-92.
36. Richard IH, McDermott MP, Kurlan R, Lyness JM, Como PG, Pearson N, et al. A randomized, double-blind, placebo-controlled trial of antidepressants in Parkinson disease. Neurology. 2012;78(16):1229-36.
37. Barone P, Poewe W, Albrecht S, Debieuvre C, Massey D, Rascol O, et al. Pramipexole for the treatment of depressive symptoms in patients with Parkinson's disease: a randomized, double-blind, placebo-controlled trial. Lancet Neurol. 2010;9(6): 573-80.

38. Pahwa R, Stacy MA, Factor SA, Lyons KE, Stocchi F, Hersh BP, et al. Ropinirole 24-hour prolonged release: randomized, controlled study in advanced Parkinson disease. Neurology. 2007;68(14):1108-15.
39. Barone P, Santangelo G, Morgante L, Onofrj M, Meco G, Abbruzzese G, et al. A randomized clinical trial to evaluate the effects of rasagiline on depressive symptoms in non-demented Parkinson's disease patients. Eur J Neurol. 2015;22(8):1184-91.
40. Kulisevsky J, Pascual-Sedano B, Barbanoj M, Gironell A, Pagonabarraga J, García-Sánchez C. Acute effects of immediate and controlled-release levodopa on mood in Parkinson's disease: a double-blind study. Mov Disord. 2007;22(1):62-7.
41. Dobkin RD, Menza M, Allen LA, Gara MA, Mark MH, Tiu J, et al. Cognitive-behavioral therapy for depression in Parkinson's disease: a randomized, controlled trial. Am J Psychiatry. 2011;168(10):1066-74.
42. Makkos A, Pál E, Aschermann Z, Janszky J, Balázs É, Takács K, et al. High-frequency repetitive transcranial magnetic stimulation can improve depression in Parkinson's disease: a randomized, double-blind, placebo-controlled study. Neuropsychobiology. 2016;73(3):169-77.
43. Popeo D, Kellner CH. ECT for Parkinson's disease. Med Hypotheses. 2009;73(4):468-9.
44. Pontone GM, Williams JR, Anderson KE, Chase G, Goldstein SA, Grill S, et al. Prevalence of anxiety disorders and anxiety subtypes in patients with Parkinson's disease. Mov Disord. 2009;24(9):1333-8.
45. Dissanayaka NN, Sellbach A, Matheson S, O'Sullivan JD, Silburn PA, Byrne GJ, et al. Anxiety disorders in Parkinson's disease: prevalence and risk factors. Mov Disord. 2010;25(7):838-45.
46. Shiba M, Bower JH, Maraganore DM, McDonnell SK, Peterson BJ, Ahlskog JE, et al. Anxiety disorders and depressive disorders preceding Parkinson's disease: a case-control study. Mov Disord. 2000;15(4):669-77.
47. Leentjens AFG, Dujardin K, Pontone GM, Starkstein SE, Weintraub D, Martinez-Martin P. The Parkinson Anxiety Scale (PAS): development and validation of a new anxiety scale. Mov Disord. 2014;29(8):1035-43.
48. Singhal BS, Lalkaka JA, Sheth A. Management of anxiety and depression in Parkinson's Disease. In: Mizuno Y, Fisher A, Hanin I (Eds). Mapping the Progress of Alzheimer's and Parkinson's Disease. Springer, Boston: Advances in Behavioral Biology; 2002;51. pp. 417-22.
49. Ludwig CL, Weinberger DR, Bruno G, Gillespie M, Bakker K, LeWitt PA, et al. Buspirone, Parkinson's disease, and the locus ceruleus. Clin Neuropharmacol. 1986;9(4):373-8.
50. Starkstein SE, Merello M, Jorge R, Brockman S, Bruce D, Power B. The syndromal validity and nosological position of apathy in Parkinson's disease. Mov Disord. 2009;24(8):1211-6.
51. Pagonabarraga J, Kulisevsky J, Strafella AP, Krack P. Apathy in Parkinson's disease: clinical features, neural substrates, diagnosis, and treatment. Lancet Neurol. 2015;14(5):518-31.
52. Thobois S, Lhommee E, Klinger H, Ardouin C, Schmitt E, Bichon A, et al. Parkinsonian apathy responds to dopaminergic stimulation of D_2/D_3 receptors with piribedil. Brain. 2013;136 (Pt 5):1568-77.
53. Devos D, Moreau C, Maltete D, Lefaucheur R, Kreisler A, Eusebio A, et al. Rivastigmine in apathetic but dementia and depression-free patients with Parkinson's disease: a double-blind, placebo-controlled, randomized clinical trial. J Neurol Neurosurg Pschiatry. 2014;85(6):668-74.

CHAPTER 10

Impulse Control Disorders in Parkinson's Disease

Roopa Rajan, Seetha Lekshmi B

INTRODUCTION

Parkinson's disease (PD) is typically defined by the troublesome motor problems that characterize—bradykinesia, rigidity, and tremor at rest along with postural instability.[1] However, a multitude of nonmotor symptoms were known to be associated with PD since its earliest descriptions. Nonmotor symptoms in PD are many and diverse, affecting the domains of neuropsychiatry, cognition, autonomic functions, pain, and sleep to name a few. Nonmotor symptoms may be PD-related; they may also be brought out or worsened by the medications used for treatment of PD. Since its introduction in the late 1960s, behavioral changes were noticed in levodopa-treated PD patients.[2] Certain patients exhibited behaviors like drug seeking and others involved in meaningless repetitive tasks which simulated "punding" in cocaine abusers.[3] Impulse control disorder (ICD) are one among the behavioral and psychiatric manifestations in PD.

Impulse control disorder comprises a constellation of disorders that are characterized by pleasurable behaviors performed excessively and are commonly associated with an inability to suppress internal urges.[4] The major forms of ICD seen in PD include pathological gambling (PG), hypersexuality (HS), compulsive buying/shopping (CB), and binge eating (BE). Other manifestations of impulsive and compulsive behaviors are termed as impulse control related behaviors (ICRB). These nonmotor symptoms are often difficult to evaluate and treat. ICDs have been included in the diagnostic and statistical manual of mental disorders (DSM-V) as a dysregulation of self-emotional and behavioral control. It is important to watch for the emergence of ICDs in PD patients due to their potential for serious social, psychic, legal, and financial consequences.

EPIDEMIOLOGY

Although ICDs are commonly encountered in PD patients treated with dopaminergic agents, some studies report their occurrence in drug naïve-PD patients and in the general population. ICDs may be underestimated in the general population and reported frequencies vary from 0.2% to 5.3%.[4] The wide range of variability may be explained by different genetic, ethnic, and cultural backgrounds, in addition to the different assessment tools used. Two large studies [DOMINION and ICARUS (Impulse Control disorders And the association of neuRopsychiatric symptoms, cognition and qUality of life in ParkinSon disease)] involving >1,000 patients, identified the frequency of ICD to be 17.1–28.6% in PD patients.[5,6] The prevalence of ICD remained relatively stable during longitudinal follow-up in the ICARUS study, ranging between 29.3% and 26.5% at 1 year and 2 year follow-up. In the longitudinal, multicentric DIGPD study, 5-year cumulative incidence of ICD was 46%.[7] Majority of the patients who developed ICD in these studies were on treatment, particularly with dopamine agonists. However, it has been reported that nearly 20% of newly diagnosed treatment naïve PD patients may show some symptoms suggestive of ICD.[8] It is still debated whether the mere presence of PD itself confers enhanced risk for the development of ICDs or exposure to dopaminergic agents is essential to its occurrence.

The prevalence of ICDs and ICRB in PD varies among populations and few Asian studies reported ranges between 2% and 35%.[5,9] These were largely single-centered, hospital based studies. A multidisciplinary clinic-based study done in South India assessed 305 patients for ICD/ICRB and at least one ICRB or ICD was diagnosed in 96 patients (31.6%) among which punding was the most common (15.7%), followed by CB (8.2%). Punding behaviors involved making newspaper cuttings of pictures of celebrities or arranging and rearranging clothes, utensils, and furniture for several hours of the day, which differed from the classic punding behaviors reported in Western populations. Two or more ICRBs were observed in 7.5%. Premorbid ICD was reported by 6.6%, which were exacerbated in 65% after starting on a dopamine agonist.[9] Another study from North India screened 299 PD patients and found at least one ICD in 24.8% and ICRB in 42.8%.[10] Here too, punding was the most common behavior (12.4%) followed by HS (11.0%), hobbyism (9.4%), and CB (8.4%).

RISK FACTORS

The strongest risk factor for development of ICD in PD is exposure to dopaminergic medications.[11] Among the dopaminergic drugs, dopamine agonists (pramipexole, ropinirole, cabergoline, bromocriptine, rotigotine, apomorphine) in particular have been implicated in the development of ICD. ICDs are about 2.7 times more likely to be present in patients treated with a dopamine agonist drug compared to those not exposed to such medications.[5] The nonergot dopamine agonists, pramipexole, and ropinirole have consistently shown the strongest association with ICD across studies. There is no difference between pramipexole and ropinirole in the tendency to develop ICD.[12] Longer acting preparations of dopamine agonists do not seem to reduce the risk of developing ICD. Apart from dopamine agonists, other dopaminergic drugs are also associated with ICD. Levodopa is associated with development of ICD, though the risk with dopamine agonists is almost double that of levodopa. Higher dopamine agonist and overall levodopa equivalent daily doses were associated with higher risk of ICD.[13] In addition to the dopaminergic drugs, male gender, young age at onset, and predominant left sided parkinsonism are possible additional risk factors (**Table 1**). A dose-matched study however, failed to establish the significance of these factors in PD population.[11]

Not all PD patients exposed to therapeutic doses of dopamine agonists develop ICD and hence additional factors such as personality traits and genetic factors have been implicated. Patients with ICD are thought to have novelty seeking personality traits at baseline.[11] Among genetic factors, dopamine, serotonin, and N-methyl-D-aspartate (NMDA) receptor encoding genes have been studied for association with PD. Genetic polymorphisms in *DRD1, DRD2,* and *GRIN2B* were associated with ICD in Malaysian PD patients.[14] *DRD3* and *GRIN2B* variants were associated with ICD in Korean PD patients.[14,15] In Indian PD patients, the *DRD3*p. Ser9Gly (rs6280) polymorphism was associated with ICD.[16] In a prospective study with whole exome data, various candidate genes were assessed for ICD risk and *OPRK1, HTR2A,* and *DDC* variants were shown to be the strongest genetic predictive factors.[17]

TABLE 1: Risk factors for ICD in PD.

Drugs	• Dopamine agonists (pramipexole, ropinirole, and rotigotine), apomorphine, levodopa, and amantadine* • Higher risk with higher doses of dopamine agonist and/or total LEDD
Deep brain stimulation	New onset ICDs after STN-DBS, often self-limiting
Psychological traits/Psychiatric disease	Novelty seeking personality trait, depression, anxiety, substance use disorder, and family history of substance/alcohol use disorder
Genetic factors*	*DRD3, GRIN2B, HTR2A, OPRK1, DDC, DRD1, and DRD2*
Clinical features of PD	Young age at onset, male gender, and prolonged disease duration

*putative risk factors.

(*DRD3:* dopamine receptor D3 gene; *GRIN2B:* glutamate N-methyl-D-aspartate receptor type 2B gene; *HTR2A:* serotonin receptor type 2A gene; ICD: impulse control disorders; LEDD: levodopa equivalent daily dosage; PD: Parkinson's disease; STN-DBS: subthalamic nucleus deep brain stimulation)

The effect of subthalamic nucleus deep brain stimulation (STN-DBS) on ICD has been studied recently.[18] STN-DBS has interesting effects on ICD, patients with pre-existing ICD prior to surgery often experience remission in symptoms commensurate with the dopaminergic medication reduction postoperatively.[19] On the other hand, patients may experience new onset ICD after STN-DBS, these are usually in the 1st year postsurgery and are self-limiting in most cases.[20]

PATHOPHYSIOLOGY

The mesolimbic pathways are implicated in the pathophysiology of ICD. These pathways are some of the most important reward response systems in the human brain and are heavily dopaminergic innervated. Prolonged exposure to exogenous dopaminergic agents may result in overstimulation of the circuitry, eventually culminating into the development of ICD.[21] Though the pathophysiology behind ICD is incompletely understood, it has been postulated as a phased process of priming induction-establishment.[21] In the priming phase, the pathophysiological changes associated with PD, specifically selective dopaminergic denervation of the dorsal rather than ventral striatum creates a favorable background for ICDs to develop. The ventral striatum has rich connections to the limbic system and higher representation of dopamine D3 type receptors.[22] On ventral striatal overstimulation may induce ICD on exposure to dopamine agonists, particularly those with higher D3 affinity like pramipexole. Finally, in the establishment phase, there is impaired negative feedback from the dopamine depleted and dysfunctional frontostriatal circuits. It is postulated that genetic variants such as the gain-of-function *DRD3* variant reported in Indian patients, may increase the risk of ICD by enhancing the sensitivity of D3 receptors to dopaminergic stimulation.[16]

Another hypothesis explains the development of ICD in relation to the phasic and tonic dopamine release model.[23] Phasic dopamine surge occurs in response to unexpected rewards, which gets suppressed in the absence of expected rewards whereas in response to expectation of rewards there is tonic release of dopamine. In patients with PD this reward response mechanism is modulated by extrinsic dopaminergic drug administration. In the presence of extrinsic dopamine, the phasic dopamine suppression to lack of an expected reward may be blunted, resulting in impaired negative feedback to punishment. In combination with enhanced positive feedback in expectation of reward, these dysfunctional responses may blunt the ability to suppress pleasurable yet disruptive behaviors.[24,25]

The nucleus accumbens (Nac) plays a major role in integrating afferent information from the ventral subiculum of the hippocampus (vSub), the medial prefrontal cortex (mPFC), and the basolateral amygdala (BLA) (**Fig. 1**).[21] The hippocampal afferents (vSub) provide spatial, context-specific information, and the cortical drive to persist with a rewarding activity.[26] The mPFC afferents subserve behavioral flexibility by facilitating attentional shifting away from a nonrewarding stimulus and thus, response inhibition.[27] The afferent input from the BLA provides affective information specific to the task at hand, while simultaneously activating the mPFC to shift attention when an aversive emotional outcome or punishment is encountered. Cortical glutamatergic inputs from all the three input pathways are excitatory on the Nac medium spiny neurons (MSNs) and stimulates GABA-ergic efferent activity via a direct striatonigral-thalamic pathway or an indirect ventral pallidal-STN-nigral pathway to the mediodorsal thalamus.[28] The effect of dopamine on this system is dependent on its phasic or tonic release from the ventral tegmentum.[29] The net effect of increased phasic ventral tegmental dopamine release, as occurs in while an unexpected reward is received, is modulation of the cortical afferent activity on the NAc in favor of the hippocampal drive, via D1 receptor and NMDA receptor mediated LTP along with simultaneous D2 receptor mediated LTD in the mPFC-NAc pathway.[30] On the other hand, tonic decreases in dopamine release as occurs following an aversive stimulus or punishment, results in a net decrease in dopamine. In the presence of persistent dopaminergic stimulation, these tonic decreases may be blunted, altering the dynamics in favor of ICD development.

DIAGNOSIS AND SUBTYPES

The four classical ICDs in PD include PG, HS, CB, and BE. Punding, hobbyism, walkabout, hoarding, and compulsive medication use completes the spectrum of ICDs-RD.[4,23,31-37] Validated screening tools such as the modified Minnesota Impulse Disorders Interview (mMIDI) and Questionnaire for Impulsive-Compulsive Disorders in Parkinson's Disease (QUIP) can be used in the clinic to screen for ICD symptoms.[38,39] Diagnosis rests upon meeting several well laid out criteria, which are different for the various ICD subtypes.

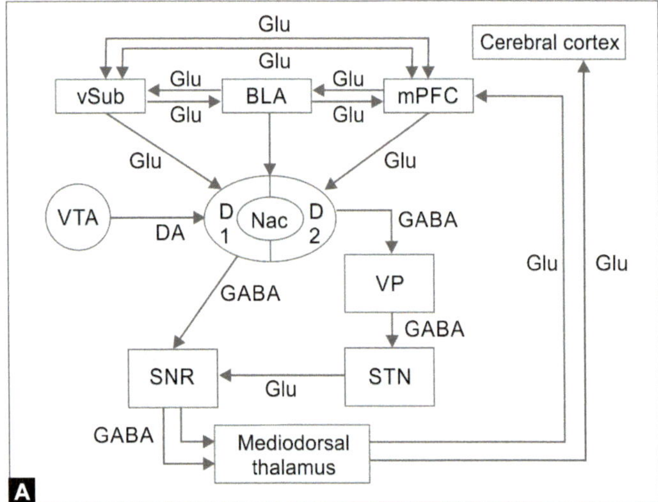

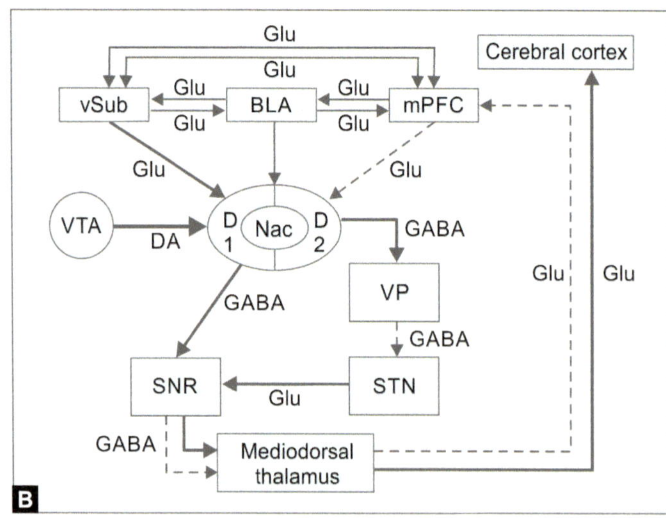

Note: The lines highlighted in bold represent increased activity in the circuit and the dotted lines a decrease in activity.

(BLA: basolateral amygdala; DA: Dopamine; Glu: glutamate; mPFC: medial prefrontal cortex; Nac: nucleus accumbens; SNR: substantia nigra; STN: subthalamic nucleus; Vsub: ventral subiculum of the hippocampus; VTA: ventral tegmental area; VP: ventral pallidum)

FIGS. 1A AND B: Schematic representation of the afferent and efferent connections of the nucleus accumbens relevant to decision making in normal state (A) and in the presence of elevated ventral striatal Dopamine (B) as in PD patients medicated with dopaminergic drugs.

Pathological gambling is diagnosed as per the DSM-V and is defined as a persistent and recurrent problematic gambling behavior. This involves preoccupation with gambling, spending increasing amounts of money in spite of losses, and unsuccessful attempts at cutting down gambling behavior. Patients often try to hide the problem and these behaviors result in difficulties in maintaining relationships, professional, or educational pursuits. In societies where there are legal barriers to access gambling, variant behaviors such as excessive buying of lottery tickets may be seen. Taking into account the similarities to drug addiction, PG was recently removed from ICDs and incorporated to a new category of "substance-related and addictive disorders" in the DSM-V.[4,23,32,34-36] CB is defined as repetitive and excessive buying of articles that are not needed or in excess of quantities than needed.[40] It is different from the closely related phenomenon of kleptomania, as compulsive buyers usually pay for their purchases with grave financial implications. Patients often describe an irresistible urge or anxiety that is relieved only when a purchase is made. HS is defined as increased preoccupation with sexual thoughts or activities and excessive demands for sex from partners. Patients may also engage in associated behaviors such as exhibitionism and paraphilia. Compulsive eating is defined by an inability to control the urge to eat, resulting in eating food in amounts greater than required to alleviate hunger.[41] Patients often indulge in frequent snacking in between meals and even at night time. Weight gain is often a serious consequence of this behavior.

Impulsive-compulsive-related behaviors have distinct clinical presentations from the four major ICDs and are often considered a milder phenotype of ICD. Punding involves repetitive behaviors such as collecting specific items, arranging and re-arranging objects excessively, or taking objects apart again and again. Punding becomes a problem when the subjects neglect their physiological needs and their social or professional responsibilities. Some punders retain insight regarding the futility of their behavior, but are unable to control the urge to perform it. Some report performing the repetitive activity as enjoyable and may become irritated when interrupted; others report no joy or satisfaction while carrying out the activity.[42] Hobbyism pertains to higher-level repetitive behaviors such as sports, gardening, drawing, painting or other artistic endeavors that are done repetitively to the exclusion of other physical and daily responsibilities. Walkabout is a form of ICRB characterized by excessive aimless wandering. Some patients develop hoarding which is the acquisition of a large number of items with no value in real life without discarding them.

Dopamine dysregulation syndrome (DDS) is a unique compulsive behavior that is considered under the spectrum of ICD. It is characterized by compulsive and excessive use of dopaminergic medication beyond the doses needed for optimal control of motor or nonmotor symptoms.[43] High potency and short-acting dopaminergic medications (levodopa and subcutaneous apomorphine) are often preferred. Patients exhibit classical addiction behaviors such as hoarding, lying about overuse, and irritability or anger when asked to reduce the overuse. Excessive medication use may result in levodopa-induced dyskinesias and additional psychiatric symptoms. The risk factors for DDS are similar to that of classical ICD young-onset PD, male gender, past, and family history of psychiatric disease.[44,45]

MANAGEMENT

The mainstay of treatment of ICDs is to withdraw or reduce the inciting agent, often a dopamine agonist.[46] Education of the patients and caregivers regarding the symptoms of ICD is essential at the time of initiating dopaminergic therapy, especially dopamine agonists. This along with regular screening on follow-up visits will enable early detection and treatment. In individual cases, behavioral or environmental approaches such as limiting access to money, credit cards, food, and monitoring cell phone or internet usage can be advised. Patients reporting troublesome ICD or ICRB will need reduction in the doses of dopamine agonists. Some respond to dose reduction while others require complete withdrawal of the drug for remission of symptoms. Withdrawal of dopamine agonist may result in worsening of motor symptoms, in which case levodopa dose can be increased or an additional drug such as catechol-O-methyltransferase (COMT) inhibitor (entacapone) or monoamine oxidase (MAO) inhibitor (rasagiline and selegiline) added. Other strategies that have been tried include switching to transdermal rotigotine or apomorphine subcutaneous infusion but the evidence of benefit is insufficient and these medications are also known to induce ICD.[47] A placebo-controlled study did not find any benefit of addition of naltrexone on ICD resolution.[48] Some patients with ICD may have psychiatric comorbidities such as anxiety and depression which may be worsening the behaviors and contributing to a poor quality of life overall. In such situations, psychiatric medications including antidepressants, antipsychotics, and anxiolytics may be added. In the absence of psychiatric indications, these drugs do not seem to help control ICD. Cognitive behavioral therapy may be useful in selected patients with ICD. DBS has inconsistent effects on ICD as discussed earlier. In patients with ICD who are otherwise candidates for STN-DBS due to motor fluctuations and dyskinesias, medication withdrawal after STN-DBS may help in symptom resolution.[49]

DOPAMINE AGONIST WITHDRAWAL SYNDROME

Withdrawal or reduction of dopamine agonists may precipitate the dopamine agonist withdrawal syndrome (DAWS).[50] DAWS consists of psychiatric manifestations such as anxiety, depression, restlessness, agitation, and autonomic symptoms like sweating and postural hypotension. It is similar to withdrawal symptoms reported with other drugs such as cocaine and amphetamines. Nearly one-fifth of patients withdrawing dopamine agonists may experience such symptoms. Those receiving higher total levodopa equivalent daily dosage of drugs and higher dopamine agonist doses are at higher risk. DAWS may occur irrespective of the rate of tapering and can appear at the onset of tapering or later. Symptoms may be severe enough to mandate reintroduction of dopamine agonist, albeit at a lower dose.

CONCLUSION

Impulse control disorders are an important and perhaps under-reported nonmotor symptom of PD. Given the strong association with medications, especially dopamine agonist medications, educating the patient, and caregiver about these symptoms is mandatory, along with frequent screening questions during review visits. Timely diagnosis and management, often by withdrawal of the causative medication, is essential to prevent serious physical, psychosocial, financial, and legal effects.

REFERENCES

1. Postuma RB, Berg D, Adler CH, Bloem BR, Chan P, Deuschl G, et al. The new definition and diagnostic criteria of Parkinson's disease. Lancet Neurol. 2016;15(6):546-8.
2. Lawrence AD, Evans AH, Lees AJ. Compulsive use of dopamine replacement therapy in Parkinson's disease: reward systems gone awry? Lancet Neurol. 2003;2(10):595-604.
3. Friedman JH. Punding on levodopa. Biol Psychiatry. 1994;36(5):350-1.
4. Weintraub D, David AS, Evans AH, Grant JE, Stacy M. Clinical spectrum of impulse control disorders in Parkinson's disease. Mov Disord. 2015;30(2):121-7.
5. Weintraub D, Koester J, Potenza MN, Siderowf AD, Stacy M, Voon V, et al. Impulse control disorders in Parkinson disease: a cross-sectional study of 3090 patients. Arch Neurol. 2010;67(5):589-95.
6. Antonini A, Barone P, Bonuccelli U, Annoni K, Asgharnejad M, Stanzione P. ICARUS study: prevalence and clinical features of impulse control disorders in Parkinson's disease. J Neurol Neurosurg Psychiatry. 2017;88(4):317-24.
7. Corvol J-C, Artaud F, Cormier-Dequaire F, Rascol O, Durif F, Derkinderen P, et al. Longitudinal analysis of impulse control disorders in Parkinson disease. Neurology. 2018;91(3): e189-201.
8. Smith KM, Xie SX, Weintraub D. Incident impulse control disorder symptoms and dopamine transporter imaging in Parkinson disease. J Neurol Neurosurg Psychiatry. 2016;87(8):864-70.
9. Sarathchandran P, Soman S, Sarma G, Krishnan S, Kishore A. Impulse control disorders and related behaviors in Indian patients with Parkinson's disease. Mov Disord. 2013; 28(13):1901-2.
10. Sharma A, Goyal V, Behari M, Srivastva A, Shukla G, Vibha D. Impulse control disorders and related behaviours (ICD-RBs) in Parkinson's disease patients: Assessment using "Questionnaire for impulsive-compulsive disorders in Parkinson's disease" (QUIP). Ann Indian Acad Neurol. 2015;18(1):49-59.
11. Voon V, Sohr M, Lang AE, Potenza MN, Siderowf AD, Whetteckey J, et al. Impulse control disorders in Parkinson disease: a multicenter case--control study. Ann Neurol. 2011;69(6): 986-96.
12. Grall-Bronnec M, Victorri-Vigneau C, Donnio Y, Leboucher J, Rousselet M, Thiabaud E, et al. Dopamine Agonists and Impulse Control Disorders: A Complex Association. Drug Saf. 2018;41(1):19-75.
13 Weintraub D, Siderowf AD, Potenza MN, Goveas J, Morales KH, Duda JE, et al. Association of Dopamine Agonist Use with Impulse Control Disorders in Parkinson's Disease. Arch Neurol. 2006;63(7):969-73.
14. Zainal Abidin S, Tan EL, Chan S-C, Jaafar A, Lee AX, Abd Hamid MHN, et al. DRD and GRIN2B polymorphisms and their association with the development of impulse control behaviour among Malaysian Parkinson's disease patients. BMC Neurol. 2015;15:59.
15. Lee JY, Lee EK, Park SS, Lim JY, Kim HJ, Kim JS, et al. Association of DRD3 and GRIN2B with impulse control and related behaviors in Parkinson's disease. Mov Disord. 2009;24(12): 1803-10.
16. Krishnamoorthy S, Rajan R, Banerjee M, Kumar H, Sarma G, Krishnan S, et al. Dopamine D3 receptor Ser9Gly variant is associated with impulse control disorders in Parkinson's disease patients. Parkinsonism Relat Disord. 2016;30:13-7.
17. Kraemmer J, Smith K, Weintraub D, Guillemot V, Nalls MA, Cormier-Dequaire F, et al. Clinical-genetic model predicts incident impulse control disorders in Parkinson's disease. J Neurol Neurosurg Psychiatry. 2016;87(10):1106-11.
18. Michael Schüpbach WM. Impulsivity, impulse control disorders, and subthalamic stimulation in Parkinson's disease. Basal Ganglia. 2012;2(4):205-9.
19. Merola A, Romagnolo A, Rizzi L, Rizzone MG, Zibetti M, Lanotte M, et al. Impulse control behaviors and subthalamic deep brain stimulation in Parkinson disease. J Neurol. 2017;264(1):40-8.
20. Amami P, Dekker I, Piacentini S, Ferré F, Romito LM, Franzini A, et al. Impulse control behaviours in patients with Parkinson's disease after subthalamic deep brain stimulation: de novo cases and 3-year follow-up. J Neurol Neurosurg Psychiatry. 2015;86(5):562-4.

21. Lee JY, Jeon BS. Maladaptive Reward-Learning and Impulse Control Disorders in Patients with Parkinson's Disease: A Clinical Overview and Pathophysiology Update. J Mov Disord. 2014;7(2):67-76.
22. Brewer JA, Potenza MN. The Neurobiology and Genetics of Impulse Control Disorders: Relationships to Drug Addictions. Biochem Pharmacol. 2008;75(1):63-75.
23. Marques A, Durif F, Fernagut P-O. Impulse control disorders in Parkinson's disease. J Neural Transm (Vienna). 2018;125(8): 1299-312.
24. Frank MJ, Seeberger LC, O'reilly RC. By carrot or by stick: cognitive reinforcement learning in parkinsonism. Science. 2004;306(5703):1940-3.
25. Kéri S, Moustafa AA, Myers CE, Benedek G, Gluck MA. {alpha}-Synuclein gene duplication impairs reward learning. Proc Natl Acad Sci U S A. 2010;107(36):15992-4.
26. Ambroggi F, Ishikawa A, Fields HL, Nicola SM. Basolateral amygdala neurons facilitate reward-seeking behavior by exciting nucleus accumbens neurons. Neuron. 2008;59(4): 648-61.
27. Kalivas PW, Volkow N, Seamans J. Unmanageable motivation in addiction: a pathology in prefrontal-accumbens glutamate transmission. Neuron. 2005;45(5):647-50.
28. Macpherson T, Morita M, Hikida T. Striatal direct and indirect pathways control decision-making behavior. Front Psychol. 2014;5:1301.
29. Grace AA. Phasic versus tonic dopamine release and the modulation of dopamine system responsivity: a hypothesis for the etiology of schizophrenia. Neuroscience. 1991;41(1): 1-24.
30. Goto Y, Grace AA. Dopaminergic modulation of limbic and cortical drive of nucleus accumbens in goal-directed behavior. Nat Neurosci. 2005;8(6):805-12.
31. Weintraub D, Claassen DO. Impulse Control and Related Disorders in Parkinson's Disease. Int Rev Neurobiol. 2017;133:679-717.
32. Bhattacharjee S. Impulse control disorders in Parkinson's disease: Review of pathophysiology, epidemiology, clinical features, management, and future challenges. Neurol India. 2018;66(4):967-75.
33. Cossu G, Rinaldi R, Colosimo C. The rise and fall of impulse control behavior disorders. Parkinsonism Relat Disord. 2018;46(Suppl 1):S24-9.
34. Jiménez-Urbieta H, Gago B, de la Riva P, Delgado-Alvarado M, Marin C, Rodriguez-Oroz MC. Dyskinesias and impulse control disorders in Parkinson's disease: From pathogenesis to potential therapeutic approaches. Neurosci Biobehav Rev. 2015;56:294-314.
35. Maloney EM, Djamshidian A, O'Sullivan SS. Phenomenology and epidemiology of impulsive-compulsive behaviours in Parkinson's disease, atypical Parkinsonian disorders and non-Parkinsonian populations. J Neurol Sci. 2017;374:47-52.
36. Zhang Y, He AQ, Li L, Chen W, Liu ZG. Clinical characteristics of impulse control and related disorders in Chinese Parkinson's disease patients. BMC Neurol. 2017;17(1):98.
37. Ramírez Gómez CC, Serrano Dueñas M, Bernal O, Araoz N, Sáenz Farret M, Aldinio V, et al. A Multicenter Comparative Study of Impulse Control Disorder in Latin American Patients With Parkinson Disease. Clin Neuropharmacol. 2017;40(2): 51-5.
38. Chamberlain SR, Grant JE. Minnesota Impulse Disorders Interview (MIDI): Validation of a structured diagnostic clinical interview for impulse control disorders in an enriched community sample. Psychiatry Res. 2018;265:279-83.
39. Weintraub D, Hoops S, Shea JA, Lyons KE, Pahwa R, Driver-Dunckley ED, et al. Validation of the questionnaire for impulsive-compulsive disorders in Parkinson's disease. Mov Disord. 2009;24(10):1461-7.
40. McElroy SL, Keck PE, Pope HG, Smith JM, Strakowski SM. Compulsive buying: a report of 20 cases. J Clin Psychiatry. 1994;55(6):242-8.
41. Nirenberg MJ, Waters C. Compulsive eating and weight gain related to dopamine agonist use. Mov Disord. 2006;21(4): 524-9.
42. Evans AH, Katzenschlager R, Paviour D, O'Sullivan JD, Appel S, Lawrence AD, et al. Punding in Parkinson's disease: its relation to the dopamine dysregulation syndrome. Mov Disord. 2004;19(4):397-405.
43. Warren N, O'Gorman C, Lehn A, Siskind D. Dopamine dysregulation syndrome in Parkinson's disease: a systematic review of published cases. J Neurol Neurosurg Psychiatry. 2017;88(12):1060-4.
44. Giovannoni G, O'Sullivan JD, Turner K, Manson AJ, Lees AJ. Hedonistic homeostatic dysregulation in patients with Parkinson's disease on dopamine replacement therapies. J Neurol Neurosurg Psychiatry. 2000;68(4):423-8.
45. Pezzella FR, Colosimo C, Vanacore N, Di Rezze S, Chianese M, Fabbrini G, et al. Prevalence and clinical features of hedonistic homeostatic dysregulation in Parkinson's disease. Mov Disord. 2005;20(1):77-81.
46. Samuel M, Rodriguez-Oroz M, Antonini A, Brotchie JM, Ray Chaudhuri K, Brown RG, et al. Management of impulse control disorders in Parkinson's disease: Controversies and future approaches. Mov Disord. 2015;30(2):150-9.
47. Ramirez-Zamora A, Gee L, Boyd J, Biller J. Treatment of impulse control disorders in Parkinson's disease: Practical considerations and future directions. Expert Rev Neurother. 2016;16(4):389-99.
48. Papay K, Xie SX, Stern M, Hurtig H, Siderowf A, Duda JE, et al. Naltrexone for impulse control disorders in Parkinson disease: a placebo-controlled study. Neurology. 2014;83(9):826-33.
49. Kim A, Kim YE, Kim HJ, Yun JY, Yang HJ, Lee WW, et al. A 7-year observation of the effect of subthalamic deep brain stimulation on impulse control disorder in patients with Parkinson's disease. Parkinsonism Relat Disord. 2018;56:3-8.
50. Vitale C, Amboni M, Erro R, Picillo M, Pellecchia MT, Barone P, et al. Parkinson's disease management and impulse control disorders: current state and future perspectives. Expert Rev Neurother. 2019;19(6):495-508.

CHAPTER **11**

Sleep in Parkinson's Disease

Preeti Devnani, Nikita Changlani, Rachael Fernandes

INTRODUCTION

"...the sleep becomes much disturbed. The tremulous motions of the limbs occur during sleep, and augment until they awaken the patient, and frequently with much agitation and alarm..."

—(*An essay on the Shaking Palsy, James Parkinson, 1817*).

Parkinson's disease (PD) is manifested by resting tremor, rigidity, bradykinesia, and postural instability. Though traditionally described with motor manifestations is currently recognized for its debilitating nonmotor manifestations and multisystem involvement such as autonomic dysregulation, cognitive impairment, constipation, mood, and sleep disturbances. These often grossly impair quality of life and functional outcome. Prevalence of sleep disorders in patients with PD is 2–3.5 times higher than that in healthy controls. About 60–98% of patients with PD has sleep disturbances such as sleep fragmentation, excessive daytime sleepiness (EDS), restless leg syndrome (RLS), parasomnias, disturbed sleep/wake patterns, circadian rhythm disorders, rapid eye movement (REM) behavior disorder (RBD), and sleep-disordered breathing.[1] Involuntary daytime sleep "attacks" may occur due to medications that are used to treat PD. Sleep disturbances, such as RBD, are known to predate the motor manifestations for decades.

Sleep quality is known to impact attention and executive function. Patients with RBD exhibit impairment to perform tasks of executive,[2,3] memory, and visuospatial function,[3] proposing that manifestation of RBD indicates a more rapid cognitive decline.

PATHOPHYSIOLOGY OF SLEEP DISTURBANCES IN PARKINSON'S DISEASE

In PD, there is a reduction of dopamine-producing neurons leading to dopamine depletion in substantia nigra (SN) and in the nigrostriatal pathway to the caudate and putamen.[4] The relative over-activity of the indirect pathway functionally disinhibits the subthalamic nucleus (STN). Decreased inhibition of the direct pathway causes additional disinhibition of the output nuclei [globus pallidus internus (GPi) and substantia nigra pars reticulata (SNr)]. Increased output from GPi causes increased inhibition of the thalamus and reduced excitatory input to the motor cortex. There is increasing evidence that the genetic and environmental insults leading to PD commonly lead to abnormal forms of a normal protein, α-synuclein, which seem to contribute to cell death.[5] Neurodegenerative changes in central sleep regulatory centers in the forebrain thalamus and SN that occur in PD contribute to sleep disturbances. Degenerative changes in PD may directly affect sleep/wake mechanisms. Neurotransmitters that mediate non-REM (NREM) and REM sleep mediate sleep functions such as norepinephrine, serotonin, dopamine, γ-aminobutyric acid (GABA), and glycine are variably damaged in PD. Lesions in the arousal pathway result in EDS, often with a narcolepsy-like phenotype. Motor disability, painful dystonia, restless legs, mood disturbances, and vivid dreaming impair sleep quality in PD. Dopaminergic medications dosage and timing of administration can alter sleep quality and daytime alertness.

Positron emission tomography (PET) imaging of dopamine transporters (DATs) were performed in 41 patients. Striatal dopaminergic depletion were not significantly correlated with any of the various nonmotor symptoms in PD.[6]

SLEEP MANIFESTATIONS IN PARKINSON'S DISEASE

Excessive Daytime Sleepiness and Parkinson's Disease

Excessive daytime sleepiness in patients with PD is three to four fold more prevalent than in healthy controls, affecting about 21–76% of patients. EDS symptoms can fluctuate over the course of PD and significantly impacts quality of life and daytime functioning. It can mimic certain narcolepsy type symptoms, such as abrupt onset of REM sleep and sleep attacks. These can be objectively demonstrated as reduced mean sleep latency and sleep onset REMs on multiple sleep latency testing. The etiology of EDS in PD is thought to be multifactorial. EDS can be worsened by dopaminergic medications, comorbid mood disturbances, and nonrestorative sleep. Medications that alter sleep parameters include antidepressants, antipsychotics, and diuretics. These patients have underlying circadian rhythm abnormalities and expected physiological changes in sleep. While the pathophysiology of these changes is not definite, cerebrospinal fluid phosphorylated tau/total tau ratio, and subsequent autonomic dysfunction may be contributing factors. PD patient with EDS exhibits alterations in brain structure and function. It is unclear whether EDS is a potential manifestation of more severe brain stem neurodegeneration.

Excessive daytime sleepiness may be associated with an increased risk of cognitive decline. Among 4,894 elderly people, those who felt sleepy during the daytime had an increased risk of cognitive decline 8 years later.[6]

Sleep Attacks

Sleep attacks are sudden onset of sleep episodes that could occur in patients with PD. The incidence of these sleep attacks has been reported to be 3.8–22.8%. Patients with PD often decide to reduce driving due to perception of declining ability to drive.[7] A significant contributing factor to these sleep attacks in patients with PD other than poor quality night-time sleep is dopaminergic medications as dopamine agonists and levodopa/carbidopa combinations.

Insomnia

The prevalence of insomnia in patients with PD varies from 27 to 80%. Common manifestations of insomnia are sleep fragmentation (74–88%) and early awakenings (terminal insomnia; 40%).[8] In addition to PD pathophysiology, motor symptoms (particularly inability to turn over in bed and foot cramps), medications, mood disorders, pain, physical disability (lack of exercise), and poor sleep hygiene contribute to the clinical presentation of insomnia in patients with PD. Research has shown that doxepin and nonpharmacologic treatment such as cognitive behavioral therapy with bright light therapy substantially improve insomnia in PD.[9]

Restless Leg Syndrome and Parkinson's Disease

Restless leg syndrome is characterized as an urge to move the legs associated with uncomfortable sensations, motor restlessness, worsening at rest with at least partial relief by activity, and circadian variation (URGE diagnostic criteria: International Restless Legs Study Group). Sleep disturbances, periodic limb movement in sleep (PLMS), a positive family history, and favorable clinical response to dopaminergic drugs support the diagnosis. RLS tends to present in mid to later life with a prevalence of 2.7–10% in Western populations.[10,11] Several clinical studies have shown an association between RLS and PD.[12-14] PD symptoms preceded the RLS symptoms in approximately 70% of patient. Nomura et al. reported only 10 (7.9%) patients with RLS among 126 PD patients.[15] PD patients with RLS were older and had a higher prevalence of depression than those without RLS, less likely to have a family history of RLS, and had lower serum ferritin levels. It has been postulated that there is a possible masking effect of dopaminergic therapy when assessing for RLS in PD. A recent study of 11 patients with 2 *Parkin* mutations and 11 sex-matched patients with idiopathic PD found the prevalence of RLS to be 45% and 0%, respectively ($p = 0.04$), providing stronger evidence of an association with *Parkin* mutation.[16,17] No differences in the clinical phenotype were found between RLS patients with and without a *Parkin* mutation. The dopaminergic neuronal cell loss in the ventrolateral part of the substantia nigra pars compacta (SNPC) are thought to contribute to the motor symptoms and link PD and RLS. Variability in lesion patterning might explain why some patients with PD may develop RLS. Also notable are significant increases in tyrosine hydroxylase in the SN in PD but not in the putamen in RLS.[18] RLS can be an accompaniment of several other pathological conditions. Uremia, low ferritin, neuropathy, and myelopathy can present with secondary

RLS. Treatment of the underlying disease in these conditions may substantially alleviate RLS. RLS in PD can further contribute to poor night-time sleep by potentially promoting hyperarousal episodes.

RAPID EYE MOVEMENT SLEEP BEHAVIOR DISORDER AND PARKINSON'S DISEASE

Rapid eye movement sleep behavior disorder, which is characterized by dream-enacted, sometimes violent and aggressive behaviors was first reported by Schenck and his colleagues in 1986. In 1965, Jouvet et al. showed that cats with bilateral pontine tegmental lesions developed "Oneiric behavior" (dream related behavior) similar to RBD in humans. In 1970s, Hishikawa's group had also described peculiar sleep state in alcoholics similar to RBD.

During REM sleep there is characteristically muscle atonia. In RBD, this muscle atonia is absent during REM sleep. RBD occurs in 25–65% of patients with PD and antedates onset of motor findings of PD by several years in 20–30% of cases. However, <1% of patients with PD complain about RBD symptoms to their primary care physician before receiving a diagnosis of PD. RBD in PD patients is associated with faster motor progression in patients with greater synuclein and dopaminergic pathology and with higher risk of cognitive decline in patients with greater synuclein and amyloid pathology.

The prevalence of patients with PD in India varies greatly depending upon the geographical area from a relatively low of 14–41/100,000 in non-Parsi communities to an exceptionally high of 328/100,000 in Parsi communities.[19] In a case-control study conducted in north India, 26 (19.4%) of 134 patients had RBD.[20] Patients with RBD had significantly higher prevalence of insomnia, nocturnal awakening, early morning awakenings, and snoring. Most clinical events were brief and confined to vocalization or limb movements.

NONRAPID EYE MOVEMENT PARASOMNIAS AND PARKINSON'S DISEASE

Occurrences of NREM parasomnia behavior (NPB) are manifestations of a continuum of the intricate pathophysiology of arousal disorders involving dysfunction of cortical and subcortical motor control during sleep in PD. NPBs might be due to the combination of structural [i.e., neurodegeneration and functional (drug-induced) dysfunction]. Adult onset sleepwalking or somnambulism usually appears to be a late manifestation of moderate to severe PD. Confusional arousals, somniloquy, sleep eating, and sexsomnia can occur in patients with PD.

Total of 26 out of 417 (6%) PD patients reported sleepwalking and also features of RBD, suggesting the presence of parasomnia overlap disorder.

ASSESSMENT AND MANAGEMENT OF SLEEP PROBLEMS IN PATIENTS WITH PARKINSON'S DISEASE

The Parkinson's Disease Sleep Scale (PDSS) Numerical scoring and its modified version (PDSS-2), and the Scales for Outcomes in PD-Sleep (SCOPA-S) for sleep disturbances are specifically developed, validated, and employed for screening for PD. PDSS is a visual analog scale addressing 15 commonly reported symptoms associated with sleep disturbance. It is a reliable and easily administered questionnaire measuring sleep disturbances. This includes the following:

- Overall quality of night's sleep
- Sleep onset and maintenance insomnia
- Nocturnal restlessness
- Nocturnal psychosis
- Nocturia
- Nocturnal motor symptoms
- Sleep refreshment
- Daytime dozing

Parkinson's Disease Sleep Scale, along with Epworth Sleepiness Scale (ESS) (a widely accepted sleepiness scale), is an "easy to apply" instrument for identifying sleep-related problems in PD. In addition, for specific assessment for RBD, the RBD clinical questionnaire can be used.

TREATMENT STRATEGIES

Nonpharmacological Management of Insomnia

Cognitive behavior therapy and sleep-hygiene measures, particularly, restricting excessive time in bed and avoiding evening naps are cornerstones of management. Light is an important "zeitgeber" of the sleep-wake cycle and many elderly individuals and individuals with chronic illness have reduced exposure to bright light. Exposure to bright light entrains the body to normal cycles of light and dark with normalization of sleep circadian rhythm.[21,22]

Pharmacotherapy

Optimum treatment by medications for sleep must be individualized, depending on sleep onset, maintenance, or early morning awakening symptomatology.

Medications such as hypnotics (e.g., zolpidem and eszopiclone-newer benzodiazepine receptor agonist) are helpful in addressing insomnia but preferably avoided in concomitant untreated sleep apnea patients.

Hypnotic drugs, often prescribed for sleep disorders, worsen daytime sedation and the risk of falls and are therefore less suitable for PD patients.[23] Melatonin may benefit subjective sleep disturbances in PD patients, but objective improvement of sleep quality is minimal.

Ramelteon, a melatonin receptor agonist, is useful in sleep initiation insomnia. Sedating antidepressants (e.g., mirtazapine and trazodone) are useful in insomnia. Side effects that include urinary retention, effect on blood pressure, and the potential for appearance of extrapyramidal symptoms are to be observed with caution.

Clonazepam may be a good option for the treatment of maintenance insomnia (i.e., sleep fragmentation) due to PLMS or if RBD is present.

If insomnia is due to motor disability of PD, evening dose of controlled-release levodopa to improve mobility improves insomnia and improving subjective sleep quantity. Memantine has been shown to be useful in the other nocturnal behavioral abnormalities in PD patients with dementia.[24]

Sustained Release versus Immediate Release Formulations

Use of sustained release formulations improves nocturnal symptoms in advanced PD with sleep disturbances. Use of rotigotine (RTG) for nocturnal dysfunction in PD has been suggested in several open-label studies, in the RECOVER study which was the first one to use the PDSS-2 as a core primary outcome measure, no significant impact on daytime somnolence was observed. In the NIGHT-PD study, RTG transdermal patch showed benefit in sleep dysfunction and nocturia in PD.

Impact of Surgery

Patients with PD have reported the emergence of RLS after STN deep brain stimulation (DBS).[25] In a study conducted in 17 patients undergoing STN DBS, six patients were diagnosed with RLS preoperatively and no new cases emerged after the surgery.[26] Although STN DBS improves overall sleep quality and RLS symptoms, case reports of parasomnia overlap syndrome have been reported post DBS.[27]

MANAGEMENT OF EXCESSIVE DAYTIME SLEEPINESS

Behavioral interventions such as scheduled naps, scheduling alerting activities in evening hours, sunlight exposure on awakening, timed dosage administration of dopaminergic drugs, and judicious usage of sedating drugs help to address EDS.

Modafinil, a wake-promoting medication promoting alertness and enhancing cognition through dopamine, hypocretin, histamine, epinephrine, GABA, and glutamate pathways is used in primary hypersomnia of central origin and narcolepsy. Meta-analysis of three trials showed modafinil usage to have a significant reduction in sleepiness, as assessed by the ESS (–2.24 points, 95% CI –3.90 to –0.57, $p < 0.05$). In one study, treatment with caffeine was associated with a nonsignificant improvement of 1.71 points in ESS (95% CI –3.57 to 0.13).[28]

In a small trial, nocturnally administered sodium oxybate, increased slow-wave sleep as a percentage of total sleep time and improved subjective night-time and day-time sleep complaints in patients with PD.[29]

Sleep Disturbances: The Caregiver Burden

Caring for patients with PD and poor health related quality of life in patients with PD increase the strain in caregivers. Self-perceived bad night-time sleep in spouses (27%) was related to the severity of PD and poor sleep quality in patients with PD.[30,31]

CONCLUSION

Patients with PD have been shown to have poor sleep efficiency and sleep fragmentation, resulting in negative neurocognitive outcomes related to severe sleep deprivation. EDS may be confounded by dopaminergic medications. The heterogeneity of sleep disturbances that impacts the clinical burden of PD is frequently undiagnosed. Sleep disorders in PD are common and amenable to treatment. A lower clinical threshold to identify and appropriately intervene would help maximize the impact of "sleep benefit" i.e., motor improvement on awakening as well as long-term cognitive and functional gain.

REFERENCES

1. Mondragón-Rezola E, Arratíbel-Echarren I, Ruiz-Martínez J, Martí-Massó JF. Sleep disorders in Parkinson's disease: insomnia and sleep fragmentation, daytime hypersomnia, alterations to the circadian rhythm and sleep apnea syndrome. Rev Neurol. 2010;50(Suppl 2):S21-6.
2. Sinforiani E, Zangaglia R, Manni R, Cristina S, Marchioni E, Nappi G, et al. REM sleep behavior disorder, hallucinations, and cognitive impairment in Parkinson's disease. Mov Disord. 2006;21(4):462-6.

3. Vendette M, Gagnon JF, Decary A, Massicotte-Marquez J, Postuma RB, Doyon J, et al. REM sleep behavior disorder predicts cognitive impairment in Parkinson disease without dementia. Neurology. 2007;69(19):1843-9.
4. Alexander GE. Biology of Parkinson's disease: pathogenesis and pathophysiology of a multisystem neurodegenerative disorder. Dialogues Clin Neurosci. 2004;6(3):259-80.
5. Stefanis L. α-Synuclein in Parkinson's Disease. Cold Spring Harb Perspect Med. 2012;2(2):a009399.
6. Jaussent I, Bouyer J, Ancelin ML, Berr C, Foubert-Samier A, Ritchie K, et al. Excessive sleepiness is predictive of cognitive decline in the elderly. Sleep. 2012;35(9):1201-7.
7. Chung SJ, Lee JJ, Ham JH, Ye BS, Lee PH, Sohn YH. Striatal Dopamine Depletion Patterns and Early Non-Motor Burden in Parkinsons Disease. PLoS One. 2016;11(8):e0161316.
8. Ylikoski A, Martikainen K, Partinen M. Parkinson's disease and restless legs syndrome. Eur Neurol. 2015;73(3-4):212-9.
9. Stolwyk RJ, Scally KA, Charlton JL, Bradshaw JL, Iansek R, Georgiou-Karistianis N. Self-Regulation of Driving Behavior in People with Parkinson Disease. Cogn Behav Neurol. 2015;28(2):80-91.
10. Rothdach AJ, Trenkwalder C, Haberstock J, Keil U, Berger K. Prevalence and risk factors of RLS in an elderly population: the MEMO study. Memory and Morbidity in Augsburg Elderly. Neurology. 2000;54(5):1064-8.
11. Allen RP, Walters AS, Montplaisir J, Hening W, Myers A, Bell TJ, et al. Restless legs syndrome prevalence and impact: REST general population study. Arch Intern Med. 2005;165(11):1286-92.
12. Ondo WG, Vuong KD, Jankovic J. Exploring the relationship between Parkinson disease and restless legs syndrome. Arch Neurol. 2002;59(3):421-4.
13. Garcia-Borreguero D, Odin P, Serrano C. Restless legs syndrome and PD: a review of the evidence for a possible association. Neurology. 2003;61(6):S49-55.
14. Banno K, Delaive K, Walld R, Kryger MH. Restless legs syndrome in 218 patients: associated disorders. Sleep Med. 2000;1(3):221-9.
15. Nomura T, Inoue Y, Miyake M, Yasui K, Nakashima K. Prevalence and clinical characteristics of restless legs syndrome in Japanese patients with Parkinson's disease. Mov Disord. 2006;21(3):380-4.
16. Adel S, Djarmati A, Kabakci K, Pichler I, Eskelson C, Lohnau T, et al. Co-occurrence of restless legs syndrome and Parkin mutations in two families. Mov Disord. 2006;21(2):258-63.
17. Limousin N, Konofal E, Karroum E, Lohmann E, Theodorou I, Dürr A, et al. Restless legs syndrome, rapid eye movement sleep behavior disorder, and hypersomnia in patients with two parkin mutations. Mov Disord. 2009;24(13):1970-6.
18. Peeraully T, Tan EK. Linking restless legs syndrome with Parkinson's disease: clinical, imaging and genetic evidence. Transl Neurodegener. 2012;1(1):6.
19. Bharucha NE, Bharucha EP, Bharucha AE, Bhise AV, Schoenberg BS. Prevalence of Parkinson's disease in the Parsi community of Bombay, India. Arch Neurol. 1988;45(12):1321-3.
20. Vibha D, Shukla G, Goyal V, Singh S, Srivastava AK, Behari M. RBD in Parkinson's disease: A clinical case control study from North India. Clin Neurol Neurosurg. 2011;113(6):472-6.
21. Thorpy MJ. Sleep disorders in Parkinson's disease. Clin Cornerstone. 2004;6(1):S7-15.
22. Dowling GA, Mastick J, Colling E, Carter JH, Singer CM, Aminoff MJ. Melatonin for sleep disturbances in Parkinson's disease. Sleep Med. 2005;6(5):459-66.
23. Xiang W, Sun YQ, Teoh HC. Comparison of nocturnal symptoms in advanced Parkinson's disease patients with sleep disturbances: pramipexole sustained release versus immediate release formulations. Drug Des Devel Ther. 2018;12:2017-24.
24. Levin OS, Batukaeva LA. Efficacy of memantine in Parkinson's disease with dementia. Zh Nevrol Psikhiatr Im S S Korsakova. 2008;108(12):16-23.
25. Kedia S, Moro E, Tagliati M, Lang AE, Kumar R. Emergence of restless legs syndrome during subthalamic stimulation for Parkinson disease. Neurol. 2004;63(12):2410-2.
26. Chahine LM, Ahmed A, Sun Z. Effects of STN DBS for Parkinson's disease on restless legs syndrome and other sleep-related measures. Parkinsonism Relat Disord. 2011;17(3):208-11.
27. Bargiotas P, Muellner J, Schuepbach WMM, Bassetti CL. Parasomnia overlap disorder, Parkinson's disease and subthalamic deep brain stimulation: three case reports. BMC Neurol. 2017;17(1):137.
28. Rodrigues TM, Castro Caldas A, Ferreira JJ. Pharmacological interventions for daytime sleepiness and sleep disorders in Parkinson's disease: Systematic review and meta-analysis. Parkinsonism Relat Disord. 2016;27:25-34.
29. Ondo WG, Perkins T, Swick T, Hull KL Jr, Jimenez JE, Garris TS, et al. Sodium oxybate for excessive daytime sleepiness in Parkinson disease: an open-label polysomnographic study. Arch Neurol. 2008;65(10):1337-40.
30. Happe S, Berger K; FAQT Study Investigators. The association between caregiver burden and sleep disturbances in partners of patients with Parkinson's disease. Age Ageing. 2002;31(5):349-54.
31. Kelly DH, McGinley JL, Huxham FE, Menz HB, Watts JJ, Iansek R, et al. Health-related quality of life and strain in caregivers of Australians with Parkinson's disease: An observational study. BMC Neurol. 2012;12:57.

CHAPTER 12

Dysautonomia in Parkinson's Disease

Sujith Ovallath, Rinsha Rafeeqe

INTRODUCTION

Parkinson's disease (PD) is characterized by motor and nonmotor clinical features out of which motor symptoms like tremor, bradykinesia, postural instability, and rigidity are most prevalent and disabling for the patients. Behavioral, sleep or perceptual dysfunction as well as dysautonomia constitute the nonmotor symptoms of PD. Deficits in cardiovascular, gastrointestinal (GI), genitourinary, and thermoregulatory functions constitute autonomic features in PD.[1] This has been mentioned by James Parkinson in his historic description of parkinsonism as "mysterious sympathetic influence" in connection with the autonomic nervous system.[2]

Dysautonomias reflect a primary abnormality of autonomic systems or of regulation of those systems. Both types of primary as well as secondary autonomic abnormality seem to occur in PD. There is mounting evidence that PD affects a chain of neurons in autonomic pathways. Consequently, autonomic physiology may serve as a window into nonmotor PD progression and allow the development of mechanistically-based treatment strategies for several nonmotor features of PD.[3]

Dysautonomia develops as the disease advances, affecting the quality of life and the course of treatment of PD. One of the most crucial differential diagnoses for dysautonomia is multiple system atrophy and progressive supranuclear palsy. PD affected patients with comorbidities like diabetes are more prone for secondary dysautonomia. Autonomic dysfunction is seen in case of many drug interactions especially psychotropic drugs with their vast effects such as anticholinergic, adrenergic, and other effects.[4]

The autonomic manifestations in PD can present as mainly affect cardiovascular manifestation, bowel dysfunction, lower urinary tract dysfunction, or sexual dysfunction.

PATHOPHYSIOLOGY

Autonomic nervous system can be divided into central autonomic networks, sympathetic pathways, parasympathetic pathways, and the enteric nervous system. The autonomic function is controlled by central autonomic networks, linking the neocortex, diencephalon, and brainstem.[4] The somatic and autonomic nervous systems are integrated by the nucleus tractus solitarius (NTS) and maintain homeostasis with projections to the hypothalamus, limbic structures, and descending autonomic tracts.[5] PD pathology is characterized by intraneuronal inclusions which contain alpha (α)-synuclein known as Lewy bodies (Lewy-related pathology). α-synuclein is a presynaptic protein thought to involve in maintaining synaptic integrity and regulate dopamine synthesis. PD pathology is caused by α-synuclein aggregation which in turn is responsible for neurodegeneration. α-synuclein degeneration was demonstrated in a chain of neurons forming autonomic pathways including: The hypothalamus, preganglionic parasympathetic projection neurons in the dorsal motor nucleus of the vagus and preganglionic and postganglionic sympathetic projection neurons. α-synucleinopathy was also found in several end organs including the submandibular gland, lower esophagus, duodenum, pancreas, bronchus, larynx, epicardium, adrenal medulla, parathyroid, and ovary.

CARDIOVASCULAR SYSTEM

Patients with PD frequently have symptoms or signs consistent with cardiovascular dysautonomia. Numerous sympathetic neuroimaging studies have shown that most patients with PD have at least some loss of sympathetic innervation of the heart, and results of long-term follow-up. Concentrations of radioactivity have been noted after injection of different sympathoneural imaging agents, including ^{123}I-metaiodobenzylguanidine, 6-^{18}F-fluorodopamine, and ^{11}C-hydroxyephedrine.[6] A histological loss of neurons and Lewy bodies in peripheral parts of the sympathetic nervous system, for example, in the sympathetic ganglia or a loss in tyrosine hydrolase color in the epicardium area can also be found in PD patients. Damage or destruction of postganglionic sympathetic efferents is the main origin of dysautonomia. Parallel to cardiac denervation, there is histological loss of neurons and Lewy bodies in peripheral parts of sympathetic nervous system.

Orthostatic Hypotension

Orthostatic hypotension (OH) can be defined as fall in blood pressure of ≥20 mm Hg systolic or 10 mm Hg diastolic when moving from supine to standing. It is present in up to 52% of PD patients.[7] How OH in PD happens is a subject of debate but thought mostly as a consequence of sympathetic denervation of the vasculature, as cardiac sympathetic denervation does not impair orthostatic tolerance. In normal persons, baroreflex-mediated sympathetic activation causing vasoconstriction maintains blood pressure in the standing posture. This compensatory vasoconstriction is absent or attenuated in patients with PD, resulting in OH. Interestingly, OH can occasionally precede the development of PD. Other factors like insufficient water intake, diabetes, and medications like amantadine, levodopa, and selegiline can also contribute to orthostatic fall in blood pressure. In advanced dysautonomia, supine hypotension can also be a feature.

Heart Rate Variability

Heart rate variability (HRV) is also is an important diagnostic tool to screen for individuals at risk for PD. Some HRV variables, namely the standard deviation of the R-R intervals (SDNN), the very-low frequency (VLF) and low frequency (LF) spectral components, and the LF/HF ratio, are found to be decreased in patients with PD. Details of autonomic testing are described in **Table 1**.

TABLE 1: Autonomic changes in Parkinson's disease.

	Test	*Results in PD*	*Impression*
Cardiovascular system	Valsalva in baroreflex in SBP[9]	Lower compensatory increase in SBP[8]	Sympathetic deficiency
	Respiratory sinus arryhthmia (measured during valsalva, deep breathing, standing up or hand grip)	• Premature ventricular contractions • Sympathetic deficiency in baroreflex	Lower compensatory increase
		Lower hear rate variability influence[10,11]	Parasympathetic deficiency in vagal
Skin/Sweat gland	Sympathetic skin response	Lower amplitude and longer latency[12-16]	Sympathetic deficiency in distal extremities
	Thermoregulatory sweat test QSART sympathetic deficiency	• 10e40% anhidrosis[17,18] • Normal or lower sweat response[19,20]	Cutaneous sympathetic deficiency
	Microneurography	Lower skin sympathetic peroneal nerve activity[21]	Post-ganglionic cutaneous sympathetic deficiency
Urinary tract	Urodynamic testing	Reduced bladder capacity, detrusor overactivity, external sphincter relaxation[22]	Parasympathetic dysfunction in nigrostriatal and ventral-tegmental-mesolimbic systems
Gastrointestinal tract	Colonic scintigraphy	Longer colonic transit time[22]	Parasympathetic dysfunction in enteric network and vagus
	Esophageal manometry and scintigraphy	Esophageal dysmotolity[23]	Parasympathetic dysfunction in vagus motor pathways
	Gastric scintigraphy	Delayed gastric emptying time[24]	Parasympathetic dysfunction in vagus motor pathways
Pupil	Electrogastrography parasympathetic tone	More time with gastric dysrhythmia[25]	Relatively lower gastric
	Light reflex pupillography	Lower constriction velocity[26]	Lower parasympathetic function from the Edinger–Westphal nucleus

(SBP: systolic blood pressure; QSART: quantitative sudomotor axon-reflex test)

SKIN AND SWEAT GLANDS

Both hyperhidrosis and reduced sweating have been reported in PD. Sweating is controlled by sympathetic signals originating in preoptic sweat center in hypothalamus. The sympathetic fibers synapse with neurons in the intermediolateral cell columns of the spinal cord. This is further connected to unmyelinated postganglionic class C fibers in the paravertebral ganglia that form peripheral nerves to reach the sweat glands.[27] Skin biopsies done in PD patients have demonstrated lower cutaneous autonomic innervation in blood vessels, sweat glands, and arrector pili muscle.[28] The sympathetic skin response (SSR) is recorded by electrodes on the palmar and plantar surfaces and thermoregulatory sweat testing (TST) and the quantitative sudomotor axon-reflex test (QSART) are useful test for autonomic skin involvement.[12,17,18,29-31] It has been determined that excessive sweating in PD may occur as a compensatory reaction to lower sympathetic function in the extremities.[32]

URINARY TRACT

Urinary symptoms are very common and observed in up to 60% of PD patients. Nocturia, urgency, frequency, incontinence, and difficulty in voiding, attributable to bladder overactivity are frequently observed in PD.[22] The innervation of bladder is primarily through the parasympathetic pelvic nerve and the urethra is through the sympathetic hypogastric nerve and somatic pudendal nerve. PD neuropathology has been found in preganglionic and postganglionic sympathetic neurons as well as sacral parasympathetic nuclei. α-synuclein deposits are seen in the sacral spinal cord, pelvic plexus, and genitourinary tract in PD. Urodynamic studies performed in PD patients have demonstrated abnormalities in PD include reduced bladder capacity, detrusor overactivity, external sphincter relaxation, detrusor weakness and mild urethral obstruction,[33,34] reflecting parasympathetic and somatic dysfunction.

GASTROINTESTINAL SYSTEM

The autonomic innervation of the GI tract is by the enteric nervous system. Both Auerbach's and Meissner's plexuses are found to contain Lewy-related pathology in PD, most frequently in the lower esophagus.[22] There are several causes that can contribute to bowel dysmotility in PD. Low intake of fiber, lack of exercise, anticholinergics, and other medications can contribute. Lewy-related pathology has also been seen in the submandibular glands, stomach, small intestine, colon, and rectum in PD. Then pathology is found to follow a rostrocaudal gradient with the submandibular glands being most affected in density of α-synuclein staining, and the rectum the least.[22] In PD, 50% report lower GI symptoms such as constipation, diarrhea, and fecal incontinence.[35] In PD, constipation occurs from decreased colonic transport and disturbed defecation. Colonic transit time is increased in almost 80% of PD patients,[24] and most patients find it difficult defecate completely resulting in constipation. The bowel abnormality starts several years prior to the onset of motor symptoms of PD. In normal individuals, as rectal pressure increases, anal pressure decreases to allow passage of stool. Both rectal pressure and anal pressure increase together in 65% of PD patients.

The synucleinopathy in upper GI tract results in drooling, esophageal dysmotility, and delayed gastric emptying. Salivary production is reduced in PD, but drooling can occur due to different mechanisms. It may be due to reduced swallowing which may reflect involvement of cranial autonomic ganglia or brainstem salivary nuclei. Esophageal dysmotility is due to the impairments in vagal motor pathways. Delayed gastric emptying and gastric retention result in nausea, early satiety, and abdominal distention. Researchers have demonstrated evidence of parasympathetic dysfunction throughout the entire GI tract in PD.[36,37]

PUPILLARY CHANGES

Lewy-related pathology has been demonstrated in the Edinger–Westphal nucleus, hypothalamus, amygdala, hippocampus, and cerebral cortex.[38] Sympathetic predominance results in dilatation, while parasympathetic activity constricts the pupil.

TREATMENT

Finally, it is recognized that neuropathology of PD is not restricted to the substantia nigra or even the central dopaminergic system, but may involve the retina, peripheral autonomic nervous system and the olfactory nerves. Although various etiologies are present for autonomic symptoms in PD patients, in this chapter we will focus on the evaluation and treatment of autonomic disturbances associated with PD. For an optimal management of autonomic symptoms in PD, it requires both pharmacological and nonpharmacological approaches, and is usually only partially controlled with conventional dopaminergic therapies.

Nonpharmacological approaches for autonomic symptoms in PD have been shown in **Table 2**.

The symptoms of OH are as a result of reduced cerebral perfusion when upright. OH can be defined as a fall in systolic blood pressure below 20 mm Hg and a fall in diastolic pressure below 10 mm Hg within 3 minutes of active standing or head-up tilt. Cerebral hypoperfusion

TABLE 2: Nonpharmacological approaches for autonomic symptoms in Parkinson's disease.

Symptom	*Approach*[39]
Orthostatic hypotension and intolerance	• Avoid rapid positional changes and Valsalva maneuvers • Adopt physical countermaneuvers when required • Use tight stockings and abdominal compression bands • Use head-up body tilt (>30° incline during night), a 2–2.5 L of water and 8 g of sodium chloride daily intake • Avoid meal rich in carbohydrates and alcohol in order to avoid postprandial hypotension • Avoid exposure to warm temperature and vigorous physical exercises
Sialorrhea	• Using tactile cue for swallowing as chewing gums or candies • Adopt behavioral modification program for swallowing
Constipation	• Practice moderate physical exercise • Adequate water intake • Use of symbiotic yogurt and bulking agents
Hyperhidrosis and seborrhea	Dandruff shampoo topical applications
Weight loss	• Dietary management and energy-dense oral nutritional supplements intake

results in lightheadedness, visual disturbances or syncope in severe cases, are the typical symptoms seen in OH. It is seen that some patients are very tolerant, and do not experience any symptoms despite very low blood pressures, this is probably as a result of cerebral autoregulatory vasodilatation. In other organs, hypoperfusion in the heart can be result in angina pectoris while renal hypoperfusion may lead to oliguria and renal failure. Reduced perfusion of neck muscles results in pain affecting suboccipital and shoulder regions. Weakness, lethargy, and fatigue can occur as nonspecific symptoms seen in patients with OH. Documentation of circadian changes in blood pressure during sleep patients with autonomic failure and OH, together with a low diurnal blood pressure is aggravated by nocturnal polyuria and natriuresis. However, in many cases, OH is more likely to occur after tilting than on standing. It is often delayed by longer than the recommended 3 minutes; therefore, an evaluation of OH in PD should include blood pressure measurements before and after tilting at 60° for about 5 minutes.

Before initiating any pharmacological intervention, patients with PD and autonomic failure should be informed about various precipitating events. Patients should avoid rapid changes in position, especially from supine or sitting to standing and they should wait a few seconds before standing up. A daily intake of 2–2.5 L of water and at least 8 g of salt should be encouraged. Avoid straining during micturition or defecation. Different physical countermaneuvers, such as leg-crossing, bending forward, placing a foot on a chair can be applied at the onset of presyncopal symptoms. Tight stockings will prevent venous pooling, or abdominal compression bands can help in increasing the venous return thus preventing symptomatic OH. Since OH is often worsened after heavy meals, presumably because of splanchnic vasodilatation, avoiding of large meals rich in carbohydrates and alcohol consumption can prevent associated postprandial hypotension. PD patients with OH should also be aware that exposure to warm temperatures or during physical exertion of vigorous exercise may result in hyperhidrosis, dehydration, and OH. Finally, use of drugs with bradycardiac and vasodilatory properties could result in severe hypotension and should be avoided.

Symptom and Its Treatment[39]

- *Orthostatic hypotension and intolerance*:
  - Plasma volume expander: Fludrocortisone (starting dosage: 0.1 mg daily, slow titration up to larger dosages); desmopressin (10–40 mg nasal spray or 100–400 mg orally at bedtime).
  - Vasoactive agents: Etilefrine (15 mg daily); midodrine (30 mg daily); L-DOPS (droxidopa) (300 mg three times daily); indomethacin (50 mg three times daily); octreotide (subcutaneously starting with 100 mg daily).
- *Sialorrhea*:
  - Anticholinergics: Glycopyrrolate (1–2 mg in two or three divided doses); atropine (0.5 mg drop of solution sublingually once a day), inhalation with ipratropium bromide.
  - Adrenoreceptor agonists: Clonidine (0.15 mg daily).
  - Botulinum toxin: Serotype A
  - Radiotherapy
- *Constipation*:
  - Laxatives: Macrogol (1–3 standard doses daily); lubiprostone (48 mg daily)
  - Serotoninergic agents: Cisapride (5 mg twice daily); mosapride citrate (15 mg daily); tegaserod (6 mg twice daily)
  - Acetylcholinesterase inhibitors: Pyridostigmine (60 mg orally three times daily, up to 360 mg daily)
  - Dopaminergic agents
  - Botulinum toxin: Serotype A (two sites—puborectalis muscle injections of 30–100 U Botox)
  - Sacral nerve stimulation
- *Urinary frequency and urgency*:
  - Dopaminergic agents
  - Anticholinergics: Oxybutynin (5 mg three to four times daily or 1 patch twice a week); tolterodine

(2 mg three times daily); solifenacin (5–10 mg daily); darifenacin (7.5–15 mg daily)
  - Adrenoreceptor antagonists
  - Botulinum toxin: Serotype A (200 U injection into the detrusor muscle), deep brain stimulation-subthalamic nucleus (DBS-STN)
- *Sexual dysfunction*:
  - Dopaminergic agents: Apomorphine (sublingual at dosages of 2 or 4 mg daily); pergolide mesylate (3 mg daily)
  - DBS-STN phosphodiesterase-5 inhibitors: Sildenafil citrate (50 mg and titrated up to 100 mg); tadalafil (10 mg titrated up to maximum 20 mg/day) taken prior to sexual activity.
  - Testosterone (5 mg of testosterone topical gel administered daily); prostaglandin E1 (intracavernosal administration, gradually dosage increment)
  - Penile prosthesis
- *Hyperhidrosis and seborrhea*:
  - Aluminum chloride hexahydrate (10–12% axilla, 20% palmar-plantar, 10% craniofacial)
  - Anticholinergics: Glycopyrrolate (0.5–4% topical preparations)
  - Iontophoresis
  - Botulinum toxin: Serotype A
- *Weight loss*:
  - Percutaneous endoscopic gastrostomy

CONCLUSION

Symptoms of abnormal autonomic nervous system function occur commonly in PD. Orthostatic symptoms and signs are common in PD and mostly occur as a side effect of treatment with levodopa, a later stage in the disease progression, if prominent and early with the disease consideration to a different etiology, such as multiple system atrophy should be entertained. Instead, patients with PD and OH have clear evidence for baroreflex failure and loss of sympathetic innervation, most noticeably in the heart. In contrast, patients with multiple system atrophy have intact cardiac sympathetic innervation. Postmortem studies confirm this distinction. Because PD involves postganglionic sympathetic noradrenergic lesions, the disease seems to be not only a movement disorder with dopamine loss in the nigrostriatal system of the brain, but also a dysautonomic disorder with norepinephrine loss in the sympathetic nervous system of the heart.

REFERENCES

1. Zesiewicz TA, Baker MJ, Wahba M, Hauser RA. Autonomic nervous system dysfunction in Parkinson's disease. Curr Treat Options Neurol. 2003;5(2):149-60.
2. Ziemssen T, Reichmann H. Cardiovascular autonomic dysfunction in Parkinson's disease. J Neurol Sci. 2010;289(1-2): 74-80.
3. Jain S. Multi-organ autonomic dysfunction in Parkinson disease. Parkinsonism Relat Disord. 2011;17(2):77-83.
4. Koike Y, Takahashi A. Autonomic dysfunction in Parkinson's disease. Eur Neurol. 1997;38(Suppl 2):8-12.
5. Micieli G, Tosi P, Marcheselli S, Cavallini A. Autonomic dysfunction in Parkinson's disease. Neurol Sci. 2003;24(1):s32-4.
6. Raffel DM, Koeppe RA, Little R, Wang CN, Liu S, Junck L, et al. PET measurement of cardiac and nigrostriatal denervation in Parkinsonian syndromes. J Nucl Med. 2006;47(11):1769-77.
7. Low PA. Prevalence of orthostatic hypotension. Clin Auton Res. 2008;18(Suppl 1):8-13.
8. Goldstein DS. Dysautonomia in Parkinson's disease: neurocardiological abnormalities. Lancet Neurol. 2003;2(11):669-76.
9. Haensch CA, Jorg J. Beat-to-beat blood pressure analysis after premature ventricular contraction indicates sensitive baroreceptor dysfunction in Parkinson's disease. Mov Disord. 2006;21(4):486-91.
10. Kallio M, Haapaniemi T, Turkka J, Suominen K, Tolonen U, Sotaniemi K, et al. Heart rate variability in patients with untreated Parkinson's disease. Eur J Neurol. 2000;7(6): 667-72.
11. Mihci E, Kardelen F, Dora B, Balkan S. Orthostatic heart rate variability analysis in idiopathic Parkinson's disease. Acta Neurol Scand. 2006;113(5):288-93.
12. Orimo S, Ozawa E, Nakade S, Sugimoto T, Mizusawa H. 123-I-metaiodobenzylguanidine myocardial scintigraphy in Parkinson's disease. J Neurol Neurosurg Psychiatry. 1999;67(2): 189-94.
13. Schestatsky P, Ehlers JA, Rieder CR, Gomes I. Evaluation of sympathetic skin response in Parkinson's disease. Parkinsonism Relat Disord. 2006;12(8):486-91.
14. Braune HJ, Korchounov AM, Schipper HI. Autonomic dysfunction in Parkinson's disease assessed by sympathetic skin response: a prospective clinical and neurophysiological trial on 50 patients. Acta Neurol Scand. 1997;95(5):293-7.
15. Zakrzewska-Pniewska B, Jamrozik Z. Are electrophysiological autonomic tests useful in the assessment of dysautonomia in Parkinson's disease? Parkinsonism Relat Disord. 2003;9(3): 179-83.
16. Hirashima F, Yokota T, Hayashi M. Sympathetic skin response in Parkinson's disease. Acta Neurol Scand. 1996;93(2-3):127-32.
17. Sandroni P, Ahlskog JE, Fealey RD, Low PA. Autonomic involvement in extrapyramidal and cerebellar disorders. Clin Auton Res. 1991;1(2):147-55.
18. Lipp A, Sandroni P, Ahlskog JE, Fealey RD, Kimpinski K, Iodice V, et al. Prospective differentiation of multiple system atrophy from Parkinson disease, with and without autonomic failure. Arch Neurol. 2009;66(6):742-50.

19. Sharabi Y, Li ST, Dendi R, Holmes C, Goldstein DS. Neurotransmitter specificity of sympathetic denervation in Parkinson's disease. Neurology. 2003;60(6):1036-9.
20. Kawada M, Tamada Y, Simizu H, Yanagishita T, Yamashita N, Ishida N, et al. Reduction in QSART and vasoactive intestinal polypeptide expression in the skin of Parkinson's disease patients and its relation to dyshidrosis. J Cutan Pathol. 2009;36(5):517-21.
21. Shindo K, Iida H, Watanabe H, Ohta E, Nagasaka T, Shiozawa Z. Sympathetic sudomotor and vasoconstrictive neural function in patients with Parkinson's disease. Parkinsonism Relat Disord. 2008;14(7):548-52.
22. Sakakibara R, Uchiyama T, Yamanishi T, Shirai K, Hattori T. Bladder and bowel dysfunction in Parkinson's disease. J Neural Transm (Vienna). 2008;115(3):443-60.
23. Cersosimo MG, Benarroch EE. Neural control of the gastrointestinal tract: implications for Parkinson disease. Mov Disord. 2008;23(8):1065-75.
24. Hardoff R, Sula M, Tamir A, Soil A, Front A, Badarna S, et al. Gastric emptying time and gastric motility in patients with Parkinson's disease. Mov Disord. 2001;16(6):1041-7.
25. Sakakibara Y, Asahina M, Suzuki A, Hattori T. Gastric myoelectrical differences between Parkinson's disease and multiple system atrophy. Mov Disord. 2009;24(11):1579-86.
26. Fotiou DS, Tsiptsios I, Lithari C, Nakou M, Karlovasitou A. Cholinergic deficiency in Alzheimer's and Parkinson's disease: evaluation with pupillometry. Int J Psychophysiol. 2009;73: 143-9.
27. Braak H, Sastre M, Bohl JR, de Vos RA, Del Tredici K. Parkinson's disease: lesions in dorsal horn layer I, involvement of parasympathetic and sympathetic pre- and postganglionic neurons. Acta Neuropathol. 2007;113(4):421-9.
28. Dabby R, Djaldetti R, Shahmurov M, Treves TA, Gabai B, Melamed E, et al. Skin biopsy for assessment of autonomic denervation in Parkinson's disease. J Neural Transm. 2006;113(9):1169-76.
29. Ikemura M, Saito Y, Sengoku R, Sakiyama Y, Hatsuta H, Kanemaru K, et al. Lewy body pathology involves cutaneous nerves. J Neuropathol Exp Neurol. 2008;67(10):945-53.
30. Miki Y, Tomiyama M, Ueno T, Haga R, Nishijima H, Suzuki C, et al. Clinical availability of skin biopsy in the diagnosis of Parkinson's disease. Neurosci Lett. 2010;469(3):357-9.
31. Thaisetthawatkul P, Boeve BF, Benarroch EE, Sandroni P, Ferman TJ, Petersen R, et al. Autonomic dysfunction in dementia with Lewy bodies. Neurology. 2004;62(10):1804-9.
32. Schestatsky P, Valls-Sole J, Ehlers JA, Rieder CR, Gomes I. Hyperhidrosis in Parkinson's disease. Mov Disord. 2006;21(10): 1744-8.
33. Oyanagi K, Wakabayashi K, Ohama E, Takeda S, Horikawa Y, Morita T, et al. Lewy bodies in the lower sacral parasympathetic neurons of a patient with Parkinson's disease. Acta Neuropathol. 1990;80(5):558-9.
34. Beach TG, Adler CH, Sue LI, Vedders L, Lue L, White Iii CL, et al. Multi-organ distribution of phosphorylated alpha-synuclein histopathology in subjects with Lewy body disorders. Acta Neuropathol. 2010;119(6):689-702.
35. Jost WH, Schrank B. Defecatory disorders in de novo Parkinsonians—colonic transit and electromyogram of the external anal sphincter. Wien Klin Wochenschr. 1998;110(15): 535-7.
36. Levine ME. Sickness and satiety: physiological mechanisms underlying perceptions of nausea and stomach fullness. Curr Gastroenterol Rep. 2005;7(4):280-8.
37. Hunter S. The rostral mesencephalon in Parkinson's disease and Alzheimer's disease. Acta Neuropathol. 1985;68(1):53-8.
38. Mochizuki A, Komatsuzaki Y, Shoji S. Association of Lewy bodies and glial cytoplasmic inclusions in the brain of Parkinson's disease. Acta Neuropathol. 2002;104(5):534-7.
39. Mostile G, Jankovic J. Treatment of dysautonomia associated with Parkinson's disease. Parkinsonism Relat Disord. 2009;15: S224-32.

CHAPTER 13

Non-motor Fluctuations in Parkinson's Disease

Daniel J van Wamlen, Valentina Leta, K Ray Chaudhuri, Alexander Storch

INTRODUCTION

In this chapter, we will address the phenomenology of non-motor fluctuations (NMF), which can occur alongside, but also rarely, independent of motor fluctuations in Parkinson's disease (PD). Thus far, three clinical categories of NMF have been described (neuropsychiatric, autonomic, and sensory/pain fluctuations) and all appear to have a negative impact on quality of life of PD patients. NMF are widely seen in most patients who exhibit fluctuations in motor response after long-term levodopa treatment. Yet the general awareness of NMF remains low and NMF are often not considered in routine clinical consultations. Although there is increasing evidence on the treatment of non-motor symptoms (NMS) in PD which would also address NMF by default, little is known about the specific management of the range of NMF which, as such, remains a clear unmet need.

The concept of fluctuations in clinical response to levodopa is well-recognized, although classically these fluctuations are linked to motor function. There is a wide range of treatments and strategies that have been proposed to manage levodopa-related fluctuations such as peak-dose and diphasic dyskinesias, wearing-off, and off-related dystonia.[1] However, more recently, the need to manage NMF, which might occur both in conjunction with, but also independent, of motor fluctuations has been recognized. The phenomenon of NMF is not new and one of the first comprehensive descriptions of NMF was provided by Quinn in 1998, who gave an overview of several key NMS to show fluctuations; he described fluctuations in pain with concepts such as off-related pain, beginning and end-of-dose pain, and peak-dose pain, clearly underlining the close link of this key NMS with motor fluctuations.[2] In addition, he noted that over two-thirds of PD patients on levodopa treatment experience mood fluctuations, consisting of any combination of depression, anxiety and panic, irritability, and apathy, occurring during off-periods, and euphoria and hypersexuality during the on-period. He additionally summarized several studies showing changes in cognitive state coinciding with motor fluctuations.[2] Other studies around this time reported a dose-responsive correlation between levodopa and emotional manifestations,[3,4] but also that bradykinesia severity and mood shifting was not concordant,[5] suggesting that NMF can occur independently from motor fluctuations.

The more modern concept of NMF as a heterogeneous and complex group of fluctuations, including fluctuations of neuropsychiatric, autonomic, and sensory symptoms with a complex variation in patterns have been described by Storch and colleagues as part of the NoMoFlu study group.[6,7] Furthermore, NMF are now seen as not obligatorily occurring together with motor fluctuations and have been shown to cause a greater degree of disability and distress than motor fluctuations in some patients.[7-10] Indeed, several authors have suggested that patients with both motor fluctuations and NMF have worse quality of life than those with motor fluctuations alone.[11]

PREVALENCE

One of the early studies to report about prevalence of NMF in PD was performed by Raudino. The author described that in a cohort of 47 PD patients, of whom 38 had motor fluctuations, 60% also reported NMF which were classified as autonomic, sensory, and cognitive.[12] More recent studies have shown strong variations in prevalence rates for NMF in general ranging between 17% and 100% of patients who experience motor fluctuations.[7,8,11,13-17] Although NMF are present together with motor fluctuations in most patients, they rarely occur independently and/or even in the absence of motor fluctuations.[18,19] Since these data largely come from cross-sectional studies, it remains unknown whether NMF develop independently of motor fluctuations or- and this is much more likely due to the proposed similar pathophysiology of both types of fluctuations-whether NMF occur not independent of motor fluctuations but only before the motor fluctuations during the development of the disease to the advanced disease stage characterized by levodopa-induced complications in some patients due to unknown reasons. This latter view is supported by the longitudinal clinical data provided by Kim and colleagues showing that in over 300 patients with a disease of just over 2 years, 50% developed fluctuations of either a motor or non-motor nature within 3 years of follow-up. Of these fluctuators, over half developed both motor fluctuations and NMF at the same time, while the rest of them developed motor fluctuations first. Only a very small minority (2.8% of the fluctuators) developed NMF first.[20]

Recent studies report an influence of disease progression on NMF frequency and severity, e.g., Storch and colleagues have recently shown that NMF were dependent on Hoehn and Yahr stage with increasing NMS severity in both motor off-state and motor on state, but decreasing frequency and amplitude of motor and NMF with disease progression.[6] Indeed, in patients with Hoehn and Yahr stage 5, no significant NMF could be observed.[6] These results are in close agreement with another study on late-stage PD showing minor motor and NMF.[21,22]

PATHOPHYSIOLOGICAL MECHANISMS

Unlike for motor fluctuations, the pathophysiological basis of the development of NMF remains largely enigmatic. As many NMF follow the same patterns as motor fluctuations, it might be presumed that—at least in part—the mechanisms underlying NMF are related to dopaminergic neurotransmission. The development of motor fluctuations has been linked to pulsatile dopaminergic stimulation[23] as a consequence of the short half-life of levodopa and the progressive reduction of dopamine storage capacity due to the degeneration of dopaminergic neurons in the *substantia nigra*.[24-26] This link is exemplified by the improvement of NMS, such as apathy and pain, after intake of dopaminergic medication.[3,5,27,28] Moreover, similar risk factors exist for both NMF and motor fluctuations, such as early-onset PD, longer disease duration, female gender, and higher dopaminergic dose.[14,17,29] However, as it is known that NMS are not necessarily linked to motor symptoms or their fluctuation[17,30] and NMF can occur independently of motor fluctuations[7,31] other nondopaminergic pathways are likely to play a role in NMF. The degeneration of these latter neurotransmitter pathways is likely to result in complex interactions with dopaminergic neurotransmission, ultimately the most likely cause for NMF.[32]

On the other hand, physiological factors may play a role in NMF patterns. For instance, the body's master clock, the hypothalamic suprachiasmatic nuclei, may exert their physiological 24 hour pattern[33] on NMF as well. Although comprehensive studies on diurnal patterns of NMS are largely lacking, some evidence is available for motor symptoms in PD and the healthy population. More specifically, diurnal patterns in motor activity in healthy people have been shown in several studies.[34-36] Consistently, Stewart and colleagues identified that diurnal fluctuations were present in dopaminergic treatment-resistant motor symptoms of PD, including postural instability and gait initiation deficits.[36] Other factors that could influence NMF include diurnal changes in basal ganglia dopamine receptor sensitivity which is under the control of the suprachiasmatic nuclei.[37,38] Similarly, blood-brain barrier penetrance for several types of medication shows diurnal variation,[39] which might explain the waxing-and-waning patterns of motor symptoms—and NMF—in PD.

Recent data from the Chaudhuri group provide evidence for an even longer time frame for NMS changes by showing seasonal differences in Non-motor Symptoms Scale (NMSS) total scores with the highest scores during the winter months and lowest during summer months.[40] In addition, differences in the burden of cardiovascular, perceptual, and miscellaneous symptoms were observed between summer and winter months.[40] Such variations are not likely to be related to dopaminergic medication and are probably related to physiological circannual patterns imposed by the body's masterclock,[41] although the concept of seasonal fluctuations requires further exploration.

TYPES OF NON-MOTOR FLUCTUATIONS

Non-motor fluctuations can generally be divided into three broad categories: Neuropsychiatric, autonomic, and sensory manifestations (**Table 1**).[32,42] Of the NMF, neuropsychiatric fluctuations are most common in about half of patients. Symptoms include fluctuations in, e.g., cognition, attention span, depressive feelings, anxiety, and apathy.[17,32] Autonomic fluctuations are reported by 24–90% of PD patients with NMF, and include symptoms such as sweating, light-headedness, abdominal discomfort, and urinary urgency.[17,32] Finally, sensory fluctuations relate to, e.g., visual disturbances, different types of pain, and restless legs syndrome.[7,32] NMS that are most closely linked to motor wearing-off are anxiety and panic attacks, mood changes, cognitive slowing, and pain (**Fig. 1**).[43]

Neuropsychiatric Fluctuations

Neuropsychiatric fluctuations are the most frequent, and perhaps most disabling, of the NMF and occur in half of patients with neuropsychiatric NMS.[19] Of the neuropsychiatric NMF, anxiety, and mood fluctuations appear to have the greatest impact on quality of life.[7] Other common NMF, often coinciding with motor fluctuations, involve fluctuations in motivation and cognition.[44-47] Also apathy is a key NMF, with apathy during off-periods and excessive motivation and impulse control disorder during on-periods.[48] Many of the neuropsychiatric symptoms are mainly present during off-periods (82%),[32] and particularly anxiety, tiredness, and slowing of mental processes being frequent during motor off-periods.[8,27] On the other hand, impulsivity, hyperactivity, and euphoria/mania are more frequently observed in the on-state (**Table 1**).[8,49] Hallucinations, sometimes considered as classical for the hyperdopaminergic state, can occur both during on and off-state, even in early PD patients.[50]

TABLE 1: Non-motor fluctuations in Parkinson's disease and their relation to motor fluctuations.

Type of non-motor fluctuation	*Mainly related to motor state*	*Response to dopaminergic treatment*
Neuropsychiatric:		
• Depressive symptoms	OFF > ON	Yes
• Apathy	OFF > ON	Limited
• Fatigue	OFF > ON	Limited
• Panic attacks	OFF > ON	Yes
• Anxiety	OFF > ON	Yes
• Cognitive performance	OFF > ON	Yes
• Drowsiness	OFF > ON	Yes
• Attention	OFF > ON	Yes
• Impulse control behavior	ON > OFF	Yes (reduction)
Autonomic:		
• Light-headedness	OFF > ON	Limited
• Abdominal discomfort	OFF	Yes
• Constipation	OFF > ON	Yes
• Urinary urgency	OFF > ON	Yes
• Hyperhidrosis	OFF > ON	Limited
• Dysphagia	OFF > ON	Limited
• Stridor	OFF	Yes
Sensory:		
• Diffuse pain	OFF > ON	Yes
• Sensory pain	OFF > ON	Yes
• Dysesthesia	OFF > ON	Yes
• Visual disturbances	OFF > ON	Limited
• Restless legs syndrome	OFF	Yes

Source: Modified from Chou et al.[42]

Autonomic Fluctuations

Although autonomic symptoms are very frequent in PD,[51] the prevalence of autonomic NMF remains largely unclear. It has been estimated that between 29% and 94% of patients with NMF present with at least some autonomic symptoms.[16-19] Symptoms such as dyspnea, hyperhidrosis, cardiovascular symptoms, constipation, and urinary urgency coincide with the motor off-state,[2,8,16,17,52] and some of these symptoms improve with dopaminergic medication.[53,54] On the other hand, Storch and colleagues showed that autonomic symptoms did not show a variation coinciding with motor fluctuation and overall reported only minor changes in autonomic symptom severity.[7]

Sensory and Pain Fluctuations

Pain in PD is often associated with the motor off-state,[8,16,17] and it is at least partly improved by the administration of dopaminergic medication.[55] Especially, leg motor restlessness appears to be a common NMF as it is reported in up to 54% of patients with NMF.[8] Sensory symptoms, on the other hand, appear to be less common and occur in about 25% of patients with NMF.[18] Pathologically, two mechanisms are likely to underpin painful NMF: (1) On the

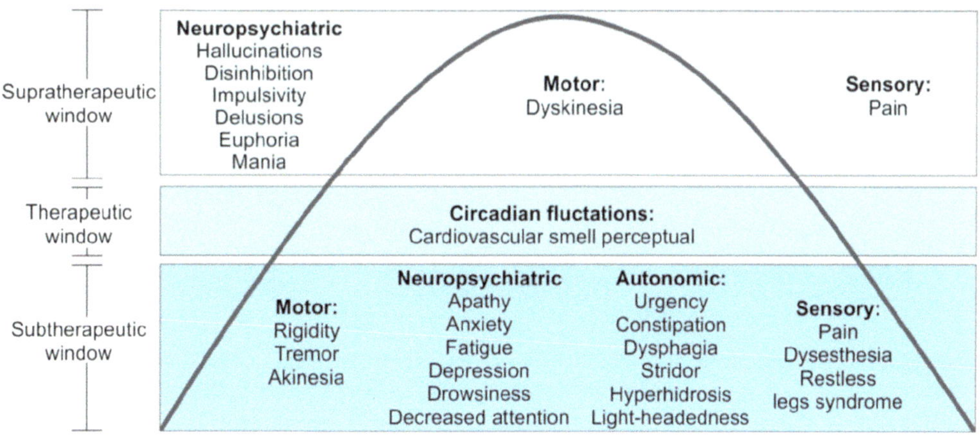

FIG. 1: Non-motor fluctuations in Parkinson's disease.

one hand pain may be related to a muscular component with increased rigidity and dystonia during motor off-state, and (2) on the other hand, spontaneous pain attributed to dysfunction in sensory striatal cortical afferents due to dopamine depletion may be involved.[56,57]

MANAGEMENT OF NON-MOTOR FLUCTUATIONS

Assessment of Non-motor Fluctuations

Although the evidence for the treatment of NMS in PD has taken a turn for the better as evident from the recent Movement Disorder Society (MDS) evidence based guidelines,[58] there is still very little evidence guiding the management of NMF. The first step in treating NMF remains proper identification (**Fig. 2**). Unfortunately, so far only three tools have been developed for the specific assessment of NMF: The non-motor fluctuation assessment (NOMOFA),[59] the Neuropsychiatric Fluctuations Scale (NFS),[60] and the NMF subsection of the MDS-NMS.[61] All scales are relatively new and have not undergone extensive clinicometric validation or validation of use in clinical practice. The MDS-NMS currently has the best validation data and its eight items related to NMF show good metric properties.[61] The Movement Disorders Society Task Force has recommended both the wearing-off questionnaires (WOQ), WOQ-19 and WOQ-9, containing motor and non-motor aspects of wearing-off, for screening in PD, but the focus of both scales is on motor aspects, rather than non-motor aspects, and, as such, may not be ideal as a screening tool for NMF.[62]

Treatment of Non-motor Fluctuations

Once NMF have been established, the main aim of their treatment is probably focused on continuous, non-pulsatile, dopaminergic stimulation (**Fig. 2**).[63] The available evidence suggests that NMF tend to at least partially respond to changes in dopaminergic therapy, similar to motor responses.[27] As such, continuous dopaminergic therapy should be pursued as much as possible, with use of extended release dopaminergic preparations, and the possible introduction of levodopa sparing strategies. Examples of this include the use of rotigotine transdermal patch, where a recent posthoc analysis of the RECOVER trial has shown that it improved NMSS domains of pain, sleep/fatigue, and mood/apathy.[64] According to the recently published MDS update on treatment for NMS of PD, patients with NMF dominated by pain may benefit from the initiation of rotigotine transdermal patch.[58] Moreover, the addition of monoamine oxidase B or catechol-O-methyltransferase inhibitors may represent an alternative therapeutic strategy by prolonging levodopa's elimination half-life, although they can lead to fluctuations in levodopa plasma levels.[65,66] Furthermore, it is becoming increasingly

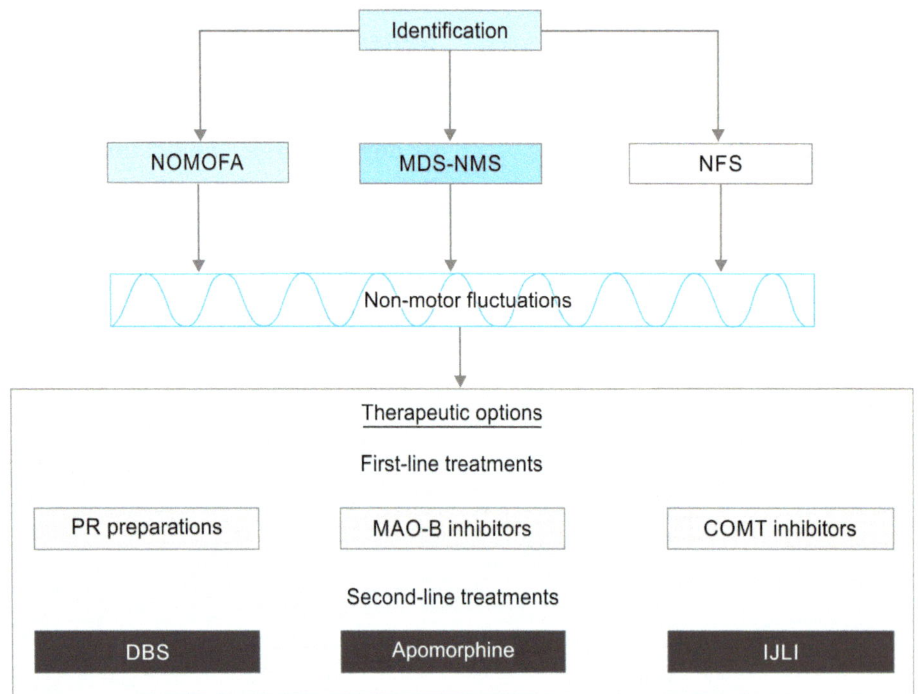

(COMT: catechol-O-methyltransferase; DBS: deep brain stimulation; IJLI: intrajejunal levodopa infusion; MAO-B: monoamine oxidase B; MDS-NMS: Movement Disorders Society Non-motor Scale; NFS: Neuropsychiatric Fluctuations Scale; NOMOFA: non-motor fluctuation assessment; PR; prolonged released)

FIG. 2: Treatment strategies for non-motor fluctuations in Parkinson's disease.

clear that nondopaminergic dysfunction is also involved in the development of some NMS[67] and, as such, a combined dopaminergic and nondopaminergic approach should be used to address NMF.[68] No studies, however, have so far looked into the use of nondopaminergic medication specifically for NMF in PD.

Once the conservative treatment options mentioned above have failed to improve NMF, advanced therapies may be considered, especially in the case of NMF occurring together with motor fluctuations. Regarding NMS clear evidence for the effectiveness of advanced therapies was provided by the two EuroInf studies. Here, subcutaneous apomorphine infusion and intrajejunal levodopa infusion (IJLI) both improved non-motor symptom burden and improvement of the sleep/fatigue, gastrointestinal, urinary, and sexual domains of the NMSS.[69] Also deep brain stimulation was able to improve NMS, but the profile of improvement was distinct from the infusion therapies and improvement was less pronounced.[70] It should be noted, however, that NMF have not been included as outcome measures in clinical trials or other studies, and, as such, only indirect evidence of NMF improvement is available.

CONCLUSION

Non-motor fluctuations can be distressing and appear to be a fairly constant companion of motor fluctuations and in some cases more troublesome with a negative effect on quality of life. Isolated NMF are difficult to diagnose and thus, often missed in clinical practice leading to inadequate management. Recent efforts at producing scales to measure NMF in clinical practice, such as the MDS-NMS (including NMF subscale), NMF assessment, and Neuropsychiatric Fluctuations Scale, may improve awareness, diagnosis, and thus, refine management.

REFERENCES

1. Ray Chaudhuri K, Poewe W, Brooks D. Motor and Nonmotor Complications of Levodopa: Phenomenology, Risk Factors, and Imaging Features. Mov Disord. 2018;33(6):909-19.
2. Quinn NP. Classification of fluctuations in patients with Parkinson's disease. Neurology. 1998;51(2 Suppl 2):S25-9.
3. Maricle RA, Nutt JG, Carter JH. Mood and anxiety fluctuation in Parkinson's disease associated with levodopa infusion: preliminary findings. Mov Disord. 1995;10(3):329-32.
4. Menza MA, Sage J, Marshall E, Cody R, Duvoisin R. Mood changes and "on-off" phenomena in Parkinson's disease. Mov Disord. 1990;5(2):148-51.
5. Maricle RA, Nutt JG, Valentine RJ, Carter JH. Dose-response relationship of levodopa with mood and anxiety in fluctuating Parkinson's disease: a double-blind, placebo-controlled study. Neurology. 1995;45(9):1757-60.
6. Storch A, Rosqvist K, Ebersbach G, NoMoFlu-PD Study Group, Odin P. Disease stage dependency of motor and non-motor fluctuations in Parkinson's disease. J Neural Transm (Vienna). 2019;126(7):841-51.
7. Storch A, Schneider CB, Wolz M, Sturwald Y, Nebe A, Odin P, et al. Nonmotor fluctuations in Parkinson disease: severity and correlation with motor complications. Neurology. 2013;80(9):800-9.
8. Witjas T, Kaphan E, Azulay JP, Blin O, Ceccaldi M, Pouget J, et al. Nonmotor fluctuations in Parkinson's disease: frequent and disabling. Neurology. 2002;59(3):408-13.
9. Rieu I, Houeto JL, Pereira B, De Chazeron I, Bichon A, Chereau I, et al. Impact of Mood and Behavioral Disorders on Quality of Life in Parkinson's disease. J Parkinsons Dis. 2016;6(1):267-77.
10. Muller B, Assmus J, Herlofson K, Larsen JP, Tysnes OB. Importance of motor vs. non-motor symptoms for health-related quality of life in early Parkinson's disease. Parkinsonism Relat Disord. 2013;19(11):1027-32.
11. Rodriguez-Violante M, Ospina-Garcia N, Davila-Avila NM, Cruz-Fino D, Cruz-Landero A, Cervantes-Arriaga A. Motor and non-motor wearing-off and its impact in the quality of life of patients with Parkinson's disease. Arq Neuropsiquiatr. 2018;76(8):517-21.
12. Raudino F. Nonmotor off in Parkinson's disease. Acta Neurol Scand. 2001;104(5):312-5.
13. Rahmani M, Benabdeljlil M, Bellakhdar F, Faris MEA, Jiddane M, Bayad KE, et al. Deep Brain Stimulation in Moroccan Patients With Parkinson's Disease: The Experience of Neurology Department of Rabat. Front Neurol. 2018;9:532.
14. Picillo M, Palladino R, Moccia M, Erro R, Amboni M, Vitale C, et al. Gender and nonmotor fluctuations in Parkinson's disease: A prospective study. Parkinsonism Relat Disord. 2016;27:89-92.
15. Lohle M, Hermann W, Hausbrand D, Wolz M, Mende J, Beuthien-Baumann B, et al. Putaminal Dopamine Turnover in de novo Parkinson's Disease Predicts Later Neuropsychiatric Fluctuations but not other major health outcomes. J Parkinsons Dis. 2019;9(4):693-704.
16. Hillen ME, Sage JI. Nonmotor fluctuations in patients with Parkinson's disease. Neurology. 1996;47(5):1180-3.
17. Gunal DI, Nurichalichi K, Tuncer N, Bekiroglu N, Aktan S. The clinical profile of nonmotor fluctuations in Parkinson's disease patients. Can J Neurol Sci. 2002;29(1):61-4.
18. Brun L, Lefaucheur R, Fetter D, Derrey S, Borden A, Wallon D, et al. Non-motor fluctuations in Parkinson's disease: prevalence, characteristics and management in a large cohort of parkinsonian outpatients. Clin Neurol Neurosurg. 2014;127:93-6.
19. Seki M, Takahashi K, Uematsu D, Mihara B, Morita Y, Isozumi K, et al. Clinical features and varieties of non-motor fluctuations in Parkinson's disease: a Japanese multicenter study. Parkinsonism Relat Disord. 2013;19(1):104-8.

20. Kim A, Kim HJ, Shin CW, Kim A, Kim Y, Jang M, et al. Emergence of non-motor fluctuations with reference to motor fluctuations in Parkinson's disease. Parkinsonism Relat Disord. 2018;54: 79-83.
21. Fabbri M, Coelho M, Abreu D, Guedes LC, Rosa MM, Costa N, et al. Do patients with late-stage Parkinson's disease still respond to levodopa? Parkinsonism Relat Disord. 2016;26:10-6.
22. Fabbri M, Coelho M, Guedes LC, Chendo I, Sousa C, Rosa MM, et al. Response of non-motor symptoms to levodopa in late-stage Parkinson's disease: Results of a levodopa challenge test. Parkinsonism Relat Disord. 2017;39:37-43.
23. Lim EW, Aarsland D, Ffytche D, Taddei RN, van Wamelen DJ, Wan YM, et al. Amyloid-beta and Parkinson's disease. J Neurol. 2019;266(11):2605-19.
24. Olanow CW, Obeso JA, Stocchi F. Continuous dopamine-receptor treatment of Parkinson's disease: scientific rationale and clinical implications. Lancet Neurol. 2006;5(8):677-87.
25. Cilia R, Akpalu A, Sarfo FS, Cham M, Amboni M, Cereda E, et al. The modern pre-levodopa era of Parkinson's disease: insights into motor complications from sub-Saharan Africa. Brain. 2014;137(Pt 10):2731-42.
26. Hirsch E, Graybiel AM, Agid YA. Melanized dopaminergic neurons are differentially susceptible to degeneration in Parkinson's disease. Nature. 1988;334(6180):345-8.
27. Stacy MA, Murck H, Kroenke K. Responsiveness of motor and nonmotor symptoms of Parkinson disease to dopaminergic therapy. Prog Neuropsychopharmacol Biol Psychiatry. 2010;34(1):57-61.
28. Defazio G, Berardelli A, Fabbrini G, Martino D, Fincati E, Fiaschi A, et al. Pain as a nonmotor symptom of Parkinson disease: evidence from a case-control study. Arch Neurol. 2008;65(9):1191-4.
29. Chaudhuri KR, Schapira AH. Non-motor symptoms of Parkinson's disease: dopaminergic pathophysiology and treatment. Lancet Neurol. 2009;8(5):464-74.
30. Chaudhuri KR, Yates L, Martinez-Martin P. The non-motor symptom complex of Parkinson's disease: a comprehensive assessment is essential. Curr Neurol Neurosci Rep. 2005;5(4):275-83.
31. Ossig C, Sippel D, Fauser M, Gandor F, Jost WH, Ebersbach G, et al. Assessment of Nonmotor Fluctuations Using a Diary in Advanced Parkinson's disease. J Parkinsons Dis. 2016;6(3): 597-607.
32. Martinez-Fernandez R, Schmitt E, Martinez-Martin P, Krack P. The hidden sister of motor fluctuations in Parkinson's disease: A review on nonmotor fluctuations. Mov Disord. 2016;31(8): 1080-94.
33. Schwartz WJ, Klerman EB. Circadian Neurobiology and the Physiologic Regulation of Sleep and Wakefulness. Neurol Clin. 2019;37(3):475-86.
34. van Hilten JJ, Hoogland G, van der Velde EA, Middelkoop HA, Kerkhof GA, Roos RA. Diurnal effects of motor activity and fatigue in Parkinson's disease. J Neurol Neurosurg Psychiatry. 1993;56(8):874-7.
35. van Hilten JJ, Kabel JF, Middelkoop HA, Kramer CG, Kerkhof GA, Roos RA. Assessment of response fluctuations in Parkinson's disease by ambulatory wrist activity monitoring. Acta Neurol Scand. 1993;87(3):171-7.
36. Stewart J, Bachman G, Cooper C, Liu L, Ancoli-Israel S, Alibiglou L. Circadian dysfunction and fluctuations in gait initiation impairment in Parkinson's disease. Exp Brain Res. 2018;236(3):655-64.
37. Ikeda E, Matsunaga N, Kakimoto K, Hamamura K, Hayashi A, Koyanagi S, et al. Molecular mechanism regulating 24-hour rhythm of dopamine D3 receptor expression in mouse ventral striatum. Mol Pharmacol. 2013;83(5):959-67.
38. Akhisaroglu M, Kurtuncu M, Manev H, Uz T. Diurnal rhythms in quinpirole-induced locomotor behaviors and striatal D2/D3 receptor levels in mice. Pharmacol Biochem Behav. 2005;80(3):371-7.
39. Cuddapah VA, Zhang SL, Sehgal A. Regulation of the Blood-Brain Barrier by Circadian Rhythms and Sleep. Trends Neurosci. 2019;42(7):500-10.
40. van Wamelen DJ, Podlewska AM, Leta V, Smilowska K, Rizos A, Martinez-Martin P, et al. Slave to the rhythm: Seasonal differences in non-motor symptoms in Parkinson's disease. Parkinsonism Relat Disord. 2019;63:73-6.
41. Lincoln G. A brief history of circannual time. J Neuroendocrinol. 2019;31(3):e12694.
42. Chou KL, Stacy M, Simuni T, Miyasaki J, Oertel WH, Sethi K, et al. The spectrum of "off" in Parkinson's disease: What have we learned over 40 years? Parkinsonism Relat Disord. 2018;51: 9-16.
43. Stacy M. The wearing-off phenomenon and the use of questionnaires to facilitate its recognition in Parkinson's disease. J Neural Transm (Vienna). 2010;117(7):837-46.
44. Nissenbaum H, Quinn NP, Brown RG, Toone B, Gotham AM, Marsden CD. Mood swings associated with the 'on-off' phenomenon in Parkinson's disease. Psychol Med. 1987;17(4):899-904.
45. Racette BA, Hartlein JM, Hershey T, Mink JW, Perlmutter JS, Black KJ. Clinical features and comorbidity of mood fluctuations in Parkinson's disease. J Neuropsychiatry Clin Neurosci. 2002;14(4):438-42.
46. Richard IH, Justus AW, Kurlan R. Relationship between mood and motor fluctuations in Parkinson's disease. J Neuropsychiatry Clin Neurosci. 2001;13(1):35-41.
47. Friedenberg DL, Cummings JL. Parkinson's disease, depression, and the on-off phenomenon. Psychosomatics. 1989;30(1):94-9.
48. Sierra M, Carnicella S, Strafella AP, Bichon A, Lhommee E, Castrioto A, et al. Apathy and Impulse Control Disorders: Yin & Yang of Dopamine Dependent Behaviors. J Parkinsons Dis. 2015;5(3):625-36.
49. Storch A, Schneider CB, Klingelhofer L, Odin P, Fuchs G, Jost WH, et al. Quantitative assessment of non-motor fluctuations in Parkinson's disease using the Non-Motor Symptoms Scale (NMSS). J Neural Transm (Vienna). 2015;122(12):1673-84.
50. Pagonabarraga J, Martinez-Horta S, Fernandez de Bobadilla R, Perez J, Ribosa-Nogue R, Marin J, et al. Minor hallucinations occur in drug-naive Parkinson's disease patients, even from the premotor phase. Mov Disord. 2016;31(1):45-52.
51. Jost WH. Autonomic dysfunctions in idiopathic Parkinson's disease. J Neurol. 2003;250(Suppl 1):128-30.
52. Stacy M, Bowron A, Guttman M, Hauser R, Hughes K, Larsen JP, et al. Identification of motor and nonmotor wearing-off in Parkinson's disease: comparison of a patient questionnaire versus a clinician assessment. Mov Disord. 2005;20(6):726-33.

53. Goetz CG, Lutge W, Tanner CM. Autonomic dysfunction in Parkinson's disease. Neurology. 1986;36(1):73-5.
54. Pursiainen V, Korpelainen JT, Haapaniemi TH, Sotaniemi KA, Myllyla VV. Blood pressure and heart rate in Parkinsonian patients with and without wearing-off. Eur J Neurol. 2007;14(4):373-8.
55. Ford B. Pain in Parkinson's disease. Mov Disord. 2010;25 (Suppl 1):S98-103.
56. Juri C, Rodriguez-Oroz M, Obeso JA. The pathophysiological basis of sensory disturbances in Parkinson's disease. J Neurol Sci. 2010;289(1-2):60-5.
57. Tinazzi M, Recchia S, Simonetto S, Tamburin S, Defazio G, Fiaschi A, et al. Muscular pain in Parkinson's disease and nociceptive processing assessed with CO2 laser-evoked potentials. Mov Disord. 2010;25(2):213-20.
58. Seppi K, Ray Chaudhuri K, Coelho M, Fox SH, Katzenschlager R, Perez Lloret S, et al. Update on treatments for nonmotor symptoms of Parkinson's disease-an evidence-based medicine review. Mov Disord. 2019;34(2):180-98.
59. Kleiner-Fisman G, Martine R, Lang AE, Stern MB. Development of a non-motor fluctuation assessment instrument for Parkinson disease. Parkinsons Dis. 2011;2011:292719.
60. Schmitt E, Krack P, Castrioto A, Klinger H, Bichon A, Lhommee E, et al. The Neuropsychiatric Fluctuations Scale for Parkinson's Disease: A Pilot Study. Mov Disord Clin Pract. 2018;5(3):265-72.
61. Martinez-Martin P, Schrag A, Weintraub D, Rizos A, Rodriguez-Blazquez C, Chaudhuri KR. Pilot Study of the International Parkinson and Movement Disorder Society-sponsored Non-motor Rating Scale (MDS-NMS). Mov Disord Clin Pract. 2019;6(3):227-34.
62. Antonini A, Martinez-Martin P, Chaudhuri RK, Merello M, Hauser R, Katzenschlager R, et al. Wearing-off scales in Parkinson's disease: critique and recommendations. Mov Disord. 2011;26(12):2169-75.
63. van Wamelen DJ, Grigoriou S, Chaudhuri KR, Odin P. Continuous Drug Delivery Aiming Continuous Dopaminergic Stimulation in Parkinson's Disease. J Parkinsons Dis. 2018;8(s1):S65-72.
64. Kassubek J, Chaudhuri KR, Zesiewicz T, Surmann E, Boroojerdi B, Moran K, et al. Rotigotine transdermal system and evaluation of pain in patients with Parkinson's disease: a post hoc analysis of the RECOVER study. BMC Neurol. 2014;14:42.
65. Leta V, Jenner P, Chaudhuri KR, Antonini A. Can therapeutic strategies prevent and manage dyskinesia in Parkinson's disease? An update. Expert Opin Drug Saf. 2019;18(12):1203-18.
66. Leta V, van Wamelen DJ, Sauerbier A, Jones S, Parry M, Rizos A, et al. Opicapone and Levodopa-Carbidopa Intestinal Gel Infusion: The Way Forward Towards Cost Savings for Healthcare Systems? J Parkinsons Dis. 2020;10(4):1535-9.
67. Titova N, Qamar MA, Chaudhuri KR. The Nonmotor Features of Parkinson's Disease. Int Rev Neurobiol. 2017;132:33-54.
68. Franke C, Storch A. Nonmotor Fluctuations in Parkinson's Disease. Int Rev Neurobiol. 2017;134:947-71.
69. Martinez-Martin P, Reddy P, Katzenschlager R, Antonini A, Todorova A, Odin P, et al. EuroInf: a multicenter comparative observational study of apomorphine and levodopa infusion in Parkinson's disease. Mov Disord. 2015;30(4):510-6.
70. Dafsari HS, Martinez-Martin P, Rizos A, Trost M, Dos Santos Ghilardi MG, Reddy P, et al. EuroInf 2: Subthalamic stimulation, apomorphine, and levodopa infusion in Parkinson's disease. Mov Disord. 2019;34(3):353-65.

SECTION

4

DIAGNOSTIC TESTS IN MOVEMENT DISORDERS

CHAPTER 14

Movement Disorders: Role of Imaging

Meher Ursekar, Rima Ramesh Sansi

INTRODUCTION

Movement disorders with Parkinsonian features are commonly encountered in clinical practice. An estimated 10 million people in the world and 1% of those over 60 years are afflicted with Parkinson's disease (PD).[1] Thorough clinical evaluation along with structural imaging such as magnetic resonance imaging (MRI) and functional imaging techniques like positron emission tomography/single-photon emission computed tomography (PET/SPECT) can aid in the differentiation as well as prognostication of these disorders which show considerable clinical overlap thus, allowing selection of suitable therapy.

CLASSIFICATION

Movement disorders are best classified according to clinical presentation into akinetic-rigid and hyperkinetic disorders (**Box 1**).[2]

Box 1 Classification of movement disorders.

Akinetic-rigid syndromes: Parkinsonism

Degenerative:

- Idiopathic Parkinson's disease
- Atypical Parkinsonian syndrome (APS)
  - Progressive supranuclear palsy (PSP)
  - Multiple system atrophy (MSA)
  - Corticobasal degeneration (CBD)
  - Spinocerebellar ataxia (SCA), types 2, 3, 17

Symptomatic:

- Drugs, toxins, normal pressure hydrocephalus, prion infections, and trauma

Hyperkinetic syndromes

Jerky syndromes:

- Myoclonus including excessive startle
- Tics including ballismus
- Chorea

Nonjerky hyperkinetic syndromes:

- Dystonia including athetosis
- Tremor

IMAGING TECHNIQUES

Computed Tomography

The role of computed tomography (CT) is limited in the evaluation of movement disorders especially in their chronic phases. However, it finds a role in the assessment of a patient with acute-onset of a movement disorder, viz.—hemiballism due to hemorrhage or infarct of the red nucleus as well as in patients who present with "symptomatic" Parkinsonism. In addition, CT may be helpful in some cases of striatonigral calcinosis where the deposition may be remarkably symmetrical,[3] mimicking neurodegeneration with brain iron accumulation (NBIA), which makes it difficult to distinguish the two conditions on MRI.

Conventional Magnetic Resonance Imaging

The multiplanar capabilities and the high spatial as well as contrast resolution of MRI make it a robust tool for ruling out structural neuroparenchymal abnormalities which may result in "symptomatic" Parkinsonism. MRI is useful in pattern recognition and identification of characteristic regional distribution in the loss of volume of specific central nervous system (CNS) structures that typify some movement disorders. The atrophy patterns are best assessed on T1-weighted (T1-W) volumetric spoiled gradient (VSG) echo or fluid-attenuated inversion recovery (FLAIR) images where the high signal intensity of neuroparenchyma contrasts with the low signal intensity of cerebrospinal fluid (CSF). Further, T2-W images also play a significant role in the assessment of these conditions. T2 high signal abnormalities correspond to areas of gliosis, demyelination, or Wallerian degeneration whereas low T2 signal intensity areas represent regions of ferrugination (abnormal iron accumulation). This type of contrast is more conspicuous at increasing strengths of magnet and in gradient echo T2* imaging. Diffusion tensor imaging (DTI) and diffusion tensor tractography (DTT) can facilitate visualization of selective degeneration of individual major white matter (WM) fiber systems in the brainstem and cerebellum.

Diffusion Magnetic Resonance Imaging

Diffusion-weighted (DW) imaging and DTI help in the evaluation of chemical and physical properties of gray matter (GM) and WM microstructures. Several studies have utilised quantitative parameters such as apparent diffusion coefficient (ADC) in movement disorders and indices derived from DTI such as mean diffusivity (MD) and fractional anisotropy (FA) for the diagnosis of movement disorders.

Magnetization Transfer Magnetic Resonance Imaging

Difference in the signal intensities with and without magnetization transfer (MT) is used to calculate MT ratio (MTR), which is a measure of microstructural integrity and have the capability of revealing subcortical WM and GM abnormalities in several movement disorders.

IMAGING FINDINGS IN SPECIFIC DISORDERS

Idiopathic Parkinson's Disease

Idiopathic Parkinson's Disease (IPD) is characterized by intraneuronal Lewy body inclusions in substantia nigra compacta resulting in nigral degeneration and loss of nigrostriatal projection fibers which is associated with striatal dopamine deficiency in the posterior putamen. The nondopamine deficient syndromes are not associated with these pathophysiological mechanisms while the atypical Parkinsonian disorders such as progressive supranuclear palsy (PSP), multiple system atrophy (MSA), and corticobasal degeneration (CBD) are linked with striatal dopamine deficiency but with non-Lewy body pathologies.

Conventional MRI is usually normal in early IPD and its chief role is to rule out mimics such as bilateral subdural hematoma, normal pressure hydrocephalus, or any intracranial tumor. Studies have shown that transcranial ultrasound may detect increased echogenicity from the lateral margin of the midbrain in patients with PD, though it suffers from poor specificity. Further, this technique is operator dependent, is subjective in nature and may thus, show interobserver variance. Finally, patients with excessive tremor are not suitable for this examination as movement artifacts impede optimal evaluation of images.

Atrophy of the lentiform nucleus is a feature of APSs and DW sequences may demonstrate increased ADCs in 90–100% patients with clinically probable MSA and PSP whereas ADCs in the putamen are normal in PD.[4-6] The flowchart presented in **Flowchart 1** summarizes the role of structural and functional imaging in diagnosing different Parkinsonian syndromes.[7] Given the scope of the chapter, we will limit further discussion only to structural imaging of these disorders.

Nigrosome 1 within the posterior-thirds of substantial nigra returns high signal on susceptibility-weighted imaging (SWI/T2*) imaging and is surrounded anteriorly, medially, and laterally by low signal intensity resembling the classic split tail of a swallow. In advanced IPD, the high-signal intensity of nigrosome is reduced or absent and thus, the swallow tail sign is absent. Two underlying mechanisms have been proposed, viz.: increased iron content or decreased neuromelanin content.[8]

Progressive Supranuclear Palsy

Several 2D morphometric indices have been proposed to overcome the subjectivity of visual perception of midbrain atrophy which is a characteristic feature of PSP. These include reduction in anteroposterior diameter of the midbrain which gives rise to an appearance on axial cross-sectional images of the "Mickey Mouse Sign" (**Fig. 1**). The A-P diameter is measured in the axial plane at the level of the superior colliculus, from the interpeduncular fossa to the intercollicular groove, and <12 mm is considered abnormal.[9,10] Loss of the lateral convex profile of the midbrain has been termed the "Morning Glory Sign" (**Flowchart 1**).[11] Midbrain-to-pons surface area ratio, measured on mid-sagittal T1-W images is another useful metric. It is reduced to ~0.12 (normal ~24)[12] and is the most accurate index to distinguish PSP from multisystem atrophy-P (in which there is atrophy of both, the mid brain and the pons) (**Fig. 2**). Midbrain atrophy with flattening of its rostral convex profile and relative preservation of the basis pontis produces an appearance that has led some

Tremor, stiffness, or slowness suggestive of Parkinsonism

T1 and T2-W MRI to detect structural lesions

Abnormal

Secondary Parkinsonism to be considered (cerebral infarction, hydrocephalus, granuloma, tumor, toxic/traumatic brain injury)

Normal

Transcranial ultrasound to detect midbrain echogenicity

Normal/Abnormal

DAT SPECT or PET/ F-Dopa PET/DTBZ PET to detect striatal dopamine deficiency

Normal

Nondopamine deficient syndromes (drug induced PD, benign tremor, and psychogenic)

Abnormal

Typical features

Atypical features

Trial of dopaminergic medication

Poor response

DW MRI to detect increased striatal ADC/FDG PET to detect striatal glucose hypometabolism

Good response

Normal

Abnormal

Probable Parkinson's disease

Probable atypical Parkinsonian syndrome (MSA/PSP/CBD)

(ADC: apparent diffusion coefficient; DW: diffusion-weighted; FDG: florodeoxyglucose; MRI: magnetic resonance imaging; PET: positron emission tomography; SPECT: single-photon emission computed tomography)

FLOWCHART 1: Imaging algorithm for Parkinson's disease (PD), dopamine transporter (DAT), dihydrotetrabenazine (DTBZ).

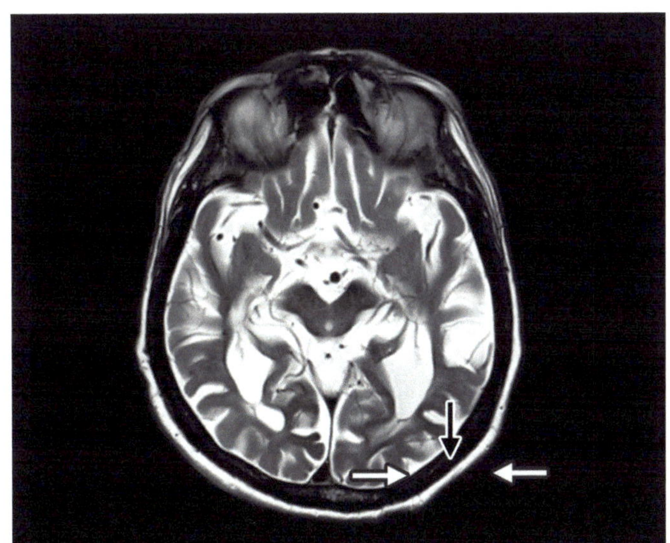

FIG. 1: Mickey Mouse Sign: Reduced anteroposterior diameter of midbrain tegmentum, measured from interpeduncular fossa to intercollicular grove (black arrow) and Morning Glory Sign: Loss of lateral convexity of midbrain (white arrow).

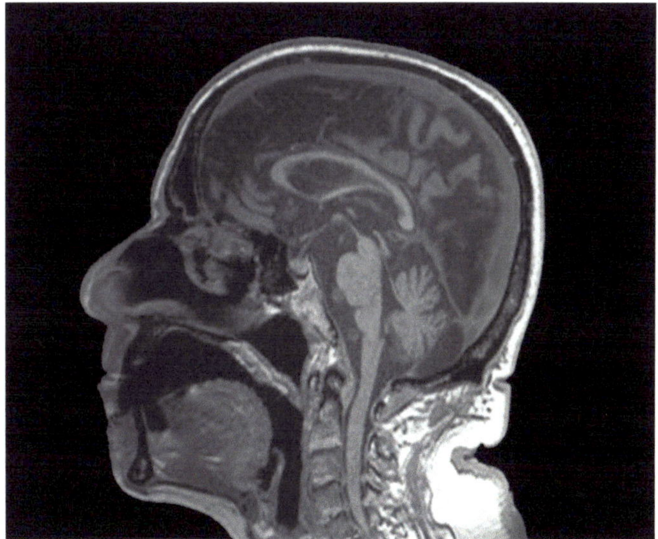

FIG. 2: Reduced mid-sagittal midbrain-pons area ratio to approximately 12 (normal~24). Most accurate metric helps to distinguish progressive supranuclear palsy (PSP) from multiple system atrophy-parkinsonian type (MSA-p) which shows atrophy of both midbrain and pons.

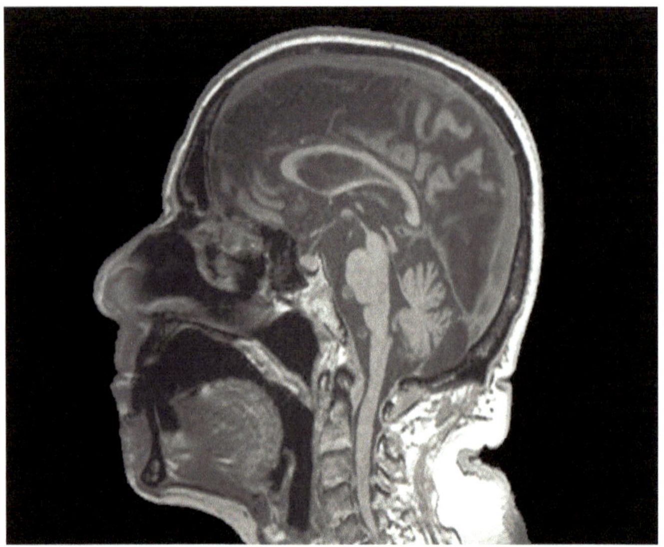

FIG. 3: Humming bird sign/penguin sign: Midbrain atrophy with flattening of its rostral convex profile and relative preservation of pons.

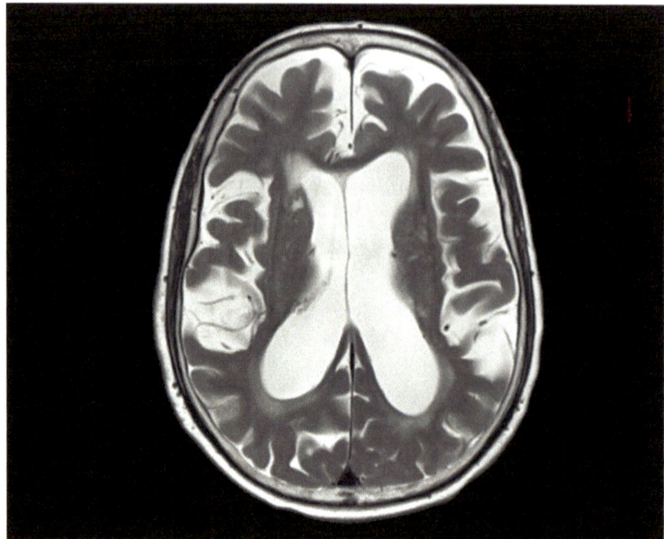

FIG. 4: Axial T2-W image showing putaminal atrophy.

Japanese authors, to suggest that it resembles a "humming bird" with its long thin beak[13] or a "standing king penguin" with a small head corresponding to the midbrain and a disproportionate large body corresponding to the relatively preserved pons (**Fig. 3**).[12]

The likelihood of PSP in patients with unclassifiable Parkinsonism can be predicted by using the Magnetic Resonance Parkinsonism Index (MRPI). The width of the superior cerebellar peduncle (SCP) must be measured in an oblique coronal plane on T1-W VSG echo images along with the width of the middle cerebellar peduncle (MCP) on sagittal T1-W VSG echo images. By averaging the values from the right and left sides, mean SCP and MCP widths are calculated. The P/M ratio is obtained as the ratio of area of pons (P) and midbrain (M) as measured on mid-sagittal T1-W VSG echo sequence. The index is then calculated by multiplying the P/M ratio by the MCP width to the SCP width ratio:[14,15]

$$(P/M) \times (MCP/SCP)$$

A value of >13.55 is abnormal and strongly suggests that such patients will go on to develop PSP. Other features include T2 high signal abnormalities in the midbrain tectum, pontine tegmentum, and inferior olivary nucleus.

The diffusion-weighted imaging (DWI) reveals remarkably higher regional ADC (rADC) values in the globus pallidus and putamen in patients with PSP possibly suggesting an ongoing striatal degeneration.

Multiple System Atrophy

Multiple system atrophy encompasses a group of neurodegenerative disorders with shared histological features, viz.: Striatonigral degeneration with or without autonomic dysfunction (Shy–Drager syndrome) and sporadic olivopontocerebellar atrophy (OPCA). On the basis of predominating symptoms, patients are classified as having either the Parkinsonian type of MSA (MSA-P) or cerebellar type type (MSA-C). From the imaging standpoint, there are a few features that distinguish the two entities.

In MSA-P the abnormalities are confined to the putamen. Putaminal atrophy when present helps to distinguish this from IPD (**Fig. 4**). Putaminal T2 hypointensity may also be seen. However, it is a nonspecific sign as it may be seen in Wilson's disease (WD), PSP and NBIA, and other acquired conditions. Slit-like T2 hyperintensity along the lateral margins of the putamina may also be observed. Similar finding may also be seen in IPD and has also been reported in healthy individuals at 3 tesla imaging.[16]

Patients with MSA-C show diffuse T2 high signal abnormality in the transverse pontine fibers, middle cerebellar peduncles, cerebellar WM, attributable to atrophy of the pontocerebellar and fibers with sparing of the corticospinal tracts, and superior cerebellar peduncles.[17] This combination of preserved and altered T2 signal of WM tracts produces the characteristic "hot cross bun" sign in the basis pontis on the T2-axial images. This sign is highly sensitive for MSA-C, being reported in 80% of cases,[18] however, it is not specific as it may be seen in several subtypes of spinocerebellar ataxias, paraneoplastic degeneration from a testicular tumor, progressive multifocal leukoencephalopathy, bilateral middle cerebellar peduncle infarction, leptomeningeal metastasis from breast cancer, fragile X tremor ataxia syndrome (FXTAS), cerebrotendinous xanthomatosis, and variant Creutzfeldt–Jakob disease.[19-25]

The combination of increased ADC in putamen and globus pallidus and increased ADC and decreased FA in the pons and middle cerebellar peduncles may help distinguish MSA-P from PD and PSP. MTR is also reduced in the putamen in MSA compared with PD and healthy controls.

Corticobasal Degeneration

As the symptomatology of CBD is nonspecific, MRI finds a central role in its diagnosis by demonstrating a characteristic brain atrophy pattern. There is asymmetric atrophy with secondary widening of cortical sulci, with a predilection for the parietal lobes, anterior middle and posterior inferior frontal, and paracentral regions. Associated atrophy of the ipsilateral cerebral peduncle is observed.[26,27] The subcortical WM in the regions of affectation may demonstrate FLAIR high signal abnormality, attributable to neuronal degeneration, especially demyelination secondary to axonal loss. The basal ganglia do not reveal any atrophy or signal alteration.[26] In a minority of patients the atrophy may be symmetrical.

HUNTINGTON CHOREA

Huntington's disease (HD) is an inherited neurodegenerative disorder caused by expansion of trinucleotide CAG sequence in the *huntington* gene (HTT), located on chromosome 4.[27,28] The most consistent neuroimaging feature is noteworthy and progressive striatal atrophy, the volume loss of the striatum corresponding with age of onset of disease, duration of illness as well as with CAG repeat length.[29-31] Putaminal atrophy correlates with the severity of motor disturbances cognitive as well as Mini-Mental Status Examination Scores are inversely correlated with caudate atrophy.[32,33] Caudate atrophy can be quantified by comparing intercaudate distance (CC) to frontal horn (FH) and calvarial width [inner table (IT)]. Normal FH/CC ratio is 2-3 and CC/IT ratio is 0.03–0.14. In HD, FH/CC ratio is decreased while CC/IT ratio is increased.

As the disease progresses there is cortical loss that progresses from dorsal to ventral cortical regions. Widespread WM loss is also detected and underlines the role of structural connectivity degradation in the pathogenesis of this disorder. Resting state functional MRI (fMRI) studies are able to demonstrate abnormal functional network connectivity and thus, have a role in quantifying neuronal dysfunction as well as assessment of disease progression. Differential diagnosis include Wilson disease and Leigh's disease both of which involve WM, cerebellum, and brainstem. Other differentials include Hallervorden-Spatz syndrome, carbon monoxide poisoning, and hypoglycemic encephalopathy.

FRAGILE X TREMOR ATAXIA SYNDROME

Fragile X tremor ataxia syndrome presents as a sporadic condition and MRI has a fundamental role in its diagnosis.[34] MRI demonstrates symmetrical T2 high signal abnormality in peridentate WM and middle cerebellar peduncles. Similar signal abnormalities are also observed in periventricular deep WM and corpus callosum; however, the signal intensity and shape of the pons are preserved[35] with diffuse supra- and infratentorial atrophy. Atrophy of midbrain and low signal intensity in the basal ganglia may be observed in some cases accounting for the extrapyramidal symptoms.[36]

WILSON'S DISEASE

It is a rare inborn error of copper metabolism with an autosomal recessive pattern of inheritance. MRI of the brain is nearly always abnormal in patients with neurological disturbances. On FLAIR images, a thin hyperintense signal abnormality is noted in the claustrum known as the "bright claustrum" sign. Another imaging feature is the "face of the giant panda" characterized by T2 hyperintense signal abnormality in the midbrain tegmentum with normally hypointense red nuclei (forming the eyes), preserved signal intensity of pars reticularis of substantia nigra (constituting the ears), and low signal intensity of the superior colliculus (chin). Face of miniature panda may be seen in the pons and is constituted by the hypointensity of central tegmental tract and medial longitudinal fasciculus (eyes), hyperintensity of aqueduct opening into fourth ventricle (mouth), and superior cerebellar peduncles (cheeks). The combination of the aforementioned signs is termed as "double panda sign".

Similar imaging features may be observed in Leigh's disease, hypoxic ischemic encephalopathy, methanol poisoning, Japanese B encephalitis, and extrapontine myelinolysis. The characteristic clinical manifestation of these disease entities distinguish them from WD.

PANTOTHENATE-KINASE-ASSOCIATED NEURODEGENERATION (NEURODEGENERATION WITH BRAIN IRON ACCUMULATION I)

Conventional MRI may demonstrate the "eye of tiger sign", in the medial portion of the globus pallidi, representing T2 high signal intensity surrounded by T2 hypointense signal abnormality attributable to iron deposition, reactive gliosis, and axonal swelling (spheroids).[37] This sign was present in patients with PANK2 mutations codifying for pantothenate kinase 2 enzyme, however, it was not present in patients

TABLE 1: Magnetic resonance imaging (MRI) features of IPD and APS.

MRI technique		*Imaging feature*	*Significance*
IPD	SWI/T2*	Split tail sign of swallow-loss of nigrosome high signal intensity	Diagnostic accuracy of >90% for Parkinson's disease and dementia with Lewy body
PSP	T1(Sag)	Midbrain to pons surface area ratio (~0.12)	Distinguishes PSP from MSA-P (most accurate index)
	T1(Sag)	Loss of convex upper border of midbrain	Distinguishes PSP from IPD
	T1(Ax)	Reduction in A-P diameter (~<12) and Mickey Mouse Sign	Distinguishes PSP from MSA, IPD, and CBD
	T1(Ax)	Loss of lateral convex margin of midbrain tegmentum and Morning Glory Sign	Distinguishes PSP from MSA, IPD, and CBD
	Oblique T1 (Cor) and T1 (Sag)	MRPI (>13.5)	Helps to predict PSP in patients with unclassifiable IPD
MSA	T2/PD (Ax)	Hot cross bun	Distinguishes MSA-C from PSP and IPD
	T2/PD (Ax)	Putaminal atrophy	Distinguishes MSA-P from IPD
CBD	T1	Asymmetric cortical atrophy	Likely to suggest CBD more than MSA or PSP
	T2	High signal intensity in SCWM	Neuronal degeneration

(APS: atypical Parkinsonian syndrome; CBD: corticobasal degeneration; IPD: idiopathic Parkinson's disease; MRPI: Magnetic Resonance Parkinsonism Index; MSA-P: multiple system atrophy-parkinsonian type; PD: Parkinson's disease; PSP: progressive supranuclear palsy; SCWM: subcortical white matter; SWI: susceptibility-weighted imaging)

without PANK2 mutations[38] and also in patients with other types of NBIA. This sign is nonspecific and similar signal abnormalities have also been reported in PSP, CBD, early-onset levodopa responsive PD,[39] Parkinsonian variant of MSA[40] as well as in pallidal necrosis caused by carbon monoxide (CO) intoxication (**Table 1**).[41] Further, it is also known to change[39] or disappear overtime.[42]

CONCLUSION

Structural and functional imaging techniques add to the specificity in the diagnosis and are useful when combined with the clinical evaluation, in differentiating amongst various movement disorders that are encountered in clinical practice.

REFERENCES

1. de Lau LM, Breteler MM. Epidemiology of Parkinson's disease. Lancet Neurol. 2006;5(6):525-35
2. Abdo WF, van de Warrenburg BP, Burn DJ, Quinn NP, Bloem BR. The clinical approach to movement disorders. Nat Rev Neurol. 2010;6(1):29-37.
3. Kobari M, Nogawa S, Sugimoto Y, Fukuuchi Y. Familial idiopathic brain calcification with autosomal dominant inheritance. Neurology. 1997;48(3):645-9.
4. Zecca L, Casella L, Albertini A, Bellei C, Zucca FA, Engelen M, et al. Neuromelanin can protect against iron-mediated oxidative damage in system modeling iron overload of brain aging and Parkinson's disease. J Neurochem. 2008;106(4):1866-75.
5. Schocke MF, Seppi K, Esterhammer R, Kremser C, Jaschke W, Poewe W, et al. Diffusion-weighted MRI differentiates the Parkinson variant of multiple system atrophy from PD. Neurology. 2002;58(4):575-80.
6. Seppi K, Schocke MF, Esterhammer R, Kremser C, Brenneis C, Mueller J, et al. Diffusion-weighted imaging discriminates progressive supranuclear palsy from PD, but not from the Parkinson variant of multiple system atrophy. Neurology. 2003;60(6):922-27.
7. Nicoletti G, Lodi R, Condino F, Tonon C, Fera F, Malucelli E, et al. Apparent diffusion coefficient measurements of the middle cerebellar peduncle differentiate the Parkinson variant of MSA from Parkinson's disease and progressive supranuclear palsy. Brain. 2006;129(Pt 10):2679-87.
8. Brooks DJ. Imaging approaches to Parkinson disease. J Nucl Med. 2010;51(4):596-609.
9. Righini A, Antonini A, De Notaris R, Bianchini E, Meucci N, Sacilotto G, et al. MR imaging of the superior profile of the midbrain: differential diagnosis between progressive supranuclear palsy and Parkinson disease. AJNR Am J Neuroradiol. 2004;25(6):927-32.
10. Josephs KA. Frontotemporal lobar degeneration. Neurol Clin. 2007;25(3):683-96.
11. Adachi M, Kawanami T, Ohshima H, Sugai Y, Hosoya T. Morning glory sign: a particular MR finding in progressive supranuclear palsy. Magn Reson Med Sci. 2004;3(3):125-32.

12. Oba H, Yagishita A, Terada H, Barkovich AJ, Kutomi K, Yamauchi T, et al. New and reliable MRI diagnosis for progressive supranuclear palsy. Neurology. 2005;64(12):2050-5.
13. Kato N, Arai K, Hattori T. Study of the rostral midbrain atrophy in progressive supranuclear palsy. J Neurol Sci. 2003;210 (1-2):57-60.
14. Morelli M, Arabia G, Salsone M, Novellino F, Giofrè L, Paletta R, et al. Accuracy of magnetic resonance parkinsonism index for differentiation of progressive supranuclear palsy from probable or possible Parkinson disease. Mov Disord. 2011;26(3):527-33.
15. Morelli M, Arabia G, Novellino F, Salsone M, Giofrè L, Condino F, et al. MRI measurements predict PSP in unclassifiable parkinsonisms: a cohort study. Neurology. 2011;77(11):1042-7.
16. Lee WH, Lee CC, Shyu WC, Chong PN, Lin SZ. Hyperintense putaminal rim sign is not a hallmark of multiple system atrophy at 3T. AJNR Am J Neuroradiol. 2005;26(9):2238-42.
17. Savoiardo M, Strada L, Girotti F, Zimmerman RA, Grisoli M, Testa D, et al. Olivopontocerebellar atrophy: MR diagnosis and relationship to multisystem atrophy. Radiology. 1990;174(3):693-6.
18. Watanabe H, Saito Y, Terao S, Ando T, Kachi T, Mukai E, et al. Progression and prognosis in multiple system atrophy: an analysis of 230 Japanese patients. Brain. 2002;125(Pt 5):1070-83.
19. Lee YC, Liu CS, Wu HM, Wang PS, Chang MH, Soong BW. The 'hot cross bun' sign in the patients with spinocerebellar ataxia. Eur J Neurol. 2009;16(4):513-6.
20. Jain RS, Nagpal K, Tejwani S. 'Hot-cross bun' and 'inverse trident sign' in progressive multifocal leukoencephalopathy with HIV seropositivity. Neurol India. 2014;62(3):341-2.
21. Ishikawa H, Kawada N, Taniguchi A, Odachi K, Mizutani A, Asahi M, et al. Paraneoplastic neurological syndrome due to burned-out testicular tumor showing hot cross-bun sign. Acta Neurol Scand. 2016;133(5):398-402.
22. Pan Z, Yang G, Yuan T, Wang Y, Pang X, Gao Y, et al. 'Hot cross bun' sign with leptomeningeal metastases of breast cancer: a case report and review of the literature. World J Surg Oncol. 2015;13:43.
23. Roh SY, Jang HS, Kim YH. Hot cross bun sign following bilateral pontine infarction: a case report. J Mov Disord. 2013;6(2):37-9.
24. Jain RS, Sannegowda RB, Agrawal A, Hemrajani D, Jain R, Mathur T. 'Hot cross bun' sign in a case of cerebrotendinous xanthomatosis: a rare neuroimaging observation. BMJ Case Rep. 2013;2013:bcr2012006641.
25. Kamm C, Healy DG, Quinn NP, Wüllner U, Moller JC, Schols L, et al. The fragile X tremor ataxia syndrome in the differential diagnosis of multiple system atrophy: data from the EMSA Study Group. Brain. 2005;128(Pt 8):1855-60.
26. Koyama M, Yagishita A, Nakata Y, Hayashi M, Bandoh M, Mizutani T, et al. Imaging of corticobasal degeneration syndrome. Neuroradiology. 2007;49(11):905-12.
27. Taki M, Ishii K, Fukuda T, Kojima Y, Mori E. Evaluation of cortical atrophy between progressive supranuclear palsy and corticobasal degeneration by hemispheric surface display of MR images. AJNR Am J Neuroradiol. 2004;25(10):1709-14.
28. A novel gene containing a trinucleotide repeat that is expanded and unstable on Huntington's disease chromosomes. The Huntington's Disease Collaborative Research Group. Cell. 1993;72(6):971-83.
29. Rosas HD, Goodman J, Chen YI, Jenkins BG, Kennedy DN, Makris N, et al. Striatal volume loss in HD as measured by MRI and the influence of CAG repeat. Neurology. 2001;57(6): 1025-8.
30. Rosas HD, Koroshetz WJ, Chen YI, Skeuse C, Vangel M, Cudkowicz ME, et al. Evidence for more widespread cerebral pathology in early HD: an MRI-based morphometric analysis. Neurology. 2003;60(10):1615-20.
31. Aylward EH, Li Q, Stine OC, Ranen N, Sherr M, Barta PE, et al. Longitudinal change in basal ganglia volume in patients with Huntington's disease. Neurology. 1997;48(2):394-9.
32. Harris GJ, Pearlson GD, Peyser CE, Aylward EH, Roberts J, Barta PE, et al. Putamen volume reduction on magnetic resonance imaging exceeds caudate changes in mild Huntington's disease. Ann Neurol. 1992;31(2):69-75.
33. Harris GJ, Aylward EH, Peyser CE, Pearlson GD, Brandt J, Roberts-Twillie JV, et al. Single photon emission computed tomographic blood flow and magnetic resonance volume imaging of basal ganglia in Huntington's disease. Arch Neurol. 1996;53(4):316-24.
34. Brunberg JA, Jacquemont S, Hagerman RJ, Berry-Kravis EM, Grigsby J, Leehey MA, et al. Fragile X premutation carriers: characteristic MR imaging findings of adult male patients with progressive cerebellar and cognitive dysfunction. AJNR Am J Neuroradiol. 2002;23(10):1757-66.
35. Ginestroni A, Guerrini L, Della Nave R, Tessa C, Cellini E, Dotti MT, et al. Morphometry and ^{1}H-MR spectroscopy of the brain stem and cerebellum in three patients with fragile X-associated tremor/ataxia syndrome. AJNR Am J Neuroradiol. 2007;28(3):486-8.
36. Scaglione C, Ginestroni A, Vella A, Dotti MT, Nave RD, Rizzo G, et al. MRI and SPECT of midbrain and striatal degeneration in fragile X-associated tremor/ataxia syndrome. J Neurol. 2008;255(1):144-6.
37. McNeill A, Birchall D, Hayflick SJ, Gregory A, Schenk JF, Zimmerman EA, et al. T2* and FSE MRI distinguishes four subtypes of neurodegeneration with brain iron accumulation. Neurology. 2008;70(18):1614-9.
38. Hayflick SJ, Hartman M, Coryell J, Gitschier J, Rowley H. Brain MRI in neurodegeneration with brain iron accumulation with and without PANK2 mutations. AJNR Am J Neuroradiol. 2006;27(6):1230-3.
39. Desai SV, Bindu PS, Ravishankar S, Jayakumar PN, Pal PK. Relaxation and susceptibility MRI characteristics in Hallervorden-Spatz syndrome. J Magn Reson Imaging. 2007; 25(4):715-20.
40. Chang MH, Hung WL, Liao YC, Lee YC, Hsieh PF. Eye of the tiger-like MRI in parkinsonian variant of multiple system atrophy. J Neural Transm. 2009;116(7):861-6.
41. Prockop LD, Chichkova RI. Carbon monoxide intoxication: an updated review. J Neurol Sci. 2007;262(1-2):122-30.
42. Baumeister FAM, Auer DP, Hortnagel K, Freisinger P, Meitinger T. The eye-of-the-tiger sign is not a reliable disease marker for Hallervorden-Spatz syndrome. Neuropediatrics. 2005;36(3):221-2.

CHAPTER 15

Nuclear Imaging in Movement Disorders

Vikram R Lele, Priyanka Korepu

PARKINSONISM

Classification: Most common type of movement disorder is further classified into three groups (**Flowchart 1**).

1. Primary and idiopathic Parkinsonism (80%) (genetic or sporadic)
2. Atypical Parkinsonism:
   i. Progressive supranuclear palsy (PSP)
   ii. Lewy body dementia (LBD)
   iii. Corticobasal degeneration (CBD)
   iv. Multisystem atrophy (MSA): (MSAc) cerebellar type or (MSAp) Parkinson type
3. Secondary Parkinsonism:
   i. Drug-induced Parkinsonism: Neuroleptic drugs
   ii. Toxic: Manganese (Mn), carbon monoxide (CO) poisoning, 1-methyl-4-phenyl-1,2,3,6-tetrahydro-pyridine (MPTP), cyanide
   iii. Vascular Parkinsonism
   iv. Posthypoxic
   v. Postencephalitic-tumor, infection, and normal pressure hydrocephalus (NPH)
   vi. Post-traumatic
   vii. Other neurodegenerative disorders

INTRODUCTION AND THE NEED FOR MOLECULAR IMAGING

Early differentiation between Parkinson disease (PD) and atypical Parkinsonian syndromes (APS) is helpful for prognostication and treatment optimization. An early and correct differential diagnosis of Parkinsonism is of utmost importance given the excellent treatment options and prognosis in patients without nigrostriatal degeneration [e.g., drug-induced Parkinsonism and essential tremor (ET)] and the limited responsiveness to levodopa and faster progression to disability and death in patients with APS compared to PD.[1,2] Diagnosis of these entities is still largely dependent on a detailed history and thorough neurological examination. However, postmortem studies suggest that the clinical diagnosis of PD is incorrect in about 25% of patients.[3] Frequent misdiagnosis includes secondary Parkinsonism and APS such as MSA, PSP, and CBD. In turn, cumulative clinicopathological data suggest that about 30% of MSA and PSP and up to 74% of CBD patients are not correctly diagnosed even at late stage.[4] The symptoms of PD do not manifest till there is a loss

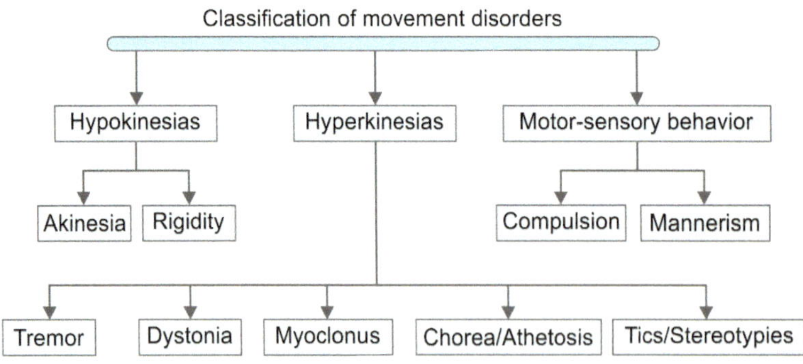

FLOWCHART 1: Classification of movement disorders.

of approximately 50% of nigral neurons or 80% of striatal dopamine.[5]

Routine laboratory studies are not helpful in the diagnosis of PD and their use should be reserved for patients with atypical features. Structural neuroimaging studies such as computed tomography (CT) and conventional magnetic resonance imaging (MRI) have a limited role in the evaluation of Parkinsonian syndromes and other movement disorders because they are generally normal in early stages and subsequent scans in later stages of disease may show diagnostic changes on MRI.

Against this background, single-photon emission computed tomography (SPECT) and positron emission tomography (PET) are used with two aims: First, to identify patients with progressive nigrostriatal degeneration, which is the common pathological feature in PD, MSA, PSP, and CBD. Secondly, to differentiate these patient groups.

Accurate diagnosis of neurodegenerative Parkinsonism can be achieved by imaging nigrostriatal function.[6-8] However, dopaminergic imaging does not differentiate between PD, MSA, PSP, and CBD. Instead, [^{18}F]-FDG (2-fluoro-2-deoxy-glucose) PET has gained acceptance as the method of choice here. It surpasses the diagnostic accuracies of other common techniques.[9]

IMAGING MODALITIES IN NUCLEAR MEDICINE: PET AND SPECT

The underlying principle of PET and SPECT is to image and quantify a physiological function or molecular target of interest in vivo by noninvasively assessing the spatial and temporal distribution of the radiation emitted by an intravenously injected target-specific radiotracer. Importantly, PET and SPECT tracers are administered in a nonpharmacological dose (micrograms or less), so they neither disturb the underlying system nor cause pharmacological or behavioral effects. Because of their ability to visualize molecular targets and functions on a macroscopic level with unsurpassed sensitivity, down to picomolar concentration, PET and SPECT are also called molecular imaging techniques.

In PET, a positron-emitting radiotracer (mostly FDG—half-life—110 min) is injected. The emitted positron travels a short distance in tissue (effective range <1 mm for common PET nuclides) before it encounters an electron, yielding a pair of two 511-keV annihilation photons emitted in opposite directions. This photon pair leaving the body is detected quasi-simultaneously (within a few nanoseconds) by scintillation detectors of the PET detector rings that surround the patient's head. The spatial resolution of modern PET systems is about 3-5 mm.[10]

Single-photon emission computed tomography employs gamma-emitting radionuclides that decay by emitting a single gamma ray. Typical radionuclides employed for neurological SPECT are technetium-99m (^{99m}Tc; half-life = 6.02 h) and iodine-123 (^{123}I; half-life = 13.2 h). Gamma cameras are used for SPECT acquisition, whereby usually two or three detector heads rotate around the patient's head to acquire two dimensional planar images of the head from multiple angles. The SPECT possesses a considerably lower sensitivity than PET. Thus, rapid temporal sampling (image frames of seconds to minutes) as a prerequisite for pharmacokinetic analyses is the strength of PET, whereas a single SPECT acquisition usually takes 20–30 minutes. Furthermore, the spatial resolution of modern SPECT is only about 7–10 mm deteriorating with increasing distance between object and collimator. Thus, SPECT is more susceptible to partial volume effects than PET, which can be a particular drawback when it comes to imaging small structures or lesions (e.g., brain tumors). The important advantages of SPECT over PET are the lower costs and broad availability of SPECT systems and radionuclides. Modern day's imaging systems are hybrid systems such as PET/CT or PET/MRI and SPECT/CT for better attenuation correction and image localization.

IMAGING DOPAMINERGIC SYSTEM

Dopamine Synthesis

The PET tracer 3,4-dihydroxy-6-[^{18}F]-fluoro-L-phenylalanine {[^{18}F]-DOPA} evaluates the first step in dopaminergic transmission, namely dopamine synthesis, which takes place in the presynaptic dopaminergic neurons. It is taken up into neurons by an active transport system and is converted to [^{18}F] dopamine by aromatic L-amino-acid decarboxylase (AADC), which represents the rate-limiting step in dopamine synthesis in dopaminergic neurons. As such, [^{18}F]-DOPA uptake reflects the synthetic ability of dopaminergic neurons to produce dopamine through AADC (**Table 1**). However, [^{18}F]-DOPA tends to underestimate loss.

Storage in Synaptic Vesicles

The dopamine produced at the synaptic level is stored in synaptic vesicles by the vesicular monoamine transporter type 2 (VMAT2), which is responsible for translocating monoamine neurotransmitters from the cytoplasm into vesicles. In the central nervous system, VMAT2 is expressed exclusively by monoaminergic neurons. Over 95% of striatal VMAT2, transporters are associated with dopaminergic terminals and striatal VMAT2 density is a linear function of the nigrostriatal neuron number. PET radiotracer (^{11}C)dihydrotetrabenazine [(^{11}C)DTBZ] is a specific ligand of VMAT2 and is used as an in vivo marker of nigrostriatal dopaminergic system integrity (**Fig. 1**).

TABLE 1: A brief summary of agents and their targets.

Targets	*SPECT-RP*	*PET RP*	*Changes in PD patients*
• Aromatic L-amino acid decarboxylase (AADC) • Dopamine metabolism and storage		• [^{18}F]-DOPA • [^{18}F]-Fluorodopamine	Reduced striatal binding in PD patients
VMAT2 receptor (vesicle storage)		• (^{11}C) • [^{18}F]-AV133 [^{18}F-FP-DTBZ]	Reduced striatal binding in PD patients
DAT receptor uptake (Presynaptic)	• ^{123}I-FP-CIT • ^{123}I-β-CIT • ^{123}I-altropane • ^{99m}Tc-TRODAT-1	• (^{11}C)-MP • (^{11}C) and [^{18}F]-CFT • (^{11}C)-PE2I • [^{18}F]-FP-PE2I • (^{11}C)-RTI32	Reduced striatal binding in PD patients
• Dopamine receptors (Postsynaptic) • D2 • D1	• ^{123}I-IBZM • ^{123}I-IBF • ^{123}I-Epidpride	• (^{11}C) and [^{18}F]-raclopride • [^{18}F]-DMFP • [^{18}F]-Fallypride • (^{11}C)-FLB456 • (^{11}C)-PHNO • (^{11}C) SCH23390	• Altered receptor number in PD • Increased in early untreated disease • Decreases slightly on treatment initiation
Other pathways:			
Beta-amyloid		• (^{11}C)-PIB • [^{18}F]-Av45 • Florbetapir, florbetaben, flutemetamol	Identifies amyloid pathology in p/w Parkinson's dementia
Glucose metabolism		[^{18}F]-FDG	• PD-specific network patterns • Atypical/Parkinson plus versus idiopathic PD differentiation
• PBR-activated microglia • Brain inflammation		PK11195	Increased inflammation in PD patients
Myocardial sympathetic innervations	^{123}I or ^{131}I MIBG	[^{18}F]-FMBG	Reduced cardiac sympathetic innervation in PD

(DAT: dopamine transporter; DOPA: dihydroxyphenylalanine; FDG: 2-fluoro-2-deoxy-glucose; MIBG: metaiodobenzylguanidine; PBR: peripheral-type benzodiazepine receptor; PD: Parkinson disease; PET: positron emission tomography; RP: radiopharmaceutical; SPECT: single-photon emission computed tomography; VMAT2: vesicular monoamine transporter type 2)

Presynaptic Membrane Dopamine Transporters

Dopamine transporter (DAT) is a sodium chloride-dependent transmembrane protein localized to the presynaptic nigrostriatal cell surface. It plays a critical role in the regulation of the extracellular dopamine concentration and has been considered a marker of dopamine terminal innervations. Dopamine reuptake through the DAT is the primary mechanism of dopamine removal from the region of the synaptic cleft. A decrease in DAT density indicates decreased amount of presynaptic terminals that produce dopamine. Among many DAT-specific tracers used in PET and SPECT imaging, the cocaine analogs, are the most widely used in clinical practice due to their affinity to DAT and ability to assess decreased DAT density, which may precede clinical symptoms in PD. Many SPECT and PET tracers are used as discussed below to evaluate DAT in PD.

Postsynaptic Dopamine Receptors

Dopamine released into the synaptic cleft binds mainly to the postsynaptic striatal D2 receptors, and the binding capacity of these receptors can be measured by PET tracer like (^{11}C)-raclopride. It showed that striatal dopamine D2 binding to the postsynaptic dopaminergic receptors was either normal or increased in PD patients. This increase has been interpreted as a compensatory reaction to the reduction of striatal dopaminergic terminals. D2 receptor upregulation is most evident at early stages

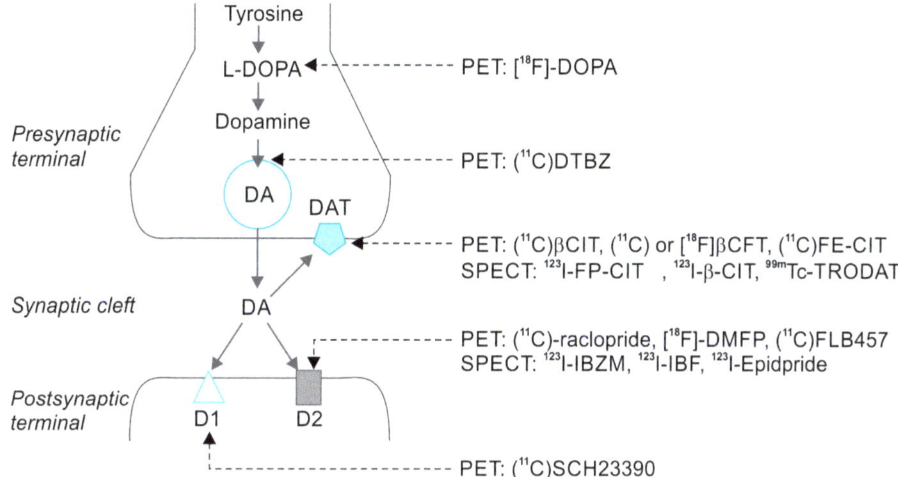

(DAT: dopamine transporter; DTBZ: dihydrotetrabenazine; L-DOPA: L-3,4-dihydroxyphenylalanine; PET: positron emission tomography; SPECT: single-photon emission computed tomography)

FIG. 1: Nigrostriatal dopaminergic synapse and targets of PET and SPECT ligands. Tyrosine is converted to L-DOPA by tyrosine hydroxylase. L-DOPA is then converted to dopamine (DA) which is gathered into vesicles by vesicular monoamine transporter type 2 (VMAT2) and from which it is released into the synaptic cleft. Dopamine binds to D1 and D2 receptors on the postsynaptic membrane. Some dopamine re-enters the presynaptic terminal via dopamine transporters.

and contralateral to the clinically most affected side and is usually the site of onset in PD. On the other hand, the increase in postsynaptic D2 receptor binding could also be due to loss of endogenous dopamine, thereby unloading the postsynaptic receptors and ultimately increasing uptake of (^{11}C)-raclopride or similar PET tracers in these receptors.

Metabolic Imaging

In addition to loss of dopaminergic neurons, damage to subcortical structures alters the functional connectivity across brain regions in a disease-specific manner as discussed below. [^{18}F]-FDG is the PET tracer used to assess cerebral glucose metabolism.

Neuroinflammation

Currently there are no tracers that bind Lewy body inclusions in vivo but the glial reaction to the presence of pathology can be detected with PET. Microglial cells are normally in a resting state, but become activated in response to any local disturbance, such as inflammation, trauma, ischemia, tumor, and neurodegeneration. In PD, the loss of dopamine neurons is linked with activation of microglia within the substantia nigra, which might in turn promote degeneration of nigral neurons as the disease progresses. Mitochondria of activated microglia express peripheral benzodiazepine sites that bind the PET tracer (^{11}C) {1-[2-chlorophenyl]-N-methyl-N-[1-methylpropyl]-3-isoquinoline-carboxamide [(^{11}C)PK11195]}. Imaging with (^{11}C)PK11195 showed higher tracer uptake in midbrain, striatum, pallidum, and frontal cortex of PD patients compared to age-matched healthy subjects. Moreover, midbrain (^{11}C)PK11195 binding was inversely correlated with DAT levels in the posterior putamen and positively correlated with the severity of motor impairment.[11]

Dopamine Transporter Imaging Agents

Both PET and SPECT have been used as in vivo methods to evaluate neuronal loss in PD.[12,13] Although PET provides higher resolution and better quantitative capacity than SPECT, SPECT is more practical as a routine procedure. Several ^{123}I-labeled DAT SPECT imaging agents based on cocaine or the closely-related tropane derivatives have been reported.[14] These studies indicated that this technique might be useful in identifying individuals in the preclinical and asymptomatic phase of the disease. However, because of the limited availability and relatively high cost of ^{123}I, few ^{123}I-labeled DAT ligands have been routinely applied for DAT imaging. ^{99m}Tc has a suitable energy and half-life for imaging, is relatively inexpensive, and is readily obtainable. Imaging with ^{99m}Tc-labeled ligands would therefore be more suitable for routine use. Several ^{99m}Tc-labeled tropanes have been reported,[15] among which, a ^{99m}Tc-labeled tropane derivative, [2-[[2-[[[3-(4-chlorophenyl)-8-methyl-8-azabicyclo[3,2,1] oct-2-yl]methyl](2-mercaptoethyl)amino]ethyl]-amino] ethanethiolato(3-)-N2,N2',S2,S2]oxo-[1R-(exo-exo)]-[^{99m}Tc]-technetium (^{99m}Tc-TRODAT-1), has been intensively studied and has already shown promise in humans and other primates.[16]

Scan Protocol for TRODAT Single-photon Emission Computed Tomography

No fasting is required for the scan. ^{99m}Tc-TRODAT (20–25 mCi) was injected intravenously to the patients and brain SPECT scan was acquired 4 hours later. Initial scan was done within half an hour of injection to look at the distribution of radiopharmaceutical in the body. Brain SPECT-CT images are taken using low energy high resolution (LEHR) collimator 3–4 hours post injection. The scan duration was for 30 minutes. Sedation was given to the patients whenever required after taking informed consent and explaining about the fasting requirements.

Dopamine Transporter Scan Interpretation

Dopamine transporter scans were classified as normal or abnormal based on visual analysis (**Table 2**).

Abnormal scans were further classified based on degree of dopaminergic deficit seen (semiquantitative analysis based step 10/GE cool color scale) and which part of striatum is affected, viz. putamen or caudate or both.

Abnormal scans	Mild dopaminergic deficit
	Moderate dopaminergic deficit
	Severe dopaminergic deficit

METABOLIC IMAGING IN PARKINSONIAN SYNDROMES

Today's PET systems are either constructed as hybrid PET/CT or, more recently, PET/MRI systems. Here, the primary focus is on PET studies using the glucose analog, [^{18}F]-FDG to assess cerebral glucose metabolism. With the rate of glucose metabolism being closely related to maintenance of ion gradients and transmitter turnover (in particular, glutamate), [^{18}F]-FDG represents an ideal tracer for assessment of neuronal function and its changes.[17] After uptake in cerebral tissue by specific glucose transporters, [^{18}F]-FDG is phosphorylated by hexokinase. Since [^{18}F]-FDG-6-P is neither a substrate for transport back out of the cell nor it can be metabolized further, it is irreversibly trapped in cells. Therefore, the distribution of [^{18}F]-FDG in tissue imaged by PET closely reflects the regional distribution of cerebral glucose metabolism and, thus, neuronal function. Using appropriate pharmacokinetic models and a plasma input function {i.e., [^{18}F]-FDG concentration in arterial or arterialized venous plasma}, the absolute cerebral metabolic rate of glucose (CMRglc in μmol/min/100 g tissue) can be estimated. In the case of [^{18}F]-FDG, absolute quantification is usually not necessary for routine clinical studies, since the diagnostic information can often be obtained from the typical pattern of [^{18}F]-FDG uptake or relative estimates of regional glucose metabolism gained by normalizing regional [^{18}F]-FDG uptake to the uptake of a suitable reference region unaffected by disease.

TABLE 2: Scan interpretation of dopamine transporter.

Scan findings	*Scan results*
Bilateral equal uptake of tracer in both the striatum	Normal
Reduction in uptake of tracer (dopaminergic deficit) in either striatum	Abnormal

Patient Preparation and Scanning

Patients were fasting for at least 4 hours prior to FDG PET/CT brain and plain water was allowed. Each patient was injected with 111–185 MBq (3–5 mCi) of [^{18}F]-FDG intravenously followed by a rest period of 60 minutes with eyes open in a silent and dimly lit isolation room with minimal auditory stimulation after which the scan is done. Scan duration is for 8 minutes. Sedation was given to the patients whenever required.

Image Analysis

Visual Reading

2-fluoro-2-deoxy-glucose-PET images were displayed as a series of transaxial slices scaled to a common maximum in standard color scale (step 10 scale) and graded as mild, moderate, and severe hypometabolism in different regions of the brain as follows—bilateral frontal, parietal, medial and lateral temporal, and occipital regions, anterior and posterior cingulate gyrus and precuneus, midbrain, striatum, thalamus, cerebellum, and sensorimotor cortex. A particular pattern is seen in each of the clinical condition as mentioned below. Computer-assisted analysis can also be used depending on the availability of the software.

Diagnostic Criteria of Idiopathic Parkinson's Disease and Atypical Parkinsonian Syndromes on FDG Brain PET-CT Based on the Data Published in Literature[18]

- Parkinson disease is characterized by a posterior temporoparietal, occipital, and sometimes frontal hypometabolism (especially in PD with cognitive impairment) and relative hypermetabolism of putamen, pallidum, thalamus sensorimotor cortex, pons, and cerebellum.
- Multisystem atrophy patients show a marked hypometabolism of (posterior) putamen, pons, and cerebellum, which may be more pronounced in striatum or in pons and cerebellum, depending on

the predominant side of degeneration and, thus, clinical presentation (striatonigral/MSA-P and olivopontocerebellar/MSA-C, respectively).

- In case of PSP, regional hypometabolism is consistently noted in medial, dorsal, and ventrolateral frontal areas [i.e., anterior cingulate gyrus, supplementary motor area (SMA), precentral gyrus, and premotor to posterior prefrontal areas], caudate, thalamus, and upper brain stem.
- Finally, CBD is characterized by highly asymmetric hypometabolism of frontoparietal areas, striatum, and thalamus contralateral to the most affected body side. Cortical hypometabolism may be pronounced in parietal cortex and usually extends across the sensorimotor cortex into the cingulate gyrus and premotor to posterior prefrontal areas.

Literature review showed several studies which showed an excellent concordance between the imaging diagnosis by FDG-PET and clinical diagnosis of Parkinsonian syndromes on an individual case to case basis—Brajkovic et al.[19]—92% concordance, Tripathi et al.[20]—91.7% concordance, and Eckert et al.[21]—85.4% concordance. Clinical diagnosis at 2 years of follow-up was used as a gold standard in the above studies based on the published clinicopathological data which shows a very high concordance [99% positive predictive value (PPV)] between clinical diagnosis after atleast 2 years of follow-up by a movement disorder neurologist and the findings at postmortem examination.[22]

Dopaminergic (DAT) imaging cannot differentiate between idiopathic and APS but is helpful in differentiating Parkinsonian syndrome patients from those without any nigrostriatal degeneration (e.g., drug-induced Parkinsonism and ET). It is important as the clinical management of these conditions differs significantly.[23]

There are a few studies in literature which investigated and concluded that dopaminergic imaging might be helpful to detect Parkinsonism cases even in prodromal stages (prior to the onset of motor symptoms).[24]

Ponsen et al. demonstrated that 10% of hyposmic patients who had abnormal DAT binding at baseline developed PD at 2 years of follow-up and this figure rose to 12.5% at 5 years of follow-up.[25] Another prospective study showed that idiopathic RBD [rapid eye movement (REM) sleep behavior disorder] patients exhibited decreased DAT binding and faster rates of DAT-binding decline compared to healthy controls. After 3 years of follow-up, 15% of RBD patients, who also had the lowest DAT binding at baseline, had developed PD.[26] A recent report on sequential biomarker assessment of population-based hyposmia screening in a first and DAT imaging in a second step—the Parkinson At-Risk Syndrome (PARS) study—reported decreased radiotracer binding using DAT-SPECT to be present in 11% of hyposmic compared with 1% of normosmic participants. Also male sex and constipation were predictive for a DAT-deficit such that combining all these factors increased the percentage of subjects with a DAT deficit to 40%.[27]

HYPERKINETIC MOVEMENT DISORDERS

Tremors

Essential tremor: A bilateral, largely symmetric postural, or kinetic tremor involving the hands and forearms and sometimes the head.

Orthostatic tremor (OT): High frequent tremor in the legs that mainly occurs when patients are standing still.

Imaging:

- Increased regional cerebral blood flow (rCBF) and glucose metabolism in *cerebellum, sensorimotor cortex, and thalamus*
- Dopaminergic system imaging: Normal

Chorea

Rapid, semipurposeful, graceful, dance-like nonpatterned involuntary movements involving distal, or proximal muscle groups.

Imaging:

- [^{18}F]-2-fluoro-2-deoxy-glucose PET studies in patients with neurodegenerative disorders with chorea (specifically HD, SCA17, DRPLA, McLeod syndrome, and ChAc) demonstrate progressive glucose hypometabolism in the striatum in addition to reduced striatal D1 and D2 receptor binding.
- In contrast, striatal hypermetabolism was found in cases of chorea of transient etiologies (hyperthyroidism, polycythemia vera, and Sydenham's chorea). It suggests different pathophysiological mechanisms in transient versus chronic/progressive/neurodegenerative etiologies of chorea.[28]

Tics

Clinical hallmark of Gilles de la Tourette syndrome (TS)—relatively brief and intermittent involuntary movements (motor tic) and sounds (phonic tic).

Imaging:

- Regional rCBF PET and SPECT findings mostly correlated with hypoperfusion of the caudate nucleus and cingulate cortex.

Myoclonus

Brief muscles jerk; occur in many neurologic/non-neurologic disorders.

Imaging:

- Hypoperfusion and/or hypometabolism of the frontoparietal cortex was found in patients with negative epileptic myoclonus, Alzheimer's disease, CBD, Creutzfeldt-Jakob disease, fatal familial insomnia, and posthypoxic myoclonus.
- Decreased rCBF and/or glucose metabolism in the cerebellum and thalamus.

Dystonia

Dystonia is a syndrome characterized by sustained muscle contractions causing distorted voluntary movements or abnormal postures.

Dopa-responsive dystonia (DRD) is another form of idiopathic torsion dystonia characterized by early-onset and diurnal fluctuations. Clinical features include dystonia, variable degrees of Parkinsonism, and an excellent and sustained response to levodopa.

Imaging features:

- Presynaptic dopaminergic imaging helps to differentiate DRD patients from Parkinsonism, as DRD patients generally have normal uptake levels while PD patients show striatal uptake reductions.
- On [^{18}F]-FDG PET, dystonia patients typically show increased metabolism in the lentiform nucleus, basal ganglia, and associated outflow pathways to the sensorimotor cortex along with regions involved in motor performance.
- Dopa-responsive dystonia patients show a distinct metabolic pattern characterized by relative increases in the dorsal midbrain, cerebellar vermis, and supplementary motor area, evidencing covarying decrements in the putamen, lateral premotor, and motor cortical regions. This metabolic pattern is not expressed in dystonia gene carriers of the *DYT1* or *DYT6* gene mutation, thereby supporting the hypothesis of a different pathophysiology for DRD.[11]

ACKNOWLEDGMENT

I am thankful to Dr Vivek Mathew James and Dr Aashish Gambhir for their support and assistance in compiling the images and table in this chapter.

CONCLUSION

To summarize, nuclear medicine (PET and SPECT) serves as a problem solving tool to the clinician/neurophysician in cases of diagnostic dilemma whether it is parkinsonism or not and also to differentiate between types of atypical parkinsonian syndromes, especially in the early stages of disease when MRI will be normal.

REFERENCES

1. Kempster PA, Williams DR, Selikhova M, Holton J, Revesz T, Lees AJ. Patterns of levodopa response in Parkinson's disease: A clinico-pathological study. Brain. 2007;130(8):2123-8.
2. O'Sullivan SS, Massey LA, Williams DR, Silveira-Moriyama L, Kempster PA, Holton JL, et al. Clinical outcomes of progressive supranuclear palsy and multiple system atrophy. Brain. 2008;131(5):1362-72.
3. Tolosa E, Wenning G, Poewe W. The diagnosis of Parkinson's disease. Lancet Neurol. 2006;5(1):75-86.
4. Ling H, O'Sullivan SS, Holton JL, Revesz T, Massey LA, Williams DR, et al. Does corticobasal degeneration exist? A clinicopathological re-evaluation. Brain. 2010;133(7):2045-57.
5. Agid Y. Parkinson's disease: pathophysiology. Lancet. 1991;337 (8753):1321-4.
6. Benamer HTS, Patterson J, Grosset DG, Booij J, de Bruin K, van Royen E, et al. Accurate differentiation of parkinsonism and essential tremor using visual assessment of [^{123}I]-FP-CIT SPECT imaging: The [^{123}I]-FP-CIT study group. Mov Disord. 2000;15(3):503-10.
7. Benítez-Rivero S, Marín-Oyaga VA, García-Solís D, Huertas-Fernández I, García-Gómez FJ, Jesús S, et al. Clinical features and ^{123}I-FP-CIT SPECT imaging in vascular parkinsonism and Parkinson's disease. J Neurol Neurosurg Psychiatry. 2013;84(2):122-9.
8. Marshall VL, Reininger CB, Marquardt M, Patterson J, Hadley DM, Oertel WH, et al. Parkinson's disease is overdiagnosed clinically at baseline in diagnostically uncertain cases: A 3-year European multicenter study with repeat [^{123}I]FP-CIT SPECT. Mov Disord. 2009;24(4):500-8.
9. Meyer PT, Hellwig S. Update on SPECT and PET in parkinsonism-Part 1: Imaging for differential diagnosis. Curr Opin Neurol. 2014;27(4):390-7.
10. Phelps ME, Hoffman EJ, Mullani NA, Ter-Pogossian MM. Application of annihilation coincidence detection to transaxial reconstruction tomography. J Nucl Med. 1975;16(3): 210-24.
11. Berti V, Pupi A, Mosconi L. PET/CT in diagnosis of movement disorders. Ann N Y Acad Sci. 2011;1228:93-108.
12. Booij J, Tissingh G, Winogrodzka A, van Royen EA. Imaging of the dopaminergic neurotransmission system using single-photon emission tomography and positron emission tomography in patients with parkinsonism. Eur J Nucl Med. 1999;26(2):171-82.
13. Innis RB, Seibyl JP, Scanley BE, Laruelle M, Abi-Dargham A, Wallace E, et al. Single photon emission computed tomographic imaging demonstrates loss of striatal dopamine transporters in Parkinson disease. Proc Natl Acad Sci USA. 1993;90(24): 11965-9.

14. A multicenter assessment of dopamine transporter imaging with DOPASCAN/SPECT in parkinsonism. Parkinson study group. Neurology. 2000;55(10):1540-7.
15. Meltzer PC, Blundell P, Jones AG, Mahmood A, Garada B, Zimmerman RE, et al. A technetium-99m SPECT imaging agent which targets the dopamine transporter in primate brain. J Med Chem. 1997;40(12):1835-44.
16. Huang WS, Lin SZ, Lin JC, Wey SP, Ting G, Liu RS. Evaluation of Early-Stage Parkinson's disease with 99mTc-TRODAT-1 Imaging. J Nucl Med. 2001;42(9):1303-8.
17. Sokoloff L. Relation between physiological function and energy metabolism in the central nervous system. J Neurochem. 1977;29(1):13-26.
18. Meyer PT, Frings L, Rücker G, Hellwig S. (18)F-FDG PET in Parkinsonism: Differential Diagnosis and evaluation of cognitive impairment. J Nucl Med. 2017;58(12):1888-98.
19. Brajkovic L, Kostic V, Sobic-Saranovic D, Stefanova E, Jecmenica-Lukic M, Jesic A, et al. The utility of FDG-PET in the differential diagnosis of Parkinsonism. Neurol Res. 2017;39(8):675-84.
20. Tripathi M, Dhawan V, Peng S, Kushwaha S, Batla A, Jaimini A, et al. Differential diagnosis of parkinsonian syndromes using F-18 fluorodeoxyglucose positron emission tomography. Neuroradiology. 2013;55(4):483-92.
21. Eckert T, Barnes A, Dhawan V, Frucht S, Gordon MF, Feigin AS, et al. FDG PET in the differential diagnosis of parkinsonian disorders. Neuroimage. 2005;26(3):912-21.
22. Hughes AJ, Daniel SE, Ben-Shlomo Y, Lees AJ. The accuracy of diagnosis of parkinsonian syndromes in a specialist movement disorder service. Brain. 2002;125(4):861-70.
23. Catafau AM, Tolosa E, DaTSCAN Clinically Uncertain Parkinsonian Syndromes Study Group. Impact of dopamine transporter SPECT using 123I-Ioflupane on diagnosis and management of patients with clinically uncertain parkinsonian syndromes. Mov Disord. 2004;19(10):1175-82.
24. Mahlknecht P, Seppi K, Poewe W. The concept of prodromal Parkinson's disease. J Parkinsons Dis. 2015;5(4):681-97.
25. Ponsen MM, Stoffers D, Wolters EC, Booij J, Berendse HW. Olfactory testing combined with dopamine transporter imaging as a method to detect prodromal Parkinson's disease. J Neurol Neurosurg Psychiatry. 2010;81(4):396-9.
26. Iranzo A, Valldeoriola F, Lomeña F, Molinuevo JL, Serradell M, Salamero M, et al. Serial dopamine transporter imaging of nigrostriatal function in patients with idiopathic rapid-eye-movement sleep behaviour disorder: a prospective study. Lancet Neurol. 2011;10(9):797-805.
27. Jennings D, Siderowf A, Stern M, Seibyl J, Eberly S, Oakes D, et al. Imaging prodromal Parkinson disease: The Parkinson Associated Risk Syndrome Study. Neurology. 2014;83(19): 1739-46.
28. Ehrlich DJ, Walker RH. Functional neuroimaging and chorea: a systematic review. J Clin Mov Disord. 2017;4(1):8.

CHAPTER 16

Electrophysiological Evaluation of Movement Disorders: An Overview

Shweta Prasad, Robert Chen, Pramod Kumar Pal

INTRODUCTION

Electrophysiological diagnostic procedures play a critical role in the diagnostic workup for movement disorders.[1] They are primarily used for (1) confirming and characterizing a clinically-diagnosed movement disorder, (2) providing a diagnosis when clinical characterization and diagnosis is difficult, (3) differentiating organic from functional, (4) presurgical evaluation of surgical treatment of tremor, and (5) understanding the pathophysiology of various movement disorders. **Box 1** shows examples of clinical settings when a movement disorder specialist may refer a patient for an electrophysiological evaluation.

This review will briefly outline the evaluation of patients with tremor, myoclonus, and dystonia using basic electrophysiological techniques commonly employed for evaluation of movement disorders.

TREMOR

Electrophysiological evaluation of tremor provides objective, reproducible information, and often aids in identifying the origin of the tremor.[1] Although the importance of electrophysiology for tremor was well established, the recent consensus criteria on tremor by the International Parkinson and Movement Disorder Society has laid special emphasis on electrophysiology,[2] wherein, electrophysiology plays a role in defining an axis-1 syndrome and elucidating an axis-2 etiology. Electrophysiological characterization of tremor provides information about tremor frequency, pattern of muscle activation, duration and amplitude of muscle bursts, and the presence of mechanical, mechanical-reflex, or central components of tremor.[3] Apart from a definite utility in the characterization of organic tremors, electrophysiology often plays a critical role in the diagnosis of functional tremors.

Box 1 Common reasons for referral by movement disorders specialists for an electrophysiological evaluation.

- For characterization of abnormal or bizarre movements: Are they tremor, ataxia, myoclonus, tic, asterixis, dystonia, etc.?
- For characterization of tremor, especially to determine the frequency
- To differentiate between organic and psychogenic tremor, myoclonus, and dystonia
- In the following situations where patients present with:
  - Rest as well on postural and action tremor of hands: Do they have Parkinson's disease, essential tremor, or both?
  - Inability to stand because of tremulousness of legs: Do they have orthostatic tremor?
  - Multiple sclerosis and tremulous upper limbs: Are the movements tremor, ataxia or a combination? How likely are they to benefit from surgery?
  - Cervical dystonia and tremor of head: Do they have dystonic head tremor or superimposed essential tremor?
  - A sudden onset tremor, which, fluctuates, is variable, distractible, changes in body parts involved: Is this psychogenic tremor?
  - Spontaneous or stimulus-sensitive jerks of a part of body or whole body: Is it myoclonus (cortical, subcortical, brainstem, or spinal), tics, functional movement disorder or exaggerated startle reflex (physiologic or pathologic)?
  - Features of akinetic-rigid syndrome and spontaneous and/or stimulus-sensitive myoclonus: Do they have multiple system atrophy, corticobasal degeneration, or Parkinson's disease with myoclonus?

METHODS OF ELECTROPHYSIOLOGICAL ASSESSMENT OF TREMOR

Characterization of tremor requires recording of the movement and muscles involved in production of the movement. In an ideal setting in order to record all six degrees of freedom, i.e., three for rotation and three for translations in a three-dimensional space, a triaxial accelerometer and gyroscope are necessary, in addition to a multichannel surface electromyogram (EMG) for each limb. However, this is not a practical setup and in most clinical settings, a one-axis accelerometer in combination with two-channel EMG is adequate.

Surface EMG: Electrodes are usually placed in pairs, in order to cover the agonist and antagonist muscles involved in tremor. Electrodes may be placed in a belly-belly or tendon-belly arrangement along the longitudinal axis of the muscle.

Accelerometer: Usually secured with the recording axis aligned with the dominant tremor axis. The protocol for recording a tremor varies slightly based on the joint and limb being recorded.

Recording a Tremor

The amplifier should have a sampling frequency of at least 1,000 Hz and filter settings should be as follows:[3]

- *Electromyogram*: High pass—10–20 Hz, low pass—250 Hz
- *Accelerometer*: High pass—2 Hz, low pass—30 Hz

Prior to placing electrodes, the appropriate muscle should be selected by palpating the limb to identify the site of maximum movement and skin should always be thoroughly cleaned in order to reduce artefacts and impedance (ideal <10 kΩ).

Methods of recording an upper limb and lower limb tremor are described in **Boxes 2** and **3**.[3,4]

Processing of Data

Data obtained from recording a tremor is typically in the time domain, i.e., change in either voltage or acceleration over time (**Flowchart 1**). Although data in the frequency domain is more relevant to tremor, time domain data must also be reviewed to ascertain burst pattern, burst duration, interburst interval, and frequency (**Fig. 1**). Conversion of data from time domain to frequency domain requires a fourier transformation,[5] which provides a power spectrum demonstrating the relative power of different frequencies within the recorded signal.[6] Following transformation, analysis should be performed to ascertain components involved in generation of tremor—mechanical, mechanical-reflex, and central (**Fig. 1**).[3]

Apart from analyzing the time and frequency domains of data, coherence, i.e., whether the phase difference

Box 2 Method of recording an upper limb tremor.

- The patient should be seated with forearms pronated and resting on the armrest; rather than on the lap in order to isolate the limb as much as possible and reduce signal contamination
- Tremor should be recorded in each of the following positions for at least 30–60 s
- Rest: Forearm supported by armrest; and wrists dangling freely in the air
- Posture: The hand should be extended beyond the armrest; and the wrist should be extended against gravity while resting the forearm on the armrest
- Action tremor: Slow (<2 Hz) flexion and extension of the hand at the wrist. This movement has to be slow in order to differentiate this movement from the tremor
- Specific positions and tasks which historically produce a tremor should also be assessed in addition to the above positions
- Loading refers to the technique of strapping weights (1, 1.5, or 2 lb) on the dorsum of the hand in order to separate peripheral and central components of tremor, and to investigate functional tremor
- Cognitive tasks such as mental arithmetic may be employed to elicit as well as modulate a tremor
- When a functional origin is suspected, the following additional steps should be performed:
    - Performing slow and fast voluntary movements with the contralateral hand (such as opening and closing a fist, pronation and supination of forearm, tapping thumb and index finger or tapping a finger on table), or performing rapid tongue movements, etc. This procedure helps to determine whether the tremor frequency can be entrained by the frequency of the voluntary movement
    - Distractibility of the tremor should be assessed when cognitive tasks are being performed
    - Additional tests such as tapping of contralateral hand at different frequencies (1,3,5 Hz), response to ballistic movements, tonic activation (co-activation sign), coherence testing, and loading should be performed

Box 3 Method of recording a lower limb tremor.

- A lower limb tremor is typically recorded to confirm or exclude a clinical diagnosis of orthostatic tremor
- Continuous recordings should be obtained in the following positions:
    - Sitting with feet firmly planted on the ground, and with legs stretched out horizontally
    - Sitting to standing position
    - Standing with feet comfortably apart
    - If possible, when the patient is walking
    - Modulation of tremor when weight bearing on lower limbs is altered, e.g., when leaning on arms and pushing forward onto the table

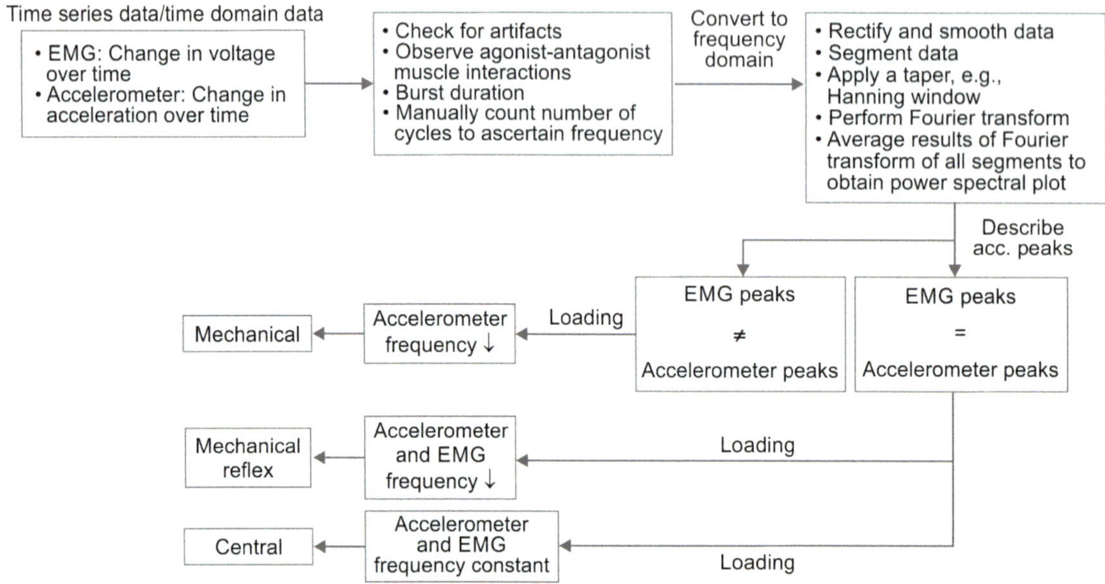

(EMG: electromyography)

FLOWCHART 1: Electrophysiological evaluation of tremor.

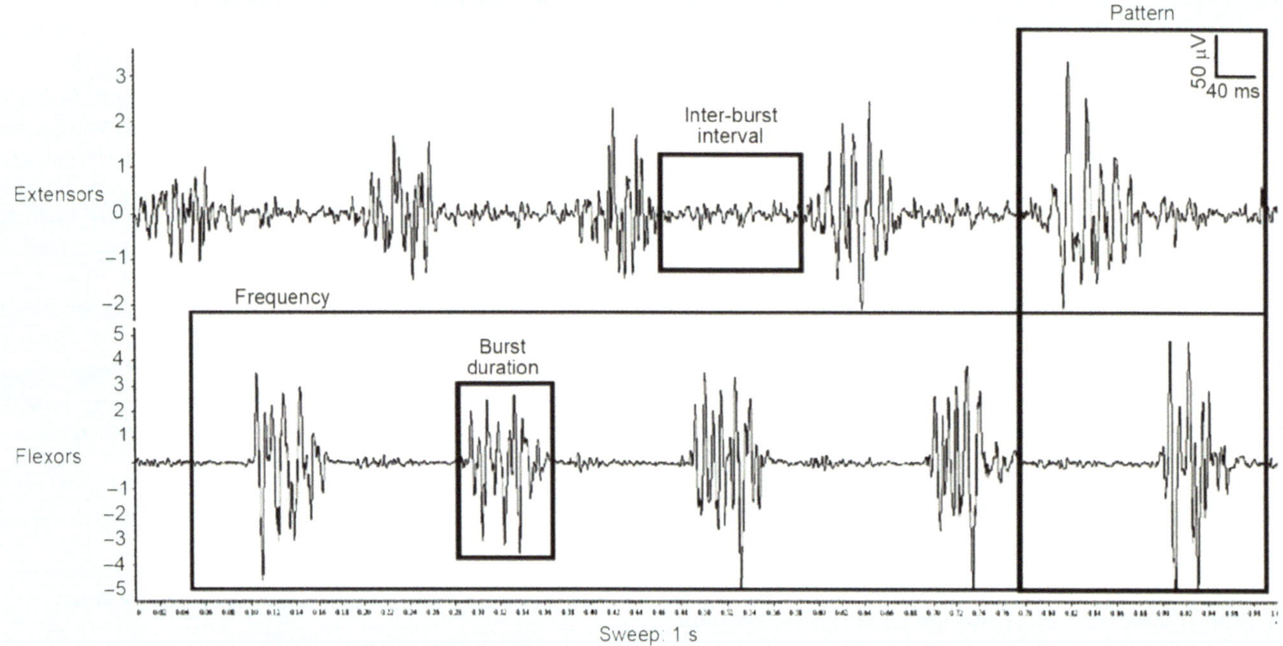

FIG. 1: Surface electromyogram (EMG) recording of a tremor showing the main features that should be observed—burst pattern, burst duration, interburst interval, and frequency.

of two signals is constant, can also be evaluated. This is obtained by dividing the cross spectrum of both signals by the autospectrum of each signal.[7] A value of zero implies no coherence, whereas one suggests perfect coherence.

INTERPRETATION OF DATA

Results obtained from electrophysiology should be evaluated in association with other clinical features and history. Electrophysiological findings of the most common tremor syndromes are described below in **Table 1**.

Physiological and Enhanced Physiological Tremor

A physiological tremor is frequently observed in normal individuals and typically has only a mechanical component (6–12 Hz), although a central component (8–12 Hz) has also been described.[8] There is usually no correlation with

EMG. An enhanced physiological tremor is predominantly high frequency (8–12 Hz), low amplitude postural tremor which is commonly observed under conditions of stress, fatigue, anxiety, or hypoglycemia.[9] These may often be aggravated by drugs, hyperthyroidism, and alcohol withdrawal. This type of tremor may have all three components, i.e., mechanical, mechanical-reflex, and central, and a reduction in tremor frequency can be observed with loading.

Essential tremor

Essential tremor (ET) is typically a clinical diagnosis and electrophysiology commonly shows a 4–12 Hz central and mechanical component (**Fig. 2**), the latter of which can be separated by loading.[10] Patients with ET plus may also have a rest tremor which is usually the same frequency as the action component. An inverse relation between tremor frequency and age has been reported in ET.[11] In several cases, it may be difficult to clinically differentiate between ET and enhanced physiological tremors. In such situations, as mentioned earlier, loading may be beneficial. Although cocontraction between agonist and antagonist muscles is often associated with ET, alternating contractions may also be seen.[12]

TABLE 1: Characteristics of common tremor syndromes.

Tremor syndrome	*Predominant activation patterns*	*Frequency (Hz)*
Physiological tremor	Posture	6–12
Enhanced physiological tremor	Posture	8–12
Essential tremor	Posture and kinetic	4–12
Parkinsonian tremor	Rest	4–7
Orthostatic tremor		
OT	Posture (standing)	13–18
Slow OT	Posture (standing)	≤12
Functional tremor	Variable	6–11
Dystonic tremor	Posture	4–7
Cerebellar tremor	Intention	<5
Holmes tremor	Rest, posture, and intention	<4.5–5
Palatal tremor	Rest	0.5–5
Neuropathic tremor	Posture and kinetic	3–6

(OT: orthostatic tremor)

Parkinsonian Tremor

Parkinson's disease (PD) is classically associated with a "pill rolling" rest tremor which typically has a frequency between 4 and 7 Hz, although higher frequencies have been described. Alternating contraction of the agonist and antagonist muscles is commonly described; however, cocontraction may also occur. A patient with PD may have (1) a typical Parkinsonian rest tremor plus a postural/kinetic tremor with same frequency as his rest tremor (difference ≤1.5 Hz) and often there is a pause in the tremor during the transition from rest to posture, i.e., "re-emergence" (**Fig. 3**); (2) a postural/kinetic tremor in addition to rest tremor, but with different frequency (difference >1.5 Hz); (3) or rarely only postural/kinetic tremor (4-9 Hz) without rest tremor.[13,14] A postural tremor with a frequency different to that of the rest tremor with no re-emergence may be dopamine unresponsive.[14]

Benign tremulous parkinsonism is an entity characterized by tremor dominance with minimal and slow progression of Parkinsonian symptoms.[15] The tremor in this condition is electrophysiologically similar to PD, however, response to levodopa is variable.[16]

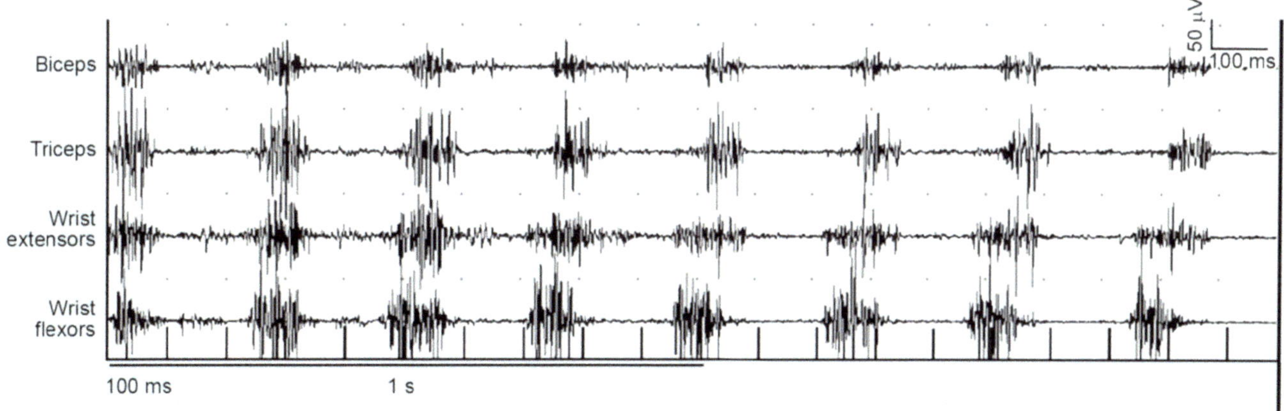

FIG. 2: Surface electromyogram (EMG) recording of an essential tremor demonstrating a 5 Hz tremor with cocontraction of agonist and antagonist muscles.

Orthostatic Tremor

This is a rare tremor syndrome characterized by a high frequency symmetric lower limb tremor that is activated when standing, is absent while sitting or lying down, and reduces by walking or leaning (**Fig. 4**). Based on tremor frequency, orthostatic tremor (OT) may be subdivided into OT (13–18 Hz) and slow OT (≤12 Hz).[17] However, frequencies as high as 23 Hz have been reported.[18] A single central oscillator rather than two has been suggested in OT, and this is the only nonfunctional tremor with right-left coherence. OT should be differentiated from orthostatic myoclonus, the frequency of which is slower (3–7 Hz).

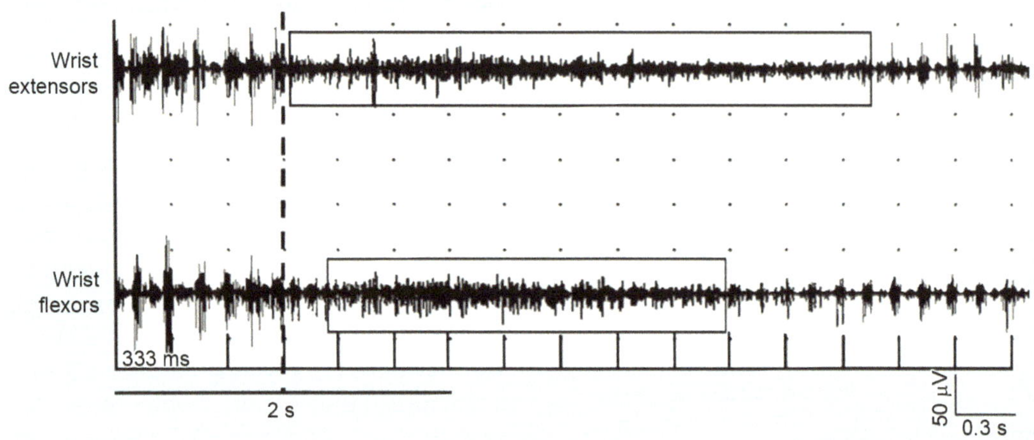

FIG. 3: Surface electromyogram (EMG) recording of a tremor in Parkinson's disease demonstrating re-emergence of the rest tremor. Dashed line signifies the transition from rest to posture and boxes signify the latency before re-emergence.

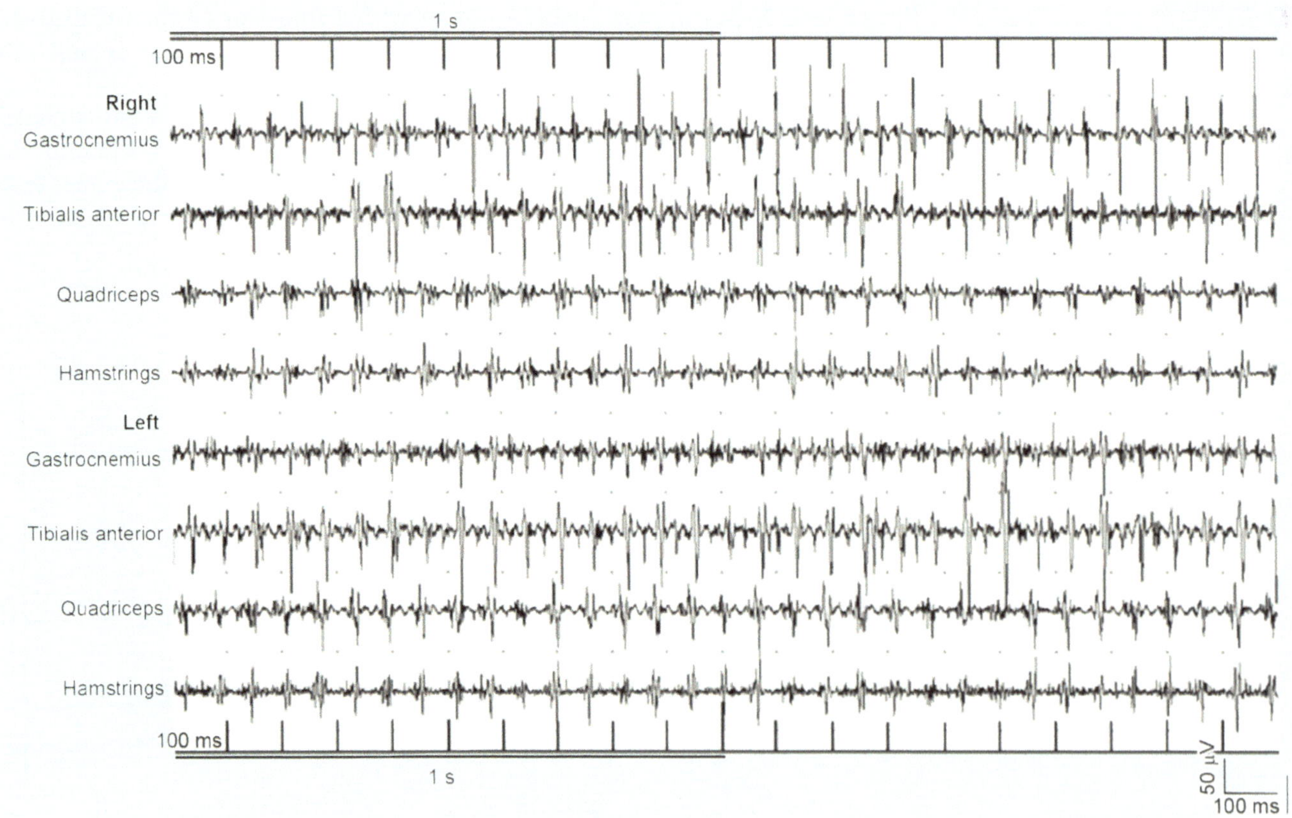

FIG. 4: Surface electromyogram (EMG) recording of an orthostatic tremor recorded while the patient was standing revealed a 15–16 Hz synchronous tremor.

Functional Tremor

A functional tremor is often suspected in a sudden onset, unclassifiable tremor with unusual clinical combinations of activation patterns, and changing characteristics—amplitude, frequency, direction, and body part.[19] The frequency of functional hand tremors may range between 6 and 11 Hz. In addition to routine tremor recording specific maneuvers should be performed to ascertain distractibility, entrainability, and variability (**Box 2, Figs. 5 and 6**). "Coactivation sign" which consists of voluntary contraction of agonist and antagonist muscles of the tremulous joint before the tremor begins has been described in functional tremors, and can be recorded during electrophysiology.[20] In addition, as described in **Box 2**, tests such as tapping of contralateral hand at different frequencies (1, 3, and 5 Hz), response to ballistic movements, tonic activation (coactivation sign), coherence testing, and loading should also be performed. Although individual tests may have low sensitivity in functional tremor, a combination of multiple tests provides higher sensitivity and specificity for the diagnosis of functional tremor.[21] Electrophysiological characteristics of functional tremor are listed in **Box 4**.

Other Tremor Syndromes

Dystonic Tremor

Two types of tremor are known to coexist with dystonia, (1) Dystonic tremor: A tremor in the dystonic body part, i.e., dystonic muscle contraction, and (2) Tremor associated with dystonia: The tremor is not in the dystonic body part.[22] A dystonic tremor is typically irregular, with varying amplitude and may have an irregular frequency (<7 Hz). The presence of geste antagoniste and null point may be helpful in diagnosing a dystonic tremor.[2]

Cerebellar Tremor

Low frequency (<5 Hz) intention tremors which occur due to lesions in the cerebellothalamic pathway. Syndromic associations are needed to ascertain the diagnosis.

Holmes Tremor

This is a low frequency (<4.5–5 Hz) combination of rest, postural, and intention tremor. Usually occurs following damage around the red nucleus, i.e., to the dentato-rubro-thalamo-cortical tract or lesions in the brainstem, cerebellum, or thalamus.[2]

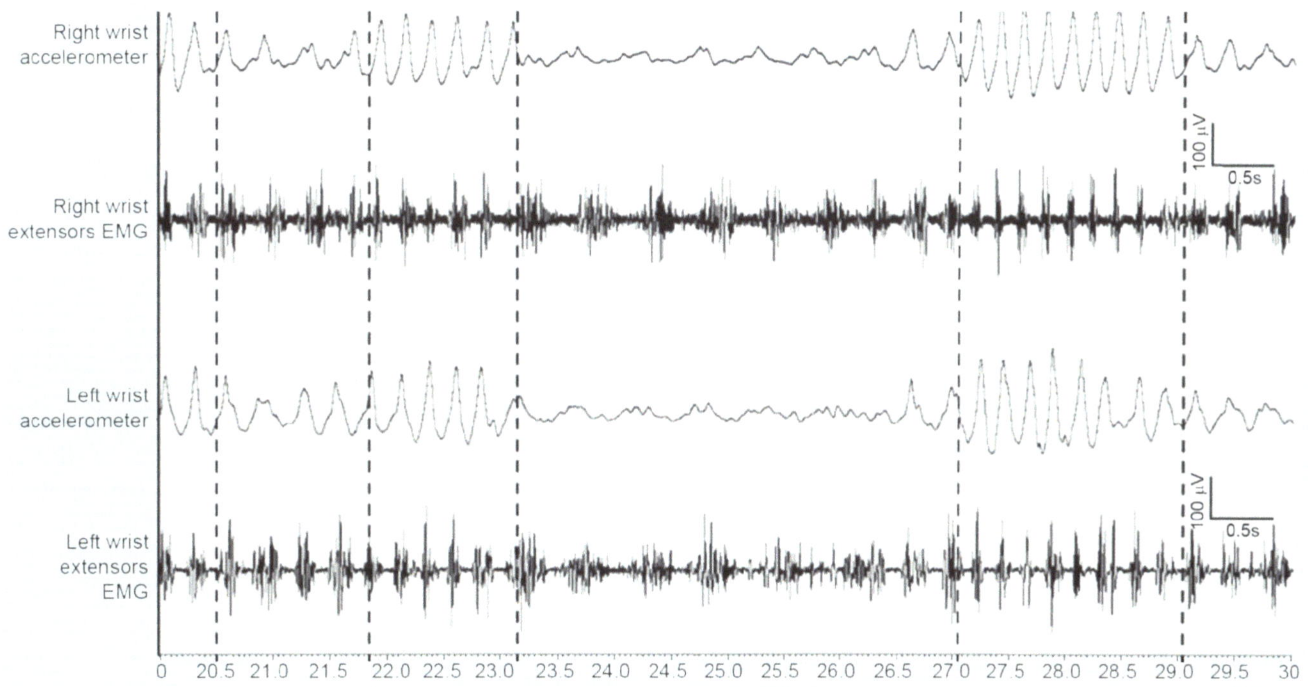

(EMG: electromyogram)

FIG. 5: Accelerometric and surface EMG recording of a functional tremor reveals the presence of variable frequencies over the course of a 10 seconds recording.

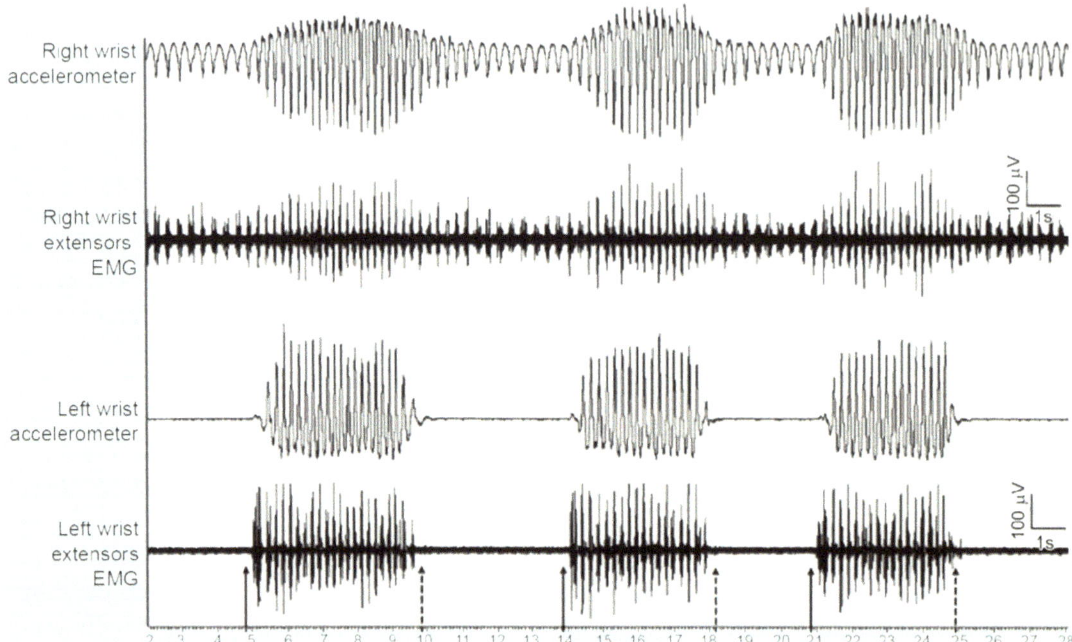

(EMG: electromyogram)

FIG. 6: Accelerometric and surface EMG recording of a functional tremor demonstrating entrainment. The subject has a 4 Hz right hand tremor, which gets entrained to the voluntary movements of the left hand which has a higher frequency of 6–7 Hz. Solid arrow signifies the onset of voluntary movements of the left hand and the dashed arrow signifies cessation of the movement.

Box 4 Electrophysiological characteristics of functional tremor.

- Usually low frequency tremor, *not >11 Hz*
- *Inability to maintain* a voluntary oscillatory limb movement at the *same frequency* for any length of time
- Power spectrum analysis may show *dissipated/variable tremor frequency* (organic tremor usually has a well-defined peak frequency)
- Distraction can change the amplitude and frequency of tremor
- EMG equivalent of clinical coactivation sign can often be observed. In patients with functional hand tremor, a tonic coactivation phase of the wrist flexor and extensor muscles was observed approximately 300 ms before the reciprocal alternating tremor bursts develop
- Usually the duration of tremor *bursts* is longer (>70 ms) than that seen in organic tremor
- *Absence* of *frequency dissociation* (simultaneous occurrence in separate muscles groups of tremors with different frequencies)
- There is increase in tremor amplitude with peripheral loading (unlike in organic tremor) as additional cocontraction of muscles is needed to maintain the reflex activity
- Tremor can be *entrained* (when asked to tap out a beat with the limb contralateral to the tremulous limb, tremor in the latter either dissipates, or shifts to the frequency of tapping)
- High coherence is seen between the frequency spectra of voluntary activity and the "involuntary tremor"
- Inability to tap the hand at specified frequencies

Palatal Tremor

Palatal tremor is characterized by a rhythmic 0.5–5 Hz tremor. Essential palatal tremor typically presents with symptoms of ear click and is attributed to contractions of the tensor veli palatine muscle. The magnetic resonance imaging (MRI) is usually normal in this condition. Symptomatic palatal tremor is secondary to lesions in the dentato-olivary pathway and is typically combined with ataxia.[2]

Neuropathic Tremor

This is predominantly an action tremor, rarely observed at rest with a frequency between 3 and 6 Hz.[23] It is typically observed in demyelinating inflammatory neuropathies and some hereditary neuropathies. It is thought to arise secondary to central processing of mistimed and distorted peripheral input which may be secondary to impaired proprioception in neuropathy.[24]

Task Specific Tremors

These are tremors commonly restricted to and associated with a specific task, for e.g., writing. In such cases, the tremor usually beings when the task is initiated and ends when the task is stopped. The most commonly reported is primary writing tremor wherein a 4–5 Hz, alternating contraction tremor predominantly occurs with the act of writing. It may be subclassified into type A, where the

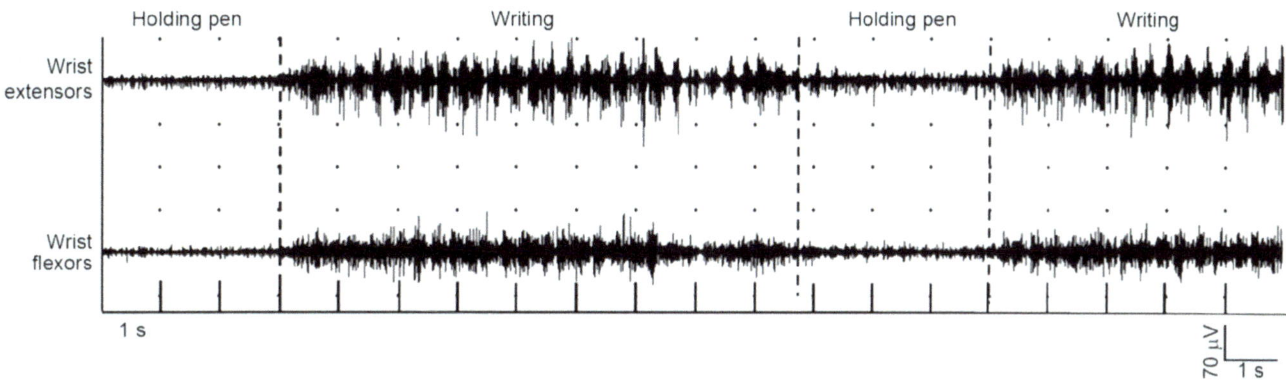

FIG. 7: Surface electromyogram (EMG) recording of a primary writing tremor. The subject has no tremor while holding the pen and develops a tremor upon starting to write. The tremor subsides when he stops writing.

tremor appears only during writing (**Fig. 7**), and type B, where the tremor appears once the hand position used in writing is observed and persists through the act of writing.[25]

MEASUREMENT OF BALLISTIC ARM MOVEMENTS

Ballistic movements may be used to quantify abnormalities of movement pattern during voluntary goal directed movement of a joint, usually a proximal joint. Analysis of ballistic joint movements are useful to quantify cerebellar dysfunction.[26] In healthy subjects, there is a characteristic triphasic EMG burst pattern involving the antagonistic muscle pair: The first agonist burst initiates and accelerates movement, the following antagonist burst decelerates the movement, and finally the second agonist burst dampens the oscillations induced by this decelerating process.[27] In cerebellar dysfunction, there is increased movement overshoot, delayed muscle activations within the triphasic EMG, and an asymmetry of the velocity profile characterized by a shortened deceleration phase.[27] In patients of ET with additional intention tremor, there are abnormalities of the triphasic pattern and kinematics parameters consistent with a disturbed cerebellar timing function.[27]

MYOCLONUS

Myoclonus can be characterized according to the locations affected as focal, multifocal, or generalized, and whether it is spontaneous or triggered by sensory stimulus (reflex myoclonus). It may also be classified based on its origin as cortical, subcortical, brainstem, and spinal.

Cortical Myoclonus

Cortical myoclonus may be epileptic or nonepileptic in origin. Epileptic cortical myoclonus is usually part of an epileptic syndrome and electroencephalogram (EEG) in such patients tends to show additional epileptic features such as spikes, polyspikes, and spike-and-wave discharges.[28] Electrophysiology plays a key role in identifying these subtypes since each subtype is associated with a specific range of EMG burst durations (**Table 2**).

Cortical myoclonus is characterized by jerks of short duration which are most prominent distally in the limbs. These movements tend to increase with voluntary actions. Surface EMG of affected limbs tends to show 30–40 ms bursts which are comprised of single or several compound muscle action potentials (**Fig. 8**).[19] EEG back-averaging may reveal time locked discharges from the contralateral primary motor cortex which precede the EMG discharge or silence by 20–40 ms.[29] In some cases, cortical myoclonus may be stimulus sensitive which is suggestive of increased excitability of the sensorimotor cortex. This is reflected in increased somatosensory evoked potential (SEP) amplitudes. In cortical myoclonus, N20 potential is usually normal and the subsequent components, i.e., P25 and N35 may have increased amplitudes. If the amplitude between P25 and N35 is larger than 10 µV, it is considered a giant SEP and is suggestive of cortical myoclonus.[29] Paired stimulation with an interstimulus interval <100 ms usually reduces the cortical SEP responses. In patients with cortical myoclonus without giant SEP, decreased attenuation of SEP by paired stimulation may be used to demonstrate a cortical origin.[29] Long latency reflex (LLR) and cutaneous muscular reflex (CMR) can also be used to study stimulus sensitive myoclonus. LLR or CMR responses occurring at rest are abnormal. LLR-I, which refers to the response that occurs approximately 40 ms after median nerve stimulation, may

TABLE 2: Electrophysiological characteristics of different subtypes of myoclonus.

Myoclonus subtype	*Electrophysiological characteristics*
Cortical myoclonus	30–40 ms EMG bursts
	Positive EEG back-averaging
	Giant somatosensory evoked potentials
	Long latency reflex: Enlarged LLR-I
	May be stimulus sensitive
	Cutaneous muscular reflex:
	• MSA: Exaggerated E2 • CBS: Increased amplitude, and short latency of E2
Subcortical (myoclonus dystonia)	EMG burst 100–300 ms
	Absence of giant SEP
	Absence of short-latency discharge from EEG back-averaging
Brainstem (reflex) myoclonus	Variable EMG burst duration
	May be stimulus sensitive
	Simultaneous rostral and caudal muscle recruitment and activation
Spinal myoclonus	
Segmental	EMG burst duration >1,000 ms
	Irregular or semi rhythmic bursts
Propriospinal	EMG burst duration >1,000 ms
	Synchronous activity of truncal flexor and extensor muscles
	Poorly consistent bursts
	High conduction velocity (>16 m/s)

(CBS: corticobasal syndrome; LLR: long latency reflex; MSA: multiple system atrophy)

be enlarged in cortical reflex myoclonus, even in the absence of giant SEP. In multiple system atrophy, the E2 response of the CMR, which refers to the long latency excitation component of the CMR which usually occurs 60 ms after stimulation, is exaggerated and increased amplitude with short latency of E2 is observed in corticobasal syndrome.[30]

Myoclonus may also be negative, wherein electrophysiology shows a transient interruption in muscle contraction which shows as a silent period lasting 50–120 ms.[31] Usually negative myoclonus is of cortical origin, however, it may also be subcortical in case of toxic-metabolic encephalopathy associated asterixis.[31] In epileptic negative myoclonus, the EMG silence may be time locked to an epileptic EEG abnormality.

Subcortical Myoclonus

This is a nonspecific term used to describe myoclonus which lacks features suggestive of cortical, brainstem, or spinal myoclonus. Myoclonus-dystonia is often described under this heading. It lacks the classical features of cortical or brainstem myoclonus and is characterized by multifocal, focal, and generalized jerks which may be either brief or long duration, along with spasms. They may be stimulus sensitive with exaggerated response to sensory stimuli. Transcranial magnetic stimulation (TMS) shows normal intracortical facilitation and inhibition[32] and enlarged SEPs are absent.

Brainstem Myoclonus

Brainstem myoclonus is also known as reticular myoclonus. This may present as periodic, stimulus sensitive, generalized jerks, and affecting proximal limb flexors. The pattern of muscle recruitment typically starts in the trapezius or sternocleidomastoid, then spreads rostrally to the orbicularis oculi and caudally to limb muscles.[33] The startle reflex is a normal brainstem-mediated response triggered by sudden stimuli. The EMG burst durations may be between 150 and 400 ms and the spread follows a rostral-caudal pattern of muscle recruitment.[34] Usually this reflex shows habituation after repeated stimulation. However, in hyperekplexia, subjects have exaggerated response which does not habituate. Hyperekplexia can be differentiated from reticular myoclonus based on longer EMG bursts, long latencies in distal limbs, and absence of spontaneous jerks.[34]

Spinal Myoclonus

Two types of spinal myoclonus have been described: Spinal segmental myoclonus and propriospinal myoclonus.[31] Spinal segmental myoclonus usually has long (>1,000 ms) irregular or semirhythmic bursts, is limited to few contiguous myotomes, and is secondary to focal spinal lesions. Propriospinal myoclonus is suggested to be secondary to abnormal spread of an impulse along the propriospinal pathway. Typically, the recruitment begins at a myotome and then spreads rostrally and caudally (**Fig. 9**). Patients may present with arrhythmic flexion jerks in the truncal axial muscles, knees, and hips. The organicity of propriospinal myoclonus is debatable with several reports of functional myoclonus presenting as propriospinal myoclonus. Electrophysiology of an organic propriospinal myoclonus usually shows synchronous activity of truncal flexor and extensor muscles, longer (>1,000 ms) poorly consistent bursts, and high conduction velocity (>16 m/s).[35]

Functional Myoclonus

Variability in order of muscle recruitment, normal LLR, absence of short latency cortical discharge with EEG back averaging, and presence of Bereitschaftspotential (BP) or beta event-related desynchronization are suggestive of a functional myoclonus. BP is premovement potential

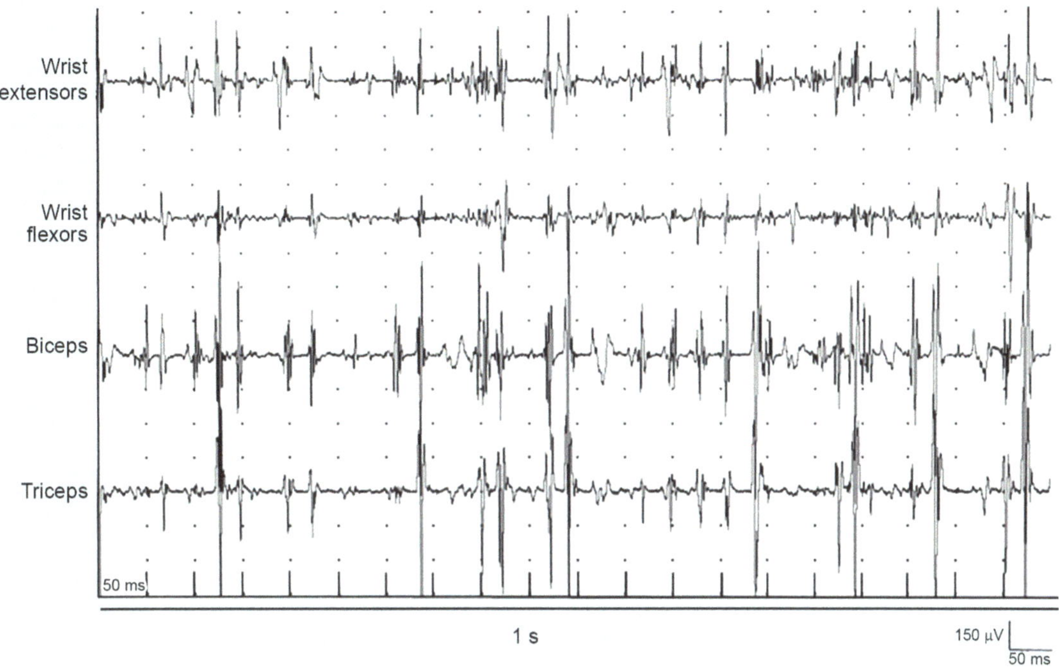

FIG. 8: Surface electromyogram (EMG) recording of cortical myoclonus. The recording shows irregular, high frequency, and short duration bursts.

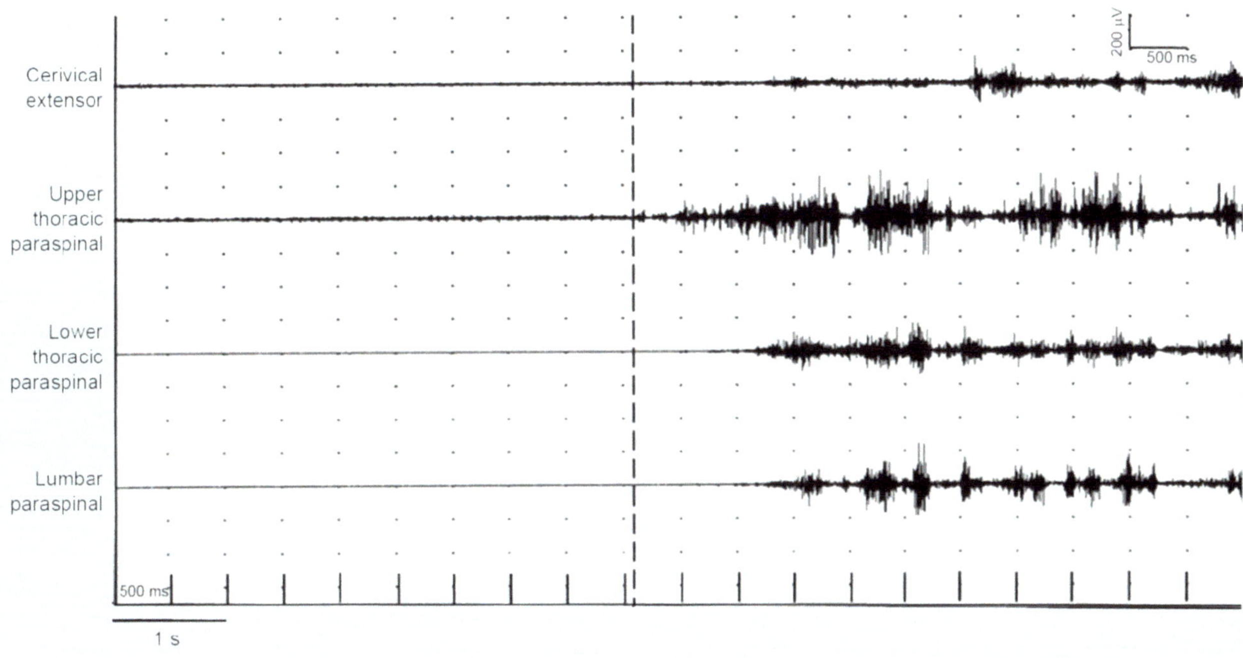

FIG. 9: Surface electromyogram (EMG) recording of propriospinal myoclonus. The recording shows bursts from paraspinal muscles which start in the upper thoracic paraspinal muscles following a change in posture (sitting to standing—dashed line). The muscle activity spreads to lower thoracic and lumbar paraspinal muscles, followed by cervical extensor muscles.

recorded by jerk locked back averaging (**Fig. 10**). Self-initiated voluntary movements are usually preceded by a slow rising negative potential about 1–1.5 seconds prior to the movement and this potential has two phases, early and late. The late phase which rises rapidly suggests the involvement of the premotor cortex including

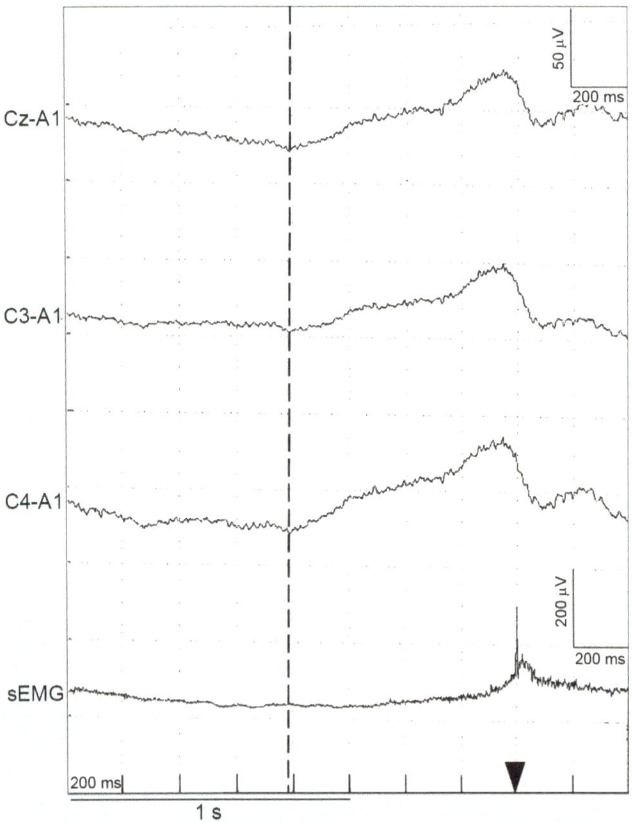

FIG. 10: Bereitschaftspotential observed in all electroencephalogram (EEG) channels, and starts about 800 ms prior to the surface electromyogram activity (sEMG). Dashed line represents the onset of the BP and the arrow represents muscle activity.

supplementary motor area in the preparation of movement. Premovement potentials are difficult to record in very rapid movements, i.e., >1 every 3–5 seconds. Although BP is not ideal for diagnosing functional jerks with very low or very high frequencies, the presence of the BP prior to the onset of jerks and the absence of BP prior to an intended wrist extension are highly diagnostic of functional jerks.[36] Often tic disorders may also demonstrate a short BP and this should be interpreted with caution.

DYSTONIA

Dystonia is electrophysiologically characterized by cocontractions of agonist and antagonist muscles with overflow of contractions to muscles not associated with the task.[37] These observations may be due to impaired inhibition. Reduced reciprocal inhibition in the spinal cord and enhanced blink reflex have also been reported in dystonia.[38] TMS studies have demonstrated a reduction in short interval intracortical inhibition, silent period and surround inhibition, suggestive of decreased cortical inhibition.[38] However, these findings are not specific for dystonia. Surface EMG and occasionally needle EMG recordings are beneficial to identify overactive muscles prior to administering botulinum toxin.

Functional Dystonia

Distinguishing between organic and functional dystonia is often challenging and a few electrophysiological measurements may aid in the differentiation. Abnormally high plasticity will be elicited on paired associative stimulation in organic dystonia in comparison to functional dystonia.[39] In organic blepharospasm, an enhanced R2 blink reflex recovery curve may be observed, whereas, this is normal in functional blepharospasm.[40]

MISCELLANEOUS

Stiff person syndrome (SPS) is characterized by excessive axial rigidity and exaggerated reflex spasms to exteroceptive stimuli. EMG is a crucial component of the diagnostic workup as it demonstrates characteristic continuous motor unit activity of paraspinal muscles.[41] This muscle activity resolves with sleep and following administration of benzodiazepines. Exteroceptive reflexes are exaggerated, tend to habituate poorly, and spread as reflex spasms into muscles uninvolved in the reflex. Polysynaptic reflexes tend to also be enhanced and begin with a characteristic pattern of one or several myoclonic jerks which occur at short intervals (50–70 ms). These are synchronous in antagonistic muscle pairs and are followed by prolonged tonic activation of muscles which are clinically visualized as spasms.[42]

CONCLUSION

Electrophysiology is an invaluable adjunct to clinical evaluation and plays a significant role in accurate phenomenological delineation and diagnosis of movement disorders. In addition, electrophysiological studies play a critical role in furthering the pathophysiological understanding of movement disorders.

REFERENCES

1. Chen KS, Chen R. Principles of Electrophysiological Assessments for Movement Disorders. J Mov Disord. 2020;13(1): 27-38.
2. Bhatia KP, Bain P, Bajaj N, Elble RJ, Hallett M, Louis ED, et al. Consensus Statement on the classification of tremors, from the task force on tremor of the International Parkinson and Movement Disorder Society. Mov Disord. 2018;33(1):75-87.
3. Vial F, Kassavetis P, Merchant S, Haubenberger D, Hallett M. How to do an electrophysiological study of tremor. Clin Neurophysiol Pract. 2019;4:134-42.

4. Elble RJ, McNames J. Using portable transducers to measure tremor severity. Tremor Other Hyperkinet Mov. 2016;6:375.
5. Hallett M. Overview of human tremor physiology. Mov Disord. 1998;13(Suppl 3):43-8.
6. Cohen MX. Analyzing neural time series data: theory and practice. United Kingdom: MIT press; 2014.
7. Halliday DM, Rosenberg JR, Amjad AM, Breeze P, Conway BA, Farmer SF. A framework for the analysis of mixed time series/point process data-theory and application to the study of physiological tremor, single motor unit discharges and electromyograms. Prog Biophys Mol Biol. 1995;64(2-3): 237-78.
8. Raethjen J, Pawlas F, Lindemann M, Wenzelburger R, Deuschl G. Determinants of physiologic tremor in a large normal population. Clin Neurophysiol. 2000;111(10):1825-37.
9. Deuschl G, Raethjen J, Lindemann M, Krack P. The pathophysiology of tremor. Muscle Nerve. 2001;24(6):716-35.
10. Haubenberger D, Hallett M. Essential Tremor. N Engl J Med. 2018;379(6):596-7.
11. Calzetti S, Baratti M, Gresty M, Findley L. Frequency/amplitude characteristics of postural tremor of the hands in a population of patients with bilateral essential tremor: implications for the classification and mechanism of essential tremor. J Neurol Neurosurg Psychiatry. 1987;50(5):561-7.
12. Milanov I. Clinical and electromyographic examinations of patients with essential tremor. Can J Neurol Sci. 2000;27(1): 65-70.
13. Deuschl G, Bain P, Brin M. Consensus statement of the Movement Disorder Society on Tremor. Ad Hoc Scientific Committee. Mov Disord. 1998;13(Suppl 3):2-23.
14. Dirkx MF, Zach H, Bloem BR, Hallett M, Helmich RC. The nature of postural tremor in Parkinson disease. Neurology. 2018;90(13):e1095-e103.
15. Josephs KA, Matsumoto JY, Ahlskog JE. Benign tremulous parkinsonism. Arch Neurol. 2006;63(3):354-7.
16. Kano O, Okonogi S, Hanashiro S, Miura K, Ikeda K, Iwasaki Y. Levodopa-responsive benign tremulous parkinsonism. Case Rep Neurol. 2013;5(2):139-42.
17. Hassan A, Ahlskog JE, Matsumoto JY, Milber JM, Bower JH, Wilkinson JR. Orthostatic tremor: Clinical, electrophysiologic, and treatment findings in 184 patients. Neurology. 2016;86(5): 458-64.
18. Piboolnurak P, Yu QP, Pullman SL. Clinical and neurophysiologic spectrum of orthostatic tremor: case series of 26 subjects. Mov Disord. 2005;20(11):1455-61.
19. Brown P, Thompson PD. Electrophysiological aids to the diagnosis of psychogenic jerks, spasms, and tremor. Mov Disord. 2001;16(4):595-9.
20. Deuschl G, Koster B, Lucking CH, Scheidt C. Diagnostic and pathophysiological aspects of psychogenic tremors. Mov Disord. 1998;13(2):294-302.
21. Schwingenschuh P, Saifee TA, Katschnig-Winter P, Macerollo A, Koegl-Wallner M, Culea V, et al. Validation of "laboratory-supported" criteria for functional (psychogenic) tremor. Mov Disord. 2016;31(4):555-62.
22. Elble RJ. Defining dystonic tremor. Curr Neuropharmacol. 2013;11(1):48-52.
23. Hess CW, Pullman SL. Tremor: clinical phenomenology and assessment techniques. Tremor Other Hyperkinet Mov (N Y). 2012;2.
24. Deuschl G, Bergman H. Pathophysiology of nonparkinsonian tremors. Mov Disord. 2002;17(Suppl 3):S41-8.
25. Bain PG, Findley LJ, Britton TC, Rothwell JC, Gresty MA, Thompson PD, et al. Primary writing tremor. Brain. 1995;118 (Pt 6):1461-72.
26. Koster B, Deuschl G, Lauk M, Timmer J, Guschlbauer B, Lucking CH. Essential tremor and cerebellar dysfunction: abnormal ballistic movements. J Neurol Neurosurg Psychiatry. 2002;73(4):400-5.
27. Flament D, Hore J. Movement and electromyographic disorders associated with cerebellar dysmetria. J Neurophysiol. 1986;55(6):1221-33.
28. Zutt R, Elting JW, Tijssen MAJ. Tremor and myoclonus. Handb Clin Neurol. 2019;161:149-65.
29. Shibasaki H, Hallett M. Electrophysiological studies of myoclonus. Muscle Nerve. 2005;31(2):157-74.
30. Chen R, Ashby P, Lang AE. Stimulus-sensitive myoclonus in akinetic-rigid syndromes. Brain. 1992;115(Pt 6):1875-88.
31. Kojovic M, Cordivari C, Bhatia K. Myoclonic disorders: a practical approach for diagnosis and treatment. Ther Adv Neurol Disord. 2011;4(1):47-62.
32. Li JY, Cunic DI, Paradiso G, Gunraj C, Pal PK, Lang AE, et al. Electrophysiological features of myoclonus-dystonia. Mov Disord. 2008;23(14):2055-61.
33. Beudel M, Elting JWJ, Uyttenboogaart M, van den Broek MWC, Tijssen MAJ. Reticular Myoclonus: It really comes from the brainstem! Mov Disord Clin Pract. 2014;1(3):258-60.
34. Brown P, Rothwell JC, Thompson PD, Britton TC, Day BL, Marsden CD. The hyperekplexias and their relationship to the normal startle reflex. Brain. 1991;114(Pt 4):1903-28.
35. Erro R, Bhatia KP, Edwards MJ, Farmer SF, Cordivari C. Clinical diagnosis of propriospinal myoclonus is unreliable: an electrophysiologic study. Mov Disord. 2013;28(13):1868-73.
36. van der Salm SM, Tijssen MA, Koelman JH, van Rootselaar AF. The bereitschaftspotential in jerky movement disorders. J Neurol Neurosurg Psychiatry. 2012;83(12):1162-7.
37. Sanger TD, Chen D, Fehlings DL, Hallett M, Lang AE, Mink JW, et al. Definition and classification of hyperkinetic movements in childhood. Mov Disord. 2010;25(11):1538-49.
38. Hallett M. Neurophysiology of dystonia: The role of inhibition. Neurobiol Dis. 2011;42(2):177-84.
39. Quartarone A, Rizzo V, Terranova C, Morgante F, Schneider S, Ibrahim N, et al. Abnormal sensorimotor plasticity in organic but not in psychogenic dystonia. Brain. 2009;132(Pt 10):2871-7.
40. Aramideh M, Ongerboer de Visser BW. Brainstem reflexes: electrodiagnostic techniques, physiology, normative data, and clinical applications. Muscle Nerve. 2002;26(1):14-30.
41. Sarva H, Deik A, Ullah A, Severt WL. Clinical Spectrum of Stiff Person Syndrome: A Review of Recent Reports. Tremor Other Hyperkinet Mov (NY). 2016;6:340.
42. Armon C, McEvoy KM, Westmoreland BF, McManis PG. Clinical neurophysiologic studies in stiff-man syndrome: use of simultaneous video-electroencephalographic-surface electromyographic recording. Mayo Clin Proc. 1990;65(7):960-7.

CHAPTER 17

Assessment of Cognition and Behavior in Parkinson's Disease

Urvashi Shah

INTRODUCTION

In 1817, James Parkinson in An essay on the Shaking Palsy, described motor symptoms as the primary clinical characteristics of Parkinson's disease (PD) stating that, *"senses and intellect (being) uninjured"*.[1] However, subsequent observations challenged this assumption and Charcot wrote that *"mind is clouded and memory affected"*.[2] The notion of PD being a motor disorder still predominated and only in the 1980's, formal neuropsychological assessments were used to establish patterns of the cognitive and behavioral issues.[3] The magnitude and spectrum are widespread and heterogeneous. About 20–50% are estimated to have mild cognitive impairment (MCI) or specific executive dysfunction in the early phase of illness[4] and up to 80% develop dementia in the long-term.[5] Behavioral issues are estimated to occur in more than half of all PD patients in some form of neuropsychiatric morbidity—mood issues (depression and anxiety), psychosis (hallucinations and delusions), apathy, and impulse control disorders (ICDs).[6]

The significant nonmotor cognitive and behavior issues represent a major morbidity that remains poorly understood, unacknowledged, and largely unaddressed. Yet, they are a source of significant burden for the patients and caregivers, a major unmet need and challenge in PD.[7] Hence, it is critical that treating clinicians understand the issues, elicit the same in clinical interviews, and systematically evaluate to guide and refer patients and families for management.

COGNITIVE ISSUES

There is considerable variability in the presentation of cognitive impairment—type/number of domains affected, severity, and progression rate. There is a continuum of impairment ranging from PD-MCI in the early stages to PD-dementia (PD-D) in the advanced stages. However, not all with PD-MCI convert to PD-D, some remain stable with MCI and some revert to normal.[8]

Underlying the varied presentation is a complex factors making it difficult to delineate a single cognitive phenotype. Autopsy studies typically show cortical-limbic degeneration and deposition of Lewy bodies and neurites whose core constituent is abnormal α-synuclein. However, basal ganglia pathology and Alzheimer's disease-related amyloid beta (Aβ) pathology may also coexist. Cardiovascular disease adds a vascular cognitive burden and multiple neurotransmitters deficiencies (dopaminergic plus cholinergic, serotonergic, and noradrenergic) has also been found. Finally, other nonmotor symptoms [rapid eye movement (REM) sleep disorders and mood issues] also impact cognition.[9]

Cognitive Phenotype

Cognitive evaluations identified mainly nonamnestic domains and a primary executive dysfunction, frontal-striatal phenotype in early phase of disease was suggested wherein dopamine depletion affected dopaminergic inputs to the frontal lobe. This phenotype was unlikely to progress to dementia. The dual syndrome hypothesis postulated an additional visual spatial and semantic fluency dysfunction, the posterior cortical phenotype, wherein cholinergic deficits and Lewy bodies increased likelihood of progressing to dementia.[10] Currently, the focus is on understanding the progression continuum from PD-MCI to PD-D. MCI, an intermediate stage between normal aging and dementia-related changes explains MCIs found on objective testing that do not interfere with activities of daily living, but can progress to a dementia in a subset of patients. PD-MCI is a recent construct with a more heterogeneous presentation. It is in the foreground of research as with advancements in disease modifying drugs, it may be useful to diagnose and intervene early to delay or prevent progression. An early diagnosis also facilitates counseling and rehabilitation planning.[11] In a large subset of patients with advancing illness, the cognitive impairment gradually progresses to involve more domains, interfering with activities of daily life and developing into PD-D.

COGNITIVE ASSESSMENT

Clinical History

The first level of evaluation is eliciting or recognizing cognitive issues presented as subjective cognitive complaints (SCC) by the patient and family. Certain key domains are affected and frequently reported as SCC (**Table 1**).

Cognitive Testing

There are a number of standardized assessment tools available but in PD the tools have to be carefully selected for the following reasons:

- In elderly PD patients, the reported cognitive complaints may be due to normal aging. It is critical that the cognitive tests have stringent age/education, culture specific, normative data, or well-defined impairment cutoff scores to interpret test performance as normal aging or impairment.
- The predominant motor symptoms are confounders. Cognitive tests that have manual dexterity and a speed component may not assess the true cognitive ability as the scores reflect the compromised motor ability. Important to select relatively "motor-free" tasks.
- Nonmotor symptoms (depression, apathy, sleep issues, and fatigue) may interfere with ability to perform adequately on the cognitive tests. Understanding the impact of nonmotor symptoms on ability to perform on tests for the interpretation of test results.

The Movement Disorder Society (MDS) Task Force in 2007 and 2012 has published clinical criteria, recommendations for testing, descriptors, and cutoff score criteria.[12,13] Test batteries include global cognitive screens/scales and tests assessing five domains (attention and working memory, executive function, memory, language, and visual spatial). Two levels of testing with different criteria are recommended. Level I is a brief test battery, easily administered by clinicians, but has less diagnostic certainty. Level II is a comprehensive battery recommended for characterizing the disorder and use in research settings. However, it is time/expertise intensive and should be administered and interpreted by trained professionals with understanding of neuropsychology (**Table 2**).

Diagnosis Criteria

Movement Disorder Society Criteria for Parkinson's Disease-Mild Cognitive Impairment Diagnosis[13]

- **Clinical Criteria:**
    - Established PD diagnosis based on United Kingdom PD Brain Bank criteria
    - Subjective report of gradual cognitive decline by the patient, relatives, or observed by clinician
    - Decreased scores on objective neuropsychological testing as compared to age and education normative/control data

TABLE 1: Cognitive domains and subjective complaints.

Cognitive domain	*Domain descriptor*	*Subjective cognitive complaints (SCC)*
Attention:		
• Focused attention	Selective focus and ignoring other competing stimuli	Distracted and needs repeated instructions
• Sustained attention	Attending to a task for a longtime.	Short attention span and poor concentration
Working memory	Temporary storage and information manipulation	Difficulty with multitasking
Executive function	Initiating, planning, organizing, problem solving, and goal setting	Difficulties starting a task, organizing and planning the day, executing activities, and solving complex problems. Needs prompt and cues
Memory	Learning and recalling	Difficulty recalling events, names, appointments, messages, etc. Recall improves if cues or choices are provided
Language	Naming objects, generating words, and comprehending	Difficulty finding the right words, forming thoughts, communicating, and following complex conversations
Visual spatial	Estimating distances, depth, and finding routes	Difficulty parking a car and finding places

TABLE 2: Examples of cognitive tests.[#14,15]

Cognitive domains	*Screens/Scales/Tests*
Global cognitive screens	• Mini-Mental State Examination (MMSE)[16*] • Mattis Dementia Rating Scale (MDRS)[17**] • Montreal Cognitive Assessment (MoCA)[18] • Addenbrooke Cognitive Examination-III (ACE III)[19]
Parkinson's disease specific global cognitive scales	• Scales for Outcomes in Parkinson Disease-Cognition (SCOPA-COG)[20] • Parkinson Disease-Cognitive Rating Scale (PD-CRS)[21] • Mini-Mental Parkinson (MMP)[22] • Parkinson's Disease Dementia-Short Screen (PDD-SS)[23]
Attention and working memory	• Serial subtraction[16*] (MMSE) • Months reversed* • Letter number sequencing and coding** [Wechsler Adult Intelligence Scale (WAIS-IV)] • Digit span** • Stroop test**
Executive function: • Verbal fluency • Concept formation • Cognitive flexibility/ Set shifting • Planning/Problem solving	• Phonemic/Lexical fluency* • Similarities** • Wisconsin Card Sorting Test ** • Trails B** • Tower of London**
Memory	• Three Word Recall[16*] (MMSE) • Auditory Verbal Learning Test (AVLT)** • (Free recall and cued recall) • Prose Recall Test**
Visual spatial	• Copy overlapping pentagons[16*] (MMSE) • Clock Copy** • Judgment of Line Orientation Test ** • Cube analysis, fragmented letters, VOSP tests**
Language	Boston Naming Test **

#Details in References 14 and 15.

*Movement Disorder Society (MDS) Task Force Recommendation for Level I Evaluation.

**MDS Task Force Recommendation for Level II Evaluation.

- ○ Cognitive issues not significant enough to interfere with simple daily life activities, but may mildly compromise complex activities.
- ○ Cognitive changes are not due to other factors (metabolic, head injury, stroke, medications, etc.) or other nonmotor comorbidities (depression, fatigue, sleep disorders, etc.)
- **Test Criteria (Table 3)**

TABLE 3: Test impairment criteria.*

	Level I	*Level II*
Global cognitive ability	Impairment on global cognitive screens OR	
Five domains test battery: (Working memory, attention, executive function, memory, and visual spatial)	Impairment in at least two tests on the limited battery that has <2 tests per domain or <5 domains assessed	Impairment in at least two tests (same domain or one in each domain) on a comprehensive battery with two tests in each domain and all five domains assessed

*Impairment is defined as test performance 1–2 standard deviation (SD) below appropriate norms/significant decline in serial testing/ significant decline as compared to premorbid level of functioning.

The level II comprehensive battery is recommended for subtype classification:

- Parkinson's disease-MCI single domain: Impairments in two tests of a single-specified domain.
- Parkinson's disease-MCI multiple domain: Impairments in at least one test in two or more specified domains. The classification is further elaborated as:
- Amnestic MCI single domain (aMCIsd): Two memory tests impaired and all other domains unimpaired.
- Nonamnestic MCI single domain (naMCIsd): Two tests impaired in any one domain other than the memory domain.
- Amnestic MCI multiple domain (aMCImd): At least one test impaired in the memory domain and one test in any other domain.
- Nonamnestic MCI multiple domain (naMCImd): Two tests impaired in two different domains other than the memory domain.

Multiple domain subtypes, amnestic and nonamnestic, are more likely to convert to PD-D in the long-term. A higher rate of about 50% converting to dementia is estimated when the more stringent 2 standard deviation (SD) impairment criteria is used to diagnose PD-MCI at baseline.[24]

Movement Disorder Society Criteria for Parkinson's Disease—Dementia Diagnosis[25]

- Clinical criteria:
  - ○ The symptoms must occur within an established PD diagnosis. There is an overlap between pathological and clinical features of PD-D and Lewy

body dementia (LBD) and both are regarded as two entities of the same spectrum of Lewy body disease. For the purposes of clinical diagnosis and management, the two are distinguished by the time point of symptom appearance. When dementia symptoms appear after the onset of motor symptoms or in the context of an established PD diagnosis, it is diagnosed as PD-D; but if the dementia symptoms appear prior to or in 1 year of the motor symptoms, the diagnosis of LBD is considered.
    - In PD-D the cognitive impairment interferes with daily life functioning, over and above those imposed by motor problems.
- Test criteria: Impairment in at least two out of the four core cognitive domains (attention, executive function, memory, and visual spatial function) with relatively preserved core language functions and the most common impairment being in the executive function.

BEHAVIORAL ISSUES

People with PD are vulnerable for developing mood and behavior issues due to multiple factors:[26] (1) Complex pathophysiology of the illness and multiple neurotransmitter deficiencies; (2) Medication related-side effects of dopaminergic agents; (3) Deep brain stimulation (DBS)-related effects; and (4) Psychosocial burden of living with a chronic, progressive, and incurable illness (**Flowchart 1**).

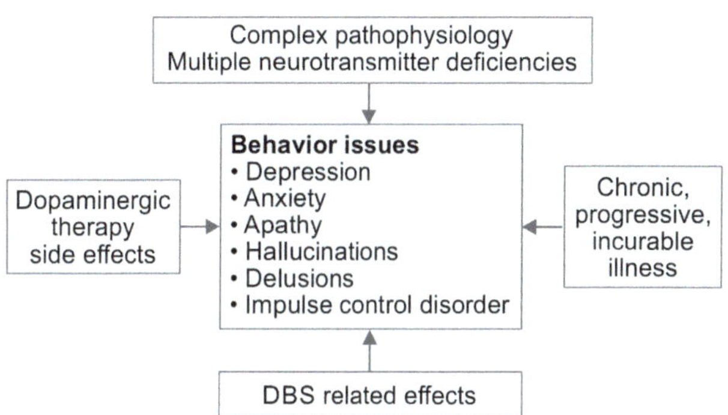

(DBS: deep brain stimulation)

FLOWCHART 1: Complex pathophysiology: Multiple neurotransmitter deficiencies.

Types of Disorders[26]

Depression and Anxiety

Mood issues are common and a number of scales are used to evaluate depression and anxiety in PD. However, there are certain PD specific challenges that result in misinterpretation of scores and confound the diagnosis of depression:

- Overlap of certain PD symptoms (fatigue, sleep disturbances, loss of appetite, decreased attention/concentration, and psychomotor slowing) with symptoms of depression. Somatic symptoms associated with depression are commonly seen in PD even when there is no depression.
- Apathy in PD results in decreased interest and participation. This mimics symptom of lack of pleasure (anhedonia) seen in depression.
- In PD-D, cognitive impairments result in slowing and decreased participation also seen in depression.
- Perception of low mood depends on whether the patient is in the "ON" or "OFF" period. In the challenging "OFF" phase there is a greater tendency to report mood issues and evaluation of mood should be in the "ON" period.

Hence, at times, scores on the depression scale may be high even in the absence of depression. It is important that in such situations, the diagnosis is based on an expert clinical interview using diagnostic and statistical manual of mental disorders (DSM) criteria.

Apathy[27]

Apathy is a core symptom in PD, seen in up to 40% of the patients. The key symptom is loss of motivation and also lack of goal directed behaviors, loss of interest, indifference, decreased participation, poor initiation, and emotional blunting resulting in decreased social interactions. There is overlap of symptoms with features of depression and cognitive decline. The pathophysiology is the core dysfunction of PD involving the limbic dopaminergic system and the frontal subcortical pathways. Apathy also occurs when there is dopamine agonists withdrawal symptoms (DAWS) and after DBS with dopamine agonists (DA) reduction.

Psychosis in Parkinson's Disease

The most common features of psychosis are illusions (misperception of actual objects), delusions (fixed, false beliefs), and hallucinations (sensory experience in absence of external stimuli). Historically, these symptoms became more prevalent after the advent of L-DOPA and DA treatments, as drug induced psychiatric states.[28] The most common are the vivid, visual hallucinations involving persons, objects, or animals.[29] In the early stages there may be preserved insight and hallucinations are nonthreatening and may not perturb the patient. When benign they do not need treatment and patients develop coping strategies. However, in later stages, there may be loss of insight causing significant distress. The malignant and psychotic hallucinations are treated with atypical antipsychotics and identified risk factors are advanced disease, older age, cognitive impairments, and depression.[30] Delusions are less common but are extremely distressing for the patients and caregivers and often center on themes of paranoid suspiciousness about spouse infidelity referred to as Othello syndrome.[31]

Impulse Control Disorders

"Impulse control and related disorders (ICDs-RD) encompass a heterogeneous group of disorders that involve pleasurable behaviors performed repetitively, excessively, and compulsively."[32]

Patients feel an uncontrollable urge, inability to resist temptation, sense of reward, and no concerns of negative consequences or potential harm to self and family. The behaviors impact personal and professional life and are a source of considerable stress to the family. The main types of ICDs are pathological gambling, hypersexual disorders, binge eating, and compulsive buying. Other related disorders include perseveration/repetition of certain odd behaviors—punding (repetitive purposeless behaviors), hobbyism (repetitive participation in sports and arts), walkabout (excessive aimless walking), hoarding (storing and unwilling to discard), and dopamine dysregulation syndrome (DDS) (compulsive and excessive medication use). Dysregulation of the mesocorticolimbic reward pathways is hypothesized as the underlying pathology. However, a significant association between use of DA and presence of ICDs has been observed. DAs have a preferential affinity for the D2 and D3 dopamine receptors in the limbic and ventral striatum regions involved in the reward pathways and "overstimulation" due to DAs may result in increase in impulsivity and ICDs.[32]

ASSESSMENT OF BEHAVIOR DISORDERS

Several scales and questionnaires have been developed to evaluate behavior issues in PD but the consensus is that most of the scales are not optimal. It is important to understand that these scales are not diagnostic instruments and were primarily created for detection and measuring severity of a symptom. The gold standard for evaluation of behavior issues remains an in-depth, expert structured interview that uses established clinical criteria (DSM). However, since the issues in PD remain poorly understood and often unreported it is important that the clinician detects their presence using the instruments and then refers to an expert for diagnosis and management. Several scales have been critically examined by the MDS Rating Scale Task Force, American Academy of Neurology (AAN), and National Institutes of Health (NIH) expert groups. Their recommendations and other commonly used scales are tabled below (**Table 4**).[33-35]

TABLE 4: Examples of Mood and Behavior Scales.

Behavior issues	*Recommended screening scales*
Mood • Depression[36]	• Hamilton Rating Scale for Depression (HAM-D), • Beck Depression Inventory (BDI) • Montgomery–Asberg Depression Rating Scale (MADRS) • Hospital Anxiety and Depression Scale (HADS) • Geriatric Depression Scale (GDS) • Zung Self-Rating Depression Scale (SDS) • Cornell Scale for Depression in Dementia (CSDD)
Mood • Anxiety[37]	• Beck Anxiety Inventory (BAI) • Hospital Anxiety and Depression Scale—Subscale Anxiety • Hamilton Anxiety Rating Scale (HARS) • Parkinson Anxiety Scale (PAS)
Apathy[38]	• Apathy Scale (AS) • Lille Apathy Rating Scale (LARS)
Psychosis[39] • Hallucinations/ Delusions	• Neuropsychiatric Inventory (NPI) • Brief Psychiatric Rating Scale (BPRS) • Positive and Negative Syndrome Scale (PANSS) for Schizophrenia (PANSS) • Scale for the Assessment of Positive Symptoms • Parkinson Psychosis Questionnaire (PPQ) • Scale for Evaluation of Neuropsychiatric Disorders in Parkinson's disease (SEND-PD) • Rush Hallucination Inventory
Impulse control disorders[40]	• Questionnaire for Impulsive-Compulsive Disorders in Parkinson's Disease (QUIP) • Parkinson's Disease-Rating Scale (QUIP-RS) • Ardouin Scale of Behavior in Parkinson's Disease (ASBPD) • Impulse Control Disorders and Related Conditions Questionnaire (ICDRC)

EVALUATION IN INDIA

Evaluating cognition and behavior in India is challenging due to significant cultural, education, and socioeconomic diversity but some tests with Indian normative data are now available.[41] However, in several Indian PD studies, either level I screening tools [Mini-Mental State Examination (MMSE)] or Parkinson's disease specific cognitive scales Scales for Outcomes in Parkinson Disease-Cognition (SCOPA-COG)] have been used. Level II comprehensive neuropsychological evaluations are rare and across studies there is no uniformity in type of tools, norms, or scoring criteria used (**Table 5**). MMSE that is frequently used does not have a test for executive function and is of limited value in PD. For behavior

TABLE 5: Cognitive assessment–Indian Studies.

Indian Studies (Cognitive evaluation and results)	Test protocol	Score analysis (Scores comparison with normative data/ cutoff scores/normal control data/other patient data)
Krishnan et al., 2006[42]	• Addenbrooke Cognitive Examination • Wisconsin Card Sorting Test • Trail Making Test A and B	Indian Normative Data (Score comparison between three diseases patient groups)
Singh and Behari, 2006[43]	• Hindi Mini-Mental State Examination • Verbal memory: ○ Rey Auditory Verbal Learning Test Visual memory: ○ Benton Visual Retention Test ○ Form Sequence Learning	• Cutoff Score • Control "other" patient group
Adhikari et al., 2012[44]	Kolkata Cognitive Screening Battery	Indian Normative Data
Sanyal et al., 2014[45]	Mini-Mental State Examination: • 15 item Boston Naming Test • SCOPA-COG • Memory Word List • Construction Praxis	Healthy and Normal Control Group (NC)
Das et al., 2016[46]	Mini-Mental State Examination: • SCOPA-COG	Comparison of scores between: • Young versus late-onset • Tremor versus postural instability and gait disorder (PIGD) • Mild versus moderate motor impairment
Pal et al., 2018[47]	• Mini-Mental State Examination • Domain Specific Assessment ○ *Memory*: Word and Picture Recall Computerized tests ○ *Executive function*: Stroop Test ○ *Attention*: Digit Span Forward Test ○ *Psychomotor speed*: Trail Making A ○ *Visuospatial*: Trail Making B ○ *Language*: Sentence Repetition	Healthy and Normal Control Group
Chaudhary et al., 2018[48]	SCOPA-COG	Comparison of scores between "young versus late-onset groups"

(SCOPA-COG: Scales for Outcomes in Parkinson Disease-Cognition)

evaluations as well, a wide variety of scales has been used (**Table 6**). Scales may be self-answered, informant, or observer rated and should be selected based on patient education level, reliability of informant, or observer expertise. There are no national guidelines for selecting the evaluation tools suited for our population and it is important that a Task Force be commissioned to create India specific protocols.

SUMMARY

Cognitive and behavior issues in PD are now occupying center stage in PD research due to the growing recognition that these nonmotor issues significantly impact quality of life and are a major burden for caregivers. The cognitive progression continuum from MCI to dementia underscores the need for early identification and intervention. The realization of the complex relationship between PD dopaminergic medications and neuropsychiatric symptoms underlines the need to identify the problems early and modify any medication related issues. A number of PD specific tools and criteria have been developed but there is considerable heterogeneity in tests used across centers. There is a need to create a uniform, India specific protocol for valid and reliable evaluation of cognitive and behavioral problems in PD.

TABLE 6: Neuropsychiatric assessment in Indian studies.

Studies	*Scales*
Harbishettar V et al., 2005[49]	• Mini-International Neuropsychiatric Interview (MINI) • Y-BOCS Symptom Checklist
Singh and Behari, 2006[43]	Hamilton Depression Rating Scale (HAM-D)
Sarathchandran P et al., 2013[50]	• Minnesota Impulsive Disorder Interview • Barratt Impulsivity Scale • Eysenck Personality Inventory • Beck Depression Inventory (BDI) • Hospital Anxiety and Depression Scale
Amar BR et al., 2014[51]	Neuropsychiatric Inventory (NPI)
Sanyal et al., 2014[45]	Montgomery–Asberg Depression Rating Scale (MADRS)
Rai et al., 2015[52]	• Mini-International Neuropsychiatric Interview (MINI) • Beck's Depression Inventory (BDI), • Brief Psychiatric Rating Scale (BPRS), • Hamilton Rating Scale for Anxiety (HAM-A),
Das et al., 2016[46]	• SCOPA-Psychiatric Complications (SCOPA-PC) • Beck's Depression Inventory (BDI) (Bengali translation)

(SCOPA: Scales for Outcomes in Parkinson Disease-Cognition)

REFERENCES

1. Parkinson J. An Essay on the Shaking Palsy: 1817. J Neuropsychiatry Clin Neurosci. 2002;14(2):223-36.
2. Walusinski O. Jean-Martin Charcot and Parkinson's disease: Teaching and teaching materials. Rev Neurol (Paris). 2018;174(7-8):491-505.
3. Lees AJ, Smith E. Cognitive deficits in the early stages of Parkinson's disease. Brain. 1983;106(2):257-70.
4. Sollinger AB, Goldstein FC, Lah JJ, Levey AI, Factor SA. Mild cognitive impairment in Parkinson's disease: subtypes and motor characteristics. Parkinsonism Relat Disord. 2010;16(3): 177-80.
5. Hely MA, Reid WG, Adena MA, Halliday GM, Morris JG. The Sydney multicenter study of Parkinson's disease: the inevitability of dementia at 20 years. Mov Disord. 2008;23(6):837-44.
6. Anderson KE. Behavioral disturbances in Parkinson's disease. Dialogues Clin Neurosci. 2004;6(3):323-32.
7. Goldman JG, Vernaleo BA, Camicioli R, Dahodwala N, Dobkin RD, Ellis T, et al. Cognitive impairment in Parkinson's disease: a report from a multidisciplinary symposium on unmet needs and future directions to maintain cognitive health. NPJ Parkinsons Dis. 2018;4:19.
8. Weil RS, Costantini AA, Schrag AE. Mild Cognitive Impairment in Parkinson's Disease—What Is It? Curr Neurol Neurosci Rep. 2018;18(4):17.
9. Halliday GM, Leverenz JB, Schneider JS, Adler CH. The neurobiological basis of cognitive impairment in Parkinson's disease. Mov Disord. 2014;29(5):634-50.
10. Williams-Gray CH, Evans JR, Goris A, Foltynie T, Ban M, Robbins TW, et al. The distinct cognitive syndromes of Parkinson's disease: 5 year follow-up of the CamPaIGN Cohort. Brain. 2009;132(11):2958-69.
11. Weil RS, Costantini AA, Schrag AE. Mild Cognitive Impairment in Parkinson's Disease-What Is It? Curr Neurol Neurosci Rep. 2018;18(4):17.
12. Dubois B, Burn D, Goetz C, Aarsland D, Brown RG, Broe GA, et al. Diagnostic procedures for Parkinson's disease dementia: recommendations from the movement disorder society task force. Mov Disord. 2007;22(16):2314-24.
13. Litvan I, Goldman JG, Tröster AI, Schmand BA, Weintraub D, Petersen RC, et al. Diagnostic Criteria for Mild Cognitive Impairment in Parkinson's Disease: Movement Disorder Society Task Force Guidelines. Mov Disord. 2012;27(3):349-56.
14. Lezak MD, Howieson DB, Loring DW. Neuropsychological Assessment. New York: Oxford University Press; 2004.
15. Kulisevsky J, Pagonabarraga J. Cognitive impairment in Parkinson's disease: tools for diagnosis and assessment. Mov Disord. 2009;24(8):1103-10.
16. Folstein MF, Folstein SE, McHugh PR. "Mini-mental state". A practical method for grading the cognitive state of patients for the clinician. J Psychiatr Res. 1975;12(3):189-98.
17. Mattis S. Dementia Rating Scale: Professional manual. Psychological Assessment Resources; 1988.
18. Gill DJ, Freshman A, Blender JA, Ravina B. The Montreal cognitive assessment as a screening tool for cognitive impairment in Parkinson's disease. Mov Disord. 2008;23(7):1043-6.
19. Reyes MA, Perez-Lloret S, Roldan Gerschcovich R, Martin ME, Leiguarda R, Merello M. Addenbrooke's Cognitive Examination validation in Parkinson's disease. Eur J Neurol. 2009;16(1): 142-7.
20. Marinus J, Visser M, Verwey NA, Verhey FRJ, Middelkoop HAM, Stiggelbout AM, et al. Assessment of cognition in Parkinson's disease. Neurology. 2003;61(9):1222-8.

21. Pagonabarraga J, Kulisevsky J, Llebaria G, Garcia-Sanchez C, Pascual-Sedano B, Gironell A. Parkinson's disease-cognitive rating scale: A new cognitive scale specific for Parkinson's disease. Mov Disord. 2008;23(7):998-1005.
22. Mahieux F, Michelet D, Manifacier MJ, Boller F, Fermanian J, Guillard G. Mini-Mental Parkinson: first validation study of a new bedside test constructed for Parkinson's disease. Behav Neurology. 1995;8(1):15-22.
23. Pagonabarraga J, Kulisevsky J, Llebaria G, Garcia-Sanchez C, Pascual-Sedano B, Martinez-Corral M, et al. PDD-Short Screen: A brief cognitive test for screening dementia in Parkinson's disease. Mov Disord. 2010;25(4):440-6.
24. Hoogland J, Boel JA, de Bie RMA, Geskus RB, Schmand BA, Dalrymple-Alford JC, et al. Mild cognitive impairment as a risk factor for Parkinson's disease dementia. Mov Disord. 2017;32(7):1056-65.
25. Emre M, Aarsland D, Brown R, Burn DJ, Duyckaerts C, Mizuno Y, et al. Clinical Diagnostic Criteria for Dementia Associated with Parkinson's Disease. Mov Disord. 2007;22(12):1689-707.
26. Anderson KE. Behavioral disturbances in Parkinson's disease. Dialogues Clin Neurosci. 2004;6(3):323-32.
27. Dujardin K, Sockeel P, Devos D, Delliaux M, Krystkowiak P, Destée A, et al. Characteristics of apathy in Parkinson's disease. Mov Disord. 2007;22(6):778-84.
28. Factor SA, Molho ES, Podskalny GD, Brown D. Parkinson's disease: drug-induced psychiatric states. Adv Neurol. 1995;65:115-38.
29. Holroyd S, Currie L, Wooten GF. Prospective study of hallucinations and delusions in Parkinson's disease. J Neurol Neurosurg Psychiatry. 2001;70(6):734-8.
30. Aarsland D, Larsen JP, Cummins JL, Laake K. Prevalence and clinical correlates of psychotic symptoms in Parkinson's disease: a community-based study. Arch Neurol. 1999;56(5):595-601.
31. Graff-Radford J, Ahlskog JE, Bower JH, Josephs KA. Dopamine agonists and Othello's syndrome. Parkinsonism Relat Disord. 2010;16(10):680-2.
32. Gatto EM and Aldinio V. Impulse Control Disorders in Parkinson's Disease. A Brief and Comprehensive Review. Front. Neurol. 2019;10:351.
33. Ravina B, Marder K, Fernandez HH, Friedman JH, McDonald W, Murphy D, et al. Diagnostic criteria for psychosis in Parkinson's disease: report of an NINDS, NIMH work group. Mov Disord. 2007;22(8):1061-8.
34. Fernandez HH, Aarsland D, Fenelon G, Friedman JH, Marsh L, Troster AI, et al. Scales to Assess Psychosis in Parkinson's Disease: Critique and Recommendations. Mov Disord. 2008;23(4):484-500.
35. Martinez-Martin P, Leentjens AF, de Pedro-Cuesta J, Chaudhuri KR, Schrag AE, Weintraub D. Accuracy of Screening Instruments for Detection of Neuropsychiatric Syndromes in Parkinson's Disease. Mov Disord. 2016;31(3):270-9.
36. Schrag A, Barone P, Brown RG, Leentjens AF, McDonald WM, Starkstein S, et al. Depression rating scales in Parkinson's disease: critique and recommendations. Mov Disord. 2007;22(8):1077-92.
37. Leentjens AF, Dujardin K, Marsh L, Martinez-Martin P, Richard IH, Starkstein SE, et al. Anxiety rating scales in Parkinson's disease: critique and recommendations. Mov Disord. 2008;23 (14):2015-25.
38. Leentjens AF, Dujardin K, Marsh L, Martinez-Martin P, Richard IH, Starkstein SE, et al. Apathy and anhedonia rating scales in Parkinson's disease: critique and recommendations. Mov Disord. 2008;23(14):2004-14.
39. Miyasaki JM, Shannon K, Voon V, Ravina B, Kleiner-Fisman G, Anderson K, et al. Practice parameter: evaluation and treatment of depression, psychosis, and dementia in Parkinson disease (an evidence-based review): report of the Quality Standards Subcommittee of the American Academy of Neurology. Neurology. 2006;66(7):996-1002.
40. Izzo VA, Donati MA, Ramat S, Primi C. Impulse control disorders in Parkinson's disease: A systematic review on the psychometric properties of the existing measures. PLoS One. 2019;14(6):e0217700.
41. Porrselvi AP, Shankar V. Status of Cognitive Testing of Adults of India. Ann Indian Acad Neurol. 2017;20(4):334-40.
42. Krishnan S, Mathuranath PS, Sarma S, Kishore A. Neuropsychological functions in progressive supranuclear palsy, multiple system atrophy and Parkinson's disease. Neurol India. 2006;54(3):268-72.
43. Singh S, Behari M. Verbal and visual memory in patients with early Parkinson's disease: effect of levodopa. Neurol India. 2006;54(1):33-7.
44. Adhikari S, Basu J, Das SK, Misra AK. Effects of age, stage of disease, and educational level on cognitive dysfunction in non-demented idiopathic Parkinsonism: A preliminary report. Ind Psychiatry J. 2012;21(1):32-8.
45. Sanyal J, Banerjee TK, Rao VR. Dementia and cognitive impairment in patients with Parkinson's disease from India: a 7-year prospective study. Am J Alzheimers Dis Other Demen. 2014;29(7):630-6.
46. Das D, Biswas A, Roy A, Sauerbier A, Bhattacharyya KB. Cognitive impairment in idiopathic Parkinson's disease. Neurol India. 2016;64(3):419-27.
47. Pal A, Pegwal N, Kaur S, Mehta N, Behari M, Sharma R. Deficit in specific cognitive domains associated with dementia in Parkinson's disease. J Clin Neurosci. 2018;57:116-20.
48. Chaudhary S, Joshi D, Pathak A, Mishra VN, Chaurasia R, Gupta G. Comparison of Cognitive Profile in Young-and Late-onset Parkinson's Disease Patients. Ann Indian Acad Neurol. 2018;21(2):130-2.
49. Harbishettar V, Pal PK, Reddy YC, Thennarasu K. Is there a relationship between Parkinson's disease and obsessive-compulsive disorder? Parkinsonism Relat Disord. 2005;11(2): 85-8.
50. Sarathchandran P, Soman S, Sarma G, Krishnan S, Kishore A. Impulse control disorders and related behaviors in Indian patients with Parkinson's disease. Mov Disord. 2013;28(13):1901-2
51. Amar BR, Yadav R, Reddy YC, Pal PK. A clinical profile of patients with Parkinson's disease and psychosis. Ann Indian Acad Neurol. 2014;17(2):187-92.
52. Rai NK, Goyal V, Kumar N, Shukla G, Srivastava AK, Singh S, et al. Neuropsychiatric co-morbidities in non-demented Parkinson's disease. Ann Indian Acad Neurol. 2015;18(1):33-8.

CHAPTER 18

Rating Scales in Movement Disorders

Rukmini Mridula Kandadai, Swetha Reddy Tandra, Suryaprabha Turaga, Rupam Borgohain

INTRODUCTION

Scales are essential in any disease to objectively quantify the illness, disability, handicap, and its impact on patient's lifestyle. They should be universally applicable and should be sensitive to pick minor changes in the course of disease. In the field of movement disorders also, scales are essential to clearly define the presence and severity of various aspects of the disease and to study their impact on quality of life. Additionally, the use of scales has also become a part of the diagnostic criteria of certain disorders. Few commonly used scales in Parkinsonian disorders, tremors, dystonia, and ataxia are discussed below.

PARKINSONIAN DISORDERS

Parkinson's Disease

Parkinson's disease (PD) is the prototype of hypokinetic movement disorders and is characterized by a constellation of motor and nonmotor symptoms (NMS). The disease is heterogeneous in its manifestations and thus it becomes important to define and categorize all aspects of the disease to get an overall picture of the impairment of the individual patient. Unified scales as well as scales for individual aspects have been made and each has its own strengths and lacunae. Scales concentrating on motor symptoms are discussed first followed by scales for NMS.

Motor Symptoms

Hoehn and Yahr Scale (Table 1)

It is an easy and commonly used system for describing the progression of motor symptoms of PD. Originally formulated by Melvin Yahr and Margaret Hoehn in 1967, it had stages 1 through 5. In the 1990s, a modified Hoehn and Yahr scale was proposed with the addition of stages 1.5 and 2.5 to help describe the intermediate course of the disease.[1]

H and Y scale is the most commonly and widely used scale in assessing PD. The ease of application, short time it takes to complete and the overview of motor and functional disability it envisions, makes it practical for research and patient care. The scale has been used in assessing natural history of disease and the impact

TABLE 1: Hoehn and Yahr scale.

Stage	*Hoehn and Yahr scale*	*Modified Hoehn and Yahr scale*
1	Unilateral involvement only usually with minimal or no functional disability	Unilateral involvement only
1.5		Unilateral and axial involvement
2	Bilateral or midline involvement without impairment of balance	Bilateral involvement without impairment of balance
2.5		Mild bilateral disease without recovery on pull test
3	Bilateral disease: Mild-to-moderate disability with impaired postural reflexes and physically independent	Mild-to-moderate bilateral disease; some postural instability; and physically independent
4	Severely disabling disease and still able to walk or stand unassisted	Severe disability and still able to walk or stand unassisted
5	Confinement to bed or wheelchair unless aided	Wheelchair bound or bedridden unless aided

of levodopa. The conversion from stage 2 to stage 3 denotes the start of progressive impairment in cognition, motor disability, lesser response to drugs, and overall poorer outcome. Clinimetric assessment has shown the scale to have validity and reliability at least in the midranges.[1]

The scale is limited however by its basis only on motor symptoms, non-linearity in describing progression, and its mixing of impairment and disability. The scale in research settings is useful primarily for defining inclusion/exclusion criteria.

Unified Parkinson's Disease Rating Scale

The Unified Parkinson's Disease Rating Scale (UPDRS) was developed in 1987 as an effort to incorporate elements from then existing scales to provide a comprehensive but efficient and flexible means to monitor PD-related disability and impairment. This consists of four parts—part I: mentation, behavior, and mood; part II: activities of daily living; part III: motor; part IV: complications of treatment. Overall the time taken to administer the scale is around 15–30 minutes and can be shortened if part I and part II are filled in by the patient themselves.[2]

This scale is easy to use and widely utilized. It has been relied on, for various drugs and surgical therapies trials and the US and European regulatory agencies rely on it for new drug approvals. It has also been used for assessing the Parkinsonian features of other diseases such as progressive supranuclear palsy (PSP) and diffuse Lewy body disease (DLBD). The score has been shown to increase with disease progression (part III ~7 points/year) and is responsive to therapeutic intervention. Within the scale, part II which measures the activities of daily living correlates with part III of the scale measuring motor impairment. But the scale has its limitations. Part I can be used only as a screening assessment of mood, behavior, and cognition and cannot effectively determine the amount of impairment. Some of nonmotor aspects such as bradyphrenia, anxiety, sleep disorders, dysautonomia, and fatigue cannot be assessed using UPDRS. There is no clear demarcation in the UPDRS scores which can identify overall mild, moderate, and severe disease. The scores in the UPDRS are not uniform with yes/no questions on motor fluctuations and complications of therapy and others with range of severity. The options are more structured toward moderate and severe disease and may be less sensitive for evaluating progress and drug responses in early disease.[2]

Movement Disorder Society-Unified Parkinson's Disease Rating Scale

A task force was sponsored in 2001 to critique the UPDRS and they modified the existing scale to form Movement Disorder Society-UPDRS.[2] This scale has a uniform rating of all parameters assessed into slight, mild, moderate, and severe. Although it has four parts similar to UPDRS, the part I—(nonmotor aspects of experiences of daily living) deals with more aspects of NMS and has incorporated assessment of anxiety, sleep disorders, constipation, urinary disturbances, and fatigue as well as dopamine dysregulation syndrome. Similarly, few additions have been made in other parts of the scale. Part I and part II can be filled by the patients themselves or by their attendants. The part III has been modified to add certain aspects such as toe tapping and freezing of gait. The tremor is classified better and the scale systematically categorizes the tremor using its amplitude as an objective measure. The scale has been translated and validated into various languages for use in different parts of the world.[2]

Dyskinesias

While the part IV of UPDRS deals with dopa induced dyskinesias, it is a poor scale for objective quantification of dyskinesias. The Rush Dyskinesias Rating Scale and the Abnormal Involuntary Movement Scales (AIMS) are more reliable scales, and the recently developed scales Parkinson Disease Dyskinesia Scale (PDYS-26), and the Unified Dyskinesia Rating Scale (UDysRS) have excellent clinimetric properties and appear to provide a reliable and valid assessment tool of dyskinesia in PD.[3]

Nonmotor Symptoms

Nonmotor symptoms are not covered well under UPDRS and require other scales to quantify them. NMS Quest and Nonmotor Symptoms Scale (NMSS) are two scales used to quantify the entire NMS as a whole.

Nonmotor symptoms Quest is a 30 items questionnaire which has yes/no answers.[4] This instrument does not provide an overall score of disability; instead, it is designed to draw attention to the presence of NMS and to prompt health professionals to initiate further investigation.

In contrast to the screening questionnaire, the NMSS is a 30 items scale divided into nine domains; cardiovascular, sleep/fatigue, mood/cognition, perceptual problems, attention/memory, gastrointestinal, urinary, sexual function, and miscellaneous.[5] Quantification of symptoms is based on a multiple of severity (0–3) and frequency scores (0–4).[5]

Scales have been made to assess individual NMS in detail, e.g., Scales for Outcomes of Parkinson's disease (SCOPA)-Cognition and Montreal Cognitive Assessment (MoCA) for cognition,[6] Hospital Anxiety and Depression Scale (HADS), Montgomery–Asberg Depression Rating Scale (MADRS) for depression,[7] Neuropsychiatric Inventory (NPI), SCOPA-Psychiatric Complications (SCOPA-PC) for psychosis,[8] Questionnaire for Impulsive-Compulsive Disorders (QUIP), and Rating Scale (QUIP-RS) for impulsive control disorders (ICD) and ICD-related behaviors,[9] SCOPA-autonomic symptoms (SCOPA-AUT) for overall assessment of autonomic disorders,[10]

SCOPA-sleep and Epworth Sleepiness Scale (ESS) for sleep.[11] King's Parkinson's Disease Pain Scale as well as King's Parkinson's Disease Pain Questionnaire are scales recently developed to comprehensively assess the type of pain, severity, and its impact on quality of life as well as its relationship to levodopa.[12,13] Individual scales have been used for assessing restless leg syndrome, olfactory loss, apathy, gastrointestinal, and sexual impairments in specific trials and studies.

Quality of Life

Individual scales can identify the presence or absence of certain aspects of PD but the impact on quality of life can be studied by scales such as PDQ-39, and Schwab and England activities of daily living scale.[14]

The Schwab and England activities of daily living scale is a 0–100% staging system, in which 100% stands for completely independent and 0% for a vegetative state.

The PDQ-39 is the most widely used PD specific measure of health status. It contains 39 questions, covering eight aspects of quality of life.[14] The instrument was developed on the basis of interviews with people diagnosed with the disease and has been widely validated. Each item scores from 0 (never) to 4 (always). Subscale scores and a summary index representing the global health-related quality of life (HRQoL) can be calculated, with higher scores representing worse HRQoL. The PDQ-39 has been shown to have good internal consistency and stability with satisfactory content validity. Other scales such as SCOPA-Psychosocial questionnaires (SCOPA-PS) have been found to be useful as a cross-cultural multiple language unified scale for quality of life assessment.[15]

Atypical Parkinsonian Diseases

Most atypical Parkinsonian patients are usually evaluated using UPDRS for assessing their motor functions and absence of response with levodopa on the scale is a strong pointer for diagnosis of atypical Parkinsonian syndromes.

Unified Multiple System Atrophy Rating Scale (UMSARS) was developed in 2004 and comprises of four subsections—part I: historical, 12 items; part II: motor examination, 14 items; part III: autonomic examination; and part IV: global disability scale.[16] The UMSARS has integrated assessment of Parkinsonian, cerebellar, and autonomic aspects and was found to have a high internal consistency and inter-rater reliability. The scale takes around 30–45 minutes to perform and is a good semiquantitative scale for use.

Progressive Supranuclear Palsy Rating Scale (PSPRS) was devised in 2007.[17] The scale has 28 items in six categories: Daily activities (by history), behavior, bulbar, ocular motor, limb motor, and gait/midline. Each item is either scored from 0 to 2 (six items) or 0 to 4 (22 items) with a maximum score of 100. Inter-rater reliability is good. Mean rate of progression is 11.3 (±11.0) points/year. The PSPRS score is a good independent predictor of subsequent survival and gait function.

The Natural History and Neuroprotection in Parkinson Plus Syndromes (NNIPPS)-Parkinson Plus Scale is a recent scale designed to study the disease progression in both disorders and studies 15 clinically relevant dimensions, including activity of daily living/mobility, axial bradykinesia, limb bradykinesia, rigidity, oculomotor, cerebellar, bulbar/pseudobulbar, mental, orthostatic, urinary, limb dystonia, axial dystonia, pyramidal, myoclonus, and tremor.[18] It has a good internal consistency, inter-rater reliability, and was found to be a sensitive tool to record change.

Assessment of corticobasal syndrome or DLBD is done by combining scales for movement disorders (UPDRS) and cognitive assessment.

TREMORS

Various scales have been used for assessing tremor severity in patients with essential tremor.

The Fahn-Tolosa-Marin Tremor Rating Scale (TRS) is a widely used clinical rating scale for tremor, rating severity of tremor by body part from 0 (none) to 4 (severe).[19] The scale is divided into three parts. Part A assesses examiner-reported tremor location/severity (amplitude); Part B assesses examiner-reported ability to perform specific motor tasks/functions (writing, drawing, and pouring with dominant and nondominant hands); and Part C assesses patient-reported functional disability resulting from the tremor (speaking, eating, drinking, hygiene, dressing, writing, working, and social activities).

In 1993, Bain et al., formulated a numerical (0–10) visual analog scale to rate postural and rest tremor of the limbs, voice, and head which correlated well with the impact of tremor on daily functions.[20]

The Washington Heights-Inwood Genetic Study of Essential Tremor (WHIGET) TRS,[21] revised in 2001 is a 23-item videotaped examination that assesses rest, postural, and kinetic tremor severity. Rated tasks include arm extension, pouring water between cups, drinking from a spoon, drinking from a cup, drawing Archimedes spirals, and touching a finger to the nose.

The Essential Tremor Rating Assessment Scale (TETRAS) is a recent scale developed by the tremor research group utilizing a half-point interval 0–4 scale. The scale measures the excursion of a body part due to tremor and is scored on specific amplitude measurements in cm. It has a good inter-rater and intra-rater reliability for head and upper extremity tremor.

Other measures include accelerometer-based assessments of tremor and quality of life assessment scale

QUEST (quality of life in essential tremor). QUEST is a brief, 30-item, and essential tremor specific QoL scale with excellent reliability and has five scales: Physical, psychosocial, communication, hobbies/leisure, and work/finance.[22]

DYSTONIA

The Burke-Fahn-Marsden Dystonia Rating Scale (BFMDRS) devised in 1985 is one of the first widely used scales to assess generalized dystonia patients. It has a motor part assessing dystonia and a part assessing the resulting disability. The motor subscale evaluates two clinical features of dystonia (severity and provoking factors) in eight body regions (eyes, mouth, neck, and the four limbs) and one functional area (speech and swallowing). Severity ranges from 0 (no dystonia) to 4 (severe dystonia). The provoking factors assess the situation under which dystonia occurs and range from 0 (no dystonia) to 4 (dystonia at rest). These two features, severity and provoking factors, are multiplied and then scores are summed, except for the eyes, mouth, and neck which are halved before summing. The resulting maximum total score on the BFM severity is 120. The BFMDRS section on disability assesses the effects of dystonia on ADL (speech, handwriting, feeding, eating/swallowing, hygiene, dressing, and walking) and the total maximum score is 30. The disadvantage of the scale is that it is not very sensitive in picking up changes in mild disease and does not distinguish between proximal and distal segments.[23]

The Unified Dystonia Rating Scale (UDRS) includes a more detailed assessment of separate body areas with specific ratings for proximal and distal limbs and does not mix bodily inspection with functional variables such as speech and swallowing. 14 body areas are evaluated for dystonia severity and duration. Severity rating is specific for each body region and varies from 0 (no dystonia) to 4 (extreme dystonia); duration also ranges from 0 to 4 and assesses whether dystonia occurs at rest or with action, and whether it is predominantly of maximal or submaximal intensity. The total UDRS score is the sum of the severity and duration factors with a maximum total of 112.[23]

The Global Dystonia Rating Scale (GDS) evaluates the severity of dystonia in the same 14 body areas as the UDRS. The GDS ranges from 0 (no dystonia) to 10 (severe dystonia). There are no modifying factors in the GDS and the total score is the sum of all the body area scores with a maximum of 140.[23]

The above scales are applicable for generalized dystonia. Individual scales have been formulated to assess focal or segmental dystonia, e.g., Toronto Western Spasmodic Torticollis Rating Scale (TWSTRS) comprised of three separate subscales: Motor severity, disability, and pain due to dystonia are used for cervical dystonia, Blepharospasm Disability Index (BSDI) for blepharospasm, Writer's Cramp Rating Scale (WCRS), AIMS, or the Extrapyramidal Symptoms Rating Scale (ESRS) for tardive dyskinesias.[23] Apart from these scales, Short-Form Health Survey (SF-36), PDQ-39, and Cervical Dystonia Impact Profile (CDIP-58) are some of the scales used to assess quality of life in patients with dystonia.[23]

ATAXIA

As is the case for dystonia, various scales have been developed for assessing ataxia to assess severity, disease stage, and the impact of medications.

The International Cooperative Ataxia Rating Scale (ICARS) is an outcome measure, formulated in 1997 by the committee of the World Federation of Neurology for quantification of impairment due to cerebellar ataxia. The scale is scored out of 100 with 19 items and four subscales of posture and gait disturbance (seven items, 34 points); limb kinetic function (seven items, 52 points); speech disorder (two items, eight points); and oculomotor disorder (three items, six points). Higher scores indicate higher levels of impairment. It has been validated for spinocerebellar and Friedreich's ataxia.[24]

Scale for the Assessment and Rating of Ataxia (SARA): This is a shorter scale with eight items, gait, stance, sitting, speech disturbance, finger-finger test, nose-finger test, fast alternating hand movements, and heel-shin slide, yielding a total score of 0 (no ataxia) to 40 (most severe ataxia).[24]

Modified International Cooperative Ataxia Rating Scale (MICARS): The 120-point scale has seven additional tests to the ICARS—in kinetic function, speech disorders, and oculomotor function.[24]

Brief Ataxia Rating Scale (BARS) was developed in 2009 in an attempt to both reduce redundancies of the ICARS and to shorten and simplify the administration of ataxia outcome measures.[24]

Friedreich's Ataxia Rating Scale (FARS) is a semiquantitative ataxia and nonataxia assessment scale.[24] It has four domains: (1) Functional staging (0–6, overall mobility); (2) ADL (0–36); (3) Neurological assessment of bulbar, upper and lower limbs, peripheral nerve, and upright stability/gait functions (maximum scores of 11, 36, 16, 26, and 28, total of 117); and (4) Quantitative timed activities—PATA rate (the number of repetitions of the word "PATA" in a 10-second interval using a tape recorder), nine-hole pegboard (9HPT), and timed 25-feet walk (T25FW). This scale has a good correlation with ICARS.

Other quantitative ataxia scales—Coordination Ability and Tremor System (CATSYS 2000), The Ataxia Functional Composite Scale (AFCS), Composite Cerebellar Functional Score (CCFS) and its Writing Version, and The Spinocerebellar Ataxia Functional Index (SCAFI) are more sensitive in picking up smaller changes and may be more useful in class II trials.[24]

OTHER DISORDERS

Various scales have been formulated for individual diseases like The Unified Huntington's disease Rating Scale (UHDRS),[25] a research tool which has been developed by the Huntington's study group to provide a uniform assessment of the clinical features and course of HD. The components of the UHDRS are: Motor assessment, cognitive assessment, behavioral assessment, independence scale, functional assessment, and total functional capacity (TFC). Similarly a recent scale has been formulated for Wilson's disease-Global Assessment Scale for Wilson's Disease (GAS for WD) that grades the multisystemic manifestations of the disease and has two tiers.[26] Tier 1 scores the global disability in four domains: Liver, cognition and behavior, motor, and osseomuscular. Tier 2 is multidimensional scale for a fine-grained evaluation of the neurological dysfunction. Universidade Federal de Minas Gerais (UFMG) Sydenham's Chorea Rating Scale (USCRS) is a scale used for assessing Sydenham's chorea.[27] A unified scale for assessing various aspects of pantothenate kinase-associated neurodegeneration (PKAN)-Disease Rating Scale (PKAN-DRS) was recently developed for assessing dystonia, Parkinsonism, and other neurological signs.[28]

CONCLUSION

Scales are important in movement disorders as they can quantify the disease, help in studying its natural course, and can pick up changes with interventions, thus helping in identifying relevant treatment options.

REFERENCES

1. Goetz CG, Poewe W, Rascol O, Sampaio C, Stebbins GT, Counsell C, et al. Movement Disorder Society Task Force report on the Hoehn and Yahr staging scale: status and recommendations. Mov Disord. 2004;19(9):1020-8.
2. Goetz CG, Fahn S, Martinez-Martin P, Poewe W, Sampaio C, Stebbins GT, et al. Movement Disorder Society-sponsored revision of the Unified Parkinson's Disease Rating Scale (MDS-UPDRS): Process, format, and clinimetric testing plan. Mov Disord. 2007;22(1):41-7.
3. Colosimo C, Martínez-Martín P, Fabbrini G, Hauser RA, Merello M, Miyasaki J, et al. Task force report on scales to assess dyskinesia in Parkinson's disease: critique and recommendations. Mov Disord. 2010;25(9):1131-42.
4. Chaudhuri KR, Martinez-Martin P, Brown RG, Sethi K, Stocchi F, Odin P, et al. The metric properties of a novel non-motor symptoms scale for Parkinson's disease: Results from an international pilot study. Mov Disord. 2007;22(13):1901-11.
5. Martinez-Martin P, Rodriguez-Blazquez C, Abe K, Bhattacharyya KB, Bloem BR, Carod-Artal FJ, et al. International study on the psychometric attributes of the non-motor symptoms scale in Parkinson disease. Neurology. 2009;73(19):1584-91.
6. Kulisevsky J, Pagonabarraga J. Cognitive impairment in Parkinson's disease: tools for diagnosis and assessment. Mov Disord. 2009;24(8):1103-10.
7. Kuhlman GD, Flanigan JL, Sperling SA, Barrett MJ. Predictors of health-related quality of life in Parkinson's disease. Parkinsonism Relat Disord. 2019;65:86-90.
8. Visser M, Verbaan D, van Rooden SM, Stiggelbout AM, Marinus J, van Hilten JJ. Assessment of psychiatric complications in Parkinson's disease: The SCOPA-PC. Mov Disord. 2007;22(15):2221-8.
9. Evans AH, Okai D, Weintraub D, Lim SY, O'Sullivan SS, Voon V, et al. Scales to assess impulsive and compulsive behaviors in Parkinson's disease: Critique and recommendations. Mov Disord. 2019;34(6):791-8.
10. Evatt ML, Chaudhuri KR, Chou KL, Cubo E, Hinson V, Kompoliti K, et al. Dysautonomia rating scales in Parkinson's disease: sialorrhea, dysphagia, and constipation--critique and recommendations by movement disorders task force on rating scales for Parkinson's disease. Mov Disord. 2009;24(5):635-46.
11. Högl B, Arnulf I, Comella C, Ferreira J, Iranzo A, Tilley B, et al. Scales to assess sleep impairment in Parkinson's disease: critique and recommendations. Mov Disord. 2010;25(16):2704-16.
12. Chaudhuri KR, Rizos A, Trenkwalder C, Rascol O, Pal S, Martino D, et al. King's Parkinson's disease pain scale, the first scale for pain in PD: An international validation. Mov Disord. 2015;30(12):1623-31.
13. Martinez-Martin P, Rizos AM, Wetmore J, Antonini A, Odin P, Pal S, et al. First comprehensive tool for screening pain in Parkinson's disease: the King's Parkinson's Disease Pain Questionnaire. Eur J Neurol. 2018;25(10):1255-61.
14. Martinez-Martin P, Jeukens-Visser M, Lyons KE, Rodriguez-Blazquez C, Selai C, Siderowf A, et al. Health-related quality-of-life scales in Parkinson's disease: critique and recommendations. Mov Disord. 2011;26(13):2371-80.
15. Virués-Ortega J, Carod-Artal FJ, Serrano-Dueñas M, Ruiz-Galeano G, Meza-Rojas G, Velázquez C, et al. Cross-cultural validation of the Scales for Outcomes in Parkinson's Disease-Psychosocial questionnaire (SCOPA-PS) in four Latin American countries. Value Health. 2009;12(2):385-91.
16. Wenning GK, Tison F, Seppi K, Sampaio C, Diem A, Yekhlef F, et al. Development and validation of the Unified Multiple System Atrophy Rating Scale (UMSARS). Mov Disord. 2004;19(12):1391-402.
17. Golbe LI, Ohman-Strickland PA. A clinical rating scale for progressive supranuclear palsy. Brain. 2007;130(Pt 6):1552-65.
18. Payan CA, Viallet F, Landwehrmeyer BG, Bonnet AM, Borg M, Durif F, et al. Disease severity and progression in progressive supranuclear palsy and multiple system atrophy: validation of the NNIPPS--Parkinson Plus Scale. PLoS One. 2011;6(8):e22293.
19. Stacy MA, Elble RJ, Ondo WG, Wu SC, Hulihan J, TRS study group. Assessment of interrater and intrarater reliability of the Fahn-Tolosa-Marin Tremor Rating Scale in essential tremor. Mov Disord. 2007;22(6):833-8.

20. Bain PG, Findley LJ, Atchison P, Behari M, Vidailhet M, Gresty M, et al. Assessing tremor severity. J Neurol Neurosurg Psychiatry. 1993;56(8):868-73.
21. Louis ED, Barnes L, Wendt KJ, Ford B, Sangiorgio M, Tabbal S, et al. A teaching videotape for the assessment of essential tremor. Mov Disord. 2001;16(1):89-93.
22. Tröster AI, Pahwa R, Fields JA, Tanner CM, Lyons KE. Quality of life in Essential Tremor Questionnaire (QUEST): development and initial validation. Parkinsonism Relat Disord. 2005;11(6):367-73.
23. Thobois S, Taira T, Comella C, Moro E, Bressman S, Albanese A. Pre-operative evaluations for DBS in dystonia. Mov Disord. 2011;26(Suppl 1):S17-22.
24. Saute JA, Donis KC, Serrano-Munuera C, Genis D, Ramirez LT, Mazzetti P, et al. Ataxia rating scales—psychometric profiles, natural history and their application in clinical trials. Cerebellum. 2012;11(2):488-504.
25. Klempír J, Klempírova O, Spacková N, Zidovská J, Roth J. Unified Huntington's disease rating scale: clinical practice and a critical approach. Funct Neurol. 2006;21(4):217-21.
26. Aggarwal A, Aggarwal N, Nagral A, Jankharia G, Bhatt M. A novel Global Assessment Scale for Wilson's Disease (GAS for WD). Mov Disord. 2009;24(4):509-18.
27. Teixeira AL Jr, Maia DP, Cardoso F. UFMG Sydenham's chorea rating scale (USCRS): Reliability and consistency. 2005;20(5):585-91.
28. Marshall RD, Collins A, Escolar ML, Jinnah HA, Klopstock T, Kruer MC, et al. A scale to assess activities of daily living in Pantothenate Kinase-Associated Neurodegeneration. Mov Disord Clin Pract. 2019;6(2):139-49.

CHAPTER 19

Technology in Movement Disorders

Soaham Dilip Desai, Manan Mayur Mehta, Indu Ghanshyam Bhana

INTRODUCTION

Movement disorders affect individuals by causing dysfunction in the coordination of body movements. Movement disorders are assessed by clinicians using observations of patients in the clinic and listening to history of impairment in daily activities. As these disorders are variable through the day, just a single in clinic observation gives only a snapshot of the overall difficulties faced by patients. The evaluation and sharing of knowledge on movement disorders happens through images and videos. However, there are technological limitations with videography in evaluating movement disorders. The advent of novel technologies has led to their utilization in evaluation, monitoring, and rehabilitation of movement disorders. Novel technology has been predominantly used in the field of Parkinson's disease (PD). Recent collaborative research projects between innovator scientists, engineers, and physicians have also been planned in other movement disorders such as dystonia, tremor, and chorea. In this chapter, we shall describe the uses of novel technology, mainly in PD (as majority of work has been done in PD) and will also give an idea of its use in other movement disorders.

TECHNOLOGY IN PARKINSON'S DISEASE

Parkinson's disease is a progressive neurodegenerative disorder that affects the lives of patients and care givers at an exponential rate.[1] The World Health Organization (WHO) data reveals that around 7–10 million people have been affected with PD.[2,3] Affecting around 3% of the people above the age of 65 years, PD is one of the most common chronic progressive neurodegenerative diseases worldwide with patient numbers expected to increase further in future.[2] The aim of PD treatment is to make the patients independent and to improve their quality of life. Patients with Parkinson's (PWP) disease require regular follow-ups and lifelong monitoring of their symptoms, quality of life, drug effects and side effects, and motor fluctuations.

Advances in technology are being evaluated for their role in monitoring, diagnosis, remote assessment, treatment, rehabilitation, improving life quality, and large scale research.

Technology in Evaluation and Monitoring

In advanced PD, the major sources of disability for patients are features such as freezing, falls, motor fluctuations, neuropsychiatric, and autonomic dysfunction. The clinician should have a perfect idea about the patient's daily routine activities and motor fluctuations for dose optimization and scheduling. The current concept of managing PWP is by serial visits to neurologists in their clinics. Assessment of patients with PD includes history, examination use of clinical scale [Unified PD Rating Scale (International Parkinson's Disease and Movement Disorder Society (MDS)-UPDRS)], and for patients with fluctuations, the patient diary.[4] Often, patients find it difficult to fill these diaries and are also not making accurate judgment about symptoms. Clinical assessment in the clinic is of little value when the patient is having frequent motor fluctuations.[5,6] There is need for frequent visits to the clinic, that may be very inconvenient for the aged patients who are having multiple comorbidities, impaired mobility, and cognition.[7-10]

This has given rise to the thought of using novel technology for continuous assessment of PD symptoms. These include techniques analyzing electromyography (EMG) signals, electroencephalogram (EEG) signals, imaging modalities [magnetic resonance imaging (MRI) and computed tomography (CT scan)], various wearable sensors and audio sensors.

Different tools such as EMG, EEG, neuroimaging, wearable sensors, and electronic patient diaries (e-diary) help in evaluation and monitoring PD.

Electromyography

Electromyography provides information of activity of different muscles. Three important issues in PWP have been assessed using EMG over the last few years. Quantifying tremors in PWP, differentiating tremors in PD from those of patients with essential tremor (ET) and healthy controls, and identifying freezing of gait (FoG) have been assessed utilizing EMG. Tremors in PWP cause an important hindrance to daily activities, but monitoring tremors remotely using video can make it difficult. Different studies[11-16] have used nonlinear analysis techniques, morphology analysis techniques, spectral based analysis techniques, and combination of these techniques for analysis of EMG signals for differentiating PWP from healthy controls. Ruonalla *et al.* suggested an algorithm to differentiate ET and PD tremors using surface EMG of biceps brachii muscle during isometric tension. This research had shown 76% accuracy for correct diagnosis in patients with ET and 74% accuracy for PWP.[14] Bryan *et al.*[17] have provided an algorithm for predicting FoG in PWP using a dynamic neural network to detect instances of FoG. This network utilized data collected by an EMG sensor (placed on the shin of tibia) and an axial accelerometer (placed on forearm and thigh) applied to patients with PD with frequent FoG. The results suggested that instances of FoG could be predicted with 83% sensitivity and 97% specificity by this method.

Electroencephalogram

Electroencephalogram has mainly been assessed for its role in detection of FoG. Ardi AM *et al.*[18] used wavelet decomposition and pattern recognition techniques to assess FoG in PWP. They used a four-channel wireless EEG system and the sensors were placed at occipital one (O1-primary visual receiving area), parietal four (P4-navigational movement area), central zero (Cz-primary motor area), and frontal zero (Fz-supplementary motor area). They studied 26 patients with PD with significant FoG. Through the proposed classifier, the results had verified the possibility of applying the EEG in FoG detection in PWP during walking with the highest accuracy of 76.7% using the selected features.[18] However, the role of EEG has not been confirmed to be of relevant practical use as yet.

Neuroimaging Modalities

Newer neuroimaging technologies like functional MRI and positron emission tomography (PET) can detect neural structural and functional pathology. These tests are being studied to assess their role as biomarkers in preclinical PD, for early identification of PD, for differentiating PD from secondary parkinsonism and atypical parkinsonism, subtyping different nonmotor types of PD based on predominant metabolic function derangement, assessing the role of possible neuroprotective agents in terms of metabolic neurotransmitter functions and tracking disease progression serially. **Table 1** below depicts some of these approaches. Neuroimaging technologies using specific tracers to assess different metabolic pathways (e.g., serotonin, dopamine, and cholinergic system) and its function are also being assessed for their role in early diagnosis and as a marker of disease severity. A detailed evaluation of these different imaging biomarkers is beyond the scope of this chapter, focusing predominantly on the role of newer technology in Parkinsonism.

TABLE 1: Newer imaging technology in Parkinsonism[#, 1-14]

Role of imaging technology in Parkinsonism		
Early identification of prodromal PD	*Diagnosis of PD*	*Assessing progression of PD*
DaT scan can detect early striatonigral degeneration	• DaT, 18-fluorodopa, or VMAT scans can differentiate between degenerative Parkinsonian syndromes and essential tremor/secondary Parkinsonism • These cannot differentiate PD from other Parkinsonism types	Gray matter volume, caudate volume, and cortical thickness measurements can correlate with cognitive decline in PD
Transcranial ultrasound showing substantia nigra hyperechogenicity associated with PD development at 3–5 years follow-up	• fMRI can differentiate between tremor predominant and rigidity predominant subtypes of PD • Few imaging signs like "humming bird sign", "hot cross bun sign" can help identifying specific syndromes	Basal ganglia iron assessment by MRI relaxation rate *R2 can correlate with disease progression

[#] For references, please refer to supplemental data as available on accompanying CD supplement.

(DaT: dopamine transporter; fMRI: functional magnetic resonance imaging; PD: Parkinson's disease; VMAT: vesicular monoamine transporter)

Limitations of Electroencephalogram, Electromyography and Imaging

In EEG based methods, electrical activity measurement reflects only the sum total of excitatory and inhibitory postsynaptic potentials of the superficial cortical level neurons. The localization by EEG may sometimes give confusing recording due to propagation of electrical activity in the extracellular space. The electrode placement and carrying them during all routine activities are also very cumbersome for patients.[19,20] For using EMG-based methods, proper placement of electrodes along the anatomical region and knowledge of anatomy in detail are very important.[21] EMG will not be useful for recording the static movement.[22] Neuroimaging modality is good for depicting exact anatomic picture. However, as PD is a neurodegenerative disease, changes associated are more at the neurotransmitter level than gross anatomic differences, which cannot be demonstrated by neuroimaging modalities. Due to the above-mentioned disadvantages of these technological tools including EEG, EMG, and neuroimaging, more easily approachable and less cumbersome methods are needed for evaluation and monitoring PWP.

Wearable Sensors

A wearable device is an electronic gadget which is compact and can be worn over parts of the body with comfort over an extended period. It contains digital electronic sensors for recording of variables associated with various parameters such as acceleration, light flux, sound pressure, skin temperature, or blood volume. An accelerometer detects human motion and measures acceleration in motion along the reference axis. A gyroscope is useful in measuring angular rotation of body segments along the rotational axis. A magnetometer is used in combination, which measures any change in rotation of the body segment in respect to the earth's magnetic field. The combination of multimodal sensors (accelerometer, gyroscope, and magnetometer) provides quick and accurate body parts positioning. Audio sensors help in determination of speech disturbances as well.

Table 2 enlists the different ways in which wearable sensor technologies have been used in evaluation in PD.

Table 3 enlists the current research work done on the ability of wearable sensors in providing objective measures of the disease.

TABLE 2: Wearable technologies for evaluation of PD symptoms.

Different methods to evaluate PD symptoms using sensors	*Study*	*Observations*	*Reference#*
Assessment of tremor and bradykinesia in PD patients	Arash et al. carried out two studies for detecting tremor and bradykinesia using gyroscopes to measure angular velocity during patient movement	The algorithm which they provided had a high degree of correlation with the parameters related to tremor and bradykinesia assessment by UPDRS subscore	15,16
LID detection in PD	Keijsers et al. suggested a technique utilizing neural network for detection of dyskinesia and differentiating dyskinesia from the individual patient's voluntary movements. This included six triaxial accelerometers being positioned at different parts of the body while patient being engaged in ADL	The proposed efficiency of neural network classifier in differentiating dyskinesia from nondyskinesia with the recognition rate of 93.7% for arm, 99.7% for trunk, and 97.0% for leg	17
Home monitoring by web-based application	Patel et al. proposed the concept of home-monitoring utilizing wireless sensors. Here the information is transmitted to the clinicians using web-based application	The home-monitoring system composed of software services, functioning at three level: Central portal server, patient's hosts, and clinician's host level. In addition, there was also provision for video interaction between the clinician and the patient, providing information useful in PD management and drug dosage titration	18
Gait Impairment assessment	Cancela et al. utilized a method for assessment of gait impairment using five triaxial accelerometers placed on the limb and one triaxial accelerometer on the belt of patients	Various parameters of gait (step frequency, stride length, entropy, and arm swing) could be assessed for long-periods. This helped in estimating motor fluctuations and improvement in various parameters associated with medications	19

Continued

Continued

Different methods to evaluate PD symptoms using sensors	*Study*	*Observations*	*Reference#*
Rest tremor monitoring	LeMoyne et al. proposed the use of wireless accelerometer for monitoring PD rest tremor. They used two wireless accelerometers, one placed in a static position while the second one placed over dorsum of hand	This allowed wireless accelerometer application in providing a significant degree of accuracy, consistency, and reliability in quantification of waveform of PD tremor	20
Detection of freezing of gait (FoG)	Haritz et al. proposed a method for freezing detection by gait analysis using an accelerometer to measure the acceleration in three axis and a gyroscope to measure angular velocity in two axis from the three locations on the lower limb including foot, shin, and thigh	A sensor placed at the lower limbs could detect 80.8% of FoG episode correctly and heel perpendicular to the coronal plane could detect 82.7% of FoG episodes correctly using measurements of angular velocity and acceleration	21
Audio sensors	Phonation test was conducted through the use of sustained vowels and this was detected using audio sensors. Dysphonia was detected efficiently without using the articulatory or linguistic modules of running speech, which has many confusing effects	It was shown that the sustained vowel "/a/" was sufficient for voice assessment and prediction as well as monitoring of speech impairment in PD.[53-56] Studies of speech disorders in PD patients have led to the development of many speech signal processing algorithms	22–24

For references, please refer to supplemental data as available on accompanying CD supplement.

(ADL: activities of daily living; PD: Parkinson's disease; UPDRS: Unified Parkinson Disease Rating Scale; LID: Levodopa induced dyskinesia)

TABLE 3: Enlists the current research work done with use of sensors for assessment.

Study	*Country*	*Sample size*	*Assessment*	*Patient location*	*Findings*	*Reference no.#*
Pasluosta et al. (2015)	Germany	139	Postural assessment using wearable inertial sensors	In clinic	Wearable foot sensors can estimate postural instability in Parkinson disease	25
Pérez-López et al. (2016)	Spain	92	Motor assessments using an accelerometer	At home	A single belt-worn accelerometer can detect dyskinesias with >90% accuracy in persons with Parkinson disease	26
Silva de Lima et al. (2017)	Netherlands, USA, and Canada	953	Long-term motor analysis using smartwatch sensor and accelerometer	At home	Wearable sensors are feasible for collecting long-term data of daily motor activity in individuals with Parkinson disease	27
Schlachetzki et al. (2017)	Germany	291	Gait assessment using wearable sensors	In clinic	Wearable sensors are useful for quantitatively assessing gait impairment in people with Parkinson disease	28
Jeon et al. (2017)	Korea	85	Tremor severity scoring using wristwatch wearable sensor	In clinic	Machine-learning algorithms combined with wearable sensor data can score Parkinsonian tremors with >85% accuracy	29
Suppa et al. (2017)	Italy	60	Gait assessment using wearable sensors	In clinic	A wireless wearable sensor system can detect freezing of gait in patients with Parkinson disease with >98% accuracy	30
Bonora et al. (2017)	Italy	103	Postural assessment using inertial sensors	In clinic	Wearable sensors can distinguish between the ability of healthy controls and people with parkinsonism to adjust posture in response to balance shifts	31
Adams et al. (2017)	USA	56	Motor assessments using wearable sensors	In clinic and at home	Wearable sensor use is feasible and well received among individuals with movement disorders and can distinguish activity profiles of those with and without disease	32

For references, please refer to supplemental data as available on accompanying CD supplement.

Development of Electronic Patient Diaries

Over the last 20 years, PD diaries have provided valuable information into the patient's symptoms, quality of life, and therapeutic benefits. However, with the advent of new technologies, there are opportunities to capture a wider range of individualized motor, nonmotor, and circadian complex fluctuations with greater accuracy as an e-diary/tracker interface. A total of 12 PD diaries have been developed, mostly as instruments in clinical trials. Only two [Parkinson Disease Home Diary and core assessment program for surgical interventional therapies-PD (CAPSIT-PD) diary] have been designated as "recommended" by the MDS Task Force on Rating Scales. The phenomenological, contextual, and clinometric gaps identified in existing diaries as well as the potential strategies to correct them are listed in **Table 4**.

Using Technology for Remote Assessment of Patients and for Neurology Education (Teleneurology)

Large areas of the world are unable to access proper neurological care.[23] In India, nearly 1 billion people live in regions that lack a practicing neurologist who is affiliated with a major professional society.[24] More than 40% patients of PD do not see a neurologist over a 4-year period.[25] To change this situation, a new model is Telehealth, which comprises of the use of technology to provide healthcare, education, and remote monitoring.[26] Video conferencing and smartphones have increased the capabilities and availability of telehealth. Tele-neurology could benefit many chronic neurological conditions like PD in which patients have impaired mobility, cognitive functions, and driving ability. Beck *et al.* studied 195 patients with PD, where the neurologist would do remote monitoring as well as video conferencing. It was observed that there was no difference in the quality of life between in-person and virtual visits. On the contrary, virtual visits with remote specialists were preferred to usual care with local physicians.

As per a WHO report, the median number of post-graduate neurology trainees in the pipeline was between 0 and 4 per year per 10 million people in low income countries.[23] Tele-neurology is supporting these efforts to increase the capacity of neurological services in resource poor countries.[27,28] Neurologists can have continued

TABLE 4: Gaps of current (paper) diaries and strategies to address them in an e-diary.[33]

Gap of current diaries		*Strategies for correction into an e-diary*
Essential limitations	Absence of nonmotor fluctuations	Nonmotor fluctuations assessment within a diary is needed
	Incomplete definitions of OFF and ON states	• Clear definitions of motor states and expanding the repertoire of motor behaviors • Combine real-time assessments with wearable sensors and e-diary tracking
	Under-representation of partial states	• Partial states can be recognized by patients and add granularity to transitional states • OFF and ON states may be replaced with measurement of symptom and disability severity along a continuum
	Inaccurate and partial reporting of motor complications	Allow for independent recognition of peak dose and diphasic dyskinesia, and OFF-associated dystonia. Allow for separate/complementary input by spouse or other immediate caregiver
	Lack of functional assessment	Allow for quantification of functioning that accounts for the wide nature, duration, and severity of OFF periods at any "level" of fluctuation
Contextual limitations	Absent cognitive debriefing	Conduct cognitive debriefing to improve items and increase the precision of self-reported measures
	Heterogeneous frequency of assessments	Evaluate real-time assessments with or without variably spaced frequency of assessments
	Data integrity limitations	Compliance assessment and improved patient interface can be implemented with electronic diaries
	Absent medication tracking	Implement medication tracking to correlate with function and assist with management strategies
	Absent meal type and sleep quality	Implement meal tracking and sleep quality recording to determine effect on response to medications
Clinimetric limitations	Subjective information without objective measures (trackers)	Implement a smartphone based application with integrated action-dependent and action-independent (wearable sensors) symptom measures
	Heterogeneous measurement formats and validations methods	Adopt visual analog scales as measurement format and anchor metrics on patient-relevant outcomes

[#]For references, please refer to supplemental data as available on accompanying CD supplement.

Source: Adapted from Movement Disorder Society-Task Force on Technology.

medical education and interactions with their global colleagues through regular teleconferencing for clinical cases and subspecialty consultation.

Technology in Treatment of Parkinson's Disease

Advanced PD has limited options in the management plan. Surgical techniques like deep brain stimulation (DBS) are frequently adopted. DBS therapy is invasive, expensive, requiring technological expertise, infrastructure, and is not free of complications. Recent studies show that using the newer technology, less invasive methods can be adopted in achieving therapeutic goals in advanced PD.

Magnetic resonance imaging guided focused ultrasound has been used to perform thalamotomy in drug refractory tremors of PD. In this technique, the use of radiofrequency offers the possibility to perform subthalamic thermocoagulation causing pallidothalamic tractotomy with reduced risks and optimized accuracy. Magara *et al.*[29,30] studied 13 patients who underwent the ultrasonic subthalamotomy and monitored using UPDRS and global symptomatic relief in chronic therapy resistant PD patients. The study demonstrated the feasibility, safety, and accuracy of the MRI-guided focused ultrasound technique. Schlesinger *et al.*[31] also demonstrated good outcomes with less complications in this study.

Another technique is the stereotactic electrical stimulation of the prelemniscal radiation (RAPRL), a subthalamic bundle of fibers, which is an exquisite target that can be visualized easily on ventriculogram. Velasco *et al.*[32] studied 10 patients of PD, where in tetrapolar electrodes were stereotactically oriented through a frontal parasagittal approach to the RAPRL contralateral to the most prominent symptoms. Preoperative and postoperative evaluations at 3, 6, 9, and 12 months after surgery were performed using conventional PD scales and quantitative evaluations of tremor amplitude and reaction time. In all patients, temporary suppression of tremor occurred when the electrodes reached the target. The most effective stimulation was obtained when the pair of contacts was placed in the RAPRL. Long-term stimulation at 130 Hz, 0.09–0.450 ms, and 1.5–3.0 V produced significant improvement in tremor and rigidity and mild improvement in bradykinesia.

Using Technology for Large Scale Research

With the technological advances seen in the field of medicine, one can expect the future to be technology driven. Wearable devices and sensors have now been put into research studies to provide an insight into what might be achievable in future. Two large-scale studies on wearable devices in PD research are prime examples. "Smartphone-PD" was a global observational study which included healthy and PD patients and used a software downloaded on their Android smartphones.[33] A total of 457 participants were observed for >46,000 hours of data capture by sensor over a span of 6 months. These included GPS location, accelerometer, gyroscope, magnetometer, proximity, and ambient light flux. They allowed systematic tests of gait, voice, touchscreen tapping as well postural and rest tremors using the smartphones, which helped in preparing various algorithms to differentiate between drug responsiveness and nonresponsiveness as well as to quantify the responsiveness with regard to various treatments.[34] The "mPower" iPhone-based study of PD patients included 57 patients of PD, used various machine learning algorithms and assessed data from touch screen tapping sensors.[35] Medication responsiveness was also quantified using the data. The evidence for the clinical utility of the wearable device monitoring is promising. This approach provides real time objective assessment, which has the potential to bring great changes in PD management, benefiting the patients, and their caregivers.

Technology in Rehabilitation and Improving Quality of Life

Despite all the advances in treatment, PWP have affected quality of life, requiring assistance in walking, bathing, toileting, dressing, and undressing.[36] As we await further treatment options, various technological tools can help the patients and their care givers in dealing with disability to improve quality of life.

Table 5 enlists the different ways in which technology can help in rehabilitation to improve quality of life.

Using Technology to Transfer Delivery of Care at Home

Neurodegenerative disorders require constant care, and to improve PD care, most of it must be delivered at home. Home care is not new, as in the early part of the 20th century, the house call was a dominant means of providing care, with 40% of physician-patient encounters in 1930 occurring in the home.[37] Because of changing demographic, social, and technological factors, the demand for in-home care is likely to grow.

The newer care models for PD care include multidimensional methods. They include a combination of remote monitoring, self-monitoring, and multidisciplinary care, which enables a patient-centered care at home and decreasing in clinic visits (**Fig. 1**).

There could be questions on whether PWP would be able to manage the devices and handle prolonged wearable sensors. Questions of whether such data collected by wearable device lead to relevant treatment change are still unanswered. However, the initial experience is favorable provided, there are clear instructions and full participation

TABLE 5: Use of novel technology in rehabilitation and for improvement in quality of life.

Sr. No.	*Mode of novel technology*	*Rehabilitation opportunities*	*References#*
1.	Voice enabled software and ease of access devices	Intelligent personal assistant software (IPA) is a software agent which performs tasks and services for an individual, based on user input and ability to access the internet for various information (e.g. Apple's Siri, Google home, blackberry's assistant, and Amazon's Alexa/ECHO). Such devices can be helpful to PWP who experience motor disabilities	
2.	Voice enabled keyboards and oversized keyboards	Desktop computers with keyboard, adjusting as per patients need, typing by using a voice control system or those with oversized keys (four times larger) can make typing easier for PWP	
3.	Mobile phone apps	Few examples: • *Parkinson mPower app*: This app uses the sensors in iPhone to measure patients' tremor, gait, and balance to track and store this information • *DAF professional*: This is a speech therapy app for iOS and Android users. It helps PD patients to slow their rate of speech so that it sound clearer to others • *Parkinson home exercises*: This video app demonstrates exercises for PD patients and covers a wide range of movement topics such as posture, gait, balance, and flexibility. It can be downloaded from Apple store and Google play • *Parkinson's EasyCall*: This Android app helps in making phone calls easier for patients with dexterity issues	
4.	Driving and transport	Self-driven vehicles as being devised by Google and Tesla could improve the impairment in transport, experienced by PWPs	34
5.	Monitoring exercise and rehabilitation	Wearable sensors could provide real time monitoring of mechanics of motor impairments and this could help in improving exercise and rehabilitation. Hence, rehabilitation therapies can be individualized and planned based on data derived from wearable sensors	35
6.	Managing falls	During an event of a fall, devices could be used to alert the emergency medical services. Sensors can be attached to patient's shoes, slippers, necklace and even floor carpets to detect sudden movements of the body, and timely report the fall, to seek immediate medical care	36–41
7.	Managing FoG	• Using technologic advances for helping in cueing for patients of Parkinson's disease have shown promising results • LASER shoes used for cueing in PD patients could improve FoG duration as well as frequency in a study of 21 PWP.[98] • Rosenthal et al.[99] used a custom built wireless electrical stimulator worn on the waist to allow patients to walk freely. Fixed rhythmic biphasic electrical bursts were delivered during walking, such that the amplitude of the bursts was of sufficient intensity to produce a sensory response only and not motor. Nine participants with idiopathic PD performed a self-identified walking task during both control (no cue) and cueing (electrical stimulation) conditions. Cueing done by sensory electrical stimulation resulted in a reduction in the time taken to complete a walking task and in the number of FoG episodes. This study provides evidence that sensory electrical stimulation cueing delivered in a "fixed" rhythmic manner has the potential to be an effective cueing mechanism for FoG prevention	
8.	Use of assistive devices with embedded sensors	• Utensils with sensors in the handles detect tremor and steady the utensil • Laser light enabled support stick to provide additional visual cue to improve walking and gait are available in the market • A stabilizing handle is available, which can be attached to fork or spoon to provide stabilization and reduce spilling • Magnetic infused buttons on dress shirts assist patients with tremors or impaired dexterity, and help them dress and undress independently • Other products such as sock aids, one handed belts, dressing sticks, and one-handed nail clippers are also available in market	

For references, please refer to supplemental data as available on accompanying CD supplement.

(DAF: Delayed Auditory Feedback; FoG: Freezing of Gait; PD: Parkinson's disease; PWP: patients with Parkinson's)

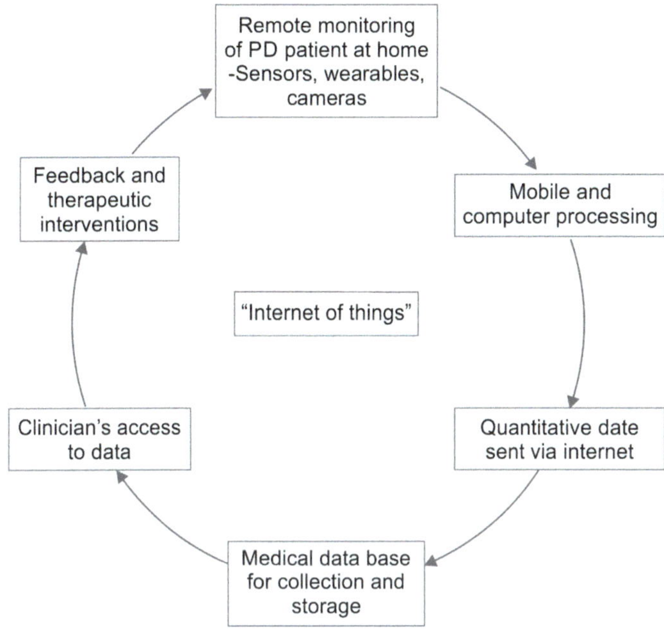

(PD: Parkinson's disease)

FIG. 1: Schematic diagram showing how "internet of things" can connect patients and doctors.

of patients.[38] As per some preliminary evidence, web-based video conferencing may offer similar clinical benefits to that of in-person care, while saving patients and caregivers 100 miles of travel and 3 hours of time per visit.[39] Multidisciplinary care including speech therapy,[40] mental healthcare, and "tele-rehabilitation"[41] can also be delivered remotely.

TECHNOLOGY IN TREMORS

Various studies have been done on transducer-based evaluation of tremors, using accelerometers, gyroscopes, EMG activity, vocal acoustic analysis, and several other methods. Transducers provide objective, precise linear measurements of tremor amplitude, frequency, and occurrence without the potential bias introduced by perceptions of patients and clinical raters. However, most of the transducers used for tremor analysis have not been developed for specific diseases. Their use and data analysis require training and a single transducer may not adequately capture the complex motion of a body part and multiple transducer use would be expensive and time consuming. Hence, these methods are still under research at present for use in tremor analysis.[42-44]

Sensor-based measures frequently will be used to complement the clinical examination and are an obvious choice when the goal is to measure tremor in the absence of a clinician. Continuous measurement of tremor using wearable devices is a promising approach to capture tremor in natural settings that are functionally relevant, but this approach has not been shown to be more sensitive to change than periodic assessments with rating scales. The utility of long-term recordings will depend on the development of valid computer algorithms for identifying and quantifying tremor against a background of other voluntary and involuntary movement.

TECHNOLOGY IN CHOREA AND HUNTINGTON'S DISEASE[45]

Chorea in patients with Huntington's disease (HD) dramatically undermines a patient's ability to perform the activities of daily living that the rest of us take for granted. The routine clinical assessment of an HD patient, at best, offers only a subjective snapshot of the patient's well-being and functional ability which hinders clinical assessments and complicates drug-development. A few research projects utilizing digital tools, biometric monitoring devices, and platforms are currently in progress. Examples of such technological approaches include:

- Q-motor, a well-qualified tapping-based motor function monitoring tool deployed in natural history studies and recent HD clinical trials.
- Teva/Intel are trying to develop a wearable-tech platform based on a sensor-equipped smartwatch and smartphone to monitor chorea in HD.
- A unique data analytics engine that continually monitors and analyzes HD hallmark motor symptoms is being evaluated.

CONCLUSION

A multitude of technology-based objective measures of Parkinsonian impairments have been developed which are quite promising for significantly changing the diagnostic, monitoring, and therapeutic landscape in PD (**Fig. 2**). These tools are relatively cheap, compact in size, reusable, have a good reproducibility, and objectively capture information enabling clinicians to have real time evaluation of patient symptoms. These technologies can have a large impact on patient diagnosis, evaluation, and monitoring even from a remote place. They can help in large scale community research and also in-patient as well as outpatient rehabilitation to improve quality of life at home. However, all these technologies and their applications have limitations. Availability of internet, computers, and smartphones is still scarce in low income countries. Most of the elderly population find it difficult to use a smartphone. Also, there is no uniformity amongst the manufacturers of these devices and wearable sensors. There is no common or uniform method of collecting, computing, and analyzing the data recorded

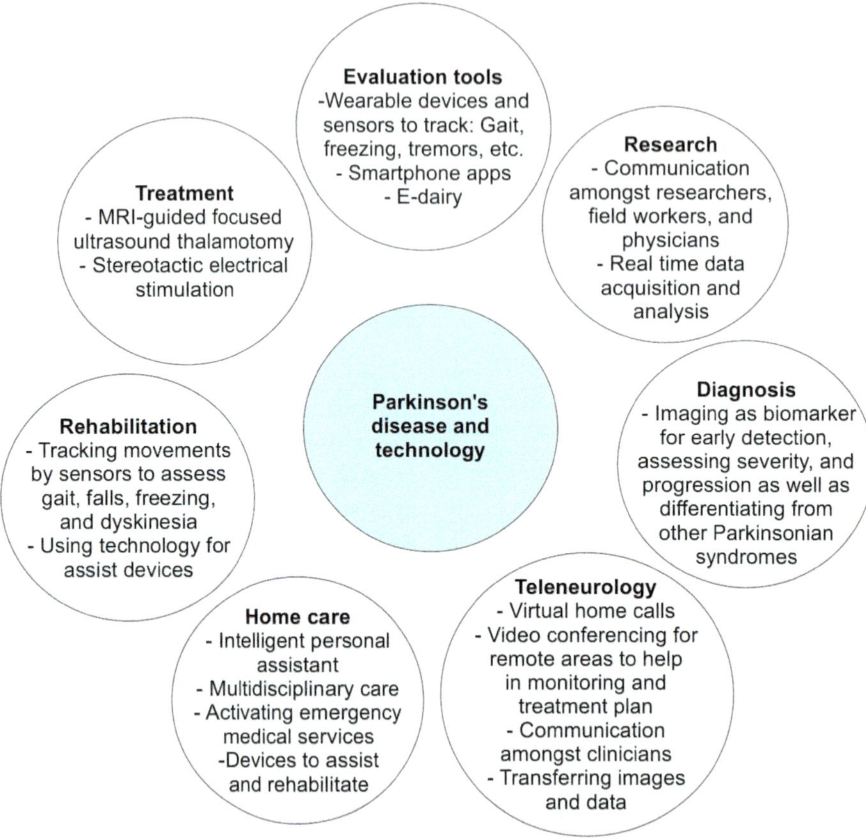

FIG. 2: Summary on newer technology in Parkinson's diease.

with newer technical devices. How this information will help in therapeutic intervention, also remains unanswered. Future studies need to address the above limitations and steps need to be taken toward making a uniform and systematic plan of care for PWP, using advanced technology.

REFERENCES

1. Lang AE, Lozano AM. Parkinson's disease. N Engl J Med. 1998;339(16):1130-43.
2. Hardman JG, Limbird LE. Goodman & Gilman's: The pharmacological basis of therapeutics. New York: McGraw Hill; 2001.
3. GBDPsD Collaborators. Global, regional, and national burden of Parkinson's disease, 1990–2016: A systematic analysis for the global burden of disease study 2016. The Lancet Neurology. 2018;17(11):939-53.
4. Goetz CG, Tilley BC, Shaftman SR, Stebbins GT, Fahn S, Martinez-Martin P, et al. Movement Disorder Society-sponsored revision of the Unified Parkinson's Disease Rating Scale (MDS-UPDRS): scale presentation and clinimetric testing results. Mov Disord. 2008;23(15):2129-70.
5. Patel S, Lorincz K, Hughes R, Huggins N, Growdon J, Standaert D, et al. A body sensor network to monitor parkinsonian symptoms: Extracting features on the nodes. In Proceedings of the 5th International Workshop on Wearable Micro and Nanosystems for Personalised Health, Valencia, Spain. 2008;2123:2123.
6. Goetz CG, Fahn S, Martinez-Martin P, Poewe W, Sampaio C, Stebbins GT, et al. Movement Disorder Society-sponsored revision of the Unified Parkinson's Disease Rating Scale (MDS-UPDRS): process, format, and clinimetric testing plan. Mov Disord. 2007;22(1):41-7.
7. Patel S, Sherrill D, Hughes R, Hester T, Huggins N, Lie-Nemeth T, et al. Analysis of the severity of dyskinesia in patients with Parkinson's disease via wearable sensors. IEEE Xplore. 2006:4.
8. Oung QW, Hariharan M, Basah SN, Yaacob S, Sarillee M, Lee HL. Use of technological tools for Parkinson's disease early detection: A review. IEEE International Conference on Control System, Computing and Engineering (ICCSCE), 2014:343-8.
9. Parkinson Study Group. Evaluation of dyskinesias in a pilot, randomized, placebo-controlled trial of remacemide in advanced Parkinson disease. Arch Neurol. 2001;58(10):1660-8.
10. Pastor-Sanz L, Pansera M, Cancela J, Pastorino M,MT Arredondo Waldmeyer. Mobile Systems as a Challenge for Neurological Diseases Management – The Case of Parkinson's Disease, Diagnostics and Rehabilitation of Parkinson's Disease, Juliana Dushanova, IntechOpen, DOI: 10.5772/16729. Available from: https://www.intechopen.com/books/diagnostics-and-rehabilitation-of-parkinson-s-disease/mobile-systems-as-a-challenge-for-neurological-diseases-management-the-case-of-parkinson-s-disease

11. Fattorini L, Felici F, Filligoi GC, Traballesi M, Farina D. Influence of high motor unit synchronization levels on non-linear and spectral variables of the surface EMG. J Neurosci Methods. 2005;143(2):133-9.
12. Meigal AI, Rissanen S, Tarvainen MP, Karjalainen PA, Iudina-Vassel IA, Airaksinen O, et al. Novel parameters of surface EMG in patients with Parkinson's disease and healthy young and old controls. J Electromyogr Kinesiol. 2009;19(3):e206-13.
13. Rissanen S, Kankaanpää M, Tarvainen MP, Nuutinen J, Tarkka IM, Airaksinen O, et al. Analysis of surface EMG signal morphology in Parkinson's disease. Physiol Meas. 2007;28(12):1507-21.
14. Ruonala V, Meigal A, Rissanen SM, Airaksinen O, Kankaanpää M, Karjalainen PA. EMG signal morphology in essential tremor and Parkinson's disease. Annu Int Conf IEEE Eng Med Biol Soc. 2013;2013:5765-8.
15. De Michele G, Sello S, Carboncini MC, Rossi B, Strambi SK. Cross-correlation time-frequency analysis for multiple EMG signals in Parkinson's disease: a wavelet approach. Med Eng Phys. 2003;25(5):361-9.
16. Sturman MM, Vaillancourt DE, Metman LV, Bakay RA, Corcos DM. Effects of subthalamic nucleus stimulation and medication on resting and postural tremor in Parkinson's disease. Brain. 2004;127(9):2131-43.
17. Cole BT, Roy SH, Nawab SH. Detecting freezing-of-gait during unscripted and unconstrained activity. Annu Int Conf IEEE Eng Med Biol Soc. 2011;2011:5649-52.
18. Handojoseno AM, Shine JM, Nguyen TN, Tran Y, Lewis SJ, Nguyen HT. The detection of Freezing of Gait in Parkinson's disease patients using EEG signals based on Wavelet decomposition. Annu Int Conf IEEE Eng Med Biol Soc. 2012;2012:69-72.
19. Smith SJ. EEG in the diagnosis, classification, and management of patients with epilepsy. J Neurol Neurosurg Psychiatry. 2005;76(Suppl 2):2-7.
20. Schomer DL, da Silva FL. Electroencephalography: basic principles, clinical applications, and related fields, 7th edition. Philadelphia: Lippincott Williams & Wilkins; 2005.
21. Rash GS. Electromyography Fundamentals. 1999;4.
22. Türker KS. Electromyography: some methodological problems and issues. Phys Ther. 1993;73(10):698-710.
23. World Health Organization. Atlas: Country Resources for Neurological Disorders 2004: results of a collaborative study of the World Health Organization and the World Federation of Neurology. Geneva: World Health Organization; 2004.
24. Ganapathy K. Distribution of neurologists and neurosurgeons in India and its relevance to the adoption of telemedicine. Neurol India. 2015;63(2):142-54.
25. Willis AW, Schootman M, Evanoff BA, Perlmutter JS, Racette BA. Neurologist care in Parkinson disease: A utilization, outcomes, and survival study. Neurology. 2011;77(9):851-7.
26. Board on Health Care Services; Institute of Medicine. The role of telehealth in an evolving health care environment: Workshop summary. Washington (DC): National Academies Press (US); 2012.
27. Misra UK, Kalita J, Mishra SK, Yadav RK. Telemedicine for distance education in neurology: preliminary experience in India. J Telemed Telecare. 2004;10(6):363-5.
28. Misra UK, Kalita J, Mishra SK, Yadav RK. Telemedicine in neurology: underutilized potential. Neurol India. 2005;53(1):27-31.
29. Beck CA, Beran DB, Biglan KM, Boyd CM, Dorsey ER, Schmidt PN, et al. National randomized controlled trial of virtual house calls for Parkinson disease. Neurology. 2017;89(11):1152-61.
30. Magara A, Bühler R, Moser D, Kowalski M, Pourtehrani P, Jeanmonod D. First experience with MR-guided focused ultrasound in the treatment of Parkinson's disease. J Ther Ultrasound. 2014;2(1):11.
31. Schlesinger I, Eran A, Sinai A, Erikh I, Nassar M, Goldsher D, et al. MRI guided focused ultrasound thalamotomy for moderate-to-severe tremor in Parkinson's disease. Parkinson's Dis. 2015;2015:219149.
32. Velasco F, Jiménez F, Pérez ML, Carrillo-Ruiz JD, Velasco AL, Ceballos J, et al. Electrical stimulation of the prelemniscal radiation in the treatment of Parkinson's disease: an old target revised with new techniques. Neurosurgery. 2001;49(2):293-306.
33. Abiola SO, Biglan KM, Dorsey ER, Harris DA, Little MA, Saria S, et al. Smartphone-PD: Preliminary results of an mHealth application to track and quantify characteristics of Parkinson disease in real-time. Technology. 2015;18:8.
34. Zhan A, Little MA, Harris DA, Abiola SO, Dorsey ER, Saria S, et al. High frequency remote monitoring of Parkinson's disease via smartphone: Platform overview and medication response detection. 2016.
35. Chaibub Neto EL, Bot BM, Perumal T, Omberg L, Guinney J, Kellen M, et al. Personalized hypothesis tests for detecting medication response in Parkinson disease patients using iPhone Sensor data. Pac Symp Biocomput. 2016;21:273-84.
36. Fukunaga H, Kasai T, Yoshidome H. Clinical findings, status of care, comprehensive quality of life, daily life therapy and treatment at home in patients with Parkinson's disease. Eur Neurol. 1997;38(Suppl 2):64-9.
37. Meyer GS, Gibbons RV. House calls to the elderly—a vanishing practice among physicians. N Engl J Med. 1997;337(25):1815-20.
38. Ferreira JJ, Godinho C, Santos AT, Domingos J, Abreu D, Lobo R, et al. Quantitative home-based assessment of Parkinson's symptoms: the SENSE-PARK feasibility and usability study. BMC Neurol. 2015;15(1):89.
39. Dorsey ER, Venkataraman V, Grana MJ, Bull MT, George BP, Boyd CM, et al. Randomized controlled clinical trial of "virtual house calls" for Parkinson disease. JAMA neurology. 2013;70(5):565-70.
40. Constantinescu G, Theodoros D, Russell T, Ward E, Wilson S, Wootton R. Treating disordered speech and voice in Parkinson's disease online: a randomized controlled non-inferiority trial. Int J Lang Commun Disord. 2011;46(1):1-16.
41. Bloem BR, de Vries NM, Ebersbach G. Nonpharmacological treatments for patients with Parkinson's disease. Mov Disord. 2015;30(11):1504-20.
42. Haubenberger D, Abbruzzese G, Bain PG, Bajaj N, Benito-León J, Bhatia KP, et al. Transducer-based evaluation of tremor. Mov Disord. 2016;31(9):1327-36.
43. Lambrecht S, Gallego JA, Rocon E, Pons JL. Automatic real-time monitoring and assessment of tremor parameters in the upper limb from orientation data. Front Neurosci. 2014;8:221.
44. Elble R, Bain P, João Forjaz M, Haubenberger D, Testa C, Goetz CG, et al. Task force report: scales for screening and evaluating tremor: critique and recommendations. Mov Disord. 2013;28(13):1793-800.
45. Papapetropoulos S. (2019). Tech Blog: Healthcare Technology in Movement Disorders. [online] Available from movementdisorders.org.; https://www.movementdisorders.org/MDS/Off-Nav/2017/Healthcare--Tech-Are-We-Ready.htm [Last accessed May, 2021].

ADDITIONAL REFERENCES TO IN TABLES TO BE MADE AVAILABLE AS ONLINE/CD APPENDIX AS SUPPLEMENTAL DATA

1. Holtbernd F, Eidelberg D. The utility of neuroimaging in the differential diagnosis of parkinsonian syndromes. Semin Neurol. 2014;34(2):202-9.
2. Cilia R, Marotta G, Benti R, Pezzoli G, Antonini A. Brain SPECT imaging in multiple system atrophy. J Neural Transm (Vienna). 2005;112(12):1635-45.
3. Lin KJ, Weng YH, Hsieh CJ, Lin WY, Wey SP, Kung MP, et al. Brain imaging of vesicular monoamine transporter type 2 in healthy aging subjects by 18F-FP-(+)-DTBZ PET. PLoS One. 2013;8(9):e75952.
4. Loane C, Politis M. Positron emission tomography neuro-imaging in Parkinson's disease. Am J Transl Res. 2011;3(4): 323-41.
5. Lozza C, Baron JC, Eidelberg D, Mentis MJ, Carbon M, Marie RM. Executive processes in Parkinson's disease: FDG-PET and network analysis. Hum Brain Mapp. 2004;22(3):236-45.
6. Henkel K, Karitzky J, Schmid M, Mader I, Glatting G, Unger JW, et al. Imaging of activated microglia with PET and [11C]PK11195 in corticobasal degeneration. Mov Disord. 2004;19(7):817-21.
7. Politis M, Su P, Piccini P. Imaging of Microglia in Patients with Neurodegenerative Disorders. Front Pharmacol. 2012;3:96.
8. Rana B, Juneja A, Saxena M, Gudwani S, Kumaran SS, Agrawal RK, et al. Regions-of-interest based automated diagnosis of Parkinson's Disease using T1-weighted MRI. Expert Systems with Applications. 2015;42(9):4506-16.
9. Schocke MF, Seppi K, Esterhammer R, Kremser C, Jaschke W, Poewe W, et al. Diffusion-weighted MRI differentiates the Parkinson variant of multiple system atrophy from PD. Neurology. 2002;58(4):575-80.
10. Focke NK, Helms G, Scheewe S, Pantel PM, Bachmann CG, Dechent P, et al. Individual voxel-based subtype prediction can differentiate progressive supranuclear palsy from idiopathic Parkinson syndrome and healthy controls. Hum Brain Mapp. 2011;32(11):1905-15.
11. Berg D, Behnke S, Seppi K, Godau J, Lerche S, Mahlknecht P, et al. Enlarged hyperechogenic substantia nigra as a risk marker for Parkinson's disease. Mov Disord. 2013;28(2):216-9.
12. Sakakibara R, Tateno F, Kishi M, Tsuyusaki Y, Terada H, Inaoka T. MIBG myocardial scintigraphy in pre-motor Parkinson's disease: a review. Parkinsonism Relat Disord. 2014;20(3):267-73.
13. Badoud S, Nicastro N, Garibotto V, Burkhard PR, Haller S. Distinct spatiotemporal patterns for disease duration and stage in Parkinson's disease. Eur J Nucl Med Mol Imaging. 2016;43(3):509-16.
14. Poston KL, Eidelberg D. FDG PET in the Evaluation of Parkinson's Disease. PET Clin. 2010;5(1):55-64.
15. Salarian A, Russmann H, Wider C, Burkhard PR, Vingerhoets FJ, Aminian K. Quantification of tremor and bradykinesia in Parkinson's disease using a novel ambulatory monitoring system. IEEE Trans Biomed Eng. 2007;54(2):313-22.
16. Salarian A, Russmann H, Vingerhoets FJ, Burkhard PR, Aminian K. Ambulatory monitoring of physical activities in patients with Parkinson's disease. IEEE Trans Biomed Eng. 2007;54(12): 2296-9.
17. Keijsers NL, Horstink MW, Gielen SC. Ambulatory motor assessment in Parkinson's disease. Mov Disord. 2006;21(1): 34-44.
18. Patel S, Chen BR, Buckley T, Rednic R, McClure D, Tarsy D, et al. Home monitoring of patients with Parkinson's disease via wearable technology and a web-based application. Annu Int Conf IEEE Eng Med Biol Soc. 2010;2010:4411-4.
19. Cancela J, Pastorino M, Arredondo MT, Pansera M, Pastor-Sanz L, Villagra F, et al. Gait assessment in Parkinson's disease patients through a network of wearable accelerometers in unsupervised environments. Annu Int Conf IEEE Eng Med Biol Soc. 2011;2011:2233-6.
20. LeMoyne R, Mastroianni T, Grundfest W. Wireless accelerometer configuration for monitoring Parkinson's disease hand tremor. Adv Parkinson's Dis. 2013;2(02):62-7.
21. Zabaleta H, Keller T, Fimbel EJ. Gait analysis in frequency domain for freezing detection in patients with Parkinson's disease. Gerontechnology. 2008;7(2).
22. Tsanas A, Little MA, McSharry PE, Spielman J, Ramig LO. Novel speech signal processing algorithms for high-accuracy classification of Parkinson's disease. IEEE. 2012;59(5):1264-71.
23. Little MA, McSharry PE, Hunter EJ, Spielman J, Ramig LO. Suitability of dysphonia measurements for telemonitoring of Parkinson's disease. IEEE. 2009;56(4):1015-22.
24. Little MA, McSharry PE, Roberts SJ, Costello DA, Moroz IM. Exploiting nonlinear recurrence and fractal scaling properties for voice disorder detection. Biomed Eng Online. 2007;6(1):23.
25. Pasluosta CF, Barth J, Gassner H, Klucken J, Eskofier BM. Pull test estimation in Parkinson's disease patients using wearable sensor technology. Annu Int Conf IEEE Eng Med Biol Soc. 2015;2015:3109-12.
26. PÈrez-LÛpez C, Sam‡ A, RodrÌguez-MartÌn D, Moreno-ArÛstegui JM, Cabestany J, Bayes A, et al. Dopaminergic-induced dyskinesia assessment based on a single belt-worn accelerometer. Artif Intell Med. 2016;67:47-56.
27. de Lima AL, Hahn T, Evers LJ, de Vries NM, Cohen E, Afek M, et al. Feasibility of large-scale deployment of multiple wearable sensors in Parkinson's disease. PloS One. 2017;12(12): e0189161.
28. Schlachetzki JC, Barth J, Marxreiter F, Gossler J, Kohl Z, Reinfelder S, et al. Wearable sensors objectively measure gait parameters in Parkinson's disease. PloS One. 2017;12(10):e0183989.
29. Jeon H, Lee W, Park H, Lee HJ, Kim SK, Kim HB, et al. Automatic classification of tremor severity in Parkinson's disease using a wearable device. Sensors. 2017;17(9):2067.
30. Suppa A, Kita A, Leodori G, Zampogna A, Nicolini E, Lorenzi P, et al. L-DOPA and Freezing of gait in Parkinson's Disease: Objective assessment through a Wearable Wireless system. Front Neurol. 2017;8:406.
31. Bonora G, Mancini M, Carpinella I, Chiari L, Ferrarin M, Nutt JG, et al. Investigation of anticipatory postural adjustments during one-leg stance using inertial sensors: evidence from subjects with Parkinsonism. Front Neurol. 2017;8:361.
32. Adams JL, Dinesh K, Xiong M, Tarolli CG, Sharma S, Sheth N, et al. Multiple wearable sensors in Parkinson and Huntington disease individuals: a pilot study in clinic and at home. Digit Biomark. 2017;1(1):52-63.
33. Movementdisorders.org. (2018). PD Diary. [online] Available at: https://www.movementdisorders.org/MDS/Resources/2018/PD-Diary.htm [Accessed 14 Dec. 2018].

34. Crizzle AM, Classen S, Uc EY. Parkinson disease and driving: an evidence-based review. Neurology. 2012;79(20):2067-74.
35. Borrione P, Tranchita E, Sansone P, Parisi A. Effects of physical activity in Parkinson's disease: A new tool for rehabilitation. World J Methodol. 2014;4(3):133-43.
36. Leddy AL, Crowner BE, Earhart GM. Functional gait assessment and balance evaluation system test: reliability, validity, sensitivity, and specificity for identifying individuals with Parkinson disease who fall. Phys Ther. 2011;91(1): 102-13.
37. Nystrˆm H, Nordstrˆm A, Nordstrˆm P. Risk of injurious fall and hip fracture up to 26 y before the diagnosis of Parkinson disease: Nested case-control studies in a nationwide cohort. PLoS Med. 2016;13(2):e1001954.
38. Spindler M, Gooneratne NS, Siderowf A, Duda JE, Cantor C, Dahodwala N. Daytime sleepiness is associated with falls in Parkinson's disease. J Parkinson's Dis. 2013;3(3):387-91.
39. Rudzińska M, Bukowczan S, Banaszkiewicz K, Stozek J, Zajdel K, Szczudlik A. Causes and risk factors of falls in patients with Parkinson's disease. Neurol Neurochir Pol. 2008;42(3):216-22.
40. Barthel C, Nonnekes J, van Helvert M, Haan R, Janssen A, Delval A, et al. The laser shoes: A new ambulatory device to alleviate freezing of gait in Parkinson disease. Neurology. 2018;90(2):e164-71.
41. Rosenthal L, Sweeney D, Cunnington AL, Quinlan LR, "Laighin G. Sensory Electrical Stimulation Cueing May Reduce Freezing of Gait Episodes in Parkinson's Disease. J Healthc Eng. 2018;2018:4684925.

SECTION

5

TREATMENT OF PARKINSON'S DISEASE

CHAPTER 20

Management of Early Parkinson's Disease

Jimmy A Lalkaka, Varhsa A Patil, Bhimsen Singhal

INTRODUCTION

Parkinson's disease (PD) is a common neurodegenerative disorder affecting about 1% of individuals over the age of 60 years and up to 4% of those over 80 years worldwide.[1] Although there is, as yet, no cure for PD, several treatment options are now available to provide adequate symptomatic relief. This article discusses the management approach to patients who present at the early stage of disease.

TIME FRAME OF EARLY PARKINSON'S DISEASE

The first few years of the disease pass by relatively smoothly with good drug response and no significant adverse effects. This phase is commonly referred to as the "honeymoon period". As the disease advances over time, motor fluctuations appear along with distressing non-motor symptoms. The time period between the onset of motor symptoms and the appearance of motor fluctuations is regarded as the "early stage" of PD. Treatment strategies during this stage often influence the long-term course of the disease.

ACCURATE DIAGNOSIS

The first step in the management of early PD is to make an accurate diagnosis. Typical idiopathic PD starts insidiously with asymmetric motor features of bradykinesia coupled with rest tremor, rigidity, and postural imbalance. The United Kingdom Parkinson's Disease Society Brain Bank criteria have a diagnostic accuracy of up to 90%.[2] However, at the early stage, a somewhat similar pattern can occur in atypical Parkinsonian syndromes such as progressive supranuclear palsy (PSP), multiple system atrophy (MSA), and corticobasal ganglionic degeneration (CBGD). Clinical clues that point to an atypical syndrome are symmetry at onset, early falls, lack of rest tremor, prominent bladder incontinence, early hallucinations and dementia, ataxia, and poor response to levodopa.

Drugs such as phenothiazines, olanzapine, risperidone, levosulpiride, metoclopramide, and lithium also cause Parkinsonism. It is mandatory to ask for prior or ongoing drug ingestion. In some cases when the diagnosis is in doubt, imaging with dopamine transporter single photon emission computed tomography (DoT SPECT) scan helps to differentiate PD (decreased putaminal tracer uptake) from drug induced Parkinsonism (normal uptake).

Young-onset patients <40 years and those with additional hyperkinetic features like dystonia, chorea, or tremor must be investigated for Wilson's disease, manganese intoxication, acanthocytosis, neuronal degeneration with brain iron accumulation (NBIA), and genetic forms of PD.

NEUROPROTECTIVE THERAPIES

Several multicenter randomized trials over the last third to fourth decades have tested drugs that could slow or halt disease progression and afford neuroprotection. The DATATOP (Deprenyl and Tocopherol Antioxidative Therapy of Parkinsonism) trial for selegiline and tocopherol failed to show any neuroprotective benefit.[3] Coenzyme Q10, rasagiline, dopamine agonists, and several others have not demonstrated any disease modifying efficacy.

A recent multicenter trial of levodopa in early PD confirmed that, though efficacious, levodopa was not neuroprotective.[4] So at present, management of early PD remains symptomatic.

DRUGS IN EARLY PARKINSON'S DISEASE

Levodopa

Levodopa is the gold standard of therapy with proven efficacy at every disease stage. It significantly reduces bradykinesia and rigidity, but its efficacy for tremor is less robust.[5] It is combined with a decarboxylase inhibitor (carbidopa or benserazide) to prevent decarboxylation in peripheral tissues and ensure adequate delivery to the brain. Levodopa is most commonly used as an immediate release (IR) formulation, though controlled release (CR) and extended release (ER) forms are also available. It is started at a low dose (50 mg once or twice a day) and gradually titrated upward to 100 mg three times a day. This slow escalation reduces the risk of early side-effects of nausea, vomiting, giddiness, and sleepiness. If nausea and vomiting occur, domperidone can be taken prior to a levodopa dose. Alternatively, levodopa can be given after meals or supplemental carbidopa (lodosyn) can be added.

The landmark "ELLDOPA" Clinical Trial (Earlier versus Later Levodopa) clearly demonstrated the efficacy of levodopa in de novo patients with early PD.[6] Long-term complications include hallucinations, orthostatic hypotension, and motor fluctuations in the form of "wearing off" (shortened duration of benefit of each levodopa dose) and dyskinesias (involuntary choreiform or dystonic movements). Recent evidence indicates that a longer duration of illness and a higher individual levodopa dose predict onset of dyskinesias and not the duration of levodopa treatment.[7,8]

Dopamine Receptor Agonists

Dopamine receptor agonists (DA) directly stimulate the striatal postsynaptic dopamine receptors, bypassing the presynaptic dopaminergic neurons. They also have a longer half-life than levodopa.[9] The ergot agonists include bromocriptine, cabergoline, lisuride, and pergolide. They are now rarely used because of their propensity to cause pulmonary and cardiac valvular fibrosis. The nonergot agonists include ropinirole, pramipexole, piribedil, rotigotine, and apomorphine.

Ropinirole and pramipexole are the most commonly used oral agonists in early PD. Rotigotine is applied as a transdermal patch once a day. Apomorphine is not used in early PD. Double blind, placebo-controlled trials have established the efficacy of ropinirole, pramipexole, and rotigotine in improving motor symptoms of early PD.[10-12] Given as monotherapy, pramipexole and ropinirole also delayed the onset of dyskinesias over a 3–5 year period compared to levodopa.[10,11] However, these benefits are offset by troublesome side-effects. They include ankle edema, cognitive impairment, hallucinations, somnolence and sudden sleep attacks, and impulse control disorders (ICD). The DA have a higher drop-out rate in clinical trials compared to levodopa. ICD such as compulsive shopping and gambling, binge eating, hypersexuality, and punding occurred in >40% of patients treated with pramipexole or ropinirole, usually early in the course of treatment.[13] They were more likely to occur in younger men with obsessive-compulsive traits or a family history of addiction.

Monoamine Oxidase Type B Inhibitors

Selegiline and rasagiline selectively and irreversibly inhibit the monoamine oxidase type B (MAO-B) enzyme which metabolizes levodopa, thus prolonging its duration of action. They improve motor symptoms of early PD, but not to the same extent as levodopa or dopamine agonist.[14] They can cause confusion, orthostatic hypotension, and disturbed sleep. Combination with selective serotonin reuptake inhibitors (SSRIs) rarely cause the "serotonin syndrome".[15] Daily dose should not exceed 10 mg for selegiline and 1 mg for rasagiline for fear of causing a hypertensive crisis by MAO-A inhibition. Safinamide is a relatively new MAO-B inhibitor which has shown good efficacy in early PD in two placebo-controlled double-blind studies.[16,17]

Amantadine

Amantadine is an N-methyl-D-aspartate receptor antagonist with additional anticholinergic and dopaminergic activity. It produces mild motor improvement in early disease and is sometimes used as monotherapy. Dosing is typically 100 mg 1–3 times a day. However, its use is limited by adverse effects—confusion, psychosis, livedo reticularis, and orthostatic hypotension.[18] It can also uncommonly cause myoclonus and seizures. Its main use in PD remains as an antidyskinetic agent in advanced disease.

Trihexyphenidyl

Trihexyphenidyl has a particular benefit on tremor.[18] It has largely been replaced by other drugs due to its anticholinergic adverse effects, notably dry mouth, cognitive impairment, orthostatic hypotension, constipation, urinary retention, and glaucoma.

Levodopa/Carbidopa/Entacapone

Entacapone is a catechol-O-methyltransferase (COMT) inhibitor which increases the duration of action of a levodopa dose. The levodopa/carbidopa/entacapone combination pill (LCE) in early PD resulted in improved UPDRS (Unified Parkinson Disease Rating Scale) motor scores, but there was an increased incidence of side-effects, notably dyskinesia.[19,20] Hence, LCE does not have much role to play in early PD.

TREATMENT STRATEGIES IN EARLY PARKINSON'S DISEASE

When the patient is first informed about the disease, he/she is often devastated. An important task for the physician at this stage is to patiently explain the various aspects of the disease and what to expect over the course of time. This must be done in a positive reassuring way, so that the patient and family members accept the situation and are motivated to live well.

Nonpharmacological Therapy

The benefits of adopting a healthy lifestyle must be emphasized at this stage. A good night's sleep, healthy eating habits, and regular walks are recommended, as is physical therapy. The latter includes supervised physiotherapy, progressive resistance training, treadmill exercises, fixed cycling, occupational therapy, and allied disciplines like yoga, tai chi, boxing, and dance and music therapy. Few randomized clinical trials and many anecdotal reports confirm that physical conditioning significantly improves motor function and promotes a feeling of well-being.[21,22] Patients with hypophonia benefit with speech therapy using the Lee Silverman voice technique.[23] Alternative therapies such as acupuncture and cannabis-based treatments are often chosen by patients. Their use is still under investigation.

When to Start Treatment?

Making the diagnosis of PD does not necessarily mean starting medication immediately. If symptoms are mild and do not interfere with daily routine activities or job efficiency, then one can adopt a wait and watch approach. Ideally, the patient should be a part of the decision-making process. Pharmacotherapy should be started when the patient's symptoms cause functional impairment in daily activities or impaired productivity at the workplace or if a severe rest tremor is a source of social embarrassment.

Selection of Initial Drug

The selection of the initial drug in a de novo patient requires some thought. One size does not fit all. Treatment must be individualized. Factors to be taken into consideration are age of the patient, occupation, severity of the disease, phenomenology of motor symptoms, efficacy of the drug, adverse effects, presence of comorbidities, cost factor, and patient preference. In most cases, patients are started on levodopa, DA, or MAO-B inhibitor.

In elderly subjects 70 years and above, the choice is relatively easy. Levodopa is the drug of choice because dopamine agonists and MAO-B inhibitors have increased risk of cognitive impairment, hallucinations, and orthostatic hypotension in this age group.

Younger patients <50 years of age with early PD and relatively mild symptoms can be started on a DA or MAO-B inhibitor. The rationale for this choice is that though levodopa is the most efficacious drug, concerns have been raised about its long-term complications of wearing-off and dyskinesia. This is particularly so with higher levodopa starting doses.[7,8] The IR preparation of pramipexole and ropinirole with a shorter duration of action can be used three times a day for more rapid control of symptoms, while the ER once daily formulation is preferred for better compliance. If one DA is not tolerated, it can be switched to the other, often successfully.

However, when motor impairment is severe, levodopa should be preferred even in younger patients. Similarly, in a young busy executive with a demanding job and hectic lifestyle, optimum motor control takes precedence over any other issue. Inadequately controlled symptoms often lead to early retirement or lost salary. Hence, levodopa is chosen as it provides the greatest motor benefit.

Trihexyphenidyl, though rarely used nowadays, is still used in a small subset of young patients with a predominant and disabling rest tremor.[18]

Existing comorbidities and traits also need consideration while initiating therapy. Cognitively impaired subjects and those with prior psychiatric illness should not be given DA as they could precipitate dementia, psychosis, or ICD. Depressed patients may benefit with DA as the latter also possesses intrinsic antidepressant activity. Pramipexole or ropinirole would also be the favored drug in patients with coexistent restless legs syndrome.[24,25]

Apropos the debate between levodopa and DA, it must be remembered that DA and MAO-B inhibitors have less robust symptom relief and a higher overall risk of adverse events than levodopa.[26] In a long-term follow-up of early PD patients, the levodopa starting group had persistent mobility benefits and improved activities of daily living 7 years later compared to the DA group. The levodopa group, however, had more dyskinesias.[26]

It is interesting to note that most patients with dyskinesias are not bothered by them. Some may not even be aware of their presence. If given a choice between immobility and dyskinesia, most patients would prefer to have the latter. Besides, if levodopa is given in a small dose from the beginning, the risk of developing dyskinesia is very small. So, the specter of dyskinesia may have been blown out of proportion.

Adjunct Therapy

Over the ensuing months, the efficacy of the initial drug begins to slowly wane. The disease is still at the early stage with no motor fluctuations. The options at this stage are as follows:

- If levodopa was the initial drug used, the physician could select one of two paths:
  i. Gradually increase the levodopa dose or
  ii. Add DA/MAO-B inhibitor to levodopa

  The second option is usually preferred. Adding another drug will improve the motor state without having to increase levodopa dose.
- If a DA was the initial drug used, the options are:
  - Gradually increase the DA dose or
  - Add a small dose of levodopa

  The dose of dopamine agonist can be gradually increased. However, increasing beyond a certain level would expose the patient to side-effects such as ICD, psychosis, cognitive decline, and orthostatic hypotension. So, addition of a small dose of levodopa at this stage without further increasing the agonist dose would be preferred.
- If MAO-B inhibitor was the initial drug, then the add-on medication could be either levodopa or DA, depending on factors mentioned above.

Virtually all patients end up requiring levodopa at some stage in early PD in order to optimize control of their symptoms.

TREATMENT OF NONMOTOR SYMPTOMS IN EARLY DISEASE

Although frequently present, nonmotor symptoms (NMS) are often under-diagnosed. They significantly affect quality of life, sometimes more than motor symptoms. Hyposmia, depression, constipation, and rapid eye movement sleep behavior disorder (RBD) may precede the onset of motor symptoms by months to years. They serve as prodromal markers.[27]

For treatment of depression, tricyclic antidepressants (nortriptyline) and selective serotonin norepinephrine reuptake inhibitors (venlafaxine) have been found efficacious.[16] Sertraline, escitalopram, and paroxetine (SSRIs) are also commonly used. The DA pramipexole also has antidepressant action, as mentioned earlier.[28]

Common measures for constipation include increased fluid intake, regular exercise, probiotics, and a high fiber diet. Polyethylene glycol (macrogol), an osmotic laxative, has shown benefit in PD-associated constipation.[29] Enema (proctoclysis or olive oil) is used in refractory constipation. Dopaminergic drugs aggravate constipation and dose adjustments may be required. Trihexyphenidyl is the biggest culprit.

In RBD, loss of atonia in rapid eye movement sleep causes the patient to physically and verbally "act out his/her dreams". At times, the limb movements are so violent that they cause injury to self or the partner. It is treated with clonazepam (0.5–1.0 mg) or melatonin (6–15 mg) at night, but high quality evidence is lacking.[30] Excessive daytime somnolence or sudden sleep attacks require reduction or withdrawal of DA. Vehicle drivers and machine operators must be cautioned about this DA side-effect.[31] Modafinil improves subjective measures of sleepiness without changing objective measures of sleep.[29]

Impulse control disorders, mentioned earlier, must be specifically inquired into. Patients do not volunteer this history because they are either embarrassed or unaware of their existence. Caregivers and family members are often the ones who disclose them. Reducing or withdrawing DA should be the first step to mitigating ICD.[13]

Surgery in Early Parkinson's Disease

Deep brain stimulation (DBS) is a surgical procedure reserved for patients with advanced disease. The EARLYSTIM trial performed DBS at the early stage of mild motor fluctuation.[32] Based on the results, the Food and Drug Administration (FDA) approved the use of DBS in PD patients of at least 4 years duration with complications not optimally controlled with medications.

However, the jury is still out regarding DBS in the early stage of illness. This procedure is not without considerable adverse events. They include complications related to surgical implantation of the device, increased risk of depression, and suicidal behavior and poor response to gait and balance problems. Besides, patient selection is even more important in this early group, because atypical Parkinsonian syndromes can mimic PD at the early stage, leading to misdiagnosis. Performing DBS in these patients would be ineffective and detrimental. It would be prudent to exercise caution before recommending early DBS.

CONCLUSION

When selecting the appropriate medication in early PD, the therapeutic efficacy of a drug must be balanced against its adverse effect profile, financial implications, and ease of administration. Patients must also be regularly screened for NMS which may go unnoticed.

Management of early PD is not only about drug therapy. It is also about opening an effective communication channel between the patient, caregiver, and healthcare provider. A motivated, happy, and well-informed patient generally fares well during the course of the disease. A multidisciplinary approach involving the neurologist, physiotherapist, speech therapist, social worker, and counsellor is the best option.

The future of PD pharmacology lies in the identification of reliable biomarkers to detect the early prodromal stage of the disease. This would ultimately lead to treatments that are both neuroprotective and neurorestorative.

REFERENCES

1. de Lau LM, Breteler MM. Epidemiology of Parkinson's disease. Lancet Neurol. 2006;5(6):525-35.
2. Jankovic J. Parkinson's disease: clinical features and diagnosis. J Neurol Neurosurg Psychiatry. 2008;79(4):368-76.
3. Shoulson I, Oakes D, Fahn S, Lang A, Langston JW, LeWitt P, et al. Impact of sustained deprenyl (selegiline) in levodopa-treated Parkinson's disease: a randomized placebo-controlled extension of the deprenyl and tocopherol antioxidative therapy of parkinsonism trial. Ann Neurol. 2002;51(5):604-12.
4. Verschuur CVM, Suwijn SR, Boel JA, Post B, Bloem BR, van Hilten JJ, et al. Randomized delayed-start trial of levodopa in Parkinson's disease. N Engl J Med. 2019;380(4):315-24.
5. Ovallath S, Sulthana B. Levodopa: history and therapeutic applications. Ann Indian Acad Neurol. 2017;20(3):185-9.
6. Fahn S. A new look at levodopa based on the ELLDOPA study. J Neural Transm Suppl. 2006;70(suppl):419-26.
7. Cilia R, Akpalu A, Sarfo FS, Cham M, Amboni M, Cereda E, et al. The modern pre-levodopa era of Parkinson's disease: insights into motor complications from sub-Saharan Africa. Brain. 2014;137(10):2731-42.
8. Espay AJ, Morgante F, Merola A, Fasano A, Marsili L, Fox SH, et al. Levodopa-induced dyskinesia in Parkinson's disease: Current and evolving concepts. Ann Neurol. 2018;84(6): 797-811.
9. Brooks DJ. Dopamine Agonists: their role in the treatment of Parkinson's disease. J Neurol Neurosurg Psychiatry. 2000;68(6):685-9.
10. Parkinson Study Group. Pramipexole vs levodopa as initial treatment for Parkinson disease: a randomized controlled trial. JAMA. 2000;284(15):1931-8.
11. Rascol O, Brooks DJ, Korczyn AD, De Deyn PP, Clarke CE, Lang AE. A five year study of the incidence of dyskinesia in patients with early Parkinson's disease who were treated with ropinirole or levodopa. N Engl J Med. 2000;342(20):1484-91.
12. Watts RL, Jankovic J, Waters C, Rajput A, Boroojerdi B, Rao J. Randomized, blind, controlled trial of transdermal rotigotine in early Parkinson disease. Neurology. 2007;68(4):272-6.
13. Garcia-Ruiz PJ, Martnez Castrillo JC, Alonso-Canovas A, Herranz Barcenas A, Vela L, Sanchez Alonso P, et al. Impulse control disorder in patients with Parkinson's disease under dopamine agonist therapy: a multicentre study. J Neurol Neurosurg Psychiatry. 2014;85(8):840-4.
14. Pahwa R, Lyons KE. Treatment of early Parkinson's disease. Curr Opin Neurol. 2014;27(4):442-9.
15. Riederer P, Laux G. MAO-inhibitors in Parkinson's disease. Exp Neurobiol. 2011;20(1):1-17.
16. Stocchi F, Arnold G, Onofrj M, Kwiecinski H, Szczudlik A, Thomas A, et al. Improvement of motor function in early Parkinson disease by safinamide. Neurology. 2004;63(4):746-8.
17. Stocchi F, Borgohain R, Onofrj M, Schapira AH, Bhatt M, Lucini V, et al. A randomized, double-blind placebo controlled trial of safinamide as add-on therapy in early Parkinson's disease patients. Mov Dis. 2012;27(1):106-12.
18. Lees AJ. Drugs for Parkinson's disease. J Neurol Neurosurg Psychiatry. 2002;73(6):607-10.
19. Hauser RA, Panisset M, Abbruzzese G, Mancione L, Dronamraju N, Kakarieka A. Double-blind trial of levodopa/carbidopa/entacapone versus levodopa/carbidopa in early Parkinson's disease. Mov Disord. 2009;24(4):541-50.
20. Stocchi F, Rascol O, Kieburtz K, Poewe W, Jankovic J, Tolosa E, et al. Initiating levodopa/carbidopa therapy with and without entacapone in early Parkinson disease: the STRIDE-PD study. Ann Neurol. 2010;68(1):18-27.
21. Schenkman M, Moore CG, Kohrt WM, Hall DA, Delitto A, Comella CL, et al. Effect of high-intensity treadmill exercise on motor symptoms in patients with de novo Parkinson disease: a phase 2 randomised clinical trial. JAMA Neurol. 2018;75(2): 219-26.
22. Corcos DM, Robichaud JA, David FJ, Leurgans SE, Vaillancourt DE, Poon C, et al. A two-year randomized controlled trial of progressive resistance exercise for Parkinson's disease. Mov Disord. 2013;28(9):1230-40.
23. Mahler LA, Ramig LO, Fox C. Evidence-based treatment of voice and speech disorders in Parkinson's disease. Curr Opin Otolaryngol Head Neck Surg. 2015;23(3):209-15.
24. Oertel WH, Stiasny-Kolster K, Bergtholdt B, Hallström Y, Albo J, Leissner L, et al. Efficacy of pramipexole in restless legs syndrome: a six-week, multicenter, randomized, double-blind study (effect-RLS study). Mov Disord. 2007;22(2):213-9.
25. Hansen RA, Song L, Moore CG, Gilsenan AW, Kim MM, Calloway MO, et al. Effect of ropinirole on sleep outcomes in patients with restless legs syndrome: meta-analysis of pooled individual patient data from randomized controlled trials. Pharmacotherapy. 2009;29(3):255-62.
26. Gray R, Ives N, Rick C, Patel S, Gray A, Jenkinson C, et al. Long-term effectiveness of dopamine agonists and monoamine oxidase B inhibitors compared with levodopa as initial treatment for Parkinson's disease (PDMED): a large, open-label, pragmatic randomised trial. Lancet. 2014;384(9949): 1196-205.
27. Siderowf A, Jennings D, Eberly S, Oakes D, Hawkins KA, Ascherio A, et al. Impaired olfaction and other prodromal features in the Parkinson At-Risk Syndrome study. Mov Disord. 2012;27(3):406-12.
28. Seppi K, Ray Chaudhuri K, Coelho M, Fox SH, Katzenschlager R, Perez Lloret S, et al. Update on treatment of nonmotor symptoms of Parkinson's disease-an evidence-based medicine review. Mov Disord. 2019;34(2):180-98.

29. Zesiewicz TA, Sullivan KL, Arnulf I, Chaudhuri KR, Morgan JC, Gronseth GS, et al. Practice Parameter: treatment of nonmotor symptoms of Parkinson's disease: report of the Quality Standard Subcommittee of the American Academy of Neurology. Neurology. 2010;74(11):924-31.
30. Howell MJ, Schenck CH. Rapid eye movement sleep behavior disorder and neurodegenerative disease. JAMA Neurol. 2015;72(6):707-12.
31. Gjerstad MD, Alves G, Wentzel-Larsen T, Aarsland D, Larsen JP. Excessive daytime sleepiness in Parkinson's disease: is it the drugs or the disease? Neurology. 2006:67(5):853-8.
32. Mestre TA, Espay AJ, Marras C, Eckman MH, Pollak P, Lang AE. Subthalamic nucleus-deep brain stimulation for early motor complications in Parkinson's disease-the EARLYSTIM trial: early is not always better. Mov Disord. 2014;29(14): 1751-6.

CHAPTER 21

Management of Advanced Parkinson's Disease

Madhuri Behari, Abhilekh Srivastava

EVOLUTION OF PARKINSON DISEASE

Parkinson disease is a neurodegenerative disorder. The usual timeline for the disease after the initial diagnosis is made is a "honeymoon period" in which the patient responds dramatically to levodopa therapy, considerably improving the symptoms and quality of life of the patients is variable. However, after the honeymoon period is over, there is onset of motor complications namely motor fluctuations and dyskinesia, leading to progressive disability.[1] In addition, symptoms such as cognitive decline, speech, and difficulty in swallowing may appear which are poorly responsive to levodopa and further worsen the quality of life of these patients.[2] Classically, advanced PD is considered as PD with onset of motor complications such as fluctuations and dyskinesias. Objectively, on the Hoehn and Yahr scale this translates roughly to stage 4 (can walk unassisted, but markedly incapacitated to perform activities of daily living) and stage 5 (confined to wheelchair or bed).[3] Nearly, 80% of the patients after 10 years of diagnosis fulfill the definition of advanced PD.[1]

MANAGEMENT OF ADVANCED PARKINSON DISEASE

Most authors define advanced PD as presence of one of the following: [4]

- Sufficient disability which impairs independent existence despite adequate levodopa therapy
- Sufficient impairment of postural reflexes resulting in requirement of caution while walking
- Presence of gait freezing
- Presence of significant postural deformity
- Presence of motor complications (i.e., fluctuations or dyskinesias) of levodopa therapy

Motor complications which are typically seen in advanced PD can be classified into two types, i.e., motor complications associated with fluctuations and dyskinesias and with nonmotor complication. Fluctuations also known as "off" states are characterized by resumption of Parkinsonian signs and symptoms including rigidity, bradykinesia, and/or freezing. Dyskinesias on the other hand consist of involuntary movements such as choreas or dystonias which are due to the effects of levodopa. Fluctuations or the off states can be either slow or sudden and random depending on the timing of reappearance of symptoms in relation to levodopa therapy. At times there can be delayed response to intake of levodopa or complete failure to respond to an ingested dose of levodopa. Dyskinesias or involuntary movements seen in the advanced stages of PD can be further typed as peak dose (involuntary movements like chorea or dystonia coinciding with peak of levodopa action) or biphasic, i.e., involuntary movements at onset or offset of levodopa action. Other types include "off" period dystonias and simultaneous dystonia and Parkinsonism. A lot of factors are responsible in the development of these motor complications such as continuous loss of dopaminergic neurons in the nigrostriatal circuit during the course of disease, delayed emptying of stomach, loss of capacity of existing cells to store glutamate, and denervation-supersensitivity of the existing dopaminergic receptors.[5]

Management of these complications of advanced PD can be divided into: (1) Noninvasive treatment options; or (2) Invasive options.

Noninvasive Treatment Options for Fluctuations or "Off" States Include

- *Optimization of levodopa dosing*[6] with most fluctuations, changes in levodopa dosing schedules, or formulations can lead to a marked improvement in symptoms. Often, patients take levodopa/carbidopa (LD/CD) preparations following heavy meals which delays the absorption of the drug and results in delayed/unpredictable action. Simple patient education to take their medicines before meals can at times solve a lot of issues with erratic medicine action for patients. At other times, controlled release formulations have longer plasma half-life and are more useful in patients with shorter duration of action of levodopa. Controlled release preparations are also useful for patients who have frequent night arousals but are too rigid/akinetic at such times to be able to turn in bed. Measures like immediate release/mouth dissolving preparations can be used for quicker onset of action of levodopa alleviating symptoms of delayed on. Another solution to enhance absorption and ensuring a quicker onset of levodopa action is giving a liquid preparation. Liquid levodopa, as this is known as, is prepared by dissolving around 10 tablets of LD/CD (100 mg/25 mg) strength with 1,000 mL of water and adding one vitamin C tablet (500 mg). The patient is instructed to keep this mixture in an opaque container and the total daily desired dose is divided into approximately10 parts (total dose requires is 1,000 mg, then 1,000/10 of 100 mL) given after every 1.5 hours. Required solution should be prepared fresh everyday. This passes through the pylorus easily and results in a quicker and predictable onset of action, counteracting symptoms of delayed or random offs.
- *Addition of monoamine oxidase-B (MAO-B) inhibitors*[7,8] *including selegiline/rasagiline*: Addition of MAO-B inhibitors prolongs the effect of ingested levodopa by inhibiting the breakdown enzyme. Due to the prolonged effect of levodopa, motor fluctuations can potentially be reduced by addition of these drugs. Two large scale trials: PRESTO and LARGO confirmed that MAO-B inhibitors reduce off time when taken along with LD/CD combinations. Selegiline can predispose to insomnias thus is preferably given in morning.
- *Addition of catechol-O-methyltransferase (COMT) inhibitors*[9] *such as entacapone*: Similar to MAO-B inhibitors, this class of drugs also inhibits breakdown of levodopa by the enzyme COMT, thus prolonging its action and reducing fluctuations. There are some concerns of addition of COMT inhibitors, may predispose or worsen dyskinesias (STRIDE-PD study), hence, these may not be a good approach for patients with coexistent dyskinesias.
- *Addition of Dopamine agonists (DAs) such as ropinirole, pramipexole, rotigotine:*[10-12] Dopamine receptor agonists are long-acting drugs, useful in the management of fluctuations, which when added to the existing LD/CD regimen can result in an improvement in off times by up to 2 hours. Pramipexole and ropinirole are similar in pharmacokinetic properties and action but some patients may preferably respond to one over the other. Rotigotine is available as a transdermal patch, thus being useful in perioperative periods or when oral intake is compromised. DA's can also leads to improvements in sleep disturbances. Peripheral edema, drowsiness, and confusion are the commonly encountered side effects. Impulse control problems such as hyperorality, hypersexuality, or gambling can be rare but troublesome side effects.
- *Other measures*: If troublesome off states persist, addition of trihexyphenidyl and amantadine can be tried singly or on combination which may be helpful in some cases.

Noninvasive Treatment Options for Treatment of Dyskinesias Include

- *Optimization of levodopa*: In patients receiving levodopa for PD almost 56% will be expected to have levodopa-induced dyskinesias (LIDs) at the end of 10 years.[13] When a patient presents with dyskinesia, careful relation should be noted to the onset of dyskinesia with timing of levodopa intake. The most common form, i.e., peak dose dyskinesias are addressed easily by reducing individual levodopa dosage at a given time and reducing frequency of administration. Measures such as liquid levodopa may be useful in the management of troublesome dyskinesias as well.
- *Addition of amantadine*:[14] It has various mechanisms of action—increases dopamine release, inhibits dopamine reuptake, and is a N-methyl-D-aspartate (NMDA) receptor antagonist as well. It is one of the few drugs that has convincingly been shown to reduce LID. However, it must be used with caution in the elderly since it can occasionally lead to hallucinations and confusional state.
- Reduction in dosage or stopping MAO-B inhibitors/COMT inhibitors
- *Other options*:
  - *Clozapine*:[15] It is an atypical antipsychotic. It has been found to be useful in management of LID and is especially helpful when patients have coexistent hallucinations. There is a small risk of agranulocytosis in patients taking clozapine, thus total leukocyte count (TLC) monitoring is a must. Agranulocytosis, however, is mostly reversible on discontinuation of the drug.
  - *Memantine*: Some reports suggest some efficacy in reducing dyskinesia by adding memantine. Useful in presence of associated dementia.

- *Dextromethorphan*: A cough suppressant has been found to be useful in suppressing dyskinesias in sporadic studies.
- *Botulinum toxin* is recommended for focal dystonias and early morning dystonias.

Invasive Treatment Options for Management of Fluctuations and Dyskinesias

- *Continuous dopaminergic stimulation*: Based on studies observing that long-acting DAs delayed or decreased the risk of fluctuations and dyskinesias, it has been proposed that continuous dopaminergic stimulation as compared to the tradition pulsatile/discontinuous therapeutic options will be beneficial in reducing the motor complications. For these the available options are:
  - *Continuous subcutaneous apomorphine infusion*:[16] Apomorphine belongs to the class of dopaminergic agonists acting on the D1/D2 receptors. It is available only as a parenteral preparation for subcutaneous use. It has a very rapid onset of action (<5 min) but has short-lasting effect. Subcutaneous apomorphine pens are currently used to inject apomorphine for sudden or random offs when patient becomes suddenly akinetic. When given through continuous subcutaneous infusion pumps, it can be used for continuous dopaminergic stimulation. Thus, patients who have a good response to a test dose of subcutaneous apomorphine and are willing to try subcutaneous infusions pumps [especially when deep brain stimulation (DBS) is contraindicated or cannot be done] are good candidates for this mode of treatment. It has been shown to improve not just the motor fluctuations but also some nonmotor symptoms such as pain, swallowing difficulties, and urinary complaints. It is contraindicated in patients with liver failure, allergies, severe dementia (mild-to-moderate is not a contraindication) and in severe troublesome dyskinesias. Cutaneous or subcutaneous reactions including bruising, subcutaneous nodules, and, rarely, necrosis or abscess formation at injection or infusion sites have been reported. Using standard aseptic precautions, use of new needles for each injection and changing the site of injection can prevent or reduce the same. Nausea (often requiring domperidone), somnolence, and hallucinations can be seen.
  - *Intraduodenal continuous levodopa infusion (duodopa)*:[17] Levodopa, in the form of a carboxymethyl cellulose gel preparation, can be used for continuous infusion via a portable pump directly delivered to duodenum/proximal jejunum through a percutaneous gastrojejunostomy tube. Since this bypasses the pylorus, it ensures predictable and consistent absorption. This, thus, reduces off time and motor fluctuations, significantly improving quality of life of patients. Also, as expected from the continuous stimulation there is no significant increase in troublesome dyskinesias with this method. Side effects, mostly related to the complications of percutaneous gastrojejunostomy, can be seen in up to 14% cases. Patients in whom DBS is contraindicated or not an option can be considered for this form of therapy.
- *Deep brain stimulation*: This has revolutionized the management of advanced PD. For further details, refer to chapter on DBS.

Management of Freezing and Other Nonmotor Symptoms of Advanced Parkinson's Disease

- *Freezing*: Freezing in PD is defined as a brief, episodic absence, or a marked reduction in forward progression of feet despite intention to walk. Freezing is a common and bothersome symptom of PD and also responsible for a large number of falls resulting in fractures. Freezing of gait is usually resistant to traditional management approaches but can be helped with the following:
  - *Visual cues*: Like lines on the floor or pieces of paper glued to the floor which can help the patient overcome freezing.
  - *Reducing off time*: Freezing which is increased in off states can be managed by reducing off time through the above-mentioned approaches.
  - *On state freezing*: Freezing during peak dose effect of levodopa is poorly responsive to treatment and can in fact worsen with strategies to motor fluctuations. There are reports that injection methylphenidate can be useful in some of these cases.
- *Cognitive decline*:[18,19] Dementia is usually a late feature of PD but after 10 years into the illness, almost 30% of patients report some symptoms of cognitive decline. Rivastigmine belonging to the class of cholinesterase inhibitors, is the only Food and Drug Administration (FDA) approved drug for the management of mild-to-moderate PD dementia (PDD). Rivastigmine can also decrease hallucinations in patients of PD with dementia and coexistent hallucinations. Gastrointestinal (GI) symptoms and slight increase in PD tremor is the common side effects. Compliance issues and GI side effects can be bypassed with transdermal route of delivery in the form of rivastigmine skin patch. Other cholinesterase inhibitors can be tried but they have not shown to have an unequivocal benefit. Another important step in management of cognitive decline in these patients is to stop any offending drug which

may cause or exacerbate confusion and cognitive decline in these patients [e.g., trihexiphenidyl, tricyclic antidepressants (TCAs), and DAs].

- *Psychosis*:[20,21] Psychosis, agitation, and hallucinations can be seen in around 30% of patients with PD. Apart from disease progression, it can also be manifestation of side effects of some antiparkinsonian medications (such as amantadine and DAs). The strongest and most effective drug in the management of psychotic symptoms in patients with PD is clozapine. However, it is linked to agranulocytosis in some patients and therefore, complete blood monitoring is a must for patients on this medicine. Other safer options include quetiapine, which is a safer albeit slightly weaker antipsychotic available for PD patients. Since it is also an atypical antipsychotic, worsening of extra-pyramidal symptoms is rare. Pimavanserin, another atypical antipsychotic acts on serotonergic receptors (5-HT2A inverse agonist) instead of dopaminergic receptors, is also available for help in management of psychosis in PD patients and since it does not act on dopamine receptors, there is no risk of worsening of PD symptoms.[22] Typical antipsychotics worsen PD symptoms are best avoided. As is the scenario in PDD, stopping medicines which worsen psychosis (such as anticholinergics, DAs, or amantadine) and ruling out coexisting acute medical illnesses (like urinary tract infection) is an important step in the management of psychosis seen in PD patients. Rivastigmine can be an option for some cases with coexistent dementia.
- *Behavioral symptoms such as depression and anxiety*:[23,24] Depression is a very common (can affect up to 40% of patients of PD) and often overlooked symptom in PD. It can be present alone or with comorbid anxiety. Like motor symptoms, these nonmotor symptoms can also fluctuate and worsen during off states. The two most common classes of drugs available for management of depression and anxiety include TCAs and selective serotonin reuptake inhibitors (SSRIs). SSRIs are safer but may worsen tremors in PD patients. TCA's with their anticholinergic actions can improve the behavioral symptoms as well as improve tremors and help in improving quality of sleep in these patients. The choice between the two depends on the individual case with careful consideration of other comorbidities. In very rare instances, nonpharmacological options such as transcranial magnetic stimulation (TMS) or electroconvulsive therapy (ECT) can be used for severe and refractory cases.[25,26] As previously mentioned, a lot of behavioral symptoms can worsen during off states, so optimization of levodopa therapy is another important step in management of these nonmotor problems.
- *Sleep-related problems*:[27,28] The common sleep-related problems encountered in PD patients of PD include—rapid eye movement (REM) sleep behavior disorder (RBD), insomnia, or excessive day time sleepiness (EDS). RBD can at times lead to harm/injury to the patient or their bed-partners. Management includes steps to improve sleep hygiene (avoid day time naps, no light stimulus in bed room, and day time exercise) and measures to safeguard the environment of the bedroom, to avoid injuring self or their bed-partner. Pharmacological therapies include low doses of clonazepam (sedative) and melatonin at bed time for insomnia and RBD. DAs such as pramipexole and transdermal rotigotine can also improve sleep-related problems in PD patients. All these therapies can, however, result in excessive day time drowsiness and need to be titrated accordingly. For excessive day time sleepiness, first step is to reduce doses of any drugs which may be resulting in sedation (dopamine agonists especially) and a trial of modafinil which can be helpful especially in patients with comorbid obstructive sleep apnea (OSA).
- *Autonomic dysfunction*: Two common manifestations of autonomic dysfunction that can be seen in advanced PD patients include:
  - *Orthostatic hypotension (OH)*:[29] Symptoms such as dizziness on standing, presyncopal symptoms, or even syncope can result from OH [fall in blood pressure (BP) on standing >20/10 mm Hg for systolic and diastolic BP, respectively as compared to supine position at 3 minutes]. Often a difficult symptom to manage, measures to improve OH include use of compression stockings, increase fluid and salt intake, small frequent meals (to reduce postprandial dizziness), use of physical counter maneuvers, and cutting down alcohol intake. Pharmacological measures that can help in OH include use of fludrocortisone (mineralocorticoid) and midodrine (alpha receptor agonist). With all these measures, supine blood pressures have to be carefully monitored to avoid supine hypertension. A new drug, a prodrug of norepinephrine, droxidopa has been found to be very useful in management of symptoms of OH with minimal side effects.
  - *Urinary disturbances*:[30] Common urinary symptoms in PD patients include urgency, increased frequency, and occasionally urge incontinence. Most of these symptoms are due to detrusor hyperactivity and rarely due to comorbid uncontrolled diabetes or urinary tract infections. If these conditions have been ruled out, symptoms of overactive bladder can be managed with antimuscarinics such as solifenacin, tolterodine, trospium chloride, or oxybutynin. In refractory cases, intradetrusor injections of

botulinum toxin may be helpful. In some cases, there are problems of urinary retention, suggesting hypoactive bladder which is mostly drug induced (such as anticholinergics—trihexyphenidyl or TCAs like amitriptyline).

  - *Sexual dysfunction:*[31] Even though erectile dysfunction (ED) is more common and an early feature of multisystem atrophy, a large number of male PD patients in the later stages experience ED, further impairing their quality of life. When present, sildenafil and other phosphodiesterase inhibitors is a relatively safe option if there is no coexistent coronary artery disease or OH. Another option is sublingual apomorphine which has been found to be beneficial in some cases. If conservative measures fail, consultation with a urologist for intrapenile injections and vacuum pumps can be considered.
  - *Other autonomic dysfunction—sweating dysfunction:*[32] Abnormal excess sweating or sweating crises can be occasionally seen in advanced PD patients This can result in both physical and social problems for these individuals. It has been observed that these episodes of excess sweating are mostly an off phenomenon and measures to reduce off periods and addition of DAs is often useful in these individuals.

- *Dysphagia and other GI symptoms:*[33,34] Dysphagia is one of the most troublesome symptoms of advanced PD. It usually is a result of marked pharyngeal muscle bradykinesia and like with other motor symptoms can significantly vary with impact of levodopa. Dysphagia is in itself a risk factor for aspiration pneumonitis and when untreated can lead to dehydration and malnutrition. Dysphagia which is a result of levodopa-related fluctuations can be managed with optimization of levodopa methods as described earlier. For other cases, alternate routes of feeding such as a nasogastric tube or a percutaneous endoscopic gastrostomy tube have to be offered to the patient for proper nutritional support. If there is associated nausea or vomiting experienced by the patient, peripheral dopamine receptor antagonist, i.e., domperidone or a serotonin receptor antagonist like ondansetron may be used. Since domperidone also increases gastric emptying and intestinal motility, it is slightly preferred over ondansetron. Other troublesome GI symptom in advanced PD includes constipation. Management of constipation includes increasing fiber in the diet and adding psyllium husk at night, laxatives such as lactulose or polyethylene glycol and removal of offending drugs such as anticholinergics. Drooling of saliva at night or day time is also one of the disturbing problems. Mostly this is a consequence of pharyngeal bradykinesia and reduced swallowing of saliva rather than an excess production. For these, various options are use of chewing gums, using peripheral anticholinergics like glycopyrrolate and if these measures fail, intraparotid botulinum toxin can be used for decreasing salivary production.
- *Pain:*[35] Pain in PD is a common nonmotor feature (seen in up to 80% of the individuals with PD), both in the early stages of disease as well as in the advanced stages during off periods—it can be very troublesome for the patient. Commonly dull pain in the extremities or aching and stiffness in the shoulder are what the patient is most troubled by. After ruling out a primary joint pathology and/or peripheral neuropathy, a trial of adjustment of antiparkinsonian medicines so as to reduce off periods, is usually helpful. If pain does not respond to this, pregabalin, gabapentin, duloxetine, or analgesics may be added to the treatment regimen for adequate relief. Another reason of pain in advanced PD is painful off period dystonias, which if does not improve with levodopa optimization therapies, can be managed with local botulinum toxin injections.
- *Other symptoms—impulse control disorders (ICD):*[36] Often an iatrogenic symptom, ICDs can be seen in up to 30% of cases. Most commonly seen as a side effect of dopaminergic agonists, these ICDs may manifest as excessive gambling, hypersexuality, or compulsive eating. Other manifestations similar to ICDs include compulsive levodopa consumption (increasing dose of levodopa intake despite side effects like dyskinesias), punding (repetitive handling of objects like constantly rearranging watches or repeatedly folding papers, etc.) These and other ICDs are often difficult to manage. The first step is to stop any agonist drugs in the patients therapeutic regimen. If symptoms do not improve, atypical antipsychotics such as quetiapine in increasing doses may be considered. SSRIs and psychotherapy may also help at times to reduce obsessive symptoms.

CONCLUSION

In summary, all patients of PD in advanced stages suffer from both motor and nonmotor complications which become more challenging than management of primary motor symptoms of PD. Management options are rather limited and need to be carefully handled. These problems are sometimes more important to treat than the basic symptoms of PD. Optimization of levodopa therapy, addition of other dopaminergic drugs, and some invasive treatment options can all be helpful. Also to remember, nonpharmacological approaches such as physiotherapy and speech therapy have an equally important role in the management of the patient and improvement in quality of life. A final thing to note is a lot of times, therapeutic regimens and drug-drug interactions may be the cause of the patient's problem, and thus removal of an offending drug, reduction of dose in some medications, and reducing the overall medications might do more benefit to the patient than trying a new pharmacologic agent. Sometimes DBS is required for their treatment.

REFERENCES

1. López IC, Ruiz PJ, del Pozo SV, Bernardos VS. Motor complications in Parkinson's disease: ten year follow-up study. Mov Disord. 2010;25(16):2735-9.
2. Hely MA, Morris JG, Reid WG, Trafficante R. Sydney Multicenter Study of Parkinson's disease: non-L-dopa-responsive problems dominate at 15 years. Mov Disord. 2005;20(2):190-9.
3. Hoehn MM, Yahr MD. Parkinsonism: onset, progression and mortality. Neurology. 1967;17(5):427-42.
4. Fahn, Stanley, Joseph Jankovic J, and Mark Hallett M, Fahn S. Principles and Practice of Movement Disorders, 2nd edition. Elsevier; 2011:141.
5. Metman LV, Konitsiotis S, Chase TN. Pathophysiology of motor response complications in Parkinson's disease: Hypotheses on the why, where, and what. Mov Disord. 2000;15 (1):3-8.
6. Ossig C, Reichmann H. Treatment strategies in early and advanced Parkinson disease. Neurol Clin. 2015;33(1):19-37.
7. Parkinson Study Group. A randomized placebo-controlled trial of rasagiline in levodopa-treated patients with Parkinson disease and motor fluctuations: the PRESTO study. Arch Neurol. 2005;62(2):241-8.
8. Rascol O, Brooks DJ, Melamed E, Oertel W, Poewe W, Stocchi F, et al. Rasagiline as an adjunct to levodopa in patients with Parkinson's disease and motor fluctuations (LARGO, Lasting effect in Adjunct therapy with Rasagiline Given Once daily, study): a randomised, double-blind, parallel-group trial. Lancet. 2005;365(9463):947-54.
9. Stocchi F, Rascol O, Kieburtz K, Poewe W, Jankovic J, Tolosa E, et al. Initiating levodopa/carbidopa therapy with and without entacapone in early Parkinson disease: the STRIDE-PD study. Ann Neurol. 2010;68(1):18-27.
10. Iida M, Miyazaki I, Tanaka K, Kabuto H, Iwata-Ichikawa E, Ogawa N, et al. Dopamine D2 receptor-mediated antioxidant and neuroprotective effects of ropinirole, a dopamine agonist. Brain Res. 1999;838(1–2):51-9.
11. Zou L, Jankovic J, Rowe DB, Xie W, Appel SH, Le W, et al. Neuroprotection by pramipexole against dopamine-and levodopa-induced cytotoxicity. Life Sci. 1999;64(15):1275-85.
12. Trenkwalder C, Kies B, Rudzinska M, Fine J, Nikl J, Honczarenko K, et al. Rotigotine effects on early morning motor function and sleep in Parkinson's disease: a double-blind, randomized, placebo-controlled study (RECOVER). Mov Disord. 2011;26(1):90-9.
13. Blanchet PJ, Allard P, Gregoire L, Tardif F, Bédard PJ, et al. Risk factors for peak dose dyskinesia in 100 levodopa-treated parkinsonian patients. Can J Neurol Sci. 1996;23(3):189-93.
14. Ferreira JJ, Katzenschlager R, Bloem BR, Bonuccelli U, Burn D, Deuschl G, et al. Summary of the recommendations of the EFNS/MDS-ES review on therapeutic management of Parkinson's disease. Eur J Neurol. 2013;20(1):5-15.
15. Fox SH, Katzenschlager R, Lim SY, Ravina B, Seppi K, Coelho M, et al. The movement disorder society evidence-based medicine review update: Treatments for the motor symptoms of Parkinson's disease. Mov Disord. 2011;26(Suppl 3):S2-41.
16. Frankel JP, Lees AJ, Kempster PA, Stern GM. Subcutaneous apomorphine in the treatment of Parkinson's disease. J Neurol Neurosurg Psychiatry. 1990;53:96-101.
17. Kurth MC, Tetrud JW, Tanner CM, Irwin I, Stebbins GT, Goetz CG, et al. Double-blind, placebo-controlled, crossover study of duodenal infusion of levodopa/carbidopa in Parkinson's disease patients with "on-off" fluctuations. Neurology. 1993;43(9):1698-703.
18. Aarsland D, Zaccai J, Brayne C. A systematic review of prevalence studies of dementia in Parkinson's disease. Mov Disord. 2005;20(10):1255-63.
19. Emre M, Aarsland D, Albanese A, Byrne EJ, Deuschl G, de Deyn PP, et al. Rivastigmine for dementia associated with Parkinson's disease. N Engl J Med. 2004;351:2509-18.
20. Aarsland D, Larsen JP, Lim NG, Janvin C, Karlsen K, Tandberg E, et al. Range of neuropsychiatric disturbances in patients with Parkinson's disease. J Neurol Neurosurg Psychiatry. 1999;67(4):492-6.
21. Merims D, Balas M, Peretz C, Shabtai H, Giladi N. Rater-blinded, prospective comparison: quetiapine versus clozapine for Parkinson's disease psychosis. Clin Neuropharmacol. 2006;29:331-7.
22. Espay AJ, Guskey MT, Norton JC, Coate B, Vizcarra JA, Ballard C, et al. Pimavanserin for Parkinson's Disease psychosis: Effects stratified by baseline cognition and use of cognitive-enhancing medications. Mov Disord. 2018;33(11):1769-76.
23. Reijnders JS, Ehrt U, Weber WE, Aarsland D, Leentjens AF. A systematic review of prevalence studies of depression in Parkinson's disease. Mov Disord. 2008;23(2):183-9.
24. Price A, Rayner L, Okon-Rocha E, Evans A, Valsraj K, Higginson IJ, et al. Antidepressants for the treatment of depression in neurological disorders: a systematic review and meta-analysis of randomised controlled trials. J Neurol Neurosurg Psychiatry. 2011;82(8):914-23.
25. Boggio PS, Fregni F, Bermpohl F, Mansur CG, Rosa M, Rumi DO, et al. Effect of repetitive TMS and fluoxetine on cognitive function in patients with Parkinson's disease and concurrent depression. Mov Disord. 2005;20(9):1178-84.
26. Borisovskaya A, Bryson WC, Buchholz J, Samii A, Borson S. Electroconvulsive therapy for depression in Parkinson's disease: systematic review of evidence and recommendations. Neurodegener Dis Manag. 2016;6(2):161-76.
27. Aurora RN, Zak RS, Maganti RK, Auerbach SH, Casey KR, Chowdhuri S, et al. Best practice guide for the treatment of REM sleep behavior disorder (RBD). J Clin Sleep Med. 2010;6(1):85-95.

28. Shen Y, Huang JY, Li J, Liu CF. Excessive Daytime Sleepiness in Parkinson's Disease: Clinical Implications and Management. Chin Med J (Engl). 2018;131(8):974-81.
29. Sánchez-Ferro A, Benito-León J, Gómez-Esteban JC. The management of orthostatic hypotension in Parkinson's disease. Front Neurol. 2013;4:64.
30. Singer C. Urinary dysfunction in Parkinson's disease. Clin Neurosci. 1998;5(2):78-86.
31. Bronner G, Vodušek DB. Management of sexual dysfunction in Parkinson's disease. Ther Adv Neurol Disord. 2011;4(6):375-83.
32. Swinn L, Schrag A, Viswanathan R, Bloem BR, Lees A, Quinn N. Sweating dysfunction in Parkinson's disease. Mov Disord. 2003;18(12):1459-63.
33. Suttrup I, Warnecke T. Dysphagia in Parkinson's Disease. Dysphagia. 2016;31(1):24-32.
34. Edwards LL, Pfeiffer RF, Quigley EMM, Hofman R, Balluff M. Gastrointestinal symptoms in Parkinson's disease. Mov Disord. 1991;6(2):151-6.
35. Sophie M, Ford B. Management of pain in Parkinson's disease. CNS Drugs. 2012;26(11):937-48.
36. Erga AH, Alves G, Larsen JP, Tysnes OB, Pedersen KF. Impulsive and Compulsive Behaviors in Parkinson's Disease: The Norwegian ParkWest Study. J Parkinsons Dis. 2017;7(1): 183-91.

CHAPTER 22

Surgical Management of Parkinson's Disease

Natasha Tipnis, Paresh K Doshi, Pettarusp M Wadia

HISTORY AND INTRODUCTION TO SURGICAL THERAPY FOR PARKINSON'S DISEASE

Surgical therapies were introduced for the treatment of movement disorders like Parkinson's disease (PD) as early as the 1940s. Lesions in the thalamus were performed well before the introduction of levodopa (L-DOPA). However, in the absence of good imaging technology such as computed tomography (CT) scans and magnetic resonance imaging (MRIs) the results were variable and these procedures faded into oblivion, more so with the introduction of L-DOPA in the 1960s.

Levodopa was a revolution in the treatment of PD. However, long-term L-DOPA therapy resulted in the development of motor fluctuations (on and off fluctuations) and dyskinesias which can be more disabling than the disease itself.

The problems with frequent drug dosing, adverse effects, and disease fluctuations coupled with newer imaging techniques led to revival of surgical therapy for PD. Initial treatment focused on lesion surgeries—pallidotomy and thalamotomy. The discovery that high frequency deep brain stimulation (DBS) could mimic the effects of ablation in an adjustable and reversible manner revived surgical treatments for movement disorders.[1-3]

SELECTING A CANDIDATE WITH PARKINSON'S DISEASE FOR DEEP BRAIN STIMULATION

Deep brain stimulation is most effective in patients who are properly selected. In a review of patients of DBS failure >30% were associated with issues related to patient selection.[4] Several factors need to be considered before determining if a patient is an appropriate candidate for DBS surgery. Firstly, it is important that the clinical diagnosis of idiopathic PD is confirmed using standard clinical criteria[5] and disorders which can mimic PD such as multiple system atrophy and progressive supranuclear palsy (PSP) are excluded by a detailed clinical evaluation. Of the cases with atypical Parkinsonism, patients with PSP-Parkinsonism phenotype (PSP-P) can have a good response to L-DOPA, may not manifest eye signs in the initial years.[6] Rapid onset and prominent axial symptoms should raise a suspicion for atypical Parkinsonism in these cases.[6,7]

Patients with PD with on-off motor fluctuations when medication intervals are short (2–3 h), troublesome dyskinesias, or have refractory tremors that are affecting the quality of life despite best medical therapy are candidates for surgery.[8-10]

Age, disease duration, response to L-DOPA, and other comorbid conditions are other important considerations when selecting a candidate for DBS (**Table 1**).[11]

An L-DOPA challenge is performed prior to surgery following a withdrawal of antidopaminergic medication for a period of at least 12 hours. A minimum 33% improvement in the motor Unified Parkinson's Disease Rating Scale (UPDRS) is the minimum requirement before considering DBS.[8,9] The L-DOPA challenge also offers the opportunity to demonstrate the extent to which the Parkinsonian symptoms would improve after surgery. One should not expect an improvement in function greater than the best "ON medication period" with the concomitant reduction of dyskinesias. Tremor is the only exception which can improve with ventrointermediate nucleus (VIM) and subthalamic nucleus (STN) DBS even it is not significantly affected by L-DOPA. Axial and gait symptoms are less likely to be impacted than appendicular symptoms.[12]

TABLE 1: Factors determining selection of patients for bilateral DBS.

Factor	*Criteria for surgical candidate*	*Remarks*
Age	Not defined and concerns beyond 70 years	• Older patients had worse axial subscores which improve to a lesser extent and significant worsening of postoperative cognitive performance in older group[54] • Quality of life improvements less in elderly patients[55]
Response to L-DOPA	>33% improvement in UPDRS III scores with L-DOPA	Response to L-DOPA mirrors the expected response postsurgery. Gait and axial symptoms are less likely to improve post STN DBS especially if not L-DOPA responsive, tremors may improve even if not responsive to L-DOPA[8]
Neuropsychological issues	No clear selection criteria, but address and treat any preoperative depression or mood disorders	Watch for depression and hypomania, cases of suicidal ideation and suicidal behavior have been reported post DBS.[56] This has been linked to rapid withdrawal of dopaminergic medication[57]
Neuropsychiatric issues	Frank dementia-contraindicated and MCI weigh options carefully	• Reduced verbal fluency noted post DBS[30,58] • 11% DBS patients had multilevel cognitive decline versus 3% in best medical treatment group.[23] No difference in GPi versus STN DBS[23]

(DBS: deep brain stimulation; GPi: globus pallidus internus; MCI: mild cognitive impairment; STN: subthalamic nucleus; UPDRS: Unified Parkinson Disease Rating Scale)

Neuropsychological evaluation is another important presurgical assessment. Patients with significant depression at a risk of suicide are at an elevated risk of surgery and may be treated appropriately prior to being reconsidered for DBS.[13] DBS for PD does not seem to cause permanent cognitive changes. However, patients who present with cognitive decline or dementia preoperatively are at a risk of further cognitive decline after surgery making it a relative contraindication. A staged procedure is an alternative to simultaneous bilateral surgery or globus pallidus internus (GPi) may be considered as a target (see below) in patients with borderline cognitive function, especially if they have significant motor disability.

TIMING OF DEEP BRAIN STIMULATION—EARLY VERSUS LATE

In most centers DBS has been offered to patients when their motor fluctuations including disabling wearing off, significant dyskinesias, or tremors start to hamper their quality of life. In most cases the average time to DBS has been 10 years or more from onset of symptoms. There has been growing enthusiasm to offer DBS earlier in the disease course as early as 5 years from disease onset in patients with an aim to enhance quality of life[14] and occupational gains.[14,15] The advantages of this strategy need to be carefully balanced with the risk of missing features of atypical Parkinsonism which may not have manifested at this stage.[6]

TARGET FOR STIMULATION AND EFFICACY DATA

Initial ablative surgeries were performed targeting the VIM of the thalamus (for tremors), pallidotomy (for dyskinesias), and motor cortex.[3] Subsequently, VIM stimulation was used to control tremors in PD.[3] VIM stimulation does not control symptoms other than tremors. This has resulted in a shift to using bilateral STN DBS for PD (**Table 2**).[16] In the last decade increasing data has shown GPi to be an alternate target with similar improvements as compared to STN DBS.[17-21] A recent meta-analysis of studies comparing STN and GPi as a target showed no difference in activities of daily living or ON medication and ON stimulation UPDRS scores in the two groups.[22] However, the OFF medication UPDRS scores tended to be significantly lower in the STN group compared to the GPi group with significantly lower L-DOPA equivalent scores in the STN group.[22] Initial data showed that patients with STN DBS have a reduction in processing speed and verbal fluency following DBS which prompted the suggestion of using GPi as a target in patients with mild-cognitively impaired (MCI).[19] The differences in cognitive performance in patients with bilateral STN versus bilateral GPi DBS are slight and the choice of target needs to be weighed carefully (**Table 2**).[23]

Subthalamic nucleus, being a smaller target, tends to require less electrical stimulation and may therefore require slightly fewer frequent battery changes.[11] STN stimulation markedly improves dyskinesias, motor fluctuations, Parkinsonian motor signs, activities of daily living, and quality of life scores as compared to patients with advanced PD on best medical treatment.[24,25] STN stimulation has also been found to reduce nonmotor fluctuations, especially sensory, dysautonomic, and cognitive fluctuations.[26] Long-term safety and efficacy of bilateral STN has been established.[27-29] In the long-term follow-up the UPDRS motor scores increase overtime indicating that DBS is a symptomatic treatment. The change was found to be more in the ON medication UPDRS scores compared to the OFF medication UPDRS scores. Improvement in rigidity and tremors were more sustained compared to bradykinesia

TABLE 2: Targets for DBS in Parkinson's disease and status.

Target	Efficacy benefit	Disadvantages	Advantages as a target	Status
STN	Bilateral STN DBS superior to best medical therapy and sham DBS[24,25]	Verbal fluency reduced and concerns of acceleration of cognitive decline	Better medication reduction, improves OFF medication UPDRS, and longer battery life	The most widely used target. Concerns in patients with pre-existing cognitive decline
GPi	No difference in activities of daily living or ON medication, ON stimulation UPDRS scores compared to STN DBS[22]	Higher battery consumption, less L-DOPA reduction, and OFF UPDRS does not reduce to the same extent	Reduces dyskinesias and verbal fluency less affected	Alternative target to STN. Some advantage in those with cognitive decline[19]
VIM	Benefits only for tremors[3]	Does not benefit other PD symptoms	Only tremors are controlled	Abandoned as a target[16]
PPN	Investigated for benefits in gait freezing and falls	Targeting the PPN region is technically challenging[59]		• Difficulty in demons-trating objective benefit[60] • Still a research target[61]

(DBS: deep brain stimulation; GPi: globus pallidus internus; PD: Parkinson's disease; PPN: pedunculopontine nucleus; STN: subthalamic nucleus; UPDRS: Unified Parkinson Disease Rating Scale; VIM: ventrointermediate nucleus)

and postural imbalance and gait disturbance (axial signs) which tended to worsen overtime indicating disease progression. [28] Long-term cognitive evaluation 8 years post DBS, revealed a similar trend of cognitive decline in the STN DBS and nonoperated group with the exception of verbal fluency which was lower in the STN DBS group.[30]

SURGICAL TECHNIQUE

Deep brain stimulation is traditionally has been performed with the patient awake so as to facilitate localization. Better imaging guidance in recent times prompted the suggestion of direct targeting under general anesthesia.[31] General anesthesia may be required in patients with severe intolerable off symptoms, children, or those with anxiety. The results of patients operated under local anesthesia versus general anesthesia were found to be comparable in a single center study.[32]

Deep brain stimulation can be undertaken is done in two steps. The first one is done awake when the electrodes are implanted in the target (STN or GPi usually, see below). The second step involves implanting the implantable pulse generator (IPG) and connecting the IPG to the implanted electrodes, usually done under general anesthesia. Both the steps may be done on the same day or more often are performed on two different days.[8]

The localization of electrodes to the appropriate target location is performed either using a stereotactic frame or more recently frameless, using advanced imaging techniques that aid the placement of electrodes in the target. Electrophysiological mapping using microelectrode recording (MER) has been widely practiced. However, advanced imaging techniques like intraoperative MRI have put the utility of MER into question.[31,33] After MER recording, intraoperative clinical assessment for efficacy and side effects of stimulation to confirm appropriate electrode placement is carried out in the operative room.

POSTOPERATIVE PROGRAMMING

Programming of the deep brain stimulator is done after surgery, usually in the OFF-medication state. The contact point or points on the electrode that best improve the motor signs are first carefully selected. For each contact or combination thereof, the current (in volts), frequency, and pulse width (spread of current) can be adjusted to best improve the clinical symptoms and signs. Adjusting the stimulator and medications after electrode implantation can take time depending on the degree of lesion effect seen in the postoperative period. Hence, it may take weeks or even months after the procedure to see the maximal clinical effect of the procedure.

The initial programming is preferably done once the lesion effect settles and rigidity, tremor, and bradykinesia can be seen in the OFF-medication phase. Programming is done in the OFF-medication phase. It consists of identifying the best contacts by doing a stepwise monopolar contact review assessing for an improvement in rigidity, bradykinesia, and tremors on each side.[34] Usually this is done by keeping the pulse width and frequency constant at default settings of 60 μs and 130 Hz, respectively. During the initial programming threshold for side effects are established and best contacts are identified on each side. Stimulation side effects determining thresholds include stimulation somatosensory (paresthesia), motor (muscle spasms, gaze/eye deviation, stimulation induced dyskinesias, or dystonia), dysautonomia, behavioral side effects (mania and depression) or nonspecific side effects (confusion and malaise).[35] Somatosensory side effects and nonspecific effects usually are transient and habituate.

Paresthesias may become permanent at higher voltages. Remaining side effects do not habituate. Stimulation induced dyskinesias usually manifest few hours or days after initial parameter adjustment.[35] The voltage is gradually increased up to the threshold with simultaneous reduction in dopaminergic medication.[34] If adequate monopolar stimulation fails to control the motor symptoms, different contact configurations can be tried including bipolar, multipolar, and interleaving patterns.[36] In cases of freezing of gait, low frequency stimulation can be beneficial.[37] The pulse width has traditionally been fixed at 60 Hz. Reduction of pulse width has been shown to expand the therapeutic window by reducing current spread to other areas, thereby improving motor outcomes.[38]

Use of directional leads has the potential to steer current toward the target limiting side effects.[36] However, the time taken for programming may significantly increase. Research is also ongoing in the technique of closed loop or adaptive DBS where local field potentials could guide the stimulation delivered to the brain thereby saving battery life and avoiding stimulation-related adverse effects.[39]

SAFETY

Risks for DBS procedures (**Table 3**) include perioperative surgical risks (postoperative confusion, intracranial and intraventricular hemorrhage, and air embolism), infection, and hardware complications[40,41] and stimulation-induced side effects including neuropsychiatric complications.[12,42,43] Incidence of postoperative confusion has ranged from 3.9 to 33%. Elderly patients, more advanced disease, longer time spent in exploration during surgery and higher number of MER trajectories are associated with a higher risk for the same.[41] In most cases the confusion resolves sometimes taking even longer than 1 week. IPG placement may have to be deferred till postoperative confusion reduces.[41] Intraventricular or intracranial hemorrhage is the most dreaded complication. Use of MER, a rigid cannula for lead insertion, hypertension are associated with a higher prevalence of hemorrhage. Proper planning of trajectories to avoid sulci, advances in MRI imaging, and strict intraoperative control of blood pressure may minimize the risk of hemorrhage.[41] Infections are another dreaded complication. Wound infection can occur beyond the 1st year of surgery and constitutes a long-term risk.[44] Some may require surgical treatment, more severe cases may require explantation of the leads and IPG and reimplantation once the infection subsides.[41] Hardware-related complication such as lead displacement and fractures are lower in PD versus dystonia (**Table 3**). However, lead malposition is a significant problem across series reducing the benefit from DBS in those cases.[41,44]

While stimulation can cause temporary side effects which determine the threshold, stimulation can also cause worsening of speech and stimulation induced dyskinesias/dystonia.[35] Speech impairment has been thought to occur due to current spread to internal capsule (strained or spastic speech) or spread to pallidofugal and thalamocortical fibers (stuttering or hypophonic). Reduction in voltage, using bipolar configuration or low frequency stimulation have been suggested.[35] To avoid stimulation induced dyskinesias gradual escalation of stimulation and simultaneous dopaminergic dose reduction are required. In some cases there are low thresholds for dyskinesias requiring different programing options (**Table 3**).

As DBS surgeries have become more frequent, rare but serious neuropsychiatric adverse events have been recognized, more so with STN stimulation.[12,42,43] Onset or worsening of depression with a small but significant risk of suicide occurs postoperatively in a small percentage of patients, often in those who were at increased risk before the procedure.[12,42,45] Careful preoperative screening and gradual withdrawal of dopamine agonists (compared to rapid withdrawal) and careful postoperative follow-up can minimize the risk. Hypomania and mania have been reported mainly due to stimulation of the ventral contacts triggering a manic episode. Change in contacts usually can resolve this devastating side effect.[46] Long-term worsening of axial symptoms and gait is a common long-term challenge following DBS. Gait freezing, festination, and postural instability often respond poorly to DBS.[47] Optimizing stimulation, combining substantia nigra pars reticulata (SNr) and STN stimulation (interleaving) and low frequency stimulation have been different strategies recommended.[35] Other less common adverse effects are mentioned in **Table 3**.

LESION SURGERIES AND THEIR CURRENT ROLE

In 1952, Irving Cooper serendipitously performed the first pallidotomy by accidentally ligating the anterior choroidal artery in a patient with postencephalitic tremors. The modern interest in lesioning surgery for PD was reviewed by Lauri Laitinen who revisited Lars Leksell pallidotomy results and advocated that the lesioning of ventroposterolateral GPi can relieve the symptoms of PD. Pallidotomy addressed all the cardinal symptoms of PD, i.e. tremors, rigidity, and bradykinesia on the contralateral side. There was some amount of motor benefit also in the initial few months, that was lost on longer follow-ups.[48] The additional benefits that pallidotomy offered was for off period pain and dyskinesias. Though the classic pallidotomy practiced by Latinen was performed using radiofrequency lesioning, several groups used radiosurgery to obtain similar results.[49] Some groups did practice thalamotomy, as it was very effective in relieving tremors, but as it did not offer any sustained long-term benefit for other Parkinsonian symptoms, it was abandoned. The movement disorder society and Evidence-Based Medicine Task Force recommend pallidotomy as an efficacious treatment for motor fluctuations and dyskinesias.[50]

TABLE 3: Risks and complications of DBS.

Side effect	*Prevalence*	*Troubleshooting*
Surgical complications (perioperative period):		
Hemorrhage (intracerebral/ventricular)	0.6–3.5%	Careful planning of trajectories and strict intraoperative control of blood pressure
Postoperative confusion/delirium[41]	3.9–33%	IPG placement may need to be deferred
Vasovagal attack[41]		Fixing frame on the OR table and in a semireclining position may help
Pneumocephalus		Oxygen with a rebreathing mask
Seizures[44]		Short-term antiepileptics may be required
Anxiety[44]		Dexmedetomidine infusion can be given safely[62]
Impaired wound healing[44]	3.1%	
Pain and headache[44]		Paracetamol
Paresthesia		
Device related:		
Lead malposition[41,44]	1.2%	Avoid shifts due to pneuomcephalus, confirm lead position with MER, stimulation, and fluoroscopy
Infection and erosion	1–8%	May need explantation and subsequent reimplantation
Lead fracture		Important to record impedance of system regularly to identify these problems early. X-rays may identify the problem. May need surgical replacements
Lead displacement		
Cable entanglement		
Cable discomfort		
Stimulator failure		Replace IPG
Battery failure		Replace IPG
Stimulation related:		
Speech impairment	14%	Reduction of amplitudes, bipolar stimulation, and low frequency stimulation[35]
Stimulation-induced dyskinesias/dystonia		Different electrode configurations, interleaving, low frequency stimulation, lower voltages[35]
Cognitive (reduction of verbal fluency)[30]		Cholinesterase inhibitors and memantine
Psychosis/Hallucinations		May need to change contact, clozapine, quetiapine, and pimavanserin can be tried
Depression and apathy[45]		Avoid rapid withdrawal of agonist, preoperative neuropsychology assessment, and early use of antidepressants, if necessary
Suicidal ideation[45,63]		
Hypomania/Mania[46]	4–15%	Change in contact (usually dorsal contacts)
Hypersexuality and impulse control disorders		DBS may improve or worsen ICDs. Mixed results from studies[47]
Blepharospasm/Apraxia or eyelid opening[64]	1.8–3%	Botulinum toxin injections to pretarsal orbicularis oculi muscle
Diplopia		Reduce stimulation
Gait disorders[35]		Optimize stimulation, interleaving, SNr and STN stimulation, and frequency modulation

(DBS: deep brain stimulation; ICD: impulse control disorders; IPG: implantable pulse generator; MER: microelectrode recording; OR: operation room; STN: subthalamic nucleus)

Subthalamic nucleus, the main target for DBS in PD, has also been an area of interest for lesioning surgeries. Amongst the few centers practicing subthalamotomy, most of them performed unilateral lesioning. The largest reported experience involved 89 patients, in whom follow-up demonstrated that from an initial 50% reduction in UPDRS on the contralateral side at 1 year, the improvement reduced to 18% at 36 months.[51] Magnetic resonance-guided focused ultrasound (MRgFUS) has been performed in an open label study in ten patients. There was around 50% improvement in motor UPDRS, in a short-term follow-up. The main side effects were gait disturbance, which resolved in few weeks.[52] There has been a similar experience with MRgFUS unilateral pallidotomy in two independent case series.[53] The lesioning procedures are irreversible by nature and hence need more precision and understanding of the anatomy. The major side effects such as hemorrhage, hemiparesis, and dysarthria are in an acceptable range in expert hands. The author Paresh K Doshi (PKD) has a personal experience (unpublished) of >100 lesional procedures, including subthalamotomy and pallidotomy for PD.[65] We have found that there is a large amount of variability in the level of response in subthalamotomy and hence the lesions have to be tailored to individual patient, based on the length of the MER recordings and intraoperative physiology. The risk of hemiballism or uncontrolled chorea is minimal.

CONCLUSION

Deep brain stimulation is a major advancement in the management of PD to improve the quality of life of patients. Not everyone is eligible and careful selection of patients is required. Presently there is not much evidence to suggest that STN is a better target than the GPi, experience of the center is likely to guide this decision till further evidence is available. Major advances in programming, electrodes like directional leads, and the possibility of on demand or adaptive DBS are likely to revolutionize this ever-advancing field.

REFERENCES

1. Benabid AL, Pollak P, Gross C, Hoffmann D, Benazzouz A, Gao DM, et al. Acute and long-term effects of subthalamic nucleus stimulation in Parkinson's disease. Stereotact Funct Neurosurg. 1994;62(1-4):76-84.
2. Benabid AL, Chabardes S, Mitrofanis J, Pollak P. Deep brain stimulation of the subthalamic nucleus for the treatment of Parkinson's disease. Lancet Neurol. 2009;8(1):67-81.
3. Benabid AL, Pollak P, Gervason C, Hoffmann D, Gao DM, Hommel M, et al. Long-term suppression of tremor by chronic stimulation of the ventral intermediate thalamic nucleus. Lancet. 1991;337(8738):403-6.
4. Okun MS, Tagliati M, Pourfar M, Fernandez HH, Rodriguez RL, Alterman RL, et al. Management of referred deep brain stimulation failures: a retrospective analysis from 2 movement disorders centers. Arch Neurol. 2005;62(8):1250-5.
5. Hughes AJ, Daniel SE, Kilford L, Lees AJ. Accuracy of clinical diagnosis of idiopathic Parkinson's disease: a clinico-pathological study of 100 cases. J Neurol Neurosurg Psychiatry. 1992;55(3):181-4.
6. Williams DR, Lees AJ. Progressive supranuclear palsy: clinicopathological concepts and diagnostic challenges. Lancet Neurol. 2009;8(3):270-9.
7. Williams DR, Lees AJ. What features improve the accuracy of the clinical diagnosis of progressive supranuclear palsy-parkinsonism (PSP-P)? Mov Disord. 2010;25(3):357-62.
8. Machado A, Rezai AR, Kopell BH, Gross RE, Sharan AD, Benabid AL. Deep brain stimulation for Parkinson's disease: surgical technique and perioperative management. Mov Disord. 2006;21(Suppl 14):S247-58.
9. Lang AE, Widner H. Deep Brain stimulation for Parkinson's disease: Patient selection and Evaluation. Mov Disord. 2002;17(Suppl 3):S94-101.
10. Okun MS, Foote KD. Parkinson's disease DBS: what, when, who and why? The time has come to tailor DBS targets. Expert Rev Neurother. 2010;10(12):1847-57.
11. Shukla AW, Okun MS. Surgical treatment of Parkinson's disease: patients, targets, devices, and approaches. Neurotherapeutics. 2014;11(1):47-59.
12. Voon V, Saint-Cyr J, Lozano AM, Moro E, Poon YY, Lang AE. Psychiatric symptoms in patients with Parkinson disease presenting for deep brain stimulation surgery. J Neurosurg. 2005;103(2):246-51.
13. Witt K, Daniels C, Reiff J, Krack P, Volkmann J, Pinsker MO, et al. Neuropsychological and psychiatric changes after deep brain stimulation for Parkinson's disease: a randomised, multicentre study. Lancet Neurol. 2008;7(7):605-14.
14. Deuschl G, Schupbach M, Knudsen K, Pinsker MO, Cornu P, Rau J, et al. Stimulation of the subthalamic nucleus at an earlier disease stage of Parkinson's disease: Concept and standards of the EARLYSTIM-study. Parkinsonism Relat Disord. 2013;19(1):56-61.
15. Schuepbach WM, Rau J, Knudsen K, Volkmann J, Krack P, Timmermann L, et al. Neurostimulation for Parkinson's disease with early motor complications. N Engl J Med. 2013;368(7):610-22.
16. Kumar R, Lozano AM, Sime E, Lang AE. Long-term follow-up of thalamic deep brain stimulation for essential and parkinsonian tremor. Neurology. 2003;61(11):1601-4.

17. Follett KA, Weaver FM, Stern M, Hur K, Harris CL, Luo P, et al. Pallidal versus subthalamic deep-brain stimulation for Parkinson's disease. N Engl J Med. 2010;362(22):2077-91.
18. Odekerken VJ, van Laar T, Staal MJ, Mosch A, Hoffmann CF, Nijssen PC, et al. Subthalamic nucleus versus globus pallidus bilateral deep brain stimulation for advanced Parkinson's disease (NSTAPS study): a randomised controlled trial. Lancet Neurol. 2013;12(1):37-44.
19. Okun MS, Fernandez HH, Wu SS, Kirsch-Darrow L, Bowers D, Bova F, et al. Cognition and mood in Parkinson's disease in subthalamic nucleus versus globus pallidus interna deep brain stimulation: the COMPARE trial. Ann Neurol. 2009;65(5):586-95.
20. Nakamura K, Christine CW, Starr PA, Marks WJ Jr. Effects of unilateral subthalamic and pallidal deep brain stimulation on fine motor functions in Parkinson's disease. Mov Disord. 2007;22(5):619-26.
21. Evidente VG, Premkumar AP, Adler CH, Caviness JN, Driver-Dunckley E, Lyons MK. Medication dose reductions after pallidal versus subthalamic stimulation in patients with Parkinson's disease. Acta Neurol Scand. 2011;124(3):211-4.
22. Xu H, Zheng F, Krischek B, Ding W, Xiong C, Wang X, et al. Subthalamic nucleus and globus pallidus internus stimulation for the treatment of Parkinson's disease: A systematic review. J Int Med Res. 2017;45(5):1602-12.
23. Rothlind JC, York MK, Carlson K, Luo P, Marks WJ Jr, Weaver FM, et al. Neuropsychological changes following deep brain stimulation surgery for Parkinson's disease: comparisons of treatment at pallidal and subthalamic targets versus best medical therapy. J Neurol Neurosurg Psychiatry. 2015;86(6):622-9.
24. Deuschl G, Schade-Brittinger C, Krack P, Volkmann J, Schafer H, Botzel K, et al. A randomized trial of deep-brain stimulation for Parkinson's disease. N Engl J Med. 2006;355(9):896-908.
25. Weaver FM, Follett K, Stern M, Hur K, Harris C, Marks WJ Jr, et al. Bilateral deep brain stimulation vs best medical therapy for patients with advanced Parkinson disease: a randomized controlled trial. JAMA. 2009;301(1):63-73.
26. Witjas T, Kaphan E, Regis J, Jouve E, Cherif AA, Peragut JC, et al. Effects of chronic subthalamic stimulation on nonmotor fluctuations in Parkinson's disease. Mov Disord. 2007;22(12):1729-34.
27. Kishore A, Rao R, Krishnan S, Panikar D, Sarma G, Sivasanakaran MP, et al. Long-term stability of effects of subthalamic stimulation in Parkinson's disease: Indian Experience. Mov Disord. 2010;25(14):2438-44.
28. Limousin P, Foltynie T. Long-term outcomes of deep brain stimulation in Parkinson disease. Nat Rev Neurol. 2019;15(4):234-42.
29. Moro E, Lozano AM, Pollak P, Agid Y, Rehncrona S, Volkmann J, et al. Long-term results of a multicenter study on subthalamic and pallidal stimulation in Parkinson's disease. Mov Disord. 2010;25(5):578-86.
30. Zangaglia R, Pasotti C, Mancini F, Servello D, Sinforiani E, Pacchetti C. Deep brain stimulation and cognition in Parkinson's disease: an eight-year follow-up study. Mov Disord. 2012;27(9):1192-4.
31. Bezchlibnyk YB, Sharma VD, Naik KB, Isbaine F, Gale JT, Cheng J, et al. Clinical outcomes of globus pallidus deep brain stimulation for Parkinson disease: a comparison of intraoperative MRI- and MER-guided lead placement. J Neurosurg. 2020:1-11.
32. Tsai ST, Chen TY, Lin SH, Chen SY. Five-Year Clinical Outcomes of Local versus General Anesthesia Deep Brain Stimulation for Parkinson's Disease. Parkinsons Dis. 2019;2019:5676345.
33. Soares MI, Soares-Dos-Reis R, Rosas MJ, Monteiro P, Massano J. Intraoperative microelectrode recording in Parkinson's disease subthalamic deep brain stimulation: Analysis of clinical utility. J Clin Neurosci. 2019;69:104-8.
34. Volkmann J, Moro E, Pahwa R. Basic algorithms for the programming of deep brain stimulation in Parkinson's disease. Mov Disord. 2006;21(Suppl 14):S284-9.
35. Picillo M, Lozano AM, Kou N, Puppi Munhoz R, Fasano A. Programming Deep Brain Stimulation for Parkinson's Disease: The Toronto Western Hospital Algorithms. Brain Stimul. 2016;9(3):425-37.
36. Shukla AW, Zeilman P, Fernandez H, Bajwa JA, Mehanna R. DBS Programming: An Evolving Approach for Patients with Parkinson's Disease. Parkinsons Dis. 2017;2017:8492619.
37. Khoo HM, Kishima H, Hosomi K, Maruo T, Tani N, Oshino S, et al. Low-frequency subthalamic nucleus stimulation in Parkinson's disease: a randomized clinical trial. Mov Disord. 2014;29(2):270-4.
38. Reich MM, Steigerwald F, Sawalhe AD, Reese R, Gunalan K, Johannes S, et al. Short pulse width widens the therapeutic window of subthalamic neurostimulation. Ann Clin Transl Neurol. 2015;2(4):427-32.
39. Arlotti M, Marceglia S, Foffani G, Volkmann J, Lozano AM, Moro E, et al. Eight-hours adaptive deep brain stimulation in patients with Parkinson disease. Neurology. 2018;90(11):e971-6.
40. Hariz MI, Rehncrona S, Quinn NP, Speelman JD, Wensing C. Multicenter study on deep brain stimulation in Parkinson's disease: an independent assessment of reported adverse events at 4 years. Mov Disord. 2008;23(3):416-21.
41. Doshi PK. Long-term surgical and hardware-related complications of deep brain stimulation. Stereotact Funct Neurosurg. 2011;89(2):89-95.
42. Smeding HM, Speelman JD, Koning-Haanstra M, Schuurman PR, Nijssen P, van Laar T, et al. Neuropsychological effects of bilateral STN stimulation in Parkinson disease: a controlled study. Neurology. 2006;66(12):1830-6.
43. Appleby BS, Duggan PS, Regenberg A, Rabins PV. Psychiatric and neuropsychiatric adverse events associated with deep brain stimulation: A meta-analysis of ten years' experience. Mov Disord. 2007;22(12):1722-8.
44. Fenoy AJ, Simpson RK Jr. Risks of common complications in deep brain stimulation surgery: management and avoidance. J Neurosurg. 2014;120(1):132-9.
45. Doshi PK, Chhaya N, Bhatt MH. Depression leading to attempted suicide after bilateral subthalamic nucleus stimulation for Parkinson's disease. Mov Disord. 2002;17(5):1084-5.
46. Kulisevsky J, Berthier ML, Gironell A, Pascual-Sedano B, Molet J, Pares P. Mania following deep brain stimulation for Parkinson's disease. Neurology. 2002;59(9):1421-4.
47. Broen M, Duits A, Visser-Vandewalle V, Temel Y, Winogrodzka A. Impulse control and related disorders in Parkinson's disease patients treated with bilateral subthalamic nucleus stimulation: a review. Parkinsonism Relat Disord. 2011;17(6):413-7.
48. Laitinen LV, Bergenheim AT, Hariz MI. Leksell's posteroventral pallidotomy in the treatment of Parkinson's disease. J Neurosurg. 1992;76(1):53-61.

49. Cahan LD, Young RF, Li F. Radiosurgical Pallidotomy for Parkinson's Disease. Prog Neurol Surg. 2018;33:149-57.
50. Fox SH, Katzenschlager R, Lim SY, Barton B, de Bie RMA, Seppi K, et al. International Parkinson and movement disorder society evidence-based medicine review: Update on treatments for the motor symptoms of Parkinson's disease. Mov Disord. 2018;33(8):1248-66.
51. Alvarez L, Macias R, Pavón N, López G, Rodríguez-Oroz MC, Rodríguez R, et al. Therapeutic efficacy of unilateral subthalamotomy in Parkinson's disease: results in 89 patients followed for up to 36 months. J Neurol Neurosurg Psychiatry. 2009;80(9):979-85.
52. Martínez-Fernández R, Rodríguez-Rojas R, Del Álamo M, Hernández-Fernández F, Pineda-Pardo JA, Dileone M, et al. Focused ultrasound subthalamotomy in patients with asymmetric Parkinson›s disease: a pilot study. Lancet Neurol. 2018;17(1):54-63.
53. Fishman PS, Elias WJ, Ghanouni P, Gwinn R, Lipsman N, Schwartz M, et al. Neurological adverse event profile of magnetic resonance imaging-guided focused ultrasound thalamotomy for essential tremor. Mov Disord. 2018;33(5):843-7.
54. Bouwyn JP, Derrey S, Lefaucheur R, Fetter D, Rouille A, Le Goff F, et al. Age Limits for Deep Brain Stimulation of Subthalamic Nuclei in Parkinson›s Disease. J Parkinsons Dis. 2016;6(2):393-400.
55. Ory-Magne F, Brefel-Courbon C, Simonetta-Moreau M, Fabre N, Lotterie JA, Chaynes P, et al. Does ageing influence deep brain stimulation outcomes in Parkinson›s disease? Mov Disord. 2007;22(10):1457-63.
56. Soulas T, Gurruchaga JM, Palfi S, Cesaro P, Nguyen JP, Fenelon G. Attempted and completed suicides after subthalamic nucleus stimulation for Parkinson›s disease. J Neurol Neurosurg Psychiatry. 2008;79(8):952-4.
57. Weintraub D, Duda JE, Carlson K, Luo P, Sagher O, Stern M, et al. Suicide ideation and behaviours after STN and GPi DBS surgery for Parkinson›s disease: results from a randomised, controlled trial. J Neurol Neurosurg Psychiatry. 2013;84(10):1113-8.
58. Fasano A, Romito LM, Daniele A, Piano C, Zinno M, Bentivoglio AR, et al. Motor and cognitive outcome in patients with Parkinson›s disease 8 years after subthalamic implants. Brain. 2010;133(9):2664-76.
59. Doshi PK, Desai JD, Karkera B, Wadia PM. Bilateral pedunculopontine nucleus stimulation for progressive supranuclear palsy. Stereotact Funct Neurosurg. 2015;93(1):59-65.
60. Lozano AM, Lipsman N, Bergman H, Brown P, Chabardes S, Chang JW, et al. Deep brain stimulation: current challenges and future directions. Nat Rev Neurol. 2019;15(3):148-60.
61. Hamani C, Lozano AM, Mazzone PA, Moro E, Hutchison W, Silburn PA, et al. Pedunculopontine Nucleus Region Deep Brain Stimulation in Parkinson Disease: Surgical Techniques, Side Effects, and Postoperative Imaging. Stereotact Funct Neurosurg. 2016;94(5):307-19.
62. Mathews L, Camalier CR, Kla KM, Mitchell MD, Konrad PE, Neimat JS, et al. The Effects of Dexmedetomidine on Microelectrode Recordings of the Subthalamic Nucleus during Deep Brain Stimulation Surgery: A Retrospective Analysis. Stereotact Funct Neurosurg. 2017;95(1):40-8.
63. Burkhard PR, Vingerhoets FJ, Berney A, Bogousslavsky J, Villemure JG, Ghika J. Suicide after successful deep brain stimulation for movement disorders. Neurology. 2004;63(11):2170-2.
64. Umemura A, Oka Y, Yamamoto K, Okita K, Matsukawa N, Yamada K. Complications of subthalamic nucleus stimulation in Parkinson›s disease. Neurol Med Chir (Tokyo). 2011;51(11):749-55.
65. Doshi PK. Radiofrequency Lesioning for Movement and Psychiatric Disorders-Experience of 107 Cases. Frontiers in Human Neuroscience. 2021;15:310.

CHAPTER 23

Neuroprotective Drugs and Restorative Therapies in Parkinson's Disease

Greg Daniel Kuhlman, Anthony E Lang OC

INTRODUCTION

A major unmet need in the treatment of Parkinson's disease (PD) is therapy that can slow, stop, or reverse progression. In this chapter, we aim to summarize the state of the field in neuroprotection and restorative therapies for PD, describe reasons for previous failures, and provide insight into potential opportunities for the future. We cannot discuss every potential therapy and targeted mechanism in detail but hope to cover the therapeutic mechanisms and agents thought to be important, innovative, and promising. Current clinical trials investigating neuroprotective and restorative therapy are summarized in **Table 1**.

Disease modification is a general term used to describe a treatment that alters the natural course of disease, encompassing both neuroprotection and restorative therapy. The concept of neuroprotection includes supporting failing compensatory mechanisms for progressive degeneration, salvaging dying neurons by removing toxic factors, improving failing metabolic disturbances, or providing trophic support. On the other hand, restorative therapy involves replacing lost or degenerating neurons. Unfortunately, as described later, to prove neuroprotection and effective restoration of degenerated neurons we would need a way to accurately measure the underlying disease process, something we currently lack.

OBSTACLES TO SUCCESS IN CLINICAL TRIALS

There are three main underlying obstacles to discovering an effective disease modification therapy (DMT) for PD: Lack of a reliable biomarker, poor understanding of the underlying pathophysiology, and timing of enrollment in clinical studies.

It is difficult to measure the underlying disease activity in PD without a reliable biomarker. This directly impacts the ability to differentiate symptomatic effects of a study drug from PD disease activity or the effects of concurrent neurodegenerative disease. As an alternative, clinical scales based on symptoms and examination are used to measure outcome. These tend to emphasize the clinical effects of the nigrostriatal dopamine system rather than the treatment-resistant motor and non-motor features which may be more debilitating (e.g., dementia and postural instability leading to falls). Moreover, when outcome measures are applied to a progressive disease where clinical milestones are reached slowly, drug dosing for a study drug is difficult without a biomarker to confirm target engagement.

What is more, most clinical trials inherently assume that all patients with "early PD" enrolled in these trials have a uniform disorder with a uniform underlying pathophysiology. However, PD is a heterogeneous disorder with multiple pathogenic mechanisms which may contribute to neurodegeneration. Candidate therapies have a variety of mechanisms of action but may not be successful in a given patient unless the therapy targets a mechanism involved in the underlying pathophysiology in that particular patient.[1] If true, then a putative agent may only be shown to be effective if given to an enriched PD population thought to specifically benefit from the agent. The underlying pathophysiology is complex and details pertinent to neuroprotective and restorative therapies will be highlighted as they pertain to the particular agents discussed later. Furthermore, the animal models used in drug development do not accurately reflect human PD and this may explain why numerous agents that appeared

TABLE 1: Neuroprotective and restorative therapies currently under study.

Mechanism of action	Drug/Therapy	Progress			Comments
		Phase 1	Phase 2	Phase 3	
Small molecule, reduce α-syn aggregation	NPT200-11/ UCB0599				NCT02606682
	Anle138b				NCT04208152
c-Abl tyrosine kinase inhibitor	Nilotinib				"NILO-PD" and "PD Nilotinib," negative study
Bcr-Abl tyrosine kinase inhibitor	K0706				NCT03655236
Reduce α-syn aggregation	Glycerol phenylbutyrate				NCT02046434
	Green tea polyphenol				NCT00461942
Increase GCase activity	Ambroxol (GCase chaperone)				"AiM-PD," PD +/- GBA mutation
					NCT02914366, PD dementia
	LTI-291				NTR7299, PD + GBA mutation
Substrate (GluCer) reduction	Venglustat				"MOVES-PD" (NCT02906020), PD + GBA mutation, study terminated early
Active α-syn immunization	PD01A				"AFF008" (NCT01568099), "AFF008A" (NCT02216188), "AFF008E" (NCT01885494), and "AFF008AA" (NCT02618941)
	PD03A				"AFF011" (NCT02267434)
	UB-312				NCT04075318
Passive α-syn immunization	PRX002/RG7935/ prasinezumab				"PASSADENA" (NCT03100149)
					"PADOVA" (NCT04777331)
	BIIB054/cinpanemab				"SPARK" (NCT03318523), negative study
	AF82422				NCT03611569
	MEDI1341				NCT03272165
L-type CaV 1.3 channel blocker	Isradipine				"STEADY-PD3," negative trial
Increase CNS urate	Inosine				"SURE-PD3" (NCT02642393), negative trial
GLP1R agonist	Exenetide				"Exenatide-PD3" (NCT04232969)
	Semaglutide				"GIPD" (NCT03659682)
	Lixisenatide				"LixiPark" (NCT03439943)
	Liraglutide				NCT02953665
Enhance mitochondrial function	Ursodeoxycholic acid				"UP" (NCT03840005)
Antioxidant, glutathione precursor	N-acetylcysteine				"NAC for PD" (NCT01470027)
Increases glutathione levels	(R)-troloxamide quinone				NCT02462603
Iron chelation	Deferiprone				"SKY" (NCT02728843)
					"FAIRPARK-II" (NCT02655315)
Copper redistribution	Cu2+(atsm)				NCT03204929
LRRK2 kinase inhibitor	DNL201				NCT03710707, PD +/- LRRK2 mutation
	DNL151				NCT04056689, PD +/- LRRK2 mutation
Myeloperoxidase inhibitor	AZD3241				
Immunomodulation	ViNeuro				NCT00517842

Continued

Continued

Mechanism of action	*Drug/Therapy*	*Progress*			*Comments*
		Phase 1	*Phase 2*	*Phase 3*	
HMG-CoA reductase inhibitor	Lovastatin				NCT03242499
	Simvastatin				"PD STAT" (NCT02787590)
Neurotrophic factor gene therapy	Convection enhanced delivery of AAV2-GDNF				NCT01621581
Dopamine synthesis enzyme gene therapy	ProSavin				
	OXB-102/AXO-Lenti-PD				NCT03720418
	VY-AADC01				NCT03065192
Cell based therapy	Fetal VM transplant				"TRANSEURO" (NCT01898390), NCT03119636, and NCT01860794
	ESC transplant				"EUROPEAN STEM-PD" and "NYSTEM-PD"
	iPSC transplant				"CiRA"

promising in preclinical studies failed when applied to patients.

Finally, at the time of clinical presentation it is estimated that there has already been a 30–50% loss of the substantia nigra pars compacta (SNpc) neurons and 60% reduction of the nigrostriatal dopamine.[2] This means substantial neurodegeneration has occurred even "early" in the disease. Perhaps if we could identify and recruit patients earlier in the disease process then a DMT would have a greater potential for successful impact. This has led the International Parkinsonism and Movement Disorders Society (MDS) to develop research criteria for prodromal PD in an attempt to better define this population for future research trials.[3] Nevertheless, this is again limited by the lack of a reliable biomarker because diagnosis at this stage is less certain and the study population may be more heterogenous.

Clinical trial design is another important aspect to consider in measuring outcome in clinical trials, but we will not be discussing this topic. Instead, the reader may reference one of many reviews on this topic.[4]

NEUROPROTECTIVE THERAPIES

A large number of putative DMTs have been studied in PD. To date, all have failed to demonstrate convincing evidence of benefit, which has been summarized elsewhere.[5] Here we will review agents and approaches currently under study, which are summarized in **Table 1**.

Alpha Synuclein

A brief discussion of alpha-synuclein (α-syn) pathophysiology is required before describing therapeutic agents that target this protein. The discoveries of an autosomal dominant form of PD caused by a mutation in the *SNCA* gene for the synaptic protein α-syn and that α-syn is a key component of Lewy pathology led to the idea that α-syn may be pathogenic in PD.[6] The α-syn protein is composed of three regions: (1) An N-terminal domain responsible for an alpha helical structure that allows α-syn to bind to membranes, (2) Central domain described as the non-amyloid beta component (NAC) domain which is involved in α-syn aggregation when it acquires a beta-sheet structure, and (3) C-terminal domain.[7] Aside from the alpha helical structure in the N-terminal domain, the protein has significant conformational plasticity, and thus has been described as "intrinsically disordered." The N- and C-terminus domains interact to prevent aggregation in the setting of conformational plasticity. These interactions and the ability of α-syn to aggregate can be impacted by genetic mutations, post-translational modification, or environmental conditions.[7] Moreover, excessive amounts of the normal protein, caused by duplications and triplications of the *SNCA* gene, can promote α-syn aggregation and result in Lewy body disease and Lewy pathology similar to point mutations in the *SNCA* gene.[8] In the monomeric form, α-syn likely functions in synaptic vesicular transport but with aggregation can form pathogenic oligomers and insoluble fibrils in the cytoplasm which accumulate in Lewy bodies.[7] α-syn aggregation can disrupt a number of organelles (including synaptic-vesicle trafficking, endoplasmic reticulum and Golgi apparatus, mitochondria, autophagy-lysosomal system, and nuclear function), interorganelle contacts (e.g., the mitochondria-associated endoplasmic reticulum membrane), and organelle dynamics (e.g., axonal transport).[9] Dysfunction of these organelles, contacts, and dynamics can lead to increased reactive oxygen species, bioenergetic failure, impaired protein degradation, stimulate inflammation, and promote apoptosis.[6,7,9,10] Many of these processes can further encourage α-syn aggregation leading to cellular dysfunction and cell death. For example, reduced lysosomal glucocerebrosidase (GCase) activity is proposed to stabilize the toxic α-syn oligomer form and thereby promote aggregation, which in turn decreases lysosomal proteolysis.[11] Lastly, α-syn may be able to spread from cell to cell and provide a seed for further α-syn aggregation in a prion-like manner. This was initially proposed based on the observation that some patients who had undergone fetal ventral mesenchymal transplant 10 years or more earlier were found postmortem to have Lewy pathology in the transplanted neurons.[12] Likewise, cell-based studies have suggested that exosome release of α-syn aggregates may be one mechanism to explain this type of spread.[13]

Some characteristics of α-syn limit putative neuroprotective agents' ability to target α-syn. For example, recent studies have characterized distinct strains of α-syn with diverse structure, toxicity, and ability to propagate.[14] There may be different strains between patients and even in different regions of the brain within the same patient.[15] This adds heterogeneity to the underlying pathophysiology. There is also a subset of the population with incidental Lewy body pathology without clinical disease, so called incidental Lewy body disease.[16] This suggests that factors other than α-syn contribute to disease. Specifically, age (e.g., leading to increased reactive oxygen species), coexisting pathology (e.g., cross-seeding of α-syn and tau), neuroinflammation (e.g., glial activation), and selective cell vulnerability (e.g., SNpc cells with highly branched axons with multiple release sites and autonomous pacemaking activity with low calcium buffering capacity) likely contribute.[9,17]

There are essentially five strategies that might ameliorate α-syn pathophysiology (**Fig. 1**): (1) Reduce production, (2) reduce aggregation, (3) increase intracellular degradation, (4) increase extracellular degradation, and (5) blocking uptake into neighboring neurons. Of note, a single therapeutic agent may employ multiple strategies.

Reduced Intracellular Alpha Synuclein Production

Silencing RNA and antisense oligonucleotide therapies have been used for other neurologic diseases and may have promise in PD but have not yet reached the human trial stage.[18] Recently, the β2-adrenoreceptor was discovered to regulate the α-syn gene and β2-adrenoreceptor agonist use was found to be associated with lower risk of PD diagnosis, while β2-adrenoreceptor antagonist use was associated with a greater risk of PD diagnosis.[19] This suggests that β2-adrenoreceptor agonist medications could be repurposed for PD to reduce α-syn production. On the other hand, as demonstrated in a subsequent study,[20] the epidemiological associations between β2-adrenoreceptor agonist and antagonist use with risk of developing PD could be explained by confounding variables because complications of smoking (chronic pulmonary obstructive disease) and tremor, respectively, are treated with these medications. Smoking is known to have a protective effect for PD, as discussed later, which could explain the protective effect of β2-adrenoreceptor agonist use, and tremor may precede PD diagnosis, which could explain the harmful effect of β2-adrenoreceptor antagonist use.

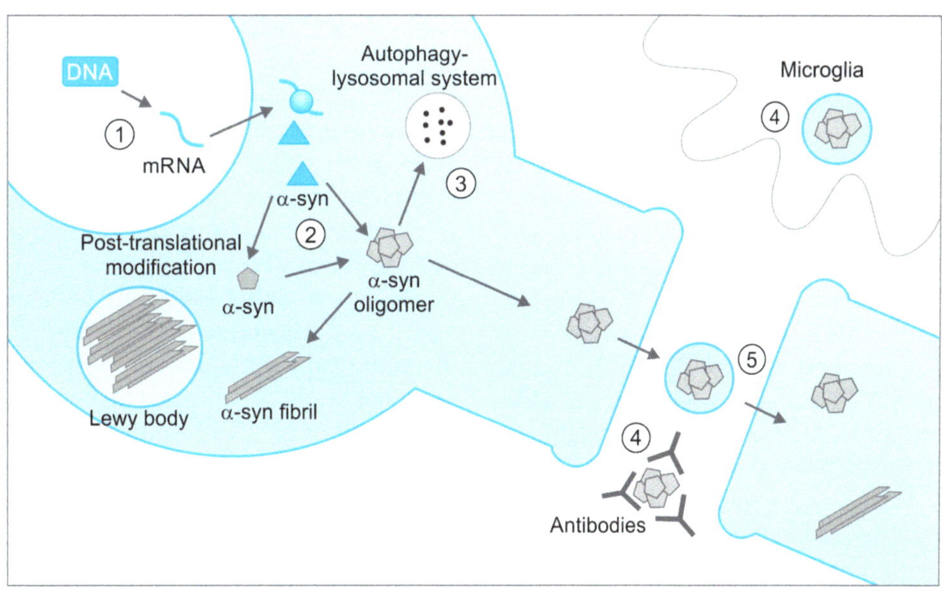

Note: This figure was modified from figure 2 in Wong et al. 2017.[9] (1) Decrease α-syn production by modifying DNA expression or mRNA translation; (2) Decrease α-syn aggregation by modifying α-syn post-translational modifications or oligomerization of pathologic α-syn species; (3) Increase degradation of α-syn by augmenting the autophagy-lysosomal system; (4) Increase extracellular α-syn degradation by activation of microglia or clearing protein directly with antibodies; (5) Decrease α-syn uptake by neighboring neurons.

(DNA: deoxyribonucleic acid; mRNA: messenger ribonucleic acid)

FIG. 1: Mechanisms of alpha synuclein targeted therapies.

Reduce Alpha Synuclein Aggregation

Small molecules have been developed for this purpose, such as NPT200-11/UCB0599. This small molecule prevents formation of oligomeric aggregates in mouse models by stabilizing the physiological structure.[21] A phase 1 trial has been completed in healthy volunteers and a phase 1 trial with PD subjects is underway. Other small molecules (anle138b and NPT088) have demonstrated ability to block aggregation of prion proteins and various toxic misfolded proteins, respectively in mouse models.[21] Anle138b is undergoing a phase 1 trial involving healthy subjects. Another approach that has been studied involves the use of intrabodies. These are fragments of full-length immunoglobulin, including the epitope specific Fv variable region, and are able to target antigens intracellularly, whereas full length antibodies cannot.[22] Two intrabodies have been developed to target α-syn including VH14, by binding to the NAC aggregation prone region, and NbSyn87, by binding to the C-terminal region.[22,23] However, these agents require viral vectors for central nervous system (CNS) delivery and the challenge will be in maintaining high levels in the CNS for a prolonged time to be effective.[23] These have not reached human clinical trials.

Nilotinib is a c-Abl tyrosine kinase inhibitor used for treatment of chronic myelogenous leukemia which garnered attention after a small open-label phase 1 trial suggested that low doses of nilotinib result in clinical benefits for subjects with PD and dementia with Lewy bodies.[24] Aberrant c-Abl is thought to phosphorylate α-syn and parkin, thereby promoting α-syn aggregation, disrupting mitochondrial homeostasis, and dysregulating the ubiquitin-proteasome system.[25] Therefore, inhibition of c-Abl may influence PD progression. A recent phase 2 trial of nilotinib showed a reasonably good safety profile and reduced levels of cerebrospinal fluid (CSF) oligomeric α-syn and phosphorylated tau which was surmised to result in increased levels of CSF dopamine metabolites.[26] Yet, nilotinib CSF/serum ratio was <1% and there was no CSF Abl inhibition. This could be explained by transporter mediated efflux of nilotinib.[27] The study authors propose that a different receptor than Abl, the discoidin domain receptor, is preferentially inhibited at lower doses which mediates the results.[26] Critics argue that low CSF oligomeric α-syn could be spurious because there was no comparison to baseline levels, dopamine metabolite levels could be explained by differences in dopaminergic medications and timing of lumbar puncture, and differences are primarily driven by statistical outliers which should caution against the pursuit of a large phase 3 trial.[28] Another phase 2 trial of nilotinib was recently completed by the Parkinson Study Group showed that nilotinib is safe and tolerable but there was no signal of clinical or biological benefit.[29] Other Abl inhibitors could be better alternatives to nilotinib. Bafetinib is better able to cross the blood brain barrier (BBB) than nilotinib but is a less specific kinase inhibitor so also poses a risk of side effects.[27] K0706 is another promising Bcr-Abl kinase inhibitor that was shown to be safe in a phase 1 trial of PD subjects[30] and is currently recruiting for a phase 2 trial.

Other small molecules with a similar proposed ability to inhibit α-syn aggregation undergoing human trials include glycerol phenylbutyrate, a nitrogen-binding agent used in inborn urea cycle disorders, and green tea polyphenols, a green tea extract. Squalamine is a naturally occurring antimicrobial aminosterol that was recently found in cell and animal studies to inhibit α-syn aggregation by displacing α-syn from the lipid membrane, which is permissive for α-syn aggregation, but has not undergone human studies.[31] However, a synthetic derivative of squalamine, ENT-01, is under study for constipation in PD (NCT03047629). Although its activity is exclusively on enteric cells, because it is not absorbed into the systemic circulation, this could hypothetically still have an impact on the CNS process.

Increase Intracellular Alpha Synuclein Degradation

The autophagy lysosomal pathway appears to be an important factor for degradation of α-syn aggregates. This is emphasized by the fact that *GBA*, the gene encoding the lysosomal enzyme GCase, is the most common genetic risk factor for PD and dementia with Lewy bodies.[32] Reduced GCase activity stabilizes the toxic α-syn oligomer form and thereby promotes aggregation, which in turn causes a decrease is lysosomal proteolysis.[11] It is reasonable to believe that agents that target GCase may be effective in PD patients with or without a *GBA* mutation because GCase activity has been shown to be decreased in PD patients without *GBA* mutations.[33]

Methods to target GCase include enzyme replacement therapy, drugs that modulate GCase activity, and substrate reduction therapy (**Fig. 2**). Unfortunately, successful enzyme replacement therapy agents used for Gaucher's disease do not effectively cross the BBB and therefore have limited utility for PD.[34] Ambroxol is a secrolytic agent used to reduce mucus production in respiratory diseases, including Gaucher's disease. Ambroxol acts as a chaperone protein that facilitates GCase folding and translocation to the lysosome thereby increasing GCase activity as has been shown in preclinical studies.[35] A recent small open-label phase 2 trial in PD subjects with and without *GBA* mutations demonstrated that a high dose of ambroxol was well tolerated, crosses the BBB, increases GCase concentration, and modulates GCase activity.[36] Further studies need to be performed to determine if this will result in clinical benefit and if this will be limited to those with a relevant *GBA* mutation. In a separate phase 2 trial, ambroxol is being investigated in patients with PD dementia. Venglustat (ibiglustat) is a substrate reducing agent that inhibits glucosylceramide synthase (GluCer) (**Fig. 2**). This was demonstrated to cross the BBB, reduce

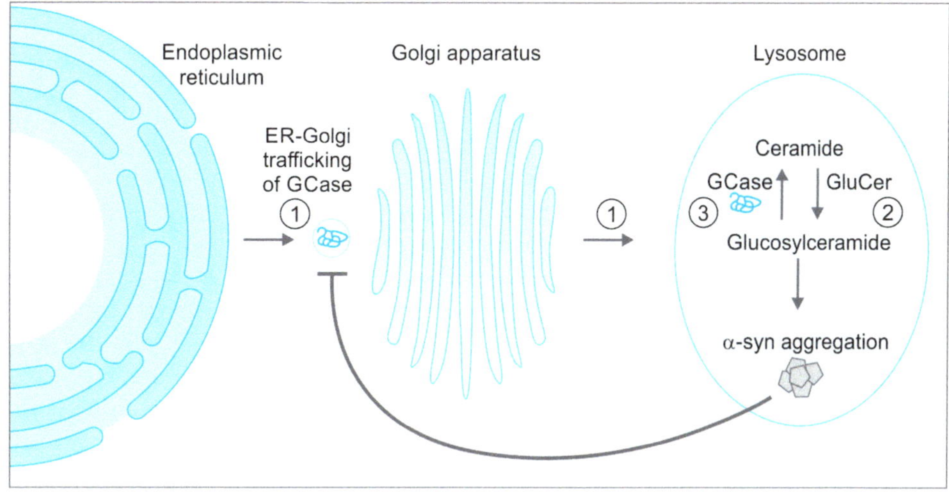

Note: This figure was modified from figure 3 in O'Hara et al. 2018.[21] (1) Improve folding and trafficking of glucocerebrosidase (GCase) to the lysosome; (2) Inhibit glucosylceramide synthase (GluCer) thereby decreasing glucosylceramide level (the substrate that promotes alpha synuclein aggregation); (3) GCase activation decreasing glucosylceramide level.

FIG. 2: Mechanisms of action of lysosomal targeted therapies.

substratein the brain, and diminish clinical manifestations in a mouse model of neuronopathic Gaucher's disease.[37] Unfortunately, a large phase 2 trial that investigated venglustat in PD patients who carry a *GBA* mutation was stopped early due to futility. However, questions have been raised about the validity of the substrate reduction strategy in *GBA1*-associated PD.[38] More recently, a small molecule named LTI-291 has been developed that penetrates the BBB and increases GCase activity (https://www.bial.com/com/bial-biotech/a-targeted-approach/). This has completed an initial phase 2a study in PD patients with *GBA* mutation which demonstrated target engagement and no serious adverse events.

Increase Extracellular Alpha Synuclein Degradation

Active immunization, a method of stimulating the host immune system to develop antibodies targeting specific proteins, and passive immunization, a method of providing exogenous antibodies targeting specific proteins, have been exciting developments in neuroprotective strategies for PD. While the prevailing thought is that these treatments work by enhancing extracellular degradation of α-syn, the mechanism of action is not completely understood. In an early animal study using an active immunization strategy, an extracellular antibody surprisingly led to decreased deposition of the intracellular α-syn protein in presynaptic terminals.[39] The authors surmised this was likely a consequence of higher lysosomal activity and microglial activation, which highlights the role of CNS inflammation in PD. The inflammatory response in neurodegenerative disorders is complex; one theory,"M1/M2 polarization," proposes the expression of proinflammatory cytokines promotes a cellular immune response (M1) which enhances neurodegeneration whereas noninflammatory cytokines promote beneficial phagocytosis and tissue remodeling (M2).[40] Microglial activation in this case is thought to lead to extracellular clearance of α-syn aggregates by phagocytosis. On the other hand, higher lysosomal activity increases intracellular α-syn degradation.[41] The antibodies may also block cell-to-cell transmission of α-syn, which possibly occurs via exocytosis.[41] Others have suggested that antibodies could be effective by decreasing the extracellular protein concentration thus creating a shift of soluble brain protein species to the periphery (the so called "peripheral sink theory").[41]

Active immunization has the advantage of being more economical than passive immunization because it does not require regular infusions. On the other hand, elderly do not respond as favorably to vaccination as younger individuals which may render this approach less effective.[42] A balance must also be struck between under-stimulating the immune system and over-stimulating the immune system leading to autoimmune complications. However, a single immunization plus a few "booster shots" may be all that is required. There are two active immunization therapies that have completed in phase 1 human clinical trials, PD01A and PD03A. Both were developed by the same company but with different antibody specificity and designed to promote a B-cell immunogenic response without a T-cell autoimmune response. In preclinical animal studies, these agents have been shown to cross the BBB, target α-syn, decrease α-syn accumulation, reduce neurodegeneration, and improve motor symptoms.[43] While results have not been published in peer-reviewed journals, the company as reported that both PD01A and

PD03A were well tolerated, aside from local skin reactions. In the PD01A studies, a series of four injections followed by "booster" injection 12 months later demonstrated that 86% of subjects generated an immune response, 55% of subjects generated serum specific antibodies, and did not result in a T cell response, which may mitigate the risk of autoimmune complications.[21,44] The company announced in January 2020 that it plans to start a phase 2 trial of PD01A (https://affiris.com/investors/#press). An additional active immunotherapy agent, named UB-312, is also pursuing a phase 1 study involving healthy participants.

The passive immunization strategy is more inconvenient and expensive since it requires regular infusions but has the advantage of bypassing the potentially senescent immune system in the elderly PD population. Two passive immunization therapies are currently in phase 2 human clinical trials, PRX002/RG7935 (prasinezumab) and BIIB054 (cinpanemab), and another, AF82422, is currently in a phase 1 trial. The phase 1 studies of PRX002, targeting the C-terminus domain of α-syn, and BIIB054, targeting the N-terminus domain of α-syn, demonstrated that these drugs were reasonably safe and reduced serum α-synin a dose dependent manner.[45,46] However, the percentage of CSF to serum drug level was only approximately 0.3–0.4% in both studies and, while changes to CSF α-syn level was not reported in the BIIB054 study, PRX002 infusions did not change CSF α-syn levels.[45,46] The prasinezumab phase 2 "PASADENA" study at 12 months did not reach the primary efficacy endpoint, although there was some signal of potential efficacy on several secondary endpoints but involves multiple longitudinal phases of study and is ongoing. This study enrolled PD patients early in their disease so there may not have been enough progression of symptoms to detect a significant difference in motor scores. This has led to a parallel phase 2b "PADOVA" study of prasinezumab that is enrolling a greater number of PD patients with more advanced disease so may be better powered to detect a significant difference in motor scores. Unfortunately, the cinpanemab phase 2 "SPARK" study was terminated at 12 months due to not reaching primary or secondary endpoints. Another passive immunization agent MEDI1341, targeting the C-terminus of α-syn, can to block extracellular α-syn spread in vitro and α-syn propagation in vivo in animal studies while achieving similar relative BBB penetration as PRX002 and BIIB054.[47] An interesting finding was that two versions of MEDI1341 were tested in animals, one version with an intact Fc interaction region (required for microglial phagocytosis) and one without, and both had a similar ability to block α-syn propagation. This suggests that microglial phagocytosis of α-syn is not required. MEDI1341 is currently in a phase 1 trial.

While immunization therapy does appear promising, there are reasons to be skeptical. This therapy likely depends on targeting extracellular α-syn which assumes that a prion-like spreading model of α-syn is a driving force in PD pathophysiology. Critics of this theory note that the pattern of Lewy pathology in PD brains often does not follow the pattern predicted by the Braak model, the distribution of Lewy pathology in PD brains is not predicted by the brain connectome, Lewy pathology, and neurodegeneration in PD do not follow a similar spatiotemporal pattern, and there is no convincing longitudinal data in PD patients to support the spreading hypothesis.[17] Also, while the C-terminus of the α-syn protein, the target of an intracellular enzyme calpain which can cleave the C-terminus of α-syn and promote toxic oligomers, is targeted by most immunization therapies,[48] it remains unknown which part of the α-syn protein or conformation of α-syn oligomer would be most effective to target. Further, it is not clear what size of oligomer should be considered "toxic", whether and which post-translational modifications promote toxicity, and if aggregation is even required to cause toxicity.[23] Also, as previously mentioned, there may be different strains of toxic α-syn between patients and even between different regions of the same brain[15] and it is unknown whether antibodies would need to be strain specific.

Reducing Uptake of Extracellular Alpha Synuclein

This strategy is at a relatively earlier stage of development. Potential mechanisms include interfering with heparin sulfate proteoglycans, needed for α-syn endocytosis to neighboring cells, and blocking cell surface proteins with high affinity for α-syn, specifically lymphocyte-activation-gene 3.[23]

Mitochondria

The discovery of 1-methyl-4-phenyl-1,2,3,6-tetrahydropyridine (MPTP) in the 1980s provided persuasive evidence that PD could be caused by a mitochondrial toxin and/or dysfunction. This is further reinforced by various PD animal models that demonstrated the critical role mitochondrial dysfunction, increased reactive oxygen species, and calcium homeostasis as well as the importance of mitochondrial homeostasis in selected genetic forms of PD (e.g., *Parkin, PINK1*, and *DJ1*).[10] Unfortunately, multiple large randomized controlled trials that investigated various agents thought to target pathophysiology involving the mitochondria have been negative. There are three agents targeting mitochondrial pathophysiology that are currently in or recently completed phase 3 clinical trials: (1) Inosine, (2) Exenatide, and (3) Isradipine.

It has been long known that certain areas of the brain are selectively vulnerable in PD. Surmeier and colleagues[17] have proposed that areas, exemplified by the dopaminergic neurons of the SNpc, share similar features that put them at risk. These areas have long and highly branched axons with a high number of terminals as well as slow rhythmic pacemaking activity with low calcium buffering capacity and cytosolic calcium oscillations. This specific type of pacemaking activity results in more oxidative stress from mitochondria which in turn, along with aging and environmental toxins, can impair mitochondrial function. The increased cytosolic calcium promotes α-syn aggregation via post-translational modification and impaired lysosomal function. Isradipine is an Food and Drug Administration (FDA) approved dihydropyridine type calcium channel blocker with the most specificity for Cav1.3 compared to other dihydropyridines, which is thought to be important for PD risk related to the pacemaking activity described above.[49] This could theoretically mitigate downstream oxidative stress, α-syn aggregation, and lysosomal dysfunction. Unfortunately, a large phase 3 study did not demonstrate benefit.[50] The authors hypothesize that the dose used, on the basis of tolerability threshold from the phase 2 study, was too low; the bioavailability in the CNS, which cannot be measured, was too low; and/or that the driving pathophysiological disease mechanism changes overtime.[50] This last point opens the possibility that isradipine may be effective in the prodromal phase but not after diagnosis.

Inosine is a precursor to uric acid, the levels of which have been shown to be inversely correlated with the development and progression of PD in multiple epidemiologic studies.[51] Uric acid is proposed to protect against neurodegeneration by its antioxidant properties but also other mechanisms such as acting as an iron chelator and antiapoptotic agent.[51] Unfortunately, the phase 3 trial investigating inosine was stopped prematurely, late in 2018, after an interim analysis demonstrated that it was unlikely to show benefit if completed. However, post-hoc analysis of the phase 2 trial showed that inosine results in a greater increase in serum and CSF urate in women.[52] If the phase 3 trial is found to be underpowered to detect a beneficial change in the subgroup of women, then using inosine in women with PD will warrant further study.

Exenatide is an FDA approved medication for diabetes mellitus that acts by stimulating the glucagon-like peptide-1 receptor (GLP1R). A multitude of mechanisms have been hypothesized to be beneficial for PD including enhanced mitochondrial biogenesis, reduced proapoptotic factors, enhanced lysosomal activity, reduced α-syn aggregation, modulation of inflammatory factors, and enhanced neuronal plasticity.[53] A phase 2 trial was performed which demonstrated a modest early-onset improvement in the MDS Unified Parkinson's Disease Rating Scale (MDS-UPDRS) part III that persisted after a washout period.[54] However, this temporal action is inconsistent with any of the mechanisms proposed above and it is possible that these results are explained by symptomatic benefit or placebo effect. Previous animal studies which demonstrated that exenatide can increase the expression of tyrosine hydroxylase, which may provide a symptomatic benefit.[55] A phase 3 trial is actively enrolling PD subjects to better examine the efficacy of exenatide. Other GLP1R agonists undergoing phase 2 trials in PD include semaglutide, lixisenatide, and liraglutide.

Other agents that target mitochondrial function are being actively studied including ursodeoxycholic acid, an FDA approved medication used for primary biliary cirrhosis, as well as N-acetylcysteine and (R)-troloxamide quinone, agents that are respectively a precursor or modifier of glutathione, an antioxidant thought to be critical in PD pathogenesis.[10]

Endogenous Heavy Metals

Increased iron deposition in the substantia nigra has been identified in postmortem studies of PD brains and low molecular weight iron can contribute to the pathophysiology by causing oxidative damage, decreasing antioxidant levels, increasing translation of α-syn, and promoting α-syn aggregation.[56] Deferiprone is an FDA approved medication used for thalassemia and works by transferring iron from cells with excessive iron to cells with deficient iron.[57] Following previous preliminary studies,[58] there are two phase 2 trials completed with results expected in 2021. Conversely, copper levels are found to be low in the substantia nigra in postmortem studies of PD brains and the repurposed radiolabeling compound Cu^{2+} complex of diacetyl*bis* [N(4)-methylthiosemi-carbazonato] [Cu^{2+}(atsm)] may selectively accumulate Cu^{2+} in areas of the brain with damaged mitochondrial electron transport chain, as occurs in PD, and inhibit nitration dependent α-syn aggregation.[59,60] A phase 1 trial investigating the use of Cu^{2+}(atsm) in PD is being pursued.

Leucine-rich Repeat Kinase 2

As noted above, the heterogeneous underlying pathophysiology in the PD population is one limitation to success in DMT trials. It would be rational to select a specific neuroprotective agent targeting a more homogenous study population identified by the presence of a relevant disease-causing mechanism. Targeting GCase in PD patients with a heterozygous *GBA* mutation is an example of this approach which is already underway (see above). Patients with leucine-rich repeat kinase 2 (*LRRK2*) mutations are an example of another opportunity to select a subtype of PD with a specific underlying pathophysiology. *LRRK2,* the most common autosomal dominant genetic cause of PD, codes for a large multifunctional protein but, unfortunately, which protein functions are relevant to disease remains unclear.[61] Interestingly, while most *LRRK2* PD cases demonstrate typical Lewy pathology, some show a bland degeneration with only cell loss and gliosis while others demonstrate primarily tau pathology similar to progressive supranuclear palsy or TDP-43 pathology.[8] This raises the concern that even within this subpopulation of PD there may be significant heterogeneous pathophysiology.

For example, those with Lewy pathology may have more dementia and autonomic dysfunction than those without.[62] The prevailing pathophysiologic theory is the "kinase activation hypothesis" caused by gain of function mutations resulting in increased tyrosine kinase activity and a variety of downstream pathologic effects.[63] This has led to the development of numerous *LRRK2* kinase inhibitors being tested in animal models tempered by discovery of renal and pulmonary toxicities.[63] Most recently, Denali therapeutics has announced successful phase 1 studies of third generation *LRRK2* kinase inhibitors DNL201 and DNL151 in PD patients with plans to advance DNL151 to an advance stage study including PD patients with and without *LRRK2* mutation.

Inflammation

The role of neuroinflammation in PD pathogenesis was first suggested in early postmortem studies of PD brains[64] and has now become an active area of research. The role of neuroinflammation in the pathophysiology of PD is complex and reviewed in detail elsewhere.[65] To summarize briefly, animal studies have demonstrated α-syn appears to be sufficient to initiate neuroinflammation, the innate immune system is critical in the neuroinflammatory process, and activation of microglia to a proinflammatory state likely proceeds neurodegeneration. Moreover, positron emission tomography (PET) ligand imaging specific to microglia has demonstrated microglial activation in PD patients, even early in the disease process.[66] A number of anti-inflammatory agents have been shown to modulate microglial activation in animal studies such as naloxone, minocycline (although there is also conflicting evidence that this may promote neurodegeneration), pioglitazone, and tacrolimus. Other agents with neuroprotective anti-inflammatory properties such as glucocorticoids, dimethyl fumarate, fasudil, and polyphenol quercetin may also be promising in the future.[10,65,67] However, large-scale human clinical studies have not been performed, with the exception of pioglitazone, which was a negative trial, and minocycline, which was found to be "non-futile" but has not been pursued further.[68,69] There has been controversial epidemiological evidence that nonsteroidal anti-inflammatory drug (NSAID) use decreases the risk of PD. One meta-analysis provided evidence specifically in favor of ibuprofen but a more recent meta-analysis failed to demonstrate this association.[70,71] Cyclo-oxygenase type II inhibition may be more relevant to PD pathophysiology[66] so perhaps specific NSAIDs such as ibuprofen, could be neuroprotective. Smaller studies of PD subjects involving AZD3241, an inhibitor of myeloperoxidase generated by microglia and sargramostim, a recombinant granulocyte macrophage colony stimulating factor, have demonstrated evidence for modulation of microglia and regulatory T-cells, respectively, which may provide a neuroprotective effect.[72,73] A clinical trial involving ViNeuro, proposed to have a variety of immunomodulating properties, was completed in 2008 but the results have not been published.

Dopaminergic Therapy

Dopaminergic medications (i.e., dopamine agonists and levodopa) are effective symptomatic treatments for PD but there have also been clinical trials which have investigated the possibility of a neuroprotective effect. Despite initial enthusiasm, there is little convincing evidence that monoamine oxidase B inhibitors (i.e., selegiline and rasagiline) have disease modifying effect. The previous investigations of monoamine oxidase B inhibitors is reviewed elsewhere.[5] Dopamine agonists have demonstrated a neuroprotective antiapoptotic effect in animal studies, but a large randomized clinical trial comparing pramipexole to placebo did not support this.[74] For levodopa, there has been conflicting evidence from animal studies with some that demonstrated a toxic effect by producing free radicals due to dopamine catabolism and others that showed a neuroprotective effect.[5] The ELLDOPA study set out to address this in a large randomized clinical trial but provided inconclusive results.[75] Namely, there appeared to be a clinical neuroprotective and/or symptomatic effect with less decline in clinical measures but a toxic effect on neuroimaging measures with decreased nigrostriatal dopamine transport ligand binding. The levodopa in EArly Parkinson's disease (LEAP) study was developed to better answer this. This 40 week delayed start study of 300 mg of levodopa with carbidopa versus placebo in patients with early clinical syndromes insufficient to interfere with activities of daily living failed to show evidence of disease modification.[76]

Nicotine, Caffeine, and Statins

Tobacco smoking and caffeine have both been associated with decreased risk of developing PD in epidemiologic studies.[77] This led to a phase 2 clinical trial investigating a nicotine patch in PD, which failed to show evidence of disease modification.[78] An alternative explanation for the decreased risk association with tobacco smoking is that PD patients in the prodromal phase are less easily addicted to nicotine resulting in decreased use.[79] Caffeine is thought to mitigate excitotoxicity through nonspecific adenosine receptor inhibition. A phase 3 clinical trial showed no improvement in PD symptoms[80] and this has not been pursued with a longer study to evaluate potential disease modifying effects. Epidemiologic studies investigating the association of statin therapy with development of PD are confounded by the primary purpose of prescribing statin therapy (i.e., dyslipidemia or cardiovascular risk factors) making their interpretation challenging.[81] Similar to GLP1R agonists described above, various mechanisms of neuroprotection in PD have been proposed including modulation of neuroinflammation and microglial activation (which may in turn impact α-syn aggregation and propagation), reduction of oxidative and nitrative stress, and promotion of neurotrophic factors independent of the impact on cholesterol.[81] Based on these proposed mechanisms, simvastatin and lovastatin are both being investigated for a neuroprotective effect in PD.

Exercise

Exercise in animal models has been shown to have numerous potentially neuroprotective effects including increased expression of anti-inflammatory cytokines, reduced proinflammatory cytokines, decreased α-syn expression, increased antioxidants, and reduced glutaminergic excitotoxicity while human studies have demonstrated neuroplastic changes such as increased serum levels of brain derived neurotrophic factor, increased corticomotor excitability, improved striatal D2 receptor binding, and changes in gray matter volume.[82] However, it is difficult to determine if these changes are simply central consequences of improved physical fitness or if this has a true neuroprotective effect on the underlying pathophysiology. This is an active area of research with little definitive evidence available to date.

Deep Brain Stimulation and Focused Ultrasound Therapy

Deep brain stimulation (DBS) has a profound symptomatic benefit for PD patients but may also have neuroprotective benefits by reducing glutaminergic excitotoxicity from the subthalamic nucleus (STN) and promoting release of neurotrophic factors[83] with evidence of neuroprotection in an α-syn animal model.[84] There is ongoing interest in evaluating this in a clinical study in early stage PD.[6] A recent study has suggested that STN DBS slows progression of rest tremor in early PD.[85] High-intensity focused-ultrasound (FUS) thalamotomy is a method of focally heating and ablating brain tissue and an established alternative therapy to DBS for symptomatic treatment of essential tremor. FUS subthalamotomy is currently being investigated in PD patients as an alternative to DBS and this may theoretically be neuroprotective for the same reasons as STN DBS.[86] In contrast, low-intensity FUS offers an alternative means of neuroprotection to temporarily, locally, and reversibly open the BBB thereby allowing other therapeutic agents access to the CNS, a common barrier to many putative neuroprotective agents. By injecting microbubbles while applying low-intensity FUS, thermal injury is avoided and alternating expansion and contraction of microbubbles is the goal, which thought to mechanically disrupt endothelial cells thereby opening the BBB.[87] This has been investigated in preclinical PD models involving use of anti-α-syn antibodies, anti-α-syn silencing RNA, and neurotrophic factors and opens up the possibility of a new focused delivery mechanism for gene therapy.[87] Excitement for this modality is tempered by uncertainties such as optimal location for therapy delivery and safety profile in humans and more research is needed.

RESTORATIVE THERAPIES

Neurotrophic Factors

Neurotrophic factors are endogenous proteins specific to populations of neurons that allow proper development, differentiation, and maintenance and may be beneficial in PD by promoting survival and restoring neuronal circuitry. The most studied neurotrophic factors in PD are glial cell line derived-neurotrophic factor (GDNF) and neurturin. To date, these have not clearly demonstrated significant neuroprotection or regeneration. One limitation is that these agents need to be delivered invasively and in close proximity to the nigrostriatal projections. The first large clinical trial delivered GDNF intraventricularly but failed to show benefit.[88] Due to concerns that GDNF did not reach the nigrostriatal neurons, a clinical trial delivering GDNF intraputaminally was pursued but this again was negative.[89] Some critics of this trial argued that it failed due to inadequate coverage of the striatum. However, a more recent trial using convection-enhanced delivery of GDNF revealed that despite improved striatal coverage compared to previous studies there remained no clinical benefit compared to placebo.[90] Given the negative results involving GDNF, next a viral-mediated gene transfer of the related neurotrophic factor neuturin, delivered to the putamen and substantia nigra, was pursued but this also did not show benefit.[91] There is now a phase 1 trial involving viral delivery of GDNF using an optimized magnetic resonance imaging (MRI)-guided convection-enhanced delivery system which is ongoing, interest in other neurotrophic factors including platelet-derived growth factor and cerebral dopaminergic neurotrophic factor,[92] and attention turned toward the prospect of FUS-delivered neurotrophic factors. There are also other explanations for previous trial failures with this modality. For example, many of the animal studies that demonstrated efficacy used a toxin-based or lesion-based animal model with delivery of the study drug soon after the initial insult to the nigrostriatal tract. However, many of the clinical studies enrolled advanced PD patients with a degree of nigrostriatal loss that may have been too severe for neurotrophic factors to have a significant impact. Indeed, advanced nigrostriatal loss may be the case in very early disease. A previous autopsy study of PD patients showed that by 4 years after diagnosis the vast majority of dopamine function marker loss (tyrosine hydroxylase and dopamine transporter) had already occurred while neurons staining for melanin are relatively preserved in the dorsal putamen.[2] This could be due to degeneration of SNpc projections or dysfunctional but potentially viable SNpc projections, either of which would impair axonal transport of trophic factors. Furthermore, the same benefit from trophic factors has not been consistently replicated in α-syn-based animal models as compared to toxin and lesion-based animal models. There is evidence that α-syn aggregation may lead to downregulation of the Ret receptor, a downstream signaling molecule critical for neurotrophic factor function,[93] which may help explain the discrepancies between the results of toxin and lesion-based animal models and α-syn-based animal models and human clinical trials.

Viral-mediated Gene Therapy

In addition to the study of viral-mediated delivery of neurotrophic factor genes, there have also been clinical studies investigating viral-mediated delivery of genes that encode enzymes involved in dopamine synthesis. A recent open label trial found that ProSavin, which encodes the rate-limiting dopamine producing enzymes tyrosine hydroxylase, aromatic L-amino acid decarboxylase (AADC), and guanosine triphosphate (GTP)-cyclohydrolase 1, was well tolerated[94] and the same pharmaceutical company has started a phase 2 study of OXB-102 (AXO-Lenti-PD) thought to have optimized expression of dopamine biosynthesis enzymes and thus improved dopamine production compared to Prosavin. Another agent, VY-AADC01, that encodes AADC is currently being studied.

Axonal Regeneration

Contrary to a long-standing and commonly held belief that CNS adult neurons cannot regenerate, researchers have shown that nigrostriatal projections can be regenerated by activating intrinsic neuronal factors that regulate axon growth during development in toxin-based animal models of PD.[95] This suggests axonal regeneration is possible but further work is needed before this can be transferred to human trials.

Cell-based Therapies

The initial most promising cell-based therapies involved transplantation of fetal ventral mesencephalic neurons. There was enthusiasm for this treatment option because of long-lasting benefit experienced by a small number of subjects in open label trials.[96] However, two National Institutes of Health funded double-blind placebo-controlled trials did not demonstrate efficacy and raised concern about the safety of this approach due to the development of dyskinesias within 1 year of transplantation, thereafter termed graft-induced dyskinesias.[97,98] The etiology of graft-induced dyskinesias is thought to be related to the presence of serotonergic neurons in the donor tissue (a result of poor tissue dissection and selection of tissue) as well as uneven striatal innervation.[99,100] These studies also suggested that immunosuppression may be important for graft survival because the later study showed that UPDRS scores were initially improved in the active treatment group but declined after immunosuppression was stopped at 6 months.[97] The TRANSEURO program is continuing to evaluate the safety and efficacy of fetal ventral mesencephalic transplantation in a longitudinal open-label study, with plans to advance this work to the use of stem cell-based therapies. Indeed, there is continued interest in using dopaminergic cells derived from embryonic stem cells (ESC) and induced pluripotent stem cells (iPSC) with early small clinical trials that have recently started (**Table 1**).[101] These options help address the limited supply of fetal mesenchymal tissue which makes application of fetal ventral mesenchymal transplant, if shown to be beneficial, impractical. ESC-based therapy has similar ethical issues as fetal tissue and is likely to require some degree of immunosuppression but produces more consistent cells compared to iPSC methods.[102] On the other hand, iPSCs can be derived from reprogramming autogenic somatic cells which would circumvent the need for immunosuppression. A recent single case report describes persistent modest improvement of posterior putaminal fluorodopa PET binding for 24 months without the use of immunosuppression.[103] This finding could indicate persistent survival of transplanted autologous iPSCs, however, similar PET changes accompanied by survival of transplanted fetal dopaminergic neurons found postmortem, has not been predictive of clinical benefit. Further, fluorodopa PET changes may be indicative of an inflammatory response to the transplant rather than cell survival. This case also highlights challenges such as the need to account for placebo effect of an invasive procedure carrying high expectations and the more costly and labor-intensive methods used for autologous iPSCs as compared to allogenic cell lines, which will limit generalizability. These cells may also carry the same genetic predisposition for PD pathology so the development of Lewy pathology in the allogenic fetal VM grafts mentioned above might occur even earlier for iPSCs.[104]

These regenerative/restorative therapies would certainly be beneficial if they can restore lost nigrostriatal dopaminergic projections and improve related motor deficits. However, even their strongest proponents acknowledge that these therapies do not address the underlying pathophysiology of PD and will therefore not address the many very disabling levodopa-resistant motor and nonmotor features of disease. In addition, successful graft mediated striatal dopamine reinnervation may not predict clinical benefit. This was recognized in one case where a patient with PD underwent fetal ventral mesencephalic transplantation without clinical benefit but had normalized nigrostriatal reinnervation demonstrated on fluorodopa PET and at postmortem analysis.[105]

CONCLUSION

We have reviewed many of the neuroprotective and restorative therapies that have been or are currently being investigated in PD as well as obstacles to success. In the future, the development of reliable biomarkers and advances in our understanding of the underlying pathophysiology will more likely lead to effective therapies that target selected subgroups of PD patients (i.e., stratified medicine) rather than expecting a "one size fits all" approach to disease modification. Examples of this may include PD patients carrying a *GBA*, *LRRK2*, or *SNCA* mutation paired with appropriate therapies (e.g., ambroxol, *LRRK2* kinase inhibitor, or anti-α-syn antibody therapy) or women with PD paired with inosine. Other therapies may be effective only if applied at appropriate stages of disease such as isradipine in prodromal PD or anti-α-syn antibody therapy in early PD. On the other hand, other fields of medicine have used combination cocktails successfully (e.g., cancer treatment and human immunodeficiency virus treatment) utilizing multiple drugs with different mechanisms of action. This approach has been all but ignored in PD but should be an important consideration in this population with heterogeneous pathophysiology. Regardless, it is hoped that one of the large advanced or up-and-coming clinical trials described above may prove successful, but with many years of equivocal or disappointing trial results with neuroprotective and regenerative therapies other avenues must continue to be explored.

REFERENCES

1. Espay AJ, Schwarzschild MA, Tanner CM, Fernandez HH, Simon DK, Leverenz JB, et al. Biomarker-driven phenotyping in Parkinson's disease: A translational missing link in disease-modifying clinical trials. Mov Disord. 2017;32(3):319-24.
2. Kordower JH, Olanow CW, Dodiya HB, Chu Y, Beach TG, Adler CH, et al. Disease duration and the integrity of the nigrostriatal system in Parkinson's disease. Brain. 2013;136(8):2419-31.
3. Berg D, Postuma RB, Adler CH, Bloem BR, Chan P, Dubois B, et al. MDS research criteria for prodromal Parkinson's disease. Mov Disord. 2015;30(12):1600-11.
4. McGhee DJM, Ritchie CW, Zajicek JP, Counsell CE. A review of clinical trial designs used to detect a disease-modifying effect of drug therapy in Alzheimer's disease and Parkinson's disease. BMC Neurol. 2016;16:92.
5. AlDakheel A, Kalia LV, Lang AE. Pathogenesis-targeted, disease-modifying therapies in Parkinson disease. Neurotherapeutics. 2014;11(1):6-23.
6. Lang AE, Espay AJ. Disease Modification in Parkinson's disease: Current Approaches, Challenges, and Future Considerations. Mov Disord. 2018;33(5):660-77.
7. Villar-Piqué A, Lopes da Fonseca T, Outeiro TF. Structure, function and toxicity of alpha-synuclein: the Bermuda triangle in synucleinopathies. J Neurochem. 2016;139(1):240-55.
8. Schneider SA, Alcalay RN. Neuropathology of genetic synucleinopathies with parkinsonism: Review of the literature. Mov Disord. 2017;32(11):1504-23.
9. Wong YC, Krainc D. α-synuclein toxicity in neurodegeneration: mechanism and therapeutic strategies. Nat Med. 2017;23(2): 1-13.
10. Ammal Kaidery N, Thomas B. Current perspective of mitochondrial biology in Parkinson's disease. Neurochem Int. 2018;117:91-113.
11. Mazzulli JR, Xu Y-H, Sun Y, Knight AL, McLean PJ, Caldwell GA, et al. Gaucher disease glucocerebrosidase and α-synuclein form a bidirectional pathogenic loop in synucleinopathies. Cell. 2011;146(1):37-52.
12. Kordower JH, Chu Y, Hauser RA, Freeman TB, Olanow CW. Lewy body-like pathology in long-term embryonic nigral transplants in Parkinson's disease. Nat Med. 2008;14(5):504-6.
13. Danzer KM, Kranich LR, Ruf WP, Cagsal-Getkin O, Winslow AR, Zhu L, et al. Exosomal cell-to-cell transmission of alpha synuclein oligomers. Mol Neurodegener. 2012;7(1):42.
14. Bousset L, Pieri L, Ruiz-Arlandis G, Gath J, Jensen PH, Habenstein B, et al. Structural and functional characterization of two alpha-synuclein strains. Nat Commun. 2013;4(1):2575.
15. Melki R. Role of different alpha-synuclein strains in synucleinopathies, similarities with other neurodegenerative diseases. J Parkinsons Dis. 2015;5(2):217-27.
16. Frigerio R, Fujishiro H, Ahn T-B, Josephs KA, Maraganore DM, DelleDonne A, et al. Incidental Lewy body disease: Do some cases represent a preclinical stage of dementia with Lewy bodies? Neurobiol Aging. 2011;32(5):857-63.
17. Surmeier DJ, Halliday GM, Simuni T. Calcium, mitochondrial dysfunction and slowing the progression of Parkinson's disease. Exp Neurol. 2017;298:202-9.
18. Leggio L, Vivarelli S, L'Episcopo F, Tirolo C, Caniglia S, Testa N, et al. microRNAs in Parkinson's Disease: From Pathogenesis to Novel Diagnostic and Therapeutic Approaches. Int J Mol Sci. 2017;18(12):2698.
19. Mittal S, Bjørnevik K, Im DS, Flierl A, Dong X, Locascio JJ, et al. β2-Adrenoreceptor is a regulator of the α-synuclein gene driving risk of Parkinson's disease. Science. 2017;357(6354):891-8.
20. Hopfner F, Wod M, Höglinger GU, Blaabjerg M, Rösler TW, Kuhlenbäumer G, et al. Use of β2-adrenoreceptor agonist and antagonist drugs and risk of Parkinson disease. Neurology. 2019;93(2):e135-42.
21. O'Hara DM, Kalia SK, Kalia LV. Emerging disease-modifying strategies targeting α-synuclein for the treatment of Parkinson's disease. Br J Pharmacol. 2018;175(15):3080-9.
22. Bhatt MA, Messer A, Kordower JH. Can intrabodies serve as neuroprotective therapies for Parkinson's disease? Beginning thoughts. J Parkinsons Dis. 2013;3(4):581-91.

23. Brundin P, Dave KD, Kordower JH. Therapeutic approaches to target alpha-synuclein pathology. Exp Neurol. 2017;298:225-35.
24. Pagan F, Hebron M, Valadez EH, Torres-Yaghi Y, Huang X, Mills RR, et al. Nilotinib Effects in Parkinson's disease and Dementia with Lewy bodies. J Parkinsons Dis. 2016;6(3):503-17.
25. Brahmachari S, Karuppagounder SS, Ge P, Lee S, Dawson VL, Dawson TM, et al. c-Abl and Parkinson's Disease: Mechanisms and Therapeutic Potential. J Parkinsons Dis. 2017;7(4):589-601.
26. Pagan FL, Hebron ML, Wilmarth B, Torres-Yaghi Y, Lawler A, Mundel EE, et al. Nilotinib Effects on Safety, Tolerability, and Potential Biomarkers in Parkinson Disease: A Phase 2 Randomized Clinical Trial. JAMA Neurol. 2020;77(3):309-317.
27. Zhang Y-K, Zhang G-N, Wang Y-J, Patel BA, Talele TT, Yang D-H, et al. Bafetinib (INNO-406) reverses multidrug resistance by inhibiting the efflux function of ABCB1 and ABCG2 transporters. Sci Rep. 2016;6(1):25694.
28. Espay AJ, Hauser RA, Armstrong MJ. The Narrowing Path for Nilotinib and Other Potential Disease-Modifying Therapies for Parkinson Disease. JAMA Neurol. 2020; 77(3):295-297.
29. Simuni T, Fiske B, Merchant K, et al. Efficacy of Nilotinib in Patients With Moderately Advanced Parkinson Disease. JAMA Neurol. 2021;78(3):312.
30. Andrew G, Faulkner R, Sadashivam V, Omidvar O, Hill J, Jagadeesan S, et al. Results of a Phase 1 Dose-Ranging Trial, and Design of a Phase 2 Trial, of K0706, a Novel C-Abl Tyrosine Kinase Inhibitor for Parkinson's Disease. (P2.8-047). Neurology. 2019;92(15).
31. Perni M, Galvagnion C, Maltsev A, Meisl G, Müller MB, Challa PK, et al. A natural product inhibits the initiation of α-synuclein aggregation and suppresses its toxicity. Proc Natl Acad Sci USA. 2017;114(6):E1009-17.
32. Sidransky E, Nalls MA, Aasly JO, Aharon-Peretz J, Annesi G, Barbosa ER, et al. Multicenter Analysis of Glucocerebrosidase Mutations in Parkinson's Disease. N Engl J Med. 2009;361(17):1651-61.
33. Parnetti L, Chiasserini D, Persichetti E, Eusebi P, Varghese S, Qureshi MM, et al. Cerebrospinal fluid lysosomal enzymes and alpha-synuclein in Parkinson's disease. Mov Disord. 2014;29(8):1019-27.
34. Schueler U, Kaneski C, Murray G, Sandhoff K, Brady RO. Uptake of mannose-terminal glucocerebrosidase in cultured human cholinergic and dopaminergic neuron cell lines. Neurochem Res. 2002;27(4):325-30.
35. McNeill A, Magalhaes J, Shen C, Chau K-Y, Hughes D, Mehta A, et al. Ambroxol improves lysosomal biochemistry in glucocerebrosidase mutation-linked Parkinson disease cells. Brain. 2014;137(5):1481-95.
36. Mullin S, Smith L, Lee K, D'Souza G, Woodgate P, Elflein J, et al. Ambroxol for the treatment of patients with Parkinson Disease With and Without Glucocerebrosidase Gene Mutations: A Nonrandomized, Noncontrolled Trial. JAMA Neurol. 2020;77(4):427-34.
37. Marshall J, Sun Y, Bangari DS, Budman E, Park H, Nietupski JB, et al. CNS-accessible Inhibitor of Glucosylceramide Synthase for Substrate Reduction Therapy of Neuronopathic Gaucher Disease. Mol Ther. 2016;24(6):1019-29.
38. Sidransky E, Arkadir D, Bauer P, Dinur T, Lopez G, Rolfs A, et al. Substrate Reduction Therapy for GBA1 -Associated Parkinsonism: Are We Betting on the Wrong Mouse? Mov Disord. 2020;35(2):228-30.
39. Masliah E, Rockenstein E, Adame A, Alford M, Crews L, Hashimoto M, et al. Effects of α-Synuclein Immunization in a Mouse Model of Parkinson's Disease. Neuron. 2005;46(6): 857-68.
40. Heneka MT, Carson MJ, Khoury J El, Landreth GE, Brosseron F, Feinstein DL, et al. Neuroinflammation in Alzheimer's disease. Lancet Neurol. 2015;14(4):388-405.
41. Braczynski AK, Schulz JB, Bach J-P. Vaccination strategies in tauopathies and synucleinopathies. J Neurochem. 2017;143(5):467-88.
42. Goodwin K, Viboud C, Simonsen L. Antibody response to influenza vaccination in the elderly: a quantitative review. Vaccine. 2006;24(8):1159-69.
43. Mandler M, Valera E, Rockenstein E, Weninger H, Patrick C, Adame A, et al. Next-generation active immunization approach for synucleinopathies: implications for Parkinson's disease clinical trials. Acta Neuropathol. 2014;127(6):861-79.
44. Zella SMA, Metzdorf J, Ciftci E, Ostendorf F, Muhlack S, Gold R, et al. Emerging Immunotherapies for Parkinson Disease. Neurol Ther. 2019;8(1):29-44.
45. Brys M, Fanning L, Hung S, Ellenbogen A, Penner N, Yang M, et al. Randomized phase I clinical trial of anti-α-synuclein antibody BIIB054. Mov Disord. 2019;34(8):1154-63.
46. Jankovic J, Goodman I, Safirstein B, Marmon TK, Schenk DB, Koller M, et al. Safety and tolerability of multiple ascending doses of PR X002/RG7935, an Anti-α-Synuclein Monoclonal Antibody, in Patients With Parkinson Disease: A randomized clinical trial. JAMA Neurol. 2018;75(10):1206-14.
47. Schofield DJ, Irving L, Calo L, Bogstedt A, Rees G, Nuccitelli A, et al. Preclinical development of a high affinity α-synuclein antibody, MEDI1341, that can enter the brain, sequester extracellular α-synuclein and attenuate α-synuclein spreading in vivo. Neurobiol Dis. 2019;132:104582.
48. Dufty BM, Warner LR, Hou ST, Jiang SX, Gomez-Isla T, Leenhouts KM, et al. Calpain-Cleavage of α-Synuclein: connecting proteolytic processing to disease-linked aggregation. Am J Pathol. 2007;170(5):1725-38.
49. Sinnegger-Brauns MJ, Huber IG, Koschak A, Wild C, Obermair GJ, Einzinger U, et al. Expression and 1,4-Dihydropyridine-Binding Properties of Brain L-Type Calcium Channel Isoforms. Mol Pharmacol. 2009;75(2):407-14.
50. The Parkinson Study Group STEADY-PD III Investigators. Isradipine versus Placebo in Early Parkinson Disease: A Randomized Trial. Ann Intern Med. 2020;172(9):591-8.
51. Yu Z, Zhang S, Wang D, Fan M, Gao F, Sun W, et al. The significance of uric acid in the diagnosis and treatment of Parkinson disease: An updated systemic review. Medicine (Baltimore). 2017;96(45):e8502.
52. Schwarzschild MA, Macklin EA, Bakshi R, Battacharyya S, Logan R, Espay AJ, et al. Sex differences by design and outcome in the Safety of Urate Elevation in PD (SURE-PD) trial. Neurology. 2019;93(14):e1328-38.
53. Athauda D, Foltynie T. Protective effects of the GLP-1 mimetic exendin-4 in Parkinson's disease. Neuropharmacology. 2018;136:260-70.
54. Athauda D, Maclagan K, Skene SS, Bajwa-Joseph M, Letchford D, Chowdhury K, et al. Exenatide once weekly versus placebo in Parkinson's disease: a randomised, double-blind, placebo-controlled trial. Lancet. 2017;390(10103):1664-75.

55. Kim KS, Park DH, Wessel TC, Song B, Wagner JA, Joh TH. A dual role for the cAMP-dependent protein kinase in tyrosine hydroxylase gene expression. Proc Natl Acad Sci U S A. 1993;90(8):3471-5.
56. Sian-Hülsmann J, Mandel S, Youdim MBH, Riederer P. The relevance of iron in the pathogenesis of Parkinson's disease. J Neurochem. 2011;118(6):939-57.
57. Cabantchik ZI, Munnich A, Youdim MB, Devos D. Regional siderosis: A new challenge for iron chelation therapy. Front Pharmacol. 2013;4:167.
58. Devos D, Moreau C, Devedjian JC, Kluza J, Petrault M, Laloux C, et al. Targeting chelatable iron as a therapeutic modality in Parkinson's disease. Antioxid Redox Signal. 2014;21(2): 195-210.
59. Hung LW, Villemagne VL, Cheng L, Sherratt NA, Ayton S, White AR, et al. The hypoxia imaging agent CuII(atsm) is neuroprotectivex and improves motor and cognitive functions in multiple animal models of Parkinson's disease. J Exp Med. 2012;209(4):837-54.
60. Donnelly PS, Liddell JR, Lim S, Paterson BM, Cater MA, Savva MS, et al. An impaired mitochondrial electron transport chain increases retention of the hypoxia imaging agent diacetylbis (4-methylthiosemicarbazonato) copperII. Proc Natl Acad Sci U S A. 2012;109(1):47-52.
61. Price A, Manzoni C, Cookson MR, Lewis PA. The LRRK2 signalling system. Cell Tissue Res. 2018;373(1):39-50.
62. Kalia LV, Lang AE, Hazrati L-N, Fujioka S, Wszolek ZK, Dickson DW, et al. Clinical correlations with Lewy body pathology in LRRK2-related Parkinson disease. JAMA Neurol. 2015;72(1): 100-5.
63. West AB. Achieving neuroprotection with LRRK2 kinase inhibitors in Parkinson disease. Exp Neurol. 2017;298:236-45.
64. McGeer PL, Itagaki S, Boyes BE, McGeer EG. Reactive microglia are positive for HLA-DR in the substantia nigra of Parkinson's and Alzheimer's disease brains. Neurology. 1988;38(8):1285-91.
65. Gelders G, Baekelandt V, Van der Perren A. Linking neuroinflammation and neurodegeneration in Parkinson's disease. J Immunol Res. 2018;2018:1-12.
66. Gerhard A, Pavese N, Hotton G, Turkheimer F, Es M, Hammers A, et al. In vivo imaging of microglial activation with [11C](R)-PK11195 PET in idiopathic Parkinson's disease. Neurobiol Dis. 2006;21(2):404-12.
67. Joshi N, Singh S. Updates on immunity and inflammation in Parkinson disease pathology. J Neurosci Res. 2018;96(3): 379-90.
68. NINDS Exploratory Trials in Parkinson Disease (NET-PD) FS-ZONE Investigators. Pioglitazone in early Parkinson's disease: a phase 2, multicentre, double-blind, randomised trial. Lancet Neurol. 2015;14(8):795-803.
69. NINDS NET-PD Investigators. A randomized, double-blind, futility clinical trial of creatine and minocycline in early Parkinson disease. Neurology. 2006;66(5):664-71.
70. Ren L, Yi J, Yang J, Li P, Cheng X, Mao P. Nonsteroidal anti-inflammatory drugs use and risk of Parkinson disease. Medicine (Baltimore). 2018;97(37):e12172.
71. Rees K, Stowe R, Patel S, Ives N, Breen K, Clarke CE, et al. Non-steroidal anti-inflammatory drugs as disease-modifying agents for Parkinson's disease: evidence from observational studies. Cochrane Database Syst Rev. 2011;11:CD008454.
72. Gendelman HE, Zhang Y, Santamaria P, Olson KE, Schutt CR, Bhatti D, et al. Evaluation of the safety and immunomodulatory effects of sargramostim in a randomized, double-blind phase 1 clinical Parkinson's disease trial. NPJ Parkinsons Dis. 2017;3(1):10.
73. Jucaite A, Svenningsson P, Rinne JO, Cselényi Z, Varnäs K, Johnström P, et al. Effect of the myeloperoxidase inhibitor AZD3241 on microglia: a PET study in Parkinson's disease. Brain. 2015;138(9):2687-700.
74. Schapira AHV, McDermott MP, Barone P, Comella CL, Albrecht S, Hsu HH, et al. Pramipexole in patients with early Parkinson's disease (PROUD): a randomised delayed-start trial. Lancet Neurol. 2013;12(8):747-55.
75. Fahn S, Oakes D, Shoulson I, Kieburtz K, Rudolph A, Lang A, et al. Levodopa and the progression of Parkinson's disease. N Engl J Med. 2004;351(24):2498-508.
76. Verschuur CVM, Suwijn SR, Boel JA, Post B, Bloem BR, van Hilten JJ, et al. Randomized Delayed-Start Trial of Levodopa in Parkinson's Disease. N Engl J Med. 2019;380(4):315-24.
77. Hernán MA, Takkouche B, Caamaño-Isorna F, Gestal-Otero JJ. A meta-analysis of coffee drinking, cigarette smoking, and the risk of Parkinson's disease. Ann Neurol. 2002;52(3):276-84.
78. Oertel W, Müller H, Schade-Brittinger C, Kamp C, Balthasar K, Articus K, et al. The NIC-PD-study—A randomized, placebo-controlled, double-blind, multi-centre trial to assess the disease-modifying potential of transdermal nicotine in early Parkinson's disease in Germany and N America. Mov Disord. 2018;33(Suppl 2).
79. Ritz B, Lee P-C, Lassen CF, Arah OA. Parkinson disease and smoking revisited: Ease of quitting is an early sign of the disease. Neurology. 2014 14;83(16):1396-402.
80. Postuma RB, Anang J, Pelletier A, Joseph L, Moscovich M, Grimes D, et al. Caffeine as symptomatic treatment for Parkinson disease (Café-PD): A randomized trial. Neurology. 2017;89(17):1795-803.
81. Carroll CB, Wyse RKH. Simvastatin as a Potential Disease-Modifying Therapy for Patients with Parkinson's disease: Rationale for Clinical Trial, and Current Progress. J Parkinsons Dis. 2017;7(4):545-68.
82. Mak MK, Wong-Yu IS, Shen X, Chung CL. Long-term effects of exercise and physical therapy in people with Parkinson disease. Nat Rev Neurol. 2017;13(11):689-703.
83. Torres N, Molet J, Moro C, Mitrofanis J, Benabid A. Neuroprotective Surgical Strategies in Parkinson's Disease: Role of Preclinical Data. Int J Mol Sci. 2017;18(10):2190.
84. Musacchio T, Rebenstorff M, Fluri F, Brotchie JM, Volkmann J, Koprich JB, et al. Subthalamic nucleus deep brain stimulation is neuroprotective in the A53T α-synuclein Parkinson's disease rat model. Ann Neurol. 2017;81(6):825-36.
85. Hacker ML, DeLong MR, Turchan M, Heusinkveld LE, Ostrem JL, Molinari AL, et al. Effects of deep brain stimulation on rest tremor progression in early stage Parkinson disease. Neurology. 2018;91(5):e463-71.
86. Foffani G, Trigo-Damas I, Pineda-Pardo JA, Blesa J, Rodríguez-Rojas R, Martínez-Fernández R, et al. Focused ultrasound in Parkinson's disease: A twofold path toward disease modification. Mov Disord. 2019;34(9):1262-73.
87. Karakatsani ME, Blesa J, Konofagou EE. Blood-brain barrier opening with focused ultrasound in experimental models of Parkinson's disease. Mov Disord. 2019;34(9):1252-61.

88. Nutt JG, Burchiel KJ, Comella CL, Jankovic J, Lang AE, Laws ER, et al. Randomized, double-blind trial of glial cell line-derived neurotrophic factor (GDNF) in PD. Neurology. 2003;60(1): 69-73.
89. Lang AE, Gill S, Patel NK, Lozano A, Nutt JG, Penn R, et al. Randomized controlled trial of intraputamenal glial cell line-derived neurotrophic factor infusion in Parkinson disease. Ann Neurol. 2006;59(3):459-66.
90. Whone A, Luz M, Boca M, Woolley M, Mooney L, Dharia S, et al. Randomized trial of intermittent intraputamenal glial cell line-derived neurotrophic factor in Parkinson's disease. Brain. 2019;142(3):512-25.
91. Warren Olanow C, Bartus RT, Baumann TL, Factor S, Boulis N, Stacy M, et al. Gene delivery of neurturin to putamen and substantia nigra in Parkinson disease: A double-blind, randomized, controlled trial. Ann Neurol. 2015;78(2):248-57.
92. Paul G, Sullivan AM. Trophic factors for Parkinson's disease: Where are we and where do we go from here? Eur J Neurosci. 2018;49(4):440-52.
93. Decressac M, Kadkhodaei B, Mattsson B, Laguna A, Perlmann T, Bjorklund A. α-Synuclein-Induced Down-Regulation of Nurr1 Disrupts GDNF Signaling in Nigral Dopamine Neurons. Sci Transl Med. 2012;4(163):163ra156.
94. Palfi S, Gurruchaga JM, Ralph GS, Lepetit H, Lavisse S, Buttery PC, et al. Long-term safety and tolerability of ProSavin, a lentiviral vector-based gene therapy for Parkinson's disease: a dose escalation, open-label, phase 1/2 trial. Lancet. 2014;383(9923):1138-46.
95. Kordower JH, Burke RE. Disease Modification for Parkinson's disease: Axonal Regeneration and Trophic Factors. Mov Disord. 2018;33(5):678-83.
96. Moriarty N, Parish CL, Dowd E. Primary tissue for cellular brain repair in Parkinson's disease: Promise, problems and the potential of biomaterials. Eur J Neurosci. 2019;49(4):472-486.
97. Olanow CW, Goetz CG, Kordower JH, Stoessl AJ, Sossi V, Brin MF, et al. A double-blind controlled trial of bilateral fetal nigral transplantation in Parkinson's disease. Ann Neurol. 2003;54(3):403-14.
98. Freed CR, Greene PE, Breeze RE, Tsai W-Y, DuMouchel W, Kao R, et al. Transplantation of Embryonic Dopamine Neurons for Severe Parkinson's Disease. N Engl J Med. 2001;344(10): 710-9.
99. Carlsson T, Winkler C, Lundblad M, Cenci MA, Björklund A, Kirik D. Graft placement and uneven pattern of reinnervation in the striatum is important for development of graft-induced dyskinesia. Neurobiol Dis. 2006;21(3):657-68.
100. Carlsson T, Carta M, Winkler C, Björklund A, Kirik D. Serotonin neuron transplants exacerbate L-DOPA-induced dyskinesias in a rat model of Parkinson's disease. J Neurosci. 2007;27(30): 8011-22.
101. Parmar M, Grealish S, Henchcliffe C. The future of stem cell therapies for Parkinson disease. Nat Rev Neurosci. 2020;21(2):103-15.
102. Stoker TB, Torsney KM, Barker RA. Emerging Treatment Approaches for Parkinson's Disease. Front Neurosci. 2018;12:693.
103. Schweitzer JS, Song B, Herrington TM, Park T-Y, Lee N, Ko S, et al. Personalized iPSC-Derived Dopamine Progenitor Cells for Parkinson's Disease. N Engl J Med. 2020;382(20):1926-32.
104. Li W, Englund E, Widner H, Mattsson B, van Westen D, Lätt J, et al. Extensive graft-derived dopaminergic innervation is maintained 24 years after transplantation in the degenerating parkinsonian brain. Proc Natl Acad Sci USA. 2016;113(23): 6544-9.
105. Kordower JH, Goetz CG, Chu Y, Halliday GM, Nicholson DA, Musial TF, et al. Robust graft survival and normalized dopaminergic innervation do not obligate recovery in a Parkinson disease patient. Ann Neurol. 2017;81(1):46-57.

CHAPTER 24

Future Directions in the Medical Therapy of Parkinson's Disease

Charulata Savant Sankhla, Mahendra Thakre

"There are things known, and there are things unknown, and in between are the doors of perception"
—Aldous Huxley

INTRODUCTION

Medical therapy for Parkinson's disease (PD) has evolved significantly and options to treat the symptoms and improve the quality of life of PD patients has grown. We, however, still lack neuroprotective or disease-modifying therapy in PD.

The major barrier to finding a cure or disease modification therapy is the heterogenicity of PD, lack of a preclinical model of sporadic PD, lack of a disease biomarker, and failure to recognize preclinical PD. A complex interplay between genes, proteins, cellular organelles, and neural networks contributes to this heterogenicity.[1]

Parkinson's disease is the consequence of changes in the neuronal cytoskeleton developing in only a few susceptible types of nerve cells.

SYMPTOMATIC TREATMENT

The management of PD depends on the time of onset, the duration of the disease, age, social situation, and the functional status of the patient. The aim is to improve the activities of daily living, and the quality of life.

The target of treatment is to improve motor function, autonomic function, cognitive rehabilitation, communicative skills, and psychiatric symptoms. All treatments currently available are symptomatic and do not slow down the disease progression.[2]

Long-term Consequences of Oral Levodopa Therapy

Levodopa (L-DOPA) was first introduced in the late 1960s and remains the gold standard for the treatment of PD even today. Response to L-DOPA is one of the criteria for the clinical diagnosis of PD.[3] Duodenum neural amino acids compete for L-DOPA uptake. Hence, it is recommended that oral L-DOPA should be taken 1 hour before or 2 hours after food.[2]

Levodopa has a short plasma half-life, hence, oral L-DOPA causes pulsatile striatal receptor stimulation. This leads to dyskinesias, troublesome motor fluctuations, and unpredictable swings from mobility to immobility. The development of dyskinesias and motor fluctuation is the major limiting factor in oral L-DOPA therapy.

Disease severity, women, tremor-dominant PD and patients with young-onset PD, carriers of autosomal recessive PD (*parkin, PINK1*, and *DJ-1*), genetic variations in dopamine receptor D2 (DRD2) gene, dopamine transporter (DAT), and opioid receptor Mu 1 (OPRM1), polymorphism Val66Met in the brain-derived neurotrophic factor (BDNF) gene and the A-allele of the catechol-O-methyltransferase (COMT) polymorphism are the risk factor for LID.[4]

Levodopa-carbidopa Intestinal Gel Therapy

Intrajejunal infusion therapy with L-DOPA is approved for the treatment of advanced PD with marked motor fluctuations.[5] L-DOPA bound to a particular matrix is constantly delivered directly into the jejunum via a percutaneous tube fixated to the abdominal wall and connected to an externally carried pump.[2] This results in a constant L-DOPA plasma level, which avoids pulsatile receptor stimulation and erratic gastric emptying. It is recommended as monotherapy. It is expensive and requires technical skills for the precise placing of the tube into the jejunal cavity. A reduction in off-time (mean off-time decreased by 4.04 hours) and an increase in on-time without troublesome dyskinesia (mean on-time without troublesome dyskinesia increased by 4.11 hours).[5] Benefits were of a greater magnitude than available medical therapies and in a similar range as reported with deep brain stimulation.[5-7] The quality of evidence for the reduction of nonmotor symptoms is low. Safety issues mainly relate to the intestinal infusion system.[6]

Levodopa-carbidopa intestinal gel (LCIG) can be used in the geriatric population. Dementia is not a contraindication for LCIG if relatives can handle the therapy, however, this may be avoided in patients with severe dementia.[8] The total daily dose of LCIG is calculated from the total dose of oral L-DOPA before initiation of LCIG therapy and the morning dose of LCIG is calculated from the morning dose of oral L-DOPA. Although L-DOPA/carbidopa intestinal gel therapy is perceived as less invasive than deep brain stimulation, there are still potentially dangerous adverse effects.

Absolute contraindications for the use of LCIG are hypersensitivity to L-DOPA, carbidopa, or any of the excipients, narrow-angle glaucoma, severe liver and renal insufficiency, severe heart failure, severe cardiac arrhythmia, and acute stroke.[8]

Device and tube-related problems are common with LCIG therapy including dislocation, occlusion, kinking, knotting, or erosion of the tube.[9]

Other patients have problems with the stoma including infection, excessive granulation tissue, or the pump itself. The most common reason for stopping therapy is repeated tube dislocation.[10] Peripheral neuropathy is common in PD and may occur with L-DOPA/carbidopa intestinal gel therapy; hyperhomocysteinemia associated with L-DOPA therapy may be responsible.[10,11]

Apomorphine

Apomorphine, the oldest dopaminergic medication used for PD over 60 years ago but was abandoned with the advent of L-DOPA. It is a potent D1 and D2 receptor agonist, rapidly absorbed after subcutaneous injection (Cmax = 20 min), and has a short half-life of 40 minutes. It works quickly when injected, the onset is usually heralded by yawning after about 5 minutes, followed by the rapid improvement of all Parkinsonian features.[10]

Apomorphine comes either as an intermittent subcutaneous injection (Pen-jet) or as prefilled syringes for continuous subcutaneous infusion. It is useful in patients with occasional disabling OFF periods requiring perhaps <2–3 injections per day.

Apomorphine failed to treat dyskinesia in clinical trials. A follow-up of 4 years in 50 patients receiving apomorphine showed 22 opted out due to suboptimal motor control. Patients on the prolonged duration of apomorphine (up to 16 h/day for 24 months) developed impulse control disorders. Other adverse effects were pathological gambling, internet addiction, compulsive eating, increased libido, and acute paranoia with attempted suicide. These effects are dopamine-mediated and ultimately led to treatment discontinuation.[12]

Sublingual Apomorphine

APL-130277 is a sublingually administered apomorphine film strip in clinical development that was recently tested for the treatment of both predictable and unpredictable off episodes. The sublingual formulation is rapidly absorbed through the oral cavity mucosa, allowing for rapid delivery.[13]

A recent phase 2 trial showed that the majority of patients had "on" within 30 minutes with a mean duration of 50 minutes. Total of 40% of patients achieved a full ON response within 15 minutes. Total of 60% remained fully ON for 90 minutes. There were no discontinuations as a result of an adverse event. The most common adverse events were dizziness (36.8%), somnolence (31.6%), and nausea (21.1%). This new sublingual route of delivery may be more practical than subcutaneous injection.[14,15]

Amantadine Extended-release Capsules

Pooled analysis of phase three trials of ADS-5102 (274 mg amantadine HCl extended-release capsules) for L-DOPA-induced dyskinesia showed a statistically significant reduction in time spent with dyskinesias, the functional impact of dyskinesias, time spent in the OFF state, and functional impact of fluctuation time for ADS-5102 versus placebo.[16]

DISEASE-MODIFYING THERAPY

The most critical unmet need in the diagnosis, treatment, and care of PD patients is to slow down or to stop the progression of the disease.

The original DATATOP (Deprenyl and Tocopherol Antioxidative Therapy of Parkinsonism) trial and subsequent extension trials showed that selegiline has significant effects early in the disease and it delays the need for dopamimetic therapy in newly diagnosed PD. However, subsequent studies showed a symptomatic benefit of selegiline. There is no convincing data to support that treatment with selegiline increases life expectancy.[17]

The delayed-start L-DOPA in early PD study (LEAP-study) and recent trials for disease-modification including the use of coenzyme Q10 [Parkinson Study Group (PSG) et al. 2014], creatine monohydrate (Kieburtz et al. 2015), pioglitazone (NINDS Exploratory Trials in PD FS-ZONE Investigators 2015), and gene therapy with neurturin (NRTN) (Olanow et al. 2015) failed to provide any evidence for disease modification.

Potential therapeutic targets are now investigated under the following categories:

- α-synuclein
- Pathogenic mechanisms distinct from α-synuclein
- *SNCA* genetic subtypes of "PD" particularly leucine-rich repeat kinase 2 (LRRK2)-related PD; and
- Interventions with possible disease-modifying effects, but not explicitly influencing the underlying PD pathobiology.

Alpha-synuclein

The etiology of PD is likely multifactorial, the protein α-synuclein is a central component to the pathogenesis of the disease. However, the mechanism by which α-synuclein causes toxicity and contributes to neuronal death remains unclear.[18]

In humans, α-synuclein is a member of a three-protein family: α-synuclein, β-synuclein, and γ-synuclein. α-synuclein is a small protein comprising 140 amino acids with three domains: a N-terminal domain (aa 1–65), a non-amyloid-β component of plaques (NAC) domain (aa 66–95), and a C-terminal domain (aa 96–140).[19]

Rare point mutations in the N-terminal domain of α-synuclein result in autosomal dominant familial PD and PD-like syndromes, presumably caused by misfolding and/or aggregation of the mutant α-synuclein protein.

Recent studies showed that the normal physiological function of α-synuclein involves roles in compartmentalization, storage, and recycling of neurotransmitters.[20]

In the past 20 years, scientific evidence supports a principal role of α-synuclein in the pathogenesis of PD. Although there is some evidence that the loss of normal α-synuclein function contributes to the disease, most animal data support a toxic process.[21]

It is likely that aggregation of α-synuclein results either from an increased release of α-synuclein and increased cell-to-cell transfer or via accumulated cellular levels of the protein.[20,22]

Several pathological factors contribute to the toxicity of α-synuclein. Firstly, the dysfunction of autophagy and ubiquitin proteasome system (UPS) are the two main pathways to clear toxic α-synuclein. This might lead to neuronal toxicities; secondly, both nitration and oxidation decrease the propensity of α-synuclein to form stable conformations, which might contribute to the progression of PD.

Currently, inflammation is implicated in studies of the pathogenesis in PD. Glial cells are responsible for neuroinflammation, and the prion-like spread of α-synuclein throughout the brain. The direct transfer of α-synuclein from neurons to astrocytes was shown in vivo using transgenic mice overexpressing human α-synuclein under a neuronal promoter (**Flowchart 1**).

Astrocytes exposed to neuronal α-synuclein had changes in the gene expression profile exhibiting an inflammatory response. Induction of proinflammatory cytokines and chemokines correlated with the extent of glial accumulation of α-synuclein. A combination of these results suggests that astroglial α-synuclein pathology is produced by direct transmission of neuronal α-synuclein aggregates, causing inflammatory responses. This transmission step is an essential mediator of pathogenic glial responses and is perceived as a new therapeutic target.[23]

There are four common ways to combat the toxicity produced by α-synuclein: (1) Decrease α-synuclein

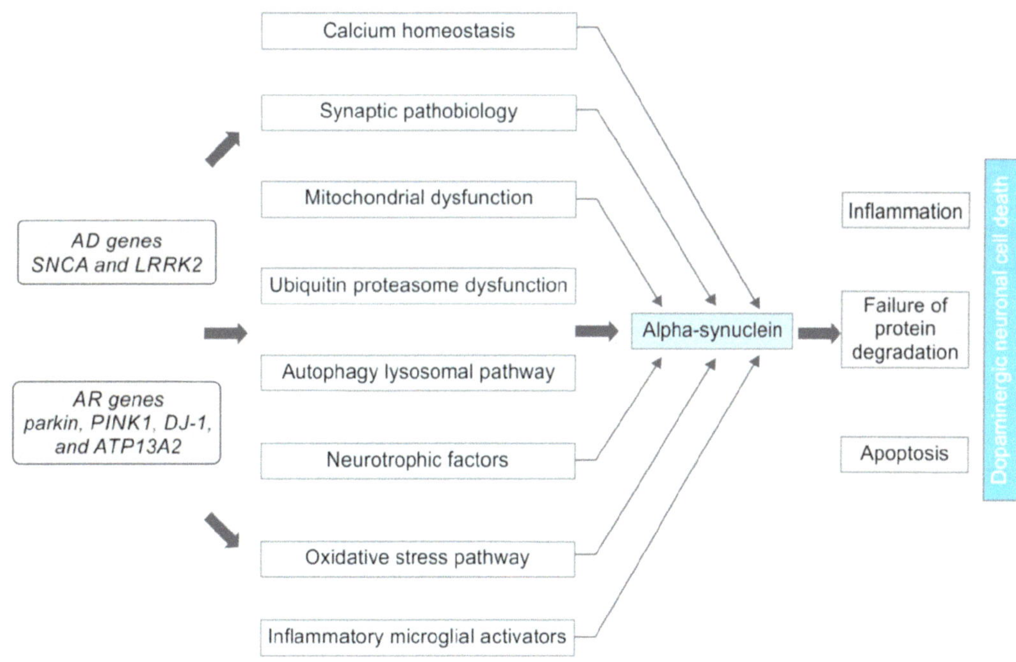

FLOWCHART 1: Proposed mechanisms resulting in cell death in Parkinson's disease (PD).

aggregation, (2) control its propagation, (3) increase its clearance, and (4) stabilize its existing settings.

Attempts to reduce α-synuclein synthesis using small interfering ribonucleic acids (siRNAs) and antisense oligonucleotides may be a future target in humans. The recent discovery that the β2-adrenoreceptor (β*2AR)* is a regulator of the α-synuclein gene and that β2AP agonists are associated with a lower incidence of PD.[24]

β2-adrenoreceptor is a regulator of the α-synuclein gene (*SNCA*). β2AR ligands modulate SNCA transcription through histone three lysine 27 acetylation of its promoter and enhancers. Over 11 years of follow-up in 4 million Norwegians, the β2AR agonist salbutamol was associated with reduced risk of developing PD [rate ratio: 0.66; 95% confidence interval (CI) 0.58–0.76]. Conversely, a β2AR antagonist correlated with increased risk.[24]

A caspase-1 inhibitor could provide neuroprotective effects on PD by reducing α-synuclein cleavage, hence, limiting its ability to form aggregates. Preventing aggregation could also be achieved using passive or active immunization approaches, such as gene-silence technologies or active protein immunization.[20]

Nilotinib is a kinase inhibitor approved for the treatment of chronic myelogenous leukemia. It has been shown to inhibit c-Abl and potentially protect against neuronal death in PD by reducing pathologic phosphorylation of both parkin and α-synuclein.[25]

Twelve patients were randomized into 150 mg ($n = 5$) or 300 mg ($n = 7$) groups and received nilotinib orally everyday for 24 weeks. This study shows that 150 mg and 300 mg doses of nilotinib appear to be safe and tolerated in patients with advanced PD. Motor and cognitive outcomes suggest a possibly beneficial effect on clinical outcomes. This small proof-of-concept study lacks a placebo group. It is warranted to evaluate the safety and efficacy of nilotinib in larger randomized, double-blind, placebo-controlled trials.[25] Recent data from NILO-PD trial suggests this agent does not show benefit in PD.[26]

The *GBA1* gene encodes the lysosomal enzyme glucocerebrosidase, the activity of which has been found to be reduced in PD patients without *GBA1* mutations, making it an interesting therapeutic target for a wider PD population.[27] In vitro and in vivo studies have reported that ambroxol increases β-glucocerebrosidase (GCase) enzyme activity and reduces synuclein levels. The recent safety study results suggest that ambroxol therapy was safe and well-tolerated.[28]

Other approaches being explored include a small stabilizing molecule designed to block misfolding of α-synuclein (NPT200-11; in phase 1 testing), treatments directed at inhibiting α-synuclein aggregation (NPT088, glycerol phenylbutyrate, squalamine), and oligomer formation (epigallocatechin gallate) (**Table 1**).[21]

TABLE 1: Mechanism of action and status of drugs.

Drug	*Mechanism of action*	*Status*
RO7046015	Passive immunization	Phase II
BIIB054	Passive immunization	Phase II
PD01A, PD03A	Active immunization	Phase I
Nilotinib	C-Abl inhibition	Phase II
NPT200-11	Inhibition of α-synuclein misfolding	Phase I
Ambroxol	Increases glucosylceramidase activity	Phase II
SAR40261	Glucosylceramide synthase inhibitor	Phase II

Unanswered Questions/Concerns Related to Alpha-synuclein-directed Therapies

Timing in the disease course of α-synuclein influencing cell death is not known; other mechanisms may precede and/or trigger α-synuclein toxicity. α-synuclein toxicity is only proven in animal models and may not be essential for neurodegeneration. α-synuclein aggregation is again not associated with neurodegeneration (e.g., *LRRK2* and *parkin*).[21]

NONSYNUCLEIN DISEASE-MODIFYING AGENTS

Caffeine

Drinking coffee is associated with a reduced risk to develop PD. There is an inverse association between caffeine intake and the risk of PD. In a systematic review and meta-analysis the relative risk for the association between caffeine intake and PD was 0.75.[29] For patients who consumed >12 ounces of coffee/day, the adjusted hazard ratio for the development of dyskinesia was 0.61 (95% CI 0.37–1.01) compared with patients who consumed <4 ounces/day.[30] Controlled data on caffeine therapy in PD are limited.

A long-term randomized controlled phase III study with a delayed start design (TEDA) has been conducted to evaluate the efficacy of caffeine 200 mg BID for 6–18 months versus placebo for motor and nonmotor aspects. Caffeine did not provide any clinically relevant improvement in motor manifestations of PD (class I evidence).[31]

Basic science data supports an effect on α-synuclein aggregation and the influence of caffeine on inflammatory processes in the gut. This needs to be further investigated in clinical trials.

Inosine

Inosine, a precursor of urate, taken orally leads to an increase of serum urate levels. The urate protected dopaminergic neurons in the rat nigrostriatal pathway against the neurotoxicity of 6-hydroxydopamine (6-OHDA) and showed that its beneficial effects might be related to its regulation on Akt/GSK3β signaling.[32]

"SURE-PD", a randomized, placebo-controlled trial of oral inosine assessing the safety of elevated serum urate from <6 mg/dL to 6.1–7.0 or 7.1–8.0 mg/dL in patients with early PD, demonstrate a dose-dependent, persistent elevation of plasma antioxidant capacity from oral inosine of potential therapeutic relevance.[33] SURE-PD III is in progress and plans to enroll 270 patients with early untreated PD.

Inosine appeared to be safe and triggered increased urate levels in serum and CSF, previously associated with decelerated disease progression.[33] It remains to demonstrate whether inosine (urate) possesses a disease-modifying potential in PD.

Nicotine

Nicotine as a potential treatment for PD has been reviewed in the past.[34] Nicotine can prevent aggregation of wild-type α-synuclein and the A53T α-synuclein mutation in the test tube.[35] In a culture system of pure human mesencephalic dopaminergic neurons (LUHMES), nicotine can reduce cell death induced by overexpression of human wild-type α-synuclein.[36] These data support a disease-modifying potential.

Based on the above-described evidence, the study nicotine-PD (NIC-PD) has been initiated, a randomized, placebo-controlled, double-blind, multicenter trial in Germany and USA that tests for a potential disease-modifying effect of transdermal (TD) nicotine treatment. TD nicotine does not slow progression in early PD. In contrast to the hypothesis, nicotine may exert an accelerating effect as evidenced by worsened Unified Parkinson's Disease Rating Scale (UPDRS) scores compared to placebo.[37]

Isradipine

Isradipine is a dihydropyridine calcium channel blocker with a relatively high affinity for Cav1.3 channels. It is approved for the treatment of hypertension. Inhibition of Cav1 channels in PD to lower cytosolic Ca^{2+} levels, mitochondrial oxidant stress, and sensitivity to toxins in neurons at risk of Lewy pathology (LP) or cell death in PD; epidemiological evidence suggests that Cav1 calcium channel blockers are associated with a lower incidence of PD.[38,39] Parkinson Study Group is conducting an ongoing 36-month phase 3 RCT (STEADY-PD III). Primary outcome measures are change in part I–III UPDRS score in the practically defined ON state; study design should allow determination of longer-term benefits including the impact on dopaminergic drug use, motor complications, and nonmotor features. Results are expected in 2019.[21]

Deferiprone

Deferiprone is a potent iron chelator. Iron plays an important role in oxidative stress; elevated levels of iron are seen in the substantia nigra pars compacta (SNc) of PD patients. Two ongoing trials evaluating potential disease-modifying effects are SKY in which 140 early (<3 years since diagnosis) stable treated PD patients are subjected to four doses of deferiprone (600–2,400 mg/day) versus placebo and FAIRPARKII which has included 338 early untreated PD patients. Patients received 30 mg/kg/day versus placebo. Primary outcome measure in SKY is change in part III Movement Disorder Society-UPDRS (MDS-UPDRS) score at 9 months. Primary outcome measures in FAIRPARKII are total MDS-UPDRS at 36 months. FAIRPARKI: small randomized double-blind delayed start (and delayed cessation) trial of 30 mg/kg/day in treated patients showed promising effects;[40] better responses in patients with lower ceruloplasmin ferroxidase activity.[21]

Many unresolved issues remain with the iron chelation approach including drug dose, lack of target engagement biomarkers, and the stage of disease chosen for patient enrollment.[41]

Exenatide

Exenatide is a synthetic version of exendin-4. It is a naturally occurring analog of human glucagon-like peptide-1 approved for the treatment of type 2 diabetes mellitus. It probably favorably modulates several crucial cellular processes including disturbances in protein synthesis, apoptosis, autophagy, mitochondrial biogenesis, and inflammation.[42]

A double-blind trial in 60 patients experiencing motor fluctuations evaluated exenatide. The primary outcome measure was off-medication motor UPDRS score at 60 weeks.[43] At 60 weeks, off-medication scores on Part III UPDRS improved significantly in the exenatide group as compared to placebo. The study concluded that exenatide had positive effects on practically defined off-medication motor scores in PARKIN-PD, which sustained beyond the period of exposure. Whether exenatide affects the underlying disease pathophysiology or induces long-lasting symptomatic effects is uncertain. Exenatide represents a significant new avenue for investigation in PD and the impact on everyday symptoms should be examined in longer-term trials.[43]

ANTI-INFLAMMATORY THERAPY

There is considerable interest in the anti-inflammatory therapies as disease-modifying drugs in PD.

Some drugs believed to modulate the immune system that have undergone preliminary studies. AZD3241 is a selective and irreversible inhibitor of myeloperoxidase, a reactive oxygen generating enzyme expressed by microglia. A recent positron-emission tomography (PET) study demonstrated a reduction of ^{11}C-PBR28 binding to translocator protein in the brain of PD patients after 6 weeks of treatment with AZD3241.[44]

A small double-blind trial of sargramostim, a recombinant granulocyte macrophage colony stimulating factor, demonstrated modest improvements in clinical, magnetoencephalography (MEG)-recorded cortical activities and regulatory T-cell number and function compared to placebo or pretreatment states.[45]

ADVANCES IN GENETICS

So far, several possible targets for the genetic treatment of PD have been identified. These targets can be classified as either disease-modifying or nondisease modifying.

The nondisease modifying treatments aimed at ailing PD symptoms is by attempting to normalize aberrant firing in the basal ganglia by expression of either dopaminergic or GABAgenic enzymes. These treatments are symptomatic and do not alter the underlying pathophysiological process.[46] ProSavin and l-amino acid decarboxylase (AADC) dopaminergic therapies are both safe and successful at reducing the need for medication in advanced PD patients.

Disease-modifying strategies revolve around stopping PD-mediated cell death and regenerating lost neurons. The most investigated approach has been the nigral overexpression of growth factors found to have neuroprotective properties. Research targeting glial cell line-derived neurotrophic factor (GDNF) family of ligands (GFLs) members [NRTN, artemin (ARTN), and persephin (PSPN)] is still ongoing, with a planned clinical study examining the putaminal overexpression of GDNF.[46] There is some evidence of restoration of the nigrostriatal pathway pathologically and on imaging. However, GDNF studies have yielded mixed results. NRT Nerebra, a GDNF analog, has also been trialed in patients with similar results to those seen with GDNF, namely promising open-label trials that have failed to translate to clinical benefit in larger trials. The cerebral dopamine neurotrophic factor (CDNF)/mesencephalic astrocyte-derived neurotrophic factor family might also be a viable alternative to the GFL family, as this family of growth factors exerts its neuroprotective effect via a different mechanism than the GFL family. The ongoing nonhuman primate (NHP) trial with CDNF versus GDNF will be most interesting. The possibility of combining nuclear receptor related 1 (Nurr1) therapy with a member of the GFL family might also be an interesting approach.[46]

STEM CELL THERAPY

Previous work has demonstrated that it is possible to successfully graft primates with nigrostriatal lesions with neurons derived from embryonic stem cells and human fetal stem cells.

The transplantation of fetal dopaminergic neurons into patients with PD different durations (mainly due to the lack and heterogeneity of donor tissue, which made standardization difficult).[47]

The use of embryonic stem cell or induced pluripotent stem cells (iPSC)derived dopaminergic (autologous) neuroblasts shows the promise of these techniques to provide clinically applicable personalized autologous cell therapy for PD.[48]

In a long-term analysis of human iPSC, cell-derived dopaminergic progenitor cells survived and functioned as midbrain dopaminergic neurons in a primate model of PD. This preclinical study using a primate model indicates that human iPS cell-derived dopaminergic progenitors are clinically applicable for the treatment of patients with PD.[49]

The difficulty of targeting the nervous system, together with extreme financial pressure, were the hindrance to stem cells trial.[50] A number of trials (NCT03119636, STEM-PD, NYSTEM PD) using ESC-derived neurons and allogenic and autologous iPSC-derived neurons have begun or expected to start over the next 2–3 years.

NEW TECHNOLOGIES FOR THE DIAGNOSIS AND CLINICAL ASSESSMENT

The use of new technology-based tools allows quantitative assessment of the motor function of PD patients. Sensors, video-assessment methods, or mobile phone applications are some of the techniques that improve the sensitivity, accuracy, and reproducibility of the evaluation of PD patients.[51]

Portable devices include inertial measurement units (IMUs). These measure the orientation, amplitude, and frequency of movement, as well as the speed of the part of the body where they are located.[51] IMUs are usually made up of accelerometers and gyroscopes, and occasionally magnetometers.[51] The Kinesia portable kinematic system (IMU) can provide greater test-retest reliability and sensitivity to change than conventional clinical ratings for measuring bradykinesia, hypokinesia, and dysrhythmia in PD patients.[52]

On the other hand, the Parkinson's KinetiGraph (PKG) provides continual monitoring of the motor status in the home environment (regarding baseline motor status, fluctuations, and benefit of treatment) using technology-based tools.

These new technology-based systems open up an unexpected range of specific and real-time data, thereby resulting in the prospect of (1) better diagnostic accuracy, (2) more sensitive monitoring of the motor and nonmotor symptoms, and (3) more precise adjustments of medical therapies.[51] However, their use is limited in routine clinical practice due to the heterogeneity of the studies, which limit the extrapolation of results and the high cost of the devices.[53,54]

The delivery and efficacy of many pharmaceutical compounds can be improved and their side effects reduced. Among drug delivery systems microparticles (MPs), nanoparticles (NPs), and hydrogels (HGs) seem to be the most effective in providing neuroprotection, although liposomes and micelles have also been investigated.[55,56] Reports on the long-term efficacy of these therapies will be available in near future.

CONCLUSION

About 200 years since the first description of PD, we are heading toward the era of explosive expansion of research data. Initial interest of symptomatic therapy has now changed to individualized treatment. The next decade in PD research will be focused on neuroprotective and disease modifying treatment. We are still at the beginning of the new horizon. The identification of monogenetic forms of PD has uncovered a role for proteasomal and mitochondrial dysfunction, oxidative stress, protein misfolding, and aberrant phosphorylation in the pathophysiology of PD. A complex interplay between genes, proteins, cellular organelles, and neural networks are the challenges for the future.

REFERENCES

1. Braak H, Braak E. Pathoanatomy of Parkinson's disease. J Neurol. 2000;247(Suppl 2):3-10.
2. Oertel W, Schulz JB. Current and experimental treatments of Parkinson disease: A guide for neuroscientists. J Neurochem. 2016;139(1):325-37.
3. Fahn S. Levodopa in the treatment of Parkinson's disease. J Neural Transm Suppl. 2006;71:1-15.
4. Aquino CC, Fox SH. Clinical spectrum of levodopa-induced complications. Mov Disord. 2015;30(1):80-9.
5. Olanow CW, Kieburtz K, Odin P, Espay AJ, Standaert DG, Fernandez HH, et al. Continuous intrajejunal infusion of levodopa-carbidopa intestinal gel for patients with advanced Parkinson's disease: A randomised, controlled, double-blind, double-dummy study. Lancet Neurol. 2014;13(2):141-9.
6. Wirdefeldt K, Odin P, Nyholm D. Levodopa-Carbidopa Intestinal Gel in Patients with Parkinson's Disease: A Systematic Review. CNS Drugs. 2016;30(5):381-404.
7. Wang L, Li J, Chen J. Levodopa-Carbidopa Intestinal Gel in Parkinson's Disease: A Systematic Review and Meta-Analysis. Front Neurol. 2018;9:620.
8. Pedersen SW, Clausen J, Gregerslund MM. Practical Guidance on How to Handle Levodopa/Carbidopa Intestinal Gel Therapy of Advanced PD in a Movement Disorder Clinic. Open Neurol J. 2012;6:37-50.
9. Antonini A, Odin P. Pros and cons of apomorphine and L-dopa continuous infusion in advanced Parkinson's disease. Parkinsonism Relat Disord. 2009;15(Suppl 4):S97-100.
10. Worth PF. When the going gets tough: How to select patients with Parkinson's disease for advanced therapies. Pract Neurol. 2013;13(3):140-52.
11. Urban PP, Wellach I, Faiss S, Layer P, Rosenkranz T, Knop K, et al. Subacute axonal neuropathy in Parkinson's disease with cobalamin and vitamin B6 deficiency under duodopa therapy. Mov Disord. 2010;25(11):1748-52.
12. Antonini A, Tolosa E. Apomorphine and levodopa infusion therapies for advanced Parkinson's disease: Selection criteria and patient management. Expert Rev Neurother. 2009;9(6):859-67.
13. Antonini A, Moro E, Godeiro C, Reichmann H. Medical and surgical management of advanced Parkinson's disease. Mov Disord. 2018;33(6):900-8.
14. Hauser RA, Olanow CW, Dzyngel B, Bilbault T, Shill H, Isaacson S, et al. Sublingual apomorphine (APL-130277) for the acute conversion of OFF to ON in Parkinson's disease. Mov Disord. 2016;31(9):1366-72.
15. Rodríguez-Blázquez C, Forjaz MJ, Lizán L, Paz S, Martínez-Martín P. Estimating the direct and indirect costs associated with Parkinson's disease. Expert Rev Pharmacoecon Outcomes Res. 2015;15(6):889-911.
16. Patni R, Johnson R, Elmer L, Isaacson S, Felt L, Tanner C, et al. Pooled analysis of phase 3 studies of ADS-5102 for levodopa-induced dyskinesia: A detailed review of MDS-UPDRS, part IV (motor complications). Parkinsonism Relat Disord. 2018;46(Suppl 2).
17. Schulz JB. Effects of selegiline and rasagiline on disease progression in Parkinson's disease. Basal Ganglia. 2012;2(4):S41-5.
18. Rocha EM, De Miranda B, Sanders LH. Alpha-synuclein: Pathology, mitochondrial dysfunction and neuroinflammation in Parkinson's disease. Neurobiol Dis. 2018;109(Pt B):249-57.
19. Jakes R, Spillantini MG, Goedert M. Identification of two distinct synucleins from human brain. FEBS Lett. 1994;345(1):27-32.
20. Reish HEA, Standaert DG. Role of α-synuclein in inducing innate and adaptive immunity in Parkinson disease. J Parkinsons Dis. 2015;5(1):1-19.
21. Lang AE, Espay AJ. Disease Modification in Parkinson's Disease: Current Approaches, Challenges, and Future Considerations. Mov Disord. 2018;33(5):660-77.
22. Samuel F, Flavin WP, Iqbal S, Pacelli C, Renganathan SDS, Trudeau LE, et al. Effects of serine 129 phosphorylation on α-synuclein aggregation, membrane association, and internalization. J Biol Chem. 2016;291(9):4374-85.

23. Lee HJ, Suk JE, Patrick C, Bae EJ, Cho JH, Rho S, et al. Direct transfer of alpha-synuclein from neuron to astroglia causes inflammatory responses in synucleinopathies. J Biol Chem. 2010;285(12):9262-72.
24. Mittal S, Bjørnevik K, Im DS, Flierl A, Dong X, Locascio JJ, et al. β2-Adrenoreceptor is a regulator of the α-synuclein gene driving risk of Parkinson's disease. Science. 2017;357(6354):891-8.
25. Pagan F, Hebron M, Valadez EH, Torres-Yaghi Y, Huang X, Mills RR, et al. Nilotinib effects in Parkinson's disease and dementia with Lewy bodies. J Parkinsons Dis. 2016;6(3):503-17.
26. Simuni T, Fiske B, Merchant K, Coffey CS, Klingner E, Caspell-Garcia C, et al. NILO-PD: A phase 2a study of nilotinib in patients with advanced and early Parkinson's disease: Final study results. Mov Disord Clin Pract. 2020.
27. Stoker TB, Barker RA. Recent developments in the treatment of Parkinson's Disease. F1000Res. 2020;9:F1000.
28. Mullin S, Smith L, Lee K, D'Souza G, Woodgate P, Elflein J, et al. Ambroxol for the Treatment of Patients with Parkinson Disease with and Without Glucocerebrosidase Gene Mutations: A Nonrandomized, Noncontrolled Trial. JAMA Neurol. 2020;77(4): 427-34.
29. Costa J, Lunet N, Santos C, Santos J, Vaz-Carneiro A. Caffeine exposure and the risk of Parkinson's disease: A systematic review and meta-analysis of observational studies. J Alzheimers Dis. 2010;20(1):S221-38.
30. Wills AMA, Eberly S, Tennis M, Lang AE, Messing S, Togasaki D, et al. Caffeine consumption and risk of dyskinesia in CALM-PD. Mov Disord. 2013;28(3):380-3
31. Postuma RB, Anang J, Pelletier A, Joseph L, Moscovich M, Grimes D, et al. Caffeine as symptomatic treatment for Parkinson disease (Café-PD): A randomized trial. Neurology. 2017;89(17):1795-803.
32. Gong L, Zhang QL, Zhang N, Hua WY, Huang YX, Di PW, et al. Neuroprotection by urate on 6-OHDA-lesioned rat model of Parkinson's disease: Linking to Akt/GSK3β signaling pathway. J Neurochem. 2012;123(5):876-85.
33. Bhattacharyya S, Bakshi R, Logan R, Ascherio A, Macklin EA, Schwarzschild MA. Oral Inosine Persistently Elevates Plasma antioxidant capacity in Parkinson's disease. Mov Disord. 2016;31(3):417-21.
34. Ascherio A, Schwarzschild MA. The epidemiology of Parkinson's disease: risk factors and prevention. Lancet Neurol. 2016;15(12):1257-72.
35. Hong DP, Fink AL, Uversky VN. Smoking and Parkinson's disease: Does nicotine affect α-synuclein fibrillation? Biochim Biophys Acta. 2009;1794(2):282-90.
36. De Andrade A, Oertel WH, Goebel J, Höllerhage M, Höglinger GU, Hengerer B. Caffeine and nicotine are protective in a new model of α-synuclein mediated cell death in vitro. Basal Ganglia. 2013;3(1):42.
37. Oertel W, Müller H, Schade-Brittinger C, Kamp C, Balthasar K, Articus K, et al. The NIC-PD-study-A randomized, placebo-controlled, double-blind, multi-centre trial to assess the disease-modifying potential of transdermal nicotine in early Parkinson's disease in Germany and N. America.
38. Ilijic E, Guzman JN, Surmeier DJ. The L-type channel antagonist isradipine is neuroprotective in a mouse model of Parkinson's disease. Neurobiol Dis. 2011;43(2):364-71.
39. Parkinson Study Group. Phase II safety, tolerability, and dose selection study of isradipine as a potential disease-modifying intervention in early Parkinson's disease (STEADY-PD). Mov Disord. 2013;28(13):1823-31.
40. Devos D, Moreau C, Devedjian JC, Kluza J, Petrault M, Laloux C, et al. Targeting chelatable iron as a therapeutic modality in Parkinson's Disease. Antioxid Redox Signal. 2014;21(2): 195-210.
41. Elkouzi A, Vedam-Mai V, Eisinger RS, Okun MS. Emerging therapies in Parkinson disease—repurposed drugs and new approaches. Nat Rev Neurol. 2019;15(4):204-223.
42. Athauda D, Foltynie T. The glucagon-like peptide 1 (GLP) receptor as a therapeutic target in Parkinson's disease: mechanisms of action. Drug Discov Today. 2016;21(5):802-18.
43. Athauda D, Maclagan K, Skene SS, Bajwa-Joseph M, Letchford D, Chowdhury K, et al. Exenatide once weekly versus placebo in Parkinson's disease: a randomised, double-blind, placebo-controlled trial. Lancet. 2017;390(10103):1664-75.
44. Jucaite A, Svenningsson P, Rinne JO, Cselényi Z, Varnäs K, Johnström P, et al. Effect of the myeloperoxidase inhibitor AZD3241 on microglia: A PET study in Parkinson's disease. Brain. 2015;138(Pt 9):2687-700.
45. Gendelman HE, Zhang Y, Santamaria P, Olson KE, Schutt CR, Bhatti D, et al. Evaluation of the safety and immunomodulatory effects of sargramostim in a randomized, double-blind phase 1 clinical Parkinson's disease trial. NPJ Parkinsons Dis. 2017;3:10.
46. Sudhakar V, Richardson RM. Gene Therapy for Parkinson's Disease. Prog Neurol Surg. 2018;33:253-64.
47. Dunnett SB, Björklund A, Lindvall O. Cell therapy in Parkinson's disease—stop or go? Nat Rev Neurosci. 2001;2(5):365-9.
48. Lindvall O. Clinical translation of stem cell transplantation in Parkinson's disease. J Intern Med. 2016;279(1):30-40.
49. Kikuchi T, Morizane A, Doi D, Magotani H, Onoe H, Hayashi T, et al. Human iPS cell-derived dopaminergic neurons function in a primate Parkinson's disease model. Nature. 2017;548(7669): 592-6.
50. Smalley E. Neural stem cell trailblazer StemCells folds. Nat Biotechnol. 2016;34(7):677-8.
51. Del Rey NL, Quiroga-Varela A, Garbayo E, Carballo-Carbajal I, Fernández-Santiago R, Monje MHG, et al. Advances in Parkinson's Disease: 200 Years Later. Front Neuroanat. 2018;12:113.
52. Heldman DA, Espay AJ, LeWitt PA, Giuffrida JP. Clinician versus machine: Reliability and responsiveness of motor endpoints in Parkinson's disease. Parkinsonism Relat Disord. 2014;20(6): 590-5.
53. Ossig C, Gandor F, Fauser M, Bosredon C, Churilov L, Reichmann H, et al. Correlation of quantitative motor state assessment using a kinetograph and patient diaries in advanced PD: Data from an observational study. PLoS One. 2016;11(8):e0161559.
54. Sánchez-Ferro Á, Elshehabi M, Godinho C, Salkovic D, Hobert MA, Domingos J, et al. New methods for the assessment of Parkinson's disease (2005 to 2015): A systematic review. Mov Disord. 2016;31(9):1283-92.
55. Garbayo E, Ansorena E, Lanciego JL, Blanco-Prieto MJ, Aymerich MS. Long-term neuroprotection and neurorestoration by glial cell-derived neurotrophic factor microspheres for the treatment of Parkinson's disease. Mov Disord. 2011;26(10):1943-7.
56. Rodríguez-Nogales C, Garbayo E, Carmona-Abellán MM, Luquin MR, Blanco-Prieto MJ. Brain aging and Parkinson's disease: New therapeutic approaches using drug delivery systems. Maturitas. 2016;84:25-31.

CHAPTER 25

Alternative and Complementary Therapies in Parkinson's Disease

Hee Jin Kim, Beomseok Jeon

INTRODUCTION

Definition of Complementary and Alternative Medicines

According to the National Center for Complementary and Integrative Health (NCCIH), complementary and alternative medicines (CAMs) are defined as practices that are not, at present, considered an integral part of conventional medicine. The word "complementary" generally refers to using a nonmainstream approach together with conventional medicine, while the word "alternative" refers to a nonmainstream approach in place of conventional medicine.[1] The NCCIH grouped complementary treatments into (1) Natural products, (2) mind and body practices, and (3) other complementary health approaches. A variety of products such as herbs, vitamins, and minerals, and probiotics are included in natural products. Mind and body practices include a large and diverse group of procedures or techniques administered or taught by a trained practitioner or teacher. Yoga, chiropractic and osteopathic manipulation, meditation, and massage therapy are the most popular mind and body practices. Others include acupuncture, relaxation techniques, Tai chi, qigong, hypnotherapy, Feldenkrais method, Alexander technique, Pilates, Rolfing Structural Integration, and Trager psychophysical integration. Other complementary health approaches may not neatly fit into either natural products or mind and body practices, for example, the practices of traditional healers, ayurvedic medicine, traditional Chinese medicine, homeopathy and naturopathy, and functional medicine.[1]

EPIDEMIOLOGY

There is a growing interest in CAMs across the globe. Despite the major advances in modern therapies for PD, CAM use is prevalent in 34–76% of patients with Parkinson's disease (PD). The frequency of CAM use for PD is 46% in India, 61% in Singapore, and 76% in Korea.[2,3] It is also high ranging from 34% to 54% in the western countries as well. In Asian countries, traditional or oriental medicine has been the most popular; while natural products such as vitamins and herbs were the most common CAM therapy for PD in the United States.[2,3] Therefore, cultural background appears to be closely related to the selection of the CAM type.

Of the sociodemographic factors, CAM use was correlated with rural location, perceived poor health, higher income, female gender, and younger age.[2] There have been conflicting results for the association of CAM use with the level of education. Some studies showed that CAM users had a higher educational level than CAM nonusers, while Kim et al. found that patients with a lower educational level tended to favor traditional oriental medicine and those with a higher educational level tended to favor traditional food and massage therapies.[2,3] Certain disease-specific factors, such as younger age at onset of PD, higher L-DOPA dose, severity of symptoms, and longer duration of PD were related to CAM use.[2,3] However, none of the sociodemographic factors or disease-specific factors were consistently associated with the use of CAMs in other studies.

MIND AND BODY PRACTICES

Acupuncture

Among the diverse spectrum of CAMs for PD, acupuncture is an intervention most often used worldwide. Acupuncture originated in China about 3,000 years ago. During the past few decades, a fair number of experimental studies showed that acupuncture has neuroprotective effects as well as symptomatic benefits in PD animal models. The suggested neuroprotective mechanisms include reduction of oxidative stress, upregulation of neurotrophic factors, modulation of neuronal activity in basal ganglia circuits, attenuation of microglial activation, and modulation of apoptosis and neuroinflammation.[4] However, the precise mechanisms of the putative neuroprotective and therapeutic effects of acupuncture are still unclear.

Many clinical trials suggested that acupuncture is effective for both motor and nonmotor symptoms such as sleep, depression, and overall quality of life (QoL).[5] Acupuncture was also shown to reduce the doses and side effect of L-DOPA when used as an adjuvant therapy to conventional medication. However, only a limited number of clinical trials used a placebo acupuncture as a control intervention. Kluger et al. found no significant differences in the benefits including mood, fatigue, sleep, and QoL between the real and sham acupuncture treatment in the randomized controlled trials (RCTs) of 94 PD patients.[6] In a review of 11 RCTs, acupuncture plus conventional drugs showed significant beneficial effects on UPDRS (Unified Parkinson's Disease Rating Scale) compared with no treatment or drug only.[7] However, there was no significant benefit of acupuncture compared with nonacupoint acupuncture, suggesting that the clinical benefits of acupuncture are possibly due to a nonspecific or placebo response to acupuncture. In the evidence-based medicine reviews published in 2011, the Movement Disorder Society concluded that there is insufficient evidence to support acupuncture as a symptomatic monotherapy, as an adjunct therapy to L-DOPA in the prevention of clinical progression and motor complications, or as treatment of motor complications.[8] In 2017, three meta-analyses were published which included RCTs that were recently published and more rigorously designed. However, they showed inconsistent results for the benefits of acupuncture on some of the PD symptoms.[9-11]

Despite the potential benefits of acupuncture for treating PD, most of the meta-analyses suggested that the evidence to support acupuncture for PD symptoms remains unclear or inconclusive due to small sample sizes and methodological flaws. Therefore, large, multicenter, and well-designed RCTs should be conducted to evaluate the clinical benefit of acupuncture including various nonmotor symptoms.

Tai Chi

Tai chi is a traditional Chinese martial art, which combines deep breathing, meditation, and slow movement with postural stability. It is one of the most widely studied alternative therapy in PD with growing popularity. The largest RCT that included 195 subjects with PD reported significant better improvements in balance, functional capacity, and falls after 24 weeks of controlled tai chi exercise compared with resistance-training or stretching groups.[12] Moreover, this improvement was maintained at 3 months after the intervention. A recent meta-analysis that included nine RCTs assessed the relative effects of tai chi to conventional therapies.[13] Of the nine RCTs, five trials used an active intervention comparator and four trials gave no intervention to the comparator group. The results support the beneficial effects of tai chi on motor functions and balance for patients with PD but not on gait or QoL. Although most trials did not systematically assessed safety, no serious adverse events were reported.

Current evidence suggests a potential benefit of tai chi for improving motor function including balance. However, additional large-scale trials with rigorous study designs are still needed to conclude whether tai chi is effective for PD because of the small sample size and methodological flaws of the prior studies.

Qigong

Qigong is a predecessor of tai chi that focuses more on meditation and internal movement of energy rather than on physical exercise. The benefits of qigong in PD have not been explored as extensively as those of tai chi. In a single-blinded RCT of 100 patients with PD, qigong for 6 months significantly improved the gait performance, functional mobility, and sleep quality compared to the control.[14] In contrast, one randomized controlled cross-over trial showed no significant benefit for either motor or nonmotor symptoms after qigong when compared with aerobic exercise.[15] Due to the limited available data and conflicting results for qigong in PD, no recommendations can be made.

Yoga

Yoga is an ancient Indian practice focusing on breathing and physical exercises, thereby combining muscle relaxation, meditation, and physical workout.[16] There are only a limited number of small RCTs using yoga interventions for PD. In a randomized pilot study of 13 subjects, yoga practice for 12 weeks significantly improved motor function and balance compared to a nonintervention control group.[17] In a RCT of 26 PD patients, a 12-week power yoga intervention improved bradykinesia, rigidity, muscle strength, mobility, activities of daily living, and overall QoL compared to a control group.[18] When a specifically designed yoga program and power training were compared, both exercises significantly improved physical performance but with no difference between the groups.[19] Currently, data are limited to make clear recommendations regarding the safety, efficacy, or feasibility of yoga in the PD population.

Massage and Manual Therapy

Massage is one of the most common forms of CAMs for PD with a usage rate varying between 7.4% and 37.7%.[20] Observational studies in subjects with PD reported improvement in gait speed and range of motion of the shoulder joint.[21,22] However, only a limited number of RCTs have investigated the effects of massage.

Neuromuscular therapy over a 4-week intervention period was more effective than music relaxation at improving the UPDRS motor score in a single-blinded RCT of 36 PD patients.[23] In another single-blinded RCT, a therapeutic Thai massage showed a significant benefit for upper limb muscle strength compared with no intervention.[24] Trager therapy is a manual therapy imparting a series of very gentle, painless, passive rocking motions to the limbs, and body. In a small pilot study, the evoked stretch response in rigid limbs decreased significantly after the Trager therapy.[25] Reflexology, a form of therapeutic massage using a series of pressure techniques to stimulate specific reflex areas on the feet and hand, improved activities of daily living, emotional well-being, and cognitive impairment in patients with PD.[26] Only one RCT investigated the benefit of the Alexander technique in a PD population.[27] Three-month massage and the Alexander technique improved the self-assessment disability scores and depression ratings in 93 PD patients compared with the no intervention group. However, there were no significant differences between the Alexander technique and massage, and no objective motor assessment was performed in this study.

Dance

In observational studies, different forms of dance have been associated with improved motor function and QoL in PD. Meta-analyses and systematic reviews found that dance was more effective than a control intervention for improving balance and motor impairment, but not for freezing of gait.[28-30] One RCT of a long-term community-based tango dancing program showed positive effects on the progression of motor symptoms as well as motor dysfunction severity, balance, and gait.[31] A few studies have reported improvement in depression, apathy, fatigue, global cognition, and executive function with dance compared to controls.[32] Regarding the QoL, Hackney and Earhart reported greater improvement in QoL with Tango compared to ballroom, tai chi, and controls, while others reported similar changes with dance and other types of exercise groups.[32]

Other forms of dance such as American ballroom may have similar benefits as Tango on motor control. Hackney and Earhart compared the effect of the Argentine tango to the waltz/foxtrot or no intervention in patients with PD.[33] Both the Tango and waltz/foxtrot showed improved measures of balance, motor ability and locomotion compared to the no intervention control, although Tango had larger effects than the waltz/foxtrot in the Timed Up and Go test as well as in the forward and backward gait features.

Further investigations with a large sample and robust methodology are needed to establish the effect of different types of dance and their long-term benefit and to determine whether dance has benefits on motor function beyond that of conventional exercise in patients with PD. Additionally, the safety of dance programs also needs to be adequately reported to ensure the appropriate implementation of dance interventions for PD.

Music Therapy

Many studies over the last few decades have reported that musical rhythm in PD treatment can improve gait, limbs co-ordination, postural control, and balance[34] although the published data on music and PD are largely observational. In a recent comprehensive systematic review that included eight RCTs (11 analyses and 241 subjects), music-based movement therapy had a positive effect on motor function and a positive trend on cognitive function and QoL.[35] Regarding the neural substrates and underlying mechanism of motor improvement, functional neuroimaging studies have suggested that rhythm and music modulate the brain activity in the dopamine pathways and dopamine release in the striatum, as well as the brain activity in the associated regions/network such as the cerebellum possibly as a compensatory/adaptive mechanism, amygdala, parietal regions, and pedunculopontine nucleus.[36]

Despite the promising clinical results of rhythm and music-based mobility training, there is insufficient evidence to support the efficacy of music therapy in subjects with PD due to the limited number of RCTs and small sample size. Additionally, whether the effects of music differ from the extent to the established effects of auditory cueing are unclear. Further studies with larger populations and a longer follow-up are needed to replicate and confirm the positive results from previous studies.

NATURAL PRODUCTS

Vitamin E

Free radicals and oxidative stress are a potential mechanism in the pathogenesis of PD. Because vitamin E is an effective free radical scavenger in the brain, its neuroprotective function is an issue for new therapeutic approaches to neurodegenerative diseases such as PD. In experimental PD studies, the effectiveness of dietary vitamin E supplementation in the prevention and treatment of clinical PD have been disappointing, with several conflicting reports.[37] In a prospective, placebo-controlled double-blind trial of 800 previously untreated patients with PD, vitamin E at a daily dose of 2,000 IU failed to delay the rate of disease progression compared with the placebo, whether administered alone or in combination with deprenyl.[38] However, one recent RCT of 60 patients with PD found that omega-3 fatty acids and vitamin E cosupplementation for 12 weeks had favorable effects on several indices of inflammation and oxidative stress as well as on the UPDRS.[39]

Coenzyme Q10

Coenzyme Q10 (CoQ10), an electron acceptor for complexes I and II, leads to decreased free radical generation and can improve the complex I activity. There have been inconsistent results regarding whether CoQ10 supplementation provides symptomatic benefits for patients with PD. However, a high-dosage of CoQ10 failed to show a therapeutic benefit in a phase III RCT of 600 patients with early PD, although CoQ10 was safe and well tolerated at dosages of 1,200–2,400 mg/day.[40] Additionally, a recent meta-analysis including eight studies with a total of 899 patients also showed no significant difference between CoQ10 and placebo on the UPDRS I, II, III, and total scores.[41]

OTHER COMPLEMENTARY HEALTH APPROACHES

Ayurveda

Ayurveda is a system of traditional medicine practices that originated in India from 5,000 to 3,000 BC.[42] An important ayurvedic medicinal plant for PD is *Mucuna pruriens* (*M. pruriens*) or velvet beans, which contain L-DOPA. *M. pruriens* have been shown to have neuroprotective effects by an antioxidant activity and by enhancing the survival of dopaminergic neurons, and have less dyskinetic potential than L-DOPA in animal models of PD.[43] Nonetheless, there have been only a limited number of clinical trials. In one pilot study with a randomized, controlled, double-blind, crossover design of eight patients with PD, patients on *M. pruriens* had a longer on-time, faster onset of action, and higher peak L-DOPA concentrations compared with an equivalent dose of L-DOPA, but had no significant difference in the UPDRS motor score and dyskinesia score.[44] Recently, a noninferiority, double-blind, randomized, controlled, crossover, phase 2b study assessed the efficacy and safety of single-dose *M. pruriens* intake in 18 patients with advanced PD.[45] Both high (17.5 mg/kg) and low dose (12.5 mg/kg) *M. pruriens* were noninferior in the motor response, on-duration and safety compared with dispersible L-DOPA/benserazide (L-DOPA at 3.5 mg/kg). High dose *M. pruriens* induced a greater efficacy and fewer dyskinesias with a more favorable tolerability profile. In contrast, another 16-week, non-inferiority, randomized, crossover, pilot study showed a less favorable tolerability to *M. pruriens* despite a similar efficacy compared with L-DOPA/carbidopa.[46]

There are other plants such as *Sida cordifolia*, *Withania somnifera* (Ashwagandha), *Hyoscyamus niger*, *Bacopa monnieri*, and Curcuma longa (turmeric) which contribute toward the ayurvedic treatment of PD.[42,43] Ayurvedic medicines other than *M. pruriens* have seldom been evaluated in clinical trials, although they are suggested to have neuroprotective effects with anti-inflammatory and antioxidative properties in the animal model of PD.

Based on the aforementioned studies, *M. pruriens* seems to offer potential as an antiparkinsonism herbal drug. However, the number of clinical trials on *M. pruriens* in PD is insufficient and the methodology of the clinical trials lacks the rigor to reach any recommendation. Besides *M. pruriens*, other ayurvedic herbs are required to validate its efficacy.

Chinese Herbal Medicine

In animal models of PD, Chinese herbs have been suggested to have neuroprotective effects for dopaminergic neurons by reducing oxidative stress, anti-inflammatory activities, and anti-apoptotic activities and improving neurotrophic activities, but also have symptomatic benefits.[47] However, the precise mechanism of the neuroprotective effects and therapeutic effects of herbal medicine are still unclear.

Many clinical studies have shown that Chinese herbal formulas as an adjunct improved both motor and non-motor symptoms and reduced the dose of dopaminergic drugs and the occurrence of dyskinesia.[48] There also have been several meta-analyses that evaluated the clinical efficacy and safety of Chinese herbal medicine. In a meta-analysis of 19 trials involving 1,371 patients with PD, Chinese herbal medicine as an adjunct therapy improved the UPDRS motor score and other subscores compared to the conventional treatment. However, there exists a publication bias for the UPDRS III and IV scores with mainly the positive results, and only 4 of the 19 trials had a placebo control. In another review of 64 trials from 15 electronic databases, 14 were placebo controlled.[49] Herbal medicine as an adjunctive therapy improved PD related outcomes and decreased the dose of antiparkinsonian drugs. However, when compared with a placebo, specific effects were not observed in favor of the herbal medicines. This study suggested that the evidence of herbal medicines in PD is not conclusive because of a huge heterogeneity in the herbal recipes and study designs between the studies. Most recently, Zhang et al. performed a meta-analysis of 27 articles involving 2,314 patients.[50] Out of 27, 23 evaluated the effect of traditional Chinese medicine plus conventional drugs versus conventional drugs alone. Compared with the controls, a significantly greater improvement in UPDRS part I, II, III, IV, and total scores were observed in patients on traditional Chinese medicine.

Despite the apparently positive findings, it is still premature to conclude the efficacy of Chinese herbal medicines for PD treatment because of the heterogeneity of the herbal recipes, publication bias, and poor methodological qualities of the clinical trials.

CONCLUSION

Patients with PD often seek CAMs due to the lack of a disease-modifying treatment and the shortcomings of traditional symptomatic medications. As the popularity of CAMs is increasingly growing, over the past 20 years, a large number of studies have been published that evaluate the benefits of CAMs. Various forms of CAMs in PD patients have reported potential benefits to relieve either motor or nonmotor symptoms or drugs-induced side effects. Above all, Tai Chi may serve as a promising CAM for PD. It has proven to be a safe and feasible intervention in improving motor function including balance for patients with PD. Similar to Tai Chi, other mind and body practices including physical intervention such as qigong, yoga, and dance seems to improve motor function, although more data is needed to corroborate this claim due to small sample size, trial design and lack of a consistent training program. Acupuncture and Chinese herbal medicines are one of the most commonly evaluated CAMs and have been used for centuries. They have been suggested to have not only symptomatic benefits but neuroprotective effects via various mechanisms. However, there is still a long way to go for the clinical usage in PD therapy due to the deficiency of high quality placebo controlled clinical trials and the lack of safety profile. Regarding other CAMs, available data are limited with mixed results.

As of now, despite widespread use and growing popularity of CAMs, evidences for efficacy and safety information are insufficient to make a recommendation. There is a need for large, multicenter, and well-designed RCTs and establishment of standardized application regimens.

Relevant conflicts of interest/financial disclosures: Nothing to report.

Funding sources for study: There are no funding sources for this study.

REFERENCES

1. National Center for Complementary and Integrative Health. (2018). Complementary, Alternative, or Integrative Health: What's In a Name? [online] Available from https://nccih.nih.gov/health/integrative-health#hed1.2018 [Last accessed May, 2021].
2. Kim HJ, Jeon B, Chung SJ. Professional ethics in complementary and alternative medicines in management of Parkinson's disease. J Parkinsons Dis. 2016;6(4):675-83.
3. Pandit AK, Vibha D, Srivastava AK, Shukla G, Goyal V, Behari M. Complementary and alternative medicine in Indian Parkinson's disease patients. J Tradit Complement Med. 2015;6(4):377-82.
4. Xiao D. Acupuncture for Parkinson's Disease: a review of clinical, animal, and functional Magnetic Resonance Imaging studies. J Tradit Chin Med. 2015;35(6):709-17.
5. Zeng BY, Zhao K. Effect of Acupuncture on the Motor and Nonmotor Symptoms in Parkinson's Disease-A Review of Clinical Studies. CNS Neurosci Ther. 2016;22(5):333-41.
6. Kluger BM, Rakowski D, Christian M, Cedar D, Wong B, Crawford J, et al. Randomized, Controlled Trial of Acupuncture for Fatigue in Parkinson's Disease. Mov Disord. 2016;31(7):1027-32.
7. Lee MS, Shin BC, Kong JC, Ernst E. Effectiveness of acupuncture for Parkinson's disease: a systematic review. Mov Disord. 2008;23(11):1505-15.
8. Fox SH, Katzenschlager R, Lim SY, Ravina B, Seppi K, Coelho M, et al. The Movement Disorder Society Evidence-Based Medicine Review Update: Treatments for the motor symptoms of Parkinson's disease. Mov Disord. 2011;26(Suppl 3):S2-41.
9. Lee SH, Lim S. Clinical effectiveness of acupuncture on Parkinson disease: A PRISMA-compliant systematic review and meta-analysis. Medicine (Baltimore). 2017;96(3):e5836.
10. Liu H, Chen L, Zhang Z, Geng G, Chen W, Dong H, et al. Effectiveness and safety of acupuncture combined with Madopar for Parkinson's disease: a systematic review with meta-analysis. Acupunct Med. 2017;35(6):404-12.
11. Noh H, Kwon S, Cho SY, Jung WS, Moon SK, Park JM, et al. Effectiveness and safety of acupuncture in the treatment of Parkinson's disease: A systematic review and meta-analysis of randomized controlled trials. Complement Ther Med. 2017;34:86-103.
12. Li F, Harmer P, Fitzgerald K, Eckstrom E, Stock R, Galver J, et al. Tai chi and postural stability in patients with Parkinson's Disease. N Engl J Med. 2012;366(6):511-9.
13. Zhou J, Yin T, Gao Q, Yang XC. A Meta-Analysis on the Efficacy of Tai Chi in Patients with Parkinson's Disease between 2008 and 2014. Evid Based Complement Alternat Med. 2015;2015:593263.

14. Xiao CM, Zhuang YC. Effect of health Baduanjin Qigong for mild to moderate Parkinson's disease. Geriatr Gerontol Int. 2016;16(8):911-9.
15. Burini D, Farabollini B, Iacucci S, Rimatori C, Riccardi G, Capecci M, et al. A randomised controlled cross-over trial of aerobic training versus Qigong in advanced Parkinson's disease. Eura Medicophys. 2006;42(3):231-8.
16. Granath J, Ingvarsson S, von Thiele U, Lundberg U. Stress management: a randomized study of cognitive behavioural therapy and yoga. Cogn Behav Ther. 2006;35(1):3-10.
17. Colgrove YS, Sharma N, Kluding P, Potter D, Imming K, VandeHoef J, et al. Effect of Yoga on Motor Function in People with Parkinson's Disease: A Randomized, Controlled Pilot Study. J Yoga Phys Ther. 2012;02(02).
18. Ni M, Mooney K, Signorile JF. Controlled pilot study of the effects of power yoga in Parkinson's disease. Complement Ther Med. 2016;25:126-31.
19. Ni M, Signorile JF, Mooney K, Balachandran A, Potiaumpai M, Luca C, et al. Comparative Effect of Power Training and High-Speed Yoga on Motor Function in Older Patients With Parkinson Disease. Arch Phys Med Rehabil. 2016;97(3):345-54.
20. Wang Y, Xie CL, Wang WW, Lu L, Fu DL, Wang XT, et al. Epidemiology of complementary and alternative medicine use in patients with Parkinson's disease. J Clin Neurosci. 2013;20(8):1062-7.
21. Donoyama N, Ohkoshi N. Effects of traditional Japanese massage therapy on various symptoms in patients with Parkinson's disease: a case-series study. J Altern Complement Med. 2012;18(3):294-9.
22. Donoyama N, Suoh S, Ohkoshi N. Effectiveness of Anma massage therapy in alleviating physical symptoms in outpatients with Parkinson's disease: a before-after study. Complement Ther Clin Pract. 2014;20(4):251-61.
23. Craig LH, Svircev A, Haber M, Juncos JL. Controlled pilot study of the effects of neuromuscular therapy in patients with Parkinson's disease. Mov Disord. 2006;21(12):2127-33.
24. Miyahara Y, Jitkritsadakul O, Sringean J, Aungkab N, Khongprasert S, Bhidayasiri R. Can therapeutic Thai massage improve upper limb muscle strength in Parkinson's disease? An objective randomized-controlled trial. J Tradit Complement Med. 2018;8(2):261-6.
25. Duval C, Lafontaine D, Hebert J, Leroux A, Panisset M, Boucher JP. The effect of Trager therapy on the level of evoked stretch responses in patients with Parkinson's disease and rigidity. J Manipulative Physiol Ther. 2002;25(7):455-64.
26. Johns C, Blake D, Sinclair A. Can reflexology maintain or improve the well-being of people with Parkinson's Disease? Complement Ther Clin Pract. 2010;16(2):96-100.
27. Stallibrass C, Sissons P, Chalmers C. Randomized controlled trial of the Alexander technique for idiopathic Parkinson's disease. Clin Rehabil. 2002;16(7):695-708.
28. Shanahan J, Morris ME, Bhriain ON, Saunders J, Clifford AM. Dance for people with Parkinson disease: what is the evidence telling us? Arch Phys Med Rehabil. 2015;96(1):141-53.
29. Lotzke D, Ostermann T, Bussing A. Argentine tango in Parkinson disease-a systematic review and meta-analysis. BMC Neurol. 2015;15:226.
30. Dos Santos Delabary M, Komeroski IG, Monteiro EP, Costa RR, Haas AN. Effects of dance practice on functional mobility, motor symptoms and quality of life in people with Parkinson's disease: a systematic review with meta-analysis. Aging Clin Exp Res. 2018;30(7):727-35.
31. Duncan RP, Earhart GM. Randomized controlled trial of community-based dancing to modify disease progression in Parkinson disease. Neurorehabil Neural Repair. 2012;26(2): 132-43.
32. McNeely ME, Duncan RP, Earhart GM. Impacts of dance on non-motor symptoms, participation, and quality of life in Parkinson disease and healthy older adults. Maturitas. 2015; 82(4):336-41.
33. Hackney ME, Earhart GM. Effects of dance on movement control in Parkinson's disease: a comparison of Argentine tango and American ballroom. J Rehabil Med. 2009;41(6): 475-81.
34. Raglio A. Music Therapy Interventions in Parkinson's Disease: The State-of-the-Art. Front Neurol. 2015;6:185.
35. Zhang S, Liu D, Ye D, Li H, Chen F. Can music-based movement therapy improve motor dysfunction in patients with Parkinson's disease? Systematic review and meta-analysis. Neurol Sci. 2017;38(9):1629-36.
36. Koshimori Y, Thaut MH. Future perspectives on neural mechanisms underlying rhythm and music based neurorehabilitation in Parkinson's disease. Ageing Res Rev. 2018;47:133-9.
37. Fariss MW, Zhang JG. Vitamin E therapy in Parkinson's disease. Toxicology. 2003;189(1-2):129-46.
38. Parkinson Study Group. Effects of tocopherol and deprenyl on the progression of disability in early Parkinson's disease. N Engl J Med. 1993;328(3):176-83.
39. Taghizadeh M, Tamtaji OR, Dadgostar E, Daneshvar Kakhaki R, Bahmani F, Abolhassani J, et al. The effects of omega-3 fatty acids and vitamin E co-supplementation on clinical and metabolic status in patients with Parkinson's disease: A randomized, double-blind, placebo-controlled trial. Neurochem Int. 2017;108:183-9.
40. Parkinson Study Group QE3 Investigators, Beal MF, Oakes D, Shoulson I, Henchcliffe C, Galpern WR, et al. A randomized clinical trial of high-dosage coenzyme Q10 in early Parkinson disease: no evidence of benefit. JAMA Neurol. 2014;71(5): 543-52.
41. Zhu ZG, Sun MX, Zhang WL, Wang WW, Jin YM, Xie CL. The efficacy and safety of coenzyme Q10 in Parkinson's disease: a meta-analysis of randomized controlled trials. Neurol Sci. 2017;38(2):215-24.
42. Gourie-Devi M, Ramu MG, Venkataram BS. Treatment of Parkinson's disease in 'Ayurveda' (ancient Indian system of medicine): discussion paper. J R Soc Med. 1991;84(8): 491-2.
43. Srivastav S, Fatima M, Mondal AC. Important medicinal herbs in Parkinson's disease pharmacotherapy. Biomed Pharmacother. 2017;92:856-63.
44. Katzenschlager R, Evans A, Manson A, Patsalos PN, Ratnaraj N, Watt H, et al. Mucuna pruriens in Parkinson's disease: a double blind clinical and pharmacological study. J Neurol Neurosurg Psychiatry. 2004;75(12):1672-7.

45. Cilia R, Laguna J, Cassani E, Cereda E, Pozzi NG, Isaias IU, et al. Mucuna pruriens in Parkinson disease: A double-blind, randomized, controlled, crossover study. Neurology. 2017;89(5):432-8.
46. Cilia R, Laguna J, Cassani E, Cereda E, Raspini B, Barichella M, et al. Daily intake of Mucuna pruriens in advanced Parkinson's disease: A 16-week, noninferiority, randomized, crossover, pilot study. Parkinsonism Relat Disord. 2018;49:60-6.
47. Song JX, Sze SCW, Ng TB, Lee CK, Leung GP, Shaw PC, et al. Anti-Parkinsonian drug discovery from herbal medicines: what have we got from neurotoxic models? J Ethnopharmacol. 2012;139(3):698-711.
48. Zeng BY. Effect and Mechanism of Chinese Herbal Medicine on Parkinson's Disease. Int Rev Neurobiol. 2017;135:57-76.
49. Kim TH, Cho KH, Jung WS, Lee MS. Herbal medicines for Parkinson's disease: a systematic review of randomized controlled trials. PLoS One. 2012;7(5):e35695.
50. Zhang G, Xiong N, Zhang Z, Liu L, Huang J, Yang J, et al. Effectiveness of traditional Chinese medicine as an adjunct therapy for Parkinson's disease: a systematic review and meta-analysis. PLoS One. 2015;10(3):e0118498.

CHAPTER 26

Multidisciplinary Approach to Parkinson's Care

Nicole D'Souza, Navaz Irani, Maria Amelia Barretto

INTRODUCTION

Parkinson's disease (PD) is a complex disorder affecting not only movement but also mood, cognitive abilities, autonomic functions, and subsequently quality of life (QoL). In the early stages of Parkinson's, pharmacological treatment is effective in controlling the symptoms and keeping patients independent. A long-term dependence on medications can, however, cause disabling side effects such as dyskinesias, motor fluctuations, confusion, and psychiatric complications.[1,2] Often in spite of optimal pharmacological treatment, patients become increasingly disabled as the disease progresses.[1,3] Furthermore, certain symptoms like on-off period, freezing and postural instability are refractory to pharmacological treatment.[4] It is for these very reasons that the emphasis is now on non-pharmacological therapies to supplement pharmacological treatment.

It is known that symptoms manifest differently in different people with Parkinson's, and every person with Parkinson's reacts differently to their symptoms and the difficulties it creates in their everyday activities. Thus, along with PD, a person's personal factors (traits, attitudes, lifestyle, etc.) and contextual factors (facilitators and barriers, family and social support, etc.) affect their functioning as well as their perception of their QoL. The biopsychosocial model given by the International Classification of Functioning, Disability and Health of the World Health Organization[5,6] (**Flowchart 1**) encourages health professionals to create a multidisciplinary framework to understand the health and health-related problems of an individual. Consequently, an approach to PD care which is multidisciplinary becomes essential.

There are several studies on inpatient and outpatient multidisciplinary treatment approach for Parkinson's.[7-9] They have shown improvements in motor function and activities of daily living,[10,11] gait parameters,[3] speech and depression[4] in patients with PD as well as the QoL of the patients[10] and their caregivers.[11] What is still lacking, however, is clear guidelines for implementation of a multidisciplinary approach as well as the standard of care for such an approach.[8,11]

MULTIDISCIPLINARY TEAM

A multidisciplinary team (MDT) has the patient and their caregivers at the center supported by healthcare professionals form varied specialities. The core members of a MDT are shown in (**Table 1**). These members should be specialized in understanding and treating PD. Along with this, the MDT members should communicate effectively with one another to develop a holistic program to achieve the shared goals of the patients.

The scope of this chapter is limited to a description of a few core MDT members. There is no rigid structure to a MDT for people with PD. Depending on the needs of the patient and their caregivers, health professionals can be included in the team as and when required.

Parkinson's Disease Nurse Specialist

A Parkinson's nurse has specialized experience, knowledge, and skills in managing Parkinson's. Over the years, their role has evolved from just dealing with a patient's personal concerns and difficulties, educating, and providing

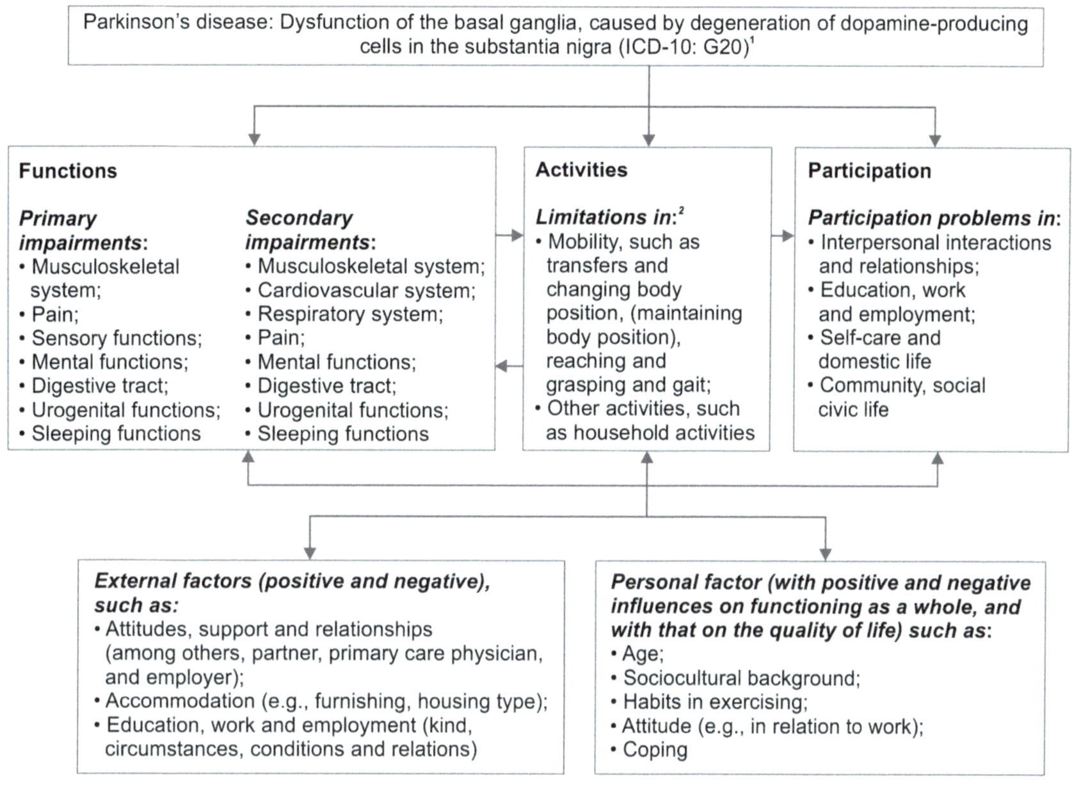

FLOWCHART 1: Global overview of impairments, limitations, and participation restrictions associated with Parkinson's disease.[6]

TABLE 1: Core members of the MDT listed by the European Parkinson's Disease Standards of Care Consensus Statement and their role in the management of people with PD.[11]

MDT member	*Role*
General practitioner	To provide day-to-day clinical management
Movement disorder specialist/neurologist	To plan and monitor treatment
Geriatrician	To provide general in- and outpatient management
PDNS	To manage care and coordinate with the hospital and community services
Physiotherapist	To maximize functional ability
Speech and language therapist	To manage difficulties with speech, communication, eating, drinking, and swallowing
Occupational therapist	To advise on measures to retain independence
Nutritionist	To ensure optimal nutrition
Psychologist	To treat depression, other mental health problems
Pharmacists	To ensure supplies of specialist medications
Complementary therapists	To provide massage and relaxation therapies

(MDT: multidisciplinary team; PD: Parkinson's disease; PDNS: Parkinson's disease nurse specialist)

emotional support to the patient and family or referring the patient to the appropriate allied health specialist or social support organization. They now assist neurologists not only in the assessment of patients but also in drug titration and monitoring the effects and side effects of medications.[12] In recent years, they have also started to play an important role in deep brain stimulation programming[13] and other advanced therapies. A Parkinson's nurse, thus, serves as a bridge between the neurologist and the patient and is becoming an integral part of a multidisciplinary approach to PD.[12] In India, certified Parkinson's disease nurse specialist (PDNS) are unavailable, however, a number of nurses have been trained extensively in-house to execute the duties of a Parkinson's nurse.

Physiotherapy

Physiotherapists (PT) play a significant role in PD right from the time of diagnosis and continues till the advanced stages of PD. The role of a PT is to maintain or increase the patient's level of functioning, decrease fall risk, prevent inactivity and secondary complications, and encourage independence in activities.[1,6] This is accomplished through a combination of physiotherapy interventions which include conventional physiotherapy (progressive strength training, balance and gait training, and fall prevention program), cueing and cognitive movement strategies, PD specific exercise programs, and complementary therapies.[14,15]

Exercise in PD has been shown to have neuroprotective effects[16] and thus is an essential part of a multidisciplinary program for PD. Several systematic reviews on the effects of conventional physiotherapy have shown improvements in physical capacity, postural deviations, balance, gait speed, step length, quality of gait, and turning.[14,17] Cueing strategies have been found to improve gait speed and stride length, help in overcoming freezing episodes, and also in improving posture and confidence in daily activities.[14,17] Cognitive movement strategies are beneficial in improving complex everyday tasks like getting up from a chair or bed. They can also be beneficial in improving a patient's ability to dual or multitask.[18]

Conventional physiotherapy, although effective, may not always focus on enjoyment and social participation. With adherence and compliance to exercise therapy being a major issue, newer therapies targeting well-being as well as enjoyment and social participation are blossoming. A novel amplitude-oriented training program called the Lee Silverman voice treatment-BIG program has shown improvements in motor function[19] as well as functional mobility as measured by the timed-up and go test and the 10 m walk test in people with PD.[20] Other complementary therapies such as dance, tai chi, hydrotherapy, robotic training, virtual reality training, whole body vibration, mental practice, aerobic training, forced cycling, treadmill training, Nordic walking, and boxing are garnering evidence supporting their use in PD.[15] Thus, physiotherapy is an essential component of a multidisciplinary approach.

Occupational Therapy

The aim of occupational therapy for people with PD is to enable meaningful performance in personal care, care of others, indoor and outdoor mobility, work-related activities, and leisure activities. Occupational therapists (OT) guide patients in learning new skills and modifying behaviors to accomplish tasks.[21] They also work with caregivers to enable them to support and aid a person with PD in their everyday tasks while caring for their own well-being.[1]

Activity limitation occurs as PD progresses compelling a person to slowly withdraw and ultimately stop pursuing certain meaningful responsibilities and activities leading to depression and a poor QoL.[22] OTs help to improve a patients skill and performance in activities through general mobility and strengthening exercises along with dexterity training.[21] When this is not sufficient to execute a task the therapist may provide a patient with compensatory strategies for their daily activities. They may also need to adapt certain tasks, manage fatigue and modify the physical environment to support the patient, and improve well-being.[1,22] In addition to this they teach self-management and cognitive behavioral strategies to help integrate these learnings into daily life activities and roles consequently diminishing the negative effect of PD on health and QoL.[22] The OT should thus work in close collaboration with the physical therapist, speech therapist, and cognitive specialist within the MDT to achieve a patients functional goals.[22]

Speech Therapy

A speech and language therapist (SLT) is concerned with improving PD patients speech and communication skills as well as ensuring safety while swallowing. In PD, the voice gradually becomes fainter and speech inarticulate. In addition to this, the presence of bradyphrenia and mental inflexibility can further disrupt the flow of speech adversely affecting a patients ability to communicate with others and consequently leading to frustration and social isolation.[23] Speech drills and exercises are usually prescribed to people with PD with the aim of improving their speech, however, more focus on the cognitive and psychosocial aspects of speech are required.[24] Instrumental aids may also be prescribed in some cases. Reviews are unable to conclude positively on the efficacy of any particular treatments for speech in PD.[23] In recent years, the Lee Silverman voice treatment—LOUD which focuses on vocal fold adduction through high-effort speech is proving to be effective in improving communication and QoL in people with PD.[25]

Dribbling of saliva and other swallowing difficulties are commonly seen in people with PD. If not treated, swallowing difficulties can lead to aspiration pneumonia and ultimately death.[26] A SLT can ensure safety while swallowing by teaching the correct head position for swallowing, swallowing techniques, and may also suggest modifications in the patients diet.

Yoga

Of the many complimentary therapies available for people with PD, the practice of yoga has steadily been gaining followers both in India and Internationally. Although yoga has various domains, in PD the asanas (postures), pranayams (breathing exercises), and meditation are most commonly practiced for therapeutic benefits. Iyengar Hatha yoga in particular has shown to be effective in people with Parkinson's in a few small sample studies with improvements noted in posture, mobility, balance, strength, flexibility, activities of daily living, mood, sleep, physiological functions, and QoL.[27-29] This form of yoga focuses primarily on postural alignment during various asanas and uses props such as ropes, bolsters, blocks, belts, chairs, and mats to help patients achieve the desired postures.[28] More quality studies are needed to prove the efficacy of yoga, however, the benefits for people with PD cannot be ignored and thus yoga should be part of a multidisciplinary approach for PD.

Psychotherapy and Neuropsychology

In recent years, there has been growing awareness about neuropsychiatric symptoms of PD and caregiver stress,[30,31] making the need for nonpharmacological mental health treatment options increasingly relevant for its management.

Psychotherapy

Neuropsychiatric symptoms of PD such as depression and anxiety affect QoL[32] and exacerbate motor symptoms.[33] Given the effectiveness of psychotherapy in the treatment of these conditions, it's significance in PD cannot be stressed enough.

Cognitive behavioral therapy (CBT), a face-to-face talk therapy which focuses on cognitive restructuring, and subsequent affect and behavior modification through therapist-facilitated self-analysis, is used for rehabilitation in mental health conditions. It has gained acceptance as an effective treatment for mood disorders including depression and related anxiety and adjustment difficulties in PD.[34] Improved QoL, coping, and eased motor decline have emerged as secondary outcomes.[35]

The role of CBT and psychology-based strategies has also been substantiated in the rehabilitation of caregiver distress and burden,[36,37] commonly seen amongst people caring for those with PD.[31]

In the management of other prevalent neuropsychiatric symptoms of PD such as apathy, psychosis, impulse control disorders, and sleep disturbances, there is preliminary evidence supporting the effectiveness of counseling and coping strategies, behavioral interventions, family interventions, and CBT.[38-41]

A 2017 review[42] shows the versatility of CBT in the protocols adapted to suit the specific treatment goals of PD, such as a focus on psychoeducation, performance and task organizers, behavioral stimulation, and relaxation. The fundamental practicality of CBT has offered itself to modified versions or contemporary variants, such as distance CBT, i.e., CBT over mediums such as phone[43] and the internet,[44] and mindfulness-based therapies.[45] These are being explored for efficacy in the coping of neuropsychiatric PD symptoms.

Neuropsychology

The cognitive profile of a person with PD could range from a relatively simple characteristic like bradyphrenia[46] to mild cognitive impairment to PD-dementia (PD-D).[47] Notwithstanding the continuum of progression, cognitive difficulties are seen in a large majority of people with PD[47,48] and it hampers functional outcomes and QoL;[49] the latter even in caregivers.[50] Thus, the relevance of the specialized field of neuropsychology emerges.

Foremost, a neuropsychological assessment will determine a customized treatment plan to accommodate the heterogeneity of cognitive impairments[51] seen in individuals with PD. Secondly, neuropsychological assessment also has critical application in pre- and post-DBS candidates to optimize the benefits of surgery and circumvent the development of neurobehavioral disorders postsurgery.[52]

In clinical practice, in the neuropsychological interventions for other conditions, the focus is on cognitive training (CT) and neuropsychological rehabilitation (NPR) seen effective in the preservation of cognitive faculties, in providing compensatory strategies to improve performance of instrumental activities of daily living (IADLs) and reducing effects of cognitive deficits, and in precluding or delaying in-patient facility admissions. In the scope of PD, more comprehensive investigations are warranted.[53]

In preliminary reports which evaluate outcomes in PD through neuroimaging and psychometric tests, CT and NPR have shown benefits in the domains of speed of processing, executive function, attention, recognition, learning, also providing evidence of the impact of CT on increasing neural plasticity, improving overall cognitive and functional performance, and reducing motor symptom effects of Parkinson's.[54-56]

However, early predementia neuropsychological interventions are warranted as compensatory neural changes are less likely to occur with progressing cognitive decline.[57]

For the rehabilitation of cognitive symptoms in PD-D, like with other types of dementia, the focus is on caregiver and/or nurse education and palliative care, as home-based or in-patient programs. Given the extent of decline in cognitive abilities, rehabilitation focuses on finding compensatory strategies to enable the person with PD to function as independently as possible.

Home-based programmes like cognitive stimulation therapy, having found utility in other dementias, are now being adapted and piloted for efficacy in PD-related cognitive impairments.[58]

The utility of mental health therapies as nonpharmacological supplements to pharmacological therapies, the growing service needs of patients with Parkinson's to manage neuropsychiatric symptoms, and the need to reduce the impact of stigma surrounding its treatment—all call for intensified investigations for mental health rehabilitation as a part of multidisciplinary treatment options in PD.

Complementary Creative Therapies

Recent clinical and academic interest is being generated by contemporary therapies which have their practical basis in traditional forms of creative or recreational pursuits such as art, dance, music, and drama. Within the scope of the multifaceted manifestations of Parkinson's, these techniques have demonstrated promising adjuncts to traditional forms of rehabilitation.

Preliminary findings for art therapy in PD suggest improvements in visuospatial tasks, as well as self-efficacy and perceptions of symptom management.[59] Clay manipulation as an art medium for symptom rehabilitation in PD has also gathered results.[60]

Music-based rehabilitation like rhythmic auditory stimulation use rhythmic-acoustic stimulation to enable intricate limb movements, in gait retraining, and in managing freezing.[61,62] However, there is no one-fits-all paradigm and the stimulus needs to be tailored to each case to avoid detrimental effects to movement and gait.[61] Speech intelligibility in severely impaired hypokinetic dysarthric speakers with PD showed improvement through rhythmic speech cueing.[63] Improvements in affective functioning and symptoms and QoL in PD through music-based therapy have also been reported.[62,64]

Dance and movement therapy (DMT) has demonstrated versatility and has been preferred to traditional forms of physiotherapy.[65,66] Its various forms—tango, jazz, waltz, ballroom—have been effective in improving PD symptoms.[65,66] In a recent pilot study done with Indian dance forms, DMT showed improvements for mood symptoms.[67] The increased motivation to use dance as a therapy is likely because dance as an activity encompasses physical activity, cognitive, and emotional stimulation, and mental and physical coordination, in addition to being an enjoyable activity in social settings.

These creative therapies provide avenues for socialization and recreation and may, therefore, promote consistent participation in therapy protocols which use them as mediums.

COMMUNITY BASED GROUP THERAPY AS A MEDIUM FOR MULTIDISCIPLINARY THERAPY FOR PARKINSON'S DISEASE

The rehabilitation options described above have proved efficacious as individual modes of therapy in Parkinson's. In clinical practice, certain challenges plague the application of individual therapy, especially in developing countries like India. These factors relate to cost of rehabilitation, availability of relevant expertise, awareness and accessibility to rehabilitation, long-term motivation to engage in and comply with individual therapy, and attitudes and stigma toward certain nonpharmacological modes of treatment.[68-70]

Research has been ongoing to overcome these barriers to individual therapy through the approach of group-based therapy. It has been found to be an economically viable option and time and labor-resourceful, besides facilitating a socially interactive, learner-optimized and socioemotionally healthy setting.[71-73] In a chronic condition like PD, these factors can prove particularly useful and resourceful as in the long-term rehabilitation of people with other chronic conditions.

Group-based therapy for PD has been used as a medium in physical therapy[74] (including Tai Chi),[75] occupational therapy,[76] psychotherapy,[77] DMT,[78] music-based therapy,[64] and have been found to improve gait and balance therapy compliance, and alleviate nonmotor symptoms, depression, and anxiety.

The Parkinson's Disease and Movement Disorder Society (PDMDS), an India-based NGO which aims to provide rehabilitation to people with Parkinson's and caregivers, has developed a model of care which is largely delivered through community-based centers pan-India. This model of care has been providing education and rehabilitation to scores of people with Parkinson's and their caregivers since 2013, through a standardized multidisciplinary 16-session written manual. The preliminary validation of the manual showed alleviation of symptoms, and patients and caregivers reported a host of perceived benefits such as better emotional well-being and social support, higher self-efficacy, improved mobility and QoL, a regained sense of independence, and better decision-making capacity.[79] Its application also found feasibility as a capacity-building paradigm in the training of allied-health professionals and individuals to deliver Parkinson's care in a group setup. This model shows potential to be replicated in other developing countries, as it has been in 13 states in India. Its successful implementation in several community-based settings is also substantiation of the efficacy of multidisciplinary group-based therapy for Parkinson's rehabilitation.

CONCLUSION

A multifaceted, progressive, and chronic illness like Parkinson's without a doubt warrants an integrated approach to its rehabilitation. The fluctuating interaction of the symptoms and its impact on overall QoL of the patient and the families indicates that there is no one-size-fits all combination and no one mode of treatment that provides a complete solution to the management of PD. Evidence of its efficacy is indicative of its application.[80]

Whether provided through individual therapy, in a group setup or in an in-patient facility, rehabilitation of PD requires the collaboration of multiple medical and rehabilitative experts to enable the patient and their family manage the web of symptoms, thus, aiding in the holistic well-being of those affected at physical, psychological, social, and functional levels and during various stages of the condition.

REFERENCES

1. Radder DLM, Sturkenboom IH, van Nimwegen M, Keus SH, Bloem BR, de Vries NM. Physical therapy and occupational therapy in Parkinson's disease. Int J Neurosci. 2017;127(10): 930-43.
2. Taylor J, Anderson WS, Brandt J, Mari Z, Pontone GM. Neuropsychiatric Complications of Parkinson's Disease Treatments: Importance of Multidisciplinary Care. Am J Geriatr Psychiatry. 2016;24(12):1171-80.
3. Wade DT, Gage H, Owen C, Trend P, Grossmith C, Kaye J. Multidisciplinary rehabilitation for people with Parkinson's disease: A randomised controlled study. J Neurol Neurosurg Psychiatry. 2003;74(2):158-62.
4. Skelly R, Lindop F, Johnson C. Multidisciplinary care of patients with Parkinson's disease. Prog Neurol Psychiatry. 2012;16(2): 10-14.
5. World Health Organization. International Classification of Functioning, Disability and Health. Geneva, Switzerland: World Health Organization; 2001.
6. KNGF Guidelines for physical therapy in patients with Parkinson's disease. Supplement to the Dutch J Physiother. 2004;114(3):19.
7. van der Marck MA, Munneke M, Mulleners W, Hoogerwaard EM, Borm GF, Overeem S, et al. Integrated multidisciplinary care in Parkinson's disease: a non-randomised, controlled trial (IMPACT). Lancet Neurol. 2013;12(10):947-56.
8. van der Marck MA, Bloem BR, Borm GF, Overeem S, Munneke M, Guttman M. Effectiveness of multidisciplinary care for Parkinson's disease: a randomized, controlled trial. Mov Disord. 2013;28(5):605-11.
9. Prizer LP, Browner N. The Integrative Care of Parkinson's Disease: A Systematic Review. J Parkinsons Dis. 2012;2(2): 79-86.
10. Guo L, Jiang Y, Yatsuya H, Yoshida Y, Sakamoto J. Group education with personal rehabilitation for idiopathic Parkinson's disease. Can J Neurol Sci. 2009;36(1):51-9.
11. Pedersen SW, Suedmeyer M, Liu LWC, Domagk D, Forbes A, Bergmann L, et al. The role and structure of the multidisciplinary team in the management of advanced Parkinson's disease with a focus on the use of levodopa-carbidopa intestinal gel. J Multidiscip Healthc. 2017;10:13-27.
12. MacMahon DG. Parkinson's disease nurse specialists: an important role in disease management. Neurology. 1999;52(7 Suppl 3):S21-5.
13. Wagle Shukla A, Zeilman P, Fernandez H, Bajwa JA, Mehanna R. DBS Programming: An Evolving Approach for Patients with Parkinson's Disease. Parkinsons Dis. 2017;2017:8492619.
14. Keus SH, Bloem BR, Hendriks EJ, Bredero-Cohen AB, Munneke M; Practice Recommendations Development Group. Evidence-based analysis of physical therapy in Parkinson's disease with recommendations for practice and research. Mov Disord. 2007;22(4):451-60.
15. Alves Da Rocha P, McClelland J, Morris ME. Complementary physical therapies for movement disorders in Parkinson's disease: a systematic review. Eur J Phys Rehabil Med. 2015;51(6):693-704.
16. Zigmond MJ, Smeyne RJ. Exercise: Is it a neuroprotective and if so, how does it work? Parkinsonism Relat Disord. 2014;20 (Suppl 1):S123-7.
17. Tomlinson CL, Herd CP, Clarke CE, Meek C, Patel S, Stowe R, et al. Physiotherapy for Parkinson's disease: a comparison of techniques. Cochrane Database Syst Rev. 2014;2014(6):CD002815.
18. Keus SH, Munneke M, Nijkrake MJ, Kwakkel G, Bloem BR. Physical therapy in Parkinson's disease: evolution and future challenges. Mov Disord. 2009;24(1):1-14.
19. McDonnell MN, Rischbieth B, Schammer TT, Seaforth C, Shaw AJ, Phillips AC. Lee Silverman Voice Treatment (LSVT)-BIG to improve motor function in people with Parkinson's disease: a systematic review and meta-analysis. Clin Rehabil. 2018;32(5):607-18.
20. Ebersbach G, Ebersbach A, Edler D, Kaufhold O, Kusch M, Kupsch A, et al. Comparing exercise in Parkinson's disease--the Berlin LSVT® BIG study. Mov Disord. 2010;25(12):1902-8.
21. Aragon A, Kings J. (2010). Occupational Therapy for People with Parkinson's: Best practice guidelines. Copyright © Parkinson's UK and College of Occupational Therapists. 2010. [online] Available from https://www.parkinsons.org.uk/sites/default/files/2017-12/otparkinsons_bestpractiseguidelines.pdf [Last accessed May, 2021].
22. Foster ER, Bedekar M, Tickle-Degnen L. Systematic Review of the Effectiveness of Occupational Therapy-Related Interventions for People with Parkinson's disease. Am J Occup Ther. 2014;68(1):39-49.
23. Herd CP, Tomlinson CL, Deane KHO, Brady MC, Smith CH, Sackley CM, et al. Comparison of speech and language therapy techniques for speech problems in Parkinson's disease. Cochrane Database Syst Rev. 2012;2012(8):CD002814.
24. Yorkston K, Baylor C, Britton D. Speech Versus Speaking: The Experiences of People With Parkinson's Disease and Implications for Intervention. Am J Speech Lang Pathol. 2017;26(2S):561-8.
25. Ramig L, Halpern A, Spielman J, Fox C, Freeman K. Speech treatment in Parkinson's disease: Randomized controlled trial (RCT). Mov Disord. 2018;33(11):1777-91.
26. Troche MS, Okun MS, Rosenbek JC, Musson N, Fernandez HH, Rodriguez R, et al. Aspiration and swallowing in Parkinson disease and rehabilitation with EMST: a randomized trial. Neurology. 2010;75(21):1912-9.
27. Roland K. Applications of yoga in Parkinson's disease: a systematic literature review. Res Rev Parkinsonism. 2014;4:1-8.
28. Colgrove YS, Sharma N, Kluding P, Potter D, Imming K, VandeHoef J, et al. Effect of Yoga on Motor Function in People with Parkinson's Disease: A Randomized, Controlled Pilot Study. J Yoga Phys Ther. 2012,2:2.
29. van Puymbroeck M, Walter A, Hawkins BL, Sharp JL, Woschkolup K, Urrea-Mendoza E, et al. Functional Improvements in Parkinson's Disease Following a Randomized Trial of Yoga. Evidence-Based Complementary and Alternative Medicine. 2018;2018:8.
30. Weintraub D, Burn DJ. Parkinson's disease: The quintessential neuropsychiatric disorder. Mov Disord. 2011;26(6): 1022-31.
31. Santos-García D, de la Fuente-Fernández R. Factors contributing to caregivers' stress and burden in Parkinson's disease. Acta Neurol Scand. 2015;131(4):203-10.

32. Barone P, Antonini A, Colosimo C, Marconi R, Morgante L, Avarello TP, et al. The PRIAMO study: A multicenter assessment of nonmotor symptoms and their impact on quality of life in Parkinson's disease. Mov Disord. 2009;24(11):1641-9.
33. Pontone GM, Bakker CC, Chen S, Mari Z, Marsh L, Rabins PV, Williams JR, Bassett SS. The longitudinal impact of depression on disability in Parkinson disease. Int J Geriatr Psychiatry. 2016;31(5):458-65.
34. Dobkin RD, Mann SL, Interian A, Gara MA, Menza M. Cognitive behavioral therapy improves diverse profiles of depressive symptoms in Parkinson's disease. Int J Geriatr Psychiatry. 2019;34(5):722-9.
35. Dobkin RD, Menza M, Allen LA, Gara MA, Mark MH, Tiu J, et al. Cognitive-behavioral therapy for depression in Parkinson's disease: a randomized, controlled trial. Am J Psychiatry. 2011;168(10):1066-74.
36. Simons G, Thompson SBN, Pasqualini MCS. An innovative education programme for people with Parkinson's disease and their carers. Parkinsonism Relat Disord. 2006;12(8):478-5.
37. Secker DL, Brown RG. Cognitive behavioural therapy (CBT) for carers of patients with Parkinson's disease: a preliminary randomised controlled trial. J Neurol Neurosurg Psychiatry. 2005;76(4):491-7.
38. Butterfield LC, Cimino CR, Salazar R, Sanchez-Ramos J, Bowers D, Okun MS. The Parkinson's Active Living (PAL) Program: A Behavioral Intervention Targeting Apathy in Parkinson's Disease. J Geriatr Psychiatry Neurol. 2017;30(1):11-25.
39. Okai D, Askey-Jones S, Samuel M, O'Sullivan SS, Chaudhuri KR, Martin A, et al. Trial of CBT for impulse control behaviors affecting Parkinson patients and their caregivers. Neurology. 2013;80(9):792-9.
40. Yang H, Petrini M. Effect of cognitive behavior therapy on sleep disorder in Parkinson's disease in China: a pilot study. Nurs Health Sci. 2012;14(4):458-63.
41. Diederich NJ, Pieri V, Goetz CG. Coping strategies for visual hallucinations in Parkinson's disease. Mov Disord. 2003;18(7):831-2.
42. Koychev I, Okai D. Cognitive-behavioural therapy for non-motor symptoms of Parkinson's disease: a clinical review. Evid Based Ment Health. 2017;20(1):15-20.
43. Dobkin RD, Menza M, Allen LA, Tiu J, Friedman J, Bienfait KL, et al. Telephone-Based Cognitive-Behavioral Therapy for Depression in Parkinson Disease. J Geriatr Psychiatry Neurol. 2011;24(4):206-14.
44. Kraepelien M, Svenningsson P, Lindefors N, Kaldo V. Internet-based cognitive behavioral therapy for depression and anxiety in Parkinson's disease—A pilot study. Internet Interventions. 2015;2(1):1-6.
45. Fitzpatrick L, Simpson J, Smith A. A qualitative analysis of mindfulness-based cognitive therapy (MBCT) in Parkinson's disease. Psychol Psychother. 2010;83(2):179-92.
46. Peavy GM. Mild cognitive deficits in Parkinson disease: Where there is bradykinesia, there is bradyphrenia. Neurology. 2010:75(12):1038-9.
47. Hobson P, Meara J. Mild cognitive impairment in Parkinson's disease and its progression onto dementia: a 16-year outcome evaluation of the Denbighshire cohort. Int J Geriatr Psychiatry. 2015;30(10):1048-55.
48. Emre M, Aarsland D, Brown R, Burn DJ, Duyckaerts C, Mizuno Y, et al. Clinical diagnostic criteria for dementia associated with Parkinson's disease. Mov Disord. 2007;22(12):1689-707.
49. Leroi I, McDonald K, Pantula H, Harbishettar V. Cognitive Impairment in Parkinson Disease: Impact on quality of life, disability, and caregiver burden. J Geriatr Psychiatry Neurol. 2012;25(4):208-14.
50. Szeto JY, Mowszowski L, Gilat M, Walton CC, Naismith SL, Lewis SJ. Mild Cognitive Impairment in Parkinson's Disease: Impact on Caregiver Outcomes. J Parkinsons Dis. 2016;6(3):589-96.
51. Litvan I, Aarsland D, Adler CH, Goldman JG, Kulisevsky J, Mollenhauer B, et al. MDS task force on mild cognitive impairment in Parkinson's disease: Critical review of PD-MCI. Mov Disord. 2011;26(10):1814-24.
52. Okun MS, Rodriguez RL, Mikos A, Miller K, Kellison I, Kirsch-Darrow L, et al. Deep brain stimulation and the role of the neuropsychologist. Clin Neuropsychol. 2007;21(1):162-89.
53. Leung IH, Walton CC, Hallock H, Lewis SJ, Valenzuela M, Lampit A. Cognitive training in Parkinson disease: A systematic review and meta-analysis. Neurology. 2015;85(21):1843-51.
54. Díez-Cirarda M, Ojeda N, Peña J, Cabrera-Zubizarreta A, Lucas-Jiménez O, Gómez-Esteban JC, et al. Increased brain connectivity and activation after cognitive rehabilitation in Parkinson's disease: a randomized controlled trial. Brain Imaging Behav. 2017;11(6):1640-51.
55. París AP, Saleta HG, de la Cruz Crespo Maraver M, Silvestre E, Freixa MG, Torrellas CP, et al. Blind randomized controlled study of the efficacy of cognitive training in Parkinson's disease. Mov Disord. 2011;26(7):1251-8.
56. Peña J, Ibarretxe-Bilbao N, García-Gorostiaga I, Gomez-Beldarrain MA, Díez-Cirarda M, Ojeda N. Improving functional disability and cognition in Parkinson disease: randomized controlled trial. Neurology. 2014;83(23):2167-74.
57. Olde Dubbelink KT, Hillebrand A, Stoffers D, Deijen JB, Twisk JW, Stam CJ, et al. Disrupted brain network topology in Parkinson's disease: a longitudinal magnetoencephalography study. Brain. 2014;137(1):197-207.
58. Leroi I, Vatter S, Carter LA, Smith SJ, Orgeta V, Poliakoff E, et al. Parkinson's-adapted cognitive stimulation therapy: a pilot randomized controlled clinical trial. Ther Adv Neurol Disord. 2019;12:1756286419852217.
59. Cucca A, Sharma K, Acosta I, Beheshti M, Berberian M, Bertish HC, et al. Can Art Therapy improve signs and symptoms of Parkinson's Disease? Preliminary Results from the "ExplorArtPD Study". Neurology. 2019;92(15):P2.8-013.
60. Bae YS, Kim DH. The Applied Effectiveness of Clay Art Therapy for Patients with Parkinson's Disease. J Evid-Based Integr Med. 2018;23:2515690X18765943.
61. Nombela C, Hughes LE, Owen AM, Grahn JA. Into the groove: Can rhythm influence Parkinson's disease? Neurosci Biobehav Rev. 2013;37(10:2):2564-70.
62. Hayashi A, Nagaoka M, Mizuno Y. Music therapy in Parkinson's disease: Improvement of Parkinsonian gait and depression with rhythmic auditory stimulation. Parkinsonism Relat Disord. 2006;12(2):S76.
63. Thaut MH, McIntosh KW, McIntosh GC, Hoemberg V. Auditory rhythmicity enhances movement and speech motor control in patients with Parkinson's disease. Funct Neurol. 2001;16(2): 163-72.
64. Pacchetti C, Mancini F, Aglieri R, Fundarò C, Martignoni E, Nappi G. Active Music Therapy in Parkinson's Disease: An Integrative Method for Motor and Emotional Rehabilitation. Psychosom Med. 2000;62(3):386-93.

65. Hackney ME, Kantorovich S, Levin R, Earhart GM. Effects of tango on functional mobility in Parkinson's disease: a preliminary study. J Neurol Phys Ther. 2007;31(4):173-9.
66. Sharp K, Hewitt J. Dance as an intervention for people with Parkinson's disease: a systematic review and meta-analysis. Neurosci Biobehav Rev. 2014;47:445-56.
67. Kunte TM, D'Souza N, Barretto M. A study of the effects of a group dance intervention program using Indian dance techniques on symptoms of Parkinson's. World Congress for Neurorehabilitation Conference, Mumbai, India; 2018.
68. Lageman SK, Mickens MN, Cash TV. Caregiver-identified needs and barriers to care in Parkinson's disease. Geriatr Nurs. 2015;36(3):197-201.
69. Ellis T, Boudreau JK, DeAngelis TR, Brown LE, Cavanaugh JT, Earhart GM, et al. Barriers to exercise in people with Parkinson disease. Phys Ther. 2013;93(5):628-36.
70. Dobkin RD, Rubino JT, Friedman J, Allen LA, Gara MA, Menza M. Barriers to Mental Health Care Utilization in Parkinson's Disease. J Geriatr Psychiatry Neurol. 2013;26(2):105-16.
71. Duncombe LW, Howe MC. Group treatment: goals, tasks, and economic implications. Am J Occup Ther. 1995;49(3):199-205.
72. Patterson F, Fleming J, Doig E. Patient perceptions of participation in group-based rehabilitation in an inpatient brain injury rehabilitation setting. Patient Educ Couns. 2019;102(1):148-54.
73. Haslam C, Haslam SA, Jetten J, Bevins A, Ravenscroft S, Tonks J. The social treatment: The benefits of group interventions in residential care settings. Psychol Aging. 2010;25(1):157-67.
74. Combs SA, Diehl MD, Chrzastowski C, Didrick N, McCoin B, Mox N, et al. Community-based group exercise for persons with Parkinson disease: a randomized controlled trial. NeuroRehabilitation. 2013;32(1):117-24.
75. Yang JH, Wang YQ, Ye SQ, Cheng YG, Chen Y, Feng XZ. The Effects of Group-Based versus Individual-Based Tai Chi Training on Nonmotor Symptoms in Patients with Mild to Moderate Parkinson's Disease: A randomized controlled pilot trial. Parkinsons Dis. 2017;2017:8562867.
76. Gauthier L, Dalziel S, Gauthier S. The benefits of group occupational therapy for Patients with Parkinson's disease. Am J Occup Ther. 1987;41(6):360-5.
77. Berardelli I, Bloise MC, Bologna M, Conte A, Pompili M, Lamis DA, et al. Cognitive behavioral group therapy versus psychoeducational intervention in Parkinson's disease. Neuropsychiatr Dis Treat. 2018;(14):399-405.
78. Duncan RP, Earhart GM. Randomized Controlled Trial of Community-Based Dancing to Modify Disease Progression in Parkinson Disease. Neurorehabil Neural Repair. 2012;26(2): 132-43.
79. Irani N, Barretto M, Mukadam N, Wandrekar J, D'Souza N, Sivaramakrishnan A. Multidisciplinary Capacity Building Module for rehabilitation and care of Parkinson's in India. World Parkinson's Congress. Portland, Oregon, USA: World Parkinson's Coalition; 2016.
80. Monticone M, Ambrosini E, Laurini A, Rocca B, Foti C. In-patient multidisciplinary rehabilitation for Parkinson's disease: A randomized controlled trial. Mov Disord. 2015;30(8):1050-8.

SECTION

6

ATYPICAL PARKINSONSIM

CHAPTER 27

Progressive Supranuclear Palsy

Sudhir V Shah, Bhagyadhan Patel, Heli S Shah

INTRODUCTION

Progressive supranuclear palsy (PSP), also known as Steele-Richardson-Olszewski syndrome, is a neurodegenerative tauopathy, primarily affecting the basal ganglia and brainstem. PSP is an atypical Parkinsonian syndrome characterized by bradykinesia, axial rigidity, impairment of vertical saccades and vertical gaze palsy ± recurrent falls ± personality changes, and cognitive impairment. Despite being considered as a Parkinsonian syndrome, unlike idiopathic Parkinson's disease (PD), PSP does not respond well to levodopa and sometimes response is only short-lived. The relentless progressive course leads to death usually from aspiration. Median survival is 5–7 years from onset and shorter in those who experience falls and dysphagia within 1 year of onset of illness. PSP is one of the most common atypical Parkinsonian syndromes as it is said to affect approximately 6 per 100,000 population worldwide with no significant bias toward gender or region.

Progressive supranuclear palsy is neuropathologically characterized by the accumulation of neurofibrillary tangles in various nuclei of the basal ganglia, cerebellum, and brainstem, the presence of which are extensively correlated with progressive neurodegeneration. The current treatment options for PSP are limited by our understanding of the disease. Various studies have suggested that biochemical changes in dopaminergic, cholinergic, and gamma-aminobutyric acid (GABA)ergic systems are all features of PSP, though no widespread studies have been able to confirm the therapeutic efficacy of drug action on these systems.[1-4]

EPIDEMIOLOGY

The prevalence of PSP varies from 2 to 6 per 100,000 population. The prevalence of PSP in the Western population has been found similar to that of the Asian population. The mean age of onset of PSP is around 65 years and its incidence increases with age. As compared to PD, the mean age at onset of PSP is around 10 years later than that of PD. PSP is presumed to be more common in males, but confirmatory data is lacking. It is reported that PSP accounts for around 6% of all Parkinsonian patients who fulfill the clinical criteria of PSP in a specialized clinic. In our experience, a significant proportion of patients with PSP tend to have sleep disorders and some of them initially present with PD-like features and later on develop PSP.[1,5-7]

CLINICAL FEATURES

The cardinal features of classical PSP consist of postural instability, early recurrent unprovoked falls, supranuclear gaze paresis, bulbar dysfunction, behavior abnormalities, cognitive dysfunction, and sleep dysfunction (**Tables 1** and **2**).[1,2,8-20]

A variety of phenotypes exist with pathology similar to that seen in classical PSP. The differences in phenotype are more prominent at the onset of illness and they tend to fade away as disease progresses (**Table 3**).

Progressive supranuclear palsy is primarily a neurodegenerative disorder, but rarely PSP-like illness has been described secondary to autoimmune encephalitis. Anti-IgLON5 antibody syndrome usually presents with

TABLE 1: Cardinal features of classical progressive supranuclear palsy (PSP).

Affected system	*Key features*
Postural instability and recurrent falls	The pattern of extrapyramidal involvement in PSP is different from that of PD. There is predominant axial more than appendicular rigidity, which leads to extended neck and broad-based stance with knees extended and arms abducted. Gait is broad based, with short steps and tendency to pivot on turning. With further progression, patients tend to fall characteristically backward even on slightest of movements. The average period from the onset to the first fall is just 16.8 months, which is significantly early as compared to other atypical Parkinsonian syndromes. Recurrent unprovoked falls can lead to multiple fractures, intracranial hematomas, and, sometimes, death
Oculomotor findings	Supranuclear ophthalmoparesis is one of the cardinal features of PSP. Gaze impairment, which improves with Doll's eye movement, is characteristic of supranuclear involvement. Impaired vertical gaze, particularly downgaze, is very typical of PSP. In early cases, gaze involvement can be demonstrated by impaired opticokinetic nystagmus and slowing of saccades in vertical direction. These patients also experience difficulty to converge, which often leads to impaired vision and reading difficulties. Vertical gaze impairment leads to spilling of food while eating and also contributes to falls
Motor involvement	Patients with PSP tend to have symmetrical bradykinesia. As mentioned above, axial rigidity dominates the clinical feature and, similar to bradykinesia, appendicular rigidity is also symmetrical. Tremors are conspicuously absent. Their presence should arouse suspicion of alternate diagnosis. Dystonia can occur in a significant proportion of patients with PSP. Blepharospasm, apraxia of eyelid opening, overcontraction of forehead muscles, retrocollis, and, sometimes, limb dystonia can occur in PSP
Frontal lobe dysfunction	Although motor features tend to dominate the clinical picture in PSP, cognitive and behavior changes are profoundly seen in PSP. These changes are seen secondary to involvement of the frontal subcortical region. Among behavior abnormalities, apathy is most common. Some patients can be anxious, agitated, disinhibited, or depressed. Cognitive dysfunction predominantly affects abstract thinking, verbal fluency, executive functions, and planning. These behavioral and cognitive features are as disabling as motor features
Pseudobulbar features	Pseudobulbar symptoms are characterized by dysarthria, dysphagia, and emotional incontinence. Speech tends to be slow, monotonous, low-pitched, and hypokinetic. In severe cases, patients can develop inability to speak due to extreme rigidity of bulbar muscles. Difficulty in swallowing, coughing while eating, and aspiration can lead to pneumonia and often requires a feeding tube
Sleep changes	Disruption of sleep architecture in the form of difficulty in falling asleep, decreased total sleep time, and frequent nocturnal awakenings has been described commonly in PSP

(PD: Parkinson's disease; PSP: progressive supranuclear palsy)

TABLE 2: Signs in progressive supranuclear palsy (PSP).

Signs	*Description*
Drunken sailor sign	Due to postural instability, patients tend to pivot on turning and are unable to take protective measures
Dirty tie sign	Downgaze palsy and rigidity of neck extensors often lead to soiling of clothes while eating
Omega sign	Tonic contraction of the corrugator muscle causing characteristic facial appearance with wrinkles in the shape of the Greek letter Ω above the root of the nose
Procerus sign	Focal dystonia of the procerus muscle causing vertical wrinkles in the glabellar region and bridge of the nose, present with both eyes open and closed, is called the procerus sign
Staring face/Mona Lisa stare	Combination of a taut face, neck in extension, fixed gaze, reduced blinking, lid retraction, overactivity of the frontalis muscle, and focal dystonia of the procerus
Round the houses sign	At a stage of PSP, when full vertical excursions are still present, some patients display an inability to produce pure vertical saccades along a straight line in the midline. Instead, they accomplish vertical saccades by moving their eyes in a lateral arc or curved trajectory called the "round the houses" sign
Gunslinger's gait/ Penguin gait	Wide-based, unsteady, and hypererect gait with knee and trunk extended and the arms slightly abducted with decreased arm swing has been likened to a Gunslinger's gait or Penguin gait
Rocket sign	There is impaired insight into postural instability and patients tend to rocket out of their chair without assistance
Applause sign	The applause sign is an inability to stop clapping after being asked to clap three times. This is not specific for PSP

TABLE 3: Salient features of progressive supranuclear palsy (PSP) phenotypes.

PSP phenotypes	Salient features
PSP with Richardson syndrome (PSP-RS)	Same as classical PSP
PSP with predominant Parkinsonism (PSP-P)	Asymmetrical onset, tremors, slower rate of progression, and moderate response to levodopa
PSP with predominant oculomotor dysfunction (PSP-OM)	Prominent supranuclear gaze involvement with minimal postural instability or cognitive features
PSP with predominant postural instability (PSP-PI)	Early postural instability without prominent oculomotor involvement
PSP with progressive gait freezing (PSP-PGF)	Early gait freezing, bradykinesia, rigidity, and unresponsiveness to dopaminergic medications
PSP with predominant frontal presentation (PSP-F)	Early frontal lobe dysfunction and then progressing to PSP at later stage
PSP with predominant speech/language disorder (PSP-SL)	Nonfluent aphasia and apraxia of speech at the onset
PSP with corticobasal syndrome (PSP-CBS)	Progressive asymmetric apraxia, dystonia, cortical sensory loss, alien limb syndrome, and levodopa unresponsiveness
Others	Rarely, combination of PSP with cerebellar degeneration (PSP-cerebellar) and upper motor involvement (PSP-primary lateral sclerosis) has been mentioned

sleep disorder, bulbar weakness, gait instability, dysautonomia, and movement disorders. However, up to 20% of patients with anti-IgLON5 antibody syndrome develop supranuclear gaze paresis (vertical and horizontal), Parkinsonism, and cognitive decline resembling PSP-like illness.

NEUROPATHOLOGY AND NEUROCHEMISTRY

The motor, behavioral, and ophthalmologic findings point toward affection of basal ganglia (globus pallidus), brainstem (superior colliculi, pedunculopontine tegmental nuclei, substantia nigra, locus coeruleus, superior cerebellar peduncle, red nucleus, reticular formation, and vestibular nuclei), and other subcortical and cortical structures (basal nucleus of Meynert and subthalamic nucleus). Histopathology reveals neuronal loss, gliosis, and deposition of tau-positive filamentous inclusions in affected areas. The presence of tufted astrocytes is considered pathognomonic of PSP. Other histopathological features include neurofibrillary tangles, neuropil threads, and coiled bodies. Deposition of tau is central to pathogenesis of PSP. The tau is encoded by microtubule-associated protein tau (MAPT), which helps to stabilize microtubules. There is disparity between 3R and 4R tau in PSP (increased 4R to 3R ratio) in PSP. The genetics linked to tauopathies such as PSP is under investigation.[1,2,21]

DIAGNOSTICS

Clinical Criteria

At present, there is no reliable serum or cerebrospinal fluid (CSF) marker available for diagnosis of PSP. Clinical features remain critical for diagnosis of PSP. Hence, clinical criteria proposed by the National Institute of Neurological Disorders and Stroke and Society for PSP (NINDS-SPSP) are widely used for its diagnosis. Sporadic occurrence of progressive PSP-related symptoms in individuals >40 years is considered mandatory for PSP. In patients who fulfill mandatory criteria, core clinical features can help in diagnosing PSP.[22]

- *Definite PSP*: Any clinical presentation with presence of neuropathological diagnosis (difficult to perform in every case)
- *Probable PSP*:
  - Presence of ocular motor dysfunction (supranuclear gaze palsy or slowing of vertical saccades) in combination with early (<3 years) postural instability or repeated unprovoked falls
  - Presence of oculomotor dysfunction with progressive gait freezing or akinetic rigid, levodopa unresponsive syndrome, or frontal/behavioral presentation
- *Possible PSP*:
  - Presence of isolated ocular motor dysfunction
  - Presence of slowing of vertical saccades and positive pull test within 3 years
  - Presence of ocular motor dysfunction in combination with speech/language disorder or corticobasal syndrome

Radiological Signs

Although PSP largely remains a clinical diagnosis, MRI remains the most useful investigation. The following features can help to differentiate PSP from other neurodegenerative disorders:[23-31]

- *Midbrain to pons ratio*: The areas of the midbrain and pons are calculated in the midsagittal image. A normal value is approximately 0.24, whereas, it is significantly reduced in PSP to <0.12 due to midbrain atrophy. It is the most sensitive radiologic sign confirming midbrain atrophy.

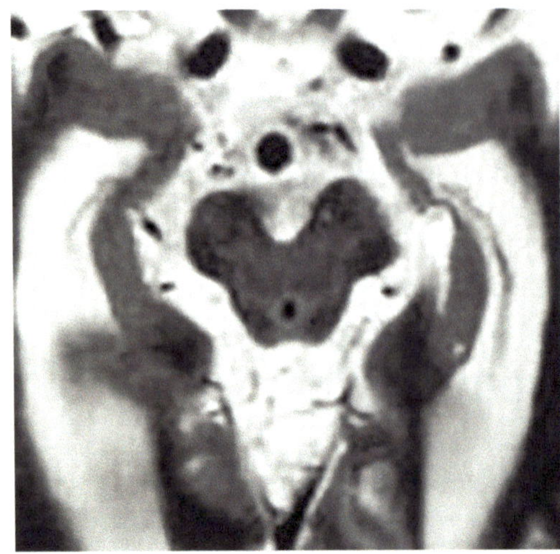

FIG. 1: T1 sagittal images show humming bird sign suggestive of midbrain atrophy.

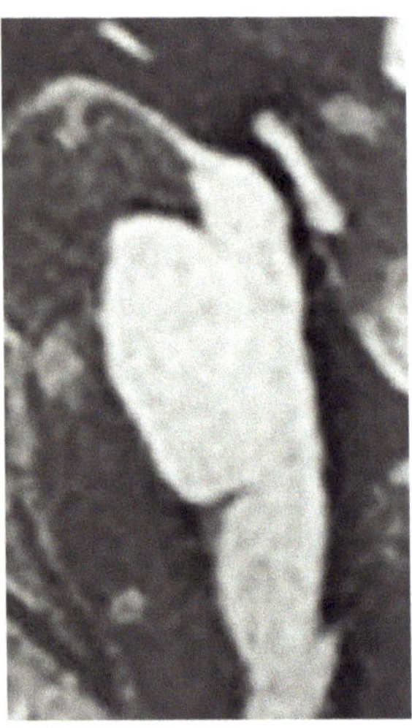

FIG. 2: T2 axial images show midbrain atrophy (Mickey Mouse sign).

- *Humming bird/Penguin sign*: The prominent atrophy of midbrain with concave upper border and preserved pons results in a profile of the brainstem (in the sagittal plane) in which the preserved pons forms the body of the bird and the atrophic midbrain, the head, with beak extending anteriorly toward the optic chiasm (**Fig. 1**).
- *Mickey Mouse or morning glory sign*: Axial MRI image of the midbrain showing selective atrophy of the midbrain tegmentum with relative preservation of the tectum and the cerebral peduncles resembling head of Mickey Mouse is called the "Mickey Mouse" sign in PSP (**Fig. 2**).
- *Magnetic resonance Parkinsonism index (MRPI)*: Selective atrophy of midbrain (M) and superior cerebellar peduncle (SCP) with sparing of pons (P) and middle cerebellar peduncle (MCP) is highlighted by MRPI. MRPI index >13.55 is seen in PSP.
- *Midbrain anteroposterior (AP) diameter*: Reduction of midbrain AP diameter at the level of superior colliculi from interpeduncular fossa to the interpeduncular groove <12 mm.

Advanced Techniques

Apart from structural imaging, advanced imaging techniques can be used to demonstrate involvement of areas other than midbrain in PSP.[1,2,23]

- *Diffusion tensor imaging (DTI)*: It shows severe involvement of putamen, caudate nucleus, midbrain, globus pallidus, and SCP as compared to PD.
- *Positron emission tomography (PET)/single-photon emission computed tomography (SPECT)*: Apart from midbrain, PET/SPECT reveals hypometabolism of bilateral frontal cortex, caudate heads, thalami, cingulate gyri, and midbrain.
- *Dopamine active transporter (DAT) imaging*: Decreased DAT binding in putamen is seen in all extrapyramidal syndromes. However, caudate involvement on DAT imaging tends to be more severe in PSP than other extrapyramidal syndromes.
- *Tau-PET imaging*: There seems to be an evolving pattern on tau-PET imaging to detect deposition of tau in basal ganglia and its circuits. However, its use in routine clinical practice needs to be validated.
- *Cerebrospinal fluid analysis*: Lower ratio of light (33 kDa) to heavy (55 kDa) tau protein in CSF favors PSP over other tauopathies. It has been validated against structural imaging of brainstem. However, for obvious reasons, its use in clinical practice is limited.

MANAGEMENT AND PROGNOSIS

The aim of management largely revolves around measures to limit the morbidity and delay mortality, as there is no specific cure for PSP at present. However, following pharmacological and nonpharmacological measures can be helpful in patients with PSP:

- *Medications*: PSP as a group largely remains unresponsive to levodopa therapy. However, early cases of PSP with Richardson syndrome (PSP-RS) and PSP with predominant Parkinsonism (PSP-P) may show modest benefit with levodopa therapy. Hence, levodopa therapy is recommended in all patients with PSP to detect responsiveness. Amantadine has been shown to benefit gait and bulbar functions in limited studies. Coenzyme Q10, cholinesterase inhibitor (rivastigmine), and antidepressants (sertraline, fluoxetine, and venlafaxine) may provide modest benefit in behavior changes and cognitive decline. Anecdotal case reports have shown improvement in ocular movements and postural instability with zolpidem to some extent. In a proportion of patients with PSP, blepharospasm and apraxia of eyelid opening may cause significant disability, which can be ameliorated by botulinum toxin injection. Selective anticholinergics such as tolterodine and solifenacin are preferred to reduce urinary frequency. Dextromethorphan and quinidine combination may be helpful in pseudobulbar symptoms. It is important to identify anti-IgLON5 syndrome and differentiate from degenerative PSP, as it is amenable to immunotherapy.

- *Nonpharmacological measures*: Measures to reduce fall, prevent injuries, and prevent aspiration are of extreme importance. These patients are dependent on all activities of daily living and, hence, require round-the-clock attention to prevent falls and subsequent injuries. As dysphagia and aspiration are leading causes of morbidity and mortality, the decision of percutaneous gastrotomy tube insertion to maintain nutrition, hydration, and prevent aspiration is critical. Overall, palliative care and symptomatic therapy remain the mainstay in the management of patients with PSP.

Overall, the prognosis of PSP is dismal. It is a relentlessly progressive disease that usually leads to a wheelchair bound state within 5 years and death within 7 years from onset of illness. However, some PSP variants such as PSP-P and PSP with progressive gait freezing (PSP-PGF) have a protracted course and a less bad prognosis than PSP-RS.[1,2]

CONCLUSION

The approach to progressive supranuclear palsy syndrome requires meticulate attention to mode of presentation, disease progression, identification of classical signs and symptoms that may provide clues to diagnosis. Growing recognition of the clinical heterogeneity within PSP spectrum, overlap, and varied phenotypes of these syndromes may further aid in early diagnosis, prognostication, measures to prevent complications (fall, trauma, and pneumonia, etc.), and hopefully, in emergence of potential disease modifying therapies in future.

REFERENCES

1. Jankovic J. Atypical Parkinsonism, Parkinsonism-plus syndromes, and secondary Parkinsonian disorders. In: Jankovic J, Hallett M, Fahn S (Eds). Principles and Practice of Movement Disorders, 2nd edition. Philadelphia: WB Saunders; 2011.
2. McFarland NR. Diagnostic Approach to Atypical Parkinsonian Syndromes. Continuum (Minneap Minn). 2016;22:1117-42.
3. Steele JC, Richardson JC, Olszewski J. Progressive supranuclear palsy. A heterogeneous degeneration involving the brainstem, basal ganglia and cerebellum with vertical gaze and pseudobulbar palsy, nuchal dystonia and dementia. Arch Neurol. 1964;10:333-59.
4. Golbe LI. Progressive Supranuclear Palsy. Curr Treat Options Neurol. 2001;3:473-7.
5. Bower JH, Maraganore DM, McDonnell SK, Rocca WA. Incidence of progressive supranuclear palsy and multiple system atrophy in Olmsted County, Minnesota, 1976 to 1990. Neurology. 1997;49:1284-8.
6. Schrag A, Ben-Shlomo Y, Quinn NP. Prevalence of progressive supranuclear palsy and multiple system atrophy: a cross-sectional study. Lancet. 1999;354:1771-5.
7. Zermansky A, Ben-Shlomo Y. Epidemiology of progressive supranuclear palsy and multiple system atrophy. In: Litvan I (Eds). Atypical Parkinsonian Disorders. United States: Humana Press; 2005.
8. Boeve BF, Silber MH, Parisi JE, Dickson DW, Ferman TJ, Benarroch EE, et al. Synucleinopathy pathology and REM sleep behavior disorder plus dementia or parkinsonism. Neurology. 2003;61:40-5.
9. Williams DR, de Silva R, Paviour DC, Pittman A, Watt HC, Kilford L, et al. Characteristics of two distinct clinical phenotypes in pathologically proven progressive supranuclear palsy: Richardson's syndrome and PSP-parkinsonism. Brain. 2005;128:1247-58.
10. Birdi S, Rajput AH, Fenton M, Donat JR, Rozdilsky B, Robinson C, et al. Progressive supranuclear palsy diagnosis and confounding features: report on 16 autopsied cases. Mov Disord. 2002;17:1255-64.
11. Williams DR, Lees AJ. What features improve the accuracy of the clinical diagnosis of progressive supranuclear palsy-parkinsonism (PSP-P)? Mov Disord. 2010;25:357-62.
12. Boxer AL, Yu JT, Golbe LI, Litvan I, Lang AE, Höglinger GU. Advances in progressive supranuclear palsy: new diagnostic criteria, biomarkers, and therapeutic approaches. Lancet Neurol. 2017;16:552-63.
13. Kurz C, Ebersbach G, Respondek G, Giese A, Arzberger T, Höglinger GU. An autopsy-confirmed case of progressive supranuclear palsy with predominant postural instability. Acta Neuropathol Commun. 2016;4:120.
14. Williams DR, Holton JL, Strand K, Revesz T, Lees AJ. Pure akinesia with gait freezing: a third clinical phenotype of progressive supranuclear palsy. Mov Disord. 2007;22:2235-41.
15. Facheris MF, Maniak S, Scaravilli F, Schüle B, Klein C, Pramstaller PP. Pure akinesia as initial presentation of PSP: a clinicopathological study. Parkinsonism Relat Disord. 2008;14:517-9.
16. Kaat LD, Boon AJW, Kamphorst W, Ravid R, Duivenvoorden HJ, van Swieten JC. Frontal presentation in progressive supranuclear palsy. Neurology. 2007;69:723-9.
17. Boeve B, Dickson D, Duffy J, Bartleson J, Trenerry M, Petersen R. Progressive nonfluent aphasia and subsequent aphasic dementia associated with atypical progressive supranuclear palsy pathology. Eur Neurol. 2003;49:72-8.

18. Josephs KA, Duffy JR. Apraxia of speech and nonfluent aphasia: a new clinical marker for corticobasal degeneration and progressive supranuclear palsy. Curr Opin Neurol. 2008;21: 688-92.
19. Koga S, Josephs KA, Ogaki K, Labbé C, Uitti RJ, Graff-Radford N, et al. Cerebellar ataxia in progressive supranuclear palsy: An autopsy study of PSP-C. Mov Disord. 2016;31:653-62.
20. Nagao S, Yokota O, Nanba R, Takata H, Haraguchi T, Ishizu H, et al. Progressive supranuclear palsy presenting as primary lateral sclerosis but lacking parkinsonism, gaze palsy, aphasia, or dementia. J Neurol Sci. 2012;323:147-53.
21. Stamelou M, de Silva R, Arias-Carrión O, Boura E, Höllerhage M, Oertel WH, et al. Rational therapeutic approaches to progressive supranuclear palsy. Brain. 2010;133:1578-90.
22. Höglinger GU, Respondek G, Stamelou M, Kurz C, Josephs KA, Lang AE, et al. Clinical diagnosis of progressive supranuclear palsy: The movement disorder society criteria. Mov Disord. 2017;32:853-64.
23. Whitwell JL, Höglinger GU, Antonini A, Bordelon Y, Boxer AL, Colosimo C, et al. Radiological biomarkers for diagnosis in PSP: Where are we and where do we need to be? Mov Disord. 2017;32:955-71.
24. Warmuth-Metz M, Naumann M, Csoti I, Solymosi L. Measurement of the midbrain diameter on routine magnetic resonance imaging: a simple and accurate method of differentiating between Parkinson disease and progressive supranuclear palsy. Arch Neurol. 2001;58:1076-9.
25. Oba H, Yagishita A, Terada H, Barkovich AJ, Kutomi K, Yamauchi T, et al. New and reliable MRI diagnosis for progressive supranuclear palsy. Neurology. 2005;64:2050-5.
26. Quattrone A, Nicoletti G, Messina D, Fera F, Condino F, Pugliese P, et al. MR imaging index for differentiation of progressive supranuclear palsy from Parkinson disease and the Parkinson variant of multiple system atrophy. Radiology. 2008;246:214-21.
27. Morelli M, Arabia G, Salsone M, Novellino F, Giofrè L, Paletta R, et al. Accuracy of magnetic resonance parkinsonism index for differentiation of progressive supranuclear palsy from probable or possible Parkinson disease. Mov Disord. 2011;26:527-33.
28. Morelli M, Arabia G, Novellino F, Salsone M, Giofrè L, Condino F, et al. MRI measurements predict PSP in unclassifiable parkinsonisms: a cohort study. Neurology. 2011;77:1042-7.
29. Massey LA, Jäger HR, Paviour DC, O'Sullivan SS, Ling H, Williams DR, et al. The midbrain to pons ratio: a simple and specific MRI sign of progressive supranuclear palsy. Neurology. 2013;80:1856-6100.
30. Longoni G, Agosta F, Kostić VS, Stojković T, Pagani E, Stošić-Opinćal T, et al. MRI measurements of brainstem structures in patients with Richardson's syndrome, progressive supranuclear palsy-parkinsonism, and Parkinson's disease. Mov Disord. 2011;26:247-55.
31. Knake S, Belke M, Menzler K, Pilatus U, Eggert KM, Oertel WH, et al. In vivo demonstration of microstructural brain pathology in progressive supranuclear palsy: a DTI study using TBSS. Mov Disord. 2010;25:1232-8.

CHAPTER 28

Multiple System Atrophy

Arup Kumar Dutta, Kamakshi Dhamija, Kalyan B Bhattacharyya

INTRODUCTION

Multiple system atrophy (MSA), a progressive neurodegenerative disease of undetermined etiology, occurs sporadically and causes Parkinsonism and cerebellar, autonomic, urinary, and pyramidal dysfunction in different patterns. Although MSA requires a clinical diagnosis, a number of tests may help in its diagnosis. MSA is subdivided into two major categories according to the predominant clinical manifestation. Predominantly Parkinsonian form of MSA (MSA-P) replaces the term striatonigral degeneration while cerebellar MSA (MSA-C) replaces the term, olivopontocerebellar atrophy (OPCA).[1,2] Many patients with striatonigral degeneration have orthostatic hypotension (OH). This combined Parkinsonism and autonomic disorder is now termed MSA-A.

Currently, there is no effective neuroprotective therapy in MSA. Symptomatic treatment is restricted largely to Parkinsonism and dysautonomia. Other features like cerebellar ataxia, are usually unresponsive to drug treatment.

HISTORICAL PERSPECTIVE

The concept of MSA has evolved over decades based on combined clinical features of Parkinsonism, cerebellar, and autonomic symptoms. Pathological findings in autopsy specimens with glial cytoplasmic inclusions (GCIs) has united these various clinical presentations/patterns into a single disease entity.

Although Menzel described the first case in 1891, it was Dejerine and Thomas in 1900 who first used the term OPCA in two sporadic cases.[3] Shy and Drager in 1960 described four cases of a "neurological syndrome with OH".[4] They defined the full syndrome comprising of OH, urinary and rectal incontinence, loss of sweating, iris atrophy, external ocular palsies, rigidity, tremor, loss of associated movements, impotence, atonic bladder, loss of rectal sphincter tone, fasciculations, wasting of distal muscles, evidence of a neuropathic lesion in the electromyogram (EMG) suggesting involvement of the anterior horn cells, and the finding of a neuropathic lesion in the muscle biopsy.

Graham and Oppenheimer in 1969 coined the term MSA, considering that clinical and pathologic features of sporadic striatonigral degeneration, with or without autonomic failure, and in some instances those of OPCA often coexist. The discovery of GCIs and α-synuclein immunostaining as a sensitive marker of MSA were major milestones in the definition of MSA as a clinicopathologic entity.

Epidemiology

Multiple system atrophy is considerably less common than PD. Its prevalence is 4–5 per 100,000. The incidence is equal among males and females.[5] The disease onset is usually in the sixth decade of life with the median age of onset being 53 years. It progresses over 10–15 years with a median survival of 9.3 years from the first symptom.[6,7]

The Parkinsonian form of MSA predominates in western hemisphere whereas, the cerebellar form predominates in the eastern part of the globe.

Evolution of Clinical Diagnostic Criteria

In 1989, Quinn[8] first proposed diagnostic criteria for MSA, and these were subsequently modified in 1994.[9] The Quinn criteria distinguish Parkinsonian and cerebellar presentations as well as three levels of diagnostic certainty (possible, probable, and definite). So far, the sensitivity and specificity of the Quinn criteria have never been prospectively determined. A retrospective validation based on postmortem verification of MSA cases demonstrated suboptimal diagnostic accuracy.[10]

In April 1998, an international consensus conference was convened to develop optimized criteria for a clinical diagnosis of MSA.[11] The MSA conference recommended three diagnostic categories of increasing certainty: Possible, probable, and definite. A definite diagnosis requires a typical neuropathological lesion pattern as well as deposition of GCIs.

The diagnosis of definite, probable and possible MSA is based on the presence of clinical features listed in **Box 1**. In addition, exclusion criteria have to be considered (**Box 2**).

Diagnostic Categories of Multiple System Atrophy

- *Possible MSA*: One criterion plus two features from separate other domains. When the criterion is Parkinsonism, a poor levodopa (L-DOPA) response qualifies as one feature (hence, only one additional feature is required).
- *Probable MSA*: Criterion—autonomic failure/urinary dysfunction plus poorly L-DOPA responsive Parkinsonism or cerebellar dysfunction.
- *Definite MSA*: Pathologically confirmed by the presence of a high density of GCIs in association with a combination of degenerative changes in the nigrostriatal and olivopontocerebellar pathways.

Box 1 Current consensus criteria for the diagnosis of multiple system atrophy, adapted from (Gilman et al. 2008).

- **Criteria for definite MSA include neuropathological findings during postmortem examination of:**
  - Widespread and abundant cerebral α-synuclein–positive glial cytoplasmic inclusions
  - Neurodegenerative changes in striatonigral or olivopontocerebellar region
- **Criteria for probable MSA include a sporadic progressive adult (>30-years-old)–onset disease characterized by:**
  - Autonomic failure involving urinary incontinence (inability to control the release of urine from the bladder with erectile dysfunction in males) or an orthostatic decrease of blood pressure within 3 min of standing by at least 30 mm Hg systolic or 15 mm Hg disatolic blood pressure
  - Poorly levodopa-responsive parkinsonism (bradykinesia with rigidity, tremor or postural instability), or
  - A cerebellar syndrome (gait ataxia with cerebellar dysarthria, limb ataxia or cerebellar oculomotor dysfunction)

Continued

Continued

- **Criteria for possible MSA include a sporadic progressive adult (>30-years-old)–onset disease characterized by:**
  - Parkinsonism (bradykinesia with rigidity tremor or postural instability), or
  - Cerebellar syndrome (gait ataxia with cerebellar dysarthria limb ataxia or cerebellar oculomotor dysfunction), and
  - At least one feature suggesting autonomic dysfunction (otherwise unexplained urinary urgency frequency or incomplete bladder emptying erectile dysfunction in males or significant orthostatic BP decline that does not meet the level required in probable MSA), and
  - At least one of the following features:
    - Babinski sign with hyperreflexia
    - Stridor
    - Rapidly progressive parkinsonism
    - Poor response to levodopa
    - Postural instability within 3 years of motor onset
    - Gait ataxia, cerebellar dysarthria, limb ataxia, or cerebellar oculomotor dysfunction
    - Dysphagia within 5 year of motor onset
    - Atrophy on MRI of putamen middle cerebellar peduncle, pons or cerebellum
    - Hypometabolism on FDG-PET in putamen, brainstem or cerebellum
    - Presynaptic nigrostriatal dopaminergic denervation on SPECT or PET

Box 2 Exclusion criteria of MSA.

- Onset after 75 years
- Family h/o ataxia, parkinsonism
- Classic pill rolling tremor
- Dementia
- Hallucinations not induced by drugs
- Clinically significant neuropathy
- White matter lesions suggesting multiple sclerosis

Exclusion criteria for the diagnosis of MSA

I. a. History symptomatic onset under 30 years of age or >75 years of age
   b. Family history of ataxia or parkinsonism, of a similar disorder systemic diseases or other identifiable causes for features listed in **Box 1**
   c. Hallucinations unrelated to medication

II. a. Physical examination DSM criteria for dementia
   b. Prominent slowing of vertical saccades or vertical supranuclear gaze palsy, classic pill rolling tremor, clinically significant neuropathy
   c. Evidence of focal cortical dysfunction such as aphasia, alien limb syndrome, and parietal dysfunction

III. Laboratory investigation: White matter lesions suggestive of multiple scerosis. Metabolic, molecular, genetic and imaging evidence of an alternative cause of features listed in **Box1**

ETIOLOGY

Multiple system atrophy is a sporadic disorder. A variety of genetic and environmental factors have been proposed to contribute to the disease pathogenesis.

Genetic Factors

Genetic predisposition to MSA was first described by Nee et al. in 1991.[12] They found higher frequencies of neurological diseases and autonomic symptoms among 148 first-degree relatives of 33 patients clinically diagnosed as having MSA compared with control subjects. Families with autosomal dominant and recessive patterns of MSA inheritance have also been reported.[13] Since the discovery of GCIs as a distinct marker for the disease, and the fact that α-synuclein was found to be a major component of GCIs, the genetic studies have revolved around this being the candidate gene. A study has shown that single nucleotide polymorphisms (SNPs) at the *SNCA* locus were significantly associated with increased risk for the development of MSA.[14] However, two other studies focusing on *SNCA* gene analysis were consistently negative for any positive association with MSA.[15]

The MSA research collaboration published an association between CoQ2 mutations and an increased risk for developing MSA. The authors postulated that theoretically CoQ2 mutations impair the mitochondrial respiratory chain and lead to less tolerance to oxidative stress, further resulting in a predisposition to MSA. However, other studies in European and Korean MSA patients failed to detect CoQ2 mutations, thereby contradicting the findings of the MSA research collaboration. Thus, currently the evidence is not strong for a causative association of CoQ2 mutations and MSA.[13] So it appears that genetic markers/links are not conclusive in causation of MSA.

Environmental and other Acquired Factors

As with Parkinson's disease (PD), alcohol and nicotine consumption is less prevalent in MSA patients than healthy controls.[16]

Some studies have hypothesized the adverse role of toxins such as mercury, methanol, carbon tetrachloride, carbon disulfide, and cyanide in causation of the disease along with the occupational solvents, plastic monomers, additives and pesticides.[17-19] Manganese has not been found to be increased in brains of patients with MSA.[17]

PATHOGENESIS

Like idiopathic Parkinson's disease (IPD) and diffuse Lewy Body Disease, MSA has been firmly established as a synucleinopathy after the discovery of α-synuclein immunostaining in the 1990s. Evidence from preclinical models and postmortem studies suggest MSA to be a primary oligodendrogliopathy. Before the α-synuclein aggregation, p25α which is an important myelin stabilizer, relocalizes into oligodendroglial soma. This leads to oligodendrocyte swelling and abnormal uptake or overexpression of α-synuclein. The interaction of P25α and α-synuclein leads to the phosphorylation and aggregation of α-synuclein into insoluble oligomers which finally takes the form of GCIs (also called Papp-Lantos bodies). These inclusions are not specific, although they are characteristics of MSA.[20] The GCIs then interfere with neuronal support and the dysfunction activates the quiescent microglial cells. There is, hence, a progressive dysfunction of oligodendrocytes that release misfolded α-synuclein into the extracellular space. The misfolded α-synuclein is taken up by neighboring neurons which then leads to formation of neuronal cytoplasmic inclusions (NCI). The toxic α-synuclein spreads in a prion-like fashion to cause multilevel neuronal dysfunction and widespread astrogliosis and atrophy, that is so characteristic of the disease. Thus, the various pathogenetic changes implicated are: (1) GCIs downhill leading to axonal α-synuclein aggregation and axonal degeneration; (2) Mitochondrial dysfunction; (3) Microgliosis; and (4) Environmental oxidative stress.[21]

Pathology of Multiple System Atrophy

The clinical patterns of the disease are related to macroscopic changes in the MSA brain.[22] There are variable changes in the cerebral cortex leading to cortical atrophy which may not be profound. In patients with the OPCA variant of the disease, atrophy of middle cerebellar peduncles (MCP) along with the pons are most marked. There are variable amounts of cell loss and gliosis, without Lewy bodies in the substantia nigra (SN), locus coeruleus, striatum, inferior olives, pontine nuclei and cerebellar Purkinje's cells, and in the intermediolateral cell columns and Onuf's nucleus in the ventral horns of the spinal cord at the second and third sacral levels.[22] Autonomic disturbances are preceded by loss of neurons in the intermediolateral column of the spinal cord.[23] Dorsal motor nucleus of vagus, vestibular nuclei, pyramidal tracts, and anterior horns may also be affected. Other medullary nuclei affected include catecholaminergic cells in the ventrolateral reticular formation[24] and cells in the arcuate nucleus. The absence of Lewy bodies distinguishes it from IPD. Putaminal atrophy shows a gray-greenish discoloration. Loss of pigment in the SN and locus coeruleus gives them a pale appearance.

Histologically, there are several features in MSA: GCIs, NCIs, neuronal nuclear inclusions (NNIs), glial nuclear inclusions (GNIs), and neuropil threads. GCIs are the most important. GCIs have been recently described in MSA with various combinations of striatonigral degeneration,

OPCA, and Shy–Drager syndrome.[25] These inclusions are not specific, although they are characteristic of MSA. This also confirms the notion that the three clinical syndromes of striatonigral degeneration, OPCA, and Shy–Drager syndrome are various manifestations of the same disease. GCIs have become a diagnostic hallmark of MSA. GCIs are found in the primary motor and other motor areas of the cerebral cortex, pyramidal, extrapyramidal, and corticocerebellar and in the supraspinal autonomic systems and their targets. Immunohistochemical studies have shown that GCIs contain α-synuclein, a synaptic protein also found in Lewy bodies in PD.[26] It has been suggested that a reduction in the solubility of α-synuclein may induce this protein to form filamentous aggregation into cytoplasmic inclusions, thus contributing to the dysfunction or death of glial cells.

Clinical Features of Multiple System Atrophy

Multiple system atrophy can cause a combination of Parkinsonian, autonomic, pyramidal, and cerebellar signs and symptoms. Like PD, MSA has a prodromal premotor phase in 20–75% of cases.[27] These symptoms include sexual dysfunction, urinary urge incontinence or retention, OH, inspiratory stridor, rapid-eye-movement sleep behavior disorder and olfactory disturbances. These features can occur months to years before the first motor symptoms of MSA appear.

When Parkinsonian features predominate, the term striatonigral degeneration is often used. In OPCA, cerebellar features are predominant. When autonomic failure predominates, the term Shy–Drager syndrome is used. These manifestations may occur in various combinations and evolve over the years/time.

Most patients with MSA are initially considered to have PD. Parkinsonian features are documented in 91% of the patients. Akinesia and rigidity predominate and is usually asymmetric. Tremor may be at rest, jerky irregular, or a classic pill rolling type.

Early and severe autonomic failure is the defining feature of MSA. Autonomic symptoms are present in 97% of patients and these may precede the motor disturbance by months or even years. An important pathological difference underlying autonomic dysfunction of PD and MSA is that in PD, the pathology for dysautonomia in PD is peripheral—ganglionic and postganglionic; while in MSA it is predominantly preganglionic/central. Most frequently affected autonomic domains in MSA are urogenital and cardiovascular. Erectile dysfunction typically occurs at disease onset in males, but this gets under-reported and has to be specifically enquired into. Females with MSA usually report genital hyposensitivity during intercourse. This is followed by appearance of urinary disturbances followed by orthostatic dysfunction. Urinary dysfunction occurs in >90% of cases. The typical symptoms include urinary urgency, frequency, urge incontinence, nocturia, and, less commonly, incomplete bladder emptying. Concomitant prostatic hypertrophy in men and perineal laxity in women may mask urological dysfunction in patients with MSA. Recurrent urinary tract infections (UTIs) are a major cause of morbidity and mortality in the MSA population.[28]

Cardiovascular involvement occurs as a result of autonomic dysfunction. The most common presentation is OH that presents as recurrent presyncope/syncope, nausea, headache, or "*coat-hanger pain*" (pain in the neck and shoulder region) on standing and is seen in 43–68% of patients, although this may also be asymptomatic. Other features of autonomic dysfunction include postprandial hypotension, supine and nocturnal hypertension, constipation, thermoregulatory dysfunction in the form of reduced sweating, cold/blue hands, and feet, and Raynaud's phenomenon.

Respiratory and sleep disturbances are also characteristic features of MSA. Respiratory involvement usually manifest as diurnal or nocturnal inspiratory stridor and is more frequent in advanced disease. The cause identified is usually atrophy of the posterior cricoarytenoid muscles resulting in failure of abduction of the vocal cords and narrowing of the airway. Sleep apnea occurs in 40% of patients. Sleep disturbances are also common and RBD is seen in 90–100% of patients. RBD is the most common sleep-related disorder in MSA and may precede the development of Parkinsonism by years.[29]

Cerebellar signs occur in about 50% of the patients. MSA of OPCA type most commonly presents with gait ataxia. Cerebellar ataxia is the predominant and presenting feature of cerebellar subtype of MSA. Typical features include an action tremulousness of hands, dysarthria, gait imbalance, wide-based gait, and nystagmus that can be spontaneous, gaze-evoked, or positional downbeat nystagmus. Oculomotor features in the form of ocular dysmetria (especially for vertical saccades) and square wave jerks can also occur.

Pyramidal signs, a mixed dysarthria with combination of hypokinetic, ataxic and spastic components,[30] nystagmus, saccadic pursuit, hypometric saccades, limitation of gaze, myoclonus, and impaired distal vibration and joint position sense are sometimes seen.

Dysphagia may become significant in the later part of the illness. Respiratory stridor may also occur. This is caused by atrophy of the posterior cricoarytenoid muscles resulting in failure of abduction of the vocal cords and narrowing of the airway.[31] In the fully developed disease, patients are permanently bed bound, almost mute and severely dysphagic and incontinent, with normal awareness. The cause of death in MSA is commonly related to development of bulbar dysfunction and dysphagia, predisposing to aspiration pneumonia.

Frank dementia is not a feature of MSA, though frontal lobe dysfunction with attention deficits are reported in one-third of cases. Emotional incontinence, depression, anxiety, panic attacks, and suicidal ideation are also common in patients with MSA. Depression can be seen as a premotor symptom of MSA in around 16% of cases. Its prevalence increases up to 60% as the disease progresses.[32]

INVESTIGATIONS

The diagnosis of MSA is primarily clinical. Neuroimaging aids in the diagnosis, and more recently, surges in development of functional neuroimaging have enhanced our diagnostic capabilities for the same.

NEUROIMAGING

Computed Tomography Head

Computed tomography (CT) has got a low sensitivity and specificity, although it may show atrophy of the brainstem, cerebellum, and rarely cerebral cortex in around 50% patients.

Magnetic Resonance Imaging Brain

Brain magnetic resonance imaging (MRI) often discloses abnormalities of the putamen or infratentorial structures. Typical signs include putaminal rim or claustrum sign, cruciform hyperintensity of pons (hot cross bun sign) and brainstem, and infratentorial atrophy.

Putaminal Rim Sign

Also known as *putaminal slit sign,* it is a relatively specific sign of MSA-P. The sign consists of putaminal atrophy that causes a hypointense signal on T2-weighted (T2W) images surrounded by a rim of hyperintensity. Hypointensity is postulated to be caused by neuronal loss, reactive astrocytosis and microgliosis. Hyperintense rim occurs due to extracellular fluid accumulation in the putaminal capsule secondary to atrophy of the nucleus. The pathophysiological process is also reflected on diffusion-weighted MRI images as in MSA-P patients, regional apparent diffusion coefficients are increased as compared to those in PD patients, although this finding cannot be used to distinguish MSA-P from progressive supranuclear palsy (PSP).[32]

Hot Cross Bun Sign

The hot cross bun sign is seen on transverse T2W image and is seen in patients with MSA-C. It is seen as a cruciform hyperintensity in the pons. The name is derived from a sweet spiced bun baked by the Christian church on the last Thursday before Easter and marked with a cross on the top with the four quarters representing the four quarters of the year. The sign is due to a selective loss of myelinated transverse pontocerebellar fibers and neurons in the pontine raphe with preservation of the pontine tegmentum and corticospinal tracts.[33] Cerebellum and MCP are also atrophied with increased signal intensity.

Other Signs

Infratentorial atrophy and signal change can be seen in the pons, MCP, and cerebellum on T2W images in MSA.

Middle cerebellar peduncle width is also useful to differentiate MSA from PD. Normal MCP width is 9.80 mm ± 0.66 mm. In PD, the average width of MCP is seen to be 9.32 mm ± 0.77 mm, while in MSA the width shrinks to 6.10 mm ± 1.18 mm.[34]

There is also evidence of substantial cortical volume loss in MSA-P, mainly comprising the cortical targets of striatal projections such as the primary sensorimotor, lateral premotor, and prefrontal cortices. Voxel-based morphometric analysis is a helpful tool for the comparison of cortical and subcortical atrophy patterns in MSA. However, the practical implications of routine use of this tool is doubtful.[32,35]

EMERGING DIAGNOSTIC RADIOLOGICAL TOOLS IN MULTIPLE SYSTEM ATROPHY

Transcranial Sonography

Transcranial sonography (TCS) appears to be a simple and innovative tool to differentiate PD from atypical Parkinsonian disorders. TCS demonstrates midbrain hyperechogenicity in the area of the SN in 80–90% of patients with PD as compared to only 10% of healthy adults and patients with atypical Parkinsonism due to MSA and PSP. Conversely, unilateral or bilateral hyperechogenicity of the lentiform nucleus can be detected in at least 70% of patients with atypical Parkinsonism due to MSA or PSP and in around one-quarter of patients with PD. "Combining a hyperechogenic lentiform nuclei (LN) with a nonmarked echogenic SN appears specific for atypical Parkinsonian patients with MSA and PSP though sensitivity is suboptimal."[35]

Functional Neuroimaging

Fluorodeoxyglucose-positron Emission Tomography Scan

This resting regional metabolic scan demonstrates decreased striatal glucose metabolism in MSA as compared to normal or raised striatal metabolism in PD.[35] There is also evidence of decreased metabolism in brainstem, cerebellum, and frontal cortices in MSA patients. Patients with MSA-C have predominant cerebellar hypometabolism, while the hypometabolism is predominantly seen in the striatum in MSA-P. The basic pathophysiology explains the different patterns of altered metabolism seen. PD is basically a nigrostriatal degeneration and, hence, a presynaptic disorder. Hence, the striatal metabolism gets increased in PD reflecting a compensatory mechanism for denervation of striatal neurons. In contrast, MSA is a striatonigral degeneration and has widespread involvement, hence, the striatal metabolism gets reduced.

Presynaptic Dopaminergic Imaging

Presynaptic dopaminergic imaging modalities are ^{18}F-fluoro-dihydroxyphenylalanine (^{18}F dopa)-PET, (^{123}I) β-carboxymethyoxy-3-β-(4-iodophenyl) tropane (^{123}I-β-CIT)- single-photon emission computed tomography (SPECT), and dopamine transporter (DAT).

^{18}F-fluoro-dihydroxyphenylalanine-PET reflects the synthetic ability of presynaptic dopaminergic neurons to produce dopamine through aromatic amino-acid decarboxylase. PD demonstrates a reduced ^{18}F dopa uptake in posterior putamen. This reduction has a well-respected anteroposterior gradient and the reduction is fairly marked in posterior putamen as compared to the caudate nucleus. In patients with clinically probable MSA-P, the function of the presynaptic dopaminergic systems is severely impaired and the uptake is reduced both in caudate nucleus as well as the putamen. A study demonstrated usefulness of this caudate-putamen index (CPI) in differentiating MSA from PD.[36] The CPI can be a useful diagnostic clue to differentiate MSA from PD as CPI (difference in the uptakes in the caudate and putamen divided by the caudate uptake) was found to be around 5.6 ± 4.6 in MSA patients while in PD, this value was 14.8 ± 5.4, reflecting relatively greater caudate involvement in MSA.

Other presynaptic imaging modalities such as ^{123}I-β-CIT SPECT and DAT demonstrate reduced striatal binding, reflecting a decreased dopaminergic synthetic ability in both the disorders,[31] but PD, by its nature, tends to show more asymmetry in ^{123}I-β-CIT uptake (however, this finding did not reach statistical difference in the study).[37]

Postsynaptic Imaging Modalities

Postsynaptic imaging involves estimation of integrity of dopaminergic D2 receptors in the striatum. This involves imaging using ^{11}C-raclopride PET and ^{123}I-IBZM SPECT. MSA shows a reduced striatal uptake, reflecting loss of postsynaptic neurons in the striatum, while in PD, the uptake is normal or raised in the striatum contralateral to the affected side of body due to presence of compensatory upregulation of postsynaptic D2 receptors in striatum. However, it is important to remember that chronic pharmacological treatment may reduce D2 receptor availability, probably due to downregulation of receptors.[35]

Imaging Cardiac Sympathetic Innervation

Most PD patients, even those without overt autonomic symptoms, show a reduced cardiac sympathetic innervation using metaiodobenzylguanidine (MIBG) scintigraphy, while this is usually normal in MSA patients. This finding indicates myocardial postganglionic sympathetic dysfunction in PD.[35]

Other Ancillary Testing

Autonomic function testing and evaluation of bladder function is obligatory in all patients with suspected MSA.

Video-urodynamic testing in MSA shows evidence of detrusor hyperreflexia, frequently combined with bladder neck incompetence, reflecting sphincter dysfunction in early stages. Later on, loss of detrusor hyperreflexia and bladder atonia ensues with incomplete bladder emptying.[32]

A pathological *sphincter EMG* showing spontaneous activity, prolonged action potential duration, as well as polyphasia is seen in many patients with probable MSA, even if there are no symptoms of urogenital failure.[32] Although there may be confounding factors for the presence of a neurogenic sphincter EMG such as chronic constipation or previous pelvic surgeries, this finding reliably differentiates MSA from PD in first 5 years of the disease. Hence, a neurogenic sphincter EMG discriminates well between the early stages of IPD and MSA-P as well as idiopathic late-onset cerebellar ataxia and MSA-C.[38,39]

Impaired stimulation of growth hormone by clonidine or arginine in MSA has been reported to discriminate both MSA-P from IPD as well as MSA-C from idiopathic late-onset cerebellar ataxia. The absence of an increase in plasma growth hormone indicates α2-adrenoreceptor loss in the hypothalamus in MSA.[36]

TREATMENT

Currently, there is no effective neuroprotective therapy in MSA. Symptomatic treatment is restricted largely to Parkinsonism and dysautonomia. Other features such as cerebellar ataxia appear to be unresponsive to drug treatment.

Treatment of Parkinsonism in Multiple System Atrophy

Practical management is largely based on empirical evidence or single randomized studies. L-DOPA is widely regarded as the antiparkinsonian therapy of choice in MSA. Despite the fact that MSA patients are commonly believed to be non- or poorly responsive to dopaminergic therapy, efficacy often lasting for up to a few years has been documented in up to 40% of cases. However, benefit is transient, leaving 90% of the MSA-P patients, L-DOPA unresponsive in the long-term. *L-DOPA responsiveness should be tested by administering escalating doses over a 3-month period up to a least 1,000 mg/day (if necessary and if tolerated).* L-DOPA-induced dyskinesias affecting orofacial and neck muscles occur in 50% of MSA-P patients, sometimes in the absence of motor benefit.[22] No controlled trials for dopaminergic agonists are available and they are often poorly tolerated by MSA patients.

Anticholinergic agents usually do not improve motor symptoms in MSA, but they may be helpful when sialorrhea is severe and disturbing.

Amantadine has been studied for motor benefit in some studies with variable results.[40,41]

Paroxetine (30 mg t.i.d.) has been shown to improve motor symptoms in a randomized double-blind placebo-controlled trial with 19 MSA patients.[42]

The studies for efficacy for neuroprotection by agents like recombinant human growth hormone (r-HGH), minocycline, and riluzole have been either inconclusive, negative, or statistically insignificant.[43-45]

At present, there is no role for deep brain stimulation procedures in the routine management of MSA patients.

Treatment of Dystonia in Multiple System Atrophy

Local injections of botulinum toxin are effective in orofacial as well as limb dystonia associated with MSA. However, severe dysphagia with the necessity of nasogastric feeding has been reported after treatment of disproportionate antecollis with botulinum toxin, and this type of treatment is not recommended currently.

Treatment for Autonomic Dysfunction in Multiple System Atrophy

Treatment for autonomic dysfunction is mainly for symptomatic management of OH, urinary dysfunction, and impotence.

Therapy for Autonomic Dysfunction

Nonpharmacological options to treat OH include sufficient fluid intake, high-salt diet, more frequent but smaller meals per day to reduce postprandial hypotension, and compression stockings.

Ingestion of approximately 0.5 L of water in <5 minutes substantially raises blood pressure in patients with autonomic failure. During the night, head-up tilt not only reduces hypertensive cerebral perfusion pressure but also increases intravascular volume up to 1 L within a week.[46]

Pharmacological therapies for OH include fludrocortisone, ephedrine, pyridostigmine, midodrine (may exacerbate urinary retention), l-threo-DOPS (a noradrenaline precursor l-threo-dihydroxyphenylserine), octreotide (somatostatin analog-may also benefit postprandial hypotension and does not adversely affect nocturnal blood pressure (BP) control, but has to be given subcutaneously), and erythropoietin.[47]

Urinary Dysfunction

Anticholinergic drugs like oxybutynin can improve symptoms of detrusor hyperreflexia or sphincter-detrusor dyssynergy. Other agents include trospium chloride, a peripherally acting quaternary anticholinergic and desmopressin (which improves nocturia). Surgical therapies for neurogenic bladder problems should be avoided in MSA, because postoperatively, a worsening bladder control is expected. With postmicturition volumes >150 mL, clean intermittent catheterization 3–4 times per day may be necessary to prevent secondary consequences.

Male Impotence

Sildenafil citrate has been shown to be effective in a randomized double-blind placebo controlled trial in patients with PD and MSA. Because it may unmask or exacerbate OH, measurement of lying and standing blood pressure before prescribing sildenafil to men with Parkinsonism is recommended.[47] Other therapeutic strategies include intracavernosal papaverine, prostaglandin E1 analog, and penile implants.

NATURAL HISTORY OF MULTIPLE SYSTEM ATROPHY

The mean survival from the onset of symptoms is 6 to 10 years with few patients surviving >15 years. Overall, the median survival period is 9.5 years. As elaborated in a study, the most common cause of death was disease-related with sudden death and infections being the most common.[48] Sudden death is notably a common cause of mortality in MSA, reported in one-third of patients. This may happen in early stages of disease while patients are still ambulatory.[43] Hence, careful screening for laryngeal stridor, neurogenic bladder dysfunction, and dysphagia remains imperative in the proper and comprehensive management of MSA patients.

Prognosis

Even in the best of hands, MSA has a poor prognosis with a mean survival of 7–9 years. Common causes of death in MSA include UTI, aspiration pneumonia, cardiopulmonary arrest, the wasting syndrome, and sudden death during sleep.

CONCLUSION

Multiple system atrophy is a mixed parkinsonian, Cerebellar and autonomic dysfunction in various combinations. It took several decade to become a distinct entity. Its diagnostic criteria and pathological basis gradually evolved over the years. Various investigations has developed to support clinical suspicision. Now it has become a separate clinico-pathological entity with a survival ranging from 6 to 10 years. No specific treatment to offer to MSA patients, only symptoms based supporting treatment is available.

Although there have been major advances in our understanding of the cellular pathology and different trials has been done for neuroprotective drugs, no curative treatment is still available.

REFERENCES

1. Daroff RB, Jankovic J, Maziotta J, Pomeroy S (Eds). Bradley's Neurology in clinical practice, 7th edition. London: Elsevier; 2016.
2. Ropper AH, Samuels MA, Klein JP. Adams and Victors Principles of neurology, 10th edition. Palatino: Cenveo publisher; 2014.
3. Dejerine J, Thomas AA. L'atrophie olivo-ponto-cerebelleuse. Nouv Iconog de la Salpetriere. 1900;13:330-70.
4. Shy GM, Drager GA. A neurological syndrome associated with orthostatic hypotension: a clinical-pathologic study. Arch Neurol. 1960;2:511-27.
5. Ben-Shlomo Y, Wenning GK, Tison F, Quinn NP. Survival of patients with pathologically proven multiple system atrophy: a meta-analysis. Neurology. 1997;48(2):384-93.
6. Wenning GK, Ben Shlomo Y, Magalhaes M, Daniel SE, Quinn NP. Clinical features and natural history of multiple system atrophy: an analysis of 100 cases. Brain. 1994;117(4):835-45.
7. Klockgether T, Ludtke R, Kramer B, Abele M, Bürk K, Schöls L, et al. The natural history of degenerative ataxia: a retrospective study in 466 patients. Brain. 1998;121(4):589-600.
8. Quinn N. Multiple system atrophy: the nature of the beast. J Neurol Neurosurg Psychiatry. 1989:78-89.
9. Quinn N. Multiple system atrophy, in movement disorders 3. In: Marsden CD, Fahn S (Eds.). London: Butterworth-Heinemann; 1994:262-81.
10. Litvan I, Booth V, Wenning GK, Bartko JJ, Goetz CG, McKee A, et al. Retrospective application of a set of clinical diagnostic criteria for the diagnosis of multiple system atrophy. J Neural Transm. 1998;105(2–3):217-27.
11. Gilman S, Low PA, Quinn N, Albanese A, Ben-Shlomo Y, Fowler CJ, et al. Consensus statement on the diagnosis of multiple system atrophy. J Auton Nerv Syst. 1998;74:189-92.
12. Nee LE, Gomez MR, Dambrosia J, Bale S, Eldridge R, Polinsky RJ. Environmental-occupational risk factors and familial associations in multiple system atrophy: a preliminary investigation. Clin Auton Res. 1991;1(1):9-13.
13. Sturm E, Stefanova N. Multiple system atrophy: genetic or epigenetic? Exp Neurobiol. 2014;23(4):277-91.
14. Scholz SW, Houlden H, Schulte C, Sharma M, Li A, Berg D, et al. SNCA variants are associated with increased risk for multiple system atrophy. Ann Neurol. 2009;65(5):610-4.
15. Hara K, Momose Y, Tokiguchi S, Shimohata M, Terajima K, Onodera O, et al. Multiplex families with multiple system atrophy. Arch Neurol. 2007;64(4):545-51.
16. Fanciulli A, Wenning GK. Multiple-system atrophy. N Engl J Med. 2015;372(3):249-63.
17. Brown RC, Lockwood AH, Sonawane BR. Neurodegenerative diseases: an overview of environmental risk factors. Environ Health Perspect. 2005;113(9):1250-6.
18. Zhou L, Jiang Y, Zhu C, Ma L, Huang Q, Chen X. Oxidative Stress and Environmental Exposures are Associated with Multiple System Atrophy in Chinese Patients. Can J Neurol Sci. 2016;43(5):703-9.
19. Hanna PA, Jankovic J, Kirkpatrick JB. Multiple system atrophy: the putative causative role of environmental toxins. Arch Neurol. 1999;56(1):90-4.
20. Rehman HU. Multiple system atrophy. Postgrad Med J. 2001;77(908):379-82.
21. Stefanova N, Bücke P, Duerr S, Wenning GK. Multiple system atrophy: an update. Lancet Neurol. 2009;8(12):1172-8.
22. Oppenheimer DR. Neuropathology of progressive autonomic failure. In: Bannister R (Ed). Autonomic failure—A textbook of clinical disorders of the autonomic nervous system. 2nd edition. Oxford: Oxford University Press; 1988:267-83.
23. Kennedy PG, Duchen LW. A quantitative study of intermediolateral column cells in motor neuron disease and the Shy-Drager syndrome. J Neurol Neurosurg Psychiatry. 1985;48(11):1103-6.
24. Benarroch EE, Smithson IL, Low PA, Parisi JE. Depletion of catecholaminergic neurons of the rostral ventrolateral medulla in multiple systems atrophy with autonomic failure. Ann Neurol. 1998;43(2):156-63.
25. Papp MI, Kahn JE, Lantos PL. Glial cytoplasmic inclusions in the CNS of patients with multiple system atrophy (striatonigral degeneration, olivopontocerebellar atrophy and Shy-Drager syndrome). J Neurol Sci. 1989;94(1–3):79-100.
26. Tu PH, Galvin JE, Baba M, Giasson B, Tomita T, Leight S, et al. Glial cytoplasmic inclusions in white matter oligodendrocytes of multiple system atrophy brains contain insoluble alpha-synuclein. Ann Neurol. 1998;44(3):415-22.
27. Jecmenica-Lukic M, Poewe W, Tolosa E, Wenning GK. Premotor signs and symptoms of multiple system atrophy. Lancet Neurol. 2012;11(4):361-8.
28. Papatsoris AG, Papapetropoulos S, Singer C, Deliveliotis C. Urinary and erectile dysfunction in multiple system atrophy (MSA). 2008;27(1):22-7.
29. Stanzani-Maserati M, Gallassi R, Calandra-Buonaura G, Alessandria M, Oppi F, Poda R, et al. Cognitive and Sleep Features of Multiple System Atrophy: Review and Prospective Study. Eur Neurol. 2014;72(5–6):349-59.
30. Kluin KJ, Gilman S, Lohman M, Junck L. Characteristics of the dysarthria of multiple system atrophy. Arch Neurol. 1996;53(6):545-8.
31. Bannister R, Gibson W, Michaels L, Oppenheimer DR. Laryngeal abductor paralysis in multiple system atrophy. A report on three necropsied cases, with observations on the laryngeal muscles and the nuclei ambigui. Brain. 1981;104(2):351-68.

32. Palma JA, Norcliffe-Kaufmann L, Kaufmann H. Diagnosis of multiple system atrophy. Auton Neurosci. 2018;211:15-25.
33. Gulati A, Virmani V, Singh P, Khandelwal N. The hot cross bun sign. Neurol India. 2009;57(1):104-5.
34. Nicoletti G, Fera F, Condino F, Auteri W, Gallo O, Pugliese P, et al. MR imaging of middle cerebellar peduncle width: differentiation of multiple system atrophy from Parkinson disease. Radiology. 2006;239(3):825-30.
35. Brooks DJ, Seppi K. Proposed neuroimaging criteria for the diagnosis of multiple system atrophy. Mov Disord. 2009;24(7): 949-64.
36. Otsuka M, Kuwabara Y, Ichiya Y, Hosokawa S, Sasaki M, Yoshida T, et al. Differentiating between multiple system atrophy and Parkinson's disease by positron emission tomography with 18F-dopa and 18F-FDG. Ann Nucl Med. 1997;11(3):251-7.
37. Pirker W, Asenbaum S, Bencsits G, Prayer D, Gerschlager W, Deecke L, et al. [123I]beta-CIT SPECT in multiple system atrophy, progressive supranuclear palsy, and corticobasal degeneration. Mov Disord. 2000;15(6):1158-67.
38. Vodusek DB. Sphincter EMG and differential diagnosis of multiple system atrophy. Mov Disord. 2001;16(4):600-7.
39. Pellecchia MT, Salvatore E, Pivonello R, Faggiano A, Barone P, De Michele G, et al. Stimulation of growth hormone release in multiple system atrophy, Parkinson's disease and idiopathic cerebellar ataxia. Neurol Sci. 2001;22(1):79-80.
40. Wenning GK, Working Group on Atypical Parkinsonism of the Austrian Parkinson's Society. Placebo-controlled trial of amantadine in multiple-system atrophy. Clin Neuropharmacol. 2005;28(5):225-7.
41. Rajrut AH, Uitti RJ, Fenton ME, George D. Amantadine effectiveness in multiple system atrophy and progressive supranuclear palsy. Parkinsonism Relat Disord. 1997;3(4): 211-4.
42. Friess E, Kuempfel T, Modell S, Winkelmann J, Holsboer F, Ising M, et al. Paroxetine treatment improves motor symptoms in patients with multiple system atrophy. Parkinsonism Relat Disord. 2006;12(7):432-7.
43. Holmberg B, Johansson JO, Poewe W, Wenning G, Quinn NP, Mathias C, et al. Safety and tolerability of growth hormone therapy in multiple system atrophy: A double-blind, placebo-controlled study. Mov Disord. 2007;22(8):1138-44.
44. Dodel R, Spottke A, Gerhard A, Reuss A, Reinecker S, Schimke N, et al. Minocycline 1-year therapy in multiple-system-atrophy: effect on clinical symptoms and [(11)C] (R)-PK11195 PET (MEMSA-trial). Mov Disord. 2010;25(1):97-107.
45. Seppi K, Peralta C, Diem-Zangerl A, Puschban Z, Mueller J, Poewe W, et al. Placebo-controlled trial of riluzole in multiple system atrophy. Eur J Neurol. 2006;13(10):1146-8.
46. Wenning GK, Stefanova N. Recent developments in multiple system atrophy. J Neurol. 2009;256(11):1791-808.
47. Flabeau O, Meissner WG, Tison F. Multiple system atrophy: current and future approaches to management. Ther Adv Neurol Disord. 2010;3(4):249-63.
48. Papapetropoulos S, Tuchman A, Laufer D, Papatsoris AG, Papapetropoulos N, Mash DC. Causes of death in multiple system atrophy. J Neurol Neurosurg Psychiatry. 2007;78(3): 327-9.

CHAPTER 29

Corticobasal Syndrome

Anil Venkatichalam, Yatin Sagvekar

INTRODUCTION

Corticobasal syndrome (CBS) is a neurodegenerative disorder that is characterized by akinetic rigid Parkinsonism, dystonia, myoclonus, cognitive decline with cortical involvement, and alien limb phenomena. It is considered to be an atypical Parkinsonian syndrome and was first described in 1967.[1] It was initially called as "corticodentatonigral degeneration with neuronal achromasia". The terminology was later modified to corticobasal degeneration (CBD),[2] based on neuropathological features. There has been a further evolution in the terminology from CBD to CBS, since there are multiple phenotypes and pathological features associated with the disorder. The heterogenous presentation of this disorder from a clinical, radiological, neuropsychological, and pathological point of view poses a major challenge for evaluation.

EPIDEMIOLOGY

Corticobasal syndrome is a challenging disorder to diagnose, as it can present with multiple phenotypes. It accounts for <5% of Parkinsonism cases that are seen in movement disorders clinics. Annual incidence is 0.62–0.92 per 100,000 population. Estimated prevalence is 4.9–7.3 per 100,000 population.[3] The exact incidence and prevalence are however unknown. The disease is prevalent worldwide and there is no racial predilection. CBS is commonly found among individuals in the sixth to eight decades of life (mean age around 65 years). Women may be more affected than men,[4] although this association is not clearly established.

CLINICAL FEATURES

The classical clinical description of CBD is an asymmetric movement disorder which is progressive with akinesia, rigidity, dystonia, focal myoclonus, ideomotor apraxia, and alien limb phenomena, generally affecting one limb.[5] Presently it is well recognized that CBD can have variable phenotypic presentations, as a result of which the term CBS is currently used. Three domains are generally affected, namely—cognitive, motor, and extrapyramidal. With disease progression, Parkinsonian features may be seen. Other domains such as oculomotor, speech, and cortical function may also be affected with disease progression.

Motor and Extrapyramidal Features

Symptoms generally start unilaterally. Initial presentation may be a dystonic presentation of hand or foot. The limb may be useless due to the development of apraxia. There is progression of symptoms, but asymmetry persists. Gait may be like Parkinson's disease (PD), mainly shuffling, short steps, and slow. Occasionally, a wide-based freezing type of gait can be present. CBS can also present as primary progressive gait freezing.[6] Early falls may be associated with the disease. Tremor is rare, but may be present. When compared to PD, tremor in CBS may be rapid and irregular. Stimulus-sensitive focal myoclonus may be present.[7] Alien limb phenomena is another important feature seen in up to 50% of cases.[8] Affected individuals complain that the limb does not feel like a part of their body and is associated with movements without voluntary control. These include movements such as simple lifting of the limb or complex motor movements such as holding and grabbing objects. Presence of alien limb phenomena should increase the suspicion of CBS.

Cognitive Impairment and Cortical Dysfunction

Cognitive impairment is characteristic of CBS. Features include dementia, behavioral changes, apraxia, and cortical sensation loss. Affected individuals can present with depression, apathy, irritability and, rarely, obsessive-compulsive features may be seen.[9] Attention and praxis are impaired. Verbal memory is less commonly affected. Visuospatial dysfunction and dysexecutive syndrome are rarely seen in CBS. Cortical dysfunction can manifest in the form of apraxia. Apraxia is inability to perform a skilled movement or a task despite having the desire and physical ability to carry it out. Commonly seen apraxias in CBS include ideomotor and ideational apraxia. Cortical sensory loss, astereognosis, and agraphaesthesia are also seen in CBS.

Speech

It is commonly affected in most patients with CBS. Dysarthria is present. Speech dysfunction may be similar to that seen in PD. Rarely pseudobulbar type of speech may be seen. CBS may also be associated with language problems such as primary progressive aphasia which is associated with nonfluent/agrammatic type of speech.[10]

Ocular Signs

Ocular signs include slow pursuit and broken saccadic eye movements. Vertical eye movements are generally normal.[11] Rarely ocular signs similar to progressive supranuclear palsy (PSP) may be seen in CBS.

PATHOLOGY

The hallmark of CBS is the presence of astrocytic plaques.[8] They represent tau accumulation in astrocytes. Astrocytic plaques are found in cortex, caudate, and putamen. They are less commonly seen in thalamus and midbrain. The other characteristic feature of CBS is ballooned neurons. Swollen cortical neurons are found in cortical layers third, fifth, and sixth. Most common locations are cingulate gyrus, amygdala, claustrum, and insular cortex.[12] However, predicting pathology in CBS can be difficult and sensitivity of clinical findings in predicting CBS pathology ranges from 26 to 56% (clinical-pathology mismatch).[13]

ROLE OF TAU

Tau is a neuronal protein that is involved in axonal transport and neuronal stabilization. Normal tau contains six isoforms that are generated by alternative messenger ribonucleic acid (RNA) splicing. This leads to formation of tau isoforms with three repeats (3R) or four repeats (4R) of tau microtubule binding domain. Normal ratio of 3R and 4R tau is equal. When this ratio is affected, it leads to neuronal degeneration. There is abnormal phosphorylation of tau which leads to impairment of axonal transport and abnormal microtubule function.[14] In CBD, there is aggregation of 4R tau isoforms.[15] Similar aggregation of 4R tau isoforms is also found in PSP.

GENETICS

Corticobasal syndrome is mainly a sporadic disease. However, CBS like presentation has been seen in patients with progranulin (PRGN) gene mutation.[16,17] Other genetic mutations associated with CBS like presentation include *MAPT* and pathogenic *C9orf72* repeat expansion.[18] There is also one case report of CBS like presentation in an individual with early onset autosomal dominant Alzheimer's disease.[19]

NEUROIMAGING

In the early stages, neuroimaging is normal.[20] With disease progression, asymmetric cortical atrophy involving the frontal and parietal regions is seen on magnetic resonance imaging (MRI).[21] Other MRI findings in CBS include corpus callosum atrophy and T2 hypointensity involving the putamen and globus pallidus.[22] Voxel based MRI morphometry shows focal atrophy involving the frontal lobe.[23]

Striatal dopamine transporter imaging (DaT scan) is abnormal in CBS. Changes are similar to PD with reduction in tracer uptake in the striatum and asymmetric uptake over the hemisphere. However, in PD reduction in uptake is more in the putamen.[24] Single-photon emission computerized tomography (SPECT) scan shows reduction in uptake in bilateral frontal and temporoparietal regions.[25] Positron emission tomography (PET) imaging shows asymmetric hypometabolism over frontoparietal region with hypometabolism over thalamus and striatum over the affected hemisphere.[26] PET imaging may be useful in differentiating CBS from other Parkinsonian disorders.[27]

DIAGNOSIS

Corticobasal syndrome is a clinical diagnosis. Diagnosis of CBS is difficult due to variable phenotypic presentations of the disease. Affected individuals may present with predominant extrapyramidal features or predominant cognitive features. It is important to differentiate CBS from other Parkinsonian disorders and dementias. **Table 1** shows the different phenotypes of CBS with clinical features.

TABLE 1: Various phenotypes of CBS with associated clinical features.

Phenotype	*Clinical presentation*
Corticobasal syndrome	Probable CBS: • Asymmetry with • Limb rigidity/akinesia, dystonia or myoclonus (at least 2 features) • Orobuccal/Limb apraxia, Cortical sensory loss, Alien limb phenomena (at least 2 features) Possible CBS: • Symmetry with • Limb rigidity/akinesia, dystonia or myoclonus (at least 1 feature) • Orobuccal/Limb apraxia, cortical sensory loss, Alien limb phenomena (at least 1 feature)
Frontal behavioural spatial syndrome	• Executive dysfunction • Behavioral changes • Visuospatial deficits (At least 2 features should be present)
Nonfluent or agrammatic variant of primary progressive aphasia	• Effortful agrammatic speech with (at least one of) • Impaired sentence comprehension • Apraxia of speech (distorted speech)
Progressive supranuclear palsy syndrome	• Axial rigidity/ akinesia • Postural instability • Behavioral changes • Urinary incontinence • Supranuclear vertical gaze palsy (At least three of the above must be present)

Phenotypes of Corticobasal Degeneration

In 2013, an expert consensus identified the various phenotypic presentations associated with pathological features suggestive of CBD. The four phenotypes of CBD identified were:

1. CBS (probable and possible)
2. Frontal behavioral spatial syndrome
3. Nonfluent or agrammatic variant of primary progressive aphasia
4. PSP syndrome

Corticobasal syndrome is commonly misdiagnosed as PD due to asymmetric presentation. However, a poor response to L-DOPA may be helpful in differentiating CBS from PD.[28] Application of clinical diagnostic criteria may be helpful for diagnosis of CBS. Neuropsychological testing and neuroimaging may be helpful for diagnosis and help to differentiate CBS from other similar disorders. There are various available clinical and research criteria that are available for diagnosis of CBS. From a clinical perspective, two criteria are commonly used. The Cambridge criteria were earlier used widely for diagnosis. This has been currently replaced by the CBS clinical criteria (**Table 2**) by Armstrong et al.[29] There are significant differences between the two criteria. In earlier stages of disease, Cambridge criteria (**Table 3**)[30] have a better applicability due to an emphasis on cognitive and language dysfunction. In the later stages, both criteria are equal for diagnosing CBS.

MANAGEMENT OF CORTICOBASAL SYNDROME

There is no treatment for CBS. Treatment is mainly targeted at symptom management and palliative care. CBS is characterized by a poor response to levodopa.[31] Other agents such as dopamine agonists and monoamine oxidase type B (MAO-B) inhibitors (selegiline and rasagiline) are ineffective for symptom management. Tremor is another issue for individuals with CBS. Topiramate, propranolol, clonazepam, or primidone may be used to control tremor. Myoclonus in CBS may respond to clonazepam. Dystonia

TABLE 2: Clinical syndromes of corticobasal degeneration as proposed by Armstrong et al.[29]

Clinical syndromes	*Onset and progression*	*Cortical dysfunction*	*Extrapyramidal dysfunction*
Probable corticobasal syndrome	• Asymmetric presentation • Insidious onset and gradual progression	At least two of: • Orobuccal/limb apraxia • Cortical sensory deficit • Alien limb phenomena (more than simple levitation)	At least two of: • Limb rigidity or akinesia • Limb dystonia • Limb myoclonus
Possible corticobasal syndrome	• Maybe symmetric onset • Insidious onset and gradual progression	At least one of: • Orobuccal/limb apraxia • Cortical sensory deficit • Alien limb phenomena (more than simple levitation)	At least one of: • Limb rigidity or akinesia • Limb dystonia • Limb myoclonus

TABLE 3: Modified Bak and Hodges criteria (Cambridge criteria).[30]

Mandatory criteria	• Insidious onset and gradual progression • No sustained response to levodopa treatment
Major criteria	• Motor features ○ Akinetic rigid syndrome • Cortical motor sensory features ○ Limb apraxia • Cognitive features ○ Speech and language impairment
Minor criteria	• Motor features ○ Focal or segmental myoclonus ○ Asymmetrical dystonia • Cortical motor sensory features ○ Alien limb phenomenon ○ Cortical sensory loss or dyscalculia • Cognitive features ○ Frontal executive dysfunction ○ Visuospatial deficits

and rigidity in CBS can be managed with baclofen or anticholinergics. Dystonic spasms and limb pain may be seen in some individuals with CBS. Dystonic spasms are difficult to treat and response to medication including botulinum toxin injections is poor.[32] Analgesics can be used for pain management. Gabapentin may be helpful for persistent limb pain.

Depression is commonly seen and should be appropriately managed with antidepressants. Selective serotonin reuptake inhibitors (SSRI) are generally used. Psychiatry consultation should be taken for symptom management and monitoring progression of depressive symptoms. Zopiclone or melatonin can be used for sleep problems. Bladder problems and urinary incontinence can be treated by drugs that can help relax the bladder or promote bladder emptying such as oxybutynin and mirabegron.

Rivastigmine or donepezil can be used for memory issues. However, the benefit of these medications is minimal in CBS. Affected individuals are sensitive to neuroleptic medication and it is better to avoid typical antipsychotics. It is advisable to start medication at lower doses and gradually increase the dose as tolerated. It is important to manage osteoporosis as individuals with CBS are at risk of falls and fractures.

Nonpharmacological techniques for management of symptoms include cognitive stimulation, physiotherapy, occupational therapy, speech and swallowing therapy, nutritional and dietary management, and palliative care. As the disease progresses, it is important to plan palliative care and advanced care management in order to enable relief of distressing symptoms associated with the disease and ensure adequate care. Care is generally provided by a team of healthcare professionals who work together. A multidisciplinary approach is useful to outline a treatment plan and enhance patient care.

CONCLUSIONS AND PROGNOSIS

Corticobasal syndrome is a progressive neurodegenerative disease. The progression to eventual mortality can vary among individual patients. Usually complications such as lower respiratory tract infections, urinary tract infections, sepsis, and complications of immobility lead to fatality. The survival ranges from 2 to 12.5 years[33] from onset, with median survival between 5.5 and 7.9 years.

REFERENCES

1. Rebeiz JJ, Kolodny EH, Richardson EP Jr. Corticodentatonigral degeneration with neuronal achromasia: a progressive disorder of late adult life. Trans Am Neurol Assoc. 1967;92:23-6.
2. Gibb WR, Luthert PJ, Marsden CD. Corticobasal degeneration. Brain. 1989;112 (Pt 5):1171-92.
3. Togasaki DM, Tanner CM. Epidemiologic aspects. Adv Neurol. 2000;82:53-9.
4. Stover NP, Wainer BH, Watts RL. Corticobasal degeneration. In: Watts RL, Koller WC (Eds). Movement Disorders: Neurologic Principles & Practice, 2nd Edition. New York: McGraw-Hill; 2004. p.763.
5. Watts R, Mirra SS, Richardson EP. Corticobasal ganglionic degeneration. In: Marsden CD, Fahn S (Eds). Movement Disorders. United Kingdom: Butterworth-Heinemann, Oxford; 1994. p. 282.
6. Factor SA, Higgins DS, Qian J. Primary progressive freezing gait: a syndrome with many causes. Neurology. 2006;66(3):411-4.
7. Carella F, Ciano C, Panzica F, Scaioli V. Myoclonus in corticobasal degeneration. Mov Disord. 1997;12(4):598-603.
8. Parmera JB, Rodriguez RD, Studart Neto A, Nitrini R, Brucki SMD. Corticobasal syndrome: A diagnostic conundrum. Dement Neuropsychol. 2016;10(4):267-75.
9. Geda YE, Boeve BF, Negash S, Graff-Radford NR, Knopman DS, Parisi JE, et al. Neuropsychiatric features in 36 pathologically confirmed cases of corticobasal degeneration. J Neuropsychiatry Clin Neurosci. 2007;19(1):77-80.
10. Josephs KA, Duffy JR. Apraxia of speech and nonfluent aphasia: a new clinical marker for corticobasal degeneration and progressive supranuclear palsy. Curr Opin Neurol. 2008;21(6):688-92.

11. Vidailhet M, Rivaud-Péchoux S. Eye movement disorders in corticobasal degeneration. Adv Neurol. 2000;82:161-7.
12. Murray R, Neumann M, Forman MS, Farmer J, Massimo L, Rice A, et al. Cognitive and motor assessment in autopsy-proven corticobasal degeneration. Neurology. 2007;68(16):1274-83.
13. Hughes AJ, Daniel SE, Ben-Shlomo Y, Lees AJ. The accuracy of diagnosis of parkinsonian syndromes in a specialist movement disorder service. Brain. 2002;125(4):861-70.
14. Wakabayashi K, Oyanagi K, Makifuchi T, Ikuta F, Homma A, Homma Y, et al. Corticobasal degeneration: etiopathological significance of the cytoskeletal alterations. Acta Neuropathol. 1994;87(6):545-53.
15. Spillantini MG, Goedert M. Tau pathology and neurodegeneration. Lancet Neurol. 2013;12(6):609-22.
16. Baizabal-Carvallo JF, Jankovic J. Parkinsonism, movement disorders and genetics in frontotemporal dementia. Nat Rev Neurol. 2016;12(3):175-85.
17. Kouri N, Carlomagno Y, Baker M, Liesinger AM, Caselli RJ, Wszolek ZK, et al. Novel mutation in MAPT exon 13 (p.N410H) causes corticobasal degeneration. Acta Neuropathol. 2014;127(2):271-82.
18. Schottlaender LV, Polke JM, Ling H, MacDoanld ND, Tucci A, Nanji T, et al. The analysis of C9orf72 repeat expansion in a large series of clinically and pathologically diagnosed cases with atypical parkinsonisms. Neurobiol Aging. 2015;36(4):1768.
19. Navarro E, Andrés De C, Guerrero C, Giménez-Roldán S. Corticobasal Syndrome in a Family with Early-onset Alzheimer's Disease Linked to a Presenilin-1 Gene Mutation. Mov Disord Clin Pract. 2015;2(4):388-94.
20. Mahapatra RK, Edwards MJ, Schott JM, Bhatia KP. Corticobasal degeneration. Lancet Neurol. 2004;3(12):736-43.
21. Hauser RA, Murtaugh FR, Akhter K, Gold M, Olanow CW. Magnetic resonance imaging of corticobasal degeneration. J Neuroimaging. 1996;6(4):222-6.
22. Savoiardo M, Grisoli M, Girotti F. Magnetic resonance imaging in CBD, related atypical parkinsonian disorders, and dementias. Adv Neurol. 2000;82:197-208.
23. Lee SE, Rabinovici GD, Mayo MC, Wilson SM, Seeley WW, DeArmond SJ, et al. Clinicopathological correlations in corticobasal degeneration. Ann Neurol. 2011;70(2):327-40.
24. Cilia R, Rossi C, Frosini D, Volterrani D, Siri C, Pagni C, et al. Dopamine Transporter SPECT Imaging in Corticobasal Syndrome. PLoS One. 2011;6(5):e18301.
25. Kreisler A, Defebvre L, Lecouffe P, Duhamel A, Charpentier P, Steinling M, et al. Corticobasal degeneration and Parkinson's disease assessed by HmPaO SPECT: the utility of factorial discriminant analysis. Mov Disord. 2005;20(11):1431-8.
26. Pardini M, Huey ED, Spina S, Kreisl WC, Morbelli S, Wassermann EM, et al. FDG-PET patterns associated with underlying pathology in corticobasal syndrome. Neurology. 2019;92(10):e1121-35.
27. Eckert T, Barnes A, Dhawan V, Frucht S, Gordon MF, Feigin AS, et al. FDG PET in the differential diagnosis of parkinsonian disorders. Neuroimage. 2005;26(3):912-21.
28. Ahlskog JE. Diagnosis and differential diagnosis of Parkinson's disease and parkinsonism. Parkinsonism Relat Disord. 2000;7(1):63-70.
29. Armstrong MJ, Litvan I, Lang AE, Bak TH, Bhatia KP, Borroni B, et al. Criteria for the diagnosis of corticobasal degeneration. Neurology. 2013;80(5):496-503.
30. Mathew R, Bak TH, Hodges JR. Screening for cognitive dysfunction in corticobasal syndrome: utility of Addenbrooke's cognitive examination. Dement Geriatr Cogn Disord. 2011;31(4):254-8.
31. Constantinescu R, Richard I, Kurlan R. Levodopa responsiveness in disorders with parkinsonism: a review of the literature. Mov Disord. 2007;22(15):2141-8.
32. Marsili L, Suppa A, Berardelli A, Colosimo C. Therapeutic interventions in parkinsonism: Corticobasal degeneration. Parkinsonism Relat Disord. 2016;22(Suppl 1):S96-100.
33. Wenning GK, Litvan I, Jankovic J, Granata R, Mangone CA, McKee A, et al. Natural history and survival of 14 patients with corticobasal degeneration confirmed at postmortem examination. J Neurol Neurosurg Psychiatry. 1998;64(2): 184-9.

CHAPTER 30

Secondary Parkinsonism

Vikram Shivkumar, Dipali Nemade, Poorna J Visa, AV Srinivasan

INTRODUCTION

Parkinsonian features were identified as early as 300 BC in ancient India and China. In AD 175, western medical literature from the popular physician Galen first described the condition with Parkinsonism symptoms under the name "shaking palsy". James Parkinson in 1817 gave a detailed explanation of this condition and Parkinson's disease (PD) was named after him. Idiopathic Parkinson's disease (IPD) constitutes 80% of patients with Parkinsonism. Classical Parkinsonian symptoms can be diagnosed with certainty, but to differentiate IPD from secondary PD may be difficult. This distinction is important as their management and prognosis vary. This review gives a brief explanation of seven types of secondary Parkinsonism.

POSTENCEPHALITIC PARKINSONISM

Encephalitis lethargica (EL), also called Von Economo's disease, has classical features of extrapyramidal symptoms (EPS) including involuntary movements, corticospinal tract signs, sleep disturbance, behavioral disorder, oculogyric crises, and respiratory disturbance.[1,2] EL patients, months or years later, are prone to develop Parkinsonian features called postencephalitic Parkinsonism (PEP).[1-3]

Etiology of Encephalitis Lethargica

The cause of EL could be due to infection or autoimmunity, but not related to influenza.[1,2,4] Since EL epidemic occurred during the same period as influenza pandemic, there was thought to be an association with both, but this was proved wrong when, on examination, EL brain specimens failed to show influenza ribonucleic acid (RNA). This was further substantiated when studies that showed positive cerebrospinal fluid (CSF) intrathecal oligoclonal bands showed CSF-polymerase chain reaction (PCR) indicative of viral encephalitis to be negative.[4-6] It was hypothesized that following group A streptococcus infection, antibodies were induced which cross reacted with components of the basal ganglia, resulting in a psychiatric and movement disorder.[4-6] Therefore, patients with EL-like syndrome following pharyngitis, whose most common cause was group A *Streptococcus*, were examined to look for autoreactive antibodies to the basal ganglia. All these patients exhibited two or more cardinal symptoms of Parkinsonism. In 95% of these patients, antibodies reactive against basal ganglia, autoantigens were found. This report suggested that the EL phenotype can occur secondary to postinfectious autoimmunity with more susceptibility to the deep gray matter neurons.[4-7]

A case was reported with fever and catatonia. Valproic acid induced Parkinsonism was suspected, but on withholding valproic acid, there was no improvement. The patient was diagnosed as PEP[2] with good response to antiparkinsonian medication.[8]

For other infection-related causes of Parkinsonism readers are requested to refer to the chapter on Infections and Movement Disorders in the same book (Chapter 43).

VASCULAR PARKINSONISM

Etiology

The term "vascular pseudoparkinsonism" was coined by Critchley in 1981, to differentiate VP from IPD, since vascular disease is not the cause for IPD.[9] Sibon et al. in 2004 described vascular Parkinsonism (VP) to include lesions such as ischemia, excitotoxic damage, postanoxic Parkinsonism, and rarely hemorrhages and arteriovenous malformations.[9] Korczyn et al. in 2015, described VP as Parkinsonism induced by stroke, nigral lesion, lacunar infarct, and basal ganglia infarct.[10] Rektor et al.[11] in 2018, classified VP into three subtypes: (1) Acute/subacute poststroke VP caused due to ischemic or hemorrhagic lesions in substantia nigra of brain, (2) Insidious onset VP, and (3) Mixed IPD[11] which included neurodegenerative Parkinsonism and cerebrovascular disease (CVD), where vascular causes contributed to Parkinsonism. Patients with increased cerebral small vessel disease such as cerebral microbleeds, lacunar infarctions, and white matter hyperintensities as seen on magnetic resonance imaging (MRI), and whose risk factors included high blood pressure, atherosclerosis, coronary artery disease, smoking, hyperhomocysteinemia, diabetes mellitus, sleep apnea, and dyslipidemia, developed Parkinsonism.[11,12]

Clinical Features

Vascular Parkinsonism has diverse clinical signs.[11] It has more lower body involvement such as gait impairment, postural instability, and loss of balance than upper limb involvement with minimal rest tremor and bradykinesia.[10,13,14] Gait is wide-based which gradually worsens with time and is accompanied by urinary difficulties, cognitive decline, and dementia.[11,13,14]

Investigative Findings

There is a discrepancy in the diagnostic criteria.[11] Small lacunes and nonconfluent white matter lesions indicating VP may not be seen on the CT scan; hence, MRI is the gold standard neuroimaging study used to diagnose VP.[11] The diagnostic findings of lower body Parkinsonism are accompanied by MRI features such as periventricular white matter lesions, presence of lacunes, and dilatation of lateral and third ventricles.[10] Studies have shown gait impairment to be associated with white matter lesions in the brain. Deep white matter hyperintensities on MRI are seen in the insidious onset subtype of VP[11] and white matter hyperintensities with lacunar infarcts are seen in mixed neurodegenerative Parkinsonism and CVD subtype of VP.[11] These two subtypes have a clinical predominant gait impairment. On the other hand, white matter lesions and lacunes are also observed in elderly with no Parkinsonism,[11] and in IPD patients with no gait impairment.[9] Therefore, these MRI findings are not sufficient for the diagnosis of VP.[10]

Single photon emission computed tomography (SPECT) imaging is used to quantify dopamine transporter (DAT) activity by its uptake of radioligand which is of different types. SPECT images using radioligand ^{123}I-FP-CIT [(^{123}I) N-ω-fluoropropyl-2β-carbomethoxy-3β-(4-iodophenyl) nortropane] showing presynaptic striatal DAT activity show a decreased uptake of dopamine markers in IPD[12] while the same extent of reduction in uptake is not seen in patients with lower body Parkinsonism. Rektor I et al. mention that the uptake of radioligand like FP-CIT visualized by SPECT (DAT scan) is abnormal in acute poststroke and mixed subtype VP, whereas, it is preserved in insidious onset VP.[11] Therefore, SPECT, MRI findings, and clinical features must be combined to diagnose VP.[10]

DRUG-INDUCED PARKINSONISM

Drug-induced Parkinsonism (DIP) is the second most common cause for Parkinsonism, the first cause being IPD. The incidence of DIP increases with age and is observed more commonly in females. With increasing age, the dopamine concentration decreases and nigral cells degenerate with time.[15-17] Neuroimaging studies show that progression of IPD is slow in younger patients than elderly, because the young IPD patients are able to maintain a more effective pre- and postsynaptic compensatory mechanism and thereby sustain a normal dopamine neurotransmission.[18] Further, the risk of developing DIP also depends on the type of offending drug, duration of exposure, rate of increasing dose, target dose, patient's vulnerability, and multiple drug treatments.[18] Clinically, DIP is identified by the presence of symmetric symptoms, no tremors and presence of bucco-linguo-masticatory dyskinesia and akathisia.[19] However, rarely, there is the presence of an asymmetric rest tremor similar to seen in IPD.[19]

Drug-induced Parkinsonism is mostly caused by a large group of antipsychotic drugs especially used to treat schizophrenia and depression. It is observed that antipsychotic drugs can induce Parkinsonism. Likewise, antiparkinsonian drugs can induce psychiatric symptoms. Psychosis seen in schizophrenia is due to increased dopaminergic activity, therefore dopamine agonists increase psychotic symptoms and antidopaminergics reduce psychotic symptoms.[15]

Treatment of Schizophrenia with Antipsychotics Induces Parkinsonism

Typical antipsychotics at therapeutically effective dosages by D2 receptor blockade produce increased prolactin levels, EPS, and in the long run cause tardive dyskinesia.[20] Atypical or second-generation antipsychotics have a lower risk of developing EPS when compared to typical or first-generation antipsychotics. Atypical antipsychotics according to "fast off D2 theory" rapidly dissociate from D2 receptors as they have low affinity for the D2 receptor. Receptor occupancy of the atypical drug wears off in 48 hours, whereas typical antipsychotics have a higher affinity and may remain attached to the D2 receptor even for 1 or 2 days after drug administration. This phenomenon in atypical antipsychotics makes the D2 receptor available for binding by endogenous dopamine, hence, low incidence of EPS.[15,17] There is also interaction between the serotonin and dopamine systems. Serotonin prevents release of dopamine from the striatum.[15] Atypical antipsychotics have a higher potency in blocking serotonin 2A receptor than the dopamine receptor,[19-21] thereby promoting dopamine release from dopamine neurons from the prefrontal cortex. This could also be the reason for low EPS.[17,20,21] The atypical antipsychotic clozapine prescribed for drug resistant negative symptoms of schizophrenia does not cause EPS, but it has a potentially fatal side effect of agranulocytosis.[19] The atypical antipsychotic quetiapine has a low risk of EPS and is safe in the elderly.[17] However, the more loosely an antipsychotic is bound to the D2 receptor, the more it ceases to show antipsychotic effects. Hence, the risk of relapse of psychotic symptoms in patients on clozapine and quetiapine. Therefore, the dosage of atypical antipsychotics such as clozapine and quetiapine will be high, whereas the dose requirement for typical antipsychotics which are tightly bound will be low to be therapeutically effective. The risk of DIP is less for second generation atypical antipsychotics. Small doses of typical antipsychotics produce the same level of EPS as high doses of atypical antipsychotics excepting clozapine.[15]

Treatment of Generalized Anxiety Disorder Using Selective Serotonin Reuptake Inhibitor and Induced Parkinsonism

Selective serotonin reuptake inhibitors (SSRI) is used to treat depression and generalized anxiety disorder (GAD). In a case report, a 29-year-old patient was diagnosed with GAD. This patient was treated with an SSRI. He later developed symptoms of Parkinsonism. He was diagnosed as DIP with GAD. So, his SSRI was stopped and he was started on the antiparkinsonian drug levodopa/carbidopa. His Parkinsonian symptoms slowly resolved. After 3 months, on weaning levodopa, he again started developing Parkinsonian features. So, he was diagnosed as irreversible DIP with GAD and continued on the antiparkinsonian drug and the tetracyclic antidepressant mirtazapine.[22] The reason for the SSRI-induced Parkinsonism could be that serotonin has an inhibitory influence on dopaminergic neurotransmission which, by producing striatal changes, causes Parkinsonian symptoms. SPECT imaging is required in this study to confirm whether the Parkinsonism developed in this case was purely due to DIP or an exacerbation of preclinical PD. The physician should be aware of DIP when a SSRI is used to treat patients.[22,23]

Diagnosis

The integrity of dopamine nigrostriatal pathway is studied using SPECT using various radioactive ligands. This allows the differentiation of IPD, VP, and DIP. In patients presenting with diverse symptoms of Parkinsonism, FP-CIT-SPECT [*N*-ω-fluoropropyl-2β-carbomethoxy-3β-(4-iodophenyl)nortropane-SPECT] can be used for a reliable and accurate differentiation of PD and VP/IPD. However, a normal DAT scan in the absence of MRI and clinical features cannot diagnose VP or DIP. Also, there is no neuropathological validation for DAT scan and so its accuracy is based on the clinical diagnosis.[22,23] Clinical diagnosis in some cases does not indicate the true diagnosis. Another imaging modality is positron emission tomography (PET) which provides images of higher resolution than the SPECT scan. Nevertheless, more DIP cases are diagnosed using SPECT scan than PET scan.[17]

Dopamine transporter radiotracer uptake in striatum is substantially decreased in PD patients, whereas in DIP, dopamine receptor blocking agents (i.e., drugs causing PD) have very low affinity for DAT; so DIP patients show normal radiotracer uptake in the striatum. In pure DIP there is symmetrical uptake of radiotracer while in drugs unmasking subclinical Parkinsonism, DAT uptake decreases asymmetrically in the striatum. So, DAT scan can be used to differentiate pure DIP from subclinical PD.[17] DIP is reversible with discontinuation of the causative drug, but DIP with subclinical parkinsonism, which may have atypical symptoms, persists.[17]

Drug-induced Parkinsonism can be caused by various other pharmacological agents including antiepileptic medication (valproate and phenytoin), antiemetics like metoclopramide, motility agents like levosulpiride, and calcium channel blockers like flunarizine. This has been covered in more detail in the Drug-induced Movement Disorder Chapter (Chapter 42).

OSMOTIC DEMYELINATION SYNDROME

Osmotic demyelination syndrome (ODS) can predispose to Parkinsonism. The presentation of ODS is varied depending on the regions of the brain affected. The most common manifestation of ODS is extrapontine myelinolysis (EPM) and central pontine myelinolysis (CPM). Both have the same pathology, association, and time course, but exhibit different clinical features.[24] On the MRI scan, CPM involves the pontine and EPM the extrapontine structures.[25] ODS commonly occurs as a result of rapid correction of hyponatremia and in those with metabolic syndrome.[25]

Fast Correction of Hyponatremia Causes Parkinsonism

A 50-year-old patient on antihypertensive medication developed hyponatremic encephalopathy. This was treated with 3% saline, after which he developed Parkinsonian symptoms. MRI of brain showed hypointense signals in the pons on T1 images and hyperintense signals in T2 images in the pons and basal ganglia, indicating demyelination.[24] Typically, ODS shows hypointense lesions in T1 images and hyperintense lesions in T2 images.[25] This patient was diagnosed as Parkinsonism secondary to ODS and so was treated with antiparkinsonian medications and improved remarkably. Demyelination occurs due to the changing osmotic forces compressing the fiber tracts. ODS is a rare occurrence of sodium correction. Therefore, restoration of sodium levels should be slow. The Parkinsonism which develops secondary to ODS is treatable and prognosis is good.[24]

Transsphenoidal Pituitary Tumor Resection Causes Parkinsonism

A 36-year-old female had undergone trans-sphenoidal pituitary resection for pituitary adenoma. Eight days later, she had symptoms due to hyponatremia. Her sodium levels were corrected, but she developed Parkinsonian symptoms. Her MRI showed hyperintensities on T2 images. She was diagnosed with isolated EPM and was treated with dopaminergic agonists with which her symptoms almost resolved. Two months later her MRI findings resolved and neurological deficit waned completely. Hyponatremia post-transsphenoidal surgery is mostly asymptomatic and rarely develops into myelinolysis.[25]

Central pontine myelinolysis and EPM happen together, with EPM occurring in 10% of the patients with CPM. Occurrence of isolated EPM is even more infrequent and can lead to Parkinsonism. CPM and EPM are difficult to diagnose with CT scan, hence, we depend on MRI findings, especially to identify EPM causing Parkinsonism. This report shows a unique link of transsphenoidal pituitary tumor resection and acute Parkinsonism which is treatable with dopamine agonist and immunotherapy.[25]

Pathophysiology of Osmotic Demyelination Syndrome

Demyelination is characterized by loss of oligodendrocytes and myelin. The hypothesis of a relationship between hyponatremia and CPM cannot be neglected. Here, the blood brain barrier (BBB) is compromised. Hyperosmotic stress induced by hyponatremia correction causes endothelial dehydration and opening of BBB. The lesions occur mainly in the pons because the myelinotoxic factor from blood responsible for demyelination is enriched in gray matter and the pons shows the greatest extent of gray and white matter admixture. The concept of hypernatremia/hyperosmolarity following rapid correction of hyponatremia is not very clear but has evolved over the years.[26] Following the quick correction of hyponatremia with hypertonic saline, the cells become dehydrated. In chronic hyponatremia apart from cells losing ions Na, K and Cl, they also lose organic osmolytes, which maintain normal protein structure and function. On correction with hypertonic saline, these ions reaccumulate in high concentration which is stressful to cells. They directly bind to proteins, causing them to denature and misfold. This interferes with normal protein structure and function of cell. The rapid correction of hyponatremia causes a sudden increase in ions, i.e., Na and Cl level and a fall in organic osmolyte level in cells which could have contributed to development of CPM.[26]

There is some evidence of apoptosis of oligodendrocytes in CPM.[27] Oligodendrocytes form myelin.[25] A necropsy study showed increased proapoptotic factor in comparison to antiapoptotic factor, indicative of apoptosis in oligodendrocytes in CPM. It is indeed curious to note that apoptosis recruits a specific potassium channel, i.e., the two-pore domain potassium channel which is necessary for homeostatic volume regulation, suggesting the possibility that osmotic stress through the activation of these ion channels can lead to the incidental stimulation of the apoptosis cascade.[27]

Disorders of Calcium Metabolism

Disorders of calcium metabolism such as hypoparathyroidism and pseudohypoparathyroidism can lead to Parkinsonism. Hyperparathyroidism is less likely to cause Parkinsonism, but there are a few reports.[28,29] They result in intracranial calcifications in a striato-pallido-dentate distribution.[30] Hypoparathyroidism can be sporadic or familial with X-linked, autosomal recessive, or dominant transmission.[31] It can also occur as a complication of thyroidectomy.[32] Pseudohypoparathyroidism is characterized by resistance to action of parathyroid hormone (PTH) at the end-organ with normal or high PTH, hypocalcemia, and hyperphosphatemia. Parkinsonism secondary to calcium metabolism disorders can be associated with seizures, cognitive, behavioral, and psychiatric symptoms.[33] The movement disorders can present in various forms including chorea, Parkinsonism, dystonia, tremor, and ataxia.[33] Neuropsychiatric symptoms may include mild memory issues, dementia, personality changes, or psychosis. Calcified areas can be easily identified on computed tomography (CT) or MRI scans. Patients might occasionally respond to levodopa but usually do not respond.

HYDROCEPHALUS CAUSING PARKINSONISM

In hydrocephalus, CSF accumulates in the ventricles increasing the intracranial pressure. Hydrocephalus causes the ventricles to dilate. The clinical presentation of Parkinsonism due to hydrocephalus is different from the classical symptoms of Parkinsonism. Hydrocephalus induced Parkinsonism along with typical PD symptoms may also show features of dorsal midbrain dysfunction such as lid retraction, convergence retraction nystagmus, light near dissociation, and forced downgaze. There have been many reports of hydrocephalus [normal pressure hydrocephalus (NPH)] symptoms resembling Parkinsonism symptoms like the gait impairment with short steps, leg rigidity, flexed posture, and impaired postural reflexes, resulting in delay in diagnosis of the underlying hydrocephalus.[34]

Pathophysiology

Dilatation of the lateral, third, and fourth ventricles applies pressure effects on periventricular structures that include the midbrain and diencephalon. This causes mechanical interruption with dopaminergic systems[34,35] which is the nigrostriatal pathway extending from the substantia nigra to the caudate nuclei and putamen,[35] and the frontal projection fibers from the basal ganglia. The gait impairment in NPH could be due to the compression of periventricular leg fibers from the frontal motor areas. Dysfunction of ascending tract cortico-striato-pallido-thalamo cortical motor loop and or nigrostriatal fibers could be because of a direct or indirect mass effect with ischemia caused due to hydrocephalus. Animal studies have shown that torsion, central herniation, direct compression of the midbrain, or its striatal efferents are caused due to enlarging third and fourth ventricles. These studies exhibit a decrease in dopamine in midbrain and striatum.[34] Ventricular dilatation could have also compressed the thalamocortical fibers which are somatotopically arranged with leg fibers medially placed, this could explain the gait and lower limb dysfunction observed in hydrocephalus. The Parkinsonism features could have been because of the disconnection between basal ganglia and supplementary motor cortex. There is the possibility that chronic hydrocephalus can lead to neurodegenerative process.[34]

While so far, we have explained how hydrocephalus can contribute to Parkinsonism, the reverse may also be true wherein Parkinsonism can predispose to hydrocephalus, several theories were put forth to substantiate this hypothesis.

Human and animal studies show neuropathological changes caused due to hydrocephalus throughout the cerebrum. The severity of the damage depends on the rate of ventricular enlargement, extent of ventriculomegaly, nearness of a structure to the ventricle, and the stage of development when the disturbance occurs.[36] Obstruction of CSF caused in hydrocephalus leads to increase in intracranial pressure and decrease in cerebral blood flow.[36] Dilatation of ventricles compresses the microvasculature. Combination of ischemic and mechanical effects causes axonal and secondary myelin damage. Ventriculomegaly causes cortical dysgenesis. Compression in the extracellular space of cortex occurs which disrupts the removal of waste products. Extracellular fluid conducts nutrients, cell, and waste product. The periventricular extracellular space of the cortex contains the waste products and depends on the capillaries to take up the extracellular fluid.[36]

Shunting in Treatment for Hydrocephalus

There are many treatments available for hydrocephalus which includes shunt. Shunt causes excess CSF from ventricle to drain into a different drainage site in the body like the peritoneum or right atrium. Commonly used types of shunt are ventriculoperitoneal shunt, ventriculoatrial shunt, and lumboperitoneal shunt. After the surgical procedure of placing a shunt the patient is continuously monitored for symptoms of complications as a late response can lead to serious consequences. The early clinical improvement seen following this procedure is due to the increase in cerebral blood flow and restoration of the extracellular fluid clearance. It is intriguing to think of remyelination of periventricular axons to occur and so the gradual improvement of symptoms, if shunting, is done soon after the development of hydrocephalus, although many authors propose a repair of neuronal and axonal damage to be unlikely.[36] Rather axonal and neuronal damage maybe the cause for permanent functional deficit. It is unclear whether myelin damage occurs primarily or secondary to axonal injury.[35,36] However, CSF shunting procedure has the risk of complications so not preferred by neurosurgeons unless absolutely required.[35,37]

TOXINS INDUCING PARKINSONISM

MPTP Causing Parkinsonism

1-Methyl-4-phenyl-4-propionpiperidine (MPPP) is an analog of the narcotic meperidine. MPTP (1-methyl-4-phenyl-1,2,3,6-tetrahydropyridine) can be inadvertently produced during the manufacture of synthetic opioid MPPP.[38] Methyl-4 phenylpyridinium (MPP+) is a toxic metabolite of MPTP. MPP+ is a neurotoxin that destroys the dopaminergic neurons in the substantia nigra. MPTP affected the nigrostriatal dopamine pathway in regions of brain similar to PD.[39] Cognitive deficits were demonstrated in MPTP patients. These cognitive alterations seen in MPTP intoxicated patients were similar to those observed in PD patients.[39]

MPTP is a Parkinsonian neurotoxin, but whether this neurotoxin produces a progressive neurodegeneration is not certain.[39] However, studies have shown a long-lasting deleterious effect exerted by MPTP.[39] MPTP exposure-induced Parkinsonism in some patients developed soon after exposure while in other patients developed only months or years later indicating a progressive neuro-degenerative process.[40]

MPTP is very lipophilic and after intravenous administration crosses the BBB. Then protoxin MPTP is converted to 1-methyl-4-phenyl-2,3-dihydropyridium (MPDP) by monoamine oxidase-B (MAO-B) which then spontaneously oxidizes to MPP+. MPP+ is taken up by the dopaminergic neurons by its high affinity to DAT and so MPP+ selectively occupies dopaminergic neurons. Within dopaminergic neurons, MPP+ is incorporated into synaptic vesicles containing dopamine. MPP+ also accumulates in mitochondria.[38] MPP+ inhibits enzymes located in the mitochondrial electron transport chain, which leads to ATP deficit, and elevated leakage of superoxide from respiratory chain. Superoxide stays in the cell in which it is produced as it cannot readily traverse cell membrane. Nitric oxide (NO) is permeable to cell membrane and NO is produced by nondopaminergic neurons present in the vicinity of dopaminergic neurons. So, NO can diffuse into neighboring dopaminergic neurons. So, if the neighboring dopaminergic neuron contains superoxide, superoxide combines with NO to form peroxynitrate which destroys the proteins, lipids, and DNA of cell and so kills the dopaminergic neurons.[38,39] The vulnerability of dopaminergic neurons to MPTP is inversely proportional to the number of astrocytes. Astrocytes protects neurons from reactive oxygen species-mediated toxicity.[38,41]

Manganese-induced Parkinsonism

Manganese (Mn) toxicity can occur from excessive inhalation of Mn, particulates in mining and welding industries.[42] It can also occur in patients with liver failure and those on total parenteral nutrition.[43,44] Mn can accumulate in the basal ganglia, specifically the globus pallidus, subthalamic nucleus, substantia nigra, and striatum and causes progressive neuronal degeneration. It can also affect the cerebellum, red nucleus, cortex, pons, and anterior horn cell of the spinal cord. It results in motor deficits and neuropsychiatric symptoms. Parkinsonism is the most common motor manifestation with bradykinesia, cogwheel rigidity, postural tremor, and postural instability. Neuropsychiatric symptoms include dementia, compulsive behaviors, hallucinations and delusions, and can even occur prior to onset of motor symptoms.[45] In contrast to PD, Mn-induced Parkinsonism is not characterized by presence of Lewy bodies. Resting tremor is less likely to occur in Mn-induced Parkinsonism. MRI brain shows characteristic bilateral hyperintensities in the globus pallidus on T1-weighted scans but is usually normal in PD. DAT scan shows diminished striatal uptake in PD but is normal in Mn-induced Parkinsonism. Mn-related Parkinsonism is less likely to respond to levodopa and these patients usually do not develop levodopa induced dyskinesias unlike patients with PD.[46]

PARKINSONISM IN GUAM

Many studies substantiated the hypothesis that amyotrophic lateral sclerosis (ALS) and Parkinsonism dementia complex (PDC) constitute a single disease entity (i.e., ALS-PDC) in the Chamorro population in Guam. In support of this hypothesis, Hirano A et al. observed that in all ALS affected patients of the Chamorro population, in addition to the typical pathological changes of ALS, neurofibrillary changes were also present.[47] In all these patients, substantia nigra was also affected. This study also showed that in 50% of PD patients in this population had spinal cord changes which were similar to those found in ALS disease.[48,49] Oskarsson et al. stated that "ALS-PDC in Guam and the western pacific is a distinct clinicopathological entity whose cause may be different from ALS."[48,49] ALS and PDC are progressive diseases and can lead to fatality, these two diseases frequently occur together and in individuals within the same families. Chamorros were the original inhabitants of Guam which is an island situated in western Pacific Ocean. Incidence of ALS and PDC was considerable in Chamorro population. In 1960, the Chamorro population constituted 50% of the total population in Guam, but by 2,000 Chamorro population constituted only 37% of the total population in Guam due to many immigrants moving and settling in Guam, marrying into the chamorro population.[50] This hybridization led to the original chamorro gene pool changing into a neo-chamorro gene pool. The incidence of ALS and PDC has decreased substantially from 1960 to 2000. Studies are conducted to find whether this reduced incidence of ALS-PDC over the period of 40 years is due to genetic factors or environmental influences. Even if there had been sufficient genetic intermixture between the Chamorro population and the immigrants, to produce a gene frequency change, and hence, a decrease in the incidence of the disease, it would require a longer generational time to take effect. Also, a genetic vulnerability to a disease would also depend on environmental influences to produce such a drastic fall in disease incidence. During this period of time from the 1960 to 2000 the island underwent modernization, so there is a possibility that modernization could have reduced the previously present environmental risk factor and hence, reduce the incidence of the disease.[49] Chris et al. states that epigenetic risk factors decreased the incidence of the disease.[49] Epigenetics is how DNA interacts with multiple small molecules present inside cells called epigenome. Epigenome can activate or deactivate genes depending upon their presence and concentration within cells. Epigenome is influenced by diet, chemical exposure, and medication. Studies have shown environmental and genetic risk factors for ALS-PDC. A study showed that hexanucleotide repeat sequence of an intron C9orf72 was not the major gene contributing to ALS-PDC in Guam.[51]

CONCLUSION

The different types of secondary Parkinsonism besides the classical symptoms of Parkinsonism also have distinguishing symptoms specific to the type of disease. However, the symptoms are not demarcated to a certain type. Neuroimaging technology along with the standard MRI study has improvised with SPECT scans which is majorly used to diagnose and differentiate types of PD. Despite these advances and the numerous studies done to characterize the different types of secondary Parkinsonism, there is still overlap in investigative findings and histopathological examination between the types and other-related conditions. It is difficult to correlate clinical symptoms with neuroimages. So, further studies are needed to be able to diagnose the type of Parkinsonism more specifically for its early identification and disease type specific treatment.

REFERENCES

1. Rail D, Scholtz C, Swash M. Post-encephalitic Parkinsonism: current experience. J Neurol Neurosurg Psychiatry. 1981;44(8): 670-6.
2. Bigman DY, Bobrin BD. Von Economo's disease and postencephalitic parkinsonism responsive to carbidopa and levodopa. Neuropsychiatr Dis Treat. 2018;14:927-31.
3. Duvoisin RC Yahr MD. Encephalitis and Parkinsonism. Arch Neurol. 1965;12:227-39.
4. Vilensky JA, Gilman S, McCall S. Does the historical literature on encephalitis lethargica support a simple (direct) relationship with postencephalitic Parkinsonism? Mov Disord. 2010;25(9):1124-30.
5. Dale RC, Church AJ, Surtees RA, Lees AJ, Adcock JE, Harding B, et al. Encephalitis lethargica syndrome: 20 new cases and evidence of basal ganglia autoimmunity. Brain. 2004;127(1): 21-33.
6. Somnier F. Autoimmune encephalitis: History & Current knowledge. Copenhagen: Statens Serum Institut; 2016.
7. Kim R, Shin CW, Kim HJ, Jeon BS. Postencephalitic parkinsonism responsive to a dopamine agonist: A case report. Parkinsonism Relat Disord. 2015;21(6):667-8.
8. Geddes JF, Hughes AJ, Lees AJ, Daniel SE. Pathological overlap in cases of parkinsonism associated with neurofibrillary tangles. A study of recent cases of postencephalitic parkinsonism and comparison with progressive supranuclear palsy and Guamanian parkinsonism-dementia complex. Brain. 1993;116(Pt 1):281-302.
9. Sibon I, Fenelon G, Quinn NP, Tison F. Vascular parkinsonism. J Neurol. 2004;251(5):513-24.
10. Korczyn AD. Vascular parkinsonism-characteristics, pathogenesis and treatment. Nat Rev Neurol. 2015;11(6):319-26.
11. Rektor I, Bohnen NI, Korczyn AD, Gryb V, Kumar H, Kramberger MG, et al. An updated diagnostic approach to subtype definition of vascular parkinsonism-Recommendations from an expert working group. Parkinsonism Relat Disord. 2018; 49:9-16.
12. Hatate J, Miwa K, Matsumoto M, Sasaki T, Yagita Y, Sakaguchi M, et al. Association between cerebral small vessel diseases and mild parkinsonian signs in the elderly with vascular risk factors. Parkinsonism Relat Disord. 2016;26:29-34.
13. Glass PG, Lees AJ, Bacellar A, Zijlmans J, Katzenschlager R, Silveira-Moriyama L. The clinical features of pathologically confirmed vascular parkinsonism. J Neurol Neurosurg Psychiatry. 2012;83(10):1027-9.
14. Gupta D, Kuruvilla A. Vascular parkinsonism: what makes it different? Postgrad Med J. 2011;87(1034):829-36.
15. Bohlega SA, Al-Foghom NB. Drug-induced Parkinson`s disease. A clinical review. Neurosciences (Riyadh). 2013;18(3):215-21.
16. Kuzuhara S. Drug-induced parkinsonism. Nihon Rinsho. 1997;55(1):112-7.
17. Shin HW, Chung SJ. Drug-induced parkinsonism. J Clin Neurol. 2012;8(1):15-21.
18. Lopez-Sendon JL, Mena MA, de Yebenes JG. Drug-induced parkinsonism in the elderly: incidence, management and prevention. Drugs Aging. 2012;29(2):105-18.
19. Kuroki T, Nagao N, Nakahara T. Neuropharmacology of second-generation antipsychotic drugs: a validity of the serotonin-dopamine hypothesis. Prog Brain Res. 2008;172:199-212.
20. Weiner DM, Burstein ES, Nash N, Croston GE, Currier EA, Vanover KE, et al. 5-hydroxytryptamine2A receptor inverse agonists as antipsychotics. J Pharmacol Exp Ther. 2001;299(1):268-76.
21. Seeman P. Atypical antipsychotics: mechanism of action. Can J Psychiatry. 2002;47(1):27-38.
22. Dixit S, Khan SA, Azad S. A Case of SSRI Induced Irreversible Parkinsonism. J Clin Diagn Res. 2015;9(2):VD01-2.
23. Lorberboym M, Djaldetti R, Melamed E, Sadeh M, Lampl Y. ^{123}I-FP-CIT SPECT imaging of dopamine transporters in patients with cerebrovascular disease and clinical diagnosis of vascular parkinsonism. J Nucl Med. 2004;45(10):1688-93.
24. Dar WR, Sofi NU, Latief M, Dar IA, Hussain M. Secondary parkinsonism due to osmotic demyelination syndrome: a case report. Egypt J Intern Med. 2015;27(4):157-9.
25. Ho PL, Chen YC, Teng CH, Wu CC, Huang P. Acute parkinsonism as an unexpected consequence of pituitary adenoma resection: A case report. Medicine (Baltimore). 2019;98(17):e15261.
26. Norenberg MD. Central pontine myelinolysis: historical and mechanistic considerations. Metab Brain Dis. 2010;25(1):97-106.
27. Martin RJ. Central pontine and extrapontine myelinolysis: the osmotic demyelination syndromes. J Neurol Neurosurg Psychiatry. 2004;75(Suppl 3):22-8.

28. Augusto CMG, de Morais NS, Santana RP, de Almeida MOP. Parkinsonism as an Atypical Manifestation of Primary Hyperparathyroidism. AACE Clin Case Rep. 2019;5(4):e244-6.
29. De Rosa A, Rinaldi C, Tucci T, Pappatà S, Rossi F, Morra VB, et al. Co-existence of primary hyperparathyroidism and Parkinson's disease in three patients: an incidental finding? Parkinsonism Relat Disord. 2011;17(10):771-3.
30. Bonazza S, La Morgia C, Martinelli P, Capellari S. Strio-pallido-dentate calcinosis: a diagnostic approach in adult patients. Neurol Sci. 2011;32(4):537-45.
31. Maeda SS, Fortes EM, Oliveira UM, Borba VC, Lazaretti-Castro M. Hypoparathyroidism and pseudohypoparathyroidism. Arq Bras Endocrinol Metabol. 2006;50:664-73.
32. Clarke BL, Brown EM, Collins MT, Juppner H, Lakatos P, Levine MA, et al. Epidemiology and Diagnosis of Hypoparathyroidism. J Clin Endocrinol Metab. 2016;101:2284-99.
33. Kostic VS, Petrovic IN. Brain Calcification and Movement Disorders. Curr Neurol Neurosci Rep. 2017;17:2.
34. Curran T, Lang AE. Parkinsonian syndromes associated with hydrocephalus: case reports, a review of the literature, and pathophysiological hypotheses. Mov Disord. 1994;9(5):508-20.
35. Chang MC, Chun MH. Secondary parkinsonism induced by hydrocephalus after subarachnoid and intraventricular hemorrhage. Neural Regen Res. 2016;11:1359-60.
36. Del Bigio MR. Neuropathological changes caused by hydrocephalus. Acta Neuropathol. 1993;85:573-85.
37. Yomo S, Hongo K, Kuroyanagi T, Kobayashi S. Parkinsonism and midbrain dysfunction after shunt placement for obstructive hydrocephalus. J Clin Neurosci. 2006;13(3):373-8.
38. Przedborski S, Jackson-Lewis V, Djaldetti R, Liberatore G, Vila M, Orolicki SBV, et al. The parkinsonian toxin MPTP: action and mechanism. Restor Neurol Neurosci. 2000;16(2):135-42.
39. Bove J, Prou D, Perier C, Przedborski S. Toxin-induced models of Parkinson's disease. NeuroRx. 2005;2(3):484-94.
40. Lev N, Melamed E, Offen D. Toxic causes of parkinsonism. Handb Clin Neurol. 2007;84:385-98.
41. Navarro JA, Heßner S, Yenisetti SC, Bayersdorfer F, Zhang L, Voigt A, et al. Analysis of dopaminergic neuronal dysfunction in genetic and toxin-induced models of Parkinson's disease in Drosophila. J Neurochem. 2014;131(3):369-82.
42. Gorell JM, Johnson CC, Rybicki BA, Peterson EL, Kortsha GX, Brown GG, et al. Occupational exposure to manganese, copper, lead, iron, mercury and zinc and the risk of Parkinson's disease. Neurotoxicology. 1999;20(2–3):239-47.
43. Hauser RA, Zesiewicz TA, Rosemurgy AS, Martinez C, Olanow CW. Manganese intoxication and chronic liver failure. Ann Neurol. 1994;36(6):871-5.
44. Bertinet DB, Tinivella M, Balzola FA, de Francesco A, Davini O, Rizzo L, et al. Brain manganese deposition and blood levels in patients undergoing home parenteral nutrition. JPEN J Parenter Enteral Nutr. 2000;24(4):223-7.
45. Calne DB, Chu NS, Huang CC, Lu CS, Olanow W. Manganism and idiopathic parkinsonism: similarities and differences. Neurology. 1994;44(9):1583-6.
46. Olanow CW. Manganese-induced parkinsonism and Parkinson's disease. Ann N Y Acad Sci. 2004;1012:209-23.
47. Hirano A, Malamud N, Elizan TS, Kurland LT. Amyotrophic lateral sclerosis and Parkinsonism-dementia complex on Guam. Further pathologic studies. Arch Neurol. 1966;15(1):35-51.
48. Oskarsson B, Horton DK, Mitsumoto H. Potential Environmental Factors in Amyotrophic Lateral Sclerosis. Neurol Clin. 2015;33(4):877-88.
49. Plato CC, Garruto RM, Galasko D, Craig UK, Plato M, Gamst A, et al. Amyotrophic lateral sclerosis and parkinsonism-dementia complex of Guam: changing incidence rates during the past 60 years. Am J Epidemiol. 2003;157(2):149-57.
50. Warren LA, Shi Q, Young K, Borenstein A, Martiniuk A. Prevalence and incidence of dementia among indigenous populations: a systematic review. Int Psychogeriatr. 2015;27(12):1959-70.
51. Dombroski BA, Galasko DR, Mata IF, Zabetian CP, Craig UK, Garruto RM, et al. C9orf72 hexanucleotide repeat expansion and Guam amyotrophic lateral sclerosis-Parkinsonism-dementia complex. JAMA Neurol. 2013;70(6):742-5.

SECTION

7

HYPERKINETIC MOVEMENT DISORDERS

CHAPTER 31

Tremors: Differential Diagnosis, Pathophysiology, and Management

Manish Mahajan, Sumit Singh

INTRODUCTION

Tremor, a rhythmic and oscillatory movement of one or more parts of the body, is undoubtedly the most common "movement disorder" (MD) encountered by neurologists. The diverse etiologies and manifestations of tremors and the clinical phenomenology makes its classification and differential diagnosis a problem.[1,2] A better understanding of the pathophysiology and the brain circuitry involved in the generation of tremor, using newer available radiological and investigative tools and development of numerous clinical scales for the standardized characterization of the tremor has contributed significantly to this process. The present communication intends to help the readers in better understanding of the diagnosis and management of tremors.

DEFINITION AND CLASSIFICATION

Tremor may be defined in a number of ways but for the sake of uniformity, recently updated International Parkinson and Movement Disorder Society (IPMDS) task force definition[2] shall be used herewith which states "tremor is an involuntary, rhythmic, and oscillatory movement of a body part."

There have been numerous attempts in the past to arrive at an effective classification of tremors. In 1981, David Marsden and colleagues[3] subclassified essential tremor (ET) into: Type I (exaggerated physiological tremor), type II (benign pathological ET), type III (severe pathological ET), and type IV (symptomatic ET). The MDS (now called the IPMDS) in 1998 published the first consensus criteria for the classification of tremors[1] followed by a revised classification scheme.[2]

The proposed system consists of two main axes: Clinical features (axis 1) and etiology (axis 2) (**Fig. 1**). There are two broad categories of tremor in axis 1: "Isolated tremor" and "combined tremor" depending upon whether there are any other neurological or relevant systemic signs. There is a possibility of shift from one category to the other overtime and the same tremor syndrome may have multiple etiologies. The recommendation is to mention all the categories in case of any evolution of the syndrome. The current scheme allows discovery of new and more accurate tremor syndromes, resulting from the ever-evolving research on the subject.

EPIDEMIOLOGY

The overall burden of tremor in the general community is not well defined due to heterogenous nature of the disease, lack of standardized questionnaires, and diagnostic criteria. Worldwide cases with mild severity may not even seek medical attention, making data collection even more difficult. This results in wide variability in the reported prevalence of tremors across different studies.[4-18] Louis and colleagues,[19] in 1995, reported the age-adjusted prevalence of 40.2 per 1,000 for ET. Tremor was also reported as the most common type of MD (14.5%) in the Bruneck Study[20] cohort (n = 706; age range of 50–89 years) with enhanced physiological tremor being the most common.[21,22] An urban community-based two-staged recent Brazilian study[23] (n = 1,186; female-to-male ratio of 1.4) an overall prevalence rate of 17.4% of tremor of all types was established in elderly population with ET (7.4%), followed by Parkinsonian tremor (5.6%) and enhanced physiological tremor (2.8%) as the main causes of tremors.[24]

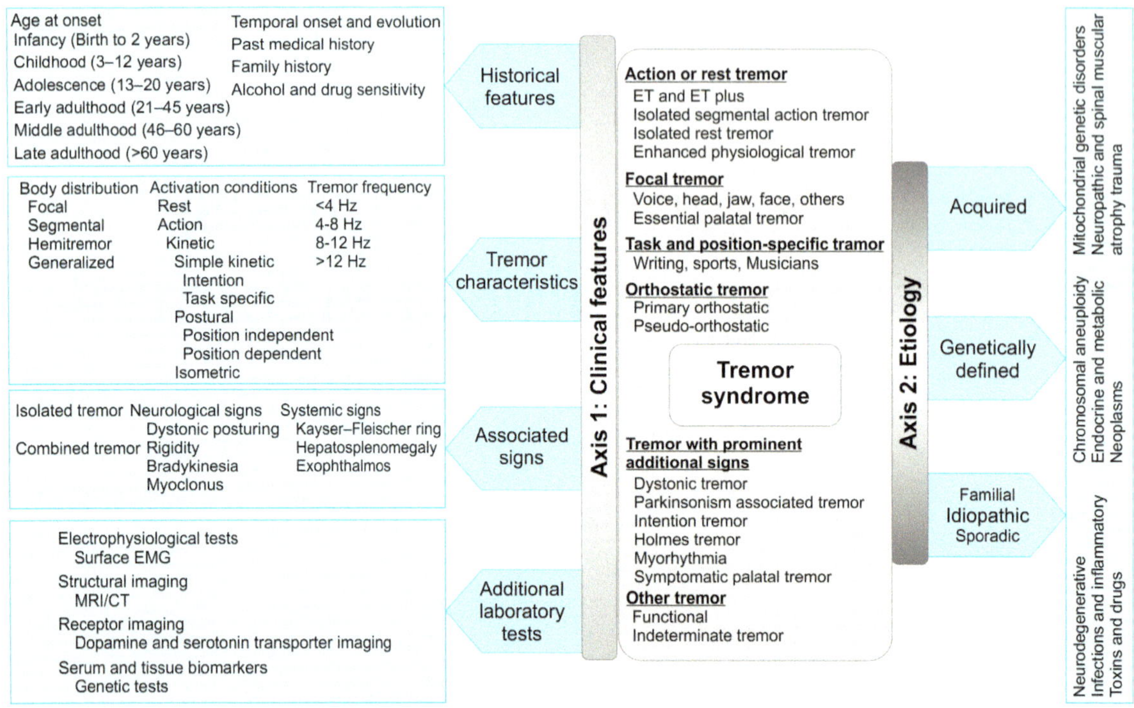

(CT: computed tomography; EMG: electromyography; ET: essential tremor; MRI: magnetic resonance imaging)

FIG. 1: Classification scheme of various tremor syndromes as per the latest International Parkinson and Movement Disorder Society (IPMDS) task force.

Earliest Indian studies from the Parsi community of Mumbai by Barucha et al.[11] in 1988 reported an exceptionally high prevalence rates of ET as 1591.7 per 100,000 with no gender difference but a significant increase with age beyond 40 years. A tertiary care teaching hospital-based study[25] (n = 106) from Delhi, stated ET as the most common tremor (59.43%) followed by dystonic tremor (DT)/task-specific tremor (21.69%), psychogenic tremor (13.20%), and alcohol-induced tremor (1.88%) with 0.94% cases of enhanced physiologic tremor, rubral tremor, thyrotoxic tremor, and drug-induced tremor each. Das and colleagues[26] had reported a prevalence of ET of 3.95 per 1,000 as compared to much lower prevalence of 0.08 per 1,000 in the rural West Bengal[27] and these observations were significantly distinct from the ones made by Gourie-Devi[28,29] from the South India.

THE ANATOMY AND PATHOPHYSIOLOGY OF TREMOR

For the development of most tremors cerebello-thalamo-cortical circuit, along with its connections with basal ganglia and brainstem nuclei, is a key pathophysiological component (**Fig. 2A**).[30] All tremors are generated both peripherally and centrally, with variable contribution from one of the four basic pathophysiological principles: Mechanical oscillations, reflex oscillations, central oscillations, or a feedback-driven oscillation.[31] The peripheral component, designated as "mechanical reflex", acts like a pendulum with a resonant frequency that is proportional to the square root of the ratio of the stiffness of the limb divided by its weight.[32,33] This is most commonly observed in the laboratory in case of enhanced physiological tremor with its characteristic lowering of frequency with addition of weight to a limb. The central component, usually referred to as the "central oscillator", has not yet been defined for any of the tremor syndromes. Both the components have a feedback-loop mechanism in place for the self-perpetuation of tremor (**Fig. 2B**).[30,32,33]

In case of Parkinson's disease (PD), the presence of many types of tremors such as rest tremors that disappears on activity, postural, re-emergent, and in some cases action or DT marks the complexity of the generation of tremor in a single patient or different individuals with the same diagnosis. The single-photon emission computed tomography (SPECT) studies have indicated that rest tremor severity correlated best with dopamine depletion in extrastriatal regions like pallidum and thalamus.[34,35] Using functional magnetic resonance imaging (fMRI), dopamine-depleted basal ganglia, and a prerequisite for the development of rest tremor (dopamine paradox of rest tremor) has been observed to be active at the onset of tremor (the switch), but the cerebellothalamic circuit shows activity corresponding with the magnitude of continuing rest tremor (dimmer).[35,36] This "dimmer-switch" model explains the improvement seen in rest tremor with either subthalamic nucleus (STN) or globus pallidus pars interna

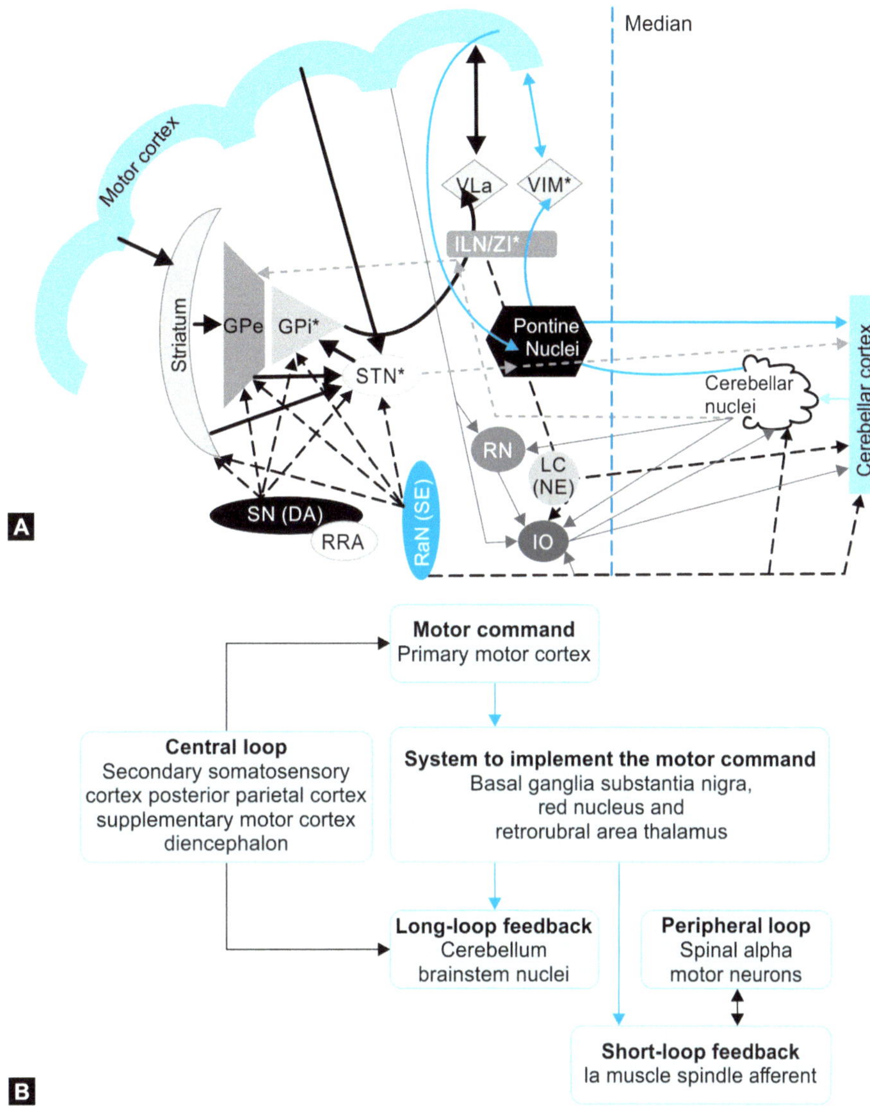

(DA: dopamine; GPe: globus pallidus pars externa; GPi: globus pallidus pars interna; ILN: interlaminar nucleus of the thalamus; IO: inferior olive; LC: locus coeruleus; NE: norepinephrine; RaN: raphe nuclei; RN: red nucleus; RRA: retrorubral area; SE: serotonin; SN: substantia nigra; STN: subthalamic nuclei; VIM: ventrointermediate nucleus of the thalamus; VLa: anterior part of the ventrolateral nucleus of the thalamus; ZI: zona incerta)

FIGS. 2A AND B: (A) The anatomy of tremor showing the basal ganglia and its connections in the bold black arrows and the cerebellar connections in the sky/light blue arrows and the light black arrows. Both the pathways are modulated by different subcortical nuclei using different neurotransmitters (black-dashed arrows) and are interconnected (gray-dashed arrows); (B) The central and the peripheral components of tremor pathogenesis and the feedback-driven oscillation model of tremors.

(GPi) or the cerebello-thalamo-cortical circuit [ventralis intermedius (VIM) nucleus of thalamus] deep brain stimulation (DBS).[30] The postural tremor of PD has been proposed to be a "resetting phenomenon" resulting from movement-induced proprioceptive input overwriting the STN oscillations in the somatosensory cortex.[37]

The pathophysiology of ET has been related to abnormal oscillatory activity within the cortico-olivo-cerebello-thalamic circuit.[30,36] Other pathological studies indicate abnormalities in cerebellar climbing fiber structure such as complex branching and reduced synaptic density along with increased Purkinje cell axonal swelling (torpedoes) in the neocerebellum, supporting the "neurodegenerative hypothesis". Another challengeable "gamma-aminobutyric acid (GABA) hypothesis" advocates the abnormal functioning of inhibitory neurotransmitter GABA, thereby disinhibiting deep cerebellar nuclei neurons ensuing overactivity in the cerebello-thalamo-cortical circuit.[30,36,38]

The pathogenesis of DT, i.e., tremor occurring in the dystonic body part, is similar to dystonia itself resulting from impaired inhibition at cortical, subcortical, and spinal level and impaired sensory motor integration. However, in case of tremor associated with dystonia (TAD), i.e., tremor involving nondystonic body part, abnormal burst firing pattern in Purkinje cells leading to functionally-distorted cerebellar output that is similar to ET has been proposed as the underlying mechanism.[39] Orthostatic tremor (OT) has been suggested to be a result of processing of the proprioceptive information in the ponto-cerebello-thalamo-cortical circuit as supported by evidence of hypermetabolism in the pontine tegmentum (relating with the tremor frequency) and hypometabolism in the mesiofrontal cortical areas especially supplementary motor area (SMA).[40] The dopaminergic deficit in the substantia nigra or the nigrostriatal fibers, observed in the [^{18}F]-fluorodopa and PET studies, is possibly contributory in the etiologically heterogenous Holmes tremor (HT).[41]

GENETICS

A positive family history in ET with an autosomal dominant inheritance pattern has been witnessed for a longtime. Linkage analyses of ET families revealed the involvement of three chromosomal regions (ETM = essential tremor monogenetic locus): ETM1 (chromosome 13q13), ETM2 (chromosome 2p24), and ETM3 (chromosome 6p23). But the findings have not been replicated across different ET families. Genome Wide Association Studies (GWAS) have found an association of ET with two single-nucleotide polymorphism (SNPs) rs 9652490 and rs 11856808, located on intron 3 of the leucine-rich repeat and immunoglobulin (Ig) domain containing 1 gene (*LINGO1*) on chromosome 15q24.3 and *SCLA1A2* gene.[42] Spinocerebellar ataxia type 12 (SCA12) is a rare form of autosomal-dominant trinucleotide repeat (expansion of CAG) ataxic disorder but is the most common type of SCA in the descendants of a single, endogamous Indian Agarwal community with tremor being the most common presentation apart from ataxia.[43]

APPROACH TO TREMORS AND DIFFERENTIAL DIAGNOSIS

As with all other neurological disorders, medical history in tremors is of paramount importance with focus on the age of onset, body areas that appear or feel tremulous, limb positions that aggravate or alleviate the tremor, presence of any other abnormal involuntary movement or neurological symptom apart from tremor, drug or dietary history (that may produce or increase the tremor), symptoms of any systemic disease especially thyroid disorder, and very importantly family history. The initial questions should be open-ended, (e.g., When do you notice the tremor?) followed by more task-specific questions, such as "Does your hand shake while you are trying to eat or write?" to ascertain the action or rest tremor (axis 1, see above). A detailed and neurological examination with focused evaluation of the area most affected is also important. The rest tremors are best observed with the body part supported but may also appear with some mental activity (such as reverse counting or mental arithmetic). The postural component is checked by asking the patient to hold his or her arms against gravity with the palms down in front and then facing one another in the midline to look for wing-beating character. In the presence of any postural component, further assessment should be made as to whether the tremor is recurrent and oscillatory, the joints that are involved, the directions in which the movement is present (e.g., for the wrist, flexion-extension, pronation-supination), whether the tremor changes its axis or plane overtime during examination, synchronicity if the tremor is bilateral, and re-emergent quality (i.e., initially absent and the time it takes to reappear). For eliciting the intentional component, performance on finger-nose-finger, heel-to-shin, and toe-to-finger testing, pouring water from one cup to the other, drawing the Archimedes spirals, or writing a sentence may be helpful. A particular note should be made for any evidence of distractibility, entrainment (when the tremor rhythm becomes synchronous with examiner's rhythm) or suggestibility which indicates a psychogenic etiology (axis 2). The frequency of the tremor, another important axis, is better studied with the help of surface electromyography (EMG) as high frequency and low amplitude component of the tremor is difficult to appreciate clinically. Lastly but importantly, head, jaw, tongue, chin, facial muscle, and voice tremors should not be missed and specifically sought.

Parkinsonian tremor is the most common cause of rest tremor. ET and enhanced physiological tremor are the most common causes of action tremor. Isolated head tremor is more likely to be dystonic rather than ET. The important differentiating features of various types of actions and rest tremor syndromes have been extensively reviewed in the literature and are summarized in **Table 1**.[44-47]

Tremor in a dystonic body part is considered to be part and parcel of the dystonia and should be labelled as DT as per the 1998 and 2017 consensus classification criteria c.f. tremor exhibited in body parts that are not dystonic, when it is currently named TAwD.[1,2] The occurrence of a *geste antagoniste* (sensory trick) found in up to 90% of patients with cervical dystonia and null-point phenomenon (decrease in tremor when body part is placed in the direction of the pull) are helpful in the differential diagnosis of head tremor.[48]

Among the various clinical scales used to quantify tremors, five tremor severity scales (the Fahn-Tolosa-Marin Tremor Rating Scale, the Bain and Findley Clinical Tremor Rating Scale, the Bain and Findley Spirography Scale, the Washington Heights-Inwood Genetic Study of Essential Tremor Rating Scale, and the Tremor Research Group Essential Tremor Rating Assessment Scale), one activities of daily living (ADL)/disability scale (the Bain and Findley Tremor ADL Scale), one quality-of-life scale (the Quality-of-Life in ET Questionnaire), and one screening instrument (the Washington Heights-Inwood Genetic Study of Essential Tremor Rating Scale, version 1) have been recently recommended by the task

TABLE 1: Differentiating features of various types of common tremor syndromes.

Characteristics	*Essential tremor*	*Enhanced physiological tremor*	*Cerebellar tremor*	*Orthostatic tremor*	*Holmes tremor*	*Parkinson disease tremor*	*Dystonic tremor*
Clinical history:							
Age of onset	Bimodal (15–20 years or between 50 and 70 years)	Not specific; Ubiquitous	Variable	Typically sixth decade	Third to fourth decade	55–75 years	Any age
Course	>3 years Slowly (young-onset) and steadily (late-onset) progressive to disability in ADLs	<3 years Fluctuating; Normalized with elimination of the cause	Variable but usually gradually progressive and disabling	Progressive worsening and disabling	Latency of 1 month to 2 years between CNS insult and onset, especially in case of stroke	Progressive	Gradually progressive
Sex distribution	Equal	No difference reported	No difference	No difference	No difference	Males > females	Females > Males
Anatomical distribution	• Upper limbs spreading to neck (most common; no-no or yes-yes type), voice, and jaw • Neck tremor more common in female	Upper limbs	Appendicular but also involves axial especially head	Legs; On standing	One upper limb (65.5%), unilateral upper and lower limb (20.7%), bilateral (13.7%); Proximal + Distal	Hands, lower limbs, jaw, tongue, or foot	• Head (may be in isolation also) or arms • Followed by the jaw, facial, or voice tremor and least the legs
Aggravating or relieving factors	• Decreased with alcohol (in 50% only, limited utility) • Neck tremor resolves on lying	Caffeine, anxiety, fatigue, hyperthyroidism, or different drugs may exacerbate	Tremor increases when approaching the target, i.e., intentional	When less severe, improves on sitting or walking	None reported	• Increased with mental activity and walking • Subsides or ceases temporarily with the voluntary activation of the muscles	• Decreases when placed in the direction of pull and vice versa • Neck tremor persist when recumbent
Family history	30–50% positive in first- or second- degree relatives	No	Yes especially in SCA	Mostly sporadic	Sporadic	Less common (1%)	Usually sporadic
Task or position specificity	No	No	No	Yes	No	No	Yes
Sensory tricks	No	No	No	No	No	No	Yes
Clinical phenomenology:							
Predominant tremor type	Kinetic	Postural	Intentional action	Postural	Three components Kinetic >Postural> Resting	Rest (May be isolated) Pill-rolling	Action > Rest; but not rhythmic or oscillatory
Other tremor types	• 50% may have intentional component in upper extremities and 10% in head • Rest tremor in 1–35%, late feature and only in arm, not legs	No intentional component	Postural, kinetic, or orthostatic	A slower, large amplitude (subharmonic) tremor may be superimposed	-	Postural and Kinetic	-

Continued

Continued

Characteristics	*Essential tremor*	*Enhanced physiological tremor*	*Cerebellar tremor*	*Orthostatic tremor*	*Holmes tremor*	*Parkinson disease tremor*	*Dystonic tremor*
Laterality and Symmetry	Bilateral but slightly asymmetrical; very rarely unilateral or marked asymmetry (5%)	Very commonly bilateral symmetrical	Usually asymmetrical	Symmetrical and synchronous	Mostly unilateral	Unilateral at onset	Asymmetrical
Postural tremor	• Yes but the amplitude is less than the kinetic tremor • Asynchronous (out-of-phase or seesaw effect) • Maximum at wrist involving flexion-extension	Amplitude much lower than ET	-	Better felt or heard with stethoscope over the legs	Present in all	• Yes with re-emergent character and kinetic component • Maximum at the metacarpophalangeal joint rather than the wrist or greater wrist rotation than flexion-extension	Dystonic posturing of the involved limb may happen during sustained posture
Re-emergent tremor	No	No	No	No	No	Yes (after few seconds; upto ~ 9 seconds)	May be present
Tremor on action	Prominent	Prominent	Intentional	No	Yes	Lessens	Prominent
Other accompanying neurological findings:							
Other soft neurological signs	• Gait ataxia (increased as compared to age-matched controls) • Memory impairment	Anxious	Scanning or dysarthric speech, nystagmus, saccadic eye abnormalities, hypotonia, dysmetria, gait ataxia	-	Hemiparesis, cranial nerve abnormalities, ataxia, hypoesthesia, dystonia	Parkinsonism Rest tremors are uncommon with MSA, CBD, and PSP	Sustained posturing Hypertrophy of dystonic muscle(s) may be seen
Head/Neck tremor	Common (late manifestation; either yes-yes or no-no type)	Never (neck tremor is always pathological)	Common	No	No	Less common	Isolated head tremor without hand involvement suggests DT
Voice tremor	More common, may be present in isolation	May be present; never isolated		No	No	Less common	Less common
Lip tremor	Rare	May be present; never isolated		No	No	Yes	Rare
Jaw tremor	Yes; More on jaw open than close	May be present; never isolated		No	No	Yes	Rare
Rigidity, hypomimia bradykinesia with decrement	No	No; even if mild ratchet like cogwheeling is present	In some SCA	Comorbid PD may be present	Rigidity in some	Yes; sequential decrement in amplitude on finger tapping Cog-wheeling present	Dystonic slowness can resemble bradykinesia

Continued

Continued

Characteristics	***Essential tremor***	***Enhanced physiological tremor***	***Cerebellar tremor***	***Orthostatic tremor***	***Holmes tremor***	***Parkinson disease tremor***	***Dystonic tremor***
Decreased arm swing	No	No		Possible	No	Yes	May be present in the dystonic limb
Handwriting	Large-angulated loops and tremulous	Tremulous	Tremulous	-	Affected	Micrographia with mild tremors	Macrographia
Abnormal posturing of head/limb	No; mild in severe and long-standing cases	No	No	No	Yes; Limb dystonia may be present	No	Yes; Head tilt
Null-point or sensory trick phenomenon	No	-	No	No	No	No	Yes
May be associated with myoclonus	Never	-		No	Reported	No	Yes
Laboratory findings:							
Tremor frequency	5–10 Hz	8–12 Hz	<5 Hz	13–18 Hz	<5 Hz	4–7 Hz	1–6 Hz, increases on active movements
Computerized tremor analysis with loading	Tremor frequency does not change with inertial loading Central neurogenic oscillation	Frequency will reduce suggesting peripherally generated mechanical reflex oscillation	Amplitude increases approaching the target	A subharmonic larger amplitude superimposed tremor may be present	-		
Functional imaging:							
Dopaminergic deficits on functional imaging	No	No	-	-	Yes	Yes	No
Response to treatment:							
Pharmacological treatment	• Propranolol, primidone (alone or combination) • Topiramate, Gabapentin, and benzodiazepines (cautiously)	• Reassurance • Beta-blockers (Propranolol in low doses) and benzodiazepines (cautiously)	Propranolol	Clonazepam, gabapentin, propranolol, primidone, carbamazepine,	Levodopa (54% responders) Botulinum toxin Quetiapine	Levodopa, anticholinergics	Botulinum toxin; levodopa response in dopa-responsive dystonia; anticholinergics, baclofen
Surgical treatment	Thalamic VIM DBS or thalamotomy or recently, focused ultrasound thalamotomy for medically refractory cases	-	Thalamic DBS in severe cases may improve the tremor but may worsen the dysmetria	Thalamic DBS	Thalamic VIM and GPi pallidotomy combination synergistically treats all three components in severe cases	Patients usually have other Parkinsonian features, requiring STN or GPi deep brain stimulation (DBS)	VIM DBS for dystonic tremor (transient benefit)

Continued

Continued

Characteristics	***Essential tremor***	***Enhanced physiological tremor***	***Cerebellar tremor***	***Orthostatic tremor***	***Holmes tremor***	***Parkinson disease tremor***	***Dystonic tremor***
Causal correlates:							
Genetics and environmental/ acquired	• Genetic risk variants have been described in *LINGO1, SLC1A2, STK32B, PPARGC1A*, and *CTNNA3* • Environmental risk factors may include higher exposure to beta-carboline alkaloids (harmane and harmine) that are present in overcooked meat	• Metabolic disturbances, such as hyperthyroidism, hypoglycemia, hyperparathyroidism, hyponatremia, hypomagnesemia, hypocalcemia, hepatic failure, and kidney failure • Exposure to drugs, including caffeine, nicotine, cocaine, theophylline, amphetamines, thyroid hormones, antidepressants (especially tricyclics, SSRIs, or SNRIs), lithium, valproic acid, amiodarone, glucocorticoids, and immunosuppressants (cyclosporine A and tacrolimus)	Lesion or dysfunction in the cerebellothalamic pathway SCA especially SCA12 in India FXTAS	-	Stroke (50%), trauma, demyelination, infective in setting of AIDS, metastatic disease, radionecrosis in pontine-midbrain region, affecting the cerebellar outflow tracts and dopaminergic nigrostriatal fibers or thalamus		-

(ADL: activities of daily living; AIDS: acquired immunodeficiency syndrome; CBD: corticobasal degeneration; DBS: deep brain stimulation; DT: dystonic tremor; FXTAS: fragile X-associated tremor/ataxia syndrome; GPi: globus pallidus pars interna; MSA: multiple system atrophy; PD: Parkinson's disease; PSP: progressive supranuclear palsy; SCA: spinocerebellar ataxia type; SSRIs: selective serotonin reuptake inhibitors; SNRIs: serotonin and norepinephrine reuptake inhibitors; STN: subthalamic nucleus; VIM: ventralis intermedius)

force from MDS on the assessment scales.[49] However, the scales vary regarding reliability, validity, or objectivity to change overtime or with therapy. Computerized or digital assessment tools studying the frequency, amplitude (more pertinent and correlating with the disability), motor unit recruitment and synchronization, and direction using accelerometer, gyroscopic data, surface EMG, or digitally acquired spiral data on a tablet, respectively with the advantages of portability, ease of acquisition, and offline analysis have been proposed for future clinical and research use.[33]

The etiological axis (axis 2) always follows axis 1 that guides the further testing, including structural and functional neuroimaging. Serum or genetic testing is based upon a syndromic diagnosis after defining the predominant tremor and is never to be used as a shot-gun approach.[44-47]

TREATMENT

Treatment of tremors is initiated when they start interfering with the ADL of the patient or when they demand it for cosmetic reasons. The management can be challenging and at times disappointing as there are only a few on-label and low-grade of evidence-based therapeutic interventions. Pharmacological and surgical treatments of various tremors are highlighted in **Table 1** and have been extensively and excellently reviewed elsewhere.[42,50-55] Use of orthotic devices or "neuroprothesis" may be considered to further improve the quality-of-life. We shall consider management options for specific tremor syndromes in the following section (see below).

ESSENTIAL TREMOR

Essential tremor is often over-diagnosed, hence, for the sake of uniformity in clinical use diagnostic criteria for ET[2] have been defined as follows:

- Isolated tremor syndrome of bilateral upper limb action tremor
- At least 3 years' duration
- With or without tremor in other locations (e.g., head, voice, or lower limbs)
- Absence of other neurological signs, such as dystonia, ataxia or Parkinsonism.

In case of the presence of any confounding factors eluded to above, it is proposed to call the syndrome as *ET plus*.[50] The 3-year duration, though more than what's needed, is probably to reduce the odds of other common differentials. Within these 3-years these tremors can otherwise be labelled as indeterminate tremor of action type unless an etiological diagnosis with the second axis is fulfilled.[2] Electrophysiological analysis, when available, by confirming the presence of central neurogenic oscillation, may help refine the diagnosis.[56] The presence of isolated tremor of voice or head, an OT with a frequency of >12 Hz, any task- or position-specific tremors and onset that is sudden with stepwise deterioration should exclude ET and ET plus.[2]

Treatments for ET can be largely categorized into three groups: Pharmacologic, other nonpharmacologic or nonsurgical treatment approaches, and surgery. Nonselective beta-blocker propranolol may be the initial pharmacological intervention. Doses up to 360 mg/day may be used but >100 mg/day are rarely tolerated; both immediate release and long-acting formulations are available and may be used; showing 55% reduction in tremor. Bronchospasm, orthostatic hypotension, bradycardia, fatigue, hypoglycemia unawareness, raised LDL, erectile dysfunction, and dysthymia are some of the known side effects. Primidone in doses up to 250–750 mg/day, gradually titrated very slowly on a weekly basis might be an equally effective alternative. Dizziness, fatigue, and malaise are common early side effects. These are the only drugs approved with level A evidence as the initial therapy to treat limb tremor in ET.[50,57] These drugs may be used alone or in combination after taking the comorbidities and side-effect profile into consideration. In ethanol-responsive ET patients, judicious use of a very small amount of alcohol (single unit) prior to select social activities, such as social dinner, may be considered.[58] However, trials of long-chain alcohol 1-octanol, its active metabolite octanoic acid, and an investigational barbiturate T2000 have not been successful in achieving their endpoints.[52] There is insufficient or no evidence of benefit for levetiracetam, amifampridine, flunarizine, trazodone, pindolol, acetazolamide, mirtazapine, nifedipine, and verapamil, so they are not currently recommended for ET.[50] Botulinum toxin type A may be considered for medically refractory ET. Unilateral or bilateral DBS of VIM nucleus of the thalamus and more recently "zona incerta" may be considered for medically refractory ET and is a safer option than unilateral surgical thalamotomy.[52,54,55,57] However, the effect of DBS has been observed to fade over around 5 years and disease progression could be responsible for this effect. Very recently, unilateral thalamic thermoablation using focused ultrasound under MRI guidance was approved by the Food and Drug Administration (FDA) for ET that is refractory to medical therapy with greater control of hand tremor and improvement in quality-of-life.[50] Behavioral therapies, relaxation techniques, and orthotics like wrist weights may be considered as adjuvant therapies.[58]

ENHANCED PHYSIOLOGICAL TREMOR

Enhanced physiological tremor is a very common bilateral upper limb action tremor that is often confused with low amplitude ET especially in the early phase of the disease. Short history (<3 years duration), electrophysiology evidence of indicating peripherally generated tremor, higher primary frequency that reduces on inertial loading, and improvement with management of the etiology help clinch the diagnosis.[2,47,51,56] Reassurance is the mainstay of the treatment, beta-blockers or benzodiazepines may be tried in lower doses cautiously.[47]

ISOLATED FOCAL TREMORS

A number of focal-isolated syndromes with voice, head, palatal, task-specific, or position-specific tremors have been described. Each one of these tremors must occur without evidence of tremor or dystonia in any other location to be labelled as "*isolated*".[2] *Voice tremor* may be part of dystonia 6 or ANO3 mutation carriers without clinical dystonia and head tremor may be seen in ET.[59,60] Subtle voice breaks may be seen due to hyperadduction or -abduction of the vocal cords resulting in the clinical picture resembling spasmodic dysphonia. *Palatal tremor* characterized by rhythmic movement of soft palate at 0.5–5 Hz is a manifestation of several syndromes. It has been further divided into two types: *Essential*, a typical-isolated tremor syndrome (with ear click, attributed to rhythmic contraction of tensor veli palatini, normal MRI of the brain, and unknown or functional etiology), and *Symptomatic*, a combined tremor syndrome (without an ear click, involving most commonly the levator veli palatini followed by other muscles innervated by brainstem nuclei, or spinal motoneurons). The latter is usually associated with olivary pseudohypertrophy and due to lesions in the Guillain–Mollaret triangle, glial fibrillary acidic protein (GFAP) or polymerase-γ mutations, or neuroferritinopathy.[61]

Intramuscular botulinum toxin type A is probably the most effective treatment for focal tremors when medications like trihexyphenidyl in a dose of up to 10 mg/day in adults and baclofen 60 mg/day or benzodiazepines have been tried.[47,51,52] Hand orthotic devices or to make the person write with the contralateral hand has also been promoted. GPi + VIM DBS may be considered in unsatisfactory response.[54,55]

PARKINSON DISEASE TREMORS

The tremor in PD is classically 4–7 Hz rest asymmetrical tremor with pill rolling character predominantly involving the hands followed by lower limbs, jaw, tongue, or foot temporarily subsiding on movement of the body part. Apart from the rest tremor, postural or kinetic tremor (or both) but with a re-emergent quality may be seen in PD. Functional brain imaging like ^{18}F-DOPA PET (^{18}F-fluoro-L-DOPA positron emission tomography) may help in the early differentiation of PD tremor from ET (**Fig. 3**).[62,63]

The rest tremor of PD require treatment when they interfere with ADLs or is a cause of social embarrassment (as with other tremor syndromes). The rest tremor in PD usually responds variably to dopaminergic therapy as compared to bradykinesia or rigidity. Anticholinergic agents such as trihexyphenidyl (2–10 mg/day) or benzhexol may be tried in these patients while warning against the neurocognitive dose-dependent side effects in elderly.[47,51] Beta-blockers may be used with modest benefit, but a Cochrane review does not support this.[64] DBS of both STN and VIM have been found to be effective, responding to increasing the frequency parameter on STN DBS programming.[47,51,54,55]

FUNCTIONAL (PSYCHOGENIC) TREMOR SYNDROME

This not so uncommon entity is characterized by inconsistent nonphysiological symptoms, sudden-onset, and a fluctuating course (± remissions) with distractibility. Usually sporadic with multiple etiologies have been reported with recommendation for a search of underlying psychiatric disorder in every case.[2] Importantly, inertial loading may produce a paradoxical increase in tremor amplitude rather than a decrease, during computerized tremor analysis. Management of this tremor is challenging with a therapeutic strategy of "retrainment" suggestion, neuropsychological interventions as and when needed.[52]

INDETERMINATE TREMOR SYNDROME

This entity is a new entry in the current classification system. It is used in case the current syndrome does not fit into a recognized category or the patient awaits evaluation for the syndrome diagnosis establishment.[2]

OTHER RARE TREMORS

Orthostatic tremor, commonly reported as unsteadiness on standing than tremor by the patients, is a high frequency tremor best elicited when the patient stands for sometime. It may be better heard using a stethoscope or recorded using surface EMG (*helicopter sign*) than visualized (**Table 1**). A subharmonic larger amplitude tremor is more disabling than the higher frequency low amplitude tremor.[65] *Primary OT* with characteristic electrophysiological characteristics may or may not be associated with dementia, PD, or SCA while a slower frequency (<13 Hz) *pseudo-OT* is usually associated with parkinsonism, SCA3, and dystonia.[2,65] Clonazepam, started at 0.5 mg in the night and gradually increased up to 2 mg 3 times/day, is the initial drug of choice followed by gabapentin, primidone, valproic acid, and carbamazepine as the second line drugs. Bilateral VIM thalamic nucleus stimulation may be tried in medication-resistant OT.[51,66]

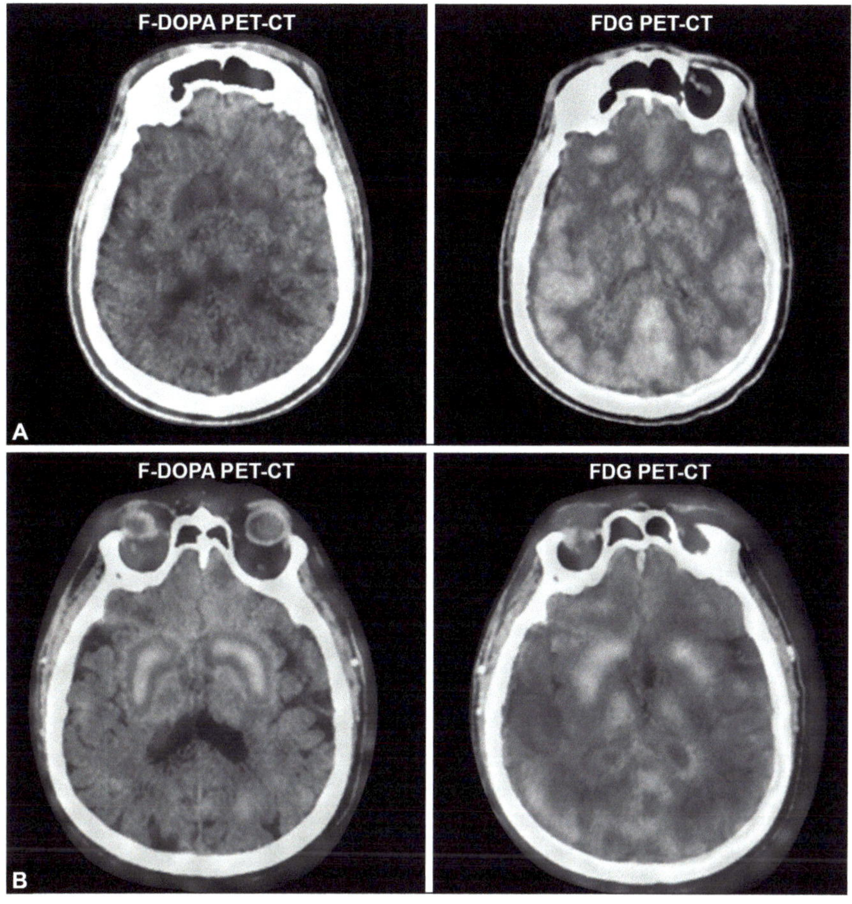

(^{18}F-DOPA-PET: 18F-fluoro-L-DOPA positron emission tomography; CT: computed tomography; ET: essential tremor; PD: Parkinson's disease)

FIGS. 3A AND B: Positive ^{18}F-DOPA-PET scan demonstrating decreased ^{18}F-DOPA uptake within the bilateral posterior greater than anterior putamen consistent with PD (3a, left panel) and uniform uptake within the bilateral caudate and putamen in a case of ET (3b, left panel). The right panel shows FDG-PET showing decreased metabolism in the striatum bilaterally in PD (3a) c.f. ET (3b). Both the patients had mildly asymmetrical (L>R) postural tremor of 3 years duration. ***(For color version, see plate 1)***

Courtesy: Dr Noaline Sinha, Consultant Nuclear Medicine, Artemis Hospital, Gurugram, India.

Holmes tremor, a slow unilateral tremor with rest, postural, and kinetic/intentional components described by Gordon Holmes in 1904, is the better nomenclature for this tremor than *rubral, mesencephalic,* or *thalamic* tremor as it may be caused by miscellaneous lesions in locations other than mesencephalon (**Table 1**).[53] Onabotulinum toxin A injected in proximal upper limb muscles, GPi DBS can be offered in selected cases.[52,53] *Drug-induced tremor* has a temporal and dose relationship with the implicated drugs is nonprogressive and does not have head tremor. Drugs may also cause rest tremors or may enhance the physiological tremors.[45] *Wilson's disease* (WD), an autosomal recessive disease that can manifest with any type of MD in young individuals, can have tremors in up to 60% of cases.[67] A proximal postural tremor, most evident when the arms are held abducted at the shoulders and flexed at the elbows known as the "wing-beating" tremor is the prototype but not the most common type of tremor in WD. Fragile **X**-associated tremor/ataxia syndrome (X-TAS) is a trinucleotide (CGG) repeat disorder involving the *FMR1* gene in elderly males who present with intention tremors and/or kinetic and postural tremors (70%) or rest tremors (10%).[47,68] Trials of N-methyl-D-aspartate (NMDA) receptor antagonist memantine and VIM DBS have been unsuccessful.[52]

CONCLUSION

The authors aim to simplify the daunting task of diagnosing, defining or classifying, and managing patients with tremor. Biochemical, neurophysiological, and neuropathological studies in primates and postmortem or brain repositories' specimens, in-vivo brain structural and functional imaging studies have contributed to the current and evolving knowledge of the pathophysiology of tremors. Newer combination evaluation techniques, including electrophysiology, have provided an important tool in the diagnostic workup of the patients. Optimization of medical treatment can provide reasonable improvement in the clinical condition of the patients. Functional stereotactic brain surgeries such as focused ultrasound ablation of STN and VIM nucleus of thalamus and phase-specific VIM DBS for ET can be used in resistant cases. Orthotic devices biofeedback, counseling, etc., can be of value in selected cases. Ongoing research in the field of tremors might provide insights in the further management options for these patients.

REFERENCES

1. Deuschl G, Bain P, Brin M. Consensus statement of the Movement Disorder Society on Tremor. Ad Hoc Scientific Committee. Mov Disord. 1998;13(3):2-23.
2. Bhatia KP, Bain P, Bajaj N, Elble RJ, Hallett M, Louis ED, et al. Consensus Statement on the classification of tremors. From the task force on tremor of the International Parkinson and Movement Disorder Society. Mov Disord. 2018;33(1):75-87.
3. Marsden CD, Obeso JA, Rothwell J. Benign essential tremor is not a single entity. In: Yahr MD (ed). Current Concepts of Parkinson Disease and Related Disorders. Amsterdam, The Netherlands: Excerpta Medica; 1983:31-46.
4. Haerer AF, Anderson DW, Schoenberg BS. Prevalence of essential tremor: results from the Copiah County study. Arch Neurol. 1982;39(12):750-1.
5. Hornabrook RW, Nagurney JT. Essential tremor in Papua, New Guinea. Brain. 1976;99(4):659-72.
6. Rautakorpi I, Takala J, Marttila RJ, Sievers K, Rinne UK. Essential tremor in a Finnish population. Acta Neurol Scand. 1982;66(1):58-67.
7. Snow B, Wiens M, Hertzman C, Calne D. A community survey of Parkinson's disease. CMAJ. 1989;141(5):418-24.
8. Acosta J, Calderon E, Obeso JA. Prevalence of Parkinson's disease and essential tremor in a village of south Spain. Neurology. 1989;39(1):181.
9. Rajput AH, Offord KP, Beard CM, Kurland LT. Essential tremor in Rochester, Minnesota: a 45-year study. J Neurol Neurosurg Psychiatry. 1984;47(5):466-70.
10. Li SC, Schoenberg BS, Wang CC, Cheng XM, Rui DY, Bolis CL, et al. A prevalence survey of Parkinson's disease and other movement disorders in the People's Republic of China. Arch Neurol. 1985;42(7):655-7.
11. Bharucha NE, Bharucha EP, Bharucha AE, Bhise AV, Schoenberg BS. Prevalence of essential tremor in the Parsi community of Bombay, India. Arch Neurol. 1988;45(8):907-8.
12. Osuntokun BO, Adeuja AO, Schoenberg BS, Bademosi O, Nottidge VA, Olumide AO, et al. Neurological disorders in Nigerian Africans: a community-based study. Acta Neurol Scand. 1987;75(1):13-21.
13. Salemi G, Savettieri G, Rocca WA, Meneghini F, Saporito V, Morgante L, et al. Prevalence of essential tremor: a door-to-door survey in Terrasini, Sicily. Neurology. 1994;44(1):61-4.
14. Chouza C, Ketzoian C, Caamano JL. Prevalence of Parkinson's disease in a population of Uruguay: preliminary results. New Trends Clin Neuropharmacol. 1994;8:122.
15. Lieberman A, Imke S, Brewer M. High prevalence of tremor in a retirement community. Neurology. 1994;44(2):A213.
16. Haimanot RT, Abebe M, Mariam AG, Forsgren L, Holmgren G, Heijbel J, et al. Community-based study of neurological disorders in Ethiopia: development of a screening instrument. Ethiop Med J. 1990;28(3):123-37.
17. Larsson T, Sjogren T. Essential tremor: a clinical and genetic population study. Acta Psychiatr Scand Suppl. 1960;36(144): 1-176.
18. Moghal S, Rajput AH, D'Arcy C, Rajput R. Prevalence of movement disorders in elderly community residents. Neuroepidemiology. 1994;13(4):175-8.
19. Louis ED, Marder K, Cote L, Pullman S, Ford B, Wilder D, et al. Differences in the prevalence of essential tremor among elderly African Americans, whites, and Hispanics in northern Manhattan, NY. Arch Neurol. 1995;52(12):1201-5.
20. Wenning GK, Kiechl S, Seppi K, Müller J, Högl B, Saletu M, et al. Prevalence of movement disorders in men and women aged 50 to 89 years (Bruneck Study cohort): a population-based study. Lancet Neurol. 2005;4(12):815-20.
21. Mancini ML, Stracci F, Tambasco N, Sarchielli P, Rossi A, Calabresi P. Prevalence of essential tremor in the territory of Lake Trasimeno, Italy: results of a population-based study. Mov Disord. 2007;22(4):540-5.
22. Louis ED, Ferreira JJ. How common is the most common adult movement disorder? Update on the worldwide prevalence of essential tremor. Mov Disord. 2010;25(5):534-41.
23. Barbosa MT, Caramelli P, Cunningham MC, Maia DP, Lima-Costa MF, Cardoso F. Prevalence and clinical classification of tremor in elderly-a community-based survey in Brazil. Mov Disord. 2013;28(5):640-6.
24. Ghosh D, Brar H, Lhamu U, Rothner AD, Erenberg G. A Series of 211 Children with Probable Essential Tremor. Mov Disord Clin Pract. 2016;4(2):231-6.
25. Shukla G, Behari M. A clinical study of non-parkinsonian and non-cerebellar tremor at a specialty movement disorders clinic. Neurol India. 2004;52(2):200-2.
26. Das SK, Banerjee TK, Roy T, Raut DK, Chaudhuri A, Hazra A. Prevalence of essential tremor in the city of Kolkata, India: a house-to-house survey. Eur J Neurol. 2009;16(7):801-7.
27. Das SK, Sanyal K. Neuroepidemiology of major neurological disorders in rural Bengal. Neurol India. 1996;44(2):47-58.
28. Gourie-Devi M, Gururaj G, Satishchandra P, Subbakrishna DK. Prevalence of neurological disorders in Bangalore, India: A community-based study with a comparison between urban and rural areas. Neuroepidemiology. 2004;23(6): 261-8.
29. Gourie-Devi M. Epidemiology of neurological disorders in India: Review of background, prevalence and incidence of epilepsy, stroke, Parkinson's disease and tremors. Neurol India. 2014;62(6):588-98.
30. Helmich RC, Toni I, Deuschl G, Bloem BR. The pathophysiology of essential tremor and Parkinson's tremor. Curr Neurol Neurosci Rep. 2013;13(9):378.
31. Deuschl G, Bergman H. Pathophysiology of nonparkinsonian tremors. Mov Disord. 2002;17(3):S41-8.

32. Hallett M. Tremor: pathophysiology. Parkinsonism Relat Disord. 2014;20(1):S118-22.
33. Hess CW, Pullman SL. Tremor: clinical phenomenology and assessment techniques. Tremor Other Hyperkinet Mov. 2012;2.
34. Rossi C, Frosini D, Volterrani D, De Feo P, Unti E, Nicoletti V, et al. Differences in nigro-striatal impairment in clinical variants of early Parkinson's disease: evidence from a FP-CIT SPECT study. Eur J Neurol. 2010;17(4):626-30.
35. Helmich RC, Janssen MJ, Oyen WJ, Bloem BR, Toni I. Pallidal dysfunction drives a cerebellothalamic circuit into Parkinson tremor. Ann Neurol. 2011;69(2):269-81.
36. Nieuwhof F, Panyakaew P, van de Warrenburg BP, Gallea C, Helmich RC. The patchy tremor landscape: recent advances in pathophysiology. Curr Opin Neurol. 2018;31(4):455-61.
37. Volkmann J, Joliot M, Mogilner A, Loannides AA, Lado F, Fazzini E, et al. Central motor loop oscillations in parkinsonian resting tremor revealed magnetoencephalography. Neurology. 1996;46(5):1359-70.
38. Hopfner F, Helmich RC. The etiology of essential tremor: Genes versus environment. Parkinsonism Relat Disord. 2018;46(1):S92-6.
39. Sarma N, Pandey S. Dystonic tremor: Definition, clinical spectrum, pathophysiology, and treatment. Ann Mov Disord. 2018;1:2-7.
40. Schöberl F, Feil K, Xiong G, Bartenstein P, la Fougére C, Jahn K, et al. Pathological ponto-cerebello-thalamo-cortical activations in primary orthostatic tremor during lying and stance. Brain. 2017;140(1):83-97.
41. Remy P, de Recondo A, Defer G, Loc'h C, Amarenco P, Planté-Bordeneuve V, et al. Peduncular 'rubral' tremor and dopaminergic denervation: a PET study. Neurology. 1995;45(3):472-7.
42. Zeuner KE, Deuschl G. An update on tremors. Curr Opin Neurol. 2012;25(4):475-82.
43. Choudhury S, Chatterjee S, Chatterjee K, Banerjee R, Humby J, Mondal B, et al. Clinical Characterization of Genetically Diagnosed Cases of Spinocerebellar Ataxia Type 12 from India. Mov Disord Clin Pract. 2017;5(1):39-46.
44. Bhidayasiri R. Differential diagnosis of common tremor syndromes. Postgrad Med J. 2005;81(962):756-62.
45. Sharma S, Pandey S. Approach to a tremor patient. Ann Indian Acad Neurol. 2016;19(4):433-43.
46. Shah B, Mall S, Chhetri R, Yadav B, Dahal P, Subedi M. A Review of Clinical Approach to a Patient with Tremor Disorder. J Alzheimers Dis Parkinsonism. 2017;7(5):386.
47. Louis ED. Tremor. Continuum (Minneap Minn). 2019;25(4): 959-75.
48. Jahanshahi M. Factors that ameliorate or aggravate spasmodic torticollis. J Neurol Neurosurg Psychiatry. 2000;68(2):227-9.
49. Elble R, Bain P, Forjaz MJ, Haubenberger D, Testa C, Goetz CG, et al. Task force report: Scales for screening and evaluating tremor: Critique and recommendations. Mov Disord. 2013;28(13):1793-800.
50. Haubenberger D, Hallett M. Essential tremor. N Engl J Med. 2018;378(19):1802-10.
51. Kamble N, Pal PK. Tremor syndromes: A review. Neurol India. 2018;66:S36-47.
52. Fasano A, Deuschl G. Therapeutic advances in tremor. Mov Disord. 2015;30(11):1557-65.
53. Raina GB, Cersosimo MG, Folgar SS, Giugni JC, Calandra C, Paviolo JP, et al. Holmes tremor: clinical description, lesion localization, and treatment in a series of 29 cases. Neurology. 2016;86(10):931-8.
54. Cury RG, Fraix V, Castrioto A, Pérez Fernández MA, Krack P, Chabardes S, et al. Thalamic deep brain stimulation for tremor in Parkinson disease, essential tremor, and dystonia. Neurology. 2017;89(13):1416-23.
55. Lake W, Hedera P, Konrad P. Deep Brain Stimulation for Treatment of Tremor. Neurosurg Clin N Am. 2019;30(2):147-59.
56. Elble RJ, Deuschl G. Tremor. In: Brown WF, Bolton CF, Aminoff M, (eds). Neuromuscular Function and Disease: Basic, Clinical and Electrodiagnostic Aspects. Philadelphia, PA: WB Saunders; 2002:1759-79.
57. American Academy of Neurology. (2019). AAN Summary of Evidence-based Guideline for Clinicians. Update: treatment of Essential tremor. [online] Available from http://www.aan.com/Guidelines/home/GetGuidelineContent/493 [Last accessed May, 2021).
58. Pal PK. Guidelines for management of essential tremor. Ann Indian Acad Neurol. 2011;14(1):S25-8.
59. Stamelou M, Charlesworth G, Cordivari C, Schneider SA, Kägi G, Sheerin UM, et al. The phenotypic spectrum of DYT24 due to ANO3 mutations. Mov Disord. 2014;29(7):928-34.
60. Xiromerisiou G, Houlden H, Scarmeas N, Stamelou M, Kara E, Hardy J, et al. THAP1 mutations and dystonia phenotypes: genotype phenotype correlations. Mov Disord. 2012;27(10): 1290-4.
61. Deuschl G, Toro C, Valls-Sole J, Zeffiro T, Zee DS, Hallett M. Symptomatic and essential palatal tremor. Clinical, physiological and MRI analysis. Brain. 1994;117(4):775-88.
62. Fasano A, Bove F, Lang AE The treatment of dystonic tremor: a systematic review. J Neurol Neurosurg Psychiatry. 2014;85(7):759-69.
63. Rinne JO. Positron emission tomography in the differential diagnosis of parkinsonism. J Mov Disord. 2009;2(2):53-7.
64. Crosby NJ, Deane KH, Clarke CE. Beta-blocker therapy for tremor in Parkinson's disease. Cochrane Database Syst Rev. 2003;1:CD003361.
65. Yaltho TC, Ondo WG. Orthostatic tremor: a review of 45 cases. Parkinsonism Relat Disord. 2014;20(7):723-5.
66. Merola A, Fasano A, Hassan A, Ostrem JL, Contarino MF, Lyons M, et al. Thalamic deep brain stimulation for orthostatic tremor: A multicenter international registry. Mov Disord. 2017;32(8):1240-4.
67. Machado A, Chien HF, Deguti MM, Cançado E, Azevedo RS, Scaff M, et al. Neurological manifestations in Wilson's disease: report of 119 cases. Mov Disord. 2006;21(12):2192-6.
68. Ure RJ, Dhanju S, Lang AE, Fasano A. Unusual tremor syndromes: know in order to recognise. J Neurol Neurosurg Psychiatry. 2016;87(11):1191-203.

CHAPTER 32

An Approach to Dystonia

Sonali Bhattad, Sanjay Pandey

INTRODUCTION

Dystonia is a hyperkinetic movement disorder and is defined by the consensus guidelines 2013 as "a movement disorder characterized by sustained or intermittent muscle contractions causing abnormal, often repetitive, movements, postures, or both.[1] Dystonic movements are typically patterned, twisting, and may be tremulous. Dystonia is often initiated or worsened by voluntary action and associated with overflow muscle activation."[1] We would like to give a brief overview of epidemiology, pathophysiology, classification of dystonia according to the axes system, clinical features, and management of dystonia through this review.

EPIDEMIOLOGY

The exact prevalence of dystonia remains unknown, but patients with dystonia represent approximately 20% of patients in the movement disorders clinic.[2,3] Prevalence of dystonia increases with age, and adult-onset focal dystonia is much more frequent than early-onset variants of dystonia, which have a prevalence of approximately 7.6/100,000 individuals.[3,4] Isolated idiopathic and genetic forms are relatively more common among the various forms of dystonia.[4]

PATHOPHYSIOLOGY

The key structures involved in the pathophysiology of dystonia are the somatosensory motor cortex, basal ganglia, brainstem, cerebellum, spinal cord and the sensory system.[5] There is a lack of inhibition and increased excitability in the above structures that lead to the facilitation of movement.[5] The striatum and cerebellum are two vital structures which have a critical role in the pathophysiology of dystonia as most dystonia-associated genes such as *GNAL*, *ANO3*, *ADCY5*, *HPCA*, and *KCTD17* are mainly expressed in the striatum whereas, others that have the highest expression in the cerebellum are *THAP1* and *KMT2B*.[6] Alterations of transcriptional regulation and dopaminergic signaling, as well as malfunctioning of the endoplasmic reticulum (ER) are due to molecular dysfunction in these dystonia genes.[6] Maladaptive plasticity is another important phenomenon proposed in the pathophysiology of dystonia, this is supported by the fact that repetitive and excessive sensory stimulation leads to dystonia.[7] The fact that dystonia is not only a motor phenomenon but also a sensory one is established by the fact of the presence of sensory tricks in cervical dystonia.[8] Therefore, the aberrancy between the various input and the output pathways, the cortical plasticity, and the sensory-motor mismatch which is exemplified using sensory tricks in the clinical settings are all held responsible for the pathogenesis of dystonia.

CLASSIFICATION OF DYSTONIA

There were various classifications proposed for dystonia in the last 20 years, but according to the recent consensus update dystonia is classified into two axes based on the clinical characteristics and etiology, respectively.[1]

The axis-I of the classifications includes clinical characteristics like:

- *Age of onset*:
  - Infancy (birth to 2 years)
  - Childhood (3–12 years)
  - Adolescence (13–20 years)
  - Early adulthood (21–40 years)
  - Late adulthood (>40 years)

Classification by age of onset of dystonia allows for more refined age categories that focus on the most likely disorders occurring in each age group.

- *Body distribution*: Classification by body region affected is clinically important because of implications for diagnosis and therapy. They can be classified as:
    - *Focal dystonias*: These are characterized by abnormal movements involving a single body part only. The various forms include: Writing dystonia (writer's cramp), cervical dystonia, blepharospasm, oromandibular dystonia, lingual dystonia, laryngeal dystonia (spasmodic dysphonia), and geniospasm.[1]
    - *Segmental dystonias*: These are characterized by abnormal movements involving two or more contiguous body parts (for example, the arm and neck), e.g., craniocervical dystonia—combination of blepharospasm as well as oromandibular, lingual, facial, laryngeal, and cervical dystonia.[1]
    - *Multifocal dystonias*: These are characterized by abnormal movements involving two or more noncontiguous body areas (for example, the right arm and the left leg).[1]
    - *Hemidystonia*: It affects one side of the body—as seen in poststroke dystonias.[1]
    - *Generalized dystonia*: It involves two or more contiguous body parts in addition to the trunk (with or without leg involvement).[1,9]
- *Temporal pattern* of disease course—distinguishes static from progressive forms.

    Diurnal variability provides descriptors on the occurrence of dystonia through the day.[1] Variability allows separating dystonia into various subdivisions like:
    - *Persistent*: Dystonia that consistently occurs under the same conditions.
    - *Action-specific*: Dystonia that occurs only during an activity or task, e.g., writer's cramp, musician's, typist's, or golfer's dystonia.

        Other variable forms of dystonia include the diurnal and paroxysmal ones.

        In the diurnal fluctuations, dystonia fluctuates during the day, with recognizable circadian variations in occurrence, severity, and phenomenology (e.g., DYT5).

        The paroxysmal dystonias are sudden self-limited episodes of dystonia usually induced by a trigger with return to preexisting neurological state. Based on the precipitating event, paroxysmal dystonia is subdivided into the kinesogenic [paroxysmal kinesigenic dyskinesia (PKD)], nonkinesogenic [paroxysmal nonkinesigenic dyskinesia (PNKD)], and exercise-induced forms [paroxysmal exercise-induced dystonia (PED)].[1,9]
- *Isolated and combined forms of dystonia*:
    - *Isolated dystonias*: Dystonia is the only motor feature, except for the presence of tremor.[1]

        DYT1 dystonia is caused by mutations in the *TOR1A* gene is the prototype of inherited isolated generalized dystonia with limb onset.[10]

        Inherited isolated syndromes with a prominent craniocervical onset: DYT6 dystonia (DYT-THAP1), DYT25 dystonia (DYT-GNAL), DYT4 (DYT-TUBB4A), DYT23 dystonia (DYT-CIZ1), and DYT24 (DYT-ANO3).[10]

        Dystonic tremor (DT) has been described as a key feature of DYT24 dystonia, appearing most commonly as head or arm tremor, and may precede the appearance of dystonic postures.[10]
    - *Combined dystonias*: Dystonia is combined with other movement disorders such as myoclonus like DYT11 (DYT-SGCE) and parkinsonism like the dopa-responsive dystonia (DYT5a, i.e., DYT/PARK-GCH1 and DYT5b, i.e., DYT/PARK-TH) and sepiapterin reductase deficiency (DYT/PARK-SPR).[10]

        The newer classification still retains the original description of generalized and focal dystonias and hence aids in appropriate planning of investigations and management.[9]

The axis-II addresses to the etiology which were based on the identifiable anatomical changes and mode of inheritance.[1] The dystonia can be further classified as inherited, acquired, or idiopathic entities.

- *Inherited dystonia*—forms of proven genetic origin—could be further differentiated into autosomal dominant, autosomal recessive, X-linked recessive, and mitochondrial forms.[1]
    - Autosomal dominant, e.g., DYT1, DYT5, DYT6, DYT11 and rapid-onset dystonia parkinsonism (DYT12), neuroferritinopathy, dentatorubral-pallidoluysian atrophy, and Huntington's disease.
    - Autosomal recessive, e.g., Wilson's disease, PKAN (NBIA1), PLAN (NBIA2), and type 2 juvenile Parkinson's disease (PARK2) and various metabolic disorders.
    - X-linked recessive, e.g., Lubag (DYT3), Lesch–Nyhan syndrome, and Mohr–Tranebjaerg syndrome.
    - Mitochondrial: Mitochondrial forms can give rise to inherited dystonias such as Leigh's syndrome or Leber's optic atrophy.[1]
- *Acquired dystonia*: The acquired dystonia is due to a known specific cause like:
    - Perinatal brain injuries
    - Infections (viral encephalitis, encephalitis lethargica, subacute sclerosing panencephalitis, human immunodeficiency virus (HIV) infection, and others)
    - *Drugs*: Levodopa and dopamine agonists, neuroleptics (dopamine receptor blocking drugs), anticonvulsants, and calcium channel blockers
    - *Toxins*: Manganese, cobalt, carbon disulfide, cyanide, methanol, disulfiram, and 3-nitropropionic acid

- *Vascular*: Ischemia, hemorrhage, and arteriovenous malformation (including aneurysm)
- *Neoplastic*: Brain tumor, and paraneoplastic encephalitis
- *Psychogenic*: Functional forms of dystonia

CLINICAL SYNDROMIC APPROACH TO DYSTONIA

A clinical syndromic approach, considering history and findings from clinical examination helps in the diagnosis of a dystonia syndrome, which in turn guides the further diagnostic workup that aims to identify the etiology.[6]

Some important phenomenological considerations that help to recognize dystonia in clinical settings are:

- Dystonic movements are caused by cocontraction of agonist and antagonist muscles that can manifest as abnormal postures that are typically mobile (not fixed) with or without twisting movements, slow writhing movements (athetosis) or with DT.[9]
- *Overflow*: It is a characteristic of dystonic movements is in which the activation of dystonic movements occurs by actions in parts of the body remote from the affected area.[9]
- *Geste antagoniste*: It is a typical feature of primary dystonia although rarely they have been described in secondary, heredodegenerative and functional (psychogenic) dystonias as well.[11] Sensory tricks or "alleviating maneuvers" are voluntary maneuvers that decrease the severity of abnormal movements or postures in patients of dystonia. Often a patient will be able to improve to some degree, the abnormal posture by touching, or even sometimes, by thinking about touching the affected body part which is explained by the "closing the loop" theory.[12]
- *Tremor in dystonia*: Tremor has been generally recognized as an important manifestation of dystonia ranging in 14–86.6% of patients.[10] There are two types of tremor described in dystonia, i.e., DT, and tremor associated with dystonia (TAWD).[13] Tremor in dystonia usually appears on posture and intention and, less commonly, at rest.[14,15] DT is clinically distinguishable by asymmetry, jerkiness, task and position specificity, and the frequent presence of null points where tremor diminishes or even disappears in certain positions of the affected body part.[16]

NONMOTOR FEATURES OF DYSTONIA

Various nonmotor symptoms like pain, neuropsychiatric abnormalities like depression, and cognitive abnormalities are described in dystonia.[17] Pain is reported in nearly 70% of patients with cervical dystonia and in up to 30% of those with focal hand dystonia or writer's cramp.[18] Depressive disorders are more frequent in cervical dystonia, blepharospasm, laryngeal dystonia, and focal hand dystonia.[19] Cognitive abnormalities are often found in combined dystonias.[17]

MANAGEMENT

Diagnostic workup: The diagnostic approach is primarily based on the clinical characteristics.[6]

Once the clinical syndrome of dystonia is defined then the investigations can be narrowed down. Various investigations described here can be useful.

- *Magnetic resonance imaging (MRI) of the brain*: It can be done to detect the iron deposition and may be useful to identify the "eye-of-the-tiger" sign in pantothenate kinase-associated neurodegeneration or the "cortical pencil lining" sign seen in neuroferritinopathy. MRI is also useful in other heredodegenerative cases, particularly Wilson's disease.[9]
- Copper and ceruloplasmin levels, white cell enzymes, acanthocytes, lactate, pyruvate, creatine kinase, and antinuclear antibody screening to look for systemic disorders causing nervous system pathology.
- Cerebrospinal fluid (CSF) analysis (analysis of pterins, dopamine and serotonin metabolites and serum and/or CSF glucose ratio) to detect dopamine synthesis pathway defects.
- The muscle or skin biopsy, or metabolic studies of blood or urine can be useful in investigating for rarer causes such as mitochondrial and metabolic disorders, as well as amino acid and lysosomal storage disorders.
- Electrophysiological studies to assess for associated myopathy or neuropathy, as indicated.
- Genetic analysis as indicated.
- Psychogenic dystonia can be diagnosed based on the established clinical criteria.

TREATMENT

Various treatment modalities are available for the treatment of dystonia ranging from pharmacological therapies to botulinum toxin injections and deep brain stimulation surgeries depending on the type of dystonia.

Pharmacological Therapies

- *Anticholinergic drugs*: Trihexyphenidyl and other anticholinergic agents are effective for the treatment of generalized and segmental dystonia rather than focal dystonia.[2] These drugs might also be helpful in patients with acute dystonic reaction and tardive dystonia.[20]

  Anticholinergic drugs have adverse effects, such as blurry vision, dry mouth, urinary retention, constipation, and cognitive impairment.[21] Therefore, starting a low dose of anticholinergic drugs and titrating slowly over several weeks often minimizes the adverse effects and improves tolerability.[22]

- *Levodopa*: Levodopa is the treatment of choice for dopa-responsive dystonias.[23]

  The pathophysiological mechanisms involved in other dystonias are not based on pathways of dopamine biosynthesis and hence levodopa has little benefit.[6]
- *Baclofen*: Baclofen, a gamma-aminobutyric acid type B (GABA-B) receptor agonist, can be used to reduce dystonic movements in some patients with dystonia.[7] The data on use of intrathecal and intraventricular baclofen infusions in patients with dystonia is reported more than the use of oral baclofen.[24]
- *Antidopaminergic drugs*: Dopamine-depleting drugs that act by inhibiting vesicular amine transporter-2 such as tetrabenazine, deutetrabenazine, and valbenazine.[25] Patients with depression should not receive this drug as there are higher chances of suicidal tendencies.[26]
- *Benzodiazepines*: Benzodiazepines (such as diazepam, clonazepam, lorazepam, and midazolam) were the most used as oral treatment agents in all types of isolated dystonia according to a cross-sectional study.[27] These drugs are used as the off-label treatment agents of dystonia by their property of muscles relaxation, although their usefulness is limited by potential adverse effects such as drowsiness and addiction.[28]

Role of Botulinum Toxin

Botulinum neurotoxin (BoNT) can be considered as a treatment option for all forms of focal and segmental dystonia.[29] It is produced by *Clostridium botulinum* and has seven immunologically distinct serotypes (named A to G), each of which is composed of a 100 kDa heavy chain and a 50 kDa light chain.[28] The types A and B are the only ones approved by the United States Food and Drug Administration (FDA) currently for therapeutic use.[30]

Botulinum neurotoxin is the first-line treatment for patients with blepharospasm and cervical dystonia (spasmodic torticollis).[31]

- *BoNT in cervical dystonia*: Class A evidence of efficacy for aboBoNT/A and rimaBoNT/B and class B evidence for onaBoNT/A and incoBoNT/A in reported in cervical dystonia.[32,33]
- *BoNT in blepharospasm*: BoNT type A (BoNT/A) is the first-line treatment if injections are placed in the pretarsal portion of the orbicularis oculi muscle.[34]
- *BoNT in other focal dystonia*: BoNT/A is probably effective for the treatment of focal upper limb dystonia and adductor spasmodic dysphonia.[35]

After long-term treatment with onaBoNT/A, only < 2% of the patients were positive for neutralizing antibodies which is a theoretical possibility that is considered exceptional.[36]

Role of transcranial magnetic stimulation (TMS): TMS enhances intracortical inhibition, a neural process deemed to be altered in dystonia. Cumulative effects can be obtained by repeated stimulation over consecutive days than single-session studies.[37]

Surgical Therapies

Ablative procedures: Pallidotomy and thalamotomy, which were commonly used for the treatment of dystonia in the past, have been essentially completely replaced by deep brain stimulation (DBS).[6]

Deep brain stimulation: DBS has great potential for different dystonia syndromes, whether idiopathic or inherited, isolated or combined.[17] It has emerged as the most effective therapy for patients with medically refractory disabling dystonia in both generalized and severe segmental and focal dystonia.[6] The two main targets of stimulation are the globus pallidus internus (GPi) and, more recently, the subthalamic nucleus (STN) for treatment of dystonia owing to their involvement in the control of motor function.[38] The most frequent complication associated with GPi-DBS is dysarthria, but parkinsonism has also been observed in some patients.[39] With STN-DBS, the complications noted are chorea, worsened handwriting, weight gain, dysarthria, shoulder pain, and depression.[40] Complications common to both the targets include incoordination, paresthesias, and perioral tingling, whereas the hardware-related complications were infection, hematoma and wire displacement that are reported.[41]

Bilateral GPi-DBS in patients with tardive dystonia has shown marked benefit with long-term follow-up.[42]

Deep brain stimulation outcomes are influenced by several features such as body distribution, age of onset, and by the relative prevalence of dystonic movements or postures.[17]

Favorable outcomes are seen in dystonias associated with *TOR1A*, *KMT2B*, and *SGCE* mutations.[6] Therefore, the genetic status is also important, with two extremes represented by DYT1 dystonia showing consistently excellent outcome and DYT12 dystonia has lack of efficacy to DBS.[17]

Magnetic resonance-guided focused ultrasound (MRgFUS): It uses ultrasonic energy that is delivered to a brain target, without the need for an incision or burr hole in the skull. The lesion is monitored in real time by MRI thermometry, which is an advantage over radiofrequency-based lesioning without hardware-related complications.[43] Whether focused ultrasound of the thalamus will have utility in the treatment of dystonia is unknown, but it has been reported to be effective in the treatment of essential tremor and Parkinson's disease.[44]

Physical treatments: Different rehabilitation strategies have been combined with BoNT to improve disability and pain in patients of dystonia.[45]

COMPLICATIONS OF DYSTONIA

Dystonic storm, also referred to as status dystonicus, is a movement disorder emergency that is a very rare complication of generalized dystonia commonly seen in the pediatric population.[46] Triggering factors include intercurrent infection and fever, discontinuation or rapid change in treatments, surgery or trauma.[46] It can be managed by controlling the triggering factors and using oral agents, such as anticholinergics, tetrabenazine, clonidine, and baclofen. Intravenous medications such as midazolam, propofol, and nondepolarizing neuromuscular blockers should be considered as supportive options. In severe cases, the use of DBS targeting the GPi as effective rescue therapy and an intrathecal baclofen pump should also be considered.[6]

Algorithm describing an approach to dystonia has been shown in **Flowchart 1**.

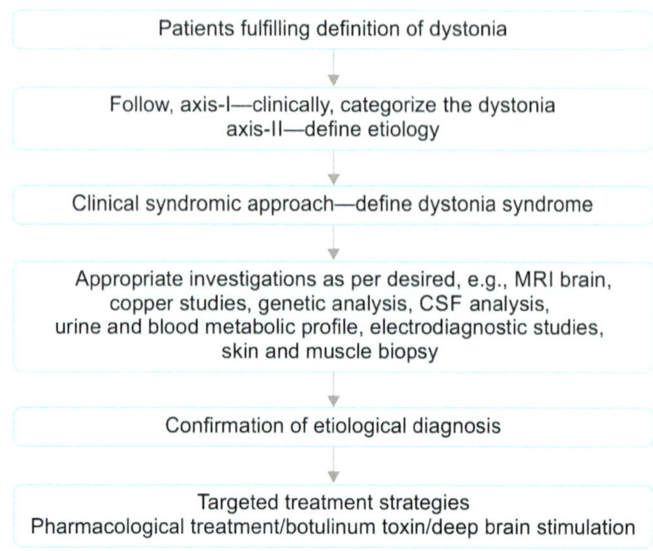

FLOWCHART 1: An approach to dystonia.

FINANCIAL DISCLOSURE/CONFLICT OF INTEREST CONCERNING THE RESEARCH RELATED TO THE MANUSCRIPT

None

FUNDING SOURCES FOR STUDY

None

ROLES OF THE AUTHORS

Sonali Bhattad and Sanjay Pandey contributed in manuscript preparation by writing the first draft, review, and critique.

FINANCIAL DISCLOSURES OF ALL AUTHORS (RELATED TO RESEARCH COVERED IN THIS CHAPTER AND FOR THE PRECEDING 12 MONTHS)

None

CONCLUSION

Dystonia is a neurological condition characterized by involuntary movements or postures due to sustained or intermittent muscle contractions. Dystonia can occur in isolation (isolated dystonia) or with additional signs (combined dystonia). The diagnosis of dystonia is largely based on clinical signs, however, the discovery of many genes underlying the isolated and combined dystonia has led to a better understanding of the pathophysiology. Pharmacotherapy including botulinum toxin remains the main treatment for focal dystonia, and deep brain stimulation has emerged as a major treatment modality for generalized dystonia.

REFERENCES

1. Albanese A, Bhatia K, Bressman SB, Delong MR, Fahn S, Fung VS, et al. Phenomenology and classification of dystonia: a consensus update. Mov Disord. 2013;28:863-73.
2. Jankovic J. Treatment of hyperkinetic movement disorders. Lancet Neurol. 2009;8:844-56.
3. Steeves TD, Day L, Dykeman J, Jette N, Pringsheim T. The prevalence of primary dystonia: a systematic review and meta-analysis. Mov Disord. 2012;27:1789-96.
4. Das SK, Banerjee TK, Biswas A, Roy T, Raut DK, Chaudhuri A, et al. Community survey of primary dystonia in the city of Kolkata, India. Mov Disord. 2007;22:2031-6.
5. Forbes PA, de Bruijn E, Nijmeijer SW, Koelman JH, van der Helm FC, Schouten AC, et al. Dynamic head-neck stabilization in cervical dystonia. Clin Biomech (Bristol, Avon). 2017;42:120-7.
6. Balint B, Mencacci NE, Valente EM, Pisani A, Rothwell J, Jankovic J, et al. Dystonia. Nat Rev Dis Primers. 2018;4:25.

7. Kroneberg D, Plettig P, Schneider GH, Kühn AA. Motor cortical plasticity relates to symptom severity and clinical benefit from deep brain stimulation in cervical dystonia. Neuromodulation. 2017;21(8):735-40.
8. Stamelou M, Edwards MJ, Hallett M, Bhatia KP. The non-motor syndrome of primary dystonia: clinical and pathophysiological implications. Brain. 2012;135:1668-81.
9. Batla A. Dystonia: a review. Neurol India. 2018;66(Suppl S1): 48-58.
10. Charlesworth G, Bhatia KP, Wood NW. The genetics of dystonia: new twists in an old tale. Brain. 2013;136(7):2017-37.
11. Thomas M, Hayflick SJ, Jankovic J. Clinical heterogeneity of neurodegeneration with brain iron accumulation (Hallervorden-Spatz syndrome) and pantothenate kinase-associated neurodegeneration. Mov Disord. 2004;19:36-42.
12. Frucht SJ. Closing the loop in cervical dystonia: a new clinical phenomenon. Tremor Other Hyperkinet Mov. 2014;4:tre-04-283-6428-1.
13. Pandey S, Sarma N. Tremor in dystonia. Parkinsonism Relat Disord. 2016;29:3-9.
14. Defazio G, Conte A, Gigante AF, Fabbrini G, Berardelli A. Is tremor in dystonia a phenotypic feature of dystonia? Neurology. 2015;84:1053-9.
15. Deuschl G. Dystonic tremor. Rev Neurol (Paris). 2003;159(10 Pt 1): 900-5.
16. Tisch S. Recent advances in understanding and managing dystonia [version 1; peer review: 2 approved]. F1000Research. 2018;7:1124.
17. Albanese A, Di Giovanni M, Lalli S. Dystonia: diagnosis and management. Eur J Neurol. 2019;26(1):5-17.
18. Kuyper DJ, Parra V, Aerts S, Okun MS, Kluger BM. Nonmotor manifestations of dystonia: a systematic review. Mov Disord. 2011;26:1206-17.
19. Berman BD, Junker J, Shelton E, Sillau SH, Jinnah HA, Perlmutter JS, et al. Psychiatric associations of adult-onset focal dystonia phenotypes. J Neurol Neurosurg Psychiatry. 2017;88:595-602.
20. Vijayakumar D, Jankovic J. Drug-induced dyskinesia, part 2: treatment of tardive dyskinesia. Drugs. 2016;76:779-87.
21. Lumsden DE, Kaminska M, Tomlin S, Lin JP. Medication use in childhood dystonia. Eur J Paediatr Neurol. 2016;20:625-9.
22. Alfradique-Dunham I, Jankovic J. Available treatment options for dystonia. Expert Opin Orphan Drugs. 2017;5:707-16.
23. Wijemanne S, Jankovic J. Dopa-responsive dystonia—clinical and genetic heterogeneity. Nat Rev Neurol. 2015;11:414-24.
24. Monbaliu E, Himmelmann K, Lin JP, Ortibus E, Bonouvrié L, Feys H, et al. Clinical presentation and management of dyskinetic cerebral palsy. Lancet Neurol. 2017;16:741-9.
25. Motta F, Antonello CE. Analysis of complications in 430 consecutive pediatric patients treated with intrathecal baclofen therapy: 14-year experience. J Neurosurg Pediatr. 2014;13:301-6.
26. Jankovic J. Dopamine depleters in the treatment of hyperkinetic movement disorders. Expert Opin Pharmacother. 2016;17:2461-70.
27. Solmi M, Pigato G, Kane JM, Correll CU. Treatment of tardive dyskinesia with VMAT-2 inhibitors: a systematic review and meta-analysis of randomized controlled trials. Drug Des Devel Ther. 2018;12:1215-38.
28. Pirazzini M, Rossetto O, Eleopra R, Montecucco C. Botulinum neurotoxins: biology, pharmacology, and toxicology. Pharmacol Rev. 2017;69:200-35.
29. Jankovic J. Botulinum toxin: state of the art. Mov Disord. 2017;32:1131-8.
30. Truong D, Dressler D, Hallet M, Zachary C. Manual of Botulinum Toxin Therapy, 2nd edition. Cambridge, UK: Cambridge University Press; 2013.
31. Albanese A, Asmus F, Bhatia KP, Elia AE, Elibol B, Filippini G, et al. EFNS guidelines on diagnosis and treatment of primary dystonias. Eur J Neurol. 2011;18:5-18.
32. Simpson DM, Hallett M, Ashman EJ, Comella CL, Green MW, Gronseth GS, et al. Practice guideline update summary: botulinum neurotoxin for the treatment of blepharospasm, cervical dystonia, adult spasticity, and headache: Report of the Guideline Development Subcommittee of the American Academy of Neurology. Neurology. 2016;86:1818-26.
33. Albanese A, Abbruzzese G, Dressler D, Duzynski W, Khatkova S, Marti MJ, et al. Practical guidance for CD management involving treatment of botulinum toxin: a consensus statement. J Neurol. 2015;262:2201-13.
34. Cakmur R, Ozturk V, Uzunel F, Donmez B, Idiman F. Comparison of preseptal and pretarsal injections of botulinum toxin in the treatment of blepharospasm and hemifacial spasm. J Neurol. 2002;249:64-8.
35. Simpson DM, Blitzer A, Brashear A, Comella C, Dubinsky R, Hallett M, et al. Assessment: botulinum neurotoxin for the treatment of movement disorders (an evidence-based review): report of the Therapeutics and Technology Assessment Subcommittee of the American Academy of Neurology. Neurology. 2008;70:1699-706.
36. Naumann M, Carruthers A, Carruthers J, Aurora SK, Zafonte R, Abu-Shakra S, et al. Meta-analysis of neutralizing antibody conversion with onabotulinum toxin A (BOTOX®) across multiple indications. Mov Disord. 2010;25:2211-8.
37. Erro R, Tinazzi M, Morgante F, Bhatia KP. Non-invasive brain stimulation for dystonia: therapeutic implications. Eur J Neurol. 2017;24:1228-e64.
38. Moro E, LeReun C, Krauss JK, Albanese A, Lin JP, Walleser Autiero S, et al. Efficacy of pallidal stimulation in isolated dystonia: a systematic review and meta-analysis. Eur J Neurol. 2017;24:552-60.
39. Schrader C, Capelle HH, Kinfe TM, Blahak C, Bäzner H, Lütjens G, et al. GPi-DBS may induce a hypokinetic gait disorder with freezing of gait in patients with dystonia. Neurology. 2011;77:483-8.
40. Mills KA, Scherzer R, Starr PA, Ostrem JL. Weight change after globus pallidus internus or subthalamic nucleus deep brain stimulation in Parkinson's disease and dystonia. Stereotact Funct Neurosurg. 2012;90:386-93.
41. Baizabal Carvallo JF, Mostile G, Almaguer M, Davidson A, Simpson R, Jankovic J. Deep brain stimulation hardware complications in patients with movement disorders: risk factors and clinical correlations. Stereotact Funct Neurosurg. 2012;90:300-6.
42. Pouclet-Courtemanche H, Rouaud T, Thobois S, Nguyen JM, Brefel-Courbon C, Chereau I, et al. Long-term efficacy and tolerability of bilateral pallidal stimulation to treat tardive dyskinesia. Neurology. 2016;86:651-9.
43. Fishman PS, Frenkel V. Treatment of movement disorders with focused ultrasound. J Cent Nerv Syst Dis. 2017;9: 1179573517705670.
44. Dallapiazza RF, Timbie KF, Holmberg S, Gatesman J, Lopes MB, Price RJ, et al. Noninvasive neuromodulation and thalamic mapping with low-intensity focused ultrasound. J. Neurosurg. 2018;128:875-84.
45. Contarino MF, Smit M, van den Dool J, Volkmann J, Tijssen MA. Unmet needs in the management of cervical dystonia. Front Neurol. 2016;7:165.
46. Allen NM, Lin JP, Lynch T, King MD. Status dystonicus: a practice guide. Dev Med Child Neurol. 2014;56(2):105-12.

CHAPTER 33

Paroxysmal Dyskinesias

Gurusidheshwar Wali, Gautam Wali

INTRODUCTION

Paroxysmal movement disorders mainly constitute of paroxysmal dyskinesias (PxDs) and episodic ataxias. Other rare conditions included in this group are orthostatic paroxysmal dystonia, benign torticollis of childhood, paroxysms with tonic conjugate deviation of the eyes and paroxysms of the tongue.

Paroxysmal dyskinesias are a rare heterogenous group of disorders characterized by episodes of abnormal involuntary movements without change in consciousness. The movements may be in the form of dystonia, chorea, ballismus, or a combination of these.[1] The episodes occur suddenly, last for a brief duration and cease spontaneously with a rapid return to interictal state. Epidemiological literature indicates that their prevalence is low. A study by Blakely and Jankovic reported that PxDs constituted 0.76% cases of all movement disorders seen at a movement disorders clinic.[2] This may be an underestimation since these disorders are likely to be underdiagnosed or misdiagnosed. Underdiagnoses is common since they are paroxysmal, brief, and often remain unwitnessed by the physician. They may be misdiagnosed as epileptic seizures, psychogenic seizures, or myotonic phenomenon. Most of these dyskinesias are idiopathic in origin while secondary cases are also described. A wide range of conditions can manifest with PxDs. These include central nervous system (CNS) disorders such as demyelination, vasculopathies, infection, trauma, anoxic brain damage, degenerative disorders, malformations, kernicterus, and migraine. Non-neurological disorders such as endocrinal, metabolic, and drug-induced conditions may also manifest as PxDs. These conditions should be suspected and investigated appropriately based on the clinical circumstances.[2,3] Recent discoveries in the molecular genetics of the primary PxDs have revealed that the various subgroups have some overlapping genetic causation. In addition, a particular gene mutation may be associated with more than one subgroup of PxD. The pathomechanism of these conditions is still unclear. This chapter will discuss various clinical aspects of PxDs along with their evolving molecular genetics. Recent developments in their cellular pathomechanisms will be highlighted.

HISTORICAL ASPECTS

Paroxysmal dyskinesia was first reported in 1892 by Shuzo Kure in a 23-year-old Japanese man who suspected it to be a case of atypical Thomsen's disease.[4] In 1901, Gowers made mention of a child with this disorder but considered it to be a form of epilepsy.[5] Modern literature on this topic has appeared since 1940 when Mount and Reback described a 23-year-old with paroxysmal dystonic movements involving the trunk and limbs. They labelled it as paroxysmal dystonic choreoathetosis.[6] Kertesz in 1967 described 10 such cases including one autopsied and used the term paroxysmal kinesigenic choreoathetosis.[7] Weber described similar cases and used the term familial dystonic choreoathetosis.[8] Lance in 1977 described a different form while reporting a family that had attacks lasting between 5 and 30 minutes and which were provoked by prolonged exercise.[9] This was recognized as an example of "intermediate type" because the attack duration was more than that of paroxysmal kinesigenic choreoathetosis but less than that of paroxysmal dystonic choreoathetosis. Demirkiran and Jankovic in 1995 proposed a revised classification of all such cases as paroxysmal kinesigenic dyskinesia (PKD), paroxysmal nonkinesigenic dyskinesia (PNKD), and paroxysmal exercise-induced dyskinesia (PED).[10] The term paroxysmal hypnogenic dyskinesia (PHD) was used to describe cases of dyskinesia associated with sleep. However, this condition is now considered as a case of autosomal dominant nocturnal frontal lobe epilepsy (ADNFLE).[11]

CLASSIFICATION

The clinical classification of the PxDs is based on the nature of the precipitating factors and duration of the attacks, more so on the former. While some attacks occur spontaneously at rest others occur following sudden movements after a period of rest and prolonged exercise. Factors such as drinking coffee or tea, stress, fatigue, menstruation, and exposure to heat or cold may provoke the occurrence of such attacks. The duration of the attacks may be either <5 minutes or >5 minutes. The defined groups may be further subdivided as primary or secondary groups on etiological basis. The classification of the primary cases used in present day practice is mentioned below along with their accepted nomenclature which is selfexplanatory.[10]

Paroxysmal kinesigenic dyskinesia: Formerly known as paroxysmal kinesigenic choreoathetosis. The episodes are commonly provoked by sudden movements after a period of rest and last <5 minutes.

Paroxysmal nonkinesigenic dyskinesia: Formerly known as paroxysmal dystonic choreoathetosis. The episodes occur spontaneously and may last for >5 minutes; at times lasting few hours.

Paroxysmal exercise-induced dyskinesia: Formerly called as the intermediate type considering the duration of the attacks which ranged between that of PKD and PNKD. They are provoked by prolonged exercise and last 5–15 minutes after the exercise is terminated.

Paroxysmal hypnogenic dyskinesia: This condition is characterized by attacks of dystonic and tonic movements that occurs in sleep lasting about a minute. This condition is believed to be a frontal lobe epilepsy recognized as ADNFLE. In view of its epileptic nature, this condition will not be discussed further in this chapter.

Exciting discoveries in the genetics of PxDs has influenced the growth of this field. The three major types of PxDs (PKD, PNKD, and PED) have been related to mutations in the proline-rich transmembrane protein 2 (*PRRT2*), myofibrillogenesis regulator 1 (*MR-1* gene, recently called as the *PNKD* gene), and glucose transporter 1 (GLUT1) (*SLC2A1*) genes, respectively. Recent reviews have stressed on the marked pleiotropy of mutations in such genes with still expanding and overlapping clinical spectra.[10,12] Erro et al.[12] have suggested an algorithm and a revised classification of these conditions based on genotype-phenotype correlation. These authors also stress the usefulness of the "trigger factor" as compared to the duration of the episodes in arriving at the proper clinical diagnosis. **Table 1** summarizes the salient clinical features of the various PxDs.

CLINICAL ASPECTS, PATHOPHYSIOLOGY, AND TREATMENT

Paroxysmal Kinesigenic Dyskinesia

Clinical information obtained through analysis of large cohorts and reviews has added significantly to our present knowledge of PKD.[1,12-15] The clinical onset of PKD is most often in the latter half of the first decade and earlier half of the second decade, although rare cases have been recorded with onset as early as 6 months and as late as 33 years. Male preponderance (4:1) is noted more often in the sporadic cases.

Typically, an attack of PKD is induced by sudden movement, more so when it is unexpected. It could also occur when there is sudden change in the speed of an ongoing activity. Nonmotor events like hyperventilation, startle, sound, and photic stimulation can provoke the attacks. The attacks increase in frequency and severity during periods of stress. An aura in the form of "crawling

TABLE 1: Salient clinical features of common primary paroxysmal dyskinesias.

Clinical features	*PKD*	*PNKD*	*PED*
Phenomenon	Dystonia/Chorea	Dystonia/Chorea	Dystonia/Chorea
Age of onset	1–20 years	Childhood	Childhood
Trigger factor	Sudden movements after a period of rest	Coffee/Alcohol/Stress	Prolonged exercise
Duration of episodes	<1 minute	10 minutes to 4 hours	5–30 minutes
Frequency of episodes	1–100/day	Variable; 1–4/day	Variable; depends upon exercise
Treatment	Antiepileptic drugs. Commonly respond to carbamazepine and phenytoin	Benzodiazepines	Poor response to AED. May respond to benzodiazepine, acetazolamide, or levodopa

(AED: antiepileptic drugs; PED: paroxysmal exercise-induced dyskinesia; PKD: paroxysmal kinesigenic dyskinesia; PNKD: paroxysmal nonkinesigenic dyskinesia)

pins and needles" may be experienced in the affected parts by almost two-thirds of the patients. Using this clue, some patients succeed in preventing or aborting the motor attacks by pressing down the affected part.

The dyskinetic attacks may be in the form of dystonia, chorea, ballismus, or a combination of these. The attacks usually occur on one side (right, left, or alternating) and at times are generalized. Majority of the attacks last few seconds to a minute and rarely up to 2 minutes. They are not associated with loss of consciousness or postictal confusion and may occur 1-20 per day and rarely up to 100 times a day. While peak frequency of the attacks is seen around puberty they gradually become less frequent and quite often cease by the age of 30 years.

Indian observations: A large family of PKD was studied in the Belgaum district of Karnataka in 1997. This family had 17 affected members out of which four had deceased. The male female ratio was 1.8:1. The clinical presentation of PKD was typical in all affected members with brief attacks of dystonic/choreic movements precipitated by sudden movements with frequency of 1-20/day. Age of onset was between 7 and 13 years. History of benign infantile convulsions was absent. Five of the affected had history of teen age tonic clonic seizures with spontaneous remission. The inheritance of the PKD was autosomal dominant spanning three successive generations. Genetics of this family revealed a second PKD locus (EKD2) on chromosome 16.[1] Relation to the *PRRT2* gene was confirmed in 2011.[16]

Pathophysiology: There has been a debate about whether the PKD is a cortical or a noncortical disorder. Several modalities of investigations have been used to solve this issue.[15] The brief duration and stereotypic nature of the attacks and their response to antiepileptic drugs favor the cortical origin of these disorders.[17] However, the phenomenology of the episodes suggests a basal ganglionic pattern. In addition, awake and sleep electroencephalograms (EEGs) fail to show ictal or intercal epileptiform discharges,[18] except in few cases.[19]

Treatment: Bruno et al. studied 121 cases with a diagnosis of idiopathic PKD. About 79% of these patients showed antiepileptic drug responsiveness.[14] Carbamazepine or phenytoin were the most commonly used drugs. Phenytoin drug dosage for PKD in children was similar to the dosage used for epileptic seizures. Adults responded well to a lower dosage of Phenytoin. In another study Hoser et al. suggested 7-15 mg/kg carbamazepine or 5 mg/kg phenytoin per day for adults.[13]

Other commonly effective drugs include topiramate and phenobarbitone. Interestingly, about 50% cases of women affected by PKD may note improvement in attack frequency during pregnancy.[14]

Paroxysmal Nonkinesigenic Dyskinesia

Paroxysmal nonkinesigenic dyskinesia (PNKD) like PKD causes periods of involuntary movements. PKND varies from PKD in terms of the duration and frequency of the attacks. PKD attacks occur daily but last only for few minutes. In contrast, PKND attacks occur few times (2-3) per year. And last for longer durations, about 1-4 hours.

Paroxysmal nonkinesigenic dyskinesia attacks are often preceded with premonitory symptoms such as tightness in one limb, involuntary movements of the mouth, and/or anxiety.[20] The movements often start from one side of the body before spreading to both sides. PKND attacks are not induced by sudden movements but rather by stress, fatigue, excitement, caffeine, or alcohol.[21] PKND forms have a childhood onset with a mean age of onset on 8 years. PKND is known to be caused by mutations in the *MR-1* gene. Genetic cases have shown a male to female ratio of 1:1 and sporadic cases a ratio of 2:1. Female patients may have a higher frequency of attacks during menstruation periods.

Pathophysiology: The pathophysiology of PNKD is not clear. Clinical, electrophysiological, imaging, and genetic studies have shed light on the same. Stress, tea, and alcohol are known to induce the episodes. Ictal and interictal EEGs are normal. However, video EEG has pointed to the involvement of the basal ganglia (caudate nuclei) in the pathophysiology. Cortical discharges are normal.[22] Ictal single-photon emission computed tomography (SPECT) studies indicated hyperperfusion of the right caudate and thalamus. Positron emission tomography (PET) studies have indicated reduced density of the presynaptic dopa decarboxylase activity in the striatum and increased density of the postsynaptic dopamine D2 receptors suggestive of chronic upregulation of postsynaptic dopa receptors.[23] Shen et al. have generated a mouse model of PNKD protein which revealed dysregulated dopamine signaling in vivo and showed that the PNKD interacts with presynaptic active zone proteins modulating neurotransmitter release.[24,25]

Treatment: Treatment of PNKD is limited and mainly aimed at avoiding the precipitating factors. Clonazepam is the drug of choice for the medical management. Drugs like haloperidol and gabapentin have been used occasionally.[20]

Paroxysmal Exercise-induced Dyskinesia

Paroxysmal exercise-induced dyskinesia is a rare form of paroxysmal movement disorder and less common than PKD and PNKD. It was first described by Lance in 1977.[9] As the name suggests, PED attacks are commonly triggered by exercises such as walking or running and in some cases exposure to cold. Rare cases have been described where passive movements, muscle vibration, and electric nerve stimulations have triggered attacks.[26] Unlike PKD, the movements are not triggered by sudden movements. The frequency of attacks varies and is dependent on the individuals physical exercise routine. On an average, the patients have 1–2 attacks per month. The attacks mostly last for 2–5 minutes on an average but can extend up to 2 hours and cease within 10 minutes after discontinuing the exercise.[27]

Dystonic movement bilaterally affecting both lower limbs and hemidystonia is the most common features.[26,27] Age of onset is mostly childhood but can range from 1–30 years. Familial and sporadic cases with autosomal dominant modes of inheritance are reported.[26] Rarely, PED presentation has been seen in idiopathic young-onset *PARKIN* Parkinson's disease patients.[28] PED has also been seen to be present in combination with rolandic epilepsy and writer's cramp (RE-PED-WC).[23]

Pathophysiology: Information about the pathophysiology of PED is limited and unclear. SPECT studies during motor attacks revealed reduced perfusion of the frontal cortex and basal ganglia and increased perfusion of the cerebellum, a SPECT pattern compatible with other forms of idiopathic and symptomatic forms of dystonia.[29] Postictal increases in homovanillic acid and 5-hydroxyindoleacetic in cerebrospinal fluid support the hypothesis of dopamine involvement in the pathophysiology of PED.[27] Recently, PED has been recognized as a result of mutations in the *GLUT1* gene.[30] Some familial cases were found to be associated with mutations in the *SLC2A1* gene. *SLC2A1* encodes the *GLUT1*. It has thus been proposed that an energy deficiency upon exertion caused by a reduced glucose transport rate is a cause of this paroxysmal movement disorder in *SLC2A1*-related cases.

Treatment: PED shows good response to benzodiazepines, levodopa, and acetazolamide but generally no response to antiepileptic drugs.

Secondary Cases of Paroxysmal Dyskinesias

Various neurological and non-neurological conditions can rarely present with PxDs. Most often, such cases are seen in adulthood and are associated with clinical or radiological clues to suggest their secondary nature. **Table 2** lists the common causes associated with secondary PxDs. Treatment of the underlying condition in addition to appropriate symptomatic treatment is necessary in such cases.

GENOTYPE PHENOTYPE CORRELATION

Elucidation of the genetic causes of PxDs has added a new dimension to the study of these disorders. The three primary PxDs (i.e., PKD, PNKD, and PED) have been related to mutations in the *PRRT2*,[31] *MR-1*,[32] and GLUT1 (*SLC2A1*)[30] genes, respectively. All groups show autosomal dominant pattern of inheritance. Recent genotype-phenotype studies reveal that there is marked pleiotropy of mutations in such genes with expanding clinical presentation and not all patients clinically presenting with either PKD, PNKD, or PED have mutations in these genes. Several new genes associated with PxDs have been identified recently. These include *ATP1A3*, *ADCY5*, *GCH1*, *PARK2*, *KCNMA1*, and *SLC16A2*.[33]

Considering these variables Erro et al. have recently described a reclassification of the PxDs and suggested an algorithm for genetic analysis.[12] **Table 3** lists the phenotypic expressions of PxDs associated genes.

TABLE 2: Common causes of secondary paroxysmal dyskinesia.

Etiological groups	*Common examples*
Immune-mediated	• Multiple sclerosis, acute disseminated encephalomyelitis, and • Hashimotos encephalopathy
Vascular	• TIAs, stroke, and Moyamoya disease
Metabolic	• Hypoglycemic/Hyperglycemic conditions • Hypocalcemia and parathyroid disorders • Hypo and hyperthyroidism
Post-traumatic	• Central trauma and peripheral trauma
Miscellaneous	• Basal ganglia calcifications • Central pontine myelinolysis • Kernicterus and encephalitis/postinfectious

(TIA: transient ischemic attack)

CELLULAR PATHOMECHANISMS OF PAROXYSMAL DYSKINESIAS

Located in human chromosome 16, *PRRT2* is the most common gene causing PKD. Most of the 70 different *PRRT2* PKD mutations are either nonsense or frameshift, causing degradation of the protein, leading to haploinsufficiency.[34] *PRRT2* gene encoded protein is widely expressed in the brain, particularly in the cerebellum, hippocampus, basal ganglia, and neocortex regions that are associated with the clinical phenotype.[34,35] *PRRT2* knockdown studies in mice suggested *PRRT2* as a presynaptic protein required for synchronous neurotransmitter release.[35] To understand the underlying disease mechanism, a recent study generated induced pluripotent stem (iPS) cell lines from skin fibroblast cells of PKD patients.[28] iPS cells can be differentiated to any desired cell type including neurons.[36] iPS cell lines were generated from three patients belonging to a consanguineous family, carrying the common c.649dupC mutation in homozygosity and heterozygosity and healthy control participants. This study showed that the loss of *PRRT2* protein in patient neurons leads causes

TABLE 3: Paroxysmal and nonparoxysmal phenomenology associated with various genes associated with paroxysmal dyskinesias.

Gene	Paroxysmal dyskinesia	Other paroxysmal disorders	Interictal abnormalities
PRRT2	PKD/PNKD/PED/ICCA/EA	BFIS/HM/FS/CAE	Cognitive deficiency
PNKD/MR1	PNKD	None	None
SLCA2A1	PED/PNKD/EA	Epilepsy/Migraine/Paroxysmal Drowsiness/Dysphoria/Pain	Microcephaly/Hypotonia/Dystonia/Chorea/Spasticity/ataxia/Cognitive deficiency
ATP1A3	PNKD/PED/EA	Epilepsy/Paroxysmal eye movements/Migraine	Cognitive deficiency/Dystonia/Chorea/Parkinsonism/Ataxia/Psychosis
ADCY5	PKD/PNKD/PED/Nocturnal PxDs	None	Dystonia/Chorea/Myoclonus/Tremor/Axial hypotonia/Orofacial myoclonus
GCH1	PED	Oculogyric crisis/RLS	General dystonia/Postural tremor/Parkinsonism/Axial hypotonia/Cerebellar features/Spastic paraperesis
PARK2	PED	None	Parkinsonism
KCNMA1	PNKD	Epilepsy	None
SLC16A2	PKD	Epilepsy	Cognitive disability/Hypotonia/Dystonia/Pyramidal signs/Pectus excavatum/Scoliosis

(BFIS: benign familial infantile seizures; CAE: childhood absence epilepsy; FS: febrile seizures; HM: hemiplegic migraine; RLS: restless legs syndrome)

hyperactivity of the voltage-dependent Na^+ channels that is essential for the rising phase of neuron action potential, thus influencing neuronal excitability. This understanding of the effect of *PRRT2* mutations in human neurons is essential to identify drug candidates that can rescue disease-specific neuronal defects in patients.

CONCLUSION

In summary the paroxysmal dyskinesias are a rare but interesting group of movement disorders that form a clinical link between non-movement disorders like epilepsy on one side and movement disorders like myoclonus on the other side. Repeated clinical examination supported by video documentation may be needed to come to a firm clinical diagnosis. Interestingly, a large number of these episodes are treatable with the use of anti-epileptic drugs. Recent genetic studies are shedding more light on the cause of these disorders and delineating them from their mimics. Cell based studies are likely to reveal their pathomechanism which in turn may lead to the development of newer strategies of management.

REFERENCES

1. Bhatia KP. Paroxysmal dyskinesias. Mov Disord. 2011;26(6):1157-65.
2. Blakeley J, Jankovic J. Secondary paroxysmal dyskinesias. Mov Disord. 2002;17:726-34.
3. Bhatia K, Schneider S. Chapter 28 Paroxysmal Dyskinesias. 2010.
4. Kato N, Sadamatsu M, Kikuchi T, Niikawa N, Fukuyama Y. Paroxysmal kinesigenic choreoathetosis: From first discovery in 1892 to genetic linkage with benign familial infantile convulsions. Epilepsy Res. 2006;70:174-84.
5. Gowers WR. Epilepsy and other chronic convulsive diseases: their causes, symptoms, and treatment. New York: William Wood & Company; 1901.
6. Mount LA, Reback S. Familial paroxysmal choreoathetosis: Preliminary Report on a Hitherto Undescribed Clinical Syndrome. Arch Neur Psych. 1940;44(4):841-7.
7. Kertesz A. Paroxysmal kinesigenic choreoathetosis. Neurology. 1967;17:680.
8. Weber MB. Familial paroxysmal dystonia. J Nerv Ment Dis. 1967;145(3):221-6.
9 Lance JW. Familial paroxysmal dystonic choreoathetosis and its differentiation from related syndromes. Ann Neurol. 1977;2(4):285-93.
10. Demirkiran M, Jankovic J. Paroxysmal dyskinesias: Clinical features and classification. Ann Neurol. 1995;38(4):571-9.
11. Sohn YH, Lee PH. Hyperkinetic Movement Disorders. In: Weiner W, Tolosa E (eds). Handbook of Clinical Neurology, 1st edition. Elsevier; 2011. pp. 367-73.
12. Erro R, Sheerin UM, Bhatia KP. Paroxysmal dyskinesias revisited: A review of 500 genetically proven cases and a new classification. Mov Disord. 2014;29(9):1108-16.
13. Gardiner AR, Jaffer F, Dale RC, Labrum R, Erro R, Meyer E, et al. The clinical and genetic heterogeneity of paroxysmal dyskinesias. Brain. 2015;138(12):3567-80.

14. Houser MK, Soland VL, Bhatia KP, Quinn NP, Marsden CD. Paroxysmal kinesigenic choreoathetosis: a report of 26 patients. J Neurol. 1999;246(2):120-6.
15. Bruno MK, Hallett M, Gwinn-Hardy K, Sorensen B, Considine E, Tucker S, et al. Clinical evaluation of idiopathic paroxysmal kinesigenic dyskinesia: new diagnostic criteria. Neurology. 2004;63(12):2280-7.
16. Valente EM, Spacey SD, Wali GM, Bhatia KP, Dixon PH, Wood NW, et al. A second paroxysmal kinesigenic choreoathetosis locus (EKD2) mapping on 16q13-q22.1 indicates a family of genes which give rise to paroxysmal disorders on human chromosome 16. Brain. 2000;123:2040-5.
17. Gardiner AR, Bhatia KP, Stamelou M, Dale RC, Kurian MA, Schneider SA, et al. PRRT2 gene mutations: From paroxysmal dyskinesia to episodic ataxia and hemiplegic migraine. Neurology. 2012;79(21):2115-21.
18. Lishman WA, Symonds CP, Whitty CW, Willison RG. Seizures induced by movement. Brain. 1962;85:93-108.
19. Sadamatsu M, Masui A, Sakai T, Kunugi H, Nanko S, Kato N. Familial paroxysmal kinesigenic choreoathetosis: an electrophysiologic and genotypic analysis. Epilepsia. 1999;40(7):942-9.
20. Bruno MK, Lee HY, Auburger GW, Friedman A, Nielsen JE, Lang AE, et al. Genotype–phenotype correlation of paroxysmal nonkinesigenic dyskinesia. Neurology. 2007;68(21):1782-9.
21. Bressman SB, Fahn S, Burke RE. Paroxysmal non-kinesigenic dystonia. Adv Neurol. 1988;50:403-13.
22. Lombroso CT, Fischman A. Paroxysmal non-kinesigenic dyskinesia: pathophysiological investigations. Epileptic Disord. 1999;1(3):187-94.
23. García MC, Intruvini S, Vazquez S, Beserra F, Rabinowicz AL. Ictal SPECT in paroxysmal non-kinesigenic dyskinesia. Case report and review of the literature. Parkinsonism Relat Disord. 2000;6(2):119-21.
24. Plant GT, Williams AC, Earl CJ, Marsden CD. Familial paroxysmal dystonia induced by exercise. J Neurol Neurosurg Psychiatry. 1984;47(3):275-9.
25. Shen Y, Ge WP, Li Y, Hirano A, Lee HY, Rohlmann A, et al. Protein mutated in paroxysmal dyskinesia interacts with the active zone protein RIM and suppresses synaptic vesicle exocytosis. Proc Natl Acad Sci USA. 2015;112(10):2935-41.
26. Bhatia KP, Soland VL, Bhatt MH, Quinn NP, Marsden CD. Paroxysmal exercise-induced dystonia: Eight new sporadic cases and a review of the literature. Mov Disord. 1997;12(6): 1007-12.
27. Bhatia KP. The paroxysmal dyskinesias. J Neurol. 1999;246: 149-55.
28. Fruscione F, Valente P, Sterlini B, Romei A, Baldassari S, Fadda M, et al. PRRT2 controls neuronal excitability by negatively modulating Na+ channel 1.2/1.6 activity. Brain. 2018;141(4):1000-16.
29. Kluge A, Kettner B, Zschenderlein R, Sandrock D, Munz DL, Hesse S, et al. Changes in perfusion pattern using ECD-SPECT indicate frontal lobe and cerebellar involvement in exercise-induced paroxysmal dystonia. Mov Disord. 1998;13(1): 125-34.
30. Suls A, Dedeken P, Goffin K, Van Esch H, Dupont P, Cassiman D, et al. Paroxysmal exercise-induced dyskinesia and epilepsy is due to mutations in SLC2A1, encoding the glucose transporter GLUT1. Brain. 2008;131(6):1831-44.
31. Chen WJ, Lin Y, Xiong ZQ, Wei W, Ni W, Tan GH, et al. Exome sequencing identifies truncating mutations in PRRT2 that cause paroxysmal kinesigenic dyskinesia. Nat Genet. 2011;43(12):1252-5.
32. Rainier S, Thomas D, Tokarz D, Ming L, Bui M, Plein E, et al. Myofibrillogenesis Regulator 1 Gene Mutations Cause Paroxysmal Dystonic Choreoathetosis. Arch Neurol. 2004;61(7): 1025-9.
33. Méneret A, Roze E. Paroxysmal movement disorders: An update. Rev Neurol (Paris). 2016;172:433-45.
34. Wu L, Tang HD, Huang XJ, Zheng L, Liu XL, Wang T,. et al. PRRT2 truncated mutations lead to nonsense-mediated mRNA decay in Paroxysmal Kinesigenic Dyskinesia. Parkinsonism Relat Disord. 2014;20(12):1399-404.
35. Valente P, Castroflorio E, Rossi P, Fadda M, Sterlini B, Cervigni RI, et al. PRRT2 Is a Key Component of the Ca^{2+}-Dependent Neurotransmitter Release Machinery. Cell Rep. 2016;15(1): 117-31.
36. Takahashi K, Tanabe K, Ohnuki M, Narita M, Ichisaka T, Tomoda K, et al. Induction of Pluripotent Stem Cells from Adult Human Fibroblasts by Defined Factors. Cell. 2007;131(5):861-72.

CHAPTER 34

Treatment of Dystonia

Utkarsh Patel, Charulata Savant Sankhla, Sanjay Pandey

INTRODUCTION

Dystonia is currently defined as a neurological syndrome characterized by involuntary, sustained, patterned and often repetitive muscle contraction of opposing muscle, causing twisting movements or abnormal postures.[1] Owing to the lack of curative therapy, the aim of currently available treatment is largely symptomatic relief. The approach is primarily aimed at improving abnormal postures and pain reduction, thereby leading to enhanced quality of life. There is a three-pronged approach of management, which includes the following: Pharmacological therapy, chemodenervation, and surgical intervention (**Flowchart 1**).

PHARMACOLOGICAL TREATMENT

Three main neurotransmitter systems (**Fig. 1**), namely cholinergic, GABAergic, and dopaminergic are critical in the medical treatment of dystonia.[2]

Medications Primarily Affecting the Cholinergic System

There are giant aspiny interneurons that release acetylcholine.[2] They constitute up to 3% of all striatal cells.[2] They act as tonically active neurons having the property of autonomous firing without synaptic activity.[3]

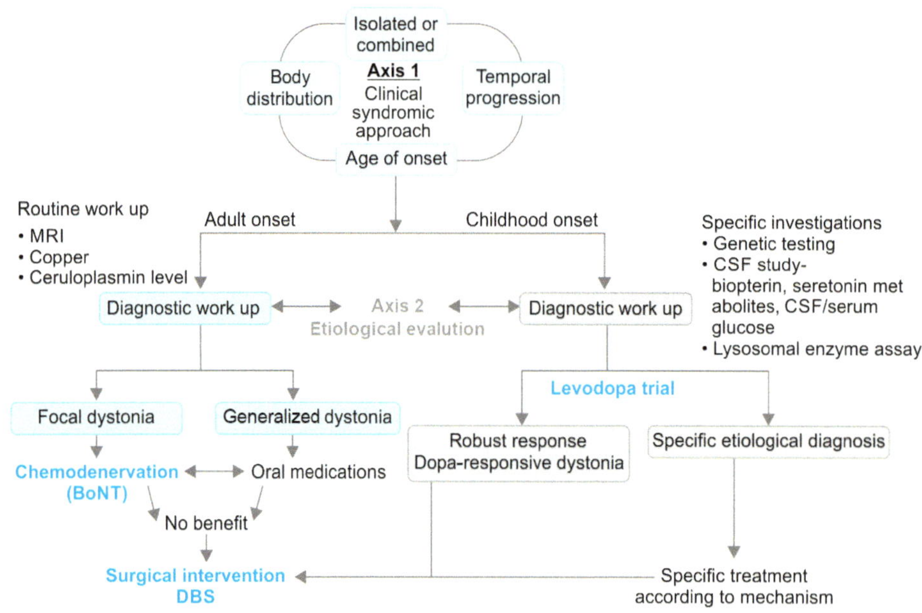

(BoNT: botulinum neurotoxin; CSF: cerebrospinal fluid; DBS: deep brain stimulation; MRI: magnetic resonance imaging)

FLOWCHART 1: Approach to diagnosis and management of dystonia.

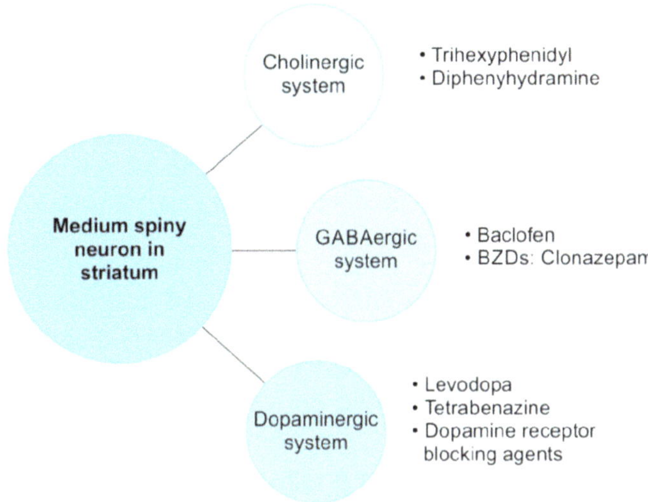

(BZDs: benzodiazepines)

FIG. 1: Major neurotransmitter systems involved in the mechanism of dystonia and drugs acting on each system.

Anticholinergic Agents

Anticholinergic medications such as trihexyphenidyl act as antagonists at postsynaptic M1 receptors and decrease hyperactivity of cholinergic interneurons.[2] Anticholinergics are considered as first-line treatment in patients with generalized dystonia.[4] These drugs might also be helpful in patients with acute dystonic reactions and tardive dystonia.[5]

Trihexyphenidyl has shown benefit in the treatment of dystonia in a prospective double-blinded study.[6] It is considered first-line therapy for dystonic tremors.[7] It is usually started at a dose of 1 mg at bedtime and slowly increased in increments of 1–2 mg every 7 days to a maximum of 100 mg/day in 3–4 divided doses.[4] Typical therapeutic doses range from 4 to 40 mg/day while children may tolerate higher doses up to 100 mg/day.[4]

Common peripheral side effects are dry mouth, urinary retention, constipation, and blurry vision. Potential central side effects are confusion, hallucination, memory impairment, and fatigue.[8] Therefore, starting a low dose of anticholinergic drugs and titrating slowly over several weeks often minimizes the adverse effects and improves tolerability.[9]

Medications Primarily Affecting the GABAergic System

Gamma-aminobutyric acid (GABA) is an inhibitory neurotransmitter in the brain and spinal cord. In patients with primary dystonia, abnormal $GABA_A$ receptor binding is seen in the motor cortex, which leads to sensory and motor disinhibition.[2]

Benzodiazepines

Benzodiazepines such as diazepam, clonazepam, lorazepam, and midazolam bind to $GABA_A$ receptors and increase the frequency of the opening of chloride channels which leads to the facilitation of inhibitory signal.[2] These drugs are used as the off-label treatment agents of dystonia by their property of muscle relaxation, although their usefulness is limited by potential adverse effects such as drowsiness and addiction. Retrospective studies have shown good results in tremor-predominant forms of dystonia, myoclonus dystonia, and blepharospasm.[4] Clonazepam is useful in the treatment of paroxysmal nonkinesigenic dyskinesia.[4] It has been shown to have benefit in 21% of patients with cervical dystonia at doses ranging from 1.5 to 12 mg/day in a retrospective study.[7]

Baclofen

Baclofen is a $GABA_B$ receptor agonist which acts at the presynaptic terminal of excitatory glutamatergic neurons and the postsynaptic sites of inhibitory interneurons in the spinal cord.[10] It can be used to reduce dystonic movements in some patients with dystonia, particularly in patients with oromandibular dystonia, and dystonic-choreoathetosis cerebral palsy with hypertonia or spasticity.[11] The data on the use of intrathecal and intraventricular baclofen infusions in patients with dystonia is reported more than the use of oral baclofen.[12]

The starting dose is 5–10 mg/day in 2–3 divided doses to be increased by 5 mg every 7 days to a maximum dose of 40 mg 3 times a day. Common side effects are sedation, dizziness, impaired coordination, fatigue, and weakness.[4] A slow taper off of the drug is advisable to avoid any withdrawal reactions such as seizure, rebound muscle rigidity, hyperpyrexia, and rhabdomyolysis.

Dopaminergic System

Levodopa

Levodopa/carbidopa is the standard of care for dopa-responsive dystonia.[4] The pathophysiological mechanisms involved in other dystonia are not based on pathways of dopamine biosynthesis and, hence, levodopa has a little benefit.[13]

It is usually started at a lower dose of 25–50 mg/day. A very good response is seen at doses ranging from 200 to 300 mg/day. A maximum dose of 600–1,000 mg/day may be tried in rare nonresponsive cases.[4] It may be used in other forms of primary dystonia, however, the response is not as dramatic as seen in dopa-responsive dystonia. If there is no improvement with a dose of 600 mg/day for 4 weeks, the drug can be stopped.

Dopamine Depleting Agents

Dopamine-depleting drugs that act by inhibiting vesicular monoamine transporter-2 (VMAT2) such as tetrabenazine, deutetrabenazine and valbenazine which are primarily used in the treatment of chorea, tics, and tardive dyskinesia might also have clinical efficacy in patients with dystonia, particularly those with tardive dystonia.[14]

A retrospective study reported that almost 70% of patients with tardive dystonia have moderate to excellent responses to the drug.[15] It has also shown some efficacy in patients with myoclonic dystonia in one case report.[15] Dosing usually begins with 12.5 mg and is slowly titrated by 12.5 mg dose every 5 days to a maximum of 100 mg/day in 3–4 divided doses.[4] Common side effects are sedation, depression, Parkinsonism, akathisia, and insomnia. Patients with depression should not receive this drug as there are higher chances of suicidal tendencies.[16]

Reserpine is another dopamine depleting agent which has an additional property of irreversible inhibition of peripheral VMAT1, leading to peripheral side effects such as dizziness and gastrointestinal upset.[4] Because of this, tetrabenazine is preferred over reserpine for the treatment of dystonia.

Dopamine Receptor Blocking Agents (Antipsychotics)

Typical antipsychotics have not been adequately studied as a treatment of dystonia. One open-label study has shown good response in 35% of the 26 patients treated chronically.[6] Common side effects are drug-induced Parkinsonism and tardive dyskinesia.

Atypical antipsychotics including clozapine and quetiapine may be useful in generalized dystonia and craniofacial dystonia.[17] Common side effects of clozapine are agranulocytosis, sedation, diabetes, and a lower threshold for seizures (**Table 1**).

CHEMODENERVATION: BOTULINUM NEUROTOXIN

Botulinum neurotoxin (BoNTs) is considered as first-line therapy for most patients with focal and segmental

TABLE 1: Some inherited dystonia with specific treatment available.

Disorder	*Clinical feature*	*Treatment*
Dopa-responsive dystonia-classic (*DYT-5A*)	• GCH-1 deficiency • Early childhood lower limb onset • Diurnal variations	Low dose levodopa/carbidopa (50–100 mg/day)
Dopa-responsive dystonia-complex (*DYT-5B*)	• TH and SRP deficiency • Infancy onset complex phenotype • Dystonia, Parkinsonism, autonomic disturbances	Levodopa/carbidopa + 5 hydroxytryptophan/ tetrahydrobiopterin
Glucose transporter type 1 deficiency	• Childhood-onset • Seizures, paroxysmal exertional dystonia	Ketogenic diet
Biotin-thiamine-responsive basal ganglia disorder	• Childhood-onset • Encephalopathy with generalized dystonia	Biotin and thiamine supplement
Wilson disease	• *ATP7B defect* • Early childhood-adulthood onset • Progressive dystonia, neuropsychiatric features, KF ring	Penicillamine, trientine, and zinc
Abetalipoproteinemia	• MTTP defect • Childhood-onset ataxia, chorea, oromandibular dystonia, and retinitis pigmentosa	Vitamin E and reduce fat diet
Aromatic L amino acid decarboxylase deficiency	• Infancy onset • Motor delay with dystonia and autonomic disturbance	Dopamine agonist and monoamine oxidase inhibitors partially help
Glutaric aciduria type 1	• GCDH deficiency • Early childhood onset encephalopathy with progressive dystonia	Lysine restriction can prevent crisis
Neurodegeneration with brain iron accumulation	• PKAN, INAD, FHAN ,BPAN, PLA2G6 • Early childhood onset • Delayed motor milestone, dystonia, Parkinsonism, and spasticity	Early iron chelation may help
Coenzyme Q10 deficiency	• Any age • Encephalopathy, seizure, and dystonia	Coenzyme Q10

(GCDH: glutaryl-CoA dehydrogenase; GCH1: GTP cyclohydrolase 1; MTTP: microsomal triglyceride transfer protein; SRP: signal recognition particle; TH: tyrosine hydroxylase)

dystonia.[4] BoNTs are derived from the bacterium *Clostridium botulinum*. It blocks the vesicular release of acetylcholine into the neuromuscular junction which leads to a decrease in involuntary activity.[18] Out of seven distinct serotypes that exist (A to G), each of which is composed of a 100 kDa heavy chain and a 50 kDa light chain.[19] Only type A and type B are used commercially. BoNT acts by the principle that its heavy chain binds to peripheral cholinergic nerve terminals and facilitates endocytosis of BoNT, following which the light chain is released into the cytoplasm and cleaves the soluble *N*-ethylmaleimide sensitive factor activating protein receptor (SNARE) proteins that are required for synaptic transmission.[19]

There are four United States Food and Drug Administration approved preparations of BoNT:

1. Onabotulinumtoxin A (onaBoNT-A): Botox©
2. Abobotulinumtoxin A (aboBoNT-A): Dysport©
3. Incobotulinumtoxin A (incoBoNT-A): Xeomine©
4. Rimabotulinumtoxin B (rimaBoNT-B): Myobloc©

There are important pharmacological differences between various BoNT preparations.[18] They differ in potency and duration of action.[18] Benefits occur after 2–7 days and last for an average of 3 months.[18]

Cranial Dystonia

Blepharospasm

Botulinum neurotoxin is considered the first-line treatment of blepharospasm.[18] OnaBoNT-A (two-class II studies) and incoBoNT-A (one class I study) injections should be considered (Level B) and aboBoNT-A may be considered (Level C) in the treatment of blepharospasm.[18] The average starting dose per eye amounts to 20 units of onaBoNT-A which is divided into four portions that are injected into the orbital portion of the orbicularis oculi around the eye.[20] If injections are placed in the pretarsal portion of the orbicularis oculis muscle with an expected success rate approaching 100%.[21]

Oromandibular Dystonia

Oromandibular dystonia can be jaw-closing, jaw-opening, or jaw-deviation dystonia. For jaw-closing dystonia, masseter and temporalis muscle is injected. The average starting dose for each muscle is around 20–25 units of onaBoNT-A.[20] For jaw opening dystonia the external (lateral) pterygoid is treated with an average starting dose of 15 units of onaBoNT-A and for the digastricus, a dose of 10 units of onaBoNT-A is normally used.[20]

Orofacial and Lingual Dystonia

Orofacial dystonia occurring with blepharospasm is known as Meige syndrome. Under electromyography (EMG) guidance, the zygomaticus major and minor, the orbicularis oris, and the buccinators are treated with an average starting dose of 5 units of onaBoNT-A for each muscle.[20] In lingual dystonia, an average starting dose of 10 units of onaBoNT-A is injected into the intrinsic tongue muscles.

Cervical Dystonia

AboBoNT-A (two class I studies) and rimaBoNT-B (three class I studies) are established as safe and effective for the treatment of cervical dystonia (Level A).[18] OnaBoNT-A (one class I and one class II study) and rimaBoNT-B (one class I study) are probably safe and effective (Level B).[18] OnaBoNT-A and rimaBoNT-B are equivalent in efficacy (two-class I comparative effectiveness studies).[18] However, there are heterogeneous outcomes noted due to differences in muscle selection, BoNT dilution and dosing, and targeting techniques (whether to use EMG or ultrasound guidance) which vary significantly among different centers.[22]

Spasmodic Dysphonia

Spasmodic dysphonia can either be adductor or abductor type. In an adductor type of spasmodic dysphonia, there is hyperadduction of vocal folds during speaking, which produces a "strain-strangled" voice. OnaBoNT-A in a dosage of 0.9 unit/0.1 mL per vocal fold is injected in bilateral thyroarytenoid muscle via a hollow-bore teflon coated EMG needle with EMG control.[20] In the abductor type, there are irregular and inappropriate abductor spasms occurring during speaking which produces breathy breaks or whispering. Posterior cricoarytenoid muscle (PCA), being the only abductor of vocal cords, is treated initially only on one side. It is injected with an average dose of 3.75 unit/0.15 mL of onaBoNT-A.[20] After 2 weeks, if the voice still has whispering quality then the contralateral PCA is injected with a dose ranging from 0.6 to 2.5 unit/0.1 mL under EMG control.[20]

Focal Hand Dystonia

For focal hand dystonia, injection of BoNT into the muscles responsible for the abnormal postures can be very effective and is often considered as the first choice.[20] There has been one class I double-blind, randomized, placebo-controlled trial that used aboBoNT-A.[23] 14 of the 20 patients receiving BoNT-A reported a beneficial effect as compared to 6 of the 19 patients in the placebo group. There have been three class II double-blind trials demonstrating efficacy with onaBoNT-A.[24-26] It's utility in musician's cramps has also been demonstrated.

After long-term treatment with onaBoNT/A, only <2% of the patients were positive for neutralizing antibodies which is a theoretical possibility that is considered exceptional.[27]

Role of Transmagnetic Stimulation

Transmagnetic stimulation enhances intracortical inhibition, a neural process deemed to be altered in dystonia. Cumulative effects can be obtained by repeated stimulation over consecutive days than single-session studies.[28]

SURGICAL THERAPIES

Ablative Procedures

Pallidotomy and thalamotomy, which were commonly used for the treatment of dystonia in the past, have been essentially completely replaced by deep brain stimulation (DBS).[13]

Deep Brain Stimulation

Deep brain stimulation has great potential for different dystonia syndromes, whether idiopathic or inherited, isolated or combined.[29] It has emerged as the most effective therapy for patients with medically refractory disabling dystonia in both generalized and severe segmental and focal dystonia.[13] The two main targets of stimulation are the globus pallidus internal (GPi) and, more recently, the subthalamic nucleus (STN) for treatment of dystonia owing to their involvement in the control of motor function.[30] The most frequent complication associated with GPi DBS is dysarthria but Parkinsonism has also been observed in some patients.[31] With STN DBS the complications noted are chorea, worsened handwriting, weight gain, dysarthria, shoulder pain, and depression.[32] Complications common to both the targets include incoordination, paresthesia's and perioral tingling, whereas the hardware-related complications were infection, hematoma, and wire displacement that are reported.[33] Bilateral GPi DBS in patients with tardive dystonia has shown marked benefit with long-term follow-up.[34] DBS outcomes are influenced by several features such as body distribution, age of onset, and by the relative prevalence of dystonic movements or postures. Favorable outcomes are seen in dystonia associated with *TOR1A*, *KMT2B*, and *SGCE* mutations.[13] Therefore, the genetic status is also important with two extremes represented by *DYT1* dystonia showing consistently excellent outcome and *DYT12* dystonia has lack of efficacy to DBS.

Magnetic Resonance Imaging-guided Focused Ultrasound

It uses ultrasonic energy that is delivered to a brain target without the need for an incision or burrhole in the skull. The lesion is monitored in real-time by magnetic resonance imaging (MRI) thermometry which is an advantage over radiofrequency-based lesioning without hardware-related complications.[35] Whether focused ultrasound of the thalamus will have utility in the treatment of dystonia is unknown, but it has been reported to be effective in the treatment of essential tremor and Parkinson's disease.[36]

Physical Treatments

Different rehabilitation strategies have been combined with BoNT to improve disability and pain in patients with dystonia.[37]

Complications of Dystonia

Dystonic storm, also referred to as status dystonicus, is a movement disorder emergency that is a very rare complication of generalized dystonia commonly encountered in the pediatric population.[38] Triggering factors may be intercurrent infection and fever, discontinuation or rapid change in treatments, surgery, or trauma.[38] It can be managed by controlling the triggering factors and the use of monotherapy or polytherapy with oral agents such as anticholinergics, tetrabenazine, clonidine, and baclofen. Intravenous medications such as midazolam, propofol, and non-depolarizing neuromuscular blockers should be considered as supportive options. In severe cases, the use of DBS targeting the GPi as effective rescue therapy and an intrathecal baclofen pump should also be considered.[13]

CONCLUSION

Management of dystonia includes pharmacotherapy with anticholinergic drugs, medications affecting GABAergic and dopaminergic system. Chemodenervation by botulinum toxin injections is a preferred treatment for focal dystonia. Surgical treatment is preferred in the generalized dystonia patients with a known favourable outcome and in focal dystonia patients who respond poorly to pharmacotherapy and chemodenervation.

REFERENCES

1. Albanese A, Bhatia K, Bressman SB, Delong MR, Fahn S, Fung VS, et al. Phenomenology and classification of dystonia: a consensus update. Mov Disord. 2013;28(7):863-73.
2. Termsarasab P, Thammongkolchai T, Frucht SJ. Medical treatment of dystonia. J Clin Mov Disord. 2016;3:19.
3. Benarroch EE. Effects of acetylcholine in the striatum. Recent insights and therapeutic implications. Neurology. 2012;79(3): 274-81.
4. Shanker V, Bressman SB. Diagnosis and management of dystonia. Continuum (Minneap Minn). 2016;22(4):1227-45.

5. Vijayakumar D, Jankovic J. Drug-induced dyskinesia, part 2: treatment of tardive dyskinesia. Drugs. 2016;76(7): 779-87.
6. Burke RE, Fahn S, Marsden CD. Torsion dystonia: a double blind, prospective trial of high-dosage trihexyphenidyl. Neurology. 1986;36(2):160-4.
7. Fasano A, Bove F, Lang AE. The treatment of dystonic tremor: a systemic review. J Neurol Neurosurg Psychiatry. 2014;85(7); 759-69.
8. Lumsden DE, Kaminska M, Tomlin S, Lin JP. Medication use in childhood dystonia. Eur J Paediatr Neurol. 2016;20(4): 625-9.
9. Alfradique-Dunham I, Jankovic J. Available treatment options for dystonia. Expert Opin Orphan Drugs. 2017;5(9):707-16.
10. Termsarasab P, Thammongkolchai T, Frucht SJ. Spinal-generated movement disorders: a clinical review. J Clin Mov Disord. 2015;2:18.
11. Monbaliu E, Himmelmann K, Lin JP, Ortibus E, Bonouvrié L, Feys H, et al. Clinical presentation and management of dyskinetic cerebral palsy. Lancet Neurol. 2017;16(9):741-9.
12. Motta F, Antonello CE. Analysis of complications in 430 consecutive pediatric patients treated with intrathecal baclofen therapy: 14-year experience. J Neurosurg Pediatr. 2014;13(3):301-6.
13. Balint B, Mencacci NE, Valente EM, Pisani A, Rothwell J, Jankovic J, et al. Author Correction: Dystonia. Nat Rev Dis Primers. 2018;4(1):37.
14. Solmi M, Pigato G, Kane JM, Correll CU. Treatment of tardive dyskinesia with VMAT-2 inhibitors: a systematic review and meta-analysis of randomized controlled trials. Drug Des Devel Ther. 2018;12:1215-38.
15. Kenney C, Hunter C, Jankovic J. Long-term tolerability of tetrabenazine in the treatment of hyperkinetic movement disorder. Mov Disord. 2007;22(2):193-7.
16. Jankovic J. Dopamine depleters in the treatment of hyper-kinetic movement disorders. Expert Opin Pharmacother. 2016; 17(18):2461-70.
17. Karp BI, Goldstein SR, Chen R, Samii A, Bara-Jimenez W, Hallett M. An open trial of clozapine for dystonia. Mov Disord. 1999;14(4):652-7.
18. Simpson DM, Hallett M, Ashman EJ, Comella CL, Green MW, Gronseth GS, et al. Practice guideline updates summary: botulinum neurotoxin for treatment of blepharospasm, cervical dystonia, adult spasticity and headache: Report of the Guideline Development Subcommittee of the American Academy of Neurology. Neurology. 2016;86(19):1818-26.
19. Pirazzini M, Rossetto O, Eleopra R, Montecucco C. Botulinum neurotoxins: biology, pharmacology, and toxicology. Pharmacol Rev. 2017;69(2):200-35.
20. Hallett M, Benecke R, Blitzer A, Comella CL. Treatment of focal dystonia with botulinum neurotoxin. Toxicon. 2009;54 (5):628-33.
21. Cakmur R, Ozturk V, Uzunel F, Donmez B, Idiman F. Comparison of preseptal and pretarsal injections of botulinum toxin in the treatment of blepharospasm and hemifacial spasm. J Neurol. 2002;249(1):64-8.
22. Albanese A, Abbruzzese G, Dressler D, Duzynski W, Khatkova S, Marti MJ, et al. Practical guidance for CD management involving treatment of botulinum toxin: a consensus statement. J Neurol. 2015;262(10):2201-13.
23. Kruisdijk JJM, Koelman JH, Ongerboer de Visser BW, de Haan RJ, Speelman JD. Botulinum toxin for writer's cramp: a randomised, placebo-controlled trial and 1-year follow-up. J Neurol Neurosurg Psychiatry. 2007;78(3):264-70.
24. Cole RA, Cohen LG, Hallett M. Treatment of musician's cramp with botulinum toxin. Med Probl Perform Art. 1991;6:137-43.
25. Tsui JK, Bhatt M, Calne S, Calne DB. Botulinum toxin in the treatment of writer's cramp: a double-blind study. Neurology. 1993;43(1):183-5.
26. Yoshimura DM, Aminoff MJ, Olney RK. Botulinum toxin therapy for limb dystonias. Neurology. 1992;42(3):627-30.
27. Naumann M, Carruthers A, Carruthers J, Aurora SK, Zafonte R, Abu-Shakra S, et al. Meta-analysis of neutralizing antibody conversion with onabotulinum toxinA (BOTOX®) across multiple indications. Mov Disord. 2010;25(13):2211-8.
28. Erro R, Tinazzi M, Morgante F, Bhatia KP. Non-invasive brain stimulation for dystonia: therapeutic implications. Eur J Neurol. 2017;24(10):1228-e64.
29. Albanese A, Di Giovanni M, Lalli S. Dystonia: diagnosis and management. Eur J Neurol. 2019;26(1):5-17.
30. Moro E, LeReun C, Krauss JK, Albanese A, Lin JP, Walleser Autiero S, et al. Efficacy of pallidal stimulation in isolated dystonia: a systematic review and meta-analysis. Eur J Neurol. 2017;24(4):552-60.
31. Schrader C, Capelle HH, Kinfe TM, Blahak C, Bäzner H, Lütjens G, et al. GPi-DBS may induce a hypokinetic gait disorder with freezing of gait in patients with dystonia. Neurology. 2011;77(5):483-8.
32. Mills KA, Scherzer R, Starr PA, Ostrem JL. Weight change after globus pallidus internus or subthalamic nucleus deep brain stimulation in Parkinson's disease and dystonia. Stereotact Funct Neurosurg. 2012;90(6):386-93.
33. BaizabalCarvallo JF, Mostile G, Almaguer M, Davidson A, Simpson R, Jankovic J. Deep brain stimulation hardware complications in patients with movement disorders: risk factors and clinical correlations. Stereotact Funct Neurosurg. 2012;90(5):300-6.
34. Pouclet-Courtemanche H, Rouaud T, Thobois S, Nguyen JM, Brefel-Courbon C, Chereau I, et al. Long-term efficacy and tolerability of bilateral pallidal stimulation to treat tardive dyskinesia. Neurology. 2016;86(7):651-9.
35. Fishman PS, Frenkel V. Treatment of Movement Disorders with Focused Ultrasound. J Cent Nerv Syst Dis. 2017;9: 1179573517705670.
36. Dallapiazza RF, Timbie KF, Holmberg S, Gatesman J, Lopes MB, Price RJ, et al. Noninvasive neuromodulation and thalamic mapping with low-intensity focused ultrasound. J Neurosurg. 2018;128(3):875-84.
37. Contarino MF, Smit M, van den Dool J, Volkmann J, Tijssen MA. Unmet needs in the management of cervical dystonia. Front Neurol. 2016;7:165.
38. Allen NM, Lin JP, Lynch T, King MD. Status dystonicus: a practice guide. Dev Med Child Neurol. 2014;56(2):105-12.

CHAPTER 35

Tics, Tourette's Syndrome, and Stereotypy

Shivam Om Mittal

TICS AND TOURETTE'S SYNDROME

INTRODUCTION

In 1885, the French neurologist Gilles de la Tourette, working under the supervision of Prof Jean Martin Charcot, described a neurological condition that he described as "*maladie des tics*". The article was based on the observation of nine individuals with features of childhood-onset, hereditability, waxing and waning severity of symptoms, and premonitory urge.[1] Tics are defined as sudden, rapid, recurrent, nonrhythmic motor movements or vocalization, generally preceded by urge. Tics are frequently observed in the pediatric population and the frequency is higher (27%) in special education populations, compared with 19.7% in a general education sample.[2] In a meta-analysis of 14 studies including 420,312 subjects, Tourette's syndrome (TS) was found to have prevalence of 1%.[3]

The most widely accepted criteria are those formulated for TS by the fifth edition of the Diagnostic and Statistical Manual of Mental Disorders (DSM-V).[4]

- Both multiple motor and one or more vocal tics are present at sometime during the illness, although not necessarily concurrently.
- The tics may wax or wane in frequency but have persisted for >1 year since first tic onset.
- Onset is before age 18 years.
- The disturbance is not attributable to the physiologic effects of a substance (e.g., cocaine) or a general medical condition (e.g., Huntington's disease and postviral encephalitis).

Patients are labelled as chronic single tic disorder or chronic multiple tic disorder if an individual exhibit one or multiple motor tic for >1 year. The most common and mildest of the idiopathic tic disorders is the transient tic disorder (TTD) of childhood. This can be differentiated from TS as TTD does not last for >1-year.

CLINICAL FEATURES

Proper history and phenomenology is the key for correct diagnosis. Although it can be challenging to differentiate between tics and other hyperkinetic disorder. Based on their phenomenology, Jankovic classified motor tics into the following: (1) Clonic, when tics involve only a single muscle or a group of muscles, causing a brief, jerking movement; (2) dystonic, when tics are slower, causing a briefly sustained abnormal posture; and (3) tonic, when tics reflect an isometric contraction, typically manifesting with a brief tension of abdominal or limb muscles.[5] Examples include blinking, eye rolling, head nodding, shoulder shrugging, and abdominal tightening. Dystonic tics include oculogyric movements, sustained mouth opening, blepharospasm, and torticollis. Complex motor tics represent more intricate co-ordinated patterns of movement involving more than one muscle group. Bending, jumping, kicking, spitting, smelling, obscene gestures (copropraxia), and elaborate repertoires of movement are examples. Phonic tics are irrelevant sounds such as sniffing, coughing, throat clearing, clicks, humming, animal sounds, or whistling. Complex phonic tics are more involved utterances including words, phrases, profanity, or racial slurs (coprolalia), repetition of others' words (echolalia), or repetition of one's own words (palilalia). The differential includes myoclonus, dystonia, athetosis, mannerisms, chorea, stereotypies, restless leg syndrome, or seizures. Sensory phenomenon of urge with improvement after the movement can also be seen in akathisia stereotypy, restless leg syndrome, and dystonia. All the hyperkinetic disorders, especially akathisia and psychogenic movements, can be suppressed but less than tics. If the movements are multifocal or they migrate, consider myoclonus and chorea as well. Tics may sometimes persist during sleep and sleep disorders can be seen in patients with tics.

Motor Symptoms

The Tourette International Consortium reported the characteristics of TS patients in a large population where the age of symptom onset ranged from 2 to 21 years, with a mean of 6.4 years and male to female ratio of 4.4:1.[6,7] The tics are most severe at 10–12 years of age and eventually improves by adolescence in about 85% of the subjects.[8,9] In another study, tics resolved completely in 50% of the patients while 40–45% patients had improvement in tics by adulthood and only 5–10% of patients continued to have tics.[10]

CLINICAL PEARLS

- Tics are sudden, repetitive, stereotyped, and nonrhythmic movements which are commonly seen in childhood.
- Tics can be either motor or phonic depending on the symptoms. Motor tics are restricted to body movements such as head jerking or facial grimacing or hand movements, etc. Phonic tics are due to repetitive movements of laryngeal, pharyngeal, nasal, or respiratory muscles.
- Tics are characterized by premonitory urge prior to the motor or phonic tic with temporary relief in the urge by the tic. Patients express premonitory urge as a sensation of internal build-up of discomfort, tightness, or paresthesia.
- Tics are generally suppressible and there is a rebound phenomenon after suppression.
- The tics tend to be exacerbated during anxiety and stress. It is possible that during stress the ability to suppress the tics is reduced.[11]
- The anatomical distribution of the tics evolves with age. Also, the frequency and severity of the symptoms fluctuates in due course.

Behavioral Features

Behavioral symptoms such as attention deficit hyperactivity disorder (ADHD) and obsessive-compulsive disorder (OCD) are commonly seen in patients with TS and often precedes motor and phonic tics as an initial manifestation of TS. OCD symptoms in children with TS became more severe at a later age and were more likely to persist than tic symptoms.[9] These comorbid behavioral conditions often interfere with learning and with academic and work performance. In a school based, community study in USA, 21% students were found to have tics and these children had prominent behavioral symptoms such as OCD, ADHD, separation anxiety, overanxious disorder, simple phobia, social phobia, agoraphobia, mania, major depression, and oppositional defiant behavior when compared to children without tics ($p < 0.05$).[12]

TOURETTE'S SYNDROMES IN ADULTS

Jankovic et al. reviewed medical records of all new TS patients who were 19 years or older on initial evaluation and comparing them with 18 years or younger patients. In the adult TS patients, 35 out of 43 (81.4%) had a history of tics with onset before the age of 18 years (mean age at onset: 8.5 ± 3.4 years), with eight (18.6%) reporting first occurrence of tics after the age of 18 years (mean age at onset: 37.8 ± 13.2 years). Only two (4.7%) patients reported tic onset after the age of 50 years.[13] These patients have different body distribution of tics with more axial involvement of motor tics such as facial and truncal area with fewer phonic tics. There was a higher prevalence of substance abuse and mood disorders with lower rates of ADHD and oppositional behavior than children with TS. Adult-onset primary dystonic tics has been described in 11 patients, where 10 patients were male and mean age of onset was 42 years. These patients also had axial involvement, involving the cranial-cervical region and the shoulders and, less frequently, the limbs.[14]

TREATMENT

Patient and their families should be educated regarding the natural course of TS. Most of the patients have complete or partial remission as they become older. If the tics are not causing any functional impairment, then watchful waiting to start treatment is acceptable.[15] There are three mainstay treatment options available need to be treatment of TS includes behavioral therapy, medical therapy, and surgical treatment.

Behavioral Therapy

Comprehensive behavioral intervention for tics (CBIT) is an individualized treatment program consisting of habit reversal training, relaxation training, and a functional intervention to address situations that sustain or worsen tics.[16] The child and adult CBIT trials demonstrated the efficacy of an eight-session protocol, though cases complicated by poor tic awareness, treatment motivation, more severe tics, or substantial clinical comorbidity may benefit from a longer course of therapy. Most children (aged 9 years or older) and adults showing an initial positive response to CBIT will maintain their treatment gains for at least 6 months. CBIT can be effective for children younger than 9 years, though there is little evidence to determine efficacy in children of this age group.[17]

Medical Therapy

A variety of drugs such as typical and atypical neuroleptics, alpha adrenergic agonists, dopamine depletors, benzodiazepines, and botulinum toxin are commonly used in the treatment of tics and other symptoms connected with TS.

Antipsychotic Medications

Haloperidol, pimozide, and aripiprazole are currently the only U.S. Food and Drug Administration (FDA) approved medications to treat tics. Other antipsychotic agents used in the treatment of TS and chronic tic disorder are fluphenazine, risperidone, tiapride, olanzapine, sulpiride, and ziprasidone.[18] A meta-analysis of antipsychotic drugs for the treatment of TS found no difference in efficacy between risperidone, haloperidol, pimozide, and ziprasidone.[19] The main advantage of atypical antipsychotics is fewer adverse effects. Typical antipsychotics may produce unacceptable adverse effects such as sedation, hyperprolactinemia, weight gain, Parkinsonism, oculogyric crisis, acute dystonia, tardive dyskinesia, and neuroleptic malignant syndrome. Fluphenazine has been reported to be efficacious as well. Patients had "moderate to marked" improvement in 80.5% of patients at initial visit and 76% at last follow-up at an optimal dose of 3.24 mg/day (range 0.5–12.0) of fluphenazine, which was continued for an average of 2.6 years (range 0.01–16.8). The most common side effects were drowsiness (26.1%), weight gain (11.6%), akathisia (8.5%), and acute dystonic reactions (7.0%). Interestingly, there were no cases of tardive dyskinesia.[20]

A systematic review of aripiprazole for TS included six randomized controlled trials and found a similar efficacy of aripiprazole and haloperidol for TS but with significantly less risk of drug-induced movement disorders with aripiprazole (1.5%) versus haloperidol (43.5%).[21] The most common adverse effects attributed to aripiprazole were nausea/vomiting (5.5%), drowsiness (3.9%), headache (3.5%), and dizziness (3.5%). Aripiprazole has become a drug of choice in treating tics and comorbidities in TS over the past decade. However, large scale trials have been missing. In a clinical trial, 133 pediatric patients were randomized in a 1:1:1 ratio to low-dose aripiprazole (5 mg/day if <50 kg; 10 mg/day if ≥50 kg), high-dose aripiprazole (10 mg/day if <50 kg; 20 mg/day if ≥50 kg), or placebo for eight.[22] High-dose aripiprazole was more effective than low-dose aripiprazole and both were superior to placebo. Importantly, tolerance was overall good and no serious adverse events or deaths occurred, indicating that oral aripiprazole is a safe and effective treatment for tics in children and adolescents.

A newer agent, ecopipam, a D_1 dopamine-receptor antagonist, has shown promising results in treatment of tics.[23] In the randomized double-blind placebo-controlled, crossover study, ecopipam showed promising results with reduction in Yale Global Tic Severity Scale (YGTSS) total tic score at 16 days ($p = 0.011$) and 30 days ($p = 0.033$). There were no weight gain, drug-induced dyskinesias, or changes in laboratory tests, electrocardiograms, vital signs, or comorbid symptoms.[24]

Dopamine Depletors

Tetrabenazine is a monoamine-depleting drug has been used for treatment of TS for a longtime.[25] In contrast with typical and atypical neuroleptics, tetrabenazine does not produce some of the adverse effects of neuroleptics such as weight gain and tardive dyskinesia. The newer agent, deutetrabenazine, an inhibitor of vesicular monoamine transporter type 2 (VMAT2) depletes presynaptic dopamine and is FDA approved for treatment in Huntington disease and tardive dyskinesia patients. This medication has been studied in an open label trial of 23 TS patients and there was a reduction in the mean YGTSS score on doses of 18–36 mg/day, and 76% of patients were "much improved" or "very much improved" compared with baseline. The reported side effects were headache, fatigue, and irritability.[26]

Noradrenergic Agents

Noradrenergic agents are classified as either presynaptic α-2 adrenergic agonists (e.g., clonidine and guanfacine) or noradrenergic reuptake inhibitors (e.g., atomoxetine). Alpha-2 agonists such as clonidine and guanfacine are considered first line medicine for patients with TS.[25] This is in spite of the fact that the level of evidence for their effectiveness is less than antipsychotics and also they are not FDA approved for the treatment of TS. As per the American Academy of Neurology (AAN) guidelines, clonidine is probably more likely helpful than placebo and guanfacine is possibly more likely helpful than placebo to reduce tic severity.[15] The most common adverse effects of clonidine and guanfacine are sedation, bradycardia and postural hypotension, and QTc prolongation with guanfacine extended release. Abrupt withdrawal of α-2 adrenergic agonists may cause rebound hypertension. In a multicentric study, "extended-release" guanfacine was not found to be beneficial when compared with placebo.[27]

Benzodiazepines

Clonazepam, the most frequently used benzodiazepine drug in TS, is effective in treating myoclonic tics. Sedation, depression, and tachyphylaxis are the most common adverse events.[28]

Botulinum Toxin

Botulinum toxin is well-established first-line treatment for several hyperkinetic movement disorders such as dystonia, hemifacial spasm, blepharospasm, etc. The use of botulinum toxin is now being extended to tremor conditions such as Parkinson's disease tremor, essential tremor, and restless leg syndrome in clinical studies.[29,30] Botulinum toxin can be helpful in simple tics involving one group of muscles, especially for dystonic and clonic tics.[28] In a Cochrane review, one randomized placebo-controlled, double-blind crossover study was included, and the authors concluded that the effect of botulinum toxin in tics is uncertain.[28]

Deep Brain Stimulation

Occasionally, TS patients experience severe and disabling symptoms refractory to conventional treatments. In these cases, deep brain stimulation (DBS) can be considered as an effective option for symptomatic control at movement disorder centers. In 1999, Vandewalle et al.[31] reported the first case of DBS with thalamic stimulation in medically refractory TS and found 90% reduction in his tics at 1 year follow-up. Since then, there are many published case reports, case series, and original peer-reviewed articles regarding DBS in TS and tic disorder patients. Dwarkanath et al. reported the first patient in India where DBS of bilateral anteromedial globus pallidus interna controlled the symptoms of TS with significant improvement of YGTSS by >72% in a patient who was refractory to medicines and behavioral therapy.[32] Doshi et al. reported two cases with good postoperative control of tics and associated obsessive-compulsive behavior with anteromedial globus pallidus interna DBS using Vercise® device, with 18 months follow-up.[33] The most common target is the centromedian-parafascicular complex of thalamus followed by globus pallidus internus. The mechanism by which DBS is effective on tics and other symptoms in TS is not yet understood. The average response, mostly from case series and prospective cohorts and only a few controlled studies, is around 40% improvement on tic severity scales.[28,34]

STEREOTYPIES

DEFINITION AND CLINICAL FEATURES

Stereotypies are defined as involuntary, repetitive, rhythmic, and nongoal-directed movements that have a pattern with predictable amplitude and location, which are partially to completely distractible and may interfere with normal functioning.[35] Stereotypies range from very simple movements to complex well-formed movements involving the arms, hands, or entire body. They can encompass movements or sounds (or a combination of both).

There are several examples such as hand-waving, rocking back and forth, fiddling with fingers, twirling objects, headbanging, lip-smacking, chewing movements, humming, self-biting, picking at skin or a bodily orifice, or hitting various parts of one's own body. Phonic stereotypies include repetitive sounds and repeated words or phrases.[36] It is not associated with any premonitory urges or building up of inner tension, and it is suppressible. While stereotypies can be stopped by distraction, the patient rarely makes a conscious effort to control the movement. Also, stereotypies are rhythmic and there is poor response to medications. These movements are associated with stress, anxiety, excitement, or fatigue.

ETIOLOGY

Stereotypies are usually seen in early childhood (<3 years), but occasionally it can be seen in adults as well.[36] Stereotypy can be due to primary or secondary etiologies. Secondary causes includes development delay, autism spectrum disorders, drug induced, basal ganglia lesions, postinfectious, paraneoplastic, psychogenic, neurodegenerative diseases such as Wilson's disease, Lesch-Nyhan, neurodegeneration with brain iron accumulation, frontotemporal dementia, neuroacanthocytosis, etc.[36,37]

TREATMENT

There are two main therapeutic options such as behavioral therapy and pharmacotherapy. Behavioral therapy is the cornerstone treatment in stereotypies such as habit reversal therapy which focuses on increasing awareness of patient's behaviors and to provide relief with strategies that replace the unwanted behavior with a less bothersome behavior. There are other behavioral therapies available as well.[38] Medical management is limited in stereotypies and most of the studies which includes small number of patients are done in patients with autism or pervasive developmental disorders. It works well in conjunction with behavioral therapy.[39] Medical treatment for stereotypies is similar to treatment of tics which includes antipsychotics, dopamine depletors and alpha-2 agonists, as discussed above. Valproic acid was also reported helpful to control stereotypic behavior in patients with autism spectrum disorders.[40]

CONCLUSION

Tics, Tourette's syndrome, and Stereotypy are group of hyperkinetic movement disorders, commonly seen in younger age group. Diagnosis is purely clinical with careful assessment of history and understanding the phenomenology of the movements. Patients with Tourette's syndrome commonly have behavioral symptoms as well. Treatment modalities include behavioral therapy such as CBIT is the first line treatment, followed by medical therapies such as dopamine antagonists, dopamine depletors, benzodiazepines, and others. Patients with disabling and severe tics, refractory of treatment, DBS could be an effective option in these patients.

REFERENCES

1. Bhattacharyya KB, Rai S. Famous people with Tourette's syndrome: Dr. Samuel Johnson (yes) & Wolfgang Amadeus Mozart (may be): Victims of Tourette's syndrome? Ann Indian Acad Neurol. 2015;18(2):157-61.
2. Kurlan R, McDermott MP, Deeley C, Como PG, Brower C, Eapen S, et al. Prevalence of tics in schoolchildren and association with placement in special education. Neurology. 2001;57(8):1383-8.
3. Robertson MM, Eapen V, Cavanna AE. The international prevalence, epidemiology, and clinical phenomenology of Tourette syndrome: a cross-cultural perspective. J Psychosom Res. 2009;67(6):475-83.
4. American Psychiatric Association. Diagnostic and statistical manual of mental disorders (DSM-5®). American Psychiatric Pub. 2013.
5. Jankovic J. Tourette syndrome. Phenomenology and classification of tics. Neurol Clin. 1997;15(2):267-75.
6. Freeman RD, Tourette Syndrome International Database Consortium. Tic disorders and ADHD: answers from a world-wide clinical dataset on Tourette syndrome. Eur Child Adolesc Psychiatry. 2007;16(Suppl 1):15-23.
7. Freeman RD, Fast DK, Burd L, Kerbeshian J, Robertson MM, Sandor P. An international perspective on Tourette syndrome: selected findings from 3,500 individuals in 22 countries. Dev Med Child Neurol. 2000;42(7):436-47.
8. Bloch MH, Leckman JF. Clinical course of Tourette syndrome. J Psychosom Res. 2009;67(6):497-501.
9. Bloch MH, Peterson BS, Scahill L, Otka J, Katsovich L, Zhang H, et al. Adulthood outcome of tic and obsessive-compulsive symptom severity in children with Tourette syndrome. Arch Pediatr Adolesc Med. 2006;160(1):65-9.
10. Hallett M. Tourette Syndrome: Update. Brain Dev. 2015;37(7): 651-5.
11. Conelea CA, Woods DW, Brandt BC. The impact of a stress induction task on tic frequencies in youth with Tourette Syndrome. Behav Res Ther. 2011;49(8):492-7.
12. Kurlan R, Como PG, Miller B, Palumbo D, Deeley C, Andresen EM, et al. The behavioral spectrum of tic disorders: a community-based study. Neurology. 2002;59(3):414-20.
13. Jankovic J, Gelineau-Kattner R, Davidson A. Tourette's syndrome in adults. Mov Disord. 2010;25(13):2171-5.
14. Erro R, Martino D, Ganos C, Damasio J, Batla A, Bhatia KP. Adult-Onset Primary Dystonic Tics: A Different Entity? Mov Disord Clin Pract. 2014;1(1):62-6.
15. Pringsheim T, Okun MS, Muller-Vahl K, Martino D, Jankovic J, Cavanna AE, et al. Practice guideline recommendations summary: Treatment of tics in people with Tourette syndrome and chronic tic disorders. Neurology. 2019;92(19):896-906.
16. Woods DW, Piacentini J, Chang S, Deckersbach T, Ginsburg G, Peterson A, et al. Managing Tourette syndrome: A behavioral intervention for children and adults therapist guide. Oxford University Press; 2008.
17. Woods DW, Miltenberger RG. A review of habit reversal with childhood habit disorders. Educ Treat Child. 1996;197-214.
18. Whittington C, Pennant M, Kendall T, Glazebrook C, Trayner P, Groom M, et al. Practitioner Review: Treatments for Tourette syndrome in children and young people -a systematic review. J Child Psychol Psychiatry. 2016;57(9):988-1004.
19. Weisman H, Qureshi IA, Leckman JF, Scahill L, Bloch MH. Systematic review: pharmacological treatment of tic disorders--efficacy of antipsychotic and alpha-2 adrenergic agonist agents. Neurosci Biobehav Rev. 2013;37(6):1162-71.
20. Wijemanne S, Wu LJC, Jankovic J. Long-term efficacy and safety of fluphenazine in patients with Tourette syndrome. Mov Disord. 2014;29(1):126-30.
21. Zheng W, Li XB, Xiang YQ, Zhong BL, Chiu HF, Ungvari GS, et al. Aripiprazole for Tourette's syndrome: a systematic review and meta-analysis. Hum Psychopharmacol. 2016;31(1):11-8.
22. Sallee F, Kohegyi E, Zhao J, McQuade R, Cox K, Sanchez R, et al. Randomized, Double-Blind, Placebo-Controlled Trial Demonstrates the Efficacy and Safety of Oral Aripiprazole for the Treatment of Tourette's Disorder in Children and Adolescents. J Child Adolesc Psychopharmacol. 2017;27(9): 771-81.
23. Gilbert DL, Budman CL, Singer HS, Kurlan R, Chipkin RE. A D1 receptor antagonist, ecopipam, for treatment of tics in Tourette syndrome. Clin Neuropharmacol. 2014;37(1):26-30.
24. Gilbert DL, Murphy TK, Jankovic J, Budman CL, Black KJ, Kurlan RM, et al. Ecopipam, a D1 receptor antagonist, for treatment of tourette syndrome in children: A randomized, placebo-controlled crossover study. Mov Disord. 2018;33(8):1272-80.
25. Pringsheim T, Doja A, Gorman D, McKinlay D, Day L, Billinghurst L, et al. Canadian guidelines for the evidence-based treatment of tic disorders: pharmacotherapy. Can J Psychiatry. 2012;57(3): 133-43.
26. Jankovic J, Jimenez-Shahed J, Budman C, Coffey B, Murphy T, Shprecher D, et al. Deutetrabenazine in Tics Associated with Tourette Syndrome. Tremor Other Hyperkinet Mov (N Y). 2016;6:422.
27. Murphy TK, Fernandez TV, Coffey BJ, Rahman O, Gavaletz A, Hanks CE, et al. Extended-Release Guanfacine Does Not Show a Large Effect on Tic Severity in Children with Chronic Tic Disorders. J Child Adolesc Psychopharmacol. 2017;27(9): 762-70.
28. Pandey S, Srivanitchapoom P, Kirubakaran R, Berman BD. Botulinum toxin for motor and phonic tics in Tourette's syndrome. Cochrane database Syst Rev. 2018;1(1):CD012285.
29. Mittal SO, Machado D, Richardson D, Dubey D, Jabbari B. Botulinum Toxin in Parkinson Disease Tremor: A Randomized, Double-Blind, Placebo-Controlled Study with a Customized Injection Approach. Mayo Clin Proc. 2017;92(9):1359-67.
30. Mittal SO, Lenka A, Jankovic J. Botulinum toxin for the treatment of tremor. Parkinsonism Relat Disord. 2019;63:31-41.

31. Vandewalle V, van der Linden C, Groenewegen HJ, Caemaert J. Stereotactic treatment of Gilles de la Tourette syndrome by high frequency stimulation of thalamus. Lancet. 1999;353(9154):724.
32. Dwarakanath S, Hegde A, Ketan J, Chandrajit P, Yadav R, Keshav K, et al. "I swear, I can't stop it!"-A case of severe Tourette's syndrome treated with deep brain stimulation of anteromedial globus pallidus interna. Neurol India. 2017;65(1):99-102.
33. Doshi PK, Ramdasi R, Thorve S. Deep brain stimulation of anteromedial globus pallidus internus for severe Tourette syndrome. Indian J Psychiatry. 2018;60(1):138-40.
34. Casagrande SCB, Cury RG, Alho EJL, Fonoff ET. Deep brain stimulation in Tourette's syndrome: evidence to date. Neuropsychiatr Dis Treat. 2019;15:1061-75.
35. Edwards MJ, Lang AE, Bhatia KP. Stereotypies: a critical appraisal and suggestion of a clinically useful definition. Mov Disord. 2012;27(2):179-85.
36. Maltete D. Adult-onset stereotypical motor behaviors. Rev Neurol (Paris). 2016;172(8–9):477-82.
37. Jankovic J, Tolosa E. Parkinson's disease and movement disorders. Lippincott, New York: Williams & Wilkins; 2007.
38. Katherine M. Stereotypic Movement Disorders. Semin Pediatr Neurol. 2018;25:19-24.
39. Aman MG, McDougle CJ, Scahill L, Handen B, Arnold LE, Johnson C, et al. Medication and parent training in children with pervasive developmental disorders and serious behavior problems: results from a randomized clinical trial. J Am Acad Child Adolesc Psychiatry. 2009;48(12):1143-54.
40. Hollander E, Soorya L, Wasserman S, Esposito K, Chaplin W, Anagnostou E. Divalproex sodium vs. placebo in the treatment of repetitive behaviours in autism spectrum disorder. Int J Neuropsychopharmacol. 2006;9(2):209-13.

CHAPTER 36

Myoclonus and Startle Syndromes

Shabbir Merchant, Mark Hallett

MYOCLONUS SYNDROME

Introduction

Myoclonus can be clinically characterized as a sudden, brief, shock-like jerk caused by either (1) an active muscle contraction, called positive myoclonus, or (2) a brief lapse of ongoing muscle contraction, known as negative myoclonus or asterixis.[1] It is important to note that myoclonic movements are simple, brief, rapid, and happen in a fairly consistent and reproducible pattern.

Characterizing myoclonus phenomenology can be challenging at times, as many different hyperkinetic movement disorders can be misconstrued as myoclonus. Certain movement disorders can coexist with myoclonus and many different movement disorders with jerk-like quality can be misdiagnosed as being myoclonic. Tic disorders, for instance, are a common movement disorder which are characterized by jerks; however, these are actually voluntary and usually partially suppressible by volition. Additionally, the sensory phenomena in tic disorders characterized by a conscious urge to move with relief of tension after the tic has occurred are typical. Many tic disorders are complex and also involve vocalizations, unlike myoclonus which are simple, rapid, and involuntary jerks. Choreiform movements may have jerk-like intrusion; however, chorea has characteristic constant flow like movements randomly distributed over the body and randomly distributed in time. Brief muscle spasms in dystonia can look like myoclonus, and myoclonus and dystonia can coexist in an autosomal dominant myoclonus-dystonia syndrome. Dystonic movements drive the involved joints into certain postures, whereas no sustained changes in muscle tone and posture are associated with myoclonic jerks. Sometimes myoclonic jerks can be rhythmic which can be misconstrued as a tremor. Functional (psychogenic) movement disorders may also mimic myoclonus; the muscle burst duration, distractibility, and presence of premotor potentials can help to differentiate them. Many different peripheral movement disorders like clonus, fasciculation, and myokymia can be misdiagnosed as myoclonic. The associated clinical findings, pattern, and amplitude of movements can be important clues for differentiation. Additionally, more than one type of myoclonic or jerk-like movement disorder can coexist in an individual and identifying them can have important therapeutic implications.[2]

Clinical Characteristics

Clinical characteristics to consider in the approach to myoclonus include the primary etiology/neurological disorder and associated neurological symptoms and signs which may have localizing value. The details of the clinical characteristics of myoclonus which include the pattern and distribution of muscle activation, stimulus sensitivity, type of stimuli which elicits the movement, and associated movement disorders may all aid in the localization and diagnosis. In terms of distribution, the whole body or most of it may be affected in a single jerk (generalized myoclonus). Many different parts of the body may be affected, not necessarily at the same time (multifocal myoclonus); or myoclonus may be confined to one particular region of the body (focal or segmental myoclonus). Myoclonic jerks may occur repetitively and rhythmically, or irregularly.[3] They may be evident at rest, on maintaining a posture, or on movement (action myoclonus). Jerks may be triggered by external stimuli (reflex myoclonus), which can be visual, auditory, or somesthetic (touch, pinprick, and muscle stretch).

Cortical myoclonus is commonly characterized by spontaneous jerks more commonly involving face and distal upper extremities. Reticular myoclonus or myoclonus of brainstem origin is commonly characterized by spontaneous total body jerks which can also be elicited by somatosensory stimulation of distal extremities. The startle reflex is characterized by a bilateral synchronous flexor response to a startling stimulus which most commonly is auditory but can also be tactile or vestibular.

Neurophysiologic Characteristics

Neurophysiologic assessment can be used to supplement the clinical examination and the physiological tests to be considered in the evaluation of myoclonus should be based on the phenomenology and clinical characteristics. A simple approach in the physiologic evaluation of myoclonus can be adopted, beginning initially with polymyography. Polymyography [recording the electromyography (EMG) burst duration, distribution, velocity of conduction of the efferent volley, pattern of spread, and stimulus sensitivity of EMG activity in affected muscles] can help categorize the pathophysiology and location in most cases of jerk-like movements.[1,4-6] Most myoclonic jerks of cortical, subcortical, and brainstem origin have very brief EMG bursts of 10–50 ms. EMG bursts in the 100 ms range are seen in some situations such as essential myoclonus.

Agonists and antagonists usually fire synchronously in myoclonus of cortical and subcortical origin. *Cortical myoclonus* is further characterized by pathologically enlarged somatosensory evoked potentials (SEPs) produced by peripheral nerve stimulation. The giant SEPs usually consist of an enlarged P_{25}/N_{33} component for the median nerve evoked potentials and is a sign of cortical hyperexcitability; the first major cortical negative peak (N_{20}) reflecting arrival of sensory volley in the cortex usually is of normal size. A cortical correlate can be back-averaged in the ongoing electroencephalography (EEG) by triggering from the EMG of the muscle jerk.[5-7] Stimuli generating giant SEPs often provoke a subsequent EMG burst of myoclonic activity (the C reflex), at a latency compatible with conduction through fast corticomotoneuronal pathways from the motor cortex to muscle, which is a correlate of cortical reflex myoclonus (**Fig. 1**). The motor volleys in cortical myoclonus activate the cranial and limb musculature in descending order via fast conducting corticospinal pathways (~100 ms). Abnormal corticomuscular and intermuscular coupling can also be a sensitive physiologic feature in cortical myoclonus.[8] The increased cortical excitability in cortical myoclonus may well be due to loss of inhibitory interneurons.[9,10] Cortical reflex myoclonus usually consists of EMG discharges, but negative cortical reflex myoclonus can also occur,[5,10-13] where a giant somatosensory cortical potential is time-locked to EMG silence. *Subcortical myoclonus* is suggested when reflex myoclonus triggered by peripheral stimuli occurs after a latency that is too short to involve cortical pathways.[14,15]

Myoclonic muscle jerks affecting axial muscles (neck, shoulders, trunk, and hips) may arise in the brainstem as an exaggerated startle response or brainstem reticular myoclonus, or in the spinal cord as propriospinal myoclonus. In *brainstem/reticular myoclonus*, there is no preceding cortical discharge. Cranial nerve muscles are usually activated in an ascending order from the XI nucleus up the brainstem; limb and axial muscles are activated in descending order. Reticular myoclonus originates in the medullary reticular formation (nucleus reticularis gigantocellularis) and most commonly attributed to brainstem hypoxic injury.[16] The physiologic differentiating characteristics of reticular myoclonus include short-duration bursts <50 ms, velocity of transmission ~50–70 m/sec, originating in the muscles innervated by lower cranial nerve nuclei with subsequent craniocaudal propagation and spontaneous jerks which can also be produced by somatosensory stimuli especially muscle stretch of the distal extremities.[6,16]

Burst durations around 70 ms are usually characteristic of startle and similar reflexes of brainstem origin (discussed in the Startle syndrome subsection of this Chapter).[2] Longer-duration bursts of >100 ms are likely dystonic, functional (psychogenic), spinal, or propriospinal. The distribution of muscles involved may suggest that it arises as a result of a lesion of a peripheral nerve, part of a plexus, a spinal root or a restricted number of segments of the spinal cord (*segmental myoclonus*). In *propriospinal myoclonus*, the first muscles activated are usually in the thoracic cord distribution, with slow upward and downward spread. The burst durations are typically longer ranging from approximately 150–450 ms (can be even longer), originating in the abdominal muscles with slow upward and downward spread at a velocity of 5–15 m/sec, limited to the spinal cord. Of note, most propriospinal myoclonus patients are deemed to be functional, but cases of organic spinal pathology have been described.[17,18] *Functional myoclonus* is suggested if stimulus-evoked jerks are of very variable latency and longer than a voluntary reaction time,[14,17,19,20] and when the Bereitschaftspotential or event relate desynchronization on the beta band is evident prior to EMG bursts on jerk-locked back-averaging of the EEG, similar to what is seen with voluntary movement.[21]

Pathophysiology of Myoclonus

Combining the clinical features of myoclonus and the results of electrophysiological investigations allows for a relatively precise localization of its site of origin in the nervous system.[1,6,7,22] The clinical and physiological characteristics also provide useful pathophysiologic

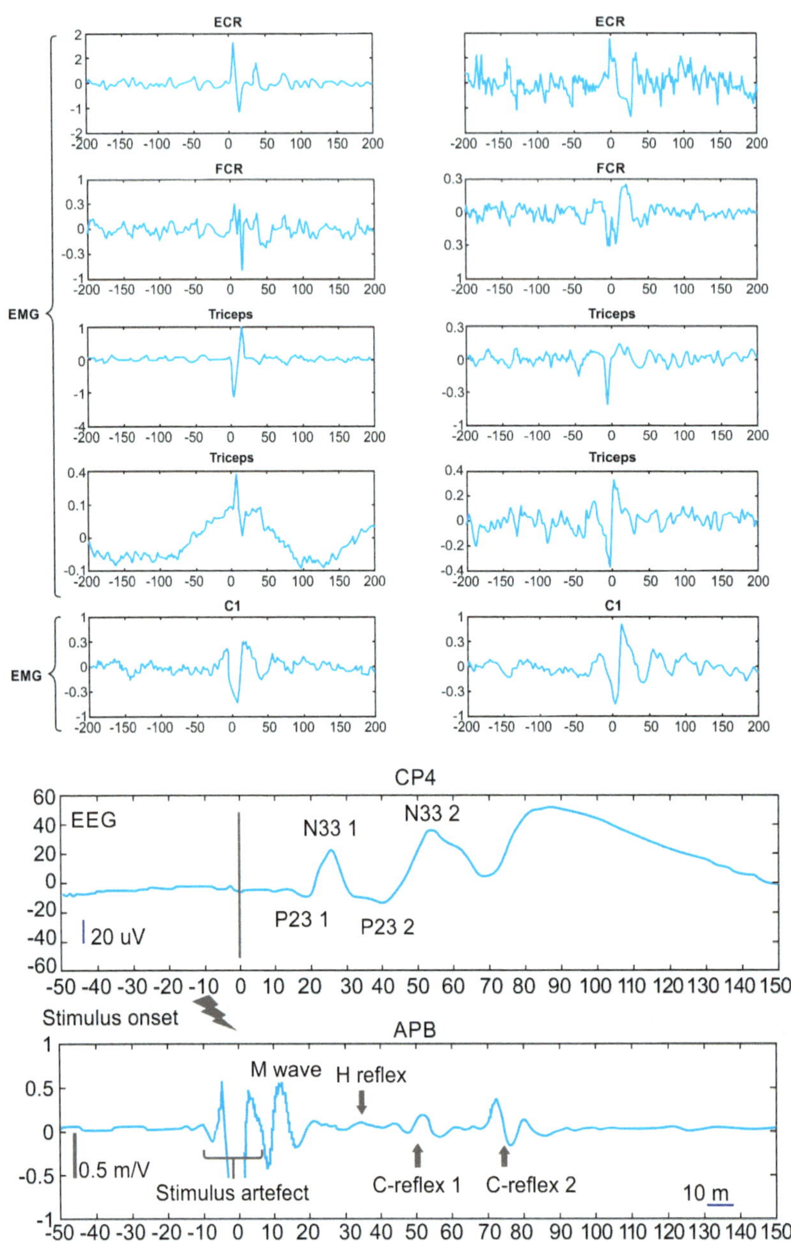

(APB: abductor pollicis brevis; ECR: extensor carpi radialis; EEG: electroencephalography; EMG: electromyography; FCR: flexor carpi radialis; SSEP: somatosensory evoked potential)

FIG. 1: Cortical myoclonus physiology; (A) EMG traces showing short-duration (<30 ms) EMG bursts in biceps-triceps and FCR-ECR pairs (simultaneous agonist-antagonist bursts) with cortical EEG spike correlate. (B) Stimulation of median nerve at rest with stimulus intensity just above motor threshold shows an initial M wave followed by an H-reflex occurring at a latency of 25–30 ms followed by a C-reflex 1 at a latency of 50 ms. A second reflex myoclonic discharge labeled as C-reflex 2 is noted around 70 ms in the EMG trace. The corresponding EEG trace is notable for a giant SSEP (increased amplitudes of the P25 and N33 components, here called P25 1 and N33 1, respectively, since they are duplicated) corresponding to the median nerve stimulation evoked responses. The EEG trace also demonstrates a giant SSEP like discharge preceding the second reflex myoclonus (C-reflex 2) discharge, as notable by the increased amplitudes of P25 2 and N33 2 components, suggestive of a hyperexcitable disinhibited cortex.

Source: Traces courtesy by Dr Felipe Vial.

insights into the generation of these abnormal movements which have therapeutic implications. On this basis, myoclonus may be shown to arise in the cerebral cortex (cortical myoclonus); in the brainstem (brainstem myoclonus); or in the spinal cord (spinal myoclonus). Rarely, lesions of spinal roots, nerve plexi, or peripheral nerves can cause myoclonus (peripheral myoclonus). Hemifacial spasm might be considered a form of peripheral myoclonus, due most often to neurovascular compression.[23]

Cortical myoclonus, characterized by fractionated and multifocal jerks predominantly involving the face and arm are suggestive of the site of origin being in the sensorimotor cortex; the face/arm have the largest homuncular representation in the cortex and one of its important functions being performance of fractionated finger movements. The conduction velocity of the efferent volley is suggestive of conduction down the spinal cord via the corticospinal pathways. Physiologic characteristics of exaggerated long loop reflexes and abnormalities in corticomuscular/intermuscular coherence are functional attributes reflecting somatotopic organization within sensorimotor cortex. Normal N_{20} component with exaggeration of the later (P25/N33) components of SEP's and abnormalities noted in cortical excitability using noninvasive brain stimulation measures such as short intracortical inhibition (SICI), interhemispheric inhibition (IHI), and intracortical facilitation (ICF) are reflective of disinhibition of sensorimotor cortex, also implicating involvement of gamma-aminobutyric acid (GABAergic) inhibitory neurons.[9,24] Some evidence also implicates cerebellum to be involved in the generation and exacerbation of cortical myoclonus based on clinical association with certain ataxia syndromes and physiologic measures implicating aberrancies in the cerebello-thalamo-cortical pathways.[25-27] These common pathophysiologic mechanisms involved in the generation of cortical myoclonus are shared by many different etiologies which result in disinhibition of the sensorimotor cortex by various mechanisms.

Brainstem myoclonus, characterized by generalized muscle jerks beginning most commonly in the muscles innervated by caudal brainstem with subsequent craniocaudal propagation, is reflective of the site of origin. The pattern of muscle activation also implicates the origin being in the brainstem reticular formation. There are three different pathophysiologic mechanisms for myoclonus of brainstem origin. One originates in caudal medullary reticular formation (nucleus reticularis gigantocellularis). The second employs pathways responsible for the startle reflex with the likely site of origin being caudal pontine reticular formation (nucleus reticularis pontis caudalis). They are both distinctive, having a separate efferent pathway as notable by the velocity of conduction of the bulbo-spinal volley; reticular myoclonus conducted at a relatively faster velocity.[16,28,29] Third is the palatal myoclonus (tremor) syndrome, which is characterized by symptomatic and essential subtypes. Symptomatic palatal myoclonus is characterized by refractory palatal movements which usually persist during sleep and stems from pathology involving the triangle of Guillain-Mollaret comprised of ipsilateral dentate nucleus, contralateral red nucleus, and inferior olivary nucleus. The likely suggested mechanism involves disinhibition of the inferior olivary nucleus with establishment of connexons between the inferior olivary neurons resulting in synchronized firing. These aberrant disinhibited signals from the inferior olives are conducted to the cerebellar cortex via climbing fibers in the inferior cerebellar peduncle, which is deemed to be the likely source of the central component of the palatal myoclonus (tremor). Essential palatal myoclonus has been deemed to be of functional origin in majority of cases; however, possible inferior olivary disinhibition from denervation hypersensitivity from poorly understood mechanisms has been considered to be a plausible explanation.[30]

Spinal cord myoclonus can be of two forms based on phenomenology; spinal segmental myoclonus affecting a restricted body part or propriospinal myoclonus characterized by generalized axial jerks or involving multiple contiguous spinal segments, which is most commonly noted to originate at the thoracic spinal level beginning in the abdominal muscles and spreading through propriospinal pathways. Lesions affecting the peripheral nerves, roots, plexi- or focal myelopathic, or space occupying lesions may produce segmental myoclonus. Most cases of propriospinal myoclonus have been deemed to be of functional origin; however, some cases of organic/symptomatic propriospinal myoclonus have been described.[17,18]

Etiology of Myoclonus

Myoclonus, originating from these different locations within the neuroaxis can be caused by many different neurologic conditions. The list of etiologies and the pathophysiologic basis of origin of myoclonus for the various etiologies is very extensive and beyond the scope of this current synthesis. A brief summary of several broad categories of etiologic classification, and their likely anatomical and pathophysiological substrate is provided here (**Table 1**).[31-35]

Certain muscle jerks like sleep jerks (hypnic jerks) and hiccups which occur under certain circumstances in normal subjects are referred to as Physiologic myoclonus. Multifocal myoclonus where no other abnormalities are identified based on neurologic assessment and other diagnostic investigations is referred to as essential myoclonus. Myoclonic jerks occurring as fragments of epilepsy or associated with epileptic disorders as a comorbidity are referred to as epileptic myoclonus. In most of these cases, the major clinical problem is epilepsy and myoclonic jerks being one of the manifestations of the epileptic attacks. Generalized or multifocal muscle jerking where an underlying identifiable neurologic disease or more commonly metabolic abnormalities are identified and referred to as symptomatic myoclonus. Functional (psychogenic) myoclonus refers to myoclonus produced as a conversion symptom.[38,39] Based on epidemiologic studies, symptomatic myoclonus was most common with

TABLE 1: Etiologic classification of myoclonus and likely anatomical localization.

Etiology	Pathophysiology/ Anatomical localization
• Physiological myoclonus (normal subjects)	
○ Sleep jerks (hypnic jerks)	Cortical/Subcortical
○ Anxiety-induced	Cortical/Subcortical
○ Exercise-induced	Cortical/Subcortical
○ Hiccup (singultus)	Subcortical/Brainstem/ Peripheral
○ Benign infantile myoclonus with feeding	Cortical/Subcortical
• Essential myoclonus (no known cause other than genetic and no other gross neurologic deficit)	
○ Hereditary (autosomal dominant and most are likely myoclonus dystonia)	Cortical/Subcortical
○ Sporadic	Cortical/Subcortical
• Epileptic myoclonus (seizures dominate and no encephalopathy, at least initially)	
○ Fragments of epilepsy	Cortical
– Isolated epileptic myoclonic jerks	Cortical
– Photosensitive myoclonus	Cortical
– Myoclonic absences in petit mal seizures	Cortical
– Epilepsia partialis continua	Cortical
○ Childhood myoclonic epilepsies	
– Infantile spasms	Cortical
– Myoclonic astatic epilepsy (Lennox–Gastaut)	Cortical
– Cryptogenic myoclonus epilepsy (Aicardi)	Cortical
– Juvenile myoclonus epilepsy of Janz	Cortical
○ Benign familial myoclonic epilepsy (Rabot)	Cortical
○ Progressive myoclonus epilepsy (Unverricht–Lundborg)	Cortical/Subcortical
• Symptomatic myoclonus (progressive or static encephalopathy dominates)	
○ Storage disease:	
– Lafora body disease	Cortical/Subcortical
– Lipidoses, e.g., GM1 and GM2 gangliosidosis, Krabbe	Cortical/Subcortical
– Ceroid-lipofuscinosis (Batten)	Cortical/Subcortical
– Sialidosis ("cherry-red spot")	Cortical/Subcortical
○ Spinocerebellar degeneration	Cortical/Subcortical with associated cerebellar disinhibition
– Unverricht–Lundborg disease	Cortical/Subcortical
– Ataxia telangiectasia	Cortical/Subcortical
– Adult-onset cerebellar ataxias	Cortical/Subcortical
– Some spinocerebellar ataxias (SCAs)	
– Multiple system atrophy-type C	
○ Basal ganglia degenerations	
– Wilson disease	Cortical/Subcortical
– Dystonia	Cortical/Subcortical
– Pantothenate kinase-associated neurodegeneration	Cortical/Subcortical
– Progressive supranuclear palsy	Cortical/Subcortical
– Multiple system atrophy-type P	Cortical/Subcortical
– Huntington disease	Cortical/Subcortical
– Corticobasal ganglionic degeneration	Cortical/Subcortical
– Dentatorubro-pallidoluysian atrophy	Cortical/Subcortical
– Parkinson disease	Cortical/Subcortical
○ Dementias	
– Creutzfeldt–Jakob disease	Cortical/Subcortical
– Alzheimer disease	Cortical/Subcortical
○ Viral encephalopathies	
– SARS-CoV-2/COVID-19[36,37]	
– Subacute sclerosing panencephalitis (SSPE)	Cortical/Subcortical
– Encephalitis lethargica	Cortical/Subcortical
– Arbor virus encephalitis	Cortical/Subcortical
– Herpes simplex encephalitis	Cortical/Subcortical
– Postinfectious encephalitis	Cortical/Subcortical
– Whipple disease	Cortical/Subcortical
• AIDS	Cortical/Subcortical
○ Autoimmune	
– Opsoclonus-myoclonus syndrome	Cortical/Subcortical/ Brainstem
• Celiac disease	Cortical/Subcortical/ Brainstem
○ Metabolic	
– Hepatic failure	Cortical/Subcortical
– Renal failure	Cortical/Subcortical
– Dialysis syndrome	Cortical/Subcortical
– Hyponatremia	Cortical/Subcortical

Continued

Continued

Etiology	*Pathophysiology/ Anatomical localization*
– Hypoglycemia	Cortical/Subcortical
– Infantile myoclonic encephalopathy	Cortical/Subcortical
– Nonketotic hyperglycemia	Cortical/Subcortical
– Mitochondrial encephalomyopathy	Cortical/Subcortical
– Multiple carboxylase deficiency	Cortical/Subcortical
– Biotin deficiency	Cortical/Subcortical
○ Toxic encephalopathies	
– Bismuth	Cortical/Subcortical
– Heavy-metal poisons	Cortical/Subcortical
– Methyl bromide, DDT	Cortical/Subcortical
– Drugs including levodopa	Cortical/Subcortical
– Serotonin syndrome (e.g., SSRIs)	Cortical/Subcortical/ Brainstem
○ Physical encephalopathies	
– Posthypoxic (Lance–Adams)	Cortical/Subcortical/ Brainstem
– Post-traumatic	Cortical/Subcortical/ Brainstem
– Heat stroke	Cortical/Subcortical/ Brainstem
– Electric shock	Cortical/Subcortical/ Brainstem/Peripheral
• Decompression injury	Cortical/Subcortical/ Brainstem
○ Focal CNS damage	
– Poststroke	Cortical/Subcortical/ Brainstem
– Post-thalamotomy	Cortical/Subcortical
– Tumor	Cortical/Subcortical/ Brainstem/Peripheral
– Trauma	Cortical/Subcortical/ Brainstem/Peripheral
– Dentato-olivary lesions (palatal myoclonus/tremor)	Brainstem
○ Functional (psychogenic)	Cortical

(AIDS: acquired immunodeficiency syndrome; CNS: central nervous system; DDT: dichlorodiphenyltrichloroethane; SSRIs: selective serotonin reuptake inhibitors)

neurodegenerative disorders being the most common etiology. Other commonly reported etiologies were epileptic myoclonus and essential myoclonus.[40,41] Functional myoclonus like many other functional neurologic syndromes is likely poorly diagnosed and under reported.[31,42,43]

STARTLE SYNDROMES

Clinical Characteristics

The startle reflex is a common physiologic response observed in healthy individuals which has been most extensively studied with auditory stimuli, though it can be elicited by visual, somatic, or vestibular stimulation.[33,44-49] Clinically, it is characterized by fairly symmetrical activation of the different muscles, originating most consistently in the muscles innervated by lower brainstem with a rostrocaudal propagation.[29,33] Exaggerated startle syndromes (hyperekplexia) consist of an excessive motor response or jump, to unexpected auditory, and sometimes, somesthetic and visual stimuli.[20,29,46,50,51] The jump consists of a blink, contortion of the face, flexion of the neck and trunk, and abduction and flexion of the arm. Such patients jump in response to sound and crash to the ground, injuring themselves without loss of consciousness.

Exaggerated startle reflexes can be characterized into "major" and "minor" subtypes. The term hyperekplexia is used mainly to define the major subtype clinically characterized by three cardinal features; generalized stiffness at birth, excessive startling, and temporary generalized stiffness after being startled. The "minor" form is mainly characterized by exaggerated, nonhabituating startling.[33,44,45] An exaggerated startle response is a component of the motor manifestations of "jumping Frenchmen" and other culturally determined startle syndromes such as Latah.[48,50] In these syndromes the startle is followed by stereotyped behaviors such as a vocalization or striking out, and it is the exaggeration of these secondary behaviors that is the most important feature.[52] Hyperekplexia must also be distinguished from startle-evoked epileptic seizures.[53]

Oligosynaptic/polysynaptic reflexes of caudal brainstem origin such as the spino-bulbo-spinal reflex (SBS reflex), trigeminocervical reflex/head retraction reflex, blink reflex, audiospinal, and vestibulospinal reflex share many phenomenological similarities with startle reflex; clinically characterized by fairly symmetrical activation of the different muscles, originating most consistently in the muscles innervated by lower brainstem with a rostrocaudal propagation, making them clinically similar.[33,54-57]

Startle and Startle-like Reflex Physiology

The distinguishing characteristics of startle and other "startle-like" reflexes of caudal brainstem origin, which are hard to discern clinically, can be identified using neurophysiological investigations. Differences can be noted in terms of the afferent stimuli which induce them, pattern of activation of different muscle groups (e.g., flexors vs. extensors), conduction velocity of the efferent volley and aberrancies in these patterns when they are abnormally exaggerated.[2,20,44,56,58,59]

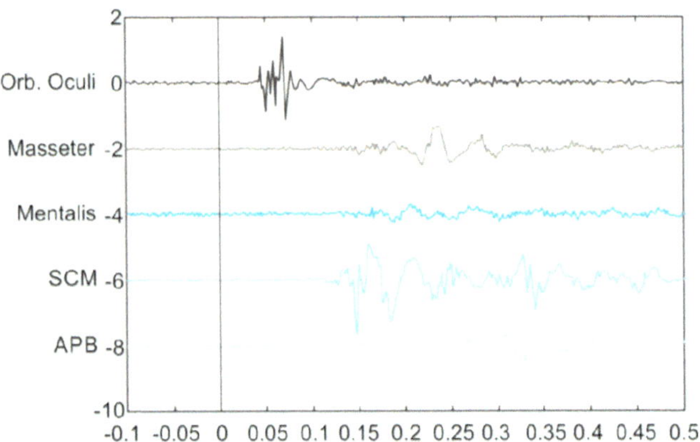

(EMG: electromyography; SCM: sternocleidomastoid; APB: abductor pollicis brevis)

FIG. 2: Rectified surface poly-EMG trace of 5 muscles (1. OrbOc: orbicularis oculi; 2. masseter; 3. mentalis; 4. SCM; 5. APB) showing an initial auditory stimulus induced blink reflex at a latency of around 35 ms followed most consistently by an "initial" SCM discharge with subsequent craniocaudal propagation at a relatively slower conduction velocity around 30 m/s. A second, very low amplitude response can be seen in the orbicularis oculi starting about the same time as the mentalis (and masseter); this likely represents the startle response proper in this muscle.

Source: Traces courtesy by Dr Felipe Vial.

The startle reflex is the most well characterized of these reflexes in humans.[33,44,46,47,49] Exaggerated startle reflexes can be characterized by features such as excessive and more widespread muscle activation, excessive EMG bursts and amplitudes, lower thresholds for response, and impaired habituation.[33,44,45] Both normal and exaggerated startle responses originate in the caudal pontine reticular formation (nucleus reticularis pontis caudalis) and transmitted via efferent pathways which are similar to the other reflexes noted above (**Fig. 2**).[33,55,56]

The SBS reflex is physiologically characterized by early and late components, most consistently provoked with stimulation of purely cutaneous nerves. The early component involves the local monosynaptic reflex arc and the afferent volley further propagates along the spinal cord via two distinct pathways of different conduction velocities. A slower conducting propriospinal pathway is limited to and has reciprocal connections within the spinal cord and another faster conducting afferent pathway has a relay center in caudal brainstem reticular formation. The efferent pathway originating in the caudal brainstem is similar to startle reflex, which gives rise to the late component of the SBS reflex. Most of our understanding about SBS reflex comes from animal studies and very little is known about the normal and exaggerated physiology of this distinctive reflex in humans.[2,55,60] The distinguishing characteristics of startle, SBS, and other "startle-like" reflexes suggest they mediate different aspects of motor and postural control. They are also distinct compared to those involved in the transmission of reticular and cortical myoclonus; which are common conditions in the clinical differential diagnosis.[7,16,47] Identifying these differences can help to localize the site of origin and understand the pathophysiology of these jerk-like movements, which may have a bearing on treatment.[2] A summary of the comparative clinical and physiologic characteristics of some of the reflexes of caudal brainstem origin and myoclonic disorders is presented in **Table 2**.[7,17,47,55,61,62]

Pathophysiology of Hyperekplexia/ Exaggerated Startle Reflex

The term "hyperekplexia" should be used for the "major" subtype of the startle syndrome. Hereditary hyperekplexia is caused by a variety of genes affecting the pre- or postsynaptic glycine receptor complex. Inhibitory glycine receptors are ligand-gated chloride channels involved in brainstem and spinal cord reflex responses. Brainstem and spinal cord disinhibition resulting from abnormalities in the functionating of these inhibitory interneurons results in hyperekplexia.[63] Mutation in the alpha-1 subunit of glycine receptor (GLRA1) complex is the most common defect in autosomal dominant hereditary hyperekplexias. Many pedigrees with autosomal recessive and compound heterozygous mutations of GLRA1 have also been reported.[35] Other mutations noted in hereditary hyperekplexia involve the beta subunit of glycine receptor (GLRB); *SLC6A5* gene encoding the presynaptic GlyT2 glycine receptor transporter; *GPHN* gene for the membrane protein gephyrin which has multiple functions including aiding the functioning of glycine and GABA receptors. *ARHGEF9* gene for collybistin is an X linked recessive mutation which causes hyperekplexia and epilepsy. Several sporadic mutations and cases with idiopathic hyperekplexia have also been reported. Pathophysiology of symptomatic exaggerated startle response can result from a large variety of etiologies affecting the brainstem and cerebral cortex, a brief summary noted in **Box 1**.[63]

TREATMENT OF MYOCLONUS AND STARTLE SYNDROMES

The drugs used to treat myoclonus generally possess anticonvulsant properties,[25,64-68] usually by enhancing GABA inhibitory activity. Unlike epilepsy where it is preferred to manage patients using monotherapy, there are good reasons for the opposite approach in the treatment of myoclonus. Based on neurophysiological evidence, antimyoclonic drugs may exert different actions on the sequence of events responsible for myoclonus, at least for those concerned with cortical myoclonus. Some drugs which decrease cortical myoclonus increase the size of the giant sensory evoked potential, while others have the opposite effect. Myoclonus thus often responds best to a combination of drugs.

TABLE 2: Summary of comparative clinical and physiologic characteristics of startle and other jerk-like movements.

	Startle reflex	*Spino-bulbo-spinal*	*Trigeminocervical reflex*	*Propriospinal myoclonus*	*Reticular myoclonus*	*Cortical myoclonus*
Phenomenology	Bilaterally synchronous flexor response to a startling stimulus	Total body jerk-like movements beginning at the level of cutaneous stimulation	Neck withdrawal and adoption of a defensive posture upon noxious stimulation in the supra/infra orbital trigeminal nerve distribution	Arrhythmic, usually flexor, brief jerks involving the trunk, hips, knees in a fairly uniform pattern	Spontaneous jerks involving the entire body which can also be evoked by somatosensory stimuli to distal extremities	Spontaneous jerks more commonly involving the face and distal upper extremities
Reflex physiology	Early eyelid blink followed most consistently by SCM with subsequent craniocaudal propagation	Early component involving segmental reflex followed by late component mediated via craniocaudal propagation originating in caudal brainstem	Early oligosynaptic component mainly characterized by drop in EMG activity in tonically active neck muscles (most consistently SCM), followed by late Splenius muscle activation mediated via polysynaptic pathways	Craniocaudal EMG discharge usually beginning at the level of the abdominal muscles; restricted to spinal cord propriospinal pathways	Craniocaudal EMG discharge beginning at the lower medulla	Cortical onset short-lasting EMG bursts (simultaneous agonist-antagonist discharge) with a cortical EEG correlate on back averaging
Afferent stimulus	Auditory; can also be elicited by visual, somatic, and vestibular stimulation	Cutaneous nerve stimulation	Noxious stimulation in trigeminal nerve distribution in the face	Spontaneous; but can be induced by tactile or auditory stimuli	Spontaneous; can be induced by somatosensory stimuli, touch or muscle stretch of distal extremities	Spontaneous; but can be triggered by tactile or other somatosensory stimuli more commonly to distal upper extremities
Pattern of muscle activation; flexors versus extensors	Mainly flexors (but extensors also noted to be activated)	Mainly flexors (but extensor activation noted; mainly based on animal studies)	Mainly neck extensors	Mainly flexors	Both flexors and extensors	Mainly involving distal upper extremities and face (which have a large cortical representation)
Site of origin	Caudal pontine reticular formation (nucleus reticularis pontis caudalis)	Medullary reticular formation	Descending tract of spinal trigeminal nucleus and spinal nucleus of accessory nerve	Limited to spinal cord (note that most cases are functional)	Medullary reticular formation (likely nucleus reticularis gigantocellularis)	Cerebral cortex
Velocity of conduction of bulbo-spinal efferent volley	~30 m/s	~30 m/s	NA	5–15 m/s	>50 m/s	~100 m/s
EMG burst duration	>70 ms	>70 ms	>70 ms	~150–450 ms (can be longer)	<50 ms	<50 ms

(EEG: electroencephalography; EMG: electromyography; SCM: sternocleidomastoid)

Box 1 Causes of exaggerated startle reflexes.

- Hereditary hyperekplexia
- Sporadic/Idiopathic hyperekplexia
- Symptomatic hyperekplexia
  - Cortical
    - Static encephalopathies
      - Children with cerebral palsy
      - Post anoxic encephalopathy
      - Post-traumsatic encephalopathy
    - Paraneoplastic
    - Multiple sclerosis
    - Infectious (Cerebral abscess/Encephalitis)
    - Structural (tumors or trauma)
    - Vascular (hemorrhage, infarct, and vascular occlusion of posterior thalamic arteries)
  - Brainstem
    - Brainstem encephalitis (e.g., sarcoid, viral encephalomyelitis, and abscess)
    - Autoimmune/Paraneoplastic (e.g., PERM, multiple sclerosis)
    - Neurodegenerative (e.g., multisystem atrophy)
    - Vascular (e.g., hemorrhage, infarction, and vascular compression)
    - Structural (e.g., trauma, and tumors)
- Neuropsychiatric or unknown physiology
  - Hexosaminidase A deficiency
  - Tourette syndrome
  - Culture-specific syndromes (e.g., jumping Frenchmen, Latah, and Myriachit)
  - Hysterical jumps
  - Anxiety disorders

Epileptic myoclonus and cortical myoclonus respond best to drugs such as sodium valproate and clonazepam, often used in combination in maximum tolerated anticonvulsant doses. Sodium valproate is the drug of choice to treat juvenile myoclonic epilepsy.[69] The initial choice of agent can be based on the underlying etiology, consideration of potential medications related side effects, and whether myoclonic jerks are the primary disabling issue or a comorbidity with refractory epilepsy. It was conventional to start with sodium valproate in patients with severe myoclonus, then to add clonazepam. If symptoms remained refractory, previously piracetam, and now more commonly levetiracetam, which has largely replaced it, can be added.[67,70] However, considering the relatively better side effect profile of levetiracetam, it is not uncommon to use it as the first agent. Tizanidine has been noted to be helpful in some patients.[71] Primidone also may be of value as an additional drug in severely affected patients, as may clobazam and acetazolamide. Zonisamide has been useful in some patients including those with myoclonus-dystonia.[72] Phenytoin, carbamazepine, lamotrigine, vigabatrin, and gabapentin may, paradoxically, worsen some types of myoclonus and should be avoided.[73] Some patients may respond to gamma-hydroxybutyric acid.[74]

Unfortunately, negative myoclonus is frequently resistant to treatment and usually persists to cause bouncy unsteady stance and gait, often with falls. Rare case reports have noted an excellent response to levetiracetam.[75,76] Epileptic negative myoclonus in atypical benign partial epilepsy of childhood can be managed with combinations of valproate, clonazepam, and corticosteroids.[77] Ethosuximide has also been found useful in some cases.[78,79]

The utility of antioxidant N-acetylcysteine and alcohol in the treatment of posthypoxic myoclonus and myoclonus in Unverricht–Lundborg disease has not been clearly established, though noted to be useful in some patients.[80,81]

Those with brainstem myoclonus seem to respond best to clonazepam.[16] Spinal and other segmental myoclonus also responds best to treatment with clonazepam or levetiracetam.[82] Some cases have responded to topiramate, valproate, serotonergic therapy, or intrathecal baclofen. Botulinum toxin can sometimes be useful for medication refractory myoclonus, especially noted to be useful for palatal myoclonus.

Essential myoclonus can sometimes be improved with alcohol, a beta-blocker such as propranolol or an anticholinergic agent.[69] Alcohol improves the myoclonus in myoclonus-dystonia syndrome, without much improvement in the associated dystonia. Most patients with essential myoclonus likely have myoclonus-dystonia. Myoclonus–dystonia can be improved with bilateral deep brain stimulation of the Globus pallidus interna (GPi). Deep brain stimulation is not ordinarily undertaken for posthypoxic myoclonus, but one case has been reported to respond to bilateral GPi stimulation.[83] Treatment with clonazepam may be very effective in some patients with exaggerated startle or hyperekplexia. Others have responded to sodium valproate or levetiracetam.

Myoclonus and jerk-like movements are a frequent presentation of functional movement disorders, and it is important to keep this in mind for the differential diagnosis. Functional movement disorders can usually be identified based on their clinical characteristics; however, clinical neurophysiology is also distinctive and can help to resolve the differential diagnosis.[6,20] A thoughtful multidisciplinary approach using a combination of antidepressant therapy, psychotherapy, and physical therapy can be useful.[84]

CONCLUSION

Myoclonus and startle syndromes are characterized as movement disorders with a 'jerk-like' phenomenology. They have several overlapping clinical characteristics and may occur in many different movement disorders. Different types of myoclonus have distinctive physiologic characteristics which requires objective clinical neurophysiology for correct categorization. Objective characterization of myoclonus can help with their localization within the neural axis, providing useful pathophysiologic insights to guide targeted workup and treatment. Startle is a normal physiologic reflex with distinctive characteristics, which can be pathologically exaggerated in certain genetic and acquired conditions.

REFERENCES

1. Shibasaki H, Hallett M. Electrophysiological studies of myoclonus. Muscle Nerve. 2005;31(2):157-74.
2. Merchant SH, Vial F, Leodori G, Fahn S, Pullman SL, Hallett M. A novel exaggerated "spino-bulbo-spinal like" reflex of lower brainstem origin. Parkinsonism Relat Disord. 2019;61:34-8.
3. Toro C, Pascual-Leone A, Deuschl G, Tate E, Pranzatelli MR, Hallett M. Cortical tremor. A common manifestation of cortical myoclonus. Neurology. 1993;43(11):2346-53.
4. Bai O, Lin P, Vorbach S, Floeter MK, Hattori N, Hallett M. A high performance sensorimotor beta rhythm-based brain-computer interface associated with human natural motor behavior. J Neural Eng. 2008;5(1):24-35.
5. Toro C, Hallett M, Rothwell JC, Asselman PT, Marsden CD. Physiology of negative myoclonus. Adv Neurol. 1995;67:211-7.
6. Merchant SHI, Vial-Undurraga F, Leodori G, van Gerpen JA, Hallett M. Myoclonus: An Electrophysiological Diagnosis. Mov Disord Clin Pract. 2020;7(5):489-499. doi: 10.1002/mdc3.12986. PMID: 32626792; PMCID: PMC7328418.
7. Hallett M, Chadwick D, Marsden CD. Cortical reflex myoclonus. Neurology. 1979;29(8):1107-25.
8. Grosse P, Guerrini R, Parmeggiani L, Bonanni P, Pogosyan A, Brown P. Abnormal corticomuscular and intermuscular coupling in high-frequency rhythmic myoclonus. Brain. 2003;126(Pt 2):326-42.
9. Hanajima R, Okabe S, Terao Y, Furubayashi T, Arai N, Inomata-Terada S, et al. Difference in intracortical inhibition of the motor cortex between cortical myoclonus and focal hand dystonia. Clin Neurophysiol. 2008;119(6):1400-7.
10. Shibasaki H. Electrophysiological studies of myoclonus. Muscle Nerve. 2000;23(3):321-35.
11. Shibasaki H. Neurophysiological classification of myoclonus. Neurophysiol Clin. 2006;36(5-6):267-9.
12. Shibasaki H. Physiology of negative myoclonus. Adv Neurol. 2002;89:103-13.
13. Tassinari CA, Rubboli G, Shibasaki H. Neurophysiology of positive and negative myoclonus. Electroencephalogr Clin Neurophysiol. 1998;107(3):181-95.
14. Thompson PD, Shibasaki H. Myoclonus in corticobasal degeneration and other neurodegenerations. Adv Neurol. 2000; 82:69-81.
15. Cantello R, Gianelli M, Civardi C, Mutani R. Focal subcortical reflex myoclonus. A clinical and neurophysiological study. Arch Neurol. 1997;54(2):187-96.
16. Hallett M, Chadwick D, Adam J, Marsden CD. Reticular reflex myoclonus: a physiological type of human post-hypoxic myoclonus. J Neurol Neurosurg Psychiatry. 1977;40(3): 253-64.
17. van der Salm SM, Erro R, Cordivari C, Edwards MJ, Koelman JHTM, van den Ende T, et al. Propriospinal myoclonus: clinical reappraisal and review of literature. Neurology. 2014;83(20):1862-70.
18. Esposito M, Erro R, Edwards MJ, Cawley N, Choi D, Bhatia KP, et al. The pathophysiology of symptomatic propriospinal myoclonus. Mov Disord. 2014;29(9):1097-9.
19. Brown P, Thompson PD. Electrophysiological aids to the diagnosis of psychogenic jerks, spasms, and tremor. Mov Disord. 2001;16(4):595-9.
20. Matsumoto J, Fuhr P, Nigro M, Hallett M. Physiological abnormalities in hereditary hyperekplexia. Ann Neurol. 1992;32(1):41-50.
21. Terada K, Ikeda A, Van Ness PC, Nagamine T, Kaji R, Kimura J, et al. Presence of Bereitschaftspotential preceding psychogenic myoclonus: clinical application of jerk-locked back averaging. J Neurol Neurosurg Psychiatry. 1995;58(6):745-7.
22. Avanzini G, Shibasaki H, Rubboli G, Canafoglia L, Panzica F, Franceschetti S, et al. Neurophysiology of myoclonus and progressive myoclonus epilepsies. Epileptic Disord. 2016;18(S2):11-27.
23. Hudson AJ, Guthmiller KB, Hyatt MN. Myoclonus following a Peripheral Nerve Block. Case Rep Anesthesiol. 2013;2013:213472.
24. Brown P, Ridding MC, Werhahn KJ, Rothwell JC, Marsden CD. Abnormalities of the balance between inhibition and excitation in the motor cortex of patients with cortical myoclonus. Brain. 1996;119(Pt 1):309-17.
25. Bhatia KP, Brown P, Gregory R, Lennox GG, Manji H, Thompson PD, et al. Progressive myoclonic ataxia associated with coeliac disease. The myoclonus is of cortical origin, but the pathology is in the cerebellum. Brain. 1995;118(Pt 5):1087-93.
26. Ganos C, Kassavetis P, Erro R, Edwards MJ, Rothwell J, Bhatia KP. The role of the cerebellum in the pathogenesis of cortical myoclonus. Mov Disord. 2014;29(4):437-43.
27. Latorre A, Rocchi L, Magrinelli F, Mulroy E, Berardelli A, Rothwell JC, et al. Unravelling the enigma of cortical tremor and other forms of cortical myoclonus. Brain. 2020;143(9):2653-63. doi: 10.1093/brain/awaa129. PMID: 32417917.
28. Frucht SJ, Leurgans SE, Hallett M, Fahn S. The Unified Myoclonus Rating Scale. Adv Neurol. 2002;89:361-76.
29. Brown P. The startle syndrome. Mov Disord. 2002;17(Suppl 2):S79-82.
30. Pearce JMS. Palatal Myoclonus (syn. Palatal Tremor). Eur Neurol. 2008;60(6):312-5.
31. Hallett M. Neurophysiologic studies of functional neurologic disorders. Handb Clin Neurol. 2016;139:61-71.
32. Erro R, Bhatia KP, Edwards MJ, Farmer SF, Cordivari C. Clinical diagnosis of propriospinal myoclonus is unreliable: an electrophysiologic study. Mov Disord. 2013;28(13):1868-73.
33. Brown P. Physiology of startle phenomena. Adv Neurol. 1995;67:273-87.
34. Tijssen MA, Vergouwe MN, van Dijk JG, Rees M, Frants RR, Brown P. Major and minor form of hereditary hyperekplexia. Mov Disord. 2002;17(4):826-30.

35. Bode A, Wood SE, Mullins JGL, Keramidas A, Cushion TD, Thomas RH, et al. New hyperekplexia mutations provide insight into glycine receptor assembly, trafficking, and activation mechanisms. J Biol Chem. 2013;288(47):33745-59.
36. Cuhna P, Herlin B, Vassilev K, Kas A, Lehericy S, Worbe Y, et al. Movement disorders as a new neurological clinical picture in severe SARS-CoV-2 infection. Eur J Neurol. 2020;27(12):e88-e90. doi: 10.1111/ene.14474. Epub 2020 Sep 14. PMID: 32786131; PMCID: PMC7436483.
37. Rábano-Suárez P, Bermejo-Guerrero L, Méndez-Guerrero A, Parra-Serrano J, Toledo-Alfocea D, Sánchez-Tejerina D, et al. Generalized myoclonus in COVID-19. Neurology. 2020;95(6):e767-e772. doi: 10.1212/WNL.0000000000009829. Epub 2020 May 21. PMID: 32439821; PMCID: PMC7455360.
38. Kapoor R, Brown P, Thompson PD, Miller DH. Propriospinal myoclonus in multiple sclerosis. J Neurol Neurosurg Psychiatry. 1992;55(11):1086-8.
39. Monday K, Jankovic J. Psychogenic myoclonus. Neurology. 1993;43(2):349-52.
40. Caviness JN. Epidemiology of myoclonus. Adv Neurol. 2002;89:19-22.
41. Caviness JN, Alving LI, Maraganore DM, Black RA, McDonnell SK, Rocca WA. The incidence and prevalence of myoclonus in Olmsted County, Minnesota. Mayo Clin Proc. 1999;74(6):565-9.
42. Yu XX, Stone J. Functional myoclonus: Time to stop jerking around with negative diagnosis. Parkinsonism Relat Disord. 2018;51:1-2.
43. Stone J, Carson A. Functional neurologic disorders. Continuum (Minneap Minn). 2015;21(3 Behavioral Neurology and Neuropsychiatry):818-37.
44. Dreissen YE, Bakker MJ, Koelman JHTM, Tijssen MA. Exaggerated startle reactions. Clin Neurophysiol. 2012;123(1):34-44.
45. Dreissen YE, Tijssen MA. The startle syndromes: physiology and treatment. Epilepsia. 2012;53(Suppl 7):3-11.
46. Brown P. Neurophysiology of the startle syndrome and hyperekplexia. Adv Neurol. 2002;89:153-9.
47. Brown P, Rothwell JC, Thompson PD, Britton TC, Day BL, Marsden CD. New observations on the normal auditory startle reflex in man. Brain. 1991;114(Pt 4):1891-902.
48. Brown P, Day BL, Rothwell JC, Thompson PD, Marsden CD. The effect of posture on the normal and pathological auditory startle reflex. J Neurol Neurosurg Psychiatry. 1991;54(10):892-7.
49. Brown P, Rothwell JC, Thompson PD, Britton TC, Day BL, Marsden CD. The hyperekplexias and their relationship to the normal startle reflex. Brain. 1991;114(Pt 4):1903-28.
50. Andermann F, Andermann E. Startle disorders of man: hyperekplexia, jumping and startle epilepsy. Brain Dev. 1988;10(4):213-22.
51. Bakker MJ, Tijssen MAJ, van der Meer JN, Koelman JHTM, Boer F. Increased whole-body auditory startle reflex and autonomic reactivity in children with anxiety disorders. J Psychiatry Neurosci. 2009;34(4):314-22.
52. Bakker MJ, van Dijk JG, Pramono A, Sutarni S, Tijssen MAJ. Latah: an Indonesian startle syndrome. Mov Disord. 2013;28(3):370-9.
53. Manford MR, Fish DR, Shorvon SD. Startle provoked epileptic seizures: features in 19 patients. J Neurol Neurosurg Psychiatry. 1996;61(2):151-6.
54. Shimamura M. Studies on a Motor Reflex with Its Reflex Center in the Bulbar Reticular Formation (Spino-Bulbo-Spinal Reflex). No To Shinkei. 1963;15:1165-72.
55. Shimamura M, Mori S, Matsushima S, Fujimori B. On the Spino-Bulbo-Spinal Reflex in Dogs, Monkeys and Man. Jpn J Physiol. 1964;14:411-21.
56. Ertekin C, Celebisoy N, Uludag B. Trigeminocervical reflexes elicited by stimulation of the infraorbital nerve: head retraction reflex. J Clin Neurophysiol. 2001;18(4):378-85.
57. Wartenberg R. Head retraction reflex. Calif Med. 1949;70(5):382.
58. Shimamura M, Aoki M, Sato T. Averaging analysis of the spino-bulbo-spinal (SBS) reflex in man. Nihon Seirigaku Zasshi. 1967;29(7):324-5.
59. Berger C, Meinck HM. Head retraction reflex in stiff-man syndrome and related disorders. Mov Disord. 2003;18(8):906-11.
60. Shimamura M. Longitudinal conduction systems serving spinal and brainstem coordination-spino-bulbo-spinal reflex. Nihon Seirigaku Zasshi. 1971;33(4):225-33.
61. Watson SR, Colebatch JG. EMG responses in the soleus muscles evoked by unipolar galvanic vestibular stimulation. Electroencephalogr Clin Neurophysiol. 1997;105(6):476-83.
62. Wright CG, Barnes CD. Audio-spinal reflex responses in decerebrate and chloralose anesthetized cats. Brain Res. 1972;36(2):307-31.
63. Bakker MJ, van Dijk JG, van den Maagdenberg AM, Tijssen MA. Startle syndromes. Lancet Neurol. 2006;5(6):513-24.
64. Agarwal P, Frucht SJ. Myoclonus. Curr Opin Neurol. 2003;16(4):515-21.
65. Papero PH, Pranzatelli MR, Margolis LJ, Tate E, Wilson LA, Glass P. Neurobehavioral and psychosocial functioning of children with opsoclonus-myoclonus syndrome. Dev Med Child Neurol. 1995;37(10):915-32.
66. Caviness JN. Treatment of myoclonus. Neurotherapeutics. 2014;11(1):188-200.
67. Caviness JN, Truong DD. Myoclonus. Handb Clin Neurol. 2011;100:399-420.
68. Chang VC, Frucht SJ. Myoclonus. Curr Treat Options Neurol. 2008;10(3):222-9.
69. Mantoan L, Walker M. Treatment options in juvenile myoclonic epilepsy. Curr Treat Options Neurol. 2011;13(4):355-70.
70. Espay AJ, Chen R. Myoclonus. Continuum (Minneap Minn). 2013;19(5 Movement Disorders):1264-86.
71. Mukand JA, Giunti EJ. Tizanidine for the treatment of intention myoclonus: a case series. Arch Phys Med Rehabil. 2004;85(7):1125-7.
72. Hainque E, Vidailhet M, Cozic N, Charbonnier-Beaupel F, Thobois S, Tranchant C, et al. A randomized, controlled, double-blind, crossover trial of zonisamide in myoclonus-dystonia. Neurology. 2016;86(18):1729-35.
73. Asconape J, Diedrich A, DellaBadia J. Myoclonus associated with the use of gabapentin. Epilepsia. 2000;41(4):479-81.
74. Arpesella R, Dallocchio C, Arbasino C, Imberti R, Martinotti R, Frucht SJ. A patient with intractable posthypoxic myoclonus (Lance-Adams syndrome) treated with sodium oxybate. Anaesth Intensive Care. 2009;37(2):314-8.
75. Gelisse P, Crespel A, Genton P, Baldy-Moulinier M. Dramatic effect of levetiracetam on epileptic negative myoclonus. Acta Neurol Scand. 2003;107(4):302-3.
76. Koh KN, Lim BC, Hwang H, Park JD, Chae JH, Kim KJ, et al. Cerebellum can be a possible generator of progressive myoclonus. J Child Neurol. 2010;25(6):728-31.

77. Yang Z, Liu X, Qin J, Zhang Y, Bao X, Chang X, et al. A study on epileptic negative myoclonus in atypical benign partial epilepsy of childhood. Brain Dev. 2009;31(4):274-81.
78. Oguni H, Uehara T, Tanaka T, Sunahara M, Hara M, Osawa M. Dramatic effect of ethosuximide on epileptic negative myoclonus: implications for the neurophysiological mechanism. Neuropediatrics. 1998;29(1):29-34.
79. Capovilla G, Beccaria F, Veggiotti P, Rubboli G, Meletti S, Tassinari CA. Ethosuximide is effective in the treatment of epileptic negative myoclonus in childhood partial epilepsy. J Child Neurol. 1999;14(6):395-400.
80. Hurd RW, Wilder BJ, Helveston WR, Uthman BM. Treatment of four siblings with progressive myoclonus epilepsy of the Unverricht-Lundborg type with N-acetylcysteine. Neurology. 1996;47(5):1264-8.
81. Genton P, Guerrini R. Effect of alcohol on action myoclonus in Lance-Adams syndrome and progressive myoclonus epilepsy. Mov Disord. 1992;7(1):92.
82. Keswani SC, Kossoff EH, Krauss GL, Hagerty C. Amelioration of spinal myoclonus with levetiracetam. J Neurol Neurosurg Psychiatry. 2002;73(4):457-8.
83. Mine J, Taketani T, Yoshida K, Yokochi F, Kobayashi J, Maruyama K, et al. Clinical and genetic investigation of 17 Japanese patients with hyperekplexia. Dev Med Child Neurol. 2015;57(4):372-7.
84. Hallett M. The most promising advances in our understanding and treatment of functional (psychogenic) movement disorders. Parkinsonism Relat Disord. 2018;46(Suppl 1):S80-2.

CHAPTER 37

Hyperekplexia and Startle Syndromes

Bhaskar Ghosh, Debjani Roy Chowdhury, Sarbani Sengupta

INTRODUCTION

The word "startle" means to give a sudden shock or surprise to a person or an animal to make somebody or something move or jump suddenly from surprise.[1] Startle response, a physiological protective response, consists of bilaterally synchronous flexion response to acoustic, tactile, and visual stimulus most marked in face and upper half of body.[2] Startle syndrome encompasses heterogeneous group of disorders characterized by either hyperstartling or startle stimulus induced other phenomenology. They can be grouped into three major categories: Hyperekplexia (HPX), neuropsychiatric disorders, and startle stimulus induced disorders. Opposite to the hyperstartling is the hypostartling, absent or reduced startle response of insignificant clinical relevance, seen in progressive supranuclear palsy and diffuse Lewy body disease.[3]

STARTLE RESPONSE

Among all the stimuli, human startle response to acoustic stimuli has been extensively studied. Required acoustic stimuli is at least 80 dB with steep rise (<5 ms).[4]

Components of physiological startle response include forward flexion of head, abduction of shoulder, flexion of elbow, pronation of forearm, clinching of fist, arrest of ongoing behavior, acceleration of heart rate, with less prominent trunk flexion and flexion of knee.[5] Normal startle response usually habituates within 1–5 trials leaving only auditory blink reflex.[2,6,7]

Physiological startle response originates in bulbopontine reticular formation especially the nucleus reticularis caudalis pontis.[5] Acoustic stimulus of startle response travel through the auditory nerve via dorsal, ventral, cochlear root nucleus (bypassing lateral lemniscus) to nuclear pontine reticularis caudalis finally via reticulospinal tract to brainstem and spinal alpha motor neuron.[8]

Startle response has two phases: (1) Early response (muscle tension reflex); and (2) Late response (orienting response). Early response is the rapid accomplishment of a defensive stance with maximum postural stability.[6,7] The late response, a period of decreased activity following first response, have a latency of 400–450 ms, lasting up to 3 seconds.[2,9] Late response of startle response could be modulated by emotional influence suggesting its cortical involvement apart from brainstem.[5]

Latency of electromyography (EMG) activity of various muscles denotes the origin and the spread of startle response. Orbicularis oculi being the first muscle to respond (latency 30–40 ms), bilateral symmetrical craniocervical muscles are involved sequentially involving upward masseter (latency 55–85 ms), downward sternocleidomastoid (latency 55–85 ms), biceps (latency 85–100 ms) with variable involvement of hamstring (latency 100–125 ms), and quadriceps (latency 130–140 ms). During habituation EMG bursts shorten and onset latencies prolong until disappear leaving the orbicularis oculi as the only muscle to respond.[5]

Startle syndrome encompasses group of disorders characterized by exaggerated startle reflex by lowering threshold, greater severity of response, resistance to habituation and likelihood of lower extremity involvement which is rare in physiological startle.[6,7,10]

CLASSIFICATION[3,5]

Startle syndromes can be classified in following groups:

- Hyperekplexia
  - Hereditary
    - Major
    - Minor
  - Sporadic
    - Major
    - Minor
  - Symptomatic
- Neuropsychiatric startle syndrome
- Startle stimulus-induced disorder

HYPEREKPLEXIA

Nowadays, HPX denotes hyperstartling with exception of patients having additional behavior or psychiatric symptoms, considered as neuropsychiatric startle syndrome.[3] HPX can be hereditary, sporadic, and symptomatic.

Hereditary Hyperekplexia

Initially, it was considered partially psychogenic (emotional stimuli) and partially epileptic (drop seizure).[11] HPX, a Greek term, was coined in 1966.[12] Till now ≥100 pedigrees and >120 sporadic cases have been identified.[3,13-16] It may be of major or minor forms.

Major Hereditary Hyperekplexia

It is characterized by three cardinal features:[12,17]

1. *Generalized stiffness at birth*: It increases during handling, disappears during sleep, gradually normalizes during first year of life. Stiff baby syndrome is now synonymous with hereditary major HPX.[3]
2. *Exaggerated startle reflex*: It is marked following unexpected auditory stimuli, persists throughout life.[2]
3. *Generalized stiffness following startle*: Short-lasting temporary generalized stiffness after being startled leading to transient arrest of movement eventually fall.[2]

Clinical Findings

Head retraction reflex is the hallmark of HPX. It is a brisk involuntary backward jerk of head, often associated with retropulsion of trunk in response to light tap to the root of nose, middle portion of upper lip, glabella, and chin with a reflex hammar.[12,18] It is a cutaneomuscular reflex composed of two excitatory components separated by an intercalated period.[19,20] The reflex is absent in normal individuals but can be seen in other neurological conditions such as cerebral palsy,[3] stiff person syndrome, and amyotrophic lateral sclerosis.[21]

Associated features include neonatal tonic cyanotic attack,[22] motor delay in first year of life with subsequent catchup,[3] sudden infant death,[3] spastic paraparesis,[3] periodic limb movement during sleep,[22] hypnogogic myoclonus,[22] stimulus-induced tonic spasm,[21] abnormal horizontal saccades,[5] inguinal, abdominal hernia, and congenital dislocation of hip due to excessive uterine contraction.[3]

Severely affected patients walk with a slow wide-based stiff gait without any ataxia. Deep tendon reflexes are normal or exaggerated with flexor plantars.[3]

Electromyography bursts are larger, long duration (especially in orbicularis oculi, sternocleidomastoid) with shorter latency compared to normal startle response. Habituation is either normal or decreased. Autonomic responses as measured by psychogalvanic response are increased.[3]

Pathogenesis and Genetics

Brainstem as the origin of HPX is supported by the following facts:

- Concentration of glycine receptor, mutation of which is the major cause of HPX, is high in brainstem and spinal cord.[3]
- Most symptomatic HPX are due to brainstem pathology.[3]
- Electromyography latencies of startle response denote its brainstem origin.[3]

Supportive evidence for cortical pathogenesis is weak contrasting with brainstem origin. Giant evoked potential has been found in very small portion of major HPX.[3]

Pathogenesis of stiffness is like due to absence of disynaptic reciprocal inhibition similar to pyramidal tract lesion though the functional test by transcranial magnetic stimulation revealed no abnormalities regarding stimulus response curves, cortical inhibition, and facilitation.[3]

Disease mostly affects postsynaptic glycine receptor, a ligand-gated chloride channel causing postsynaptic hyperpolarization and synaptic inhibition in brainstem and spinal cord. Glycine receptor, a pentametric complex consisting of alpha (α1 and α2) and β subunits, are clustered at neuronal postsynaptic membrane by gephyrin, a protein that is translocated to cell membrane by GDP-GTP exchange factor collybistin.[3] Several missense and nonsense mutation have been identified involving α, β subunits of glycine receptor, gephyrin, collybistin gene in autosomal dominant (AD), autosomal recessive (AR), or compound heterozygote HPX. Functional components of mutation include loss of α1 protein, inability to form or insert glycine receptor complex to membrane, changing the sensitivity for ligand, and channel gating abnormalities.[3]

Eighty percent of major form of HPX concerns the dominant, recessive, and compound heterozygote mutation in α1 subunit of glycine receptor (*GLRA1*) gene,[12,23,24] located on 5q33-35. Recessive inheritance of missense, nonsense, and frameshift mutation in glycine transporter 2 ($Gly\ T_2$) gene encoding the presynaptic sodium and chloride dependent transporter account for the rest 20% of major HPX cases.[24]

Minor Hereditary Hyperekplexia

This form is seen in relatives of major HPX. Differences between major and minor forms are following:

- In minor form:
  - Only exaggerated startle is present sans any stiffness either at birth or poststartle.
  - Age of onset though unclear-never neonatal, usually early infancy to puberty.[3]
  - Latency of startle response is prolonged and does not habituate.[25]
- Spinal motor excitability, as measured by reciprocal inhibition of H-reflex is disinhibited in *GLRA1* positive major form, consistent with their stiffness but normal in minor.[26]

Minor form, still an enigma, can be considered as psychological exploitation on the family members of major HPX patients. The cause of minor form is unclear. They do not show the same gene defect as in major.[25]

Sporadic Hyperekplexia

It is defined as HPX without any family history and without any established neurological cause.[3] This group has also major and minor forms.

Major Form

Resembling clinically that of the hereditary major form, sporadic form does not have any family history and tonic neonatal cyanosis, exclusively observed in hereditary major form. This group does not have a clearly defined genetic basis. *GLRA1* mutations are typically not found.[27] Occasional recessive mutations, compound heterozygosity, mutation in other postsynaptic glycinergic protein are seen.[28-32]

Minor Form

Sporadic minor form constitute acquired, idiopathic, late-onset HPX without additional neurological signs,[6,7,33] family history, childhood stiffness, or genetic basis.

Symptomatic Hyperekplexia

This group shows late-onset HPX with additional neurological signs and symptoms indicating damage to cerebral cortex, brainstem without any neonatal stiffness, and family history. Various disorders are associated with it (**Box 1**). There are some overlap between sporadic and symptomatic form especially when associated with several neurological abnormalities but not any defined syndrome.[5] It is very difficult to distinguish between symptomatic HPX and startle epilepsy especially when electroencephalogram (EEG) is normal.[5]

Approach to Hyperekplexia (Table 1)

Management of Hyperekplexia

Numerous drugs have been tried for HPX. Nevertheless clonazepam was considered to be the most effective. Mode

Box 1 Causes of symptomatic hyperekplexia.

- Cerebral palsy
- Postanoxic encephalopathy
- Paraneoplastic syndrome
- Stiff-man syndrome
- Encephalitis syndrome
- Brainstem infarction
- Posterior fossa malformation
- Medulla compression
- Multiple system atrophy

TABLE 1: Comparison of different types of HPX.[3]

Hyperekplexia	*Age of onset*	*Neonatal stiffness*	*Family history*	*Hereditary neonatal cyanosis*	*Stiffness following startle*	*Additional neuro-logical features*	*Genetic*
Hereditary major	Neonatal	+	+	+	+	±	80% GLRA1 mutation positive
Hereditary minor	Early infancy to puberty	-	+	-	-	-	Unclear
Sporadic major	Neonatal	+	-	-	+	±	GLRA1 mutation Negative Occasional postsynaptic glycine receptor mutation
Sporadic minor	Late-onset	-	-	-	-	-	No genetic basis
Symptomatic	Late-onset	-	-	-	-	+	No genetic basis

of action of clonazepam is possibly dual.[5] It may be due to its binding with high affinity benzodiazepine (BZD) binding site, closely related to gamma-aminobutyric acid (GABA) receptor, potentiating the action of GABA, a widespread inhibitory neurotransmitter. According to the second school of thought, action of clonazepam is due to the effect on modified *GLRA1*. Clinically, clonazepam reduces frequency and magnitude of startle response and reduces the frequency of fall due to transient stiffness. Dose of 0.01–0.1 mg/kg and 0.5–6 mg/day are sufficient for treatment in children and adult, respectively.[21,34] Other drugs such as sodium valproate, clobazam, and carbamazepine have been tried with variable response.[5] In hereditary HPX stiffness disappears by 1 year preferably by 5 years,[5] exaggerated startle disappears variably from infancy to adolescence,[5] usually by first and second decades of life or reappears after early disappearance.[5] Tonic neonatal cyanosis, solely found in *GLRA1* mutation positive hereditary HPX can be stopped by Vigevano maneuver, forced flexion of head and neck toward the trunk.[5]

NEUROPSYCHIATRIC STARTLE SYNDROME (BOX 2)

Culture Specific Syndrome

This group of startle-related abnormalities represents poorly understood, culture specific exploitation of physiological startle reflex characterized by nonhabituating hyperstartling provoked by loud noises, sudden commands, or by being forcefully in the side.[5] After the startle, various events occur such as screaming, throwing objects, hitting, swearing, obeying commands like "dance", "jump", and "run", imitating gesture, echolalia, coprolalia, echopraxia "forced obedience", engaging in acts that are violent, and humiliating.[5] Startles are nonhabituating with marked intensity as compared to normal startle response. Compared to the tics characterized by suppresibility, it is partially suppressible. This group of disorder are consolidated in defined social or ethnic group. Franco-Canadian Lumberjack communities: Jumping Frenchman of maine,[35,36] Acadian in Southern USA: Goosey, Ainu people of Hokkaido: Imu, Siberians: Myriachit,[37] South-East Asian women of low socioeconomic status: Latha, Batsche, Yaan, and Mali-Mali.[38,39] Vivid dreams or visual hallucination may precede the event such as sexual imagery (Latah), snakes and souls of dead (Iban Latah), White men on winged horses (South African Blacks).[5]

Box 2 Neuropsychiatric Startle syndrome.[3]

- Culture specific syndrome
  - Latah
  - Jumping Frenchman of Maine
  - Myriachit
- Startle tics
- Anxiety disorder

Startle Tic

Startle-induced reflex tic can occur as a part of Tourette's syndrome as well as independent phenomenon. Tics are characteristically preceded by inner urge, but here it is induced by startle in addition. It is controversial whether tics are provoked by startle reflex or startle is exaggerated.[22]

STARTLE STIMULUS-INDUCED DISORDER

This group of disorder encompasses neurological disorder of other domain showing excessive response other than just an excessive startle reflex due to a startling stimulus (**Box 3**).

Startle Epilepsy

It is a rare form of epilepsy comprising seizures that occur both spontaneously and induced by an unexpected stimuli (auditory, tactile, and rarely visual) and initiated by a startle.[40,41] Two groups of patients have been identified: (1) Predominant hemispheric lesion with hemiparesis and low intelligent quotient; (2) Diffuse static encephalopathy

Box 3 Startle stimulus-induced disorder.[3]

- Epilepsy:
  - Startle epilepsy, startle-provoked epileptic seizures
  - Pyridoxine-dependent epilepsy
  - Progressive myoclonus epilepsy due to different causes
- Reflex myoclonus:
  - Cortical
  - Reticular
  - Propriospinal
- Startle-induced stiffness:
  - Stiff person syndrome (SPS)
  - Jerking stiff person syndrome
  - Progressive encephalomyelitis with rigidity
  - Strychnine poisoning
  - Tetanus
- Miscellaneous:
  - Paroxysmal kinesigenic dyskinesia (PKD)
  - Cataplexy
  - Late-onset startle-induced tics
  - Creutzfeldt–Jakob disease (CJD)
  - Subacute sclerosing panencephalitis (SSPE)
  - Paraneoplastic syndromes

with marked intellectual impairment.[40] Several etiological or syndromic association such as perinatal anoxia, down syndrome, Sturge–Weber syndrome, and porencephaly are seen.[5] Seizure involves first the muscles of startle reflex, propagating to the contralateral limbs then to the ipsilateral side.[5] Semiology include characteristically tonic unilateral or bilateral posturing, forced neck turning, speech arrest, absence and atonic seizure in some instances.[5] Autonomic features, automatism, laughter, fall may be present in addition.[2] Ictal EEG shows epileptiform discharge over vertex followed by low voltage diffuse flattening starting in premotor, motor cortex spreading to frontal, and parietal region. Interictal EEG includes normal, diffuse, or focal abnormalities depending on the site of the lesion. Neuroimaging reveals frontoparietal lesion in one or both sides involving supplementary motor area in vicinity of paracentral lobule.[5] Regarding management, several antiepileptic drugs (AEDs) such as carbamazepine, sodium valproate, and levetiracetam have been studied. Pathophysiology is uncertain though provocation by startle probably represents a secondary mechanism related to kindling.[40]

Reflex Myoclonus

Cortical myoclonus is focal (multi), distal, may involve face, and main trigger being the stretching of affected limbs. EMG burst of <50 ms, giant somatosensory evoked potential (SSEP), and C reflex in SSEP are the characteristic features. Reticular and propriospinal myoclonus resembles HPX though they differ in their site of stimulus sensitivity.[3] In HPX, the stimulus sensitivity resides in mantle area contrasting with the stimulus sensitivity to limbs in reticular myoclonus, abdomen in propriospinal myoclonus with spontaneous jerks in between induced jerks.[3] In reticular myoclonus, the reflex resembles the startle reflex due to their similar origin, brainstem. But in reticular myoclonus the EMG response in the intrinsic muscles of hand and foot are not delayed relative to the more proximal limb muscle sharply contrasting to startle response.[3] In propriospinal myoclonus, the initial EMG response is in abdomen rather than cervical muscles.[3]

Startle-induced Stiffness

Startle-induced stiffness other than HPX is found in stiff person syndrome (SPS) of autoimmune, or paraneoplastic etiology characterized by continuous axial stiffness with intermittent spasm induced by sudden stimuli. Combination of stiffness and startle induced fall resembles major hereditary and sporadic HPX. The stiffness in SPS is nearly continuous contrasting with the short-lasting (1–2 seconds) poststartle stiffness in startle syndrome.[3] Exaggerated brainstem reflexes as evident by different studies are in both SPS, hereditary, or acquired HPX indicating a pathological association.[3]

In paroxysmal kinesigenic dyskinesia (PKD) the startle stimuli-induced phenomenology is choreodystonia rather than startle reflex. Cataplexy, characterized by sudden loss of muscle tone induced mostly by laughter, can occasionally occur after being startled.[3]

Exaggerated startle reflex is overshadowed by other features in Creutzfeldt–Jakob disease (CJD), subacute sclerosing panencephalitis (SSPE), and paraneoplastic syndrome.

CONCLUSION

Startle syndrome includes a wide spectrum of neurological disorder. Different variants of HPX constitute the majority of patients. It can be hereditary and sporadic, each group is subclassified to major and minor. Apart from hereditary HPX major, the genetic basis is still an enigma. Neuropsychiatric startle syndrome is a unique group with culture and geographical specificity. Symptomatic HPX and startle stimulus-induced disorder constitute a heterogeneous group of disorder.

REFERENCES

1. Hornby AS. Oxford Advanced Learner's Dictionary of Current English (5th edition). España, S.A.: Oxford University Press; 1995. p. 1164.
2. Wilkins DE, Hallett M, Wess MM. Audiogenic startle reflex of man and its relationship to startle syndromes. A review. Brain. 1986;109(3):561-73.
3. Bakker MJ, van Dijk JG, van den Maagdenberg AM, Tijssen MA. Startle syndromes. Lancet Neurol. 2006;5(6):513-24.
4. Matsumoto J, Hallett M. Startle syndromes. In: Fahn S, Marsden CD (Eds.). Movement Disorders. London: Butterworth-Heinemann; 1994. pp. 418-33.
5. Bhidayasiri R, Truong AD. Chapter 32 - Startle syndromes. Handbook of Clinical Neurology. Hyperkinetic Movement Disorders. 2011;100:421-30.
6. Brown P. The startle syndrome. Mov Disord. 2002;17(2):S79-82.
7. Brown P. Neurophysiology of the startle syndrome and hyperekplexia. Adv Neurol. 2002;89:153-9.
8. Koch M. The neurobiology of startle. Prog Neurobiol. 1999;59(2):107-28.
9. Gogan P. The startle and orienting reactions in man. A study of their characteristics and habituation. Brain Res. 1970;18(1):117-35.
10. Matsumoto J, Fuhr P, Nigro M, Hallett M. Physiological abnormalities in hereditary hyperekplexia. Ann Neurol. 1992;32:41-50.
11. Kirstein L, Silfverskiold BP. A family with emotionally precipitated drop seizures. Acta Psychiatr Neurol Scand. 1958;33(4):471-6.

12. Suhren O, Bruyn GW, Tunyman JA. Hyperexplexia, a hereditary startle syndrome. J Neurol Sci. 1966;3:577-605.
13. Doria Lamba L, Giribaldi G, De Negri E, Follo R, De Grandis E, Pintaudi M, et al. A case of major form familial hyperekplexia: prenatal diagnosis and effective treatment with clonazepam. J Child Neurol. 2007;22(6):769-72.
14. Gregory ML, Guzauskas GF, Edgar TS, Clarkson KB, Srivastava AK, Holden KR. A novel GLRA1 mutation associated with an atypical hyperekplexia phenotype. J Child Neurol. 2008;23(12):1433-8.
15. Zoons E, Ginjaar IB, Bouma PA, Carpay JA, Tijssen MA. A new hyperekplexia family with a recessive frameshift mutation in the GLRA1 gene. Mov Disord. 2012;27(6):795-6.
16. Tijssen MA, Bollen E, van Exel E, van Dijk JG. Saccadic eye movements in hyperekplexia. Mov Disord. 1995;10(6):749-53.
17. Tijssen MA, Vergouwe MN, van Dijk JG, Rees M, Frants RR, Brown P. Major and minor form of hereditary hyperekplexia. Mov Disord. 2002;17(4):826-30.
18. Shahar E, Brand N, Uziel Y, Barak Y. Nose tapping test inducing a generalized flexor spasm: a hallmark of hyperexplexia. Acta Paediatr Scand. 1991;80(11):1073-7.
19. Leon-Sarmiento FE, Arimura K, Osame M. Three silent periods in the orbiculari oculi muscles of man: normal findings and some clinical vignettes. Electromyogr Clin Neurophysiol. 2001;41(7):393-400.
20. Berger C, Meinck HM. Head retraction reflex in stiff-man syndrome and related disorders. Mov Disord. 2003;18(8): 906-11.
21. Mine J, Taketani T, Yoshida K, Yokochi F, Kobayashi J, Maruyama K, et al. Clinical and genetic investigation of 17 Japanese patients with Hyperekplexia. Dev Med Child Neurol. 2015;57(4):372-7.d
22. Dreissen YE, Tijssen MA. The startle syndromes: Physiology and treatment. Epilepsia. 2012;53(Suppl 7):3-11.
23. Chung SK, Vanbellinghen JF, Mullins JG, Robinson A, Hantke J, Hammond CL, et al. Pathophysiological mechanisms of dominant and recessive GLRA1 mutations in hyperekplexia. J Neurosci. 2010;30(28):9612-20.
24. Davies JS, Chung SK, Thomas RH, Robinson A, Hammond CL, Mullins JG, et al. The glycinergic system in human startle disease: a genetic screening approach. Front Mol Neurosci. 2010;3:8.
25. Tijssen MA, Padberg GW, van Dijk JG. The startle pattern in the minor form of hyperekplexia. Arch Neurol. 1996;53(7): 608-13.
26. Crone C, Nielsen J, Petersen N, Tijssen MA, van Dijk JG. Patients with the major and minor form of hyperekplexia differ with regards to disynaptic reciprocal inhibition between ankle flexor and extensor muscles. Exp Brain Res. 2001;140(2):190-7.
27. Shiang R, Ryan SG, Zhu YZ, Fielder TJ, Allen RJ, Fryer A, et al. Mutational analysis of familial and sporadic hyperekplexia. Ann Neurol. 1995;38(1):85-91.
28. Rees MI, Lewis TM, Vafa B, Ferrie C, Corry P, Muntoni F, et al. Compound heterozygosity and nonsense mutations in the alpha(1)-subunit of the inhibitory glycine receptor in hyperekplexia. Hum Genet. 2001;109(3):267-70.
29. Rees MI, Lewis TM, Kwok JB, Mortier GR, Govaert P, Snell RG, et al. Hyperekplexia associated with compound heterozygote mutations in the beta-subunit of the human inhibitory glycine receptor (GLRB). Hum Mol Genet. 2002;11(7):853-60.
30. Rees MI, Harvey K, Ward H, White JH, Evans L, Duguid IC, et al. Isoform heterogeneity of the human gephyrin gene (GPHN), binding domains to the glycine receptor, and mutation analysis in hyperekplexia. J Biol Chem. 2003;278(27):24688-96.
31. Forsyth RJ, Gika AD, Ginjaar I, Tijssen MA. A novel GLRA1 mutation in a recessive hyperekplexia pedigree. Mov Disord. 2007;22(11):1643-5.
32. Harvey RJ, Topf M, Harvey K, Rees MI. The genetics of hyperekplexia: more than startle! Trends Genet. 2008;24(9):439-47.
33. Hamelin S, Rohr P, Kahane P, Minotti L, Vercueil L. Late onset hyperekplexia. Epileptic Disord. 2004;6(3):169-72.
34. Dijk JM, Tijssen MA. Management of patients with myoclonus: available therapies and the need for an evidence-based approach. Lancet Neurol. 2010;9(10):1028-36.
35. Beard GM. Experiments with the "jumpers" or "jumping Frenchmen" of Maine. J Nerv Ment Dis. 1880;7:487-90.
36. Saint-Hilaire MH, Saint-Hilaire JM. Jumping Frenchmen of Maine. Mov Disord. 2001;16(3):530.
37. Hammond WA. Miryachit: a newly described disease of the nervous system, and its analogues. N Y Med J. 1884;39:191-2.
38. Chiu TL, Tong JE, Schmidt KE. A clinical and survey study of latah in Sarawak, Malaysia. Psychol Med. 1972;2(2):155-65.
39. Tanner CM, Chamberland J. Latah in Jakarta, Indonesia. Mov Disord. 2001;16(3):526-9.
40. Saenz-Lope E, Herranz FJ, Masdeu JC. Startle epilepsy: a clinical study. Ann Neurol. 1984;16(1):78-81.
41. Manford MR, Fish DR, Shorvon SD. Startle provoked epileptic seizures: features in 19 patients. J Neurol Neurosurg Psychiatry. 1996;61(2):151-6.

CHAPTER 38

Chorea, Athetosis, and Ballism

Deepa Dash, Vinay Goyal

INTRODUCTION

The terms "chorea", "athetosis", and "ballism" have been derived from Greek words meaning "to dance", "not fixed", and "to throw", respectively. Chorea, athetosis, and ballism represent a spectrum of phenomenologically-related movement disorders with shared pathophysiology and overlapping etiologies. Chorea refers to irregular, flowing, nonstereotyped, unpredictable, random, and involuntary movements that often affect the distal limbs with variable speed, timing, and direction, flowing from one body part to another. Many a times when there is mild chorea, it is difficult to differentiate it from restlessness.[1,2] Patients often try to mask the choreic movements with quasipurposive movements. Because of the coexistence of chorea, athetosis, and ballism in the same patient, they are often considered as part of the same spectrum.[3] Athetosis refers to slower, writhing movements with a sinuous quality. The term "choreoathetosis" is used when typical choreic movements coexist with athetosis. Ballism refers to involuntary movements that are proximal and large amplitude (in contrast to distal and low-amplitude contractions typical of chorea) with a flinging or kicking character. Ballism is most often unilateral (hemiballism) and although present at rest, it becomes more prominent with action. When chorea is proximal and has large amplitude, it is called ballism.

The various causes of chorea include hereditary neurodegenerative diseases, structural lesions in various deep brain structures, infectious, autoimmune disorders, metabolic etiologies, and drugs. When approaching a patient with chorea, the investigation is targeted to search for potentially reversible causes or secondary etiologies and or confirm a hereditary condition by appropriate genetic tests. There are vital clues in both history and examination to unravel the etiology of chorea.

ANATOMICAL CORRELATES

The various brain structures which have been implicated in production of chorea are the caudate nucleus, putamen, subthalamic nucleus, thalamus, and their connections. Gamma-aminobutyric acid-ergic (GABAergic) projections from globus pallidus internus (GPi) modulate activity of the motor nuclei of the thalamus, which further facilitate movement through excitatory glutamatergic projections to cortical motor areas. Activity in the GPi itself is modulated by a dual set of striatopallidal GABAergic projections, which have been termed the "direct" and "indirect" pathways. The disturbance in the balance between direct and indirect pathways in the basal ganglia circuits resulting in exaggerated dopaminergic activity will result in chorea. The alterations in the indirect pathway of basal ganglia leading to the reduced inhibitory outflow to the pallidum leads to the hyperkinetic movements seen in chorea.[4] The various etiologies which may produce this kind of disruption of the balance in the basal ganglia circuitry may be a structural lesion, neuronal degeneration of selective group of neurons, blockade of receptors of various neurotransmitters, metabolic causes, and also various autoimmune causes.

EPIDEMIOLOGY

Because of lack of community based studies, the true estimates of prevalence of chorea are unknown. Broadly based on etiology, Huntington disease (HD) is the most common causes of hereditary chorea with a prevalence estimate of 3 per 100,000 and levodopa-induced choreiform dyskinesia may be the most frequently encountered etiology of acquired chorea. Piccolo and colleagues in a case series of 51 patients with sporadic chorea who got admitted over a span of 5 years reported vascular lesions to be the most frequently encountered cause of chorea. Drugs (40%), hereditary cause (10%), and acquired immune deficiency syndrome (10%) were the other common etiologies reported in this series.[5] In children the spectrum of causes are different compared to adults with Sydenham chorea (SC) accounting for >95% of acute chorea.

CLASSIFICATION

Broadly the etiological spectrum of chorea may be categorized as primary which includes hereditary causes and secondary or acquired causes. There various clinical pointers which help in clinically differentiating hereditary chorea from acquired chorea. Time of onset and progression is the most important differentiating feature, with hereditary chorea having slow, insidious onset with relatively symmetrical involvement if limbs in contrast the acquired cause have acute to subacute onset and may have asymmetrical involvement. When there is a hemi-distribution or unilateral chorea, there is high likelihood of finding a focal structural lesion.

HEREDITARY CAUSES

The various hereditary disorders which can present as chorea as dominant phenomenology have been listed in **Box 1**. Family history can give clues to suggest the pattern of inheritance which could be autosomal dominant (AD), autosomal recessive (AR), or X-linked recessive, inheritance, and thus, helps in narrowing down the differentials in patient. However, the absence of a family history of neurological disease does not exclude a genetic disorder totally.

Box 1 Etiological classification of chorea.

- Hereditary chorea:
  - Autosomal dominant:
    - Huntington's disease (HD)
    - Huntington's disease-like 2 and other HD-like syndromes
    - *C9orf72* repeat expansions
    - Dentatorubropallidoluysian atrophy
    - Benign hereditary chorea
    - Spinocerebellar ataxia (types 2, 3, or 17)
    - Paroxysmal kinesigenic choreoathetosis
  - Autosomal recessive:
    - Ataxia-telangiectasia
    - Choreo-acanthocytosis
    - Friedreich ataxia

Continued

Continued

    - Huntington disease-like 3
    - Neuronal ceroid lipofuscinosis
    - Pantothenate kinase-associated neurodegeneration (PKAN)
    - Phenylketonuria
    - Porphyria
    - Wilson disease
    - Ataxia with oculomotor apraxia
  - X-linked
    - McLeod syndrome
    - Lesch–Nyhan disease
- Structural basal-ganglia lesions
  - Vascular chorea in stroke
  - Mass lesions (e.g., central nervous system (CNS) lymphoma and metastatic brain tumors)
  - Multiple sclerosis plaques
  - Extrapontine myelinolysis
- Autoimmune disorders:
  - Sydenham's chorea
  - Systemic lupus erythematosus
  - Chorea gravidarum
  - Antiphospholipid antibody syndrome
  - Postinfectious or postvaccinal encephalitis
  - Paraneoplastic choreas
- Infectious chorea
  - Human immunodeficiency virus (HIV) encephalopathy
  - Toxoplasmosis
  - Cysticercosis
  - Diphtheria
  - Bacterial endocarditis
  - Neurosyphilis
  - Scarlet fever
  - Viral encephalitis (mumps, measles, and varicella)
- Metabolic disorders:
  - Acute intermittent porphyria
  - Hypo-/hypernatremia
  - Hypocalcemia
  - Hyperthyroidism
  - Hypoparathyroidism
  - Hepatic/renal failure
- Toxins:
  - Alcohol intoxication or withdrawal
  - Carbon monoxide
  - Glue sniffing
  - Manganese
  - Mercury
  - Thallium
  - Toluene
- Drugs

The hereditary disorders can be categorized based on the mode of inheritance.

Autosomal dominant: The most common causes of hereditary chorea with AD inheritance include HD, HD-like (HDL) syndromes, dentatorubral-pallidoluysian atrophy (DRPLA), specific forms of spinocerebellar ataxia (SCA), neuroferritinopathy, and benign hereditary chorea (BHC).

Huntington Disease

Worldwide HD remains the most common cause of hereditary chorea. HD is caused by a cytosine-adenine-guanine (CAG) trinucleotide repeat expansion of the huntingtin (*HTT*) gene on chromosome 4p leading to an enlarged polyglutamine tract in the HTT protein.[6] The areas where there is maximal neuronal loss in HD are caudate and putamen. Adult-onset HD will present with chorea, cognitive decline, behavioral abnormality, oculomotor abnormalities which will be progressive, and will eventually lead to mortality.[7] The usual age of onset is third to fifth decade and onset before 20 years of age is considered juvenile HD. Behavioral and cognitive impairment may precede motor symptoms. Depression is common and there is higher rate of suicide rates in HD. Presenting features differ between adults and juvenile HD, with parkinsonism, dystonia, and myoclonus without prominent chorea seen in juvenile HD and is termed as "Westphal variant". Various disorders are now described as being "HDL". Of these, HDL1, HDL2, and SCA 17 show AD inheritance.

Huntington Disease-like Syndromes

Huntington's disease-like phenotype (HDL1) is disorder where in a 192-nucleotide is inserted in the region of prion protein (PRNP) encoding an octapeptide repeat in the PRNP. The HDL syndromes may present with chorea, behavioral abnormality, and cognitive dysfunction akin to HD.[8] They usually have AD inheritance, except HDL3.

C9ORF72 repeat expansions: Another important hereditary neurodegenerative condition which can present with the phenotype of HD is *C9ORF72* repeat expansions. In a recent study of 514 patients with clinically suspected HD with negative gene testing for HTT repeat expansions *C9ORF72* gene expansion was reported in 10 patients (2%).[9] Repeat expansion in the *C9orf72* gene is one of the most common causes of familial frontotemporal lobar degeneration and amyotrophic lateral sclerosis.

Benign Hereditary Chorea

Benign hereditary chorea is characterized by chorea with onset in early childhood with the peaking of symptoms by the second decade with a nonprogressive course after that. This is in contrast to HD where the disease onset is much later and has a progressive course. Also there is no reduction in life expectancy of patients with BHC and there are now studies reporting improvement in chorea as patient grows older.[10] Children may present with other neurological features such as dysarthria, axial dystonia, gait disturbance, myoclonic jerks, hypothyroidism, pulmonary infections in infancy, scholastic problems, and behavioral difficulties. Most reported patients are heterozygous for mutations in the *NKX2-1* gene (also known as the *TITF1* gene) on chromosome 14q that encodes thyroid transcription factor.

Dentatorubral Pallidoluysian Atrophy

Dentatorubral-pallidoluysian atrophy is an AD disorder because of CAG triplet expansions in the *ATN1* gene encoding atrophin-1. As expected, the expansion leads to anticipation with paternal transmission. There are wide variations in the age of onset of the disease. It should be suspected when ataxia and rigidity are accompanied by choreoathetosis, myoclonic epilepsy, and dementia. Patients present with prominent ataxia, choreoathetosis, along with cognitive decline. In patients with juvenile onset of DRPLA, myoclonic epilepsy is a prominent symptom.[11]

Spinocerebellar Ataxias

Spinocerebellar ataxias present with prominent progressive cerebellar ataxia along with other neurological features such as ophthalmoplegia, pyramidal signs, movement disorders, and cognitive dysfunction. Chorea is a prominent symptom reported in SCA types 1, 2, 3, and 17.

Neuroferritinopathy

Neuroferritinopathy is one of the disorders grouped under the broad umbrella of neurodegeneration with brain iron accumulation (NBIA). The disease is caused by the genetic mutation in the *FTL* gene which encodes for the ferritin light chain resulting in accumulation of iron in the basal ganglia. Patient present with onset in adulthood of progressive extrapyramidal feature such as chorea, dystonia, or Parkinsonism with asymmetrical involvement and cognitive impairment with the presence of action specific facial dystonia.[12] Serum ferritin may be low but presence of normal ferritin does not exclude the disease. The characteristic brain magnetic resonance imaging (MRI) demonstrates increased deposition of iron in the basal ganglia with gradient echo (T2*) signal loss and necrotic changes in the basal ganglia. In a recent study, a typical pattern of iron deposition, termed "pencil lining" with susceptibility-weighted MRI demonstrating linear areas of low signal that outline the cerebral and cerebellar cortices and other gray matter structures as if traced by a black pencil.[13]

ADCY5 mutations: *ADCY5* gene mutation can present with wide spectrum of childhood-onset hyperkinetic movement disorders. Chorea is one of the most prominent symptoms, along with other features such as facial myokymia, dystonia, and myoclonus. The clinical findings which should raise the suspicion of *ADCY5* gene mutation are the onset of symptoms in first decade, intact cognition, and prominent facial twitches. A specific feature reported is the marked fluctuations with paroxysmal attacks at night or upon waking up.[14]

Autosomal Recessive

Of the AR disorders, the important causes are chorea-acanthocytosis, Wilson disease, pantothenate kinase-associated neurodegeneration (PKAN), and ataxia-telangiectasia.

Chorea-acanthocytosis

This form of hereditary chorea presents with dominant features of chorea, dystonia, Parkinsonism, eye movement abnormalities, tics, behavioral abnormality, and intellectual decline. Although the clinical manifestations are similar to that seen in HD, the prominence of orofacial and lingual dyskinesia along with self-mutilation of lip and tongue with feeding dystonia in chorea acanthocytosis helps in clinically differentiating it from HD. Other neurological manifestation such as seizures, peripheral neuropathy, and increased levels of serum creatine kinase are common findings. The disease affects in the third decade and has relentlessly progressive course. The typical acanthocytes are present on peripheral blood films (should be sent 3–4 times) helps in the diagnosis, although their absence does not rule out the disease. The confirmatory test is the genetic testing for mutation in the *VPS13A* gene on chromosome 9 which encodes for the protein chorein.[15]

Wilson disease: Although chorea is a rare feature of Wilson disease, but should be ruled out in all patients presenting with movement disorders <40 years of age because it is a treatable disorder. The disease is caused by a mutation in the *ATP7B* gene leading to copper accumulation in various systems including brain. Common neurologic manifestations include tremor, dysarthria, ataxia, dystonia, and Parkinsonism. Investigation demonstrates low ceruloplasmin and serum copper levels, increased 24-hour urine copper excretion, and abnormal liver function tests.

Pantothenate kinase-associated neurodegeneration: PKAN is a subtype of NBIA caused by genetic mutations encoding pantothenate kinase 2 (PANK2).[16] The resultant iron deposition occurs in the basal ganglia, mostly in globus pallidus interna. Dystonia is a prominent feature along with Parkinsonism, spasticity, pigmentary retinal degeneration, and cognitive deficits. Chorea is a rarely seen.[17] Typical findings in brain MRI is "eye of the tiger" with a central focus of increased T2 signal intensity in the medial globus pallidus surrounded by a zone of hypointensity.

X-linked Diseases

The two common hereditary disorders of chorea with X-linked inheritance are McLeod syndrome and Lesch–Nyhan syndrome.

McLeod Syndrome

The syndrome has phenotype similar to chorea acanthocytosis with prominent chorea, behavioral and cognitive abnormalities, peripheral neuropathy, elevated creatine kinase (with or without clinical myopathy), and epilepsy.[18] Clinically the differentiating features form chorea-acanthocytosis are the absence of self-mutilation and typical feeding dystonia. About two-thirds of patients have cardiomyopathy and arrhythmias. McLeod syndrome is caused by a mutation on the *XK* gene causing reduction of all Kell antigens and absence of Kx antigen on red blood cells.

Lesch–Nyhan Syndrome

Lesch–Nyhan syndrome is an X-linked recessive disorder with both neurological and behavioral manifestations as presenting feature. The mutations of gene coding for the enzyme hypoxanthine-guanine phosphoribosyl transferase (HPRT) manifests with the deficiency of the enzyme which will lead to increased production of uric acid. The clinical manifestations have a wide spectrum with some patients being asymptomatic and others with the full blown neuropsychiatric features based on the amount of enzyme present. Male with this disorder present with delayed developmental milestones, subnormal cognition, along with hyperkinetic movement disorders, and symptoms because of pyramidal tract involvement. Children have self-mutilating behavior along with choreoathetosis, additionally dystonia also, is one of the dominant feature of the disease.[19]

ACQUIRED CAUSES

The spectrum of acquired causes includes vascular lesions of central nervous system, autoimmune diseases, metabolic disorders, infectious diseases, toxins, drugs, paraneoplastic syndrome, and endocrine disorders.

Vascular Lesions

Acute-onset chorea can occur due to vascular insult producing an ischemic or hemorrhagic lesion. Vascular etiology accounts for most common nonhereditary etiology of chorea in patients admitted to hospital. Vascular anomaly like Moyamoya can also present with chorea because of the involvement of the basal ganglia by the hypertrophied collateral vessels. The lesions of various brain structures which have been reported to produce chorea are subthalamic nucleus, caudate, putamen, thalamus, globus pallidus, corona radiate, subcortical white matter, and even cortex. This wide distribution suggests that chorea is a manifestation of alteration in connections of the posterolateral putamen with other structures.[20] Hematological disorders like polycythemia vera can present with chorea much before other hematological symptoms are apparent.[21] Typically it is encountered in women and presents acutely with prominent orofaciolingual involvement.

Autoimmune Disorders

Sydenham Chorea

The most common causes of chorea presenting in childhood is SC. The disease is the result of cross reactivity of antibodies of antigens of striatum with group A streptococcus. Children of age 5–15 years are affected with female dominance. Unlike other manifestations of acute rheumatic fever, SC is a delayed symptom which appears 4–6 weeks after the fever. The distribution of chorea is usually bilateral and is associated with decrease in tone, dysarthria, gait disturbance, and behavioral abnormality. In around one-third of patients the distribution may be in hemi-distribution. Usually the chorea lasts typically last 2–9 months followed by complete spontaneous resolution. A significant proportion of patients may have persistence of chorea after 2 years or may have recurrences later on. A small proportion of patients with SC may not have other manifestations of acute rheumatic fever and, thus, should undergo echocardiography to rule out carditis. There is limited utility of antistreptolysin O titer because titers usually peak much before the onset of SC symptoms. Another antibody, antideoxyribonuclease B titer is a better surrogate marker as the titers are elevated for a longer period.

Paraneoplastic Chorea

CV2/collapsin-responsive mediator protein-5 (CRMP5) antibodies induced paraneoplastic disease may present with chorea as presenting feature. This antibody is usually associated with in the small cell lung carcinoma.[22] Other neoplasms reported to have chorea as a presenting feature are breast, thymoma, lymphoma, renal cell carcinoma, and testicular cancer.[23,24]

Connective Tissue Disorders

Chorea is an uncommon manifestation of systemic lupus erythematosus (SLE). Chorea development is associated with presence of antiphospholipid antibodies in patients with SLE. Most often the chorea has unilateral distribution and is precipitated by pregnancy or usage of oral contraceptive.[25] In patients with primary antiphospholipid syndrome, chorea is reported in only 1% of patients. Chorea is an uncommon or rare manifestation of other connective tissue disorders.[26,27]

Metabolic Disorders

Hepatolenticular Degeneration

The clinical picture is heterogeneous, because patients may present with a variable combination of neurological and hepatic symptoms. Most patients have a combination of different movement disorders, but a few present with isolated chorea. MRI of the brain shows not only images compatible with cavitation in the basal ganglia (hyperintense signal on T2 and hypointense on T1) but also hyperintense T1 signal in the pallidum, putamen, and upper brainstem because of deposition of manganese.[28]

Nonketotic Hyperglycemia

One of the important causes of acute-onset chorea due to metabolic disturbance is chorea associated with nonketotic hyperglycemia. The disorder is common among the Asian population and affects females more than males. The patients usually present with unilateral or generalized chorea in combination with athetosis and or ballism. The characteristic MRI findings are hyperintense signal of the pallidum on T1 possibly indicating microhemorrhages of the pallidum. The symptoms gradually remit after the glycemic control is achieved.

Chorea Gravidarum

Chorea gravidarum encountered more often in women with a history of Sydenham's chorea or another autoimmune disorder and may be due to be a sensitization of dopamine receptors by estrogens during pregnancy. Chorea gravidarum, hyperglycemia, and other metabolic or endocrine disorders may be associated with chorea (**Box 2**).

Chorea has been reported in association with many metabolic abnormalities such as hypoglycemia, hypernatremia, hyponatremia, hypomagnesemia, and hypocalcemia. A remission of the movement disorder after correction of the metabolic abnormality suggests causal role of these abnormalities.

Box 2 Investigations in patients with chorea with possible differentials.

- Blood sample
- Blood sugar: Hyperglycemia, hypoglycemia, hypernatremia, hyponatremia, hypomagnesemia hypercalcemia, and hypocalcemia
- Blood film for acanthocytosis: Neuroacanthocytosis syndrome and Macleod syndrome
- Liver function tests: Wilson's disease and choreoacanthocytosis
- Copper studies: Wilson's disease
- Thyroid function tests: Hypothyroidism and hyperthyroidism
- Parathyroid levels: Hypoparathyroidism, hyperparathyroidism, and pseudohypoparathyroidism
- Pregnancy test: Chorea gravidarum
- Creatine phosphokinase: ChAc and McLeod syndrome
- Ceruloplasmin: Wilson's disease; aceruloplasminemia
- Ferritin: Neuroferritinopathy and Lesch–Nyhan syndrome
- Sedimentation rate: antinuclear antibodies, anti-deoxyribonucleic acid (DNA), anti-SSA, anti-SSB, anti-Ro, anti-La, etc.
- Autoimmune disease: Lupus anticoagulant, systemic lupus erythematosus, antiphospholipid antibodies, antiphospholipid syndrome, antistreptolysin O (ASO), anti-deoxyribonuclease B (anti-DNase B) titers (Sydenham's chorea)
- Human immunodeficiency virus (HIV) test: HIV/ acquired immunodeficiency syndrome (AIDS)-related infection
- Anti-gliadin antibodies: Coeliac disease
- Toxin screen: Mercury, thallium, and other toxins
- Antineuronal antibodies [anti-CRMP-5/CV2 (anti-collapsing response-mediator protein-5/CV2), anti-Hu, anti-Yo, anti-N-methyl-d-aspartate (NMDA) receptor]: Paraneoplastic syndromes
- Plasma lactate/pyruvate: Mitochondrial and other energy metabolism disorders
- Alpha-fetoprotein: Ataxia-telangiectasia, ataxia with oculomotor apraxia type 1 and 2
- Cholesterol: Ataxia with oculomotor apraxia type 1 and 2
- Erythrocyte Kx and Kell antigens: Macleod syndrome
- Genetic testing: HD, as indicated
- Magnetic resonance imaging/computed tomography (MRI/CT) + contrast: Structural lesions; iron deposition, calcification, and eye of tiger in PKAN (pantothenate kinase-associated neurodegeneration)
- Lumbar puncture: Creutzfeldt–Jakob disease; other chronic infections; lactate/pyruvate for mitochondrial and other energy metabolism disorders
- Urinary and serum organic and amino acids: Organic/amino acidopathies

Infectious Diseases

Human immunodeficiency virus (HIV) infection is the most common infective cause of chorea.[29] Hemiballism-hemichorea and tremor are the most common movement disorder in patients with HIV infection.[29] This could be due to an encephalitic presentation or other opportunistic infections or even drugs used in these settings. There reports of other infections of central nervous system (CNS) such as pyogenic meningitis, aseptic meningitis, tuberculous meningitis, Lyme disease, parasitic, or fungal infections having chorea as a part of their clinical presentation.

Drugs and Toxins

Drug-induced Chorea

A longlist of drugs has been reported to cause chorea, either as acute phenomenon or after a long-term usage (**Box 3**).

Box 3 List of drugs which have been reported to produce chorea.

- Dopamine receptor blocking agents:
  - Phenothiazines
  - Butyrophenones
  - Benzamides
- Antiparkinsonian drugs:
  - Levodopa
  - Dopamine agonists
  - Anticholinergics
- Antiepileptic drugs:
  - Phenytoin
  - Carbamazepine
  - Valproic acid
- Psychostimulants:
  - Amphetamines
  - Pemoline
  - Cocaine
- Calcium-channel blockers:
  - Cinnarizine
  - Flunarizine
  - Verapamil
- Others:
  - Lithium
  - Baclofen
  - Digoxin
  - Tricyclic antidepressants
  - Cyclosporine
  - Steroids/oral contraceptives
  - Theophylline

Some drugs require pre-existing basal ganglia abnormality to produce chorea in others no such background is required. Oral contraceptives are likely to produce chorea in patient who had previous choreic episodes because of SC or have comorbid SLE or antiphospholipid antibodies. Dopamine antagonists, on the other hand, induce dyskinesia without a pre-existing basal ganglia abnormality. The typical bucco-linguo-masticatory syndrome seen in neuroleptic tardive dyskinesia is characterized by repetitive movements of tongue twisting and protrusion, lip smacking, and chewing. Movements may improve after drug withdrawal but may also persist or worsen with time. One of the possible pathophysiology mechanisms for tardive dyskinesia is postsynaptic dopamine hypersensitivity or striatal neuroplasticity changes. Levodopa-induced chorea develops in >40% of patients with Parkinson's disease depending on age and duration and dose of levodopa treatment.[30]

MANAGEMENT OF CHOREA

The investigations which will help in reaching a diagnosis in a patient are tabulated in **Box 2**. The management of chorea targets two aspects of the disease, the etiology and the symptomatic treatment. In patients where a secondary cause is found appropriate treatment of the underlying cause or withdrawal of the offending agent will help in remission of the chorea. In hereditary chorea, currently no agent can reverse or retard the progression of chorea. The drug development approach for HD has undergone a remarkable evolution in recent years. Aside from efforts focused on symptomatic treatment, for the first time, therapies that target the HD biology are being developed to modulate disease progression. In the past decades, there have been various efforts to identify disease-modifying therapies in HD. Overall, these compounds targeted multiple downstream cellular processes and molecular targets, including oxidative stress, transcriptional dysregulation, mitochondrial dysfunction, excitotoxicity. Unfortunately, these clinical trials did not lead to the identification of a disease-modifying therapy in HD.

The field of HD therapeutics is living promising times as various disease-modifying strategies are being developed. In this Renaissance period of therapeutic development, novel interventions explore the therapeutic potential of proximal pathways in the HD cell pathogenesis, such as the synthesis of mutated variant of HTT (mHTT) and it's intracellular trafficking. The ability to inhibit the synthesis of mHTT is perhaps the therapeutic strategy with the highest potential in HD. Various mHTT-lowering approaches are under development at a preclinical phase and clinical trials have already started in some programs. Currently, the mainstay is symptomatic management of the chorea with target improving the quality of life patients.

Symptomatic Treatment

Dopamine receptor blockers are considered the most effective agents to reduce the severity of chorea. First-generation antipsychotic agents because of more potent D2-receptor blocking action have higher antichoreic action. But they are fraught with unacceptable side-effects such as sedation, acute dystonic reaction, tardive dyskinesia, and Parkinsonism. Although there are no controlled trials, open labelled reports suggest that second-generation antipsychotic drugs including olanzapine, risperidone, quetiapine, and clozapine have limited roles in the treatment of chorea.

Open-labeled reports and recent placebo-controlled trial of dopamine depleting agents like inhibitors of pre-synaptic vesicular monoamine transporter type 2 (VMAT2) such as tetrabenazine, valbenazine, and deutetrabenazine have shown efficacy and are now a first-line option for chorea associated with HD and other etiologies too.[31] Valproic acid, carbamazepine, oxcarbazepine, topiramate, levetiracetam, and gabapentin may be useful to suppress chorea in subgroup of patients.[32] Clinical experience suggests that benzodiazepines have a mild antichorea effect, but the use of such agents is poorly documented.

CONCLUSION

Chorea, athetosis, and ballism are related movement disorders which can be due to a multitude of disorders including both hereditary and acquired etiologies. A thorough work-up including a detailed family, medical, and medication history; neurologic and medical examinations; a range of laboratory tests including genetic tests; and neuroimaging will help elucidate the correct etiology. The diagnosis can be aided by giving credence to the time course, age group, and known prevalence in the population. Management should include not only symptomatic treatment of chorea but also other associated medical, neurologic, and psychiatric aspects.

REFERENCES

1. Bhidayasiri R, Truong DD. Chorea and related disorders. Postgrad Med J. 2004;80(947):527-34.
2. Cardoso F, Seppi K, Mair KJ, Wenning GK, Poewe W. Seminar on choreas. Lancet Neurol. 2006;5(7):589-602.
3. Suchowersky O, Muthipeedika J. A case of late-onset chorea. Nat Clin Pract Neurol. 2005;1(2):113-6.
4. Mink JW. The basal ganglia and involuntary movements: impaired inhibition of competing motor patterns. Arch Neurol. 2003;60(10):1365-8.
5. Piccolo I, Defanti CA, Soliveri P, Volontè MA, Cislaghi G, Girotti F. Cause and course in a series of patients with sporadic chorea. J Neurol. 2003;250(4):429-35.
6. The Huntington's Disease Collaborative Research Group. A novel gene containing a trinucleotide repeat that is expanded and unstable on Huntington's disease chromosomes. Cell. 1993;72(6):971-83.
7. Leigh RJ, Newman SA, Folstein SE, Lasker AG, Jensen BA. Abnormal ocular motor control in Huntington's disease. Neurology. 1983;33(10):1268-75.
8. Gövert F, Schneider SA. Huntington's disease and Huntington's disease-like syndromes: an overview. Curr Opin Neurol. 2013;26(4):420-7.
9. Hensman Moss DJ, Poulter M, Beck J, Hehir J, Polke JM, Campbell T, et al. C9orf72 expansions are the most common genetic cause of Huntington disease phenocopies. Neurology. 2014;82(4):292-9.
10. Armstrong MJ, Shah BB, Chen R, Angel MJ, Lang AE. Expanding the phenomenology of benign hereditary chorea: evolution from chorea to myoclonus and dystonia. Mov Disord. 2011;26(12):2296-7.
11. Egawa K, Takahashi Y, Kubota Y, Kubota H, Inoue Y, Fujiwara T, et al. Electroclinical features of epilepsy in patients with juvenile type dentatorubral-pallidoluysian atrophy. Epilepsia. 2008;49(12):2041-9.
12. Chinnery PF, Curtis AR, Fey C, Coulthard A, Crompton D, Curtis A, et al. Neuroferritinopathy in a French family with late onset dominant dystonia. J Med Genet. 2003;40(5):e69.
13. Batla A, Adams ME, Erro R, Ganos C, Balint B, Mencacci NE, et al. Cortical pencil lining in neuroferritinopathy: a diagnostic clue. Neurology. 2015;84(17):1816-8.
14. Carecchio M, Mencacci NE, Iodice A, Pons R, Panteghini C, Zorzi G, et al. ADCY5-related movement disorders: Frequency, disease course and phenotypic variability in a cohort of paediatric patients. Parkinsonism Relat Disord. 2017;41: 37-43.
15. Ueno S, Maruki Y, Nakamura M, Tomemori Y, Kamae K, Tanabe H, et al. The gene encoding a newly discovered protein, chorein, is mutated in chorea-acanthocytosis. Nat Genet. 2001;28(2):121-2.
16. Dusek P, Jankovic J, Le W. Iron dysregulation in movement disorders. Neurobiol Dis. 2012;46(1):1-18.
17. Barton B, Zauber SE, Goetz CG. Movement disorders caused by medical disease. Semin Neurol. 2009;29(2):97-110.
18. Danek A, Rubio JP, Rampoldi L, Ho M, Dobson-Stone C, Tison F, et al. McLeod neuroacanthocytosis: genotype and phenotype. Ann Neurol. 2001;50(6):755-64.
19. Jinnah HA, Visser JE, Harris JC, Verdu A, Larovere L, Ceballos-Picot I, et al. Delineation of the motor disorder of Lesch-Nyhan disease. Brain. 2006;129(5):1201-17.
20. Alarcón F, Zijlmans JC, Dueñas G, Cevallos N. Post-stroke movement disorders: report of 56 patients. J Neurol Neurosurg Psychiatry. 2004;75(11):1568-74.
21. Nazabal ER, Lopez JM, Perez PA, Del Corral PR. Chorea disclosing deterioration of polycythaemia vera. Postgrad Med J. 2000;76(900):658-9.
22. Vigliani MC, Honnorat J, Antoine JC, Vitaliani R, Giometto B, Psimaras D, et al. Chorea and related movement disorders of paraneoplastic origin: the PNS EuroNetwork experience. J Neurol. 2011;258(11):2058-68.
23. Kellinghaus C, Kraus J, Blaes F, Nabavi DG, Schäbitz WR. CRMP-5-autoantibodies in testicular cancer associated with limbic encephalitis and choreiform dyskinesias. Eur Neurol. 2007;57(4):241-3.
24. Lee EK, Maselli RA, Ellis WG, Agius MA. Morvan's fibrillary chorea: a paraneoplastic manifestation of thymoma. J Neurol Neurosurg Psychiatry. 1998;65(6):857-62.
25. Arnson Y, Shoenfeld Y, Alon E, Amital H. The antiphospholipid syndrome as a neurological disease. Semin Arthritis Rheum. 2010;40(2):97-108.
26. Benamour S, Naji T, Alaoui FZ, El-Kabli H, El-Aidouni S. Neurological involvement in Behçet's disease. 154 cases from a cohort of 925 patients and review of the literature. Rev Neurol (Paris). 2006;162(11):1084-90.
27. Venegas Fanchke P, Sinning M, Miranda M. Primary Sjogren's syndrome presenting as a generalized chorea. Parkinsonism Relat Disord. 2005;11(3):193-4.
28. Jog MS, Lang AE. Chronic acquired hepatocerebral degeneration: case reports and new insights. Mov Disord. 1995;10: 714-22.
29. Cardoso F. HIV-related movement disorders: epidemiology, pathogenesis and management. CNS Drugs. 2002;16(10):663-8.
30. Fahn S. The spectrum of levodopa-induced dyskinesias. Ann Neurol. 2000;47(4 suppl 1):S2-9.
31. Heo YA, Scott LJ. Deutetrabenazine: A Review in Chorea Associated with Huntington's Disease. Drugs. 2017;77(17):1857-64.
32. Siniscalchi A, Gallelli L, De Sarro G. Use of antiepileptic drugs for hyperkinetic movement disorders. Curr Neuropharmacol. 2010;8(4):359-66.

CHAPTER 39

Huntington's Disease and Huntington Like Disorders

Srinivas Raju D, Prashanth LK

INTRODUCTION

Chorea is a hyperkinetic movement disorder characterized by brief, abrupt, irregular, unpredictable, and non-stereotyped movements. The etiological causes for chorea are wide-ranged including various autoimmune, vascular, space occupying, metabolic, drug-induced, and genetic causes. With regards to genetic forms of chorea, Huntington's disease (HD) has almost a synonymous association with it. However, in recent years additional genes which cause HD look alike phenotypes have been described. In this chapter, the primary focus would be on HD and HD like phenocopies.

HUNTINGTON'S DISEASE

Huntington's disease is a rare neurodegenerative autosomal-dominant disorder caused by triplet repeat expansion. HD is named after George Huntington, who provided a classic account of HD in "The Medical and Surgical Reporter" (1872).[1] It is characterized by onset before midlife and a distinct phenotype of progressive movement disorders (mainly chorea, dystonia, and Parkinsonism) with cognitive, psychiatric, and behavioral symptoms often debilitating and increasing caregiver burden. HD is a trinucleotide repeat disorder with autosomal dominant inheritance. It has a strong association between repeat length and age at disease onset. Paternal transmission facilitates this anticipation phenomenon. Age at onset is also strongly linked to the clinical presentation of patients. Currently, with advanced genetics, the differential diagnosis of HD like clinical presentation is increasing and many Huntington like disorders are now being recognized. Symptomatic treatment is available and current research on disease modifying therapies are at the verge of promising outcomes.

Epidemiology

Prevalence of HD is estimated at approximately 5/100,000; it is less common among those of non-European ancestry.[2,3] Diagnosis is most often made in the third or fourth decade of life, but onset may occur from childhood through the eighth decade.[4,5] Prevalence of HD among immigrants from the Indian subcontinent was estimated to be similar to what has been observed for European populations.[6] The overall prevalence of HD in Asian was 0.40/100,000, much lower compared with that of 5.70/100,000 European, North American, and Australia.[7] It can be speculated that between 20,000 and 40,000 people are suspected to be affected with HD in Indian population and >0.2 million may be at risk. It is suggested that the prevalence of HD in India should not be underestimated.[8]

Genetics and Pathophysiology

Huntington's disease is caused by an abnormal expansion of trinucleotide repeats coding for glutamine at the N-terminus of the huntingtin protein. The expansion happen in sequences of cytosine, adenine, and guanine (CAG) in exon 1 of the HD gene, located on chromosome 4. The gene is expressed all over the body.[9] The function of huntingtin is unknown. Excitotoxicity, mitochondrial dysfunction, and dysregulation of gene expression have all been proposed as pathological mechanisms.[10-12].The HD gene is transmitted by autosomal dominant pattern of inheritance; every child of an affected subject has a 50% chance of inheriting the gene. Normally, 9–29 CAG repeats are seen. Those who have clinical symptoms of HD have a higher repeat number, around 39 or more. Most patients have a family history of HD, there also exists sporadic HD cases reported in literature.[13,14] Indian subcontinent represents one of the most ethnically and genetically diverse regions of the world. A study from National Institute of Mental Health and Neuro Sciences (NIMHANS) found that the distribution of alleles (D2642 and D4S127) in Indian HD patients are similar to West European populations and suggest that this admixture possibly occurred when British troops were located in South India during colonization.[15] In 2000, one study from Srimanth Pramanik et al. from India analyzed the distribution of CAG and adjacent CCG repeats which has also been the target of many molecular studies in the Huntingtin gene in 28 unrelated, clinically diagnosed HD patients and in normal individuals belonging to different ethnic groups. The expanded CAG repeats in patients ranged from 41 to 56, whereas in normal individuals this varied between 11 and 3. For the first time, a study has reported one four-repeat CCG allele which has not been identified in any population so far and also suggested; among the Indian population, the overall prevalence of HD may not be as high as in Western population.[16] Based on the three SNPs (rs762855, rs3856973, and rs4690073), haplogroup A was most common which corresponds to the Caucasian HD haplogroup from an Indian study by Moily et al.[8]

The characteristic neuropathological change in HD is the reduced number of medium spiny striatal neurons. The first neuropathological change takes place in the associative areas of the striatum.[17,18] Caudate changes predominate, but cell death also happen in the globus pallidus and as the disease advances, widespread atrophy occurs.[19,20]

Clinical Features

Prodromal period show motor abnormalities including mild involuntary movements and oculomotor dysfunction which predate many years before diagnosis. Early cognitive abnormalities, particularly the ability to shift cognitive sets, may antedate motor symptoms. Behavioral abnormality occurs in the prodromal period but they do not progress as overt motor and cognitive abnormalities.[21] The PREDICT-HD study identifies clinical and biological markers in premanifest individuals, motor domain scores showed greater abnormality with increase in proximity to diagnosis although bradykinesia and chorea were associated with diagnostic immediacy, also worse scores on finger tapping, tandem gait, luria, saccadic initiation, and chorea showed unique association with diagnostic probability. The course of HD is slow but progressive and is distinguished by motor and cognitive dysfunction, resulting in loss of domains related to occupation, financial management, domestic tasks, and self-care skills.[22] Gait, eye movement abnormality, dysarthria, and swallowing difficulties are seen in all patients. They progress over 10–15 years, with severe disability and death. Chorea is the hallmark of the disease, it exacerbates in the middle stages of the illness and improves as the patient becomes more debilitated, bradykinetic, and rigid. Dystonia aggravates as the disease progresses. Late-onset HD has a slower course. Juvenile-onset HD, whose symptoms occur prior to age of 20 years, has a marked clinical picture. Parkinsonism is the characteristic clinical feature, often accompanied by seizures and myoclonus. Chorea is not ominous, making a clinical diagnosis challenging when there is no family history. Psychiatric and cognitive changes can be the most prominent features, further making the diagnosis uncertain.[23] A Japanese adultonset case of HD with spasticity and cerebellar ataxia has been reported.[24] Cognitive deficits are well known symptoms of HD. Impairment of attention, visuospatial processing, and memory occurs early in the disease. The prevalence of psychiatric manifestation is reported to be 30 to >70%. Loss of energy and initiative, poor perseverance and quality of work, impaired judgment, poor self-care, and emotional blunting were all seen to be more in HD patients.[25,26] Suicide rates are increased four-fold compared with the general population. Over 25% of patients attempt suicide at some point in the illness, particularly in their fifth or sixth decade.[27] **Table 1** highlights all the symptoms with its frequency of occurrence in an Indian subgroup of 26 patients by Murgod UA et al., featuring motor, behavioral, and cognitive symptoms. Over the course of illness, HD patients go through five stages of the disease, these stages are anchored to Total Functional Capacity

TABLE 1: Symptom occurrence with percentage in Indian population.

Symptom (n = 26)	*Percentage*
Motor symptoms:	
Chorea	96.2%
Bradykinesia	96.2%
Saccadic abnormality	80.9%
Dysarthria	80.8%
Gait abnormality	73.1%
Rigidity	30.76%
Dystonia	15.4%
Behavioral symptoms:	
Irritability	73%
Depression	65.4%
Anxiety	61.5%
OCD	19.3%
Obsessions	15.4%
Compulsions	11.5%
Suicidal ideation	11.5%
Delusion	3.8%
Cognitive domain:	
Dementia	50%

(OCD: obsessive compulsive disorder)

Scores which describes occupation, finance, domestic response, activity of daily living, and in home or institutional custodial care in need.

Diagnosis and Assessment

Genetic testing for HD remains the gold standard for diagnosis of HD with repeats of 40 or more being diagnostic of HD. A gene with 36–39 repeats have a "reduced penetrance" range, which may or may not be associated with symptom onset of HD and 27–35 repeats fall into intermediate range which means the individual may not be at risk to develop HD, but their children may be at risk.

In addition to genetic testing, other ancillary tests help in HD. Somatosensory and visual evoked potentials show reduced amplitude of early cortical potentials in patients with clinical manifestation of disease as well as at risk for HD with deterioration over time.[28] Electroencephalogram (EEG) may be useful in patients with seizure. Detailed measurements on magnetic resonance imaging (MRI) of caudate volume show atrophy (**Fig. 1**), and it begins before clinical manifestation of disease and progresses over time.[29] MRI striatal volume measures should be considered as a biomarker because these measures contribute in the assessment of treatment effectiveness in HD.[30] Computed tomography brain scans may show atrophy of the head of the caudate nucleus with increased bicaudate ventricular diameter, but sensitivity of this measure is only 87.5%.[31]

The UHDRS is a useful clinical tool to follow disease progression in motor, cognitive, behavioral, and functional disability. UDHRS-For Advanced Patients (UHDRS-FAP) motor score is potentially a better instrument than the UHDRS motor score to improve disease monitoring and, subsequently, care in patients with advanced HD in long-term care facilities.[32]

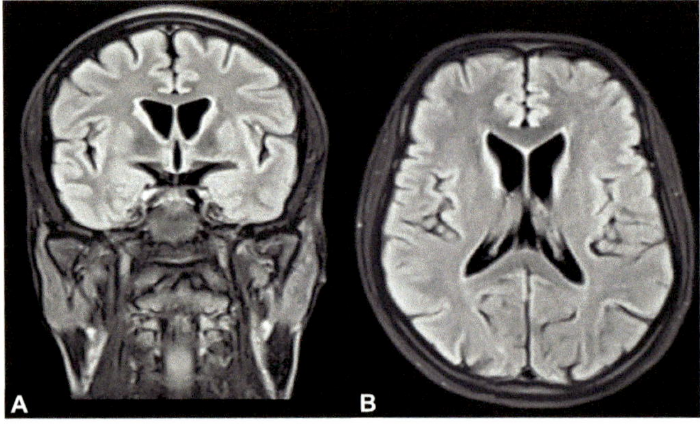

(HD: Huntington's disease; MRI: magnetic resonance imaging)

FIGS. 1A AND B: MRI coronal (A) and axial (B) FLAIR images of a 32-year-old female, familial HD with caudate atrophy.

Clinical Management

According to the American Academy of Neurology pharmacological treatment guidelines, if HD chorea requires treatment, the following received level B recommendation: Tetrabenazine (up to 100 mg/day), amantadine (300–400 mg/day), or riluzole (200 mg/day); nabilone, a synthetic cannabinoid, received level C recommendation. Data are insufficient to make recommendations regarding use of clozapine, other neuroleptics, or donepezil for HD chorea treatment (level U).[33] No clinical trials have evaluated benzodiazepines for their effect on chorea in HD. However, a small case series reported benefit from high-dose clonazepam.[34] Food and Drug Administration (FDA) has recently approved deutetrabenazine after positive results from first-HD study. In clinical practice, psychiatric treatment choices are selected as they would be for other conditions. Other molecules that have been tried for psychiatric features include amantadine, as documented in an HD case of severe perseveration,[35] and as an add-on propranolol for aggressive behavior in three HD patients.[36] Benefits have been seen with electroconvulsive therapy in six of seven cases of treatment-refractory depression in HD.[37] A single modafinil 200-mg dose increased alertness, but with no benefit on executive dysfunction (or apathy) in a double-blind, randomized, placebo-controlled cross-over study of 20 HD patients.[38] Donepezil the selective acetylcholinesterase inhibitor was associated with increased chorea, falls, irritability, and anxiety in HD patients with cognitive decline.[39] Rivastigmine had benefits in behavioral and cognitive functions in a study involving four participants with HD.[40] Deep-brain stimulation of the globus pallidus internus has been used experimentally and has been reported to be of temporary benefit in a single case reports but cannot stop the progressive neuronal death.[41] **Tables 2** and **3** summarize symptomatic treatment and therapeutic drugs in pipeline and those failed in clinical trials.

Recent Advances

Dr Kochanek unveiled the structure of huntingtin in February, 2018 at the therapeutic conference as a birthday present to HD community celebrating 25 years since the discovery of the gene. The structure announced was of the normal huntingtin protein called "wild type" but still the mutant protein structure is still unknown but it is exciting times ahead to all the research groups looking for a significant breakthrough. GENERATION-HD1 future has started recruiting for phase 3 trial of RG6042 which has raised prospects that targeting these based on Clustered Regularly Interspaced Short Palindromic Repeats (CRISPR) and antisense oligonucleotide (ASO) may have benefit in neurodegenerative disorders. Recent advances in detecting mutated huntingtin (mHTT) in cerebrospinal fluid (CSF) from HD-CSF study may also add to the feasibility of conducting early trials. Large observational studies such as

TABLE 2: Symptomatic treatment overview.

Symptom	*Drug*	*Mechanism of action*
Chorea	• Tetrabenazine • Amantadine • Riluzole • Nabilone	• Dopamine depleting agent • NMDA antagonist • Antiglutamatergic and antiexcititoxicity • Synthetic cannabinoid
Spasticity	• Baclofen • Tizanidine	Skeletal muscle relaxant
Rigidity and bradykinesia	• Levodopa • Pramipexole	• Amino acid precursor of dopamine • Dopamine agonist
Myoclonus and Seizure	• Clonazepam • Sodium valproate • levetiracetam	• Benzodiazepine • Na^+ channel blockade and increases GABA • Acts on SV2A
Bruxism	Botulinum toxin	Neuromuscular blocking agent
Dystonia	Botulinum toxin	Neuromuscular blocking agent
Psychosis	• Risperidone • Olanzapine • Quetiapine • Clozapine • Aripiprazole • haloperidol	• Atypical neuroleptic • Atypical neuroleptic • Atypical neuroleptic • Atypical neuroleptic • Atypical neuroleptic • Typical neuroleptic
Irritability, depression, anxiety, and OCD	• Citalopram • Fluoxetine • Paroxetine • Sertraline • Mirtazapine • Venlafaxine	• SSRI • SSRI • SSRI • SSRI • Presynaptic alpha-2 antagonist • SNRI
Mania	Lithium	Mood stabilizer
Sleep disturbance	• Zolpidem • Zopiclone	Hypnotics

(GABA: gamma-aminobutyric acid; NMDA: n-methyl-d-aspartate; OCD: obsessive compulsive disorder; SNRIs: serotonin–norepinephrine reuptake inhibitors; SSRI: selective serotonin reuptake inhibitor; SV2A: synaptic vesicle glycoprotein 2A)

TABLE 3: Therapeutic drug trials overview.

Drug	*Mechanism of action*	*Trial status*
Coenzyme Q10	Antioxidant	No benefit
Creatinine	Nutritional supplement and restores ATP	No benefit
Minocycline	Anti-inflammatory, antiapoptotic, and antioxidant	No benefit
Pridopidine	Dopamine-stabilizing agent	Failed to meet primary endpoint but positive results in secondary end point (UHDRS-TMS)
Latrepirdine	Antihistamine	Phase 3 NO BENEFIT
PBT2	Metalloproteinase inhibitor	Improvement in trial B cognitive test but development delayed due to side effects
Laquinimod	Immunomodulator	Phase 2 (LEGATO-HD)
Vaccinex	Monoclonal antibody	Phase 2 (SIGNAL)
PDE10A	Phosphodiesterase-10A Inhibitor	Phase 2 NO BENEFIT
BN82451	Na^+ channel blockade and antioxidant	Phase 2 completed
Cysteamine	Transglutaminase inhibitor	Benefit of TMS that is independent of chorea in a subset not taking TBZ
Selisistat	SIRT1 Inhibitor	Phase 2 promising drug
AFQ056	Metabotropic glutamate receptor 5 inhibitor	No antichorea effect but improvement in finger tapping
SRX246	Vasopressin1A receptor antagonist	Results awaited for primary outcome of tolerability

(TBZ: tetrabenazine; TMS: total motor score; UHDRS: Unified Huntington's Disease Rating Scale)

ENROLL-HD (www.enroll-hd.org) add to this information and provide rapid access to potential subjects for clinical trials. Vaccinex-SIGNAL Trial using VX15 antibody is in phase 2 trial and the results are awaited.

HUNTINGTON LIKE DISORDERS

Huntington's disease-like disorders and other phenocopies are relatively rare (**Table 4**). Only about 1% of suspected HD cases emerge as phenocopy syndromes.[42,43] Other phenocopies are not discussed in detail in this chapter, it will be elaborated in other sections of the book.

Huntington's Disease-like 1

Huntington's disease-like 1 (HDL1) is a rare presentation of autosomal dominant familial prion disease, first reported in 2001.[44] It is caused by eight (sometimes six) extra repeats of the octapeptide region in the prion protein (PrP) gene (*PRNP*). Mean-onset age is between 20 and 45 years. It resembles HD with prominent personality change, psychiatric symptoms and cognitive decline, chorea, rigidity, and dysarthria. Limb and truncal ataxia and seizures may be present.[45] The characteristic EEG features of triphasic periodic sharp wave complexes and 14-3-3 protein in

TABLE 4: Huntington disease look alikes.

Type	*Inheritance*	*Mutation*
Huntington's disease look (HDL) alike:		
HDL1	AD	PRNP
HDL2	AD	JPH3
HDL3	AR	Unknown
HDL4 or SCA17	AD	TBP
Others:		
Dentatorubral-pallidoluysian atrophy	AD	ATN1
Neuroferritinopathy	AD	FTL1
Spinocerebellar ataxia 1/2/3	AD	ATXN1/2/3
Benign hereditary chorea	AD	TITF1
C9orf72	AD	C9orf72
ADCY5	AD	ADCY5
Pantothenate kinase-associated neurodegeneration	AR	PANK2
PLA2G6-associated neurodegeneration	AR	PLA2G6
Neuroacanthocytosis	AR	VPS13A
McLeod syndrome	X linked	XK
Wilson's disease	AR	ATP7B
Friedreich ataxia	AR	FRATAXIN
Ataxia telangiectasia	AR	ATM
Ataxia with oculomotor apraxia	AR	APRATAXIN
RNF216-mediated neurodegeneration	AR	RNF216
FRRS1L chorea dementia syndrome	AR	FRRS1L

the CSF is less frequently present. Neuropathology show atrophy and prion deposition in the basal ganglia, frontal and temporal lobes, and cerebellar cortex.[45]

Huntington's Disease-like 2

Huntington's disease-like 2 (HDL2) is due to a triplet repeat expansions in the *JPH3* gene[46] on chromosome 16q24.3 seen in black South Africans of sub-Saharan decent. It resembles HD more than any other disease with similar cognitive, psychiatric, and motor features. Parkinsonism, however, may be more prominent in HDL2 compared to HD.[45] Normal alleles range from 6 to 28 triplets, whereas pathological repeat expansions range from 40 to 58 triplets.[47] Neuropathologically, both HDL2 and HD are very similar, pathologically dominated by prominent striatal and cortical atrophy with a selective loss of medium spiny neurons and astrocytic gliosis in a dorsal to ventral gradient.[48]

Huntington's Disease-like 3

Huntington's disease-like 3 (HDL3) is an autosomal recessive early-onset neurodegenerative disorder described in a Saudi Arabian family. It is characterized by mental deterioration, speech disturbance, dystonia, chorea, and other pyramidal and extrapyramidal symptoms. MRI showed progressive atrophy of the caudate nuclei bilaterally including the frontal cortex, and a link to HD was suggested by the publishers. The causative gene remains unclear, but the disease locus was mapped initially to chromosome 4p15.3, it is different from the other Huntington's like disorder from its recessive inheritance and very early-onset with a different clinical phenotype and it is still unclear whether, it has to be included under the umbrella of Huntington's like disorders.[45]

Huntington's Disease-like 4 (Spinocerebellar Ataxia Type 17)

It is an autosomal-dominant triplet repeat disorder wherein mutated *TBP* gene encodes for the TATA-box binding protein, an important general transcription initiation factor. The normal allele size ranges from 25 to 40 CAG/CAA repeats, whereas 41 to 48 CAG/CAA repeats lead to reduced penetrance and 49 and greater repeats lead to full penetrance.[49] This accounts for 0.5–1.8% of all HD-like syndromes and its age of onset is between 19 and 48 years, rarely starting during childhood.[50] Cerebellar ataxia is the prominent clinical feature (95%), it presents with a slowly progressive course, but rapid progression similar to paraneoplastic disorders or prion disease have been reported.[51] Extrapyramidal features (73%), in particular dystonia, chorea, and dementia (76%), is seen in spinocerebellar ataxia type 17 (SCA17). Additionally, pyramidal signs, epilepsy, and psychiatric disturbances are not uncommon.[44] Similar to the broad spectrum of clinical manifestations, the neuropathological findings may involve the cerebellum as well as the cerebral cortex, basal ganglia, and hippocampus.[52-54] So far SCA17 has been found to be the most common cause in HDL patients.

APPROACH TO A PATIENT WITH HUNTINGTON'S DISEASE AND HUNTINGTON LIKE DISORDERS

Based on the inheritance pattern, the age of onset and the clinical phenotypes diagnosis can be established (**Flowchart 1**). HD is the most common heritable form of chorea, if the HD gene test does not reveal pathological expansions, HDL phenocopies should be considered. However, the number of patients with an HDL syndrome in whom a molecular diagnosis can be made remains low. SCA17 seems to be the most common etiology in these patients, particularly among Caucasians, whereas in patients from South Africa, HDL2 is an important differential diagnosis. Also, HDL2 appears to mimic HD most closely. Finally, a rapid course may be suggestive of prion disease (HDL1). In

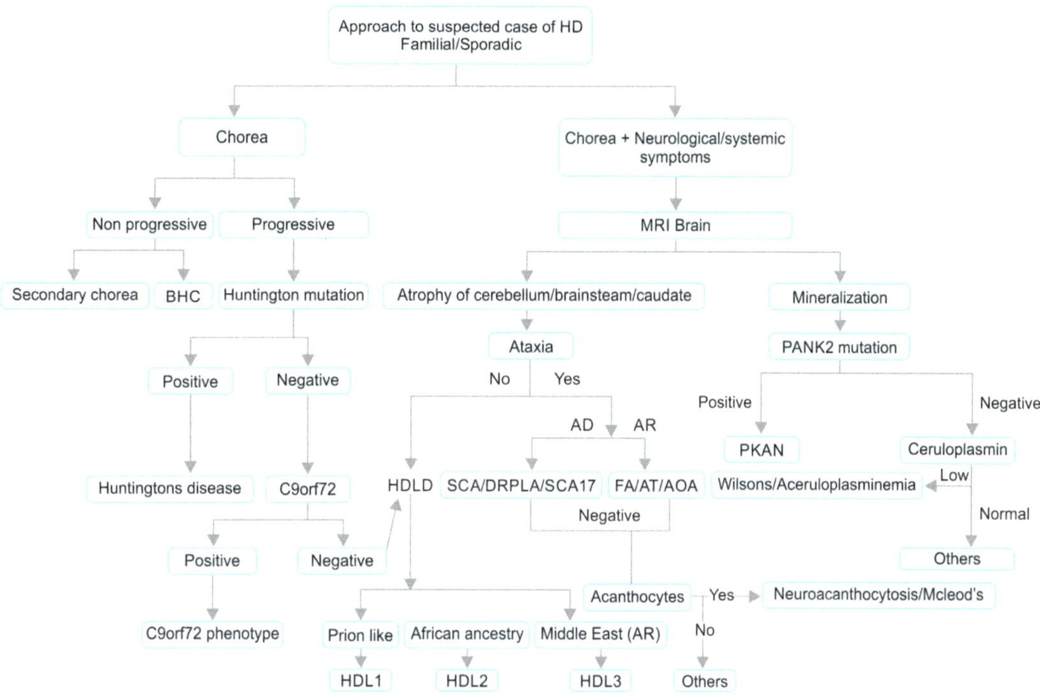

(AT: ataxia-telangiectasia; AOA: ataxia with oculomotor apraxia; BHC: benign hereditary chorea; DRPLA: dentatorubro-pallidoluysian atrophy; FA: Friedreich's ataxia; HD: Huntington's disease; HDL1: Huntington's disease-like 1; MRI: magnetic resonance imaging; PKAN: pantothenate kinase-associated neurodegeneration; SCA17: spinocerebellar ataxia type 17)

FLOWCHART 1: Approach to suspected HD.

addition to these HDL syndromes, other ataxia syndromes like autosomal dominant dentatorubro-pallidoluysian atrophy (DRPLA) and SCA 1/2/3 and autosomal recessive Friedreich's ataxia (FA), ataxia-telangiectasia (AT), and ataxia with oculomotor apraxia (AOA) can present with significant chorea. Oro-bucco-facial dystonia presentations such as neuroacanthocytosis, Mcleod's syndrome, neuroferritinopathy, and pantothenate kinase-associated neurodegeneration (PKAN) all come under the differential diagnosis. Similarly like in any other movement disorder Wilson's disease has to be ruled out. Recent literature on C9orf72 like HD presentation is abundant and it seems to be the most common among all the other diseases. Newly reported entities such as ADCY5, RNF216, and FRRS1L and its rare presentations have to be considered when common disorders are ruled out.

CONCLUSION

Chorea presenting with HD and HDLD is challenging for both the clinician and the caregiver alike, since there is no proven treatment to slow the disease progression or prevent onset of symptoms. But we are at major crossroads in finding effective therapies with promising techniques for the well being of the community in large.

REFERENCES

1. Montoya A, Price BH, Menear M, Lepage M. J Psychiatry Neurosci. 2006;31(1):21-9.
2. Hayden MR, MacGregor JM, Beighton PH. The prevalence of Huntington's chorea in South Africa. S Afr Med J. 1980;58(5):193-6.
3. Folstein SE, Chase GA, Wahl WE, McDonnell AM, Folstein MF. Huntington's disease in Maryland: clinical aspects of racial variation. Am J Hum Genet. 1987;41(2):168-79.
4. Folstein SE. Huntington Disease: A Disorder of Families. Baltimore: The Johns Hopkins Press; 1989.
5. Gilstad J, Reich SG. Chorea in an octogenarian. Neurologist. 2003;9:165-6.
6. Shiwach RS, Lindenbaum RH. Prevalence of Huntington's disease among UK immigrants from the Indian subcontinent. Br J Psychiatry. 1990;**157**:598-9.
7. Pringsheim T, Wiltshire K, Day L, Dykeman J, Steeves T, Jette N. The incidence and prevalence of Huntington's disease: A systematic review and metaanalysis. Mov Disord. 2012;27(9): 108391.
8. Moily NS, Kota LN, Anjanappa RM, Venugopal S, Vaidyanathan R, Pal P, et al. Trinucleotide repeats and haplotypes at the huntingtin locus in an Indian sample overlaps with European haplogroup A. PLoS Curr. 2014;6.

9. Strong TV, Tagle DA, Valdes JM, Elmer LW, Boehm K, Swaroop M, et al. Widespread expression of the human and rat Huntington's disease gene in brain and nonneural tissues. Nat Genet. 1993;5(3):259-65.
10. Difiglia M. Excitotoxic injury of the neostriatum: a model for Huntington's disease. Trends Neurosci. 1990;13(7):286-9.
11. Beal MF. Does impairment of energy metabolism result in excitotoxic neuronal death in neurodegenerative illnesses? Ann Neurol. 1992;31(2):119-30.
12. Nucifora FC Jr, Sasaki M, Peters MF, Huang H, Cooper JK, Yamada M, et al. Interference by huntingtin and atrophin-1 with cbp-mediated transcription leading to cellular toxicity. Science. 2001;291(5512):2423-8.
13. Dürr A, Dodé C, Hahn V, Pêcheux C, Pillon B, Feingold J, et al. Diagnosis of "sporadic" Huntington's disease. J Neurol Sci. 1995;129(1):515.
14. Davis MB, Bateman D, Quinn NP, Marsden CD, Harding AE. Mutation analysis in patients with possible but apparently sporadic Huntington's disease. Lancet. 1994;344(8924):7147.
15. Saleem Q, Muthane U, Verma IC, Brahmachari SK, Jain S. Expanding colonies and expanding repeats. The Lancet. 2002;359(9309):895-6.
16. Pramanik S, Basu P, Gangopadhaya PK, Sinha KK, Jha DK, Sinha S, et al. Analysis of CAG and CCG repeats in Huntingtin gene among HD patients and normal populations of India. Eur J Hum Genet. 2000;8:678-82.
17. Vonsattel JP, DiFiglia M. Huntington's disease. J Neuropathol Exp Neurol. 1998;57(5):369-84.
18. Middleton FA, Strick PL. Basal ganglia and cerebellar loops: motor and cognitive circuits. Brain Res Rev. 2000;31(2–3):236-50.
19. Vonsattel JP, Myers RH, Stevens TJ, Ferrante RJ, Bird ED, Richardson EP Jr. Neuropathological classification of Huntington's disease. J Neuropathol Exp Neurol. 1985;44(6):559-77.
20. Biglan K, Julian-Baros E, Yoritomo N, Ross C. Feasibility of a study of Coenzyme Q10 in pre-manifest Huntington's disease: the PREQUEL study. Neurotherapeutics. 2011;8(1):135.
21. Shoulson I, Young AB. Milestones in Huntington Disease. Mov Disord. 2011;26(6):1127-33.
22. Hedreen JC, Peyser CE, Folstein SE, Ross CA. Neuronal loss in layers V and VI of cerebral cortex in Huntington's disease. Neurosci Lett. 1991;133(2):257-61.
23. Ribai P, Nguyen K, Hahn-Barma V, Gourfinkel-An I, Vidailhet M, Legout A, et al. Psychiatric and cognitive difficulties as indicators of juvenile Huntington disease onset in 29 patients. Arch Neurol. 64(6):813-9.
24. Kageyama Y, Yamamoto S, Ueno M, Ichikawa K. A case of adultonset Huntington disease presenting with spasticity and cerebellar ataxia, mimicking spinocerebellar degeneration. Rinsho Shinkeigaku. 2003;43(1–2):16-9.
25. van Duijn E, Kingma EM, van der Mast RC. Psychopathology in verified Huntington's disease gene carriers. J Neuropsychiatry Clin Neurosci. 2007;19(4):441-8.
26. Craufurd D, Thompson JC, Snowden JS. Behavioral changes in Huntington's disease. Neuropsychiatry Neuropsychol Behav Neurol. 2001;14(4):219-26.
27. Schoenfeld M, Myers RH, Cupples LA, Berkman B, Sax DS, Clark E. Increased rate of suicide among patients with Huntington's disease. J Neurol Neurosurg Psychiatry. 1984;47(12):1283-7.
28. Lefaucheur JP, Menard-Lefaucheur I, Maison P, Baudic S, Cesaro P, Peschanski M, et al. Electrophysiological deterioration over time in patients with Huntington's disease. Mov Disord. 2006;21:1350-4.
29. Aylward EH, Codori AM, Rosenblatt A, Sherr M, Brandt J, Stine OC, et al. Rate of caudate atrophy in presymptomatic and symptomatic stages of Huntington's disease. Mov Disord. 2000;15(3):552-60.
30. Aylward EH. Magnetic Resonance Imaging Striatal Volumes: A Biomarker for Clinical Trials in Huntington's Disease. Mov Disord. 2014;29(11):1429-33.
31. Sharma P, Savy L, Britton J, Taylor R, Howick A, Patton M. Huntington's disease: a molecular genetic and CT comparison. J Neurol Neurosurg Psychiatry. 1996;60(2):206-8.
32. Winder JY, Achterberg WP, Marinus J, Gardiner SL, Roos RAC. Assessment Scales for Patients with Advanced Huntington's Disease: Comparison of the UHDRS and UHDRS-FAP. Mov Disord Clin Prac. 2018;5(5):527-33.
33. Armstrong MJ, Miyasaki JM, American Academy of Neurology. Evidence-based guideline: pharmacologic treatment of chorea in Huntington disease: report of the Guideline Development Subcommittee of the American Academy of Neurology. Neurology. 2012;79(6):597-603.
34. Peiris JB, Boralessa H, Lionel ND. Clonazepam in the treatment of choreiform activity. Med J Aust. 1976;1(8):225-7.
35. Lyketsos CG, Rosenblatt A, Rabins P. Forgotten frontal lobe syndrome or "executive dysfunction syndrome". Psychosomatics. 2004;45(3):247-55.
36. Stewart JT, Mounts ML, Clark RL Jr. Aggressive behavior in Huntington's disease: treatment with propranolol. J Clin Psychiatry. 1987;48(3):106-8.
37. Ranen NG, Peyser CE, Folstein SE. ECT as a treatment for depression in Huntington's disease. J Neuropsychiatry Clin Neurosci. 1994;6(2):154-9.
38. Blackwell AD, Paterson NS, Barker RA, Robbins TW, Sahakian BJ. The effects of modafinil on mood and cognition in Huntington's disease. Psychopharmacology (Berl). 2008;199(1):29-36.
39. Cubo E, Shannon KM, Tracy D, Jaglin JA, Bernard BA, Wuu J, et al. Effect of donepezil on motor and cognitive function in Huntington disease. Neurology. 2006;67(7):1268-71.
40. Rot U, Kobal J, Sever A, Pirtosek Z, Mesec A. Rivastigmine in the treatment of Huntington's disease. Eur J Neurol. 2002;9(6):689-90.
41. Hebb MO, Garcia R, Gaudet P, Mendez IM. Bilateral stimulation of the globus pallidus internus to treat choreathetosis in Huntington's disease: technical case report. Neurosurgery. 2006;58(2):E383.
42. Schneider SA, Walker RH, Bhatia KP. The Huntington's disease-like syndromes: what to consider in patients with a negative Huntington's disease gene test. Nat Clin Pract Neurol. 2007;3(9):517-25.
43. Wild EJ, Tabrizi SJ. Huntington's disease phenocopy syndromes. Curr Opin Neurol. 2007;20(6):681-7.
44. Moore RC, Xiang F, Monaghan J, Han D, Zhang Z, Edström L, et al. Huntington disease phenocopy is a familial prion disease. Am J Hum Genet. 2001;69(6):1385-8.
45. Schneider SA, Bird T. Huntington's Disease, Huntington's Disease Look-Alikes, and Benign Hereditary Chorea: What's New? Mov Disord Clin Pract. 2016;3(4):342-54.

46. Holmes SE, O'Hearn E, Rosenblatt A, Callahan C, Hwang HS, Ingersoll-Ashworth RG, et al. A repeat expansion in the gene encoding junctophilin-3 is associated with Huntington disease-like 2. Nat Genet. 2001;29(4):377-8.
47. Margolis RL, Holmes SE, Rosenblatt A, Gourley L, O'Hearn E, Ross CA, et al. Huntington's Disease-like 2 (HDL2) in North America and Japan. Ann Neurol. 2004;56(5):670-4.
48. Rudnicki DD, Pletnikova O, Vonsattel JP, Ross CA, Margolis RL. A comparison of huntington disease and huntington disease-like 2 neuropathology. J Neuropathol Exp Neurol. 2008;67(4): 366-74.
49. Toyoshima Y, Onodera O, Yamada M, Tsuji S, Takahashi H. Spinocerebellar ataxia type 17. In: Pagon RA, Adam MP, Ardinger HH, Wallace SE, Bean LJH, Stephens K, et al. (eds). GeneReviews. Seattle (WA): University of Washington; 1993–2020.
50. Wild EJ, Mudanohwo EE, Sweeney MG, Schneider SA, Beck J, Bhatia KP, et al. Huntington's disease phenocopies are clinically and genetically heterogeneous. Mov Disord. 2008;23(5):716-20.
51. Mehanna R, Itin I. From normal gait to loss of ambulation in 6 months: a novel presentation of SCA17. Cerebellum. 2013;12(4):568-71.
52. Rolfs A, Koeppen AH, Bauer I, Bauer P, Buhlmann S, Topka H, et al. Clinical features and neuropathology of autosomal dominant spinocerebellar ataxia (SCA17). Ann Neurol. 2003;54(3):367-75.
53. Murgod UA, Saleem Q, Anand A, Brahmachari SK, Jain S, Muthane UB. A clinical study of patients with genetically confirmed Huntington's disease from India. J Neurol Sci. 2001;190(1–2):73-8.
54. Shannon KM. Huntington's disease-clinical signs, symptoms, presymptomatic diagnosis, and diagnosis. Handb Clin Neurol. 2011;100:3-13.

SECTION

8

SECONDARY MOVEMENT DISORDERS

CHAPTER 40

Metals and Movement Disorders

Payal Shah, Vrajesh Udani

INTRODUCTION

Metals play an important role in the normal growth and metabolism of the body. They are essential for numerous physiological processes acting as cofactors for various enzymes. Accumulation of these metals in excess can occur due to excessive exposure or genetic disorders, causing toxicity by either free radical related injury, mitochondrial dysfunction, or changes in the protein structure. Excessive accumulation and deposition of metals in the brain can manifest as a movement disorder, a few of the disorders being associated with deposition of iron, copper, and manganese (Mn).

DISORDERS OF MANGANESE METABOLISM

Manganese is an essential element acting as a cofactor for lyases, isomerase, transferases, oxidoreductases, and ligases.[1] Gastrointestinal absorption and biliary excretion help in maintaining the homeostasis of Mn, a failure of which may lead to increased blood Mn levels and subsequent deposition in the brain.

The normal brain Mn levels are 5–14 ng Mn/mg protein and neurotoxicity occurs when it is increased to >3 times.

Acquired manganese toxicity[1] can occur due to:

- Occupational hazard in miners, welders, and battery manufactures
- High concentration in drinking water and parenteral nutrition
- Ephedrone ("designer" drug containing potassium permanganate) abuse
- End-stage liver disease due to impaired excretion

Hereditary Disorder of Manganese Metabolism

In 2008, the clinical features of the first hereditary disorder of Mn metabolism was described,[2] followed a few years later by a case series in which the mutation in the *SLC30A10* gene was identified.[1] This gene is predominantly expressed in the liver, brain, and gastrointestinal tract and mediates Mn efflux, as it encodes for Mn transporter. "Loss-of-function" mutations lead to reduced Mn excretion with its accumulation in liver, muscle, bloodstream, and brain. The basal ganglia are disproportionately affected resulting in a disorder characterized by a triad of progressive dystonia, polycythemia, and liver disease. This is now called hypermanganesemia with dystonia type 1 (HMNDYT1) but is also known as hypermanganesemia with dystonia, polycythemia, and cirrhosis (HMDPC).[3]

Typically, HMNDYT1 is a childhood onset disorder between 2-and 15 years of age.[1] However, recently it was shown to have an onset of <2 years in many.[3] The presentation is with a progressive dystonia/Parkinsonism syndrome with insidious, but sometimes rapid gait difficulty, limb dystonia, dysarthria, bradykinesia, and rigidity. A characteristic high stepping gait so called "cock-walk gait" has been described. Younger patients may have motor and/or speech delay and a more rapid course.[3] Spasticity rarely comes isolated.[1] Fine motor difficulties, dysdiadokokinesia, and tremors maybe prominent. Cognition is usually well preserved. By the teens, though sometimes earlier, most untreated children become wheelchair bound. A rare adult-onset form presenting primarily as a levodopa-resistant Parkinsonism has also been described.[1] An axonal neuropathy may also be seen in adults.

Liver disease may vary in severity from asymptomatic steatosis and mild increased transaminases to cirrhosis and liver failure. It may be an initial-isolated presentation without neurological disease.[3]

Polycythemia is a consistent feature and may be related to the high levels of Mn probably inducing the erythropoietin gene leading to increased levels.[1] Besides as Mn and iron compete with each other at the transporter level, iron depletion is often noted. As polycythemia may precede neurologic symptoms by several years,[3] there is a need to check Mn levels in all polycythemias of unknown cause.

Darker skin tone appears to be another sign seen, especially, in fair skinned individuals.[3]

Hypermanganesemia is universal in all described cases and probably starts in early childhood. Whole blood Mn is markedly elevated >2,000 nmol/L (normal < 320 nmol/L) in contradistinction to lower levels in acquired etiologies.[1,3] Parental carriers of this disease may also have borderline high levels.[3]

Around 14 different homozygous compound, heterozygous mutations are noted in the SLC30A10 in those tested.[1-5] Varied mutation types, often novel have been seen from different ethnic backgrounds. There seems to be a clustering of mutations in exon 1 suggesting that this might be a hotspot.[3] There seems to be no genotype-phenotype correlation as members of the same family have been observed to have variable phenotypes. However, this might be an artifact of the small numbers (~29) of patients reported till date.

Typical magnetic resonance imaging (MRI) patterns (**Fig. 1**) are T1 hyperintensity in the basal ganglia and brainstem/cerebellar white matter and dentate nucleus.[1,3,4] Typically thalamus and pons are uninvolved. T2 images are usually normal, but may have subtle hypointensities in the same region.

Treatment includes use of chelating agents like EDTA-CaNa2, given intravenously as a 5-8 day course every 4 weeks.[1,3,5] Chelation does reduce the blood Mn levels though it does not normalize. T1-weighted MRI images can be used to monitor the Mn load and these abnormalities often improve over months (**Figs. 2A** and **B**). Alternative chelating agents tried are D-penicillamine[4] and 2,3-dimercaptosuccinic acid (DMSA),[3] both of which are easily available in India. Iron supplementation may help since it competes with Mn for its intestinal absorption.[1,3]

Another gene, namely SLC98A14 was identified in 2016 in an individual with features of Mn neurotoxicity.[6] SLC98A14 codes for a Mn transporter protein required for the hepatic uptake of Mn and its subsequent biliary excretion, thus, sparing the liver, in contradistinction to HMNDYT1 (**Figs. 3A** and **B**). Loss of function mutation causes impaired biliary excretion and accumulation of Mn in the brain.[6] This disorder named HMNDYT2 has an earlier age of onset with rapid progression. Initial motor delay becomes apparent by late infancy followed by progressive dystonia and bulbar dysfunction. Serum Mn is marked elevated while iron and other trace metals are normal. Polycythemia is absent and the liver appears free of metal deposition on imaging (**Table 1**).[6] Imaging and pathological studies suggest primary involvement of globus pallidus (GP) with milder involvement of white matter and dentate nucleus (**Fig. 4**).[6-8] Response to chelation with edetate calcium disodium (EDTA-CaNa2) has been variable.[6-8] This could be attributed to different genotypes or delayed treatment after neurodegeneration has already occurred. Dietary restriction has been found to be partially effective in one individual.[7] Response can be monitored using the ratio of T1 hyperintensity of the GP to the frontal white matter—the "pallidal index".[8]

Table 1 outlines the differences between HMNDYT1 and HMNDYT2.

NEURODEGENERATION WITH BRAIN IRON ACCUMULATION

Neurodegeneration with brain iron accumulation (NBIA) denotes a group of clinically and genetically heterogeneous

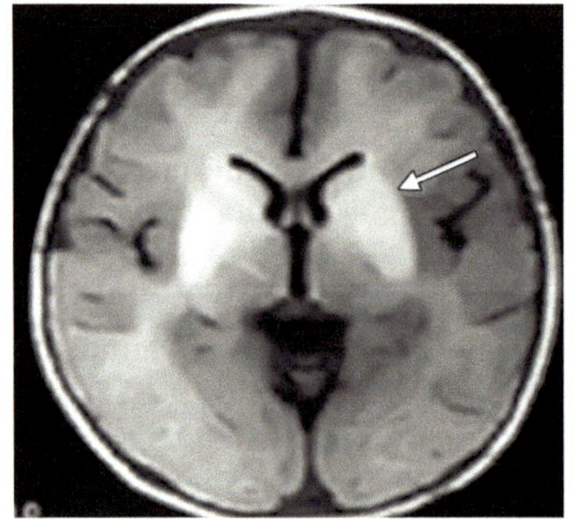

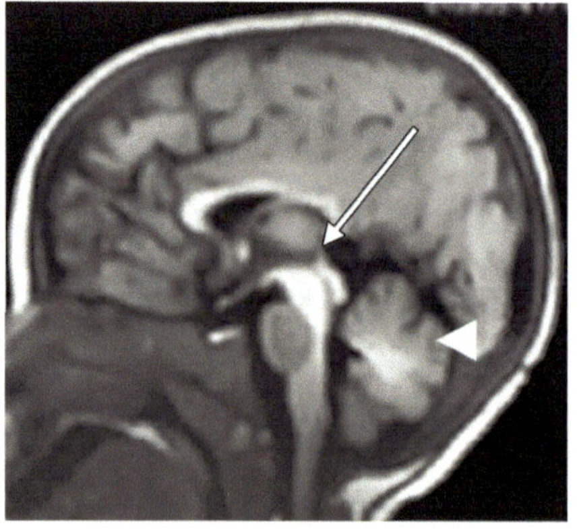

(HMNDYT1: hypermanganesemia with dystonia type 1)

FIG. 1: HMNDYT1: Typical T1 Hyperintensity in basal ganglia (short arrow), brainstem (long arrow), cerebellar white mate, and dentate nucleus (thick arrow).

Source: Modified from Zaki 2017.

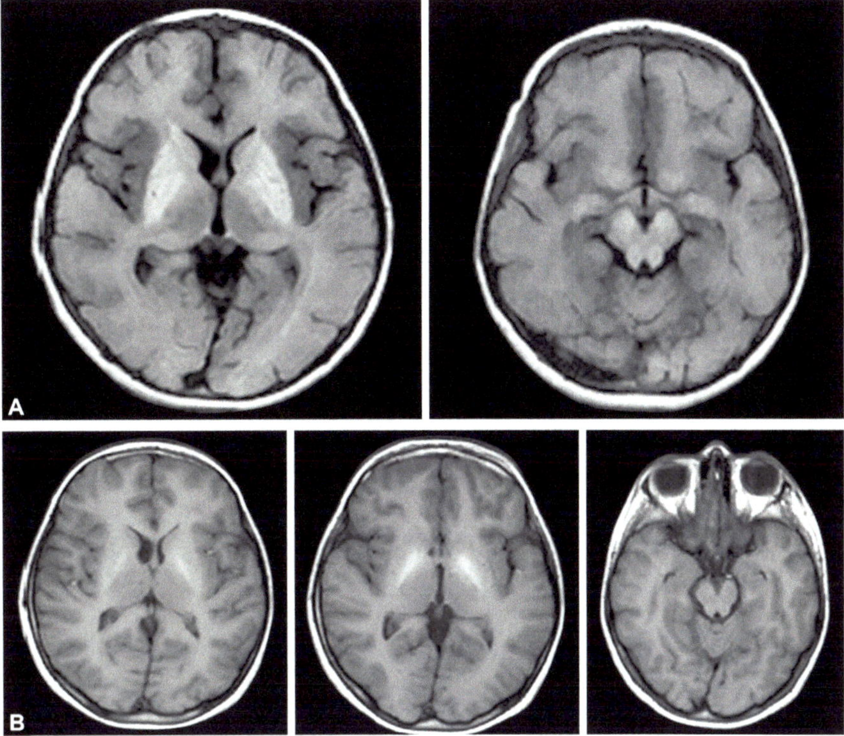

(Ca EDTA: calcium disodium ethylenediaminetetraacetic acid; HMNDYT1: hypermanganesemia with dystonia type 1)

FIGS. 2A AND B: HMNDYT1: (A) Prior to chelation with Ca EDTA. (B) 6 months after postchelation; significant decrease in T1 hyperintensity. *Source:* Modified from Tavasoli 2019.

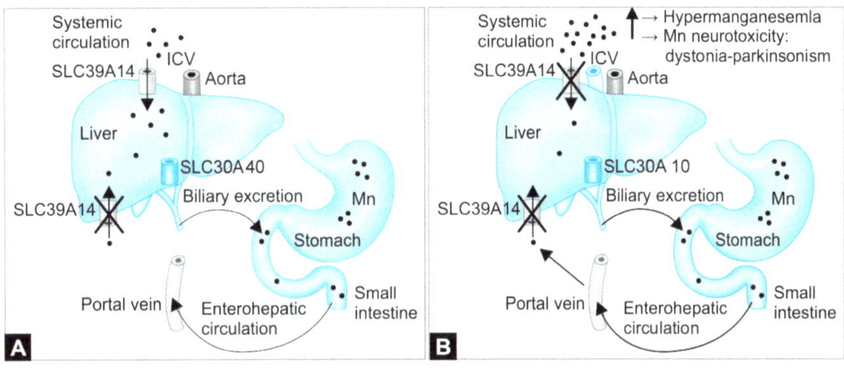

(IVC: inferior vena cava; Mn: manganese)

FIGS. 3A AND B: Proposed disease mechanism in patients with SLC39A14 mutations. (A) Under normal conditions nutritional Mn is absorbed in the duodenum and enters the enterohepatic circulation via the portal vein from which it is transported into the liver via SLC39A14, a Mn uptake transporter. Any excess Mn is rapidly removed from the systemic circulation by uptake into the liver via SLC39A14 and excreted into the bile via SLC30A10, a Mn efflux protein. (B) Dysfunction of SLC39A14 (indicated by a black X) impairs hepatic uptake of Mn for subsequent biliary excretion. Consequently, Mn accumulates in the blood and brain leading to hypermanganesemia and neurotoxicity, respectively.

disorders characterized by a combination of prominent movement disorder with imaging evidence of early deposition of iron in selectively vulnerable brain regions.[9] The pathologic hallmark along with iron deposition is the presence of axonal spheroids. Though the clinical features at onset vary widely, movement disorders with predominant dystonia in children and Parkinsonism at later ages, supervene at some stage.

Eight of the 10 known disorders are of childhood/juvenile onset and most are autosomal recessive (AR) (**Fig. 5**).[10] These are rare disorders with an estimated prevalence of 1/500,000. Rapid advances in genetics along with parallel advances in imaging has led to the ever-expanding classification of the NBIAs. Though they share clinical and imaging characteristics, most of the genes are not directly connected to iron metabolism and are primarily

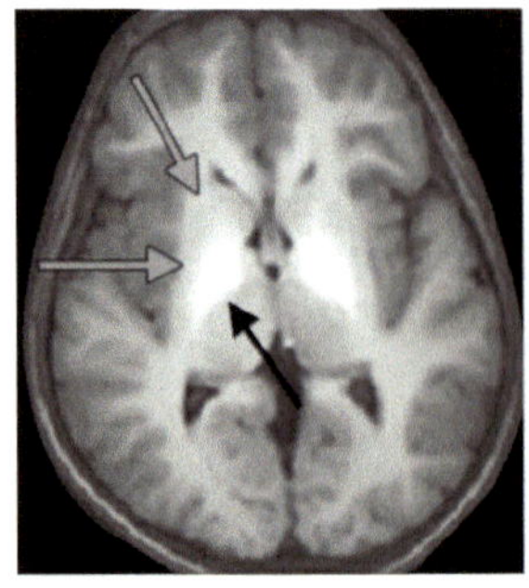
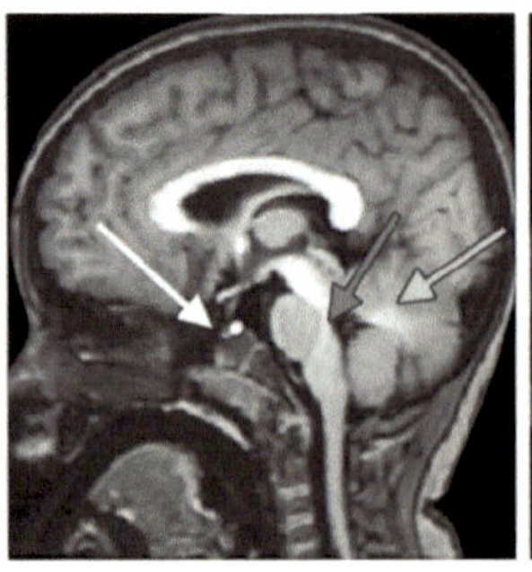
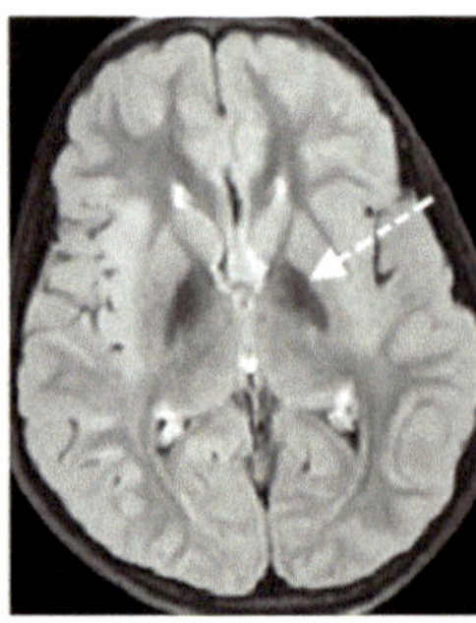

(GP: globus pallidus; HMNDYT2: hypermanganesemia with dystonia type 2)

FIG. 4: HMNDYT2: Typical T-1 hyperintensity predominantly in the globus pallidus (black arrows), brainstem (pink arrow), and dentate nucleus (gray arrow) note absence of significant change in corpus striatum (blue arrow). T2 shows GP hypointensity. ***(For color version, see plate 1)***

Source: Modified from Tuscl 2016.

NBIA subtype	Gene	Mode of inheritance	
Pantothenate kinase-associated neurodegeneration (PKAN)	*PANK2*	Autosomal recessive	Childhood
Phospholipase A2-associated neurodegeneration (PLAN)	*PLA2G6*	Autosomal recessive	
Mitochondrial membrane protein-associated neurodegeneration (MPAN)	*C19orf12*	Autosomal recessive	
Beta-propleller protein-associated neurodegeneration (BPAN)	*WDR45*	X-linked dominant	
Fatty acid hydroxylase-associated neurodegeneration (FAHN)	*FA2H*	Autosomal recessive	
Coenzyme A synthase protein-associated neurodegeneration (CoPAN)	*COASY*	Autosomal recessive	
Kufor-rakab syndrome	*ATP13A2*	Autosomal recessive	Juvenile
Woodhouse-sakati syndrome	*DCAF17*	Autosomal recessive	
Neurofernitinopathy	*FTL*	Autosomal dominant	Adult
Aceruloplasminemia	*CP*	Autosomal recessive	

Source: Modified from Hogarth 2015.

FIG. 5: The 10 forms of NBIA to date, with name, acronym, mutant gene, mode of inheritance, and age of onset.

TABLE 1: Characteristics of the hypermanganesemia syndromes.

	HMNDYT1	*HMNDYT2*
Genetics	Biallelic mutations *SLC30A10*	Biallelic mutations *SLC39A8*
Onset age	First decade	Infancy
CNS manifestations	• Dystonia/spasticity • High-stepping • "cock-walk" gait • Parkinsonism (rare)	• Dystonia; hypotonia • Spasticity, Parkinsonism • Bulbar dysfunction
Systemic manifestations	Polycythemia and chronic liver disease	None
Investigations	Increased manganese, increased hepatic enzymes, increased erythropoietin, and iron deficiency	Increased manganese
Imaging	T1-hyperintense signal globus pallidus, substantia nigra, and white matter	T2-hypointense signal globus pallidus
Treatment	Chelation, iron, and supplementation	Chelation

(CNS: central nervous system; HMDTY: hypermanganesemia with dystonia type)

involved in mitochondrial function, biochemical pathways (fatty acid metabolism), and cellular processes (autophagy/mitophagy) requiring protein products of the different NBIA genes (**Fig. 6**).

Neuroimaging abnormalities characteristics in the NBIAs are age-inappropriate evidence of iron deposition evidenced by hypointensities in the GP and substantia nigra (SN) on T2, FLAIR, and gradient -echo/susceptibility-weighted MRI images. Hypodensity on computed tomography (CT) differentiates it from calcium, which often has similar MRI.

PANTOTHENATE KINASE-ASSOCIATED NEURODEGENERATION (PKAN)

Historically, the eponym, Hallervorden–Spatz disease was the old name of the disease. However, the Julius Hallervorden and Hugo Spatz, two German neuropathologists have since been discredited for being involved in deplorable acts during Nazi rule in Germany.[11] Their names have since been dropped and pantothenate kinase-associated neurodegeneration (PKAN) is the widely accepted name since then.

This disease is the most common of the NBIAs, accounting for around 50%[10] (**Fig. 7**) and was the first be

FIG. 6: NBIA: Overview of genes and pathways involved in neurodegeneration with brain iron accumulation (NBIA). Schematic representation of a cell indicating the pathophysiologic mechanisms postulated for NBIA. Nine reported NBIA genes (white box, black outline) and their associated cellular processes are shown. Ceruloplasmin (CP) and ferritin light polypeptide (FTL) are important regulators of cellular iron homeostasis. Phospholipase A2 (PLA2G6) and fatty acid 2-hydroxylase (FA2H) are involved in lipid metabolism and membrane remodeling. Pantothenate kinase 2 (PANK2) and CoA synthase (COASY) are key enzymes in the biosynthesis of coenzyme A (CoA) utilized in a multitude of cellular processes, including the synthesis of fatty acids. WD repeat domain 45 (WDR45) and ATPase type13A2 (ATP13A2) play a role in the degradation process of autophagy. The function of the mitochondrial membrane protein C19orf12 is still unknown, but it is postulated to be associated with fatty acid biogenesis. ***(For color version, see plate 2)***

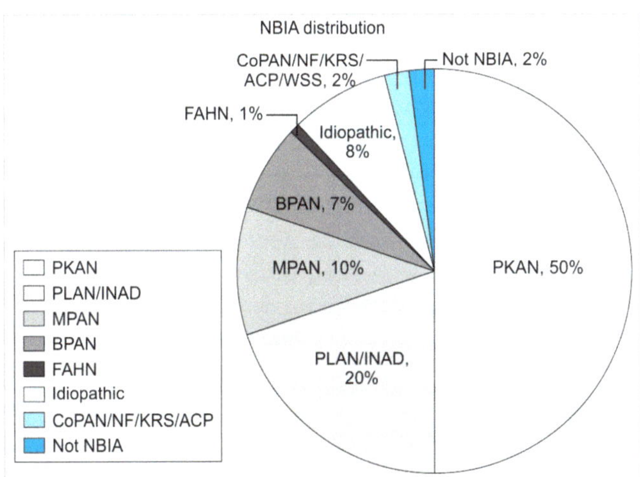

FIG. 7: NBIA—Distribution of NBIA subtypes from the North-American database.

associated with a mutation in a specific gene, pantothenate kinase 2 (*PANK-2*) in 2001. *PANK-2* is the first rate limiting step in CoA biosynthesis and catalyses the phosphorylation of vitamin B5 (pantothenate).[12] CoA is a master regulator of intermediary metabolism and is critical for several pathways. *PANK-2* in normal cells is repressed when CoA status is adequate and PKAN deficiency mimics this state leading to insufficient CoA; this leads to shutting down of pathways of intermediary metabolisms, where CoA is critical.[9] It also leads to an accumulation of neurotoxic metabolites cysteine and pantothenate. Cysteine acts as an iron chelator causing secondary iron accumulation and neuronal injury due to oxidative stress.

Pantothenate kinase-associated neurodegeneration has AR inheritance with most mutations in the *PANK-2* gene being missense, though deletions, duplications, and exon splice site variants have been identified. c.1561G>A (p.G521R) is the most common mutation identified in patients with classic PKAN.[9,13] A truncating mutation, c.215_216insA has been identified in 13/17 Indian Agrawal patients with the classic form of PKAN suggesting a founder effect.[14]

Pantothenate kinase-associated neurodegeneration presents from the more common early childhood onset "classic" form to the less frequent adolescent young adulthood onset more heterogeneous "atypical" form. This is presumably due to complete loss of gene function in the former and partial loss of function in the latter.

Classic Pantothenate Kinase-associated Neurodegeneration

The initial symptoms appear in the preschool years at around 3–4 years of age,[15] though it appeared sooner in an Indian series, where delayed walking was seen in

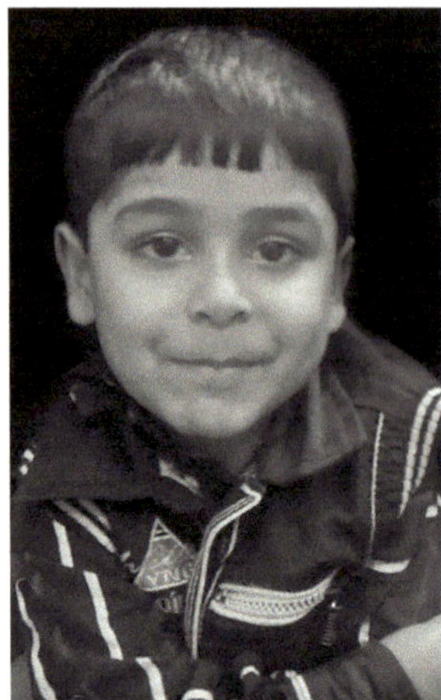
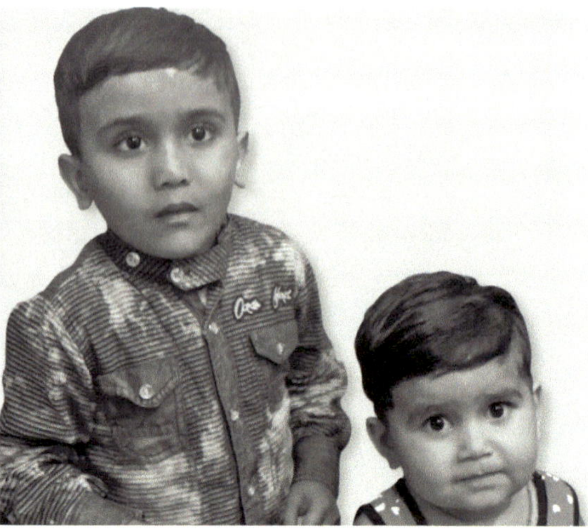

FIG. 8: One unrelated (top) and brother/sister with confirmed PKAN—both with characteristic facies (personal observation). ***(For color version, see plate 2)***

approximately 70% and was often misdiagnosed as cerebral palsy.[14] Gait imbalance and frequent falls occur probably due to subtle lower-limb dystonia. A characteristic facies seen early in our series may give a clinical clue to diagnosis (**Fig. 8**). Oromandibular and jaw opening dystonia is pathognomonic and eating-induced dystonia often become disabling. Individuals may also have spasticity, hyperreflexia, Parkinsonian features, chorea, and oculomotor abnormalities, i.e., vertical gaze paresis, hypometric saccades, and impaired pursuits. Pigmentary retinopathy is seen in about half the patients, though the Agrawal cohort always had it early and this was often asymptomatic.[14] Occasionally sectoral iris paralysis with sluggish pupillary reaction maybe seen. As the disease progress there is a decline in the cognitive function. The progression of PKAN is nonlinear and a stepwise decline is seen with intermittent periods of stability with periodic dystonic storms preceding worsening disability. Most patients are nonambulant by 15 years of age.

Atypical Pantothenate Kinase-associated Neurodegeneration

Individuals presenting with atypical features of PKAN tend to be older with a mean age of 14 years (range 1–28 years). They include all patients with nonclassic PKAN and are very heterogeneous.[15-17] Initial symptoms depend on age of onset with dystonia prominent below 20 years and Parkinsonism in later years. Mixed pictures are common. Prominent oromandibular dystonia leads to speech disturbances (palilalia, dysarthria, stuttering, and hypophonia). Other movement disorders include new-onset or worsening tics. Neuropsychiatric manifestation like obsessive-compulsive behaviors/impulsivity can be prominent though other disturbances can also occur (emotional lability, personality change, aggression, and depression). Focal symptoms like writer's cramp and localized dystonic tremors can also be the initial presentation. Cognition is little affected. There may be an initial steep decline in motor skills followed by long- periods of stability and about two-thirds remain ambulant for a longtime. Retinopathy is rare.

Neuroimaging in Pantothenate Kinase-associated Neurodegeneration

The MRI findings with an anteromedial hyperintensity surrounded by a hypointense surround in the GP, the so-called "eye of the tiger" is characteristic of PKAN and correlates well with the presence of the *PANK2* mutation.[18] What is less known, is that in those <5 years, isolated hyperintensity may predominate with little/no iron deposition (the hypointensity) which increases after 5–6 years (**Figs. 9A** to **C** and **10**).[19] Atypical PKAN has more atypical imaging findings. Also atypical "eye of the tiger" mimics can be seen in other conditions such as mitochondrial membrane protein-associated neurodegeneration (MPAN), neuroferritinopathy, carbon monoxide poisoning survivors, etc.

Neurodegeneration with brain iron accumulation 2: Phospholipase A2-associated neurodegeneration (PLAN) constitutes about 20% of all NBIA and is second only to PKAN in frequency. It affects both central and peripheral nervous systems.[10] The phospholipase-A2 gene (*PLA2G*) codes for a 85 kDa calcium independent, phospholipase A2 enzyme which plays an important role in membrane remodeling, hydrolysis of glycerophospholipids, regulation of apoptosis, and leukotriene/prostaglandin synthesis.[20,21] A spectrum of genotypic variants has been described ranging from nonsense to missense mutation, small exon deletions, copy number variants as well as splice site variants.[20-23] Though there is no clear genotype-phenotype correlations, null mutations have been found only in patients with infantile neuroaxonal dystrophy (INAD) and not the milder variants.[22,23]

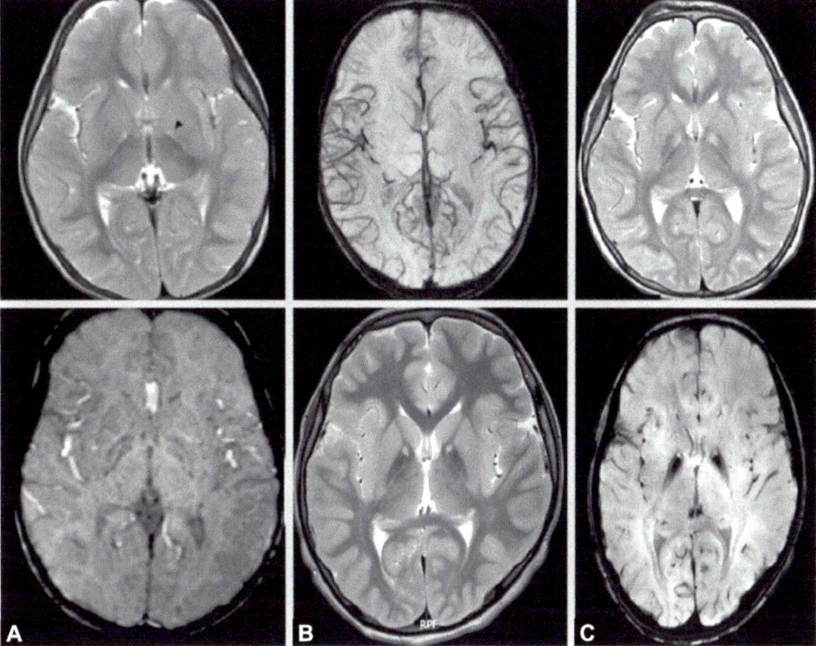

(GP: globus pallidus; SWI: susceptibility-weighted images)

FIGS. 9A TO C: (A) 2 years T2 hyperintensity in GP and no appreciable iron on SWI; (B) 3 years increasing T2 hyperintensity and early iron deposition in GP; (C) 6 years well-established "eye-of-the-tiger" with anteromedial T2 hyperintensity and surrounding hypointensity due to iron deposition.

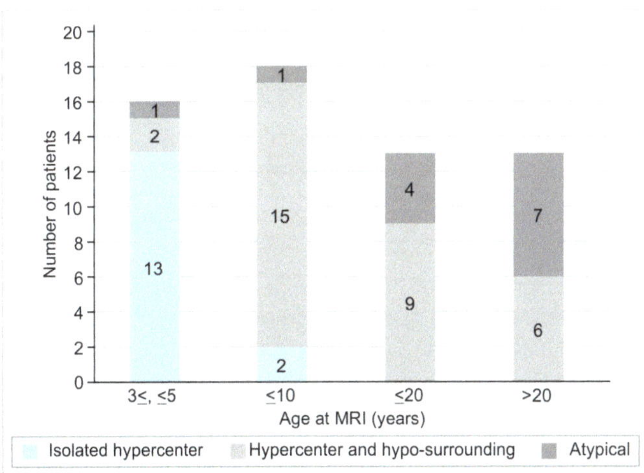

(GP: globus pallidus; MRI: magnetic resonance imaging)

FIG. 10: Age distribution of typical: "eye-of-the-tiger-" sign; "hyper-center" indicates T2 hyperintense center of GP; "hypo-surrounding": surrounding area with T2 hypointensity; atypica: atypical features.

Infantile-onset Phospholipase-A2 Associated Neurodegeneration/Infantile Neuroaxonal Dystrophy

Clinical presentation is usually between 6 months and 2.5 years of age.[22] Delayed walking is common and is followed by truncal hypotonia, motor regression, and early loss of ambulation. Spastic (70%) or hypotonic (30%) tetraparesis supervenes, along with visual impairment, nystagmus, strabismus, and optic atrophy. Later-onset may present with ataxia and later have a similar, though slower course. Death is usually inevitable by the end of first decade of life.

Magnetic resonance imaging shows cerebellar atrophy (95%) with evidence of gliosis (70%) appearing as cerebellar hyperintensity on T2/FLAIR imaging. Claval hypertrophy is fairly sensitive and specific.[21] Other findings include thinning of optic chiasm and splenium which is often vertically-oriented (**Figs. 11A** to **C**). Initially there is no/little evidence of brain iron accumulation which comes on much later with equal involvement of the globus pallidus internus (GPi) and SN (**Figs. 12A** to **D**).

Neurophysiological studies show high amplitude fast activity on the electroencephalogram (EEG). Evidence of denervation (80%) and abnormal nerve conduction studies in around a third helps in diagnosis.[21,22]

Infantile neuroaxonal dystrophy has mutations seen in approximately 75–90% although an Indian study had lower frequencies with many novel mutations.[21-23] Conjunctival and sural nerve biopsies used for diagnosis in the past, are now of historical interest.

Childhood-onset Phospholipase-A2 Associated Neurodegeneration (Atypical Neuroaxonal Dystrophy)

It is a milder variant with onset between 1.5 and 6 years of age and slower progression.[20,21,23] Initially they may have

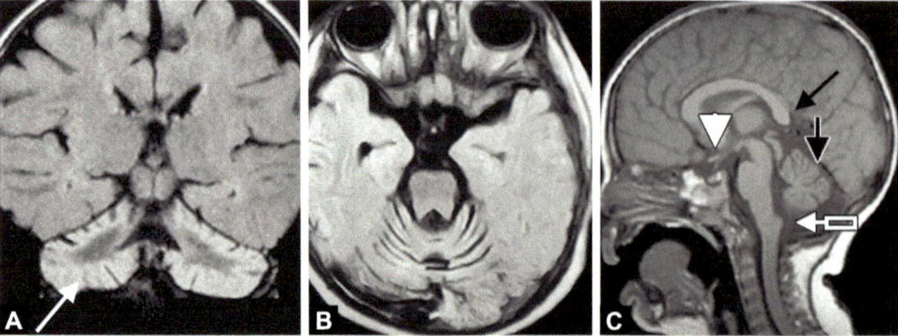

(INAD: infantile neuroaxonal dystrophy; MRI: magnetic resonance imaging)

FIGS. 11A TO C: MRI: INAD; (A) Arrow showing FLAIR hyperintensity; (B) Axial FLAIR image showing cerebellar atrophy; (C) Sagittal T1 image: cerebellar atrophy (black arrow/white outline); prominent clavum (white rectangle/small arrow); Thin optic chiasm (white arrowhead); Thin vertically-oriented splenium (black arrow).

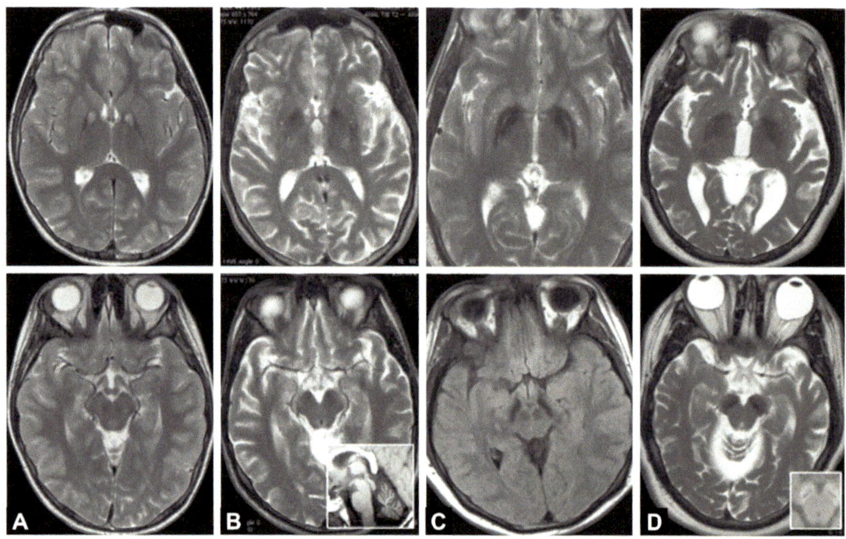

(BPAN: beta-propeller protein-associated neurodegeneration; PKAN: pantothenate kinase-associated neurodegeneration; PLAN: phospholipase-associated neurodegeneration; MPAN: mitochondrial membrane protein-associated neurodegeneration)

FIGS. 12A TO D: Magnetic resonance imaging of globus pallidus and substantia nigra in four main forms of neurodegeneration with brain iron accumulation. Axial T2-weighted imaging of globus pallidus (top series) and substantia nigra (bottom series) in (A) PKAN; (B) PLAN (inset shows cerebellar atrophy); (C) MPAN; and (D) BPAN (inset shows T1 hyperintense "halo" in cerebellar peduncles).

Source: Modified from Hayflick 2018.

language, social and behavioral deficits, and often maybe diagnosed as autistic spectrum disorder. Later motor features with gait ataxia, dysarthria, spastic tetraparesis, and progressive dystonia supervene. Optic atrophy occurs later. Intellectual disability is usual.

Magnetic resonance imaging consistently shows progressively increasing iron deposition in the GP and SN along with cerebellar atrophy.

Adult-onset Phospholipase-A2 Associated Neurodegeneration (Adult-Onset Dystonia Parkinsonism—Park14)

The presentation is in the late adolescence or early adulthood with subacute dystonia Parkinsonism.[10,20] Pyramidal signs evolve over a period of time with oculomotor abnormalities such as apraxia of eye-opening, gaze palsies, and hypometric saccades. Neurocognitive decline with psychiatric manifestations maybe seen. ^{99m}Tc-TRODAT-1 single photon emission computed tomography (SPECT) imaging suggests a defect in the dopaminergic system which may explain the initial clinical response to levodopa.

MITOCHONDRIAL MEMBRANE PROTEIN-ASSOCIATED NEURODEGENERATION

This is the third largest group of the NBIAs contributing around 10% of all. It is caused by a mutation in the *C19orf12* gene.[24,25] The function of the gene is presently unclear though it appears to be involved in fatty acid (FA) biosynthesis and amino acid degradation, thus, suggesting a relation to CoA and lipid metabolism. It is a synucleinopathy with an abundance of Lewy bodies on pathology.[25]

Typically it is of childhood-onset with a progressive spastic gait along with learning and behavior disturbances and optic atrophy. This often suggests a complicated hereditary spastic paraparesis. The later variant can come as late as 30 years and is more variable with dystonia, Parkinsonism, dementia, and psychiatric disturbances.[25]

Usually progression is slow but this may not be true in late-onset disease where it can worsen rapidly. Later axonal neuropathy/axonopathy brings on lower motor neuron signs and the combination with upper motor neuron signs may suggest amyotrophic lateral sclerosis. Cognitive dysfunction is a constant feature of this subtype.

Magnetic resonance imaging shows iron deposition in the GP and the SN (**Figs. 12A** to **D**) with atrophy of the cortex and cerebellum.

In some hyperintensity in the region of the medial medullary lamina [between GPi and globus pallidus externa (GPe)] maybe misdiagnosed as an "eye of the tiger" sign suggesting PKAN.[25]

BETA-PROPELLER PROTEIN-ASSOCIATED NEURODEGENERATION

Previously known as static encephalopathy of childhood with neurodegeneration in adulthood (SENDA), beta-propeller protein-associated neurodegeneration (BPAN) is linked to mutation in the *WDR45* gene.[26] The gene encodes for a putative autophagy protein-the beta-propeller with mutations leading to neurodegeneration. It is the only X-linked dominant NBIA and the mutant gene is most often de novo. Females are mainly affected though many males with a similar phenotype have been reported.[26]

The disease has a biphasic course. Developmental delay in early life become apparent in both motor and language skills. Seizures are common and range from few seizures requiring minimal/no treatment to a severe drug-resistant epilepsy with multiple seizure-types. Persistent severe language deficits associated with sleep disturbances, gait ataxia, and hand stereotypies are reminiscent of an atypical Rett syndrome. In late adolescence/young adulthood, neurological worsening-sometimes precipitous occurs with Parkinsonism and cognitive deterioration.[26]

Early MRIs are normal or show nonspecific but when done during the period of neurological deterioration a specific MRI feature is a bright halo on T1 surrounding the hypointense SN; a predominance of SN iron as compared to the GP is noted on T2 and susceptibility images (**Figs. 12A** to **D**).

The other NBIA disorders are rare and, hence, are summarized in **Table 2**.

Magnetic resonance imaging features often help in the differential diagnosis of the different NBIAs (**Figs. 12A** to **D**).

MANAGEMENT STRATEGIES

Symptomatic Treatments for Dystonia and Parkinsonism

- Therapies to reduce dystonia/spasticity include, high-dose trihexyphenidyl, gabapentin, clonazepam, and baclofen singly but often in combination.[27] Other less used medications include tetrabenazine, clonidine, and pregabalin.
- Levodopa may be useful in both dystonia/Parkinsonism presentations and seem to help, albeit transiently, in BPAN and MPAN[25,26] though troublesome dyskinesia and other dopa-related fluctuations occur often. Its role in PKAN is debated though a short trial may be warranted. Dopamine agonists and amantadine have also been used. The former should be used with caution as it can cause a worsening of neuropsychiatric symptoms.
- Botulinum toxin could be used for specific muscles in case of localized dystonia-related disabilities.
- Use of an intrathecal baclofen pump has been used in many developed nations but is often limited by the expense, availability, and hardware complications.
- Deep brain stimulation (DBS) generated a lot of excitement in the beginning of this century as several reports of its positive effect on dystonia and quality of life appeared.[28] However, the improvement may not be sustained[27] and if considered, one should carefully explain this to the parents.
- Thalamotomy and pallidotomy have been gradually replaced by DBS considering its irreversible nature. However, these are relatively inexpensive procedure and could be considered in selected cases where expense is a limitation.
- In dystonic storms, a common complication in PKAN, triggers like occult fractures, joint dislocations, constipation, injury elsewhere, etc., need to be actively looked for. Controlled ventilation, intensive fluid electrolyte management deep sedation with high doses of benzodiazepines is needed. Emergency DBS and bilateral pallidotomy can be lifesaving.

TABLE 2: Clinical/imaging features of the less common NBIAs.

Disease	*Onset*	*Movement Disorder*	*Pyramidal*	*Cognitive-Psychiatric*	*Other*	***Imaging***
CoPAN	Childhood	Dystonia, Parkinsonism	Spasticity	+/+OCD	Peripheral Neuropathy	T2 hypointensity GP > SN "Eye of the tiger"-like
FAHN	Childhood	Dystonia Ataxia	Spastic paraparesis++ Dysarthria	+	Optic atrophy; peripheral neuropathy seizures	• T2 hypointensity GP • White matter changes – Brainstem/ cerebellar atrophy
Kufor–Rakeb	Juvenile	Parkinsonism	Spasticity	+ Progressive	Gaze palsy; PN; and perioral myokymia	• Few have T2 hypointensity GP • Diffuse atrophy
Woodhouse-Sakati	Juvenile	Dystonia-focal chorea, dysarthria, and dysphagia		+	• Diabetes hypogonadism • Alopecia and hearing loss	• Basal ganglia T2 hypointensity • White matter changes
Neuroferritinopathy	Adult	Chorea, dystonia, and Parkinsonism		Progressive +/+	Low serum ferritin	• T2 hypointensity GP, SN, striatum, thalamus, dentate, red nucleus • Late cavitary T2 hyperintense striatal lesions
Aceruloplasminemia	Early-mid adult	• Chorea, dystonia (facial), ataxia • Parkinsonism		+/+	• Diabetes, anemia, retinopathy • Low/absent ceruloplasmin, low serum iron, copper, and elevated ferritin	Widespread T2 hypointensity GP, striatum, thalamus, SN, red nucleus, and dentate

(COASY: CoA synthase; CoPAN: COASY protein-associated neurodegeneration; FAHN: fatty acid hydroxylase-associated neurodegeneration; GP: globus pallidus; NBIAs: neurodegeneration with brain iron accumulation; OCD: obsessive-compulsive disorder; SN: substantia nigra)

Multidisciplinary Care to Improve the Quality of Life

- *Feeding and nutrition*: Due to the significant oromandibular dystonia, mastication maybe a problem and though some patients manage using dystonia-reducing "sensory tricks" many a patient will ultimately need a gastrostomy tube for fluid balance and nutrition.
- *Drooling:* Glycopyrrolate/hyoscine patches for excessive drooling or botulinum toxin injection in the salivary glands are often helpful.
- *Respiratory care:* Recurrent aspirations and skeletal abnormalities may compromise respiratory function. Regular monitoring and pulmonary hygiene are recommended.
- *Rehabilitation*: Appropriate team effort of physiotherapist, occupational therapist, speech therapist, and orthotics is required to maintain posture, promote ambulation, and prevent deformities.
- *Sleep issues:* Though it is not an issue in the early stages, pain and medication may compromise sleep as disease progresses. Relatively safe therapies for sleep induction in the form of melatonin and intermittent use of chloral hydrate maybe helpful.
- *Behavioral issues*: Children may have features of attention-deficit hyperactivity disorder (ADHD) and occasionally other psychiatric manifestations. Medications may help though the propensity of these drugs to worsen the extrapyramidal manifestations needs to be considered.

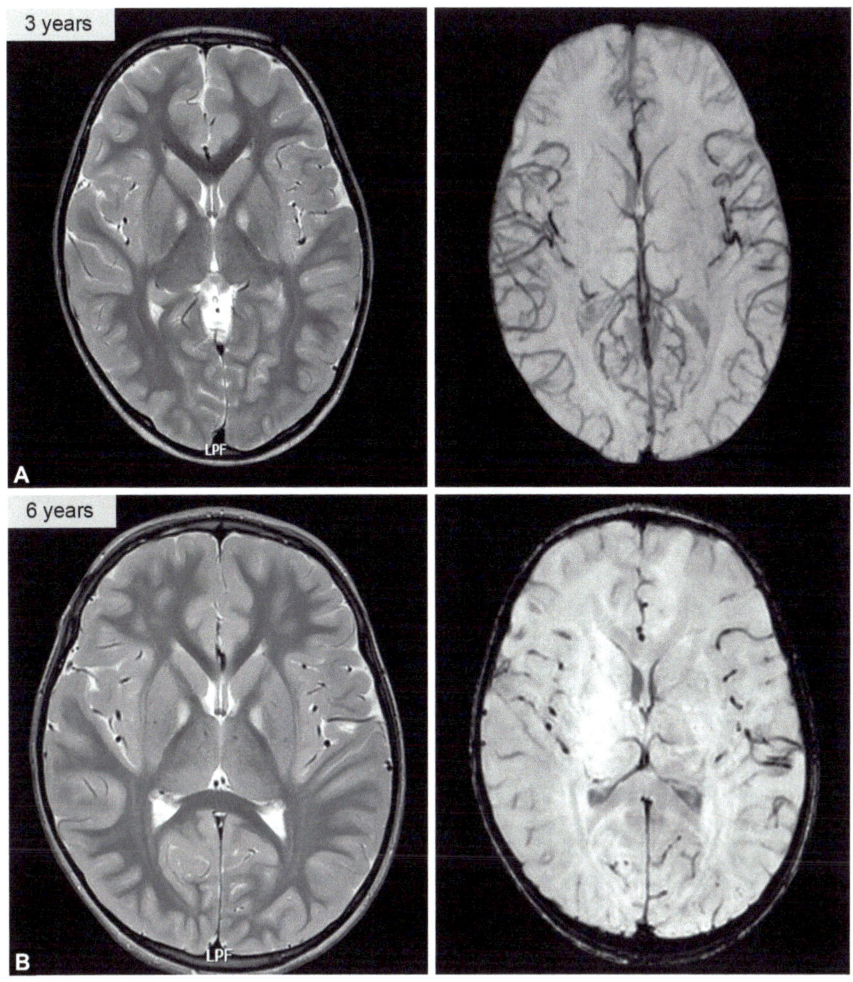

FIGS. 13A AND B: Follow-up imaging on a child given deferiprone at 3 years (A) and 6 years (B); no evidence of iron deposition.

Genetic Counseling

Since most of the NBIA disorders have AR inheritance, there is a approximately 25% risk of having an affected child in each pregnancy. All attempts should be made to identify the mutant gene in the index case for prenatal diagnosis in subsequent pregnancies.

SPECIFIC THERAPIES: PRESENT AND BEYOND

Pantothenate Kinase-associated Neurodegeneration

- *Deferiprone:* Deferiprone, an iron chelating agent, appears to decrease the iron in the GP (**Figs. 13A** and **B**) and appears to slow disease progression in a recent randomized controlled trial and open-extension follow-up.[29] However, subjective improvements were little or not at all as per parent-rating scales. However, a trial is warranted.[27]
- 4-phosphopantetheine, an intermediate metabolite in the CoA synthesis pathway bypasses the limiting step needing the *PANK-2* gene and has shown promise in mammalian models of PKAN.[30] A clinical trial is being planned.

Phospholipase A2-associated Neurodegeneration

Gene therapy is being tried as of now in a mouse model of PLAN and preliminary results appear to be encouraging (Kurian unpublished observations).

CONCLUDING REMARKS

- Disorders of manganese transport and NBIAs have been characterized phenotypically in some detail and pathophysiological mechanisms/underlying genetic variations have been worked out in many newly described disorders over the last decade.

  Important epidemiological details have emerged in PKAN where a founder mutation underlies the not uncommon prevalence of this disorder in the Indian Agrawal community.
- Characteristic imaging features help in differentiating individual disorders especially in the NBIAs.
- Chelation has already proven to be beneficial in disorders of manganese transport. We are at the threshold of treatment in both PKAN and PLAN and are in for more exciting times ahea.

REFERENCES

1. Tuschl K, Clayton PT, Gospe SM Jr, Gulab S, Ibrahim S, Singhi P, et al. Syndrome of hepatic cirrhosis, dystonia, polycythemia, and hypermanganesemia caused by mutations in SLC30A10, a manganese transporter in man. Am J Hum Genet. 2012,90(3):457-66.
2. Tuschl K, Mills PB, Parsons H, Malone M, Fowler D, Bitner-Glindzicz M, et al. Hepatic cirrhosis, dystonia, polycythaemia and hypermanganesaemia--a new metabolic disorder. J Inherit Metab Dis. 2008;31(2):151-63.
3. Zaki MS, Issa MY, Elbendary HM, El-Karaksy H, Hosny H, Ghobrial C, et al. Hypermanganesemia with dystonia, polycythemia and cirrhosis in 10 patients: Six novel SLC30A10 mutations and further phenotype delineation. Clin Genet. 2018;93(4): 905-12.
4. Mukhtiar K, Ibrahim S, Tuschl K, Mills P. Hypermanganesemia with dystonia, polycythemia and cirrhosis (HMDPC) due to mutation in the SLC30A10 gene. Brain Dev. 2016;38(9):862-5.
5. Tavasoli A, Rafsanjani KA, Hemmati S, Mojbafan M, Zarei E, Hosseini S. A case of dystonia with polycythemia and hypermanganesemia caused by SLC30A10 mutation: a treatable inborn error of manganese metabolism. BMC Pediatr. 2019; 19(1):229.
6. Tuschl K, Meyer E, Valdivia LE, Zhao N, Dadswell C, Abdul-Sada A, et al. Mutations in SLC39A14 disrupt manganese homeostasis and cause childhood-onset parkinsonism-dystonia. Nat Commun. 2016;7:11601.
7. Rodan LH, Hauptman M, D'Gama AM, Qualls AE, Cao S, Tuschl K, et al. Novel founder intronic variant in SLC39A14 in two families causing Manganism and potential treatment strategies. Mol Genet Metab. 2018;124(2):161-7.
8. Marti-Sanchez L, Ortigoza-Escobar JD, Darling A, Villaronga M, Baide H, Molero-Luis M, et al. Hypermanganesemia due to mutations in SLC39A14: further insights into Mn deposition in the central nervous system. Orphanet J Rare Dis. 2018;13(1):28.
9. Hayflick SJ, Kurian MA, Hogarth P. Neurodegeneration with brain iron accumulation. Handb Clin Neurol. 2018;147:293-305.
10. Hogarth P. Neurodegeneration with brain iron accumulation: diagnosis and management. J Mov Disord. 2015;8(1):1-13.
11. Shevell M. Hallervorden and history. N Engl J Med. 2003;348(1): 3-4.
12. Aoun M, Tiranti V. Mitochondria: A crossroads for lipid metabolism defect in neurodegeneration with brain iron accumulation diseases. Int J Biochem Cell Biol. 2015;63:25-31.
13. Hartig MB, Hörtnagel K, Garavaglia B, Zorzi G, Kmiec T, Klopstock T, et al. Genotypic and phenotypic spectrum of PANK2 mutations in patients with neurodegeneration with brain iron accumulation. Ann Neurol. 2006;59(2):248-56.
14. Udani V, Das S, Chhabria R. Panthotenate Kinase-Associated Neurodegeneration has a Founder Mutation (c.215_216insa) in Indian Agrawal Patients. Mov Disord Clin Pract. 2016;4(1): 96-9.
15. Hayflick SJ, Westaway SK, Levinson B, Zhou B, Johnson MA, Ching KHL, et al. Genetic, clinical, and radiographic delineation of Hallervorden-Spatz syndrome. N Engl J Med. 2003;348(1): 33-40.
16. Aggarwal A, Schneider S, Houlden H, Silverdale M, Paudel R, Paisan-Ruiz C, et al. Indian-subcontinent NBIA: unusual phenotypes, novel PANK2 mutations, and undetermined genetic forms. Mov Dis. 2010;25(10):1424-31.
17. Lee JH, Park J, Ryu HS, Park H, Kim YE, Hong JY, et al. Clinical Heterogeneity of Atypical Pantothenate Kinase-Associated Neurodegeneration in Koreans. J Mov Disord. 2016;9(1):20-7.
18. Hayflick SJ, Hartman M, Coryell J, Gitschier J, Rowley H. Brain MRI in neurodegeneration with brain iron accumulation with and without PANK2 mutations. AJNR Am J Neuroradiol. 2006;27(6):1230-3.
19. Lee JH, Gregory A, Hogarth P, Rogers C, Hayflick SJ. Looking Deep into the Eye-of-the-Tiger in Pantothenate Kinase-Associated Neurodegeneration. AJNR Am J Neuroradiol. 2018;39(3):583-8.
20. Guo YP, Tang BS, Guo JF. PLA2G6-Associated Neurodegeneration (PLAN): Review of Clinical Phenotypes and Genotypes. Front Neurol. 2018;9:1100.
21. Illingworth MA, Meyer E, Chong WK, Manzur AY, Carr LJ, Younis R, et al. PLA2G6-associated neurodegeneration (PLAN): further expansion of the clinical, radiological and mutation spectrum associated with infantile and atypical childhood-onset disease. Mol Genet Metab. 2014;112(2):183-9.
22. Gregory A, Westaway SK, Holm IE, Kotzbauer PT, Hogarth P, Sonek S, et al. Neurodegeneration associated with genetic defects in phospholipase A2. Neurology. 2008;71(18):1402-9.
23. Kapoor S, Shah MH, Singh N, Rather MI, Bhat V, Gopinath S, et al. Genetic Analysis of PLA2G6 in 22 Indian Families with infantile Neuroaxonal Dystrophy, Atypical Late-onset Neuroaxonal Dystrophy and Dystonia Parkinsonism Complex. PLoS One. 2016;11(5):e0155605.

24. *Hartig MB, Iuso A, Haack T, Kmiec T, Jurkiewicz E, Heim K, et al.* Absence of an Orphan Mitochondrial Protein, C19orf12, Causes a Distinct Clinical Subtype of Neurodegeneration with Brain Iron Accumulation. Am J Hum Genet. 2011;89(4):543-50.
25. Hogarth P, Gregory A, Kruer MC, Sanford L, Wagoner W, Natowicz M, et al. New NBIA subtype Genetic, clinical, pathologic, and radiographic features of MPAN. Neurology. 2013;80(3):268-75.
26. Hayflick SJ, Kruer MC, Gregory A, Haack TB, Kurian MA, Houlden HH, et al. Beta-propeller protein-associated neuro-degeneration: a new X-linked dominant disorder with brain iron accumulation. *Brain. 2013;*136(6):1708-17.
27. Hogarth P, Kurian M, Gregory A, Csanyi B, Zagustin T, Kmiec T, et al. Consensus clinical management guidelines for Pantothenate kinase-associated neurodegeneration (PKAN). Mol Genet Metab. 2017;120(3):278-87.
28. Timmermann L, Pauls KA, Wieland K, Jech R, Kurlemann G, Sharma N, et al. Dystonia in neurodegeneration with brain iron accumulation: outcome of bilateral pallidal stimulation. *Brain.* 2010;133(3):701-12.
29. Klopstock T, Tricta F, Neumayr L, Karin I, Zorzi G, Fradette C, et al. Safety and efficacy of deferiprone for pantothenate kinase-associated neurodegeneration: a randomised, double-blind, controlled trial and an open-label extension study. Lancet Neurol. 2019;18(7):631-42.
30. Jeong SY, Hogarth P, Placzek A, Gregory AM, Fox R, Zhen D, et al. 4′-Phosphopantetheine corrects CoA, iron, and dopamine metabolic defects in mammalian models of PKAN. EMBO Mol Med. 2019;11(12):e10489.

CHAPTER 41

Wilson's Disease: A Century Later

Sanjib Sinha, Arun B Taly

INTRODUCTION

Wilson's disease (WD) is an autosomal recessive disease involving a defect of copper transport by the hepatic lysosomes caused by mutations in the *ATP7B* gene. It leads to excess copper deposition in the liver, the brain, the kidneys, and the skeletal system affecting most commonly children or young adults and running an invariably fatal course if not adequately treated by decoppering therapy. Among the various inborn errors of metabolism, WD is of specific interest to physicians due to availability of effective treatment. More importantly, owing to its rarity in community and the phenotypic heterogeneity, the diagnosis is often missed or delayed. The past two decades have seen major advances in our understanding of the pathogenesis, cellular biology, and molecular genetics of the disease.[1-6]

HISTORY

Description of WD is credited to SAK Wilson who in his landmark article "progressive lenticular degeneration: A familial nervous disease associated with cirrhosis of the liver" published in 1912 issue of the brain, documented a detail description of clinical, and pathological changes in WD which hold good till date.[4,5] In 1963, the first patient with WD in India was reported.[7,8] A specialty clinic for WD at National Institute of Mental Health and Neuro-Sciences (NIMHANS), Bangalore was initiated in 1970. Since then this "WD clinic" has become a major referral and research center for WD in south India. The clinic provides care mainly to the neuropsychiatric form of WD and till date about 550 patients have been registered. Simultaneously, other regional centers from our country have shared their experience. Genetic studies on WD from India have started to appear from 2003 in the scientific literature.[9]

EPIDEMIOLOGY

The prevalence rate of WD is varied and has been reported as 12–29 per million in European populations.[10] The prevalence of WD in other Asian countries has been between 33 and 68 per million but, there are no epidemiological surveys in India.[11] Barring few exceptions,[12] most of the recent Indian literature is on neuropsychiatric form of WD.[1,13-15]

PATHOGENESIS

The major breakthrough regarding pathophysiology for WD came in 1948 when Cumings demonstrated excess of copper both in brain and liver in patients with WD. It is now known that mutations in *ATP7B*, a copper transporting protein, leads to abnormal accumulation of copper in hepatocytes and later spills into the circulation that in turn gets deposited in various organs of the body.[16,17] Excessive copper deposited in various tissues leads to free radical damage, which have been documented by detecting increased levels of serum malondialdehyde (MDA) and reduced levels of serum tocopherol in patients.[18,19] In another study, it was noted that both the pro- and anti-inflammatory cytokines were significantly elevated in patients in comparison to controls.[20] The mechanisms whereby copper deposition lead to tissue damage remain largely unanswered.[21]

GENETICS

Genetically, WD is an autosomal recessive disorder of hepatocyte copper trafficking caused by impaired function of P-type adenosine triphosphatase (ATPase), encoded by *ATP7B* gene located on chromosome 13q14 and consists of 21 exons.[16,17,22] The *ATP7B* transporter has dual synthetic and excretory roles, functioning in the transport of copper into the trans-golgi compartment, for incorporation into the plasma protein ceruloplasmin, and into the bile, for excretion of excess stores. Defective *ATP7B* function results in hepatic copper accumulation which leads to the hepatic and neurological features of WD. Until now >400 mutations in this gene have been documented from various countries. The most common *ATP7B* mutation found in patients of European origin is the histidine to glutamate substitution at amino acid 1,069 (H1069Q).[23] The genetic studies on WD in India currently are being carried out at four centers—Chandigarh, Kolkata, Vellore, and Bangalore.[24-27] The reported genetic mutations from India are variable and a large number of mutations of *ATP7B* have been documented in India including 47 novel mutations. In the study at Bangalore ($n = 102$ WD families), 36 different *ATP7B* mutations, including 13 novel ones were identified in 76/102 families. Of 36 mutations, 28 were missense, thus, making them the most prevalent mutations identified in the study. Nonsense mutations, insertion and deletion represented 3/36, 2/36, and 3/36 respectively. The haplotype analysis suggested founder effects for all the 14 recurrent mutations. This study, thus, expands the mutational landscape of *ATP7B* with a total number of 758 mutations. The most common mutations in the other three study groups are variable and include—Chandigarh group (T3305C, C2975A, 2977insA, and 3031insC-6% each), Kolkata group (C813A-19%), and Vellore group (G3182A-16% and C813A-12%).

PATHOLOGY

Liver: In the early stages of the disease, diffuse cytoplasmic copper accumulation can be seen in liver by special immunohistochemical stains for detecting copper. The initial stages of WD progress to an intermediate stage which is characterized by periportal inflammation, mononuclear cellular infiltrates, erosion of the limiting plate, lobular necrosis, and bridging fibrosis, and these features suggest hepatitis. Cirrhosis almost invariably follows with either a micronodular or a mixed macronodular-micronodular pattern. In patients with fulminant hepatic failure, parenchymal apoptosis, necrosis, and collapse might predominate often with a background of cirrhosis.[21]

Brain: In an autopsy study on brain of WD there was evidence of central pontine myelinolysis like changes, white matter cavitations, putaminal softening, ventricular dilatation, and atrophy diffuse. Histologically, there was an increase in astrocytes within the gray matter, associated with swollen glia, liquefaction, and appearances of spongiform degeneration. Neuronal loss is often accompanied by gliosis and active glial fibrillary protein. The characteristic astrocytes are Alzheimer type 1 and 2 cells. Opalski cells are distinctive for WD, and these are fairly large (35 μm diameter), with fine granular cytoplasm and slightly abnormal nuclei. These cells are thought to originate from degenerating astrocytes.[21]

Clinical Profile

The clinical manifestations of WD are protean and varied (**Box 1**). Walshe has aptly stated that no two patients of WD may have similar clinical characteristics even among the common sibship, stressing its diverse manifestations.[28]

Box 1 Clinical manifestations of Wilson's disease.

- *Hepatic*:
  - Acute hepatitis (similar to selflimiting viral hepatitis)
  - Persistently-elevated serum aminotransferases (compensated)
  - Chronic hepatitis
  - Cirrhosis (decompensated or compensated)
  - Fulminant hepatic failure (+/- hemolytic anemia)
- *Neurological*:
  - Dystonia
  - Tremor
  - Dysarthria
  - Drooling
  - Parkinsonism or akinetic-rigid syndrome
  - Gait disturbances
  - Ataxia
  - Pseudobulbar palsy
  - Chorea
  - Seizures
  - Myoclonus
  - Cognitive impairment
  - Insomnia
  - Metabolic myopathy
- *Psychiatric*:
  - Bipolar affective disorder
  - Depression
  - Neuroses
  - Personality changes
  - Schizophreniform psychosis
  - Mental retardation
- *Ophthalmic*:
  - Kayser–Fleischer (K-F) ring
  - Sunflower cataract
- *Hematological*:
  - Pallor
  - Low platelet count
  - Bleeding gums
  - Hypersplenism
  - Hematemesis
- *Other systems (rare)*:
  - Renal tubular acidosis
  - Menstrual irregularities
  - Recurrent abortion
  - Skin hyperpigmentation

TABLE 1: Clinical characteristics of Wilson's disease patients in various Indian studies.

Group	Dastur et al.[6]	Singh et al.[67]	Raiamani et al.[12]	Murthy et al.[68]	Pandit et al.[37]	Jha et al.[13]	Sinha et al.[14]	Taly et al.[1]
Year	1968	1978	1987	1988	2002	1998	2001	2007
Study period	1959–1968	1972–1975	1968–1986	1979–1986	1980–2000	1984–1993	1991–2000	1970–2000
Place of study	Bombay	Pondicherry	Vellore	Hyderabad	Pune	New Delhi	Ranchi	Bangalore
No. of cases (M:F)	23 (15:8)	08 (5:3)	30 (22:08)	12 (11:1)	124	22 (20:2)	49 (38:11)	282 (196:86)
Mean age at onset (Range)	13.4 (4–25)	13.3 (3–25)	NA (6–50)	13.3 (7–21)	8.4 (4–60)	18.5 (10–33)	13 (8–23)	15.9 (3–50)
Clinical pattern:								
• Hepatic	01	03	11	01	67	NA	-	42
• Neurological	10	03	13	10	28		34	195
• Hepatic + Neurological	02	00	--	01	00		15	10
• Musculoskeletal	03	02	06	00	00		-	06
• Psychiatric	00	00	--	00	00		-	07
• Others	05	00	--	00	10		-	07
• Asymptomatic	02	00	--	00	19		-	15

The phenotypic variability of WD often leads to delay in diagnosis, unless there is a high index of suspicion. In a large series of 307 patients of WD, evaluated at NIMHANS, Bangalore, initial misdiagnosis was recorded in 62.5% cases, leading to a mean delay of 2 years in arriving at correct diagnosis and starting treatment.[29] The salient demographic profile and types of WD across our country have been summarized in **Table 1**. The important clinical features of WD has been summarized in **Box 1**.

Though based on pathophysiology hepatic involvement occurs early in the course of WD, it may go unrecognized and may not be the first symptom for seeking clinical attention.[30] In the series published by Walshe et al. (1986), approximately 40% of patients had hepatic presentation as the first major symptom followed by neurological manifestation in 40% of patients.[31] However, subsequent international studies have emphasized neurological manifestations to be more common (60%) at presentation. Hepatic presentation is predominantly noted at younger age. Most of these patients exhibit jaundice but do not undergo investigation for WD due to rarity of the WD in the community and low index of suspicion. Hepatic symptoms range from acute fulminant hepatitis to subclinical chronic liver disease.[32] Some of these patients succumb to illness while others later in their course develop neurological symptoms. The presenting symptoms in various series have been varied and depend on the type of WD.

The neurological manifestations predominantly consists of extrapyramidal manifestations,[1] however, nonextrapyramidal manifestations such as seizures,

TABLE 2: MRI changes: Topographic distribution* (n-100).

Atrophy (%)		
Cerebral		70%
Cerebellar		52%
Brain stem		66%
Signal intensity changes (%)		
Caudate		61%
Putamen		72%
• Partial	45%	
• Whole of putamen	24%	
• Outer rim only	3%	
Globus pallidus		40%
• T2w hypointensity	34%	
• T1w hyperintensity	06%	
Internal capsule		15%
• Anterior internal capsule	4%	
• Posterior internal capsule	11%	
Thalamus		58%
• Lateral	32%	
• Diffuse	15%	
• Anterior thalamus	4%	
• Posterior thalamus	7%	
Midbrain		49%
• Diffuse	19%	
• Dorsal (tectal)	12%	
• Periaqueductal region	6%	
• Face of giant panda	12%	

Continued

Continued

Signal intensity changes (%)		
Pons		20%
• Partial (patchy)	8%	
• Ventral pons	2%	
• Dorsal pons	3%	
• Central pontine myelinolysis-like	7%	
Medulla		12%
Cerebellum		10%
• Partial	4%	
• Middle cerebellar peduncle	6%	
Cerebral white matter		25%
• Frontal	16%	
• Temporal	6%	
• Parietal	10%	
• Occipital	5%	
• Diffuse	2%	
Cortical lesions		9%
• Frontal	6%	
• Temporal	3%	
• Parietal	0%	
• Occipital	0%	
• Diffuse	1%	

*Some patients had more than one type of lesion.

cognitive decline,[29] and recurrent limb weakness[34] have also been reported. The most common presenting symptoms of WD noted from a large series of 307 patients were tremors (31.6%), dysarthria (15.6%), jaundice (12.4%), abnormal gait (8.8%), abdominal distention (7.8%), musculoskeletal symptoms (5.2%), seizures (4.9%), behavioral problems (4.6%), dystonia (3.6%), clumsiness (2.6%), drooling (2.6%), generalized weakness (2.3%), decreased scholastic performance (1.9%), changed sensorium (1.3%), bleeding symptoms (1.3%), dysphagia (0.9%), chorea (0.3%), and poor vision (0.3%).[35]

Movement disorders or involuntary movements are common in patients with WD and it could be divided into four major forms: (1) dystonic; (2) tremor; (3) Parkinsonian (akinetic-rigid); and (4) ataxic (pseudosclerotic). In a series of 282 patients by Taly et al. Parkinsonism-167, dystonia-95, and cerebellar signs-75 were common while uncommon features included chorea-24, myoclonus-9, and athetosis-6.[1] Attempts to correlate with anatomical substrate have not been successful owing to nonsystematic studies, heterogeneous patient sampling, and magnetic resonance imaging (MRI) showing equally extensive changes among others (**Figs. 1A to F**) (**Table 2**).

Psychiatric presentation of WD includes bipolar affective disorder, schizophrenia, and psychosis with cognitive decline. Involvement of frontal-subcortical circuits has

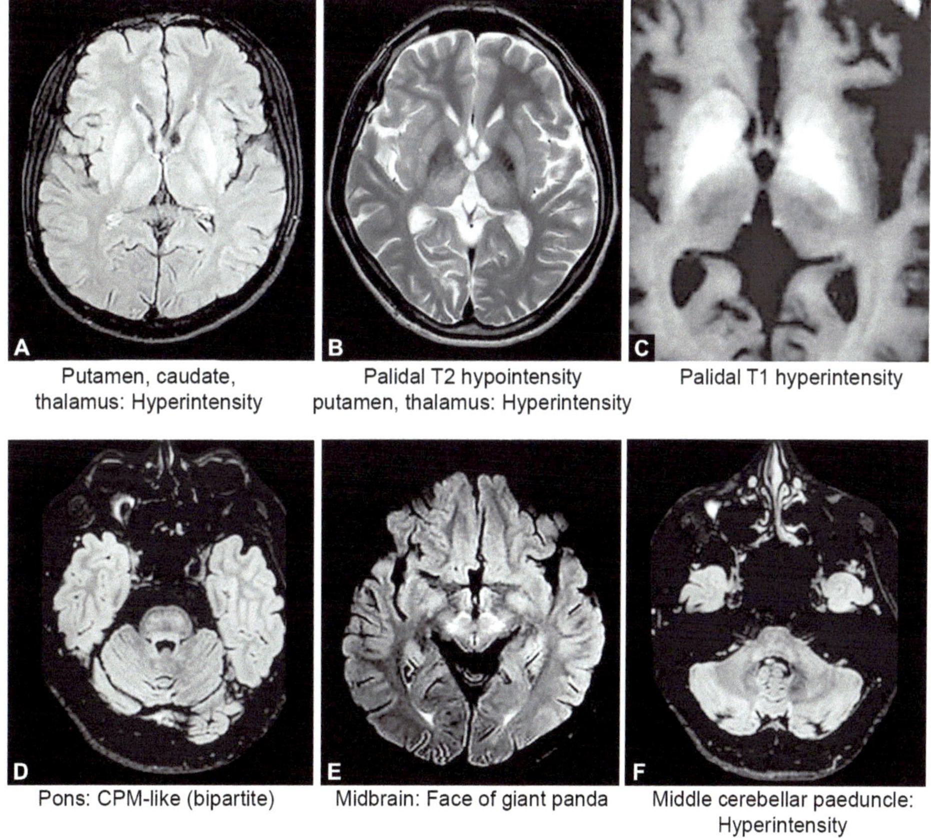

(CPM: central pontine myelinolysis; MRI: magnetic resonance imaging)

FIGS. 1A TO F: The MRI observations in patients with Wilson's disease are depicted.

been documented.[36] Psychiatric presentation of WD in India has also been noted and published as case reports,[37-39] except for a large series of patients from NIMHANS.[40,41] In the series of 350 patients with WD, 15 patients were noted to have psychiatric manifestations as the predominant symptom at the time of medical consultation. The varied psychiatric diagnosis in these patients was bipolar affective disorder, schizophrenia, and cognitive decline.[40,41] In another prospective study from the same center to look for cross-sectional psychiatric disorders in 50 patients with WD, 24% of patients fulfilled the diagnostic criteria for syndromic psychiatric diagnosis.[42]

The other less common manifestations of WD include musculoskeletal[1,6,43,44] and hematological forms.[1,45] The occurrence of malignancy associated with WD has been published in literature and include co-occurrence of retinoblastoma, hepatocellular carcinoma, basal cell carcinoma, and acute lymphoblastic leukemia. Co-occurrence of glioblastoma multiforme and WD has been documented from NIMHANS India.[46]

DIAGNOSIS

Biochemical: The prominent biochemical investigations in patients with WD are serum copper, serum ceruloplasmin, and 24 hour urinary copper studies. In addition to these, other biochemical investigations such as liver function tests, renal function tests, and hematological parameters add to the status of various organs involvement. In a study conducted at Chandigarh, to look at the copper metabolism in WD, the authors found that ceruloplasmin levels were significantly lower in patient population when compared to controls and found a good corelation between nonceruloplasmin bound copper and 24 hours urinary copper excretion.[44] In our own observation (unpublished data), data of patients where in values of all the three copper parameters were available (serum copper, ceruloplasmin, and 24 hour urinary copper), the sensitivity of serum ceruloplasmin was 88% and 24-hours urinary copper was 96%. When a combination either low ceruloplasmin or raised 24 hours urinary copper was used all but one were correctly classified from a cohort of 221 patients. In the published data of clinical profile, liver function tests were noted to be abnormal in 8–10% of patients.[1] It should be noted that ceruloplasmin being an acute phase reactant might be falsely normal in patients with acute presentation especially of hepatic form. High index of suspicion in this group of patients will lead to correct diagnosis.

Ophthalmological Evaluation

Slit lamp evaluation: Slit lamp evaluation of Kayser-Fleischer (KF) ring in patients with WD is an important diagnostic tests and forms corner stone of diagnosis. The KF ring is almost invariably present in all patients with neuropsychiatric form of WD. However, in hepatic and other forms of WD, KF ring may not be an invariable feature and could lead to misdiagnosis. The sensitivity of KF rings in large Indian studies has been 95.4%.[1] The number of patients with KF ring in various other Indian studies has been almost the same and varied between 86.6 and 97.1%.[13-15] However, KF ring in hepatic forms is less frequent and in the series of 282 patients, only 5 among 37 patients with hepatic form had KF ring.[1] Sunflower cataract is a characteristic feature of WD. However, its frequency has been very low and only a few case reports have been published.[47,48]

Electrophysiological

Electrophysiological evaluations have been carried out in WD to look for any subclinical abnormalities.

Neurophysiological evaluation: Electrophysiological evaluation to assess the neurological status including electroencephalography, visual evoked potentials, brain stem auditory evoked potentials, somatosensory evoked potentials, and nerve conduction studies have been carried out in patients with WD at NIMHANS. The somatosensory evoked potentials and nerve conduction studies have been noted to be within normal limits. However, abnormalities were noted in electroencephalogram (EEG) (41.1%), visual evoked potentials (35%), and brain stem auditory evoked potentials (42.1).[1] Earlier, Satischandra et al. had found subclinical involvement in optic nerve and caudal brain stem auditory pathways, using visual evoked potentials and brain stem auditory evoked potentials. In another study electrophysiological evaluation to study the visual pathway abnormalities in WD was carried out using electroretinography and visual evoked potentials and it demonstrated reversibility of retinal dysfunction with clinical improvement.[49-51]

In another study from NIMHANS to assess the autonomic nervous system involvement in 50 patients with WD, 13 patients had electrophysiological evidence of dysautonomia and 6 of them had clinical dysautonomia. They concluded that subclinical dysautonomia in WD is common and is due to central autonomic dysregulation and had equal involvement of both sympathetic and parasympathetic systems equally.[52-54]

Cardiac evaluation: Cardiac involvement in WD has received a scant attention in literature event though well documented.[55] In Indian literature, the only known publication on cardiac involvement in WD include evaluation of various electrocardiographic changes in WD. Fifteen among the 50 patients were noted to have an abnormality on electrocardiogram (ECG) that included sinus tachycardia, sinus bradycardia, bifid P wave, ST elevation, ST depression, T wave inversion, ventricular premature contraction, and prominent U waves.[56] They concluded that cardiac abnormalities are not rare in patients with WD and form a part of protean manifestation due to copper deposition in the myocardium.[55,56]

Imaging

X-ray evaluation has documented following abnormalities: osteoporosis, fractures, arthritis, and milkman pseudo-fractures. CT scan of brain might show variable degree of hypodensities in the basal ganglia.[1,56] Ultrasound examination is used to detect liver changes, splenomegaly, and portal hypertension.

The introduction of MRI has made dramatic inroads into the understanding of pathoanatomic correlates of clinical presentation. MRI in WD is often used as a diagnostic tool because of its significantly specific findings. There have been large number of studies on MRI from India including sequential studies with decoppering therapy.[57-64] The largest series of 100 MRIs in WD till date in world literature is from India and the salient findings were atrophy of the cerebrum (70%), brainstem (66%), and cerebellum (52%). Signal abnormalities were noted in putamen (72%), caudate (61%), thalami (58%), midbrain (49%), pons (20%), cerebral white matter (25%), cortex (9%), medulla (12%), and cerebellum (10%). The characteristic "face of giant panda" sign was noted in 12% by, feature of central pontine myelinolysis was noted in 7% and bright claustral sign in 4% of patients (**Table 2**).[58] From the same center, sequential study on MRI changes in 50 patients with WD during the course of therapy was carried out and it was noted that 70% of patients had improvement in imaging features, 20% had status quo imaging, 8% had worsening of imaging features, and in 2% there was admixture of improvement and worsening. Hence, with treatment, majority of patient show both clinical and radiological improvement.[59] Another important MRI feature in patients with WD has been the central pontine myelinolysis-like and midbrain tectal plate signal changes that can distinguish it from other extrapyramidal disorders.[60,65]

Magnetic resonance spectroscopy (MRS) is another modality of imaging to look into the ongoing biochemical changes. In a study of 40 patients and 30 controls who underwent in-vivo 2-D ^{31}P and ^{1}H MRS of basal-ganglia using an image-selected technique there was reduced breakdown and/or increased synthesis of membrane phospholipids and increased neuronal damage in basal ganglia in patients with WD.[66] There have been recent attempts to study the diffusion-weighted and tensor imaging changes in patients with WD.

THERAPEUTIC ASPECTS

The detail descriptions of WD by Wilson in 1912, ended without any therapeutic options. The diagnosis of WD was considered as an inevitable death within 5–10 years depending upon the type of presentation. It remained gloomy till Cuming's made a breakthrough in 1948, with description of deposition of copper in various body organs and suggested usage of dimercaprol (BAL) for chelating the copper. This was followed by the path-breaking discovery by Prof JM Walshe, who introduced penicillamine as decoppering therapy in 1955. Since, then drugs such as zinc, trientine, and ammonium tetrathiomolybdate have been shown to have decoppering effect and have been successfully utilized in management of WD. Liver transplantations in WD have been successfully carried out since 1982. A general approach to patients with WD is provided in the **Flowchart 1**.

The experience from Indian studies on these management issues is varied and outcomes with dimercaprol, penicillamine, potassium sulfide, and zinc have been published.[1-3,8,67-70] Recently the group of experts across India led down clinical practice and management guidelines in India.[71] Surgical interventions for unresponsive patients have also been carried out. The historical experience from the first case series published by Dastur et al. in 1968 was not encouraging. In their series of 6 patients, each received dimercaprol and penicillamine and none of them seemed to benefit from these therapies.[8] However, the recent literature has been otherwise.

Dimercaprol (BAL): Dimercaprol was the first drug introduced in successful treatment of WD. However, Dastur et al. did not find any significant improvement with the treatment in the six patients they provided.[8] Among these six patients, only three received it for >3 months. In another study by Singh et al. from Pondicherry all the 8 patients were treated with BAL and all were symptomatically better.[67] However, following success of penicillamine, the utilization of BAL has been sparse.

Penicillamine: It has been the most commonly used decoppering drug in the Indian setting. Even though penicillamine has been suggested to have significant adverse events and paradoxical worsening,[68] the same frequency has not been reported in the Indian literature.[68,70] Among the series of patients published in Indian literature, the adverse events documented were Steven Johnson syndrome-02,[67] myasthenia gravis-01,[72] and pseudoxanthoma elasticum-01.[73] Though case reports of paradoxical worsening have been noted, none of the large series published has made such observations. In our experience, only a few cases of paradoxical worsening have been noted. The probability of paradoxical worsening is significantly low if penicillamine is started on a low dose and built up to the required dosage slowly. To study the effect of penicillamine on neuromuscular junctiona a prospective study was carried over at NIMHANS involving 60 patients. Details regarding bed side fatigability tests, repetitive nerve stimulation tests, serum AchR antibodies titers during the drug naïve period and course of treatment were recorded. The authors concluded that long-term use of penicillamine

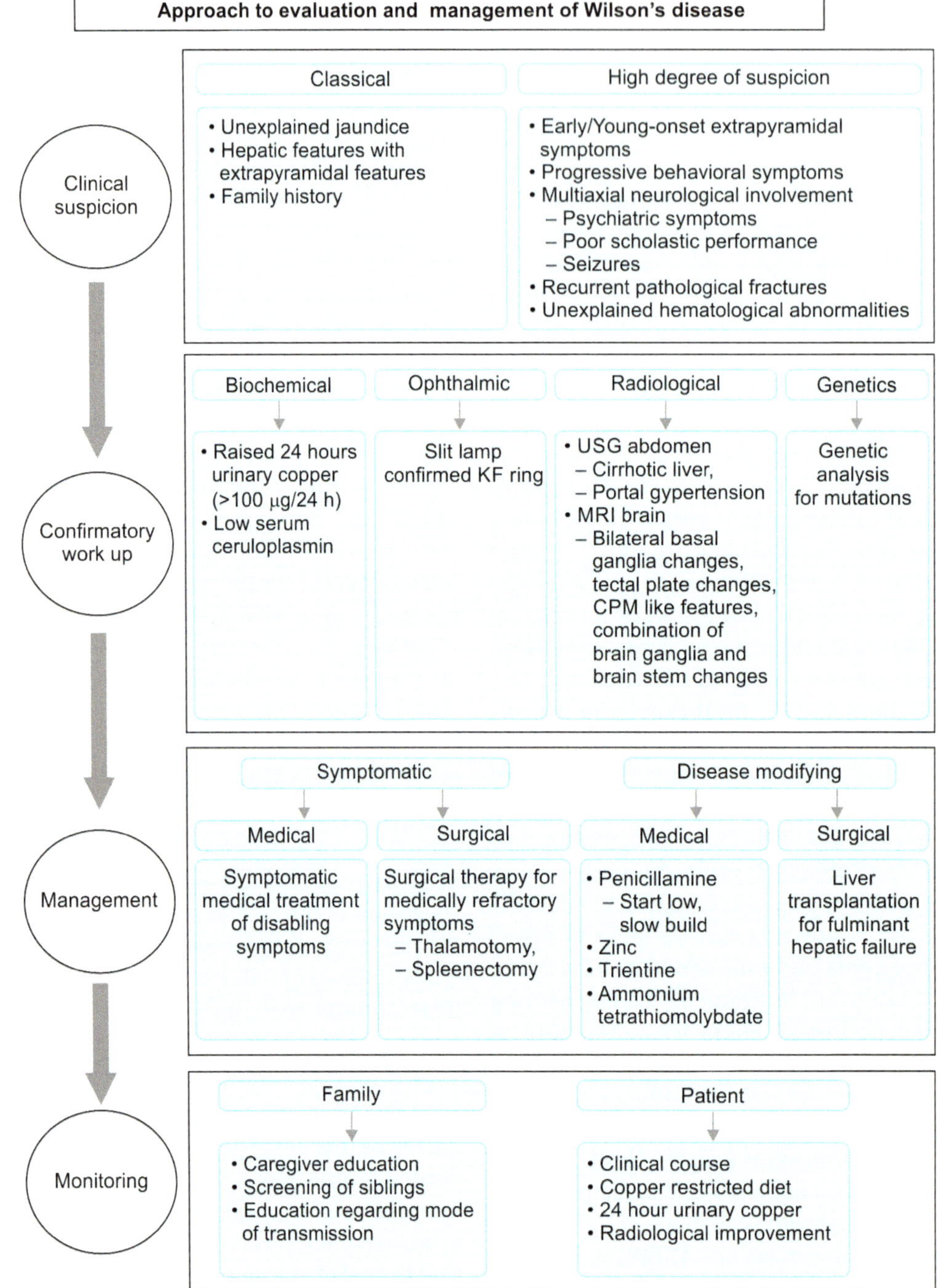

(CPM: central pontine myelinolysis; MRI: magnetic resonance imaging; USG: ultrasonography)

FLOWCHART 1: A general approach to patients with Wilson's disease.

did not produce any clinical, electrophysiological, or immunological evidence of myasthenia in patients with WD.[74] It is preferable to initiate penicillamine in a very low dosage and increase it slowly.

Zinc: It was introduced in management of WD in early 1960's. Since, then significant number of publications on its usage have been published. The most important advantage of zinc is of no or minimal side effects. Because of the minimal side effects it is also recommended as a first line drug in management of WD.

Zinc in India is gaining significant value because of economical reasons and promising recent literature. Unlike penicillamine and other decoppering agents, zinc is cheap and increases the compliance. In the first independent study of zinc therapy by Srinivasa Murthy et al. (1988), 7/8 patients who were started on maintenance zinc therapy found steady improvement.[68] In another study by Sinha et al. (2008), 45 patients who were initially on both penicillamine and zinc sulfate were later given zinc alone due to financial constraints. Among these patients during the next 2.5 years prospective evaluation no significant change in clinical status was noted while on zinc alone.[70] Hence, zinc has been proven to be effective in maintenance therapy in Indian population. In a recent study two asymptomatic siblings were started on zinc therapy. One of them became symptomatic and other had increase in 24 hours urinary copper excretion.[75] Hence, raising the possibility of failure of zinc to prevent the progression. Both these patients improved clinically and biochemically following institution of penicillamine. Overall, zinc in Indian population has been found effective for initial therapy and as a maintenance therapy. However, zinc alone as initial therapy in symptomatic patients in Indian population has not been addressed.

Trientine and ammonium tetrathiomolybdate: Trientine dihydrochloride has been used in the treatment of WD for more than three decades, but the experience in our country is very much limited. This is mainly because of high cost of the drug and non-availability. In addition lesser adverse events with penicillamine, and good therapeutic response when used in combination with zinc, its usage have been further limited. Both trientine and ammonium tetrathiomolybdate are not available in India.

Surgical modalities: Surgical therapies in WD have taken a backseat with successful treatment with medical line of management. However, a few neurological symptoms like disabling tremor could be very much resistant to treatment and may require surgical intervention over and above the medical treatment. There are very few published reports on use of surgical modalities in WD.[76,77] The most common modality being tried is thalamotomy for resistant tremors. In India, surgical management has been documented since the first series,[8] and since then a few case reports of surgical therapies in misdiagnosed cases of WD have also been documented.[29] Recently Pal and colleagues have reported successful outcome of disabling severe tremors following thalamotomy in a patient of WD.[77]

Symptomatic management of neuro Wilson's disease: Neuro WD patients will also require symptomatic management in addition to decoppering therapy, based on severity and disability of symptoms. These are varied and include—neurological and psychiatric symptoms.

Neurological symptoms: Symptomatic treatments address the issues that are clinically/subjectively bothering significantly to the patients. Neurological symptoms in WD are wide and varied and include both hypokinetic and hyperkinetic disorders. Patients can also present with seizures.

*Dystonia (**Figs. 2A to E**):* Among the various neurological symptoms, probably dystonia is the most common.[1-3] In addition to the decoppering therapy, patients with moderate to significant dystonia need to be treated for symptomatic improvement. Commonly used medications included: Trihexyphenidyl, tizanidine, baclofen, clonazepam, and tetrabenazine. Patients who have significant focal dystonia, botulinum toxin injections could be the best option. For patients with severe and generalized dystonia, deep brain stimulation (DBS), and lesionectomies of globus pallidus interna (GPI) have been done with variable benefits. Patients presenting with severe dystonic crisis may require ventilator support and central sedation.

Tremors: Tremors in WD can present in various combinations, including rest/action/postural or proximal/distal tremors. Mild tremors, which do not interfere in the activities of daily livings (ADLs), may not require any specific interventions or simple physical therapies and modifications can be useful. In patients who have tremors affecting their activities of daily living, propranolol, clonazepam, anticholinergics, topiramate, and primidone can be tried in various combinations. Pallidotomy/DBS can be considered in resistant tremors with beneficial effects.[77]

Parkinsonism: Parkinsonian symptoms in WD are treated with dopaminergic agents, including that of dopamine agonists, monoamine oxidase type-B (MAO-B) inhibitors, amantadine, and levodopa.

Seizures: Seizures are noted in about 6–8% of patients with WD with some patients presenting with seizures as initial presentations and few developing during the course of the disease. A small subgroup may develop refractory epilepsy or status epilepticus. The management of seizures remains on the standard lines like for any other seizure patients with appropriate antiepileptic medications. However, in patients with decompensated cirrhosis and active hepatic dysfunction care should be taken to avoid antiepileptics drugs with first pass metabolism in liver.

Psychiatric symptoms: Behavioral changes are frequent and many times the initial symptoms in WD. Patients can present with symptoms of poor scholastic performance, attention deficit disorder to frank psychosis, and schizophrenic personalities. Mild symptoms do improve with the proper decoppering therapies; however, patients with severe symptoms do require medical interventions. These therapies could include simple behavioral modifications to selective serotonin reuptake inhibitor (SSRI), tricyclic antidepressant (TCA), serotonin-norepinephrine reuptake inhibitor (SNRI), and atypical antipsychotics. Typical antipsychotics are avoided due to their potential to precipitate extrapyramidal symptoms. Patients with aggressive manic symptoms or significant psychosis have been treated with electroconvulsive therapies (ECT).[40-42]

Role of Liver Transplantation in Neuro Wilson's Disease

Although liver transplantation is an effective cure, there are risks associated with the procedure and the immunosuppressive therapy that follows.[78] Liver transplantation is clearly indicated for patients with acute fulminant hepatic failure and for patients with decom-

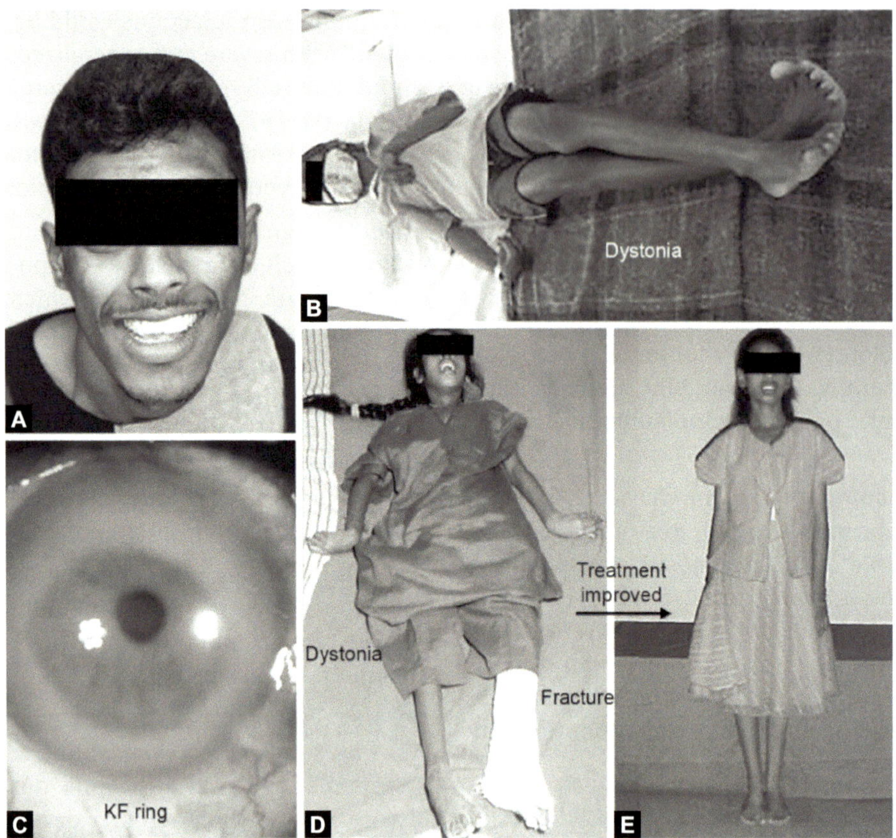

(KF: Kayser–Fleischer)

FIGS. 2A TO E: It shows various clinical features in patients with Wilson's disease. ***(For color version, see plate 3)***

pensated cirrhosis from WD. It is also indicated for patients with WD in whom medical therapy is ineffective.[79] However, in general, patients with neurological form of WD tend to have poorer outcomes as against hepatic forms of WD in relation to liver transplantation.[78-81]

Recommendations of Drug Management of Neuro Wilson's Disease

- Always "start low-go slow" during initiation of decoppering therapies.
- Penicillamine is the first line of decoppering agent. Every patient will require penicillamine, unless they have developed adverse effects to penicillamine.
- Zinc therapy is used by most centers across India and forms the main stay in long-term maintenance.
- Other decoppering agents (trientine and ammonium tetrathiomolybdate) are not available in Indian market.
- Different centers use different combinations of decoppering therapy across India. This has been attributed to various geographical/socioeconomic structures of the treating centers.
- However, primary goal of response assessment across the centers remain the clinical benefits, biochemical changes, nonceruloplasmin bound copper monitoring, and regression of MRI changes.
- Patients with significant associated neurological and psychiatric symptoms will require symptomatic therapy, in addition to decoppering therapy. Symptomatic therapy includes medications, botulinum injections, ECT, and surgical interventions (lesionectomies and DBS).
- Liver transplantation in neuro WD is limited to only very severe and nonresponding patients. However, there outcome is not similar to hepatic form.

ASSESSMENT SCALES

Assessment scales are required to monitor a disease course in longitudinal surveys which may include, clinical, biochemical, electrophysiological, imaging, or quality of life (QoL) issues. Similarly, in WD there have been various indices which have been tried to look into the clinical outcomes/stratifications (Neurological Symptom Score and Chu staging), biochemical prognostication (hepatic prognostication index), imaging prognostications (MRI Scoring Scales), and World Health Organization (WHO) QOL Scales. Recently, a new practical scale termed as Global Assessment Scale (GAS) has been introduced from Mumbai for global assessment of WD which might be useful in management and follow-up.[82,83]

Special Issues

There are several issues related to woman in WD, e.g., menstruation, pregnancy, deliveries, abortions, teratogenicity due to drugs among others. In our large series, 16 patients of WD (on treatment: 6) had conceived on 59 occasions with 30 successful pregnancies, 24 spontaneous abortions, two medical terminations of pregnancy, and three still births. Among these 16 patients, nine had history of spontaneous abortions and 12 had successful pregnancies. Hence, pregnancy does not seem to have adverse effect on the course of WD and teratogenicity was not noted in any patients on decoppering therapy. Patients with WD can be continued on decoppering therapy during the course of pregnancy with special attention.[84]

The frequency and nature of sleep abnormalities using sleep questionnaires and polysomnography (PSG) in 25 patients with WD and healthy controls have been evaluated. Sleep questionnaires detected abnormalities in 16 patients and eight controls. The study is the first of its kind in literature and revealed significant sleep disturbances in patients with WD. Studies of sleep abnormalities among patients with WD are important and the effects of treatment on sleep abnormalities in these patients in terms of QoL need to be studied.[85-87]

PROGNOSIS AND OUTCOME

The outcome of a disease in recent literature is measured by the QoL, the patient is able to reach after successful diagnosis and treatment. However, these become more and more important in the chronic disorders, where therapeutic interventions are required for lifelong. WD has come off from the shadow of being an untreatable disorder to potentially treatable disorder. However, in spite of these, therapeutic outcomes have been varied and can be broadly classified into three categories: (1) Patients who have been diagnosed, treated and have normal life, or are clinically stabilized but still have problems with QoL, (2) Patients who have relentlessly progressive course despite specific treatment, and (3) Patient who dramatically worsen and progress after long-term stable clinical course.[87]

It is believed that most of the patients with the currently available medications might lead a normal life. In a study by Prashanth et al. (2004), among the patients who were on regular follow-up, 126 of the 140 patients (90%) had good clinical outcome during the course of treatment. The authors emphasized that patients with severe illness at initial evaluation and diagnosis could also respond to the decoppering therapy and it may be difficult to differentiate between the poor and good responders at initial evaluation.[84]

A rapid progressive course is usually noted in the hepatic form of the disease, e.g., acute fulminant hepatic failure. In nonhepatic forms, the clinical course is usually indolent and relentlessly progressive, if not treated. Most of the neurological patients do respond to therapy, even when present in severe form. In the series by Prashanth et al. (2005), 50% of the patients with severe form of WD improved variably with decoppering treatment. However, it was observed that those with severe cerebral white matter signal changes may be poor responders. Some patients have very stable initial course with dramatic response to decoppering agents and later suddenly deteriorate during their clinical course, usually precipitated by poor drug compliance and sometimes by infections and stress. Once these patients start deteriorating their response to therapy may be rather poor. The exact reason for this delayed worsening remains a challenge.[88] These patients probably have very delicately maintained internal milieu and any factor which tends to change the balance leads to vicious cycle of deterioration. In another study to assess the QoL in patient with WD, it was noted that assessment of QoL gives a good supportive correlation to clinical status.[87]

CONCLUSION

Wilson's disease has an autosomal-recessive inheritance and is one of the potentially treatable inborn errors of copper metabolism caused by mutations in *ATP7B* gene. Impaired copper transportation leads to the accumulation of copper in various organs namely the brain, liver, and kidney, and consequently tissue injury and dysfunctions. Clinical manifestations are diverse and could be broadly grouped as neuropsychiatric, hepatic, and musculoskeletal.

Delayed diagnosis and treatment continue to be a major problem for patients with neurological presentations. A combination of tests is usually required to make the diagnosis that includes clinical features, estimation of serum caeruloplasmin, 24-hour urinary copper, slit lamp examination for KF rings, MRI of the brain, *ATP7B* genotyping, and hepatic copper content.

Once considered as universally fatal understating of its pathology has made a significant difference in the outcome in the last few decades. Early institution of de-coppering treatment is essential to prevent disease progression and clinical improvement. Some patients require symptomatic treatment for neuropsychiatric manifestations and occasional patients need surgery for movement disorders that are refractory to medical management. Liver transplant is the only definite treatment but has logistic issues.

Despite significant advancement in the understanding of the genetic and molecular mechanisms associated with *ATP7B* dysfunction lack of genotype-phenotype correlations, and variable clinical course and outcome remain challenging.

ACKNOWLEDGMENT

We are grateful to the staffs, residents, and faculty of various departments at NIMHANS, Bangalore for their contributions, assistance, and involvement in the care of patients and various studies spanning over four decades. Not the least, we are very thankful to our patients who consented for the research work.

REFERENCES

1. Taly AB, Meenakshi-Sundaram S, Sinha S, Swamy HS, Arunodaya GR. Wilson disease: description of 282 patients evaluated over 3 decades. Medicine (Baltimore). 2007;86:112-21.
2. Poujois A, Woimant F. Wilson's disease: A 2017 update. Clin Res Hepatol Gastroenterol. 2018;42(6):512-20.
3. Lorincz MT. Wilson disease and related copper disorders. Handbook of Clinical Neurology. Geschwind DH, Paulson HL, and Klein C (Eds). Netherland: Elsevier; 2018.pp. 280-92.
4. Wilson SA. Progressive lenticular degeneration: a familial nervous disease associated with cirrhosis of the liver. Brain. 1912;34:295-509.
5. Walshe JM. History of Wilson's disease: 1912 to 2000. Mov Disord. 2006;21(2):142-7.
6. Compston A. Progressive lenticular degeneration: a familial nervous disease associated with cirrhosis of the liver. Brain. 2009;132(8):1997-2001.
7. Wadia NH, Dastur DK. Wilson's disease in four Indian families. Neurology (Bombay). 1963;11:1.
8. Dastur DK, Manghani DK, Wadia NH. Wilson's disease in India. I. Geographic, genetic, and clinical aspects in 16 families. Neurology. 1968;8:21-31.
9. Gupta A, Neogi R, Mukherjea M, Mukhopadhyay A, Roychoudhury S, Senapati A, et al. DNA linkage based diagnosis of Wilson disease in asymptomatic siblings. Indian J Med Res. 2003;118:208-14.
10. Chu NS, Hung TP. Geographic variations in Wilson's disease. J Neurol Sci. 1993;117:1-7.
11. Arima M, Sano I. Genetic studies of Wilson's disease in Japan. Birth defects. 1968;4:54-9.
12. Pediatric Liver Study Group of India. Metabolic liver diseases in childhood: Indian scenario. Indian J Pediatr. 1999;66:S97-103.
13. Raiamani K, Sharma RN, John G, Raju JM, Ganesh A, John L. Wilson's disease in India: clinical and laboratory manifestations in thirty patients. J Assoc Physicians India. 1987;35:438-41.
14. Jha SK, Behari M, Ahuja GK. Wilson's disease: clinical and radiological features. J Assoc Physicians India. 1998;46:602-5.
15. Sinha S, Jha DK, Sinha KK. Wilson's disease in Eastern India. J Assoc Physicians India. 2001;49:881-4.
16. Bull PC, Thomas GR, Rommens JM, Forbes JR, Cox DW. The Wilson disease gene is a putative copper transporting P-type ATPase similar to the Menkes gene. Nat Genet. 1993;5: 327-37.
17. Tanzi RE, Petrukhin K, Chernov I, Pellequer JL, Wasco W, Ross B, et al. The Wilson disease gene is a copper transporting ATPase with homology to the Menkes disease gene. Nat Genet. 1993;5:344-50.
18. Sinha S, Christopher R, Prashanth LK, Vidya N, Arunodaya GR, Rao S, et al. Malondialdhyde levels in Wilson's disease? Ann Indian Acad Neurol. 2004;7:507-10.
19. Sinha S, Christopher R, Arunodaya GR, Prashanth LK, Gopinath G, Swamy HS, et al. Is low serum tocopherol in Wilson's disease a significant symptom? J Neurol Sci. 2005;228:121-3.
20. Goyal MK, Sinha S, Patil SA, Jayalekshmy V, Taly AB. Do cytokines have any role in Wilson's disease? Clin Exp Immunol. 2008;154:74-9.
21. Meenakshi-Sundaram S, Mahadevan A, Taly AB, Arunodaya GR, Swamy HS, Shankar SK. Wilson's disease: a clinico-neuropathological autopsy study. J Clin Neurosci. 2008;15: 409-17.
22. Yamaguchi Y, Heiny ME, Gitlin JD. Isolation and characterization of a human liver cDNA as a candidate gene for Wilson disease. Biochem Biophys Res Commun. 1993;197:271-7.
23. Schmidt HH. Introducing single-nucleotide polymorphism markers in the diagnosis of Wilson disease. Clin Chem. 2007;53:1568-9.
24. Kumar S, Thapa BR, Kaur G, Prasad R. Identification and molecular characterization of 18 novel mutations in the ATP7B gene from Indian Wilson disease patients: genotype. Clin Genet. 2005;67:443-5.
25. Gupta A, Aikath D, Neogi R, Datta S, Basu K, Maity B, et al. Molecular pathogenesis of Wilson disease: haplotype analysis, detection of prevalent mutations and genotype-phenotype correlation in Indian patients. Hum Genet. 2005;118:49-57.
26. Santhosh S, Shaji RV, Eapen CE, Jayanthi V, Malathi S, Chandy M, et al. ATP7B mutations in families in a predominantly Southern Indian cohort of Wilson's disease patients. Indian J Gastroenterol. 2006;25:277-82.
27. Singh N, Kallollimath P, Shah MH, Kapoor S, Bhat VK, Viswanathan LG, et al. Genetic analysis of ATP7B in 102 south Indian families with Wilson disease. PLoS One. 2019;14(5):e0215779.
28. Walshe JM, Yealland M. Wilson's disease: the problem of delayed diagnosis. J Neurol Neurosurg Psychiatry. 1992;55(8): 692-6.
29. Prashanth LK, Taly AB, Sinha S, Arunodaya GR, Swamy HS. Wilson's disease: diagnostic errors and clinical implications. J Neurol Neurosurg Psychiatry. 2004;75(6):907-9.
30. Manghani DK, Dastur DK. Wilson's disease in India. II. Biochemical and pathogenetic considerations in patients, parents, and siblings. Neurology. 1968;18(2):117-26.
31. Walshe JM, Dixon AK. Dangers of non-compliance in Wilson's disease. Lancet 1986;1(8485):845-7.
32. Brewer GJ, Yuzbasiyan-Gurkan V. Wilson disease. Medicine (Baltimore). 1992;71(3):139-64.
33. Bhave S, Bavdekar A, Pandit A. Changing pattern of chronic liver disease (CLD) in India. Indian J Pediatr. 1994;61(6):675-82.
34. Chakraborty PP, Mandal SK, Bandyopadhyay D, Bandyopadhyay R, Chowdhury SR. Recurrent limb weakness as initial presentation of Wilson's disease. Indian J Gastroenterol. 2007;26(1):36-8.
35. Singh AK. Wilson's disease: Differential improvement in neurological deficits-A prospective study of forty-three cases. Thesis submitted towards partial fulfillment for DM degree in Neurology, NIMHANS, Deemed University, NIMHANS; 1997.

36. Hegde S, Sinha S, Rao SL, Vasudev MK, Taly AB. Neuropsychological deficits and MR findings in patients with Wilson's disease. Ann Indian Acad Neurol. 2009;12:25.
37. Davis EJ, Borde M. Wilson's disease and catatonia. Br J Psychiatry. 1993;162:256-9.
38. Kumawat BL, Sharma CM, Tripathi G, Ralot T, Dixit S. Wilson's disease presenting as isolated obsessive-compulsive disorder. Indian J Med Sci. 2007;61:607-10.
39. Pandey RS, Sreenivas KN, Patil NM, Swamy HS. Dopamine beta-hydroxylase inhibition in a patient with Wilson's disease and manic symptoms. Am J Psychiatry. 1981;138:1628-9.
40. Biswas S, Paul N, Das SK. Nonmotor Manifestations of Wilson's Disease. Int Rev Neurobiol. 2017;134:1443-1459.
41. Srinivas K, Sinha S, Taly AB, Prashanth LK, Arunodaya GR, Janardhana Reddy YC, et al. Dominant psychiatric manifestations in Wilson's disease: a diagnostic and therapeutic challenge! J Neurol Sci. 2008;266(1–2):104-8.
42. Shanmugiah A, Sinha S, Taly AB, Prashanth LK, Tomar M, Arunodaya GR, et al. Psychiatric manifestations in Wilson's disease: a cross-sectional analysis. J Neuropsychiatry Clin Neurosci. 2008;20:81-5.
43. Misra AK, Biswas A, Ganguly G, Ghosh A, Das SK, Roy T. Arthropathic presentation of Wilson's disease. J Assoc Physicians India. 2004;52:246-8.
44. Kabra SK, Bagga A, Malkani I. Wilson's disease presenting with refractory rickets. Indian Pediatr. 1990;27:395-7.
45. Thapa R, Mukherjee K. Acute Wilson disease associated with beta-thalassemia. J Pediatr Hematol Oncol. 2008;30:925-7.
46. Sinha S, Prashanth LK, Mahadevan A, Satish S, Ravishankar S, Arunodaya GR, et al. Co-occurrence of Wilson's disease and glioblastoma multiforme--is it a chance association? Clin Neuropathol. 2004;23:241-4.
47. Prasad R, Kaur G, Walia BN. A critical evaluation of copper metabolism in Indian Wilson's disease children with special reference to their phenotypes and relatives. Biol Trace Elem Res. 1998;65:153-65.
48. Goyal V, Tripathi M. Sunflower cataract in Wilson's disease. J Neurol Neurosurg Psychiatry. 2000;69:133.
49. Satishchandra P, Swamy HS. Visual and brain stem auditory evoked responses in Wilson's disease. Acta Neurol Scand. 1989;79:108-13.
50. Das M, Misra UK, Kalita J. A study of clinical, MRI and multimodality evoked potentials in neurologic Wilson disease. Eur J Neurol. 2007;14:498-504.
51. Satishchandra P, Ravishankar Naik K. Visual pathway abnormalities Wilson's disease: an electrophysiological study using electroretinography and visual evoked potentials. J Neurol Sci. 2000;176:13-20.
52. Meenakshi-Sundaram S, Taly AB, Kamath V, Arunodaya GR, Rao S, Swamy HS. Autonomic dysfunction in Wilson's disease--a clinical and electrophysiological study. Clin Auton Res. 2002;12:185-9.
53. Bhattacharya K, Velickovic M, Schilsky M, Kaufmann H. Autonomic cardiovascular reflexes in Wilson's disease. Clin Auton Res. 2002;12:190-2.
54. Kumar S. Severe autonomic dysfunction as a presenting feature of Wilson's disease. J Postgrad Med. 2005;51:75-6.
55. Kuan P. Cardiac Wilson's disease. Chest. 1987;91:579-83.
56. Meenakshi-Sundaram S, Sinha S, Rao M, Prashanth LK, Arunodaya GR, Rao S, et al. Cardiac involvement in Wilson's disease-an electrocardiographic observation. J Assoc Physicians India. 2004;52:294-6.
57. Bhattacharya D. Follow up study of CT scan brain and clinical correlation in Wilson's disease. Paper submitted to NIMHANS in partial fulfillment of requirement for the award of DM degree in neurology, Deemed University, NIMHANS; 1996.
58. Sinha S, Taly AB, Ravishankar S, Prashanth LK, Venugopal KS, Arunodaya GR, et al. Wilson's disease: cranial MRI observations and clinical correlation. Neuroradiology. 2006;48:613-21.
59. Sinha S, Taly AB, Prashanth LK, Ravishankar S, Arunodaya GR, Vasudev MK. Sequential MRI changes in Wilson's disease with de-coppering therapy: a study of 50 patients. Br J Radiol. 2007;80:744-9.
60. Sinha S, Taly AB, Ravishankar S, Prashanth LK, Vasudev MK. Central pontine signal changes in Wilson's disease: distinct MRI morphology and sequential changes with de-coppering therapy. J Neuroimaging. 2007;17:286-91.
61. Saha P, Jain S, Mishra NK, Khosla A, Maheshwari MC. Extensive CT scan abnormality in Wilson's disease. J Assoc Physicians India. 1991;39:568-9.
62. Sankhyan N, Sharma S, Kalra V, Garg A, Balkrishnan P. Cystic white-matter changes in childhood Wilson's disease. Pediatr Neurol. 2008;39:281-2.
63. Thapa R, Ghosh A. 'Face of the giant panda' sign in Wilson's disease. Pediatr Radiol. 2008;38:1355.
64. Shivakumar R, Thomas SV. Teaching NeuroImages: face of the giant panda and her cub: MRI correlates of Wilson disease. Neurology. 2009;72:e50.
65. Prashanth LK, Sinha S, Taly AB, Vasudev MK. Do MRI Features distinguish Wilson's disease from other early onset extrapyramidal disorders? An analysis of 100 cases. Mov Disord. 2010;25(6):672-8.
66. Sinha S, Taly AB, Ravishankar S, Prashanth LK, Vasudev MK. Wilson's disease: ^{31}P and ^{1}H MR spectroscopy and clinical correlation. Neuroradiology. 2010;52(11):977-85.
67. Singh DS, Bisht DB, Sharma RN, Ranganathan P, Ramakrishnan S. Wilson's disease in South India. J Assoc Physicians India. 1978;26(4):217-22.
68. Murthy BS, Murthy JM, Krishnaveni A, Reddy MV, Das SM. Wilson's disease in south India and experience with zinc therapy. J Assoc Physicians India. 1988;36(7):417-9.
69. Brewer GJ, Terry CA, Aisen AM, Hill GM. Worsening of neurologic syndrome in patients with Wilson's disease with initial penicillamine therapy. Arch Neurol. 1987;44(5):490-3.
70. Sinha S, Taly AB. Withdrawal of penicillamine from zinc sulphate-penicillamine maintenance therapy in Wilson's disease: promising, safe and cheap. J Neurol Sci. 2008;264(1–2):129-32.
71. Nagral A, Sarma MS, Matthai J, Kukkle PL, Devarbhavi H, Sinha S, et al. Wilson's Disease: Clinical Practice Guidelines of the Indian National Association for Study of the Liver, the Indian Society of Pediatric Gastroenterology, Hepatology and Nutrition, and the Movement Disorders Society of India. J Clin Exp Hepatol. 2019;9(1):74-98.
72. Narayanan CS, Behari M. Generalized myasthenia gravis following use of D-pencillamine in Wilson's disease. J Assoc Physicians India. 1999;47(6):648.

73. Rath N, Bhardwaj A, Kar HK, Sharma PK, Bharadwaj M, Bharija SC. Penicillamine induced pseudoxanthoma elasticum with elastosis perforans serpiginosa. Indian J Dermatol Venereol Leprol. 2005;71(3):182-5.
74. Komal Kumar RN, Patil SA, Taly AB, Nirmala M, Sinha S, Arunodaya GR. Effect of D-penicillamine on neuromuscular junction in patients with Wilson disease. Neurology. 2004;63(5):935-6.
75. Mishra D, Kalra V, Seth R. Failure of prophylactic zinc in Wilson disease. Indian Pediatr. 2008;45(2):151-3.
76. Starikov AS. Electrical stimulation of the brain in Wilson-Konovalov hepatocerebral dystrophy (a neuromorphological and neurophysiological analysis). Neurosci Behav Physiol. 2002;32(3):255-7.
77. Pal PK, Sinha S, Pillai S, Taly AB, Abraham RG. Successful treatment of tremor in Wilson's disease by thalamotomy: A case report. Mov Disord. 2007;22(15):2287-90.
78. Schilsky ML, Scheinberg IH, Sternlieb I. Liver transplantation for Wilson's disease: indications and outcome. Hepatology. 1994;19(3):583-7.
79. Ala A, Walker AP, Ashkan K, Dooley JS, Schilsky ML. Wilson's disease. Lancet. 2007;369(9559):397-408.
80. Medici V, Mirante VG, Fassati LR, Pompili M, Forti D, Del Gaudio M, et al. Liver transplantation for Wilson's disease: The burden of neurological and psychiatric disorders. Liver Transpl. 2005;11(9):1056-63.
81. Choudhary NS, Saigal S, Saraf N, Rastogi A, Goja S, Bhangui P, et al. Outcome of living donor liver transplantation for Wilson's disease in adults: a single center experience. J Clin Exp Hepatol. 2018;8(2):132-135.
82. Prashanth LK, Sinha S, Taly AB, Mahadevan A, Vasudev MK, Shankar SK. Spectrum of epilepsy in Wilson's disease with electroencephalographic, MR imaging and pathological correlates. J Neurol Sci. 2010;291(1–2):44-51.
83. Aggarwal A, Aggarwal N, Nagral A, Jankharia G, Bhatt M.A Novel Global Assessment Scale for Wilson's Disease (GAS for WD). Mov Disord. 2009;24(4):509-18.
84. Sinha S, Taly AB, Prashanth LK, Arunodaya GR, Swamy HS. Successful pregnancies and abortions in symptomatic and asymptomatic Wilson's disease. J Neurol Sci. 2004;217(1):37-40.
85. Netto AB, Sinha S, Taly AB, Panda S, Rao S. Sleep in Wilson's disease: Questionnaire based study. Ann Indian Acad Neurol. 2011;14(1):31-4.
86. Netto AB, Sinha S, Taly AB, Panda S, Rao S. Sleep and Wilson's disease: a polysomnography-based study. Neurol India. 2010;58(6):933-8.
87. Komal Kumar RN, Taly AB, Nair KP, Sinha S, Prashanth LK, Vidya N, et al. Quality of Life in Wilson's disease. Ann Indian Acad Neurol. 2008;11(1):37-40.
88. Prashanth LK, Taly AB, Sinha S, Ravishankar S, Arunodaya GR, Vasudev MK, et al. Prognostic factors in patients presenting with severe neurological forms of Wilson's disease. QJM. 2005;98(8):557-63.

CHAPTER 42

Drug-induced Movement Disorders

Viral Ashvinbhai Barfiwala, Azad M Irani, Pettarusp Murzban Wadia

INTRODUCTION

Many pharmacological agents cause a variety of movement disorders, including dystonia, tremor, Parkinsonism, myoclonus, and dyskinesia which can be acute or chronic. These drug-induced movement disorders share a number of features, including a clear temporal relationship between drug initiation and symptom onset, a dose-effect relationship and, with the exception of tardive syndromes (TS), complete resolution of symptoms after discontinuation of the offending agent.

EPIDEMIOLOGY

Dopamine receptor blocking agents (DRBAs) such as conventional antipsychotic medications (e.g., haloperidol and chlorpromazine) and antiemetics (e.g., metoclopramide and prochlorperazine) are the most commonly implicated medications. Prevalence of neuroleptic-induced movement disorders is quite variable ranging from 29% to 74% among different studies.[1-3] In one of the recent study of patients with psychiatric disorders from India on antipsychotic agents, the prevalence of drug-induced movement disorders was found to be 5.67%.[4]

ACUTE DRUG-INDUCED MOVEMENT DISORDERS

Drug-induced movement disorders formed 11% of all acute movement disorders referred to a tertiary pediatric hospital in a prospective study in children over 10 months.[5,6] Disorders can be classified as acute such as acute dystonia, akathisia and tremors, drug-induced movement disorder emergencies, and subacute such as drug-induced Parkinsonism (DIP) (**Table 1**).

Acute Dystonia

The usual manifestations are orofacial dystonia, opisthotonus, and retrocollis (neck extension). Life-threatening laryngospasm may also occur.[7] Repeated acute dystonic reactions, in the absence of further exposure, may occur even with a single dose of DRBA. A form of subacute dystonic reaction appearing 3–10 days after starting DRBA that results in truncal lateroflexion is called the Pisa syndrome (pleurothotonus).[8]

An oculogyric crisis (OGC) may occur that is characterized by tonic conjugate ocular deviation that may last minutes to hours. The Pisa syndrome and OGC may occur both in acute and tardive dystonia.[9]

Risk factors for acute drug-induced dystonia include young age (<30 years) males, use of high potency and high dose of neuroleptics, type of underlying psychiatric illness, mental retardation, history of electroconvulsive therapy, cocaine abuse, and coexisting human immunodeficiency virus (HIV) infection.[10]

Mechanism

One hypothesis is that dopaminergic hypofunction results in a relative overactivity of cholinergic mechanisms.[11] This hypothesis is supported by a consistent amelioration of acute dystonia by anticholinergic drugs.

The other hypothesis proposes that there is paradoxic dopaminergic hyperfunction induced by DRBA through blockade of presynaptic dopamine receptors. Moreover,

TABLE 1: Acute and subacute drug-induced movement disorders.

Drug-induced movement disorder	*Key classic clinical features*	*Drugs implicated*[14]	*Treatment*	*Comments*
Acute drug-induced movement disorders:				
Acute akathisia	Subjective report of restlessness or inner tension with objective movements of the limbs with a tendency to shift body position in chair when sitting or marching when standing	DRBAs, SSRIs, and antiepileptics	Stop offending agent. Anticholinergics, low dose propranolol, clonidine, amantadine, benzodiazepines, mirtazapine, and trazodone[15,16] can be tried	
Acute dystonia[7-9]	Oculogyric crisis, orofacial dystonia, opisthotonus, and retrocollis. Laryngospasm and Pisa syndrome	DRBAs, SSRIs, methylphenidate, opioids, rivastigmine, albendazole, gabapentin, foscarnet, cetirizine, quinine, propranolol, and sevoflurane	Stop Offending agent. Anticholinergics such as benztropine, diphenhydramine, promethazine, and diazepam	Dystonic reaction may recur even after a single dose of offending drug
Acute tremors	Usually postural and kinetic tremor	SSRIs, lithium, tricyclic antidepressants, antiepileptics (valproate), bronchodilators, amiodarone, immunosuppressants (tacrolimus and cyclosporine)	Stop or reduce dose of offending drug, if not propranolol can be tried	
Drug-induced movement disorder emergencies				
Neuroleptic malignant syndrome	Fever, rigidity, mental status changes, and autonomic instability	DRBAs, prochlorperazine metoclopramide promethazine tetrabenazine lithium	Stop offending drug, hydration Control of fever Benzodiazepines, dantrolene, bromocriptine, and/or amantadine depending on severity and response to treatment[24,25]	
Serotonin syndrome	Mental status—anxiety, agitated delirium, restlessness, and disorientation, autonomic dysfunction, neuromuscular hyperactivity, rigidity, clonus in lower limbs, and tremors	SSRIs, SNRIs, TCAs MAO inhibitors lithium linezolid opioids antiepileptics (valproate and lamotrigine)	Stop offending drug, hydration. Benzodiazepines. Cyproheptadine, chlorpromazine and olanzapine in severe cases (5HT2 antagonists)	
Parkinson hyperpyrexia syndrome	Worsening of Parkinsonism with or without encephalopathy, hyperpyrexia, elevated creatinine kinase, and autonomic instability	Abrupt withdrawal of dopaminergic medication, cessation of deep brain stimulation	Resuming antiparkinsonian medications (via nasogastric tube) Apomorphine injections in severe cases	
Subacute drug-induced disorders:				
Drug-induced Parkinsonism	Symmetric Parkinsonism, temporally associated with use of offending drug or increase in dose (**Box 1**).	DRBAs, dopamine depletors, antiemetics, and calcium channel blockers (see **Table 3**)	Stop offending drug, amantadine or anticholinergics may be used. Dopaminergic agents in those with abnormal DAT scans	
Levodopa-induced dyskinesias	Peak dose or biphasic dyskinesias	Dopaminergic treatment coupled with dopaminergic neuron loss	Amantadine for peak dose dyskinesias	See Chapters on Parkinson's disease

(DAT: dopamine transporter; DRBAs: dopamine receptor blocking agents; MAO: monoamine oxidase; SSRIs: selective serotonin reuptake inhibitors; SNRI: serotonin noradrenaline reuptake inhibitors; TCAs: tricyclic antidepressants)

as the level of the DRBA decreases, sensitized postsynaptic receptors are exposed to the natural release of dopamine from presynaptic terminals.[12]

Management

Immediate treatment is cessation or withdrawal of the offending drug. Injectable anticholinergic drugs, i.e., benztropine and antihistaminic drug, i.e., diphenhydramine are particularly effective in the treatment of acute dystonia. Diazepam has also been helpful. The patients should be observed for recurrence of acute dystonia even if they receive no further DRBA.

Acute Akathisia

It is interesting that the same drugs that are supposed to calm patients can make them restless.

There are two aspects of akathisia:

1. A subjective report of restlessness or inner tension with a consequent inability to maintain a posture for several minutes, and
2. The objective manifestations of restlessness in the form of movements of the limbs, a tendency to shift body position in the chair while sitting or marching while standing.

Restless leg syndrome (RLS) can be interpreted as a focal akathisia mostly affecting legs but patients with RLS will have a clear circadian pattern, being worse in the evening. In addition, unlike RLS, periodic limb movements of sleep are not a characteristic feature in patients with akathisia.

Mechanism

One hypothesis is that DRBA cause akathisia by blocking dopamine receptors, especially, D2 receptors. The higher rates of akathisia seen with the use of high-potency D2 blocking agents support this hypothesis.[13] An alternative hypothesis proposes that DRBA antagonism of mesocortical and mesolimbic dopaminergic projections leads to akathisia.[12] Akathisia can occur after starting a dopamine receptor blocker, switching to an alternative drug or during dose escalation.[14]

Management

Initial treatment involves cessation of the offending drug. If that does not resolve the symptoms, anticholinergics, beta-blockers, i.e., propranolol (particularly in low dose), amantadine, clonidine, benzodiazepines, 5HT2A antagonists like mirtazapine[15] and trazodone[16] have been found to have variable degrees of clinical benefits in small studies with limited evidence to support their use.[14]

Acute Tremors

Drug-induced tremors are typically postural or kinetic or both. Tremors are usually symmetrical and as with other acute disorders occur acutely after dose ingestion or escalation (**Table 1**). Valproate-induced tremors, however, can occur at therapeutic doses even on a stable dose. Selective serotonin reuptake inhibitors, tricyclic antidepressants, lithium, antiepileptics, amiodarone, and bronchodilators are common drugs causing drug-induced tremors (**Table 1**).

Management

Management strategies include stopping, reducing the dose of the offending drug, or switching to an alternate drug. In cases where it may not be possible to stop the offending agent, drugs used for essential tremors namely propranolol can be beneficial.[14]

DRUG-INDUCED MOVEMENT DISORDER EMERGENCIES

Neuroleptic Malignant Syndrome

Neuroleptic malignant syndrome (NMS) is a potentially life-threatening complication related to the use of DRBAs, dopamine depleters, and antiemetic agents (**Table 1**). Incidence for NMS ranges from 0.02% to 3% among patients taking DRBAs.[17] Risk factors include use of higher doses, rapid escalation, use of parenteral therapy, and presence of acute catatonia.[18,19]

Mechanism

Central dopamine receptor blockade by DRBAs in the hypothalamus has been hypothesized to cause hyperthermia and other signs of dysautonomia.[20] Due to its effect on nigrostriatal dopamine pathways, DRBAs may lead to Parkinsonian-type symptoms such as rigidity and tremor. Other neurotransmitter systems [gamma aminobutyric acid (GABA), adrenaline, serotonin, and acetylcholine] also appear to be involved, either directly or indirectly.[21] An alternative hypothesis proposes that rigidity and muscle damage may represent a primary effect on the peripheral muscle system, perhaps from direct changes in muscle mitochondrial function.[22]

Clinical Presentation

The tetrad of distinctive clinical features includes: Fever, rigidity, mental status changes, and autonomic instability. The tetrad of symptoms typically evolves over 1–3 days. Creatinine kinase (CK) is typically

>1,000 IU/L. Other laboratory abnormalities are common but nonspecific and include leukocytosis, mild elevations of lactate dehydrogenase, alkaline phosphatase, and liver transaminases and rhabdomyolysis leading to myoglobinuria. Proposed diagnostic criteria for NMS requires the presence of hyperthermia >38.0°C on at least two occasions, CK elevation four times the upper limit of normal, blood pressure elevation ≥25% above baseline, tachycardia ≥25% above baseline, and tachypnea ≥50% above baseline.[23]

Management

Immediate withdrawal of causative DRBA, aggressive fluid management and control of fever is essential. Benzodiazepines, dantrolene, bromocriptine, and/or amantadine should be considered in a stepwise approach depending on the severity and response to treatment.[24,25]

Serotonin Syndrome

Serotonin syndrome is a clinical syndrome caused by drugs that increase serotonin activity (**Table 2**). Incidence of serotonin syndrome is thought to have increased in parallel to the increasing use of serotonergic agents in medical practice.[26]

Mechanism

Stimulation of the postsynaptic 5-HT1A and 5-HT2A receptors has been principally involved in serotonin syndrome.[27] Other neurotransmitters including adrenaline, N-methyl-d-aspartate (NMDA)/glutamate, and GABA may be involved, but the role of these agents is less clear.[28]

Clinical Presentation

Majority of the patients present within 24 hours and most within 6 hours of a change in dose or initiation of a drug.[29] Symptoms include:

- Mental status changes that include anxiety, agitated delirium, restlessness, and disorientation.
- Autonomic manifestations that include diaphoresis, tachycardia, hyperthermia, hypertension, vomiting, and diarrhea.
- Neuromuscular hyperactivity that includes tremor, muscle rigidity, myoclonus, hyper-reflexia, and bilateral Babinski sign. Hyper-reflexia and clonus are particularly common and these findings are more pronounced in the lower extremities.

Management

Causative serotonergic drug should be stopped as soon as possible. Aggressive fluid management and control of fever is essential. Benzodiazepines (e.g., lorazepam) can be used for controlling agitation as well as correcting mild increases in blood pressure and heart rate. If benzodiazepines and supportive care fail to improve agitation and correct vital signs, 5HT2 antagonists such as cyproheptadine,[30] olanzapine, and chlorpromazine can be used.[14]

TABLE 2: Drugs implicated in serotonin syndrome.[26]

Mechanism of action of drug	*Drug*
Drug that increase serotonin formation	Tryptophan
Drug that increase release of serotonin	• Amphetamines (dextroamphetamine and methamphetamine) • MDMA (ecstasy) • Amphetamine derivatives (e.g., fenfluramine) • Cocaine • Mirtazapine
Drug that impair serotonin reuptake from the synaptic cleft into the presynaptic neuron	Selective serotonin reuptake inhibitors (SSRIs): Example, citalopram, escitalopram, fluoxetine, sertraline
	Serotonin-norepinephrine reuptake inhibitors (SNRIs): Desvenlafaxine, duloxetine, and venlafaxine
	Serotonin modulators (nefazodone and trazodone)
	5-HT3 receptor antagonists (granisetron, ondansetron, and palonosetron)
	Methylphenidate and dexmethylphenidate
Drug that inhibits serotonin metabolism by inhibition of monoamine oxidase (MAO)	MAO inhibitors and nonselective (isocarboxazid and linezolid)
	MAO-A inhibitors (methylene blue and moclobemide)
	MAO-B inhibitors (rasagiline, safinamide, and selegiline)
Direct serotonin receptor agonist	Triptans
	Ergot derivatives (including dihydroergotamine, ergotamine, and methylergonovine)
Drug that increases sensitivity of postsynaptic serotonin receptor	Lithium

(MDMA: 3,4-Methylenedioxymethamphetamine)

Parkinsonism Hyperpyrexia Syndrome

Parkinsonism-hyperpyrexia syndrome is a rare fatal complication of PD. The syndrome causes significant worsening of parkinsonism with or without encephalopathy, hyperpyrexia, elevated CK and autonomic instability.[14] It can occur on abrupt withdrawal of dopaminergic medication or cessation of deep brain stimulation (DBS) due to end of life of the implantable pulse generator or explanted devices.[31,32] It can also be precipitated by an infection of metabolic disturbance. The mechanism is believed to be similar to NMS.[33]

Management

Treatment involves reinstating antiparkinsonian medication using a nasogastric tube due to dysphagia. In severe cases subcutaneous injection of apomorphine can be given intermittently or as an infusion.

SUBACUTE DRUG-INDUCED MOVEMENT DISORDERS

Drug-induced Parkinsonism

The exact prevalence and incidence of DIP are unclear because it is frequently unrecognized or misdiagnosed as PD. DIP is the second most common etiology of Parkinsonism in a large number of cohorts, after idiopathic PD.[34-36] Drug induced parkinsonism formed 2.9% of all cases with parkinonism referred to tertiarry movement disorder clinics in a large study of 14,561 patients.[37]

Parkinsonism can be induced or exacerbated by a range of medications (**Table 3**). Levosulpiride can cause rapid onset Parkinsonism occurring with a relatively low dose compared to neuroleptics.[38]

TABLE 3: Drugs causing or worsening Parkinsonism.

Drug class	*Individual drugs*
	A: Drugs likely to induce or exacerbate Parkinsonism
Typical neuroleptics	• Phenothiazine: Chlorpromazine. prochlorperazine, perphenazine, fluphenazine, and promethazine • Butyrophenones: Haloperidol • Diphenylbutylpiperidine: Pimozide • Benzamide substitutes: Sulpiride
Atypical antipsychotics	Risperidone, olanzapine, ziprasidone, and aripiprazole
Dopamine depleters	Reserpine and Tetrabenazine
Antiemetics	Metoclopramide and Levosulpiride
Calcium-channel blocker	Flunarizine and cinnarizine
	B: Drugs infrequently inducing or exacerbating Parkinsonism
Atypical antipsychotics	Clozapine and quetiapine
Mood stabilizer	Lithium
Antidepressants	Escitalopram, fluoxetine, paroxetine, and sertraline
Antiepileptics	Valproic acid and phenytoin
Antiemetics	Domperidone and itopride

The risk factors for DIP noted have included an older age, female gender, usage of high potency, high dose neuroleptics, hereditary PD, preclinical Parkinsonism, coexisting HIV infection, and coexisting tardive dyskinesias (TD).[39,40]

Clinical Presentation

Drug-induced Parkinsonism typically develops between 2 weeks and 1 month following introduction of a neuroleptic or another drug or an increase in dose. PD and DIP are often difficult to differentiate clinically (**Box 1**). DIP is generally characterized clinically as bilateral and symmetric Parkinsonism with more prominent bradykinesia and rigidity than in patients with PD.

Mechanism

Dopamine receptor blocking agents blocks postsynaptic D2 receptors in basal ganglia resulting in Parkinsonism.[12] In some cases DIP may merely be unmasking subclinical PD. This has been evidenced by both clinical[41] and pathological[42] observations. Dopamine transporter (DAT) imaging which studies presynaptic nigrostriatal deficiency is helpful in this scenario. A normal DAT study supports DIP and can predict recovery on stopping DRBA.[38,43] In a small study, 47% of patients with DIP had an abnormal DAT scan suggesting underlying preclinical or subclinical Parkinsonism unmasked by the offending drug.[38]

Management

The DRBA should be withdrawn. DIP usually resolves within weeks to months after stopping the offending drug. Cases in which DRBA cannot be withdrawn, an atypical agent like quetiapine or clozapine, should be used which has a low propensity to cause DIP. For symptomatic relief, anticholinergic agents, or amantadine can be used.[44,45] Evidence for use of levodopa or dopamine agonists in the treatment of purely DIP is limited. However, in cases

Box 1 Pearls to suspect drug-induced parkinsonism.[6]

- Subacute bilateral onset and progression of symptoms time locked to onset of medication intake. A detailed drug history is the key to suspect DIP
- Early presence of postural tremors
- Coexistence of hyperkinetic movements such as oro-buccal-lingual dyskinesia in the absence of levodopa treatment, akathisia, etc.
- Gait dysfunction such as festination and sudden transient freezing and nonmotor features such as constipation, sexual dysfunction, and hyposmia may more strongly suggest of a diagnosis of PD than DIP
- If Parkinsonism persists for >6 months after discontinuing DRBA, then underlying PD should be suspected

(DIP: drug-induced Parkinsonism; DRBA: dopamine receptor blocking agents; PD: Parkinson's disease)

with underlying preclinical or subclinical Parkinsonism (abnormal DAT scans) dopaminergic agents can cause significant symptomatic benefit.

Levodopa-induced Dyskinesias

Levodopa-induced dyskinesia occurs due to the relationship between dopaminergic loss and the resultant response to levodopa. They have been discussed in more details in the chapters on PD.

TARDIVE SYNDROME

Definition

Tardive syndrome refers to a group of disorders characterized by predominantly late-onset abnormal involuntary movements (or a sensation of restlessness causing involuntary movements) caused by exposure to DRBA and persisting for at least 1 month even after stopping the offending drug.

The American Psychiatric Association Task Force requires 3 months of exposure to a DRBA for diagnosis of TS,[46] although in patients older than 60 years, TS can occur after just 1 month of exposure to a DRBA.[47]

Clinically there are distinct types of TS that are historically referred to as TD. Unfortunately, the term TD is also used to refer to a specific type of TS characterized by oro-buccal-lingual dyskinesias. In this chapter, the tardive disorders as a whole are referred to as TS, and TD as the specific type of tardive disorder that was historically described as oral-buccal-lingual dyskinesia or classic TD.

Various TS have been described (**Table 4**). The term tardive Parkinsonism has, however, been controversial. As mentioned above DRBAs can cause DIP. However, in pure DIP the DIP resolves. In cases with persistent Parkinsonism

TABLE 4: Tardive syndromes.

Tardive syndrome	*Phenomenology*	*Symptomatic treatment*	*Comments*
Common syndromes			
Tardive dyskinesias	Stereotyped repetitive movements of the tongue, lips, and jaw. Trunk and diaphragmatic involvement, and limb involvement	Amantadine (100–300 mg/day), tetrabenazine (12.5–200 mg/day), propranolol (20–160 mg/day), ginkgo biloba (80–240 mg/day), clonazepam (0.25–6 mg/day), and GPi DBS	Stop offending drug or change to clozapine/quetiapine, if possible
Tardive dystonia	Focal, segmental, or generalized. Typical distribution—face and neck followed by the arms, trunk, and, less frequently, legs	Anticholinergics trihexyphenidyl (1–40 mg/day or higher), baclofen (10–80 mg/day), amantadine, tetrabenazine, clonazepam, ginkgo biloba, botulinum toxin, and GPi DBS	Botulinum toxin in focal dystonia
Tardive akathisia	Feeling of inner restlessness and jitteriness resulting in inability to sit or stand still	Amantadine, propranolol, and fluvoxamine[59]	
Uncommon syndromes			
Tardive myoclonus	Postural myoclonus of the upper limbs	Clonazepam	
Tardive tremor[48]	Postural and action tremors	Amantadine and tetrabenazine. Does not respond to ET or PD treatments	Worsen on DRBA withdrawal
Tardive tourettism or tardive tics[62]	Motor or vocal tics identical to Tourette's syndrome. Age of onset and exposure to DRBAs only identifying factors	Tetrabenazine	
Tardive pain[48]	Manifests with chronic pain or other unpleasant sensations in oral or genital areas. Additional TS seen in all patients described	ECT attempted, botulinum toxin to genioglossus attempted	Some it to be a focal form of tardive akathisia with severe focal sensory discomfort is interpreted as pain
Withdrawal emergent dyskinesias[47]	Choreic movements which completely resolve. No long-term oro-buccal-lingual dyskinesias. Diagnosis is usually applied retrospectively	Resolve on reinstating DRBA followed by a slow drug tapering schedule	Seen in children on discontinuation of chronic DRBA

(DRBA: dopamine receptor blocking agent; ECT: electroconvulsive therapy; ET: essential tremors; GPi DBS: bilateral globus pallidus interna deep brain stimulation; PD: Parkinson's disease; TS: tardive syndromes)

after DRBA withdrawal, DAT imaging and pathological studies supported the presence of underlying idiopathic PD.[38,42,48,49]

Tardive myoclonus, tremors, and tics are rare and have been restricted to case reports. They are discussed in **Table 4**.

Epidemiology

The main risk factor for developing TS in schizophrenia consistently has been the presence of early extrapyramidal symptoms. The association with older age was suggestive but not conclusive.[50] Recent studies on pharmacogenetics of antipsychotic adverse effects have unraveled the presence of genetic polymorphisms influencing risk of TS in patient on antipsychotic treatment. Polymorphisms in the genes coding for D2 and D3 dopamine receptors (DRD2, DRD3), catechol-O-methyl-transferase (COMT), 5-HT2A receptors (HTR2A), manganese superoxide dismutase (MnSOD), and cytochrome *P450* gene (CYP2D6) influence the risk of TD.[48]

Mechanism

The exact pathophysiology of TS is incompletely understood. In one, basal ganglia circuit activation via indirect pathway causes paucity of movements. One hypothesis is that of dopaminergic hypersensitization which states that following long-term exposure to DRBA, there is excess D2 receptor activity which inhibits the indirect pathway, resulting in hyperkinesia.[48] Another hypothesis states that the long-term blockade of D2 receptors and its subsequent hypersensitization leads to maladaptive plasticity in striatal-cortical transmission, causing an imbalance between the direct and indirect pathway which may be responsible for the persistence of symptoms even after the withdrawal of DRBA.[51] Another hypothesis is based on animal studies which has showed decreased GABA turnover and upregulation of receptors in animals with TD.[52] Oxidative stress is also a proposed mechanism causing neurotoxicity.[48] Apart from dopamine, other neurotransmitters are probably also involved in the pathogenesis of TS. Activity of 5-HT2A and 5-HT2C receptors is thought to inhibit dopamine release. Atypical antipsychotics like clozapine and quetiapine both have 5HT2A/2C antagonism which may account for dopamine release thereby accounting for the reduced risk of TS and other extrapyramidal side effects with these medication.[48]

TARDIVE DYSKINESIA

Tardive dyskinesia refers to the classic oro-buccal-lingual dyskinesias and to choreiform movements in other body parts. Some have used the term tardive stereotypy to describe the classic oro-buccal-lingual dyskinesias. However, the lack of distractibility and unpredictable nature of movements preclude it from fulfilling the defining criteria of stereotypy.[48]

Clinical Presentation

Tardive dyskinesia primarily involves stereotyped repetitive movements of the tongue, lips, and jaw resulting in a combination of tongue twisting and protrusion, lip puckering and smacking, and chewing movements. The stereotypic pattern is characteristic which differentiates it from Huntington's disease in which dyskinesia (chorea) tends to be random and unpredictable. These movements may be suppressed by voluntary actions such as putting food in the mouth or talking. Dyskinesias can involve the diaphragm or respiratory muscles resulting in hyperventilation, grunting, groaning, or dysarthria. This dyskinesia may spread to limbs causing repeated flexion and extension of the toes and foot while sitting and flexion and extension of the thighs when the patient lies down.[48]

TARDIVE DYSTONIA

Clinical Presentation

Tardive dystonia can be focal, segmental (especially in older patients), or generalized (especially in younger patients) (**Box 2**). It may involve the face-causing blepharospasm, oculogyric movements, tongue protrusions, lip retractions; the jaw causing jaw opening and closing dystonia, the neck often with retrocollis and/or laterocollis, trunk hyperextension (opisthotonos), and limb dystonia. Limb dystonia typically affects the upper limbs more often.[53-55] In a large study in India spanning 14,561 patients, 3.9% of all patients with dystonia were found be be drug induced indicating a significant burden of drug induced disorders.[37]

Box 2 Clinical features suggesting tardive dystonia versus idiopathic dystonia.

- In tardive dystonia, dystonic movements may reduce with voluntary action such as walking, whereas these dystonic movements are often exacerbated in idiopathic dystonia
- In tardive dystonia, there is usually retrocollis with backward arching of the trunk (opisthotonos) whereas in idiopathic dystonia there is laterocollis with lateral twisting of the trunk
- Oro-buccal-lingual dyskinesia or other tardive syndrome may coexist with tardive dystonia but not with idiopathic dystonia

Tardive Akathisia

Akathisia is characterized by an inner restlessness resulting in an inability to sit or stand still. Similar to acute akathisia, legs are predominantly affected. Objectively the patient may be seen marching in a place, having body rocking, crossing-uncrossing the legs while seated or rocking from one foot to the other.[48,56] Some patients may have respiratory irregularities including grunting, moaning, or even shouting.[56] Many a times, TA also have TD or tardive dystonia, so it is often difficult to attribute a given movement to one or the other.[57]

Management of Tardive Syndrome

Management of TS is challenging. Avoidance of causative drugs whenever possible would be the key. The inherent risk of TS needs to be explained and maintenance treatment reviewed at regular intervals, switching to a drug with lower risk of TS. Atypical antipsychotics should be preferred when possible to reduce the risk of TS.[48] There is no evidence to suggest that routine use of anticholinergics as a prophylactic can reduce the incidence of TS and may actually worsen cognition in these patients.[48]

While large trials for the treatment of TS are limited,[58] vesicular monoamine transporter 2 (VMAT2) inhibitors including tetrabenazine, valbenazine, and deutetrabenazine have been studied in smaller trials. Tetrabenazine has been found to be useful in TD, dystonia, akathisia, and tremors. Drowsiness, Parkinsonism, akathisia, and depression are common dose limiting side effects. Amantadine has been considered useful by the American Academy of Neurology (AAN) for the treatment of TD despite limited open label studies.[58] Propranolol at 80 mg/day has been found to be useful in a small study of TD.[48] Ginkgo biloba, an antioxidant and herbal product, has been found to improve TD, especially in those with brain-derived-neurotrophic factor (*BDNF*) gene.[48,58] Polymorphism Val66Met in the *BDNF* gene has been found to predict a good response to Ginkgo biloba in patients with TS.[59]

Benzodiazepines including clonazepam have been found to be useful in TD[58] and tardive myoclonus. Even though there is insufficient evidence, anticholinergic drugs, and baclofen can be used in tardive dystonia[54] and botulinum toxin injections can be considered in cases with focal or segmental tardive dystonia especially those with blepharospasm, oromandibular, or cervical involvement.

Tardive akathisia (TA) is usually resistant to treatment. Opioids and beta-blockers, which are used in acute akathisia, are usually not beneficial in TA. In a small case series, sigma-1 agonist, fluvoxamine has been found effective in both TD and TA.[60]

In those with severe tardive dyskinesia or dystonia refractory to treatment, surgical treatment with either pallidotomy or bilateral globus pallidus internus (GPi)-DBS can be considered. Bilateral GPi DBS has been found to be safe with an average improvement of 77.5% on the dystonia/dyskinesias rating scales across 17 studies in a meta-analysis.[61]

ILLICIT DRUGS-INDUCED MOVEMENT DISORDERS

Illicit drugs can also cause acute movement disorders (**Table 5**) which are self-limiting once exposure is stopped.[62,63]

CONCLUSION

Drug-induced movement disorders are common reversible causes of movement disorders and, hence, a detailed history of medications taken must always form a part of a neurology history taking.

DRBAs are the most frequently implicated agents and must ideally be used at the smallest effective doses and shortest effective time. Use atypical agents, wherever possible.

With pharmacology progressing, a strong suspicion must be kept in mind if any newer drug has a strong temporal relation to the onset of a movement disorder.

TABLE 5: Illicit drugs-induced movement disorders.

Agent	*Mechanism*	*Movement disorders*
Amphetamine and methamphetamine	Dopamine release and reuptake inhibition	Punding (purposeless and repetitive behaviors), tremor, dystonia choreoathetosis, and orolingual dyskinesia
Cocaine	Dopamine release and reuptake inhibition	Tremor, tics, orofacial dyskinesias, Parkinsonism, chorea, and akathisia
MDMA (Ecstasy)	5HT and dopamine release	Tremor, dystonia, and Parkinsonism
Opioids		Myoclonus

(MDMA: 3,4-methylenedioxymethamphetamine)

REFERENCES

1. Modestin J, Stephan PL, Erni T, Umari T. Prevalence of extrapyramidal syndromes in psychiatric inpatients and the relationship of clozapine treatment to tardive dyskinesia. Schizophr Res. 2000;42(3):223-30.
2. Muscettola G, Barbato G, Pampallona S, Casiello M, Bollini P. Extrapyramidal syndromes in neuroleptic-treated patients: prevalence, risk factors, and association with tardive dyskinesia. J Clin Psychopharmacol. 1999;19(3):203-8.
3. van Harten PN, Matroos GE, Hoek HW, Kahn RS. The prevalence of tardive dystonia, tardive dyskinesia, parkinsonism and akathisia The Curaçao Extrapyramidal Syndromes Study: I. Schizophr Res. 1996;19(2-3):195-203.
4. Desai N, Patel PB, Shah S, Patel TK, Shah SN, Vatsala E. Prevalence and pattern of antipsychotic induced movement disorders in a tertiary care teaching hospital in India-a cross-sectional study. Int J Psychiatry Clin Pract. 2018;22(2):101-8.
5. Dale RC, Singh H, Troedson C, Pillai S, Gaikiwari S, Kozlowska K. A prospective study of acute movement disorders in children. Dev Med Child Neurol. 2010;52(8):739-48.
6. Mehta SH, Morgan JC, Sethi KD. Drug-induced movement disorders. Neurol Clin. 2015;33(1):153-74.
7. Flaherty JA, Lahmeyer HW. Laryngeal-pharyngeal dystonia as a possible cause of asphyxia with haloperidol treatment. Am J Psychiatry. 1978;135(11):1414-5.
8. Suzuki T, Koizumi J, Moroji T, Sakuma K, Hori M, Hori T. Clinical characteristics of the Pisa syndrome. Acta Psychiatr Scand. 1990;82(6):454-7.
9. Sachdev P. Tardive and chronically recurrent oculogyric crises. Mov Disord. 1993;8(1):93-7.
10. Mohit B, D SK, Kailash B. Acute and tardive dystonia. In: KD S (ed). Drug-induced movement disorders. New York: Marcel Dekker; 2004. pp. 111-28.
11. Neale R, Gerhardt S, Liebman JM. Effects of dopamine agonists, catecholamine depletors, and cholinergic and GABAergic drugs on acute dyskinesias in squirrel monkeys. Psychopharmacology. 1984;82(1-2):20-6.
12. Marsden CD, Jenner P. The pathophysiology of extrapyramidal side-effects of neuroleptic drugs. Psychol Med. 1980;10(1):55-72.
13. Farde L, Nordström AL, Wiesel FA, Pauli S, Halldin C, Sedvall G. Positron emission tomographic analysis of central D1 and D2 dopamine receptor occupancy in patients treated with classical neuroleptics and clozapine. Relation to extrapyramidal side effects. Arch Gen Psychiatry. 1992;49(7):538-44.
14. Duma SR, Fung VS. Drug-induced movement disorders. Aust Prescr. 2019;42(2):56-61.
15. Praharaj SK, Kongasseri S, Behere RV, Sharma PS. Mirtazapine for antipsychotic-induced acute akathisia: a systematic review and meta-analysis of randomized placebo-controlled trials. Ther Adv Psychopharmacol. 2015;5(5):307-13.
16. Stryjer R, Rosenzcwaig S, Bar F, Ulman AM, Weizman A, Spivak B. Trazodone for the treatment of neuroleptic-induced acute akathisia: a placebo-controlled, double-blind, crossover study. Clin Neuropharmacol. 2010;33(5):219-22.
17. Velamoor VR. Neuroleptic malignant syndrome. Recognition, prevention and management. Drug Saf. 1998;19(1):73-82.
18. Berardi D, Amore M, Keck PE Jr, Troia M, Dell'Atti M. Clinical and pharmacologic risk factors for neuroleptic malignant syndrome: a case-control study. Biol Psychiatry. 1998;44(8): 748-54.
19. Hermesh H, Aizenberg D, Weizman A, Lapidot M, Mayor C, Munitz H. Risk for definite neuroleptic malignant syndrome. A prospective study in 223 consecutive in-patients. Br J Psychiatry. 1992;161:254-7.
20. Henderson VW, Wooten GF. Neuroleptic malignant syndrome: a pathogenetic role for dopamine receptor blockade? Neurology. 1981;31(2):132-7.
21. Spivak B, Maline DI, Vered Y, Kozyrev VN, Mester R, Neduva SA, et al. Prospective evaluation of circulatory levels of catecholamines and serotonin in neuroleptic malignant syndrome. Acta Psychiatr Scand. 2000;102(3):226-30.
22. Gurrera RJ. Is neuroleptic malignant syndrome a neurogenic form of malignant hyperthermia? Clin Neuropharmacol. 2002;25(4):183-93.
23. Gurrera RJ, Caroff SN, Cohen A, Carroll BT, DeRoos F, Francis A, et al. An international consensus study of neuroleptic malignant syndrome diagnostic criteria using the Delphi method. J Clin Psychiatry. 2011;72(9):1222-8.
24. Tsutsumi Y, Yamamoto K, Matsuura S, Hata S, Sakai M, Shirakura K. The treatment of neuroleptic malignant syndrome using dantrolene sodium. Psychiatry Clin Neurosci. 1998;52(4):433-8.
25. Bhanushali MJ, Tuite PJ. The evaluation and management of patients with neuroleptic malignant syndrome. Neurol Clin. 2004;22(2):389-411.
26. Boyer EW, Shannon M. The serotonin syndrome. N Engl J Med. 2005;352(11):1112-20.
27. Mills KC. Serotonin syndrome. A clinical update. Crit Care Clin. 1997;13(4):763-83.
28. Nisijima K, Shioda K, Yoshino T, Takano K, Kato S. Memantine, an NMDA antagonist, prevents the development of hyperthermia in an animal model for serotonin syndrome. Pharmacopsychiatry. 2004;37(2):57-62.
29. Mason PJ, Morris VA, Balcezak TJ. Serotonin syndrome. Presentation of 2 cases and review of the literature. Medicine. 2000;79(4):201-9.
30. Graudins A, Stearman A, Chan B. Treatment of the serotonin syndrome with cyproheptadine. J Emerg Med. 1998;16(4): 615-9.
31. Azar J, Elinav H, Safadi R, Soliman M. Malignant deep brain stimulator withdrawal syndrome. BMJ Case Rep. 2019;12(5):e229122.
32. Rajan R, Krishnan S, Kesavapisharady KK, Kishore A. Malignant Subthalamic Nucleus-Deep Brain Stimulation Withdrawal Syndrome in Parkinson's Disease. Mov Disord Clin Pract. 2016; 3(3):288-91.
33. Rajan S, Kaas B, Moukheiber E. Movement Disorders Emergencies. Semin Neurol. 2019;39(1):125-36.
34. Barbosa MT, Caramelli P, Maia DP, Cunningham MC, Guerra HL, Lima-Costa MF, et al. Parkinsonism and Parkinson's disease in the elderly: a community-based survey in Brazil (the Bambuí study). Mov Disord. 2006;21(6):800-8.
35. Benito-León J, Bermejo-Pareja F, Rodríguez J, Molina JA, Gabriel R, Morales JM. Prevalence of PD and other types of parkinsonism in three elderly populations of central Spain. Mov Disord. 2003;18(3):267-74.
36. Wenning GK, Kiechl S, Seppi K, Müller J, Högl B, Saletu M, et al. Prevalence of movement disorders in men and women aged 50-89 years (Bruneck Study cohort): a population-based study. Lancet Neurol. 2005;4(12):815-20.

37. Prashant LK, Kumar H, Wadia PM, Muthane U. The Spectrum Of Movement Disorders In Tertiary Care Centers In India: A Tale Of Three Cities. Annals of Indian Academy of Neurology. DOI: 10.4103/aian.AIAN_1257_20.
38. Shetty AS, Shah HJ, Lele VR, Wadia PM. Drug induced Parkinsonism: Role of functional imaging and follow up. Mov Disord. 2016;31(Suppl 2).
39. Hriso E, Kuhn T, Masdeu JC, Grundman M. Extrapyramidal symptoms due to dopamine-blocking agents in patients with AIDS encephalopathy. Am J Psychiatry. 1991;148(11):1558-61.
40. Shin HW, Chung SJ. Drug-induced parkinsonism. J Clin Neurol. 2012;8(1):15-21.
41. Goetz CG. Drug-induced Parkinsonism and idiopathic Parkinson's disease. Arch Neurol. 1983;40(5):325-6.
42. Rajput AH, Rozdilsky B, Hornykiewicz O, Shannak K, Lee T, Seeman P. Reversible drug-induced parkinsonism. Clinicopathologic study of two cases. Arch Neurol. 1982;39(10):644-6.
43. Kägi G, Bhatia KP, Tolosa E. The role of DAT-SPECT in movement disorders. J Neurol Neurosurg Psychiatry. 2010;81(1):5-12.
44. Kelly JT, Zimmermann RL, Abuzzahab FS, Schiele BC. A double-blind study of amantadine hydrochloride versus benztropine mesylate in drug-induced parkinsonism. Pharmacology. 1974;12(2):65-73.
45. Shoulson I. Carbidopa/levodopa therapy of coexistent drug-induced parkinsonism and tardive dyskinesia. Adv Neurol. 1983;37:259-66.
46. Tardive dyskinesia: summary of a Task Force Report of the American Psychiatric Association. By the Task Force on Late Neurological Effects of Antipsychotic Drugs. Am J Psychiatry. 1980;137(10):1163-72.
47. Jeste DV, Lacro JP, Palmer B, Rockwell E, Harris MJ, Caligiuri MP. Incidence of tardive dyskinesia in early stages of low-dose treatment with typical neuroleptics in older patients. Am J Psychiatry. 1999;156(2):309-11.
48. Aquino CC, Lang AE. Tardive dyskinesia syndromes: current concepts. Parkinsonism Relat Disord. 2014;20(Suppl 1):S113-7.
49. Frei K, Truong DD, Fahn S, Jankovic J, Hauser RA. The nosology of tardive syndromes. J Neurol Sci. 2018;389:10-6.
50. Tenback DE, van Harten PN, van Os J. Non-therapeutic risk factors for onset of tardive dyskinesia in schizophrenia: a meta-analysis. Mov Disord. 2009;24(16):2309-15.
51. Teo JT, Edwards MJ, Bhatia K. Tardive dyskinesia is caused by maladaptive synaptic plasticity: a hypothesis. Mov Disord. 2012;27(10):1205-15.
52. Gunne LM, Häggström JE, Sjöquist B. Association with persistent neuroleptic-induced dyskinesia of regional changes in brain GABA synthesis. Nature. 1984;309(5966):347-9.
53. Bhidayasiri R, Boonyawairoj S. Spectrum of tardive syndromes: clinical recognition and management. Postgrad Med J. 2011;87(1024):132-41.
54. Kang UJ, Burke RE, Fahn S. Natural history and treatment of tardive dystonia. Mov Disord. 1986;1(3):193-208.
55. Kiriakakis V, Bhatia KP, Quinn NP, Marsden CD. The natural history of tardive dystonia. A long-term follow-up study of 107 cases. Brain. 1998;121(Pt 11):2053-66.
56. Burke RE, Kang UJ, Jankovic J, Miller LG, Fahn S. Tardive akathisia: an analysis of clinical features and response to open therapeutic trials. Mov Disord. 1989;4(2):157-75.
57. Barnes TR, Braude WM. Akathisia variants and tardive dyskinesia. Arch Gen Psychiatry. 1985;42(9):874-8.
58. Bhidayasiri R, Fahn S, Weiner WJ, Gronseth GS, Sullivan KL, Zesiewicz TA. Evidence-based guideline: treatment of tardive syndromes: report of the Guideline Development Subcommittee of the American Academy of Neurology. Neurology. 2013;81(5):463-9.
59. Zhang XY, Zhang WF, Zhou DF, Chen DC, Xiu MH, Wu HR, et al. Brain-derived neurotrophic factor levels and its Val66Met gene polymorphism predict tardive dyskinesia treatment response to Ginkgo biloba. Biol Psychiatry. 2012;72(8):700-6.
60. Albayrak Y, Hashimoto K. Benefical effects of sigma-1 agonist fluvoxamine for tardive dyskinesia and tardive akathisia in patients with schizophrenia: report of three cases. Psychiatry Investig. 2013;10(4):417-20.
61. Mentzel CL, Tenback DE, Tijssen MA, Visser-Vandewalle VE, van Harten PN. Efficacy and safety of deep brain stimulation in patients with medication-induced tardive dyskinesia and/or dystonia: a systematic review. J Clin Psychiatry. 2012;73(11):1434-8.
62. Asser A, Taba P. Psychostimulants and movement disorders. Front Neurol. 2015;6:75.
63. Fountoulakis KN, Samara M, Siapera M, Iacovides A. Tardive Tourette-like syndrome: a systematic review. International clinical psychopharmacology. 2011;26(5):237-42.

CHAPTER 43

Infections and Movement Disorders

Niraj Kumar, Govind Madhaw

INTRODUCTION

Central nervous system (CNS) infections result in significant mortality and morbidity with meningitis and encephalitis being the most common cause of disability-adjusted life years (DALY) after stroke, migraine, and dementia in South Asia with an age-adjusted estimated global incidence of 39 and 90 per 100,000 populations, respectively.[1] Due to diverse clinical manifestations, often they create diagnostic challenges. Infections have been related to a wide spectrum of movement disorders (MDs) ranging from hyperkinetic disorders such as chorea, ballism, dystonia, tics, tremor, and myoclonus to hypokinetic disorders such as Parkinsonism. Although exact epidemiological data is lacking, a small study reported infectious causes representing 20.4% of all secondary MDs.[2] MDs have been reported in association with viruses, bacteria, mycobacterium, parasites, and prions. In a study involving 1,282 adult cases of Japanese encephalitis, dystonia was detected in 46% cases.[3] Another example suggesting a role of viral etiology in Parkinsonism is the appearance of "Parkinsonian clusters", i.e., group of individuals sharing a common environment developing Parkinsonism at greater than normal statistical rates in absence of other risk factors.[4] Bacterial infections such as streptococcal infections have been related to MDs namely Sydenham's chorea. Parasitic infections such as *Toxoplasma*, malaria, and neurocysticercosis (NCC) have been associated with ballism, choreoathetosis, and dystonia.[2]

PATHOGENESIS

Infections can result in direct neuronal damage or result in para- or postinfectious immunological damage in the CNS resulting in neurological manifestations including MDs. CNS or systemic infections result in inflammatory response characterized by increased activated microglia and inflammatory cytokines which disrupt the blood-brain barrier (BBB) and cause neuronal injury. Microbial agents, through their replication and subsequent cell lysis, may result in direct neuronal damage. Similarly, vascular inflammation can lead to loss of vascular integrity, increased permeability of cerebral vessels, and cerebral edema, ultimately resulting in neuronal damage. These mechanisms can cause chronic inflammation resulting in extensive damage to dopaminergic and related neurons leading to MD.[5] Viral agents have been shown through mechanisms of molecular mimicry to induce the aggregation and oligomerization of α-syn, leading to deposition in neuronal cells and further loss of dopaminergic neurons.[6]

The infectious agents can enter CNS either through the neural or vascular route. Three cranial nerves are having processes that innervate visceral organs and tissues that would be first contacted by viral infection including the olfactory epithelium (olfactory nerve), orofacial mucosa (trigeminal nerve), and digestive system (vagus nerve).[4] Although viruses have never been isolated from axons of these nerves, they were first seen in the regions innervated by these nerves with viruses being detected in the visceral ganglia. Detection of *A/WSN/33* strain of influenza in substantia nigra, not having any direct anatomical connection to a cranial nerve, suggests that the influenza virus may enter CNS via different mechanisms than axonal transport such as through ependymal cells lining the ventricles and shedding into cerebrospinal fluid (CSF) through the blood extravasation from penetrating capillaries or via disrupted BBB around the circumventricular organs.[7] Based on the location of

Lewy bodies and neurites initially at the olfactory bulb, gastrointestinal plexi, vagus nerve, and finally to other areas of CNS including substantia nigra, Braak suggests the possibility of infectious etiology for Parkinson's disease (PD).[8] Another hypothesis is that infectious agents may be the first "hit" in a two-hit hypothesis and this insult sensitizes the brain to a later "hit" that might not have been pathogenic in the absence of an already primed system.[8]

CLINICAL MANIFESTATIONS

Movement Disorders Related to Viral Infections

The 1918 outbreak of influenza has been linked to the development of postencephalitic Parkinsonism (PEP),[9] with a marked reduction in such cases after the 1940s. Transient tremor and gait disturbance within the 1st week of diagnosis have been reported in many patients of influenza. Risk of developing Parkinsonism high with increasing influenza attacks. An animal study reported progression of H5N1 influenza infection from peripheral to CNS. This activates innate immune response leading to transient loss of dopaminergic neurons in the substantia nigra pars compacta (SNpc) followed by persistent activation of microglia despite restoration of dopaminergic neuronal loss.[10] The dopaminergic neuron loss was not observed after vaccination or treatment with oseltamivir. Synergistic effects of influenza and the Parkinsonian toxin 1-methyl-4-phenyl-1,2,3,6-tetrahydropyridine (MPTP) have been observed in animal models.[11]

Although the frequency of encephalitis lethargica has declined dramatically, sporadic cases continued to appear with very high mortality and morbidity. The acute phase of the illness is characterized by fever, altered sensorium, and ophthalmoplegia. CSF examination typically revealed mild elevation of protein levels and pleocytosis. The presence of oligoclonal bands in the CSF of encephalitis lethargica-like cases, autoantibodies against human basal ganglia antigens and the beneficial effects of steroid therapy propose the possibility of autoimmune pathology. A significant proportion of survivors develop Parkinsonian syndrome which differs from PD by the presence of predominant dystonia, blepharospasm, oculogyric crisis, marked loss of dopamine neurons in substantia nigra, absence of Lewy bodies or neurofibrillary tangles, and poor response to levodopa. Classic extrapyramidal symptoms of bradykinesia, tremor, and "mask-like" face are a few of the overlapping features. However, cognitive disturbances such as aphasia and apraxia are rare in patients affected with PEP. The hyperkinetic subtype is characterized by the presence of generalized chorea, choreoathetosis, and dystonia. Few cases may resemble progressive supranuclear palsy.[9]

Apart from the influenza virus, Coxsackie virus[4] and hepatitis C virus (HCV)[5] have been related to Parkinsonism. PEP very similar to the influenza virus has been described with the herpes virus group namely Epstein–Barr virus (EBV), varicella-zoster virus (VZV), and less commonly with herpes simplex virus (HSV).[5]

Japanese encephalitis virus (JEV) and West Nile virus (WNV) may cause encephalitis. Endemic to India, JEV most commonly presents in the pediatric population after mosquito inoculation.[12] Clinical manifestations may range from self-limiting flu like illness to life threatening encephalitis and postencephalitic dystonia and Parkinsonism.[12] In a 3-year follow-up study of 555 suspected patients of JEV in Vietnam, several MDs were described including rest tremor, orofacial dyskinesias, choreoathetosis, mandibular dystonia, hiccups, and opsoclonus myoclonus.[13] A North Indian study by Kalita and Misra reported Parkinsonian syndrome characterized by bradykinesia, hypophonia, and axial dystonia in 70% of patients in the acute stage of illness, i.e., 1st 4 weeks after the disease onset.[14] As other manifestations regressed in subsequent months, hypophonia was a striking sequela in most patients. MDs were commonly seen in patients emerging from a coma and resolve with time. Neuroimaging revealed lentiform and thalamic involvement bilaterally. In a subsequent publication by the same authors, the involvement of the midbrain, substantia nigra, and, less commonly, cerebellum and cortical areas have been reported in magnetic resonance imaging (MRI) of the brain in patients with postencephalitis dystonia secondary to JE.[15] Das et al. reported a higher incidence of prior JEV infection among PD patients of Burdwan, a place in West Bengal state of India having several outbreaks in the last two decades.[16]

The emergence of the WNV in the USA occurred in 1999, assuming an epidemic proportion in the New York city area,[17] with meningoencephalitis being the most common presentation. Asymmetric tremors predominantly involving an upper limb, myoclonus, rigidity, bradykinesia, postural instability, opsoclonus-myoclonus, and cerebellar ataxia appear in many cases of acute WNV encephalitis patients transiently and resolve overtime.[18] Acute-onset Parkinsonian features during WNV encephalitis is a result of the WNV-induced death of dopaminergic neurons.[19] Neuropathological studies show perivascular and meningeal inflammation with neuronal loss, microglial activation, and astrocyte proliferation within the basal ganglia, thalamus, and brainstem including SNpc. Although Parkinsonian features are unrelated to MRI findings, most patients have bilateral, focal lesions in the basal ganglia, thalamus, and pons.[19] Dengue, another prominent member of the arbovirus-flavivirus group transmitted by the *Aedes* mosquito, manifests clinically with acute self-resolving febrile illness to a multisystem disease. Neurological manifestations include encephalitis, meningoencephalitis, acute-disseminated encephalomyelitis, transverse myelitis, and Guillain–Barré syndrome with rare reports of PEP.[20]

Around 60% of patients with acquired immunodeficiency syndrome (AIDS) have neurological involvement resulting from opportunistic infections (e.g., *Toxoplasma,* tuberculoma, *Cryptococcus,* JC virus, etc.), direct neuronal involvement by human immunodeficiency virus (HIV), HIV associated malignancies (primary CNS lymphoma and metastasis), or antiretroviral drugs induced adverse effects.[21] MDs have been reported as presenting symptoms in AIDS,[21] almost 3% HIV positive patients may develop MDs with hemichorea-hemiballism and tremor being most common, with loss of dopaminergic neurons in basal ganglia being the possible pathology behind the extrapyramidal features in AIDS.[22] These patients have increased susceptibility toward neuroleptics and are prone to develop drug induced dyskinesia.[22] With the introduction of highly active antiretroviral therapy (HAART), neurological complications including MDs are declining in AIDS. MDs associated with HIV encephalopathy is characterized by the early age of onset, rapid progression, bilateral upper limb involvement, poor response to levodopa along with the following additional clinical findings: dementia, seizures, oculomotor abnormalities, vacuolar myelopathy, and peripheral neuropathy.[21,22] Rest tremor is uncommon in patients with HIV infection, instead, they have postural tremor often in combination with a kinetic component. Holmes tremor (formerly called rubral or midbrain tremor) with rest, postural, and kinetic components can be seen in patients with focal midbrain lesion. HIV-associated tremor, although less troublesome for the patient, its presence is suggestive of poor prognosis.[23]

Subacute sclerosing panencephalitis (SSPE) is a progressive neurological disorder caused by persistent infection of the mutant measles virus.[24] Due to widespread immunization, it is rarely reported from Western countries. Patients belonging to the adolescent age group may present with insidious onset gradually progressive behavioral changes, myoclonus, dementia, cortical blindness, pyramidal, and extrapyramidal signs. Periodic stereotyped myoclonic jerks with a slow relaxation phase, initially involving head followed by trunk and limbs, not affect consciousness and disappear during sleep. Ataxia, dystonia, and dyskinesias may be seen in the second stage, progressing to akinetic-rigid and mute state followed by death within 1–3 years of diagnosis with the acute fulminant disease in few patients leading to death within 3 months. Brain histopathology reveals gliosis, degeneration of dendrites, demyelination, neurofibrillary tangles, infiltration of inflammatory cells, Cowdry type A inclusions, and neuronal loss.[25] The parieto-occipital region of the brain is most severely affected followed by the anterior cerebrum, subcortical structures, brainstem, and spinal cord. Electroencephalography (EEG) shows typical high amplitude long interval bilateral symmetrical periodic discharges synchronized with myoclonic jerks.[25] Antibody titer against measles is detected in plasma and CSF. Raised gamma globulin levels in CSF (10–54 μg/dL) is another characteristic feature suggestive of intrathecal synthesis of IgG. There is no satisfactory treatment available to date. Although oral isoprinosine and intrathecal interferon alfa may provide some benefit, lifelong therapy is required.[25] Prevention of this illness with effective immunization against measles is the only available option.[25]

COVID-19 pandemic has affected about 200 million people worldwide resulting in over 4 million deaths by June 2021, and the counts are still increasing.[26] Although neurological manifestations of COVID-19 are being increasingly reported, only a handful of published reports to date have described de novo movement disorders arising in the setting of COVID-19 infection.[27] The most commonly reported movement disorders are myoclonus, ataxia, and tremor appearing either during the COVID-19 illness or as a part of post-covid syndrome.[28,29,30] Parkinsonism and functional movement disorders have been reported in few patients.[31,32] Most of these cases were managed conservatively by using intravenous immunoglobulin or steroids.[27] Movement disorders may result from severe acute respiratory syndrome coronavirus 2 either directly as a manifestation of encephalitis or by the disturbed dopaminergic state due to its influence on the angiotensin-converting enzyme 2 receptors.[27,33,34] With COVID-19 pandemic being ongoing, it is likely that upcoming reports of movement disorders associated with COVID-19 will enhance our understanding in this regard.

Movement Disorders Related to Bacterial Infections

First described in the 17th century, Sydenham's chorea, the most common cause of chorea in children also referred to as St. Vitus dance, is a syndrome of neuropsychiatric, behavioral, and MD with hypotonia developing after group A beta-hemolytic *Streptococcus* infection. Being one of the diagnostic criteria of acute rheumatic fever, chorea is often self-limiting leaving behind valve dysfunction and sequela of rheumatic heart disease.[26] Recent studies had broadened this spectrum further with the inclusion of psychiatric and behavioral disorders such as anxiety, depression, attention deficit hyperactive disorders as well as poststreptococcal autoimmune basal ganglia disorders manifesting as tics, chorea, dystonia, myoclonus, opsoclonus, tremor, and stereotypies.[27] Pediatric autoimmune neuropsychiatric disorders associated with streptococcal infection (PANDAS) syndrome, first described by Swedo et al., is characterized by tic and obsessive-compulsive disorder

(OCD) secondary to autoimmune reaction against basal ganglia.[27] Affection of first degree relatives with similar movement and emotional disorders suggest the pre-existing genetic predisposition apart from infection. Movement and neuropsychiatric features are treated symptomatically. Steroid, intravenous immunoglobulin (IVIg), and even plasmapheresis have been shown to reduce the duration of illness.[26] Antibiotic prophylaxis is recommended to prevent recurrence and long-term cardiac complications in a patient with rheumatic fever and chorea, however, evidence for use of antibiotics in PANDAS and similar syndromes is still inconclusive.[26]

Helicobacter pylori seropositivity has been linked to worse motor symptoms in PD patients, either due to exacerbation of neurodegeneration or reduced anti-parkinsonian drug absorption from gastrointestinal mucosa. This was further supported by the improvement in clinical status after *H. pylori* eradication in such patients.[28] CNS involvement is reported in 63% of cases of Whipple's disease caused by *Tropheryma whipplei* with a wide range of neurological features involving cognition, behavior, hypothalamus, extrapyramidal, and oculomotor system being reported.[29] Although vertical supranuclear gaze palsy (59%), gait abnormalities (44%), ataxia (39%), oculomasticatory myorrhythmia (24%), and nonrhythmic myoclonus (15%) have been commonly reported, only 10% cases manifest the classic triad of dementia, ophthalmoplegia, and myoclonus.[29] Multiple T2 hyperintense lesions with mild contrast enhancement are seen in periventricular and periaqueductal areas. Periodic acid-Schiff (PAS) positive bacterial inclusions in small bowel biopsy and polymerase chain reaction (PCR) for bacterial nucleic acid are commonly used for diagnosis confirmation. CSF PAS staining and PCR may return positive in one-third and two-thirds cases, respectively, and brain biopsy has greater sensitivity than bowel biopsy. MD improves with antibiotics in the majority of patients, but few remain static and even worsen despite treatment.[29]

In addition to meningoencephalitis, myelitis, psychosis, seizures, polyradiculitis, cerebellar ataxia, and brain stem dysfunction, MDs comprising acute choreoathetosis, dystonia, and bradykinesia have been reported in association with acute *Mycoplasma* infection, mostly in the pediatric age group.[30]

Movement Disorders Related to Tuberculosis

Central nervous system tuberculosis is one of the most common infectious disorders with wide spectrum of clinical manifestations with MDs reported in 0.5–18.6% of cases.[31] In a 2-year follow-up study of 180 patients of tubercular meningitis (TBM) by Alarco´n et al., 30 had MD, tremor being the most common followed by dystonia, chorea, ballism, and myoclonus.[31] Patients with multiple tuberculomas, especially deep-seated and severe illness were likely to have MDs as an early neurological manifestation.[32] Although the pathogenesis of MDs had been attributed to ischemic infarction, arachnoiditis, brain edema, tuberculomas, and immune-mediated hypersensitivity reactions may also contribute.[33] In addition to basal ganglia, tuberculomas involving the thalamus, subthalamus, cerebellum, and brain stem affecting excitatory or inhibitory pathway may also cause MDs.[32] Parkinsonism may result secondary to obstructive hydrocephalus. Drugs used for the treatment of tuberculosis have been reported to cause MD. For example, the oculogyric crisis is caused by pyrazinamide.[34] Commonly used antiepileptic drugs such as phenytoin and valproate are known for extrapyramidal side effects. Similarly, concomitant use of prokinetic drugs are notorious and may cause dystonia. Nearly 85% of MD respond to antitubercular treatment (ATT).[32] However, immune mediated paradoxical worsening may complicate few cases.[35] In those not responding to ATT, surgical decompression is indicated (**Figs. 1A and B**).[34,35]

Prion Diseases

Prion, a non-nucleic acid-containing, transmissible agent that induces abnormal folding of normal cellular prion proteins in the brain, leading to brain damage. Prion diseases also known as transmissible spongiform encephalopathies affect both humans and animals, have a long incubation period but rapidly progressive once neurologic manifestations appear and are always fatal.[36]

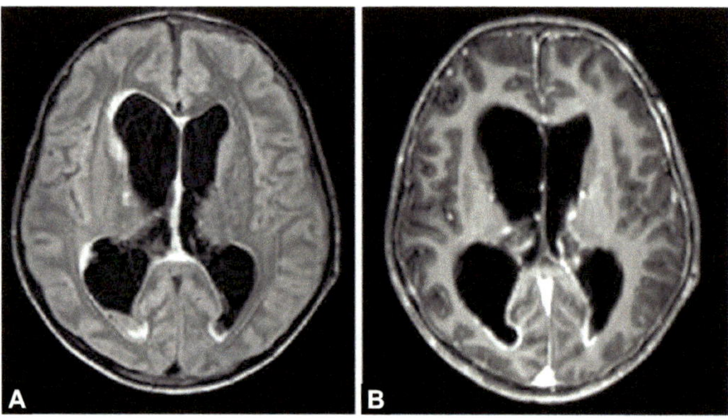

FIGS. 1A AND B: A 53-year-old male, presented with 6 months history of low grade fever, headache, progressive cognitive decline, bradykinesia, postural imbalance, and ataxia. Cerebrospinal fluid analysis showed raised protein with lymphocytic pleocytosis. Magnetic resonance image (MRI) of brain showing: (A) Asymmetrically dilated ventricles with periventricular ooze in fluid-attenuated inversion recovery (FLAIR) sequence. (B) Meningeal enhancement in T1-contrast sequence. His symptoms improved markedly with antitubercular treatment including steroids and acetazolamide.

Creutzfeldt-Jakob disease (CJD), the most important prion disease in humans has three types namely familial, sporadic, and variant CJD. Rapidly progressive dementia with myoclonus, ataxia, visual disturbances, pyramidal, and extrapyramidal symptoms are the characteristic features. Up to 90% of patients may have MDs including tremor, myoclonus, hemiballismus, Parkinsonism, and ataxia.[37] Choreoathetosis and dystonia may occur in the later stage of the disease.[38] Stimulus sensitive short interval rhythmic myoclonic jerk associated with the periodic sharp wave in EEG is most frequent hyperkinetic MD, reported in 82–100% patients.[38] CJD like pathology in brain autopsy has been reported in patients with a clinical picture of PD, corticobasal degeneration, and supranuclear palsy. Seizures although rare, appear in 8–25% of patients in the late stage of the disease, may remain resistant to antiepileptic drugs.[21] Brain MRI, particularly diffusion-weighted imaging (DWI) showing restricted diffusion in the cortical or deep nuclei gray matter (**Fig. 2B**) are characteristic of sporadic CJD. Hyperintense signal on T2 and fluid-attenuated inversion recovery (FLAIR) sequence with restriction in DWI MRI are seen in the cortical gyri (cortical ribboning), caudate, putamen, or thalamus.[36] Hyperintensity of the pulvinar nucleus in FLAIR image compared to the anterior putamen, known as classic "pulvinar sign" is characteristic of variant CJD (**Figs. 2A** to **C**).[38]

Parasitic Infestations and Movement Disorder

Cerebral malaria is the most severe form of falciparum malaria resulting in brain edema and increased mortality. Less common involvement of the thalamus, basal ganglia, and cerebellum has been described with MDs being one of the manifestations.[39,40] Opsoclonus myoclonus ataxia syndrome developing after falciparum malaria has been reported in two Indian children with normal CSF and

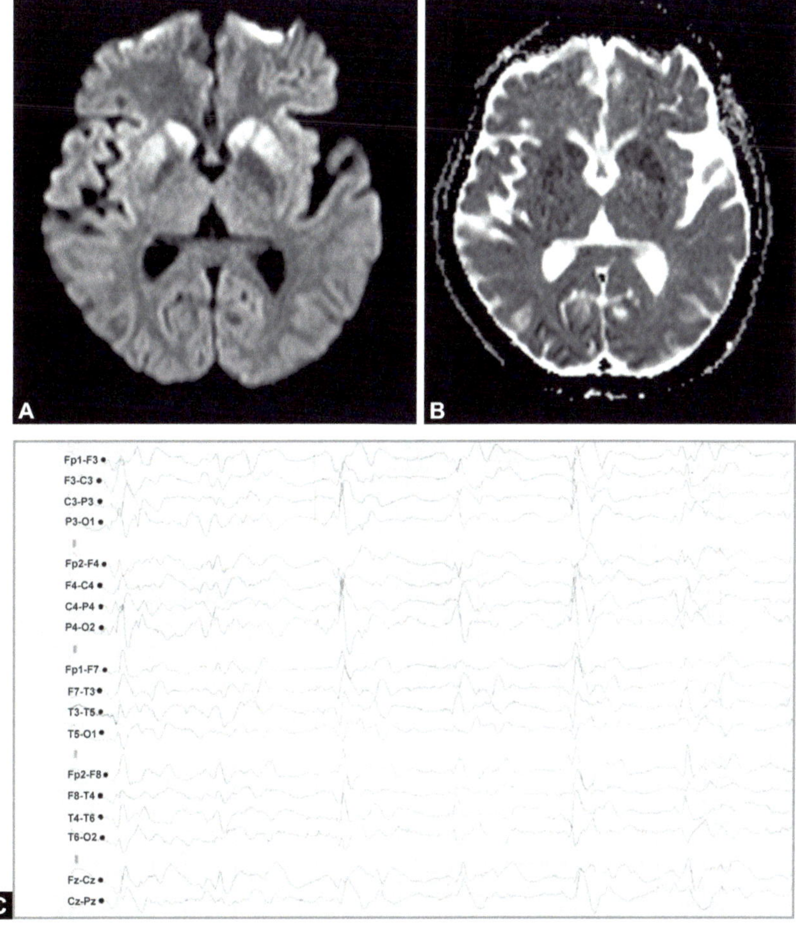

FIGS. 2A TO C: A 65-year-old male, presented with 5 months history of rapidly progressive dementia, ataxia, postural imbalance, rigidity, and myoclonus. (A) Magnetic resonance image (MRI) of brain showing hyperintensity in bilateral caudate head and putamen in FLAIR sequence, and (B) diffusion restriction in the same area in DWI sequence. (C) Electroencephalogram (EEG) showing periodic discharges at an interval of 1 second with diffuse slowing of background activity.

MRI brain, improved with high dose adrenocorticotropic hormone (ACTH) and IVIg therapy. This immune-mediated syndrome related to antibodies against neural antigens in Purkinje cells of the cerebellum, cerebral cortical neurons, and axons is also known as Kinsbourne or "dancing eyes-dancing feet" syndrome.[41]

Although seizure is the most common presentation, Parkinsonism and other MDs have been described in NCC involving basal ganglia and related structures.[42] In a study on 590 consecutive patients of NCC, 23 had MD, 15 patients had Parkinsonism, five tremors, two dystonia, and one had chorea. Cystic lesion in thalamus and putamen was found in patients with chorea and dystonia, respectively.[42] Parkinsonism has been reported in patients having ventricular cysts, hydrocephalus, or abnormal CSF findings suggestive of meningoencephalitis. While chorea, tremor, and dystonia subsided completely with anthelminthic treatment, half of the Parkinsonism patients require steroids, levodopa, and surgery in the form of cystectomy and ventriculoperitoneal shunt placement.[42,43]

TABLE 1: Clinical clues for infectious etiology in a patient with the movement disorders.

Clinical clues in a patient with movement disorder	*Organism*
History of flu-like symptoms in past with Parkinsonism	Influenza
History of acute-onset fever and altered mental state	Arbovirus and herpes virus
Immunocompromised patient and high risk behavior	HIV and opportunistic infections
History of fever with rash in childhood and improper immunization	Measles
Rapidly progressive dementia and history of cannibalism	Prions
Gastrointestinal motility disorder with dementia	Whipple's disease
Carditis and skin nodules in pediatric age group	*Streptococcus*
Fever with hepatosplenomegaly in endemic areas	Malaria
Exposure to cat	*Toxoplasma*
History of passing worms in stool, improper hand hygiene, and open land defecation practice	*Taenia solium*

DIAGNOSIS AND MANAGEMENT

Movement disorder associated with infections are peculiar in several aspects (**Box 1**). While ruling out secondary causes of MDs especially in patients with acute to subacute onset disorders, a search for systemic or neurological stigmata of infections must be made. For example, a patient of chorea may have features of carditis or skin lesion. Similarly, a patient with dystonia may have a history of febrile encephalopathy (**Tables 1** and **2**). Treatment of these disorders require specific therapy, depending on the etiology such as antiviral, antibiotics, antitubercular, or antiparasitic drugs, with or without steroids, as well as symptomatic therapy for MDs as per the phenomenology. Few cases refractory to medical management may require surgical therapy such as ventriculoperitoneal shunt for hydrocephalus, lesionectomy in case of tuberculoma, or other ring enhancing lesions, pallidotomy, or deep brain stimulation in refractory dyskinesias.

Box 1 Characteristics of movement disorders associated with infections.

- 20% of all secondary movement disorders
- MDs can be hypokinetic or hyperkinetic or mixed
- *Common phenomenologies*: Dystonia, hemichorea, hemiballismus, tremor, tics, myoclonus, paroxysmal dyskinesias, and Parkinsonism
- MRI brain often shows lesions in basal ganglia, thalamus, cerebellum, midbrain, or cortex
- Usually reversible and treatable

(MDs: movement disorders; MRI: magnetic resonance imaging)

CONCLUSION

Infection-related MDs may appear acutely during a CNS or systemic infection or weeks to months after the illness has subsided. While direct neurological involvement seems the likely pathology in former, immune-mediated neurological involvement may cause the delayed manifestation.

TABLE 2: Different microbial agents and their clinical presentation, movement disorder (MD) phenotypes, and the neuroanatomical substrate.

Organism	*Neurological syndrome*	*MD phenotype*	*Structures involved*
Influenza A	Postencephalitic syndrome	• Parkinsonism (bradykinesia, tremor, and mask like face) • No cognitive disturbances	Neuronal loss and neurofibrillary tangle in SNpc
EBV	EBV encephalitis	Akinetic rigid state, tremor, and apraxia of eyelid opening	Putaminal and caudate atrophy
VZV	Herpes zoster	Parkinsonism in the first 3 months of follow up	
JEV	Japanese encephalitis	• Rigidity, hypokinesia, masking of face, hypophonia, and tremor • Improve with time	Structural damage to thalamus, basal ganglia, and midbrain
WNV	West Nile encephalitis	• Tremor, myoclonus, rigidity, bradykinesia, and postural instability • Resolve over time	Bilateral lesion in thalamus and pons
Dengue	Dengue encephalitis	Parkinsonism (bradykinesia, tremor, and mask like face)	Transient splenial and bilateral symmetrical thalamic hyperintensity in MRI
HIV	AIDS dementia complex	Bradykinesia, postural instability, gait abnormality, masking of face, and oculomotor abnormality	α-Syn in SNpc
	HIV Parkinsonism	Bilateral onset rapid symptoms and earlier motor features	Absence of Lewy body
	Opportunistic infection (*Toxoplasma*, *Cryptococcus*, tuberculoma, and lymphoma)	Focal dystonia, hemichorea, hemiballismus, and tremor	Focal lesion in basal ganglia, thalamus, and midbrain
Measles	SSPE	Behavioral changes, dementia, cortical blindness, myoclonus, ataxia, dystonia, and akinetic rigid state	Initially parieto-occipital region, later diffuse subcortical structures and spinal cord, and Cowdry type-A inclusions
Prion	Creutzfeldt–Jakob disease (CJD)	• Rapidly progressive dementia, visual disturbances, myoclonus, ataxia, tremor, myoclonus, hemiballismus, and Parkinsonism syndromes • Choreoathetosis and dystonia	• Spongiform degeneration and prion protein deposition • Caudate and putaminal lesion in familial CJD • Pulvinar in variant CJD • Cortical ribbon in sporadic CJD
Streptococcus	Sydenham's chorea	Chorea with neuropsychiatric features, acute rheumatic fever	Autoimmune reaction against basal ganglia
	PANDAS	Tic and obsessive-compulsive disorder (OCD)	-do-
Mycoplasma	Postencephalitic syndrome	Choreoathetosis, dystonia, and bradykinesia	Bilateral striatal lesions
Mycobacterium tuberculosis	Tubercular meningitis and CNS tuberculoma	Tremor, dystonia, ballism, chorea, myoclonus, and ataxia	Edema, pressure effect, vasculitis, infarction in thalamus, basal ganglia, brainstem, cerebellum
		Parkinsonism	Multiple tuberculoma, obstructive hydrocephalus
Tropheryma whipplei	CNS whipple's disease	Vertical supranuclear gaze palsy, ataxia, myoclonus, and oculomasticatory myorhythmia	Periventricular and periaqueductal area
Malaria	Cerebral malaria	Parkinsonism and kinetic tremor	Edema of globus pallidus and cerebellum
		Opsoclonus myoclonus ataxia syndrome	Antibodies against Purkinje cells of the cerebellum
Taenia solium	Neurocysticercosis	• Parkinsonism • Dystonia and chorea	• Multiple lesion in Parkinsonism • A solitary lesion in the thalamus and putamen in others

(AIDS: acquired immunodeficiency syndrome; CNS: central nervous system; EBV: Epstein–Barr virus; HIV: human immunodeficiency virus; JEV: Japanese encephalitis virus; MRI: magnetic resonance imaging; PANDAS: pediatric autoimmune neuropsychiatric disorders associated with streptococcal infection; SNpc: substantia nigra pars compacta; SSPE: subacute sclerosing panencephalitis; VZV: varicella-zoster virus; WNV: West Nile virus)

REFERENCES

1. GBD 2016 Neurology Collaborators. Global, regional, and national burden of neurological disorders, 1990–2016: a systematic analysis for the Global Burden of Disease Study 2016. The Lancet Neurol. 2019;18(5):459-80.
2. Jhunjhunwala K, Netravathi M, Pal PK. Movement disorders of probable infectious origin. Ann Indian Acad Neurol. 2014;17(3): 292-7.
3. Muthane UB, Ragothaman M, Gururaj G. Epidemiology of Parkinson's disease and movement disordersMD in India: problems and possibilities. J Assoc Physicians India. 2007; 55:719-24
4. Jang H, Boltz DA, Webster RG, Smeyne RJ. Viral parkinsonism. Biochim Biophys Acta. 2009;1792(7):714-21.
5. Limphaibool N, Iwanowski P, Holstad MJ, Kobylarek D, Kozubski W. Infectious Etiologies of Parkinsonism: Pathomechanisms and Clinical Implications. Front Neurol. 2019;10:652.
6. Caggiu E, Paulus K, Galleri G, Arru G, Manetti R, Sechi GP, et al. Homologous HSV1 and alpha-synuclein peptides stimulate a T cell response in Parkinson's disease. J Neuroimmunol. 2017;310:26-31.
7. Takahashi M, Yamada T, Nakajima S, Nakajima K, Yamamoto T, Okada H. The substantia nigra is a major target for neurovirulent influenza A virus. J Exp Med. 1995;181(6):2161-9.
8. Hawkes CH, Del Tredici K, Braak H. Parkinson's disease: a dual-hit hypothesis. Neuropathol Appl Neurobiol. 2007;33(6): 599-614.
9. Hoffman LA, Vilensky JA. Encephalitis lethargica: 100 years after the epidemic. Brain. 2017;140(8):2246-51.
10. Jang H, Boltz D, Sturm-Ramirez K, Shepherd KR, Jiao Y, Webster R, et al. Highly pathogenic H5N1 influenza virus can enter the central nervous system and induce neuroinflammation and neurodegeneration. Proc Natl Acad Sci USA. 2009;106(33): 14063-8.
11. Sadasivan S, Sharp B, Schultz-Cherry S, Smeyne RJ. Synergistic effects of influenza and 1-methyl-4-phenyl-1, 2, 3, 6-tetrahydropyridine (MPTP) can be eliminated by the use of influenza therapeutics: experimental evidence for the multi-hit hypothesis. NPJ Parkinsons Dis. 2017;3:18.
12. Misra UK, Kalita J. Spectrum of movement disorders in encephalitis. J Neurol. 2010;257(12):2052-8.
13. Solomon T, Dung NM, Vaughn DW, Kneen R, Thao LT, Raengsakulrach B, et al. Neurological manifestations of dengue infection. Lancet. 2000;355(9209):1053-9.
14. Misra UK, Kalita J. Movement disorders in Japanese encephalitis. J Neurol. 1997;244(5):299-303.
15. Kalita J, Misra UK. Markedly severe dystonia in Japanese encephalitis. Mov Disord. 2000;15(6):1168-72.
16. Das K, Ghosh M, Nag C, Nandy SP, Banerjee M, Datta M, et al. Role of Familial, Environmental and Occupational Factors in the Development of Parkinson's Disease. Neurodegener Dis. 2011;8(5):345-51.
17. Nash D, Mostashari F, Fine A, Miller J, O'leary D, Murray K, et al. The outbreak of West Nile virus infection in the New York City area in 1999. N Engl J Med. 2001;344(24):1807-14.
18. Lenka A, Kamat A, Mittal SO. Spectrum of movement disorders in patients with neuroinvasive West Nile virus infection. Mov Disord Clin Pract. 2019;6(6):426-33.
19. Sejvar JJ, Haddad MB, Tierney BC, Campbell GL, Marfin AA, van Gerpen JA, et al. Neurologic manifestations and outcome of West Nile virus infection. JAMA. 2003;290(4):511-5.
20. Bopeththa BV, Ralapanawa U. Post encephalitic parkinsonism following dengue viral infection. BMC Res Notes. 2017;10(1):655.
21. Carroll E, Sanchez-Ramos J. Hyperkinetic movement disorders associated with HIV and other viral infections. In: Weiner WJ, Tolosa E (eds). Hyperkinetic Mov Disord. Elsevier BV; 2012:100. pp. 323-34.
22. Cardoso F. HIV-related movement disorders: epidemiology, pathogenesis and management. CNS Drugs. 2002;16(10): 663-8.
23. Arendt G, Hefter H, Hilperath F, von Giesen HJ, Strohmeyer G, Freund HJ. Motor analysis predicts progression in HIV-associated brain disease. J Neurol Sci. 1994;123(1-2):180-5.
24. Garg RK. Subacute sclerosing panencephalitis. Postgrad Med J. 2002;78(916):63-70.
25. Garg RK, Mahadevan A, Malhotra HS, Rizvi I, Kumar N, Uniyal R. Subacute sclerosing panencephalitis. Rev Med Virol. 2019;29(5):e2058.
26. Dong E, Du H, Gardner L. An interactive web-based dashboard to track COVID-19 in real time. Lancet Infect Dis 2020;20(5): 533–534.
27. Ghosh R, Biswas U, Roy D, Pandit A, Lahiri D, Ray BK, Benito-León J. De Novo Movement Disorders and COVID-19: Exploring the Interface. Movement Disorders Clinical Practice. 2021 Jul;8(5): 669-80.
28. Chan JL, Murphy KA, Sarna JR. Myoclonus and cerebellar ataxia associated with COVID-19: a case report and systematic review. J Neurol 2021.
29. Rábano-Suárez P, Bermejo-Guerrero L, Méndez-Guerrero A, Parra-Serrano J, Toledo-Alfocea D, Sánchez-Tejerina D, Santos-Fernández T, Folgueira-López MD, Gutiérrez-Gutiérrez J, Ayuso-García B, de la Aleja JG. Generalized myoclonus in COVID-19. Neurology. 2020 Aug 11;95(6):e767-72.
30. Khoo A, McLoughlin B, Cheema S, et al. Postinfectious brainstem encephalitis associated with SARS-CoV-2. J Neurol Neurosurg Psychiatry 2020;91(9):1013–1014.
31. Merello M, Bhatia KP, Obeso JA. SARS-CoV-2 and the risk of Parkinson's disease: facts and fantasy. Lancet Neurol 2021;20(2):94–5.
32. Piscitelli D, Perin C, Tremolizzo L, Peroni F, Cerri CG, Cornaggia CM. Functional movement disorders in a patient with COVID-19. Neurological Sciences. 2020 Sep;41(9):2343-4.
33. Desai I, Manchanda R, Kumar N, Tiwari A, Kumar M. Neurological manifestations of coronavirus disease 2019: exploring past to understand present. Neurological Sciences. 2021 Jan 11:1-3.
34. Aggarwal A, Adukia S, Bhatt M. Video Anthology of Movement Disorders Due to Infections in South Asia. Movement Disorders Clinical Practice. 2021 Aug;8(6):843-58.
35. Dean SL, Singer HS. Treatment of Sydenham's Chorea: A Review of the Current Evidence. Tremor Other Hyperkinet Mov (NY). 2017;7:456.
26. Squintani G, Tinazzi M, Gambarin M, Bravi E, Moretto G, Buttiglione M, et al. Post-streptococcal 'complex' movement disorders: unusual concurrence of psychogenic and organic symptoms. J Neurol Sci. 2010;288(1-2):68-71.

37. Mridula KR, Borgohain R, Chandrasekhar Reddy V, Bandaru VCh, Suryaprabha T. Association of Helicobacter pylori with Parkinson's Disease. J Clin Neurol. 2017;13(2):181-6.
38. Bally JF, Méneret A, Roze E, Anderson M, Grabli D, Lang AE. Systematic review of movement disorders and oculomotor abnormalities in Whipple's disease. Mov Disord. 2018;33(11):1700-11.
39. Beskind DL, Keim SM. Choreoathetotic movement disorder in a boy with Mycoplasma pneumoniae encephalitis. Ann Emerg Med. 1994;23(6):1375-8.
40. Alarcón F, Dueñas G, Cevallos N, Lees AJ. Movement disorders in 30 patients with tuberculous meningitis. Mov Disord. 2000;15(3):561-9.
41. Alarcón F, Maldonado JC, Rivera JW. Movement disorders identified in patients with intracranial tuberculomas. Neurologia. 2011;26(6):343-50.
42. Alarcón F, Cañizares M. Tuberculous encephalitis associated with basal ganglia lesions and movement disorders. Ecuador: Revista Ecuatoriana de Neurologí. 2015;24(1-3):42-4.
43. Wong LH, Tan E. Anti-tuberculosis medication-induced oculogyric crisis and the importance of proper history taking. Int Med Case Rep J. 2017;10:341-4.
44. Kalita J, Ranjan P, Misra UK, Das BK. Hemichorea: a rare presentation of tuberculoma. J Neurol Sci. 2003;208(1-2):109-11.
45. Geschwind MD, Wong K. Prion diseases: Geriartric Neurology. Wiley-Blackwell. 2014:267-80.
46. Rodriguez-Porcel F, Ciarlariello VB, Dwivedi AK, Lovera L, Da Prat G, Lopez-Castellanos R, et al. Movement Disorders in Prionopathies: A Systematic Review. Tremor Other Hyperkinet Mov (N Y). 2019;9.
47. Maltête D, Guyant-Maréchal L, Mihout B, Hannequin D. Movement disorders and Creutzfeldt-Jakob disease: a review. Parkinsonism Relat Disord. 2006;12(2):65-71.
48. Tamzali Y, Demeret S, Haddad E, Guillot H, Caumes E, Jauréguiberry S. Post-malaria neurological syndrome: four cases, review of the literature and clarification of the nosological framework. Malaria J. 2018;17(1):387.
49. Jayaweera DT, Vinasithambi S, Abeyawardane BY, Nimalasuriya A, Mihindukulasuriya JC, Perera SM, et al. Extrapyramidal manifestations in cerebral malaria. Ceylon Med J. 1977;22(1): 64-5.
50. Bose K, Saha S, Islam MR, Chakraborty C, Laskar M. Opsoclonus myoclonus ataxia syndrome due to falciparum malaria in two Indian children. Indian J Ophthalmol. 2016;64(11): 852-4.
51. Alarcón F, Cedeño Y, de Yébenes JG. Parkinsonism and other movement disorders in 23 cases of neurocysticercosis. Parkinsonism Relat Disord. 2017;42:47-53.
52. Bhattacharjee S, Biswas P, Mondal T. Clinical profile and follow-up of 51 pediatric neurocysticercosis cases: A study from Eastern India. Ann Indian Acad Neurol. 2013;16(4): 549-55.

CHAPTER 44

Autoimmune Movement Disorders

Dhiman Das, Kalyan B Bhattacharyya, Arup Kumar Dutta

INTRODUCTION

Autoimmune movement disorders are increasingly being recognized as a host of treatable movement disorders, as advancements of diagnostic testing and a better understanding of the pathophysiology of these disorders become apparent. The clinical approach to these disorders relies on the identification of the entity, proper diagnosis, and early institution of therapy to limit the burden of permanent neurological sequelae. The understanding that these movement disorders are associated with underlying malignancy or are a postinfectious manifestation would imply a search for these malignancies and appropriate treatment or institution of appropriate antibiotics as a part of the treatment protocol. The varied phenotypic presentations make it imperative to distinguish this group from the degenerative disorders considering the usually favorable prognosis of this group of disorders.

PATHOPHYSIOLOGY

Advanced diagnostic techniques have identified a host of antibodies in various clinical presentations but their exact pathogenic mechanism remains elusive in many instances. In elucidating the pathogenic mechanism, it is frequently observed that the potential target of these autoantibodies and their clinical presentation has a frequent parallel in genetic conditions leading to mutation of the proposed target, thus, helping us to better understand the pathogenic role of these autoantibodies. Neuronal autoantibodies are broadly classified into three groups (**Fig. 1**):

- *Neuronal surface antibodies:* These are considered pathogenic in vivo exerting their action by binding to receptors thereby causing blockade or internalization along with complement activation and inflammatory cytotoxicity.[1]
  - *N-methyl-D-aspartate receptor (NMDAR)* antibodies are a prototype surface antibody against ionotropic glutamate receptors widely expressed in the brain and pivotal for long-term synaptic plasticity[2] targeting the NR1 subunit.[3,4] Removal of the antibodies reverses the receptor internalization and residual deficits may be the result of glutamate excitotoxicity.[5] Similar symptoms may be observed with "dissociative" anesthetics such as ketamine or phencyclidine[6] or mutations of GRIN1, the gene encoding the NR1 subunit of the NMDAR.[7]
  - *Glycine receptor (GlyR) antibodies* specifically target the $\alpha1$ GlyR subunit expressed on the brainstem and spinal cord neurons, and both activate complement and cause receptor internalization via lysosomal pathways in vitro. Stiff person spectrum disorders (SPSD) and hereditary hyperekplexia, both share decreased glycinergic transmission[8,9] leading to similar clinical manifestations.
  - *Dipeptidyl-peptidase-like protein-6 (DPPX) antibodies* relate to increased central nervous system (CNS) hyperexcitability mediated by downregulation of DPPX and Kv4.2 in neuronal membranes widely expressed in the CNS and on the myenteric plexus.[10] Chronic diarrhea frequently accompanies neurologic manifestations.
  - *Voltage gated potassium channels (VGKC) antibodies:* Voltage gated potassium channels are crucial in restoring the resting membrane potential after an action potential. They are widely distributed across membranes of neurons in both the central and peripheral nervous system. The antibodies have been

Antibodies against neuronal surface antigens

Considered pathogenic as they target proteins that are accessible in vivo and, typically, play an important role in synaptic transmission, palsticity, or excitability

Examples:
Caspr2, DPPX, D2R, $GABA_AR$, $GABA_BR$, GlyR, LGI1, and NMDAR

Antibodies against intracellular synaptic antigens

Controversial role in pathogenesis (see text); their antigen could be transiently accessible during synaptic vesicle fusion and uptake

Examples:
GAD and amphiphysin

Antibodies against intracellular cytoplasmic/nuclear antigens

Considered markers of paraneoplastic syndromes with poor prognosis and treatment response, in which autoimmunity is mainly effected by cytotoxic T cells: the antigens are deemed to be inaccessible in vivo

Examples:
Hu, Yo, Ri CRMPS/CV2, Zic4, and Ma2

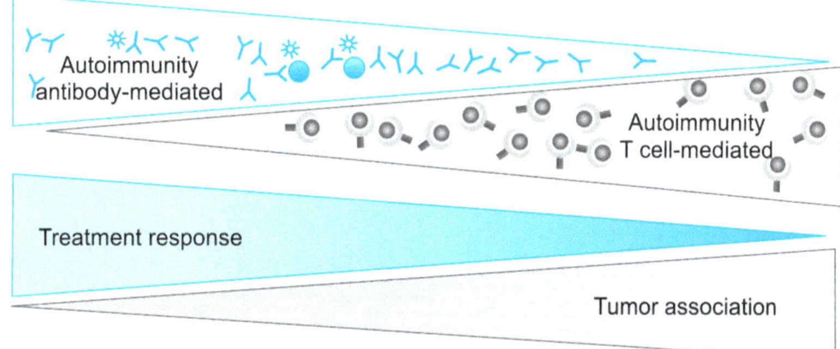

FIG. 1: The three groups of neuronal antibodies and their pathogenic roles, e.g., treatment responses and tumor associations.

Source: Reproduced with permission from BRAIN. 2018;141:13-36.

demonstrated to be targeted to two subunits of the receptor namely, leucine-rich glioma-inactivated 1 (LGI1) and contactin-associated protein-like 2 (CASPR2).[11,12] Another group of patients with VGKC antibodies but negative LGI1 and CASPR2 exists but the exact pathogenicity of these antibodies is debated. LGI1 is a secreted protein, mainly present in the hippocampus and the temporal cortex, and binds presynaptic ADAM23 to postsynaptic ADAM22 which is essential for inhibitory signal transmission. LGI1 antibodies reduce LGI1-ADAM interaction thereby reversibly reducing postsynaptic alpha-amino-3-hydroxy-5-methyl-4-isoxazole propionate (AMPA)-receptor clusters.[13] Cytoplasmic domain of Caspr2, a membrane protein expressed in the central and peripheral nervous system, is essential for potassium channel clustering at the juxtaparanodes of myelinated axons.[14] VGKC antibodies are implicated in neuromyotonia, Morvan's syndrome, and limbic encephalitis.

- *Antibodies against intracellular synaptic antigens:* Unlike the surface antigenic targets with clear established pathophysiology, in this group pathological findings substantiate a T-cell involvement thus, representing an intermediate between neuronal surface antibodies and those directed against cytoplasmic/nuclear antigens.[15,16] Anti-glutamic acid decarboxylase (GAD) antibodies have a broad phenotypic presentation ranging from SPSD, cerebellar ataxia, temporal lobe epilepsy, and limbic encephalitis to type 1 diabetes mellitus.[17]
- *Antibodies against intracellular cytoplasmic/nuclear antigens:* Their pathogenicity is debated as their target is inaccessible in vivo. It is suggested that autoreactive T cells mediate the disease process by lymphocytic infiltration and damage of neuronal structures.[18] This group of antibodies includes those against nuclear or nucleolar antigens, such as Hu or Ma, which have a diffuse expression in the CNS.

CLINICAL SPECTRUM

Among the highly variable presentation of the various antibodies, a strong index of suspicion is required for early detection and a rational approach to the patient helps halting the immune-mediated attack on the nervous system at the outset, thus, improving the prognosis. The clinical suspicion relies on the following basic principles:[19]

- Acute or subacute onset of CNS disease, often with a recognizable syndrome
- Evidence of cerebrospinal fluid (CSF) inflammation or immune activation
- Neuroimaging abnormalities evident using magnetic resonance imaging (MRI) or positron emission tomography (PET)

- Presence of CSF or serum cell surface autoantibodies with known or suspected pathogenic properties
- Evidence of reversibility with immune therapies

Autoimmune Encephalitis Associated with Movement Disorders

N-methyl-D-aspartate receptor encephalitis: It is one of the most commonly observed disorders particularly among the pediatric population where it is mostly idiopathic or may be found in children with a previous history of herpes simplex virus (HSV) encephalitis. Tumor association particularly with ovarian teratoma has been found in adult females.[20,21] The presentation may be divided into the following stages: (1) Prodromal phase with fever and headache; (2) Early stage with neuropsychiatric symptoms; (3) Late stage with stereotypy, choreoathetoid movements, dysautonomia, hypoventilation, and in some cases refractory seizures, catatonia, and mutism. Movement disorders are usually of mixed phenotype with stereotypies and perseverative behavior being very characteristic in the acute stage. Violent stereotypies are usually seen and may induce self-injuries and can range from facial movements to torsional movements involving trunk to repetitive cycling movements in limbs. In perseverative behavior, the movement is induced by a stimulus and it continues after the stimulus has been withdrawn. Akinesia is rare in children and may be late manifestations and may be more common in the adult population.[22]

Basal ganglia encephalitis (BGE): These patients present with a combination of movement disorders, psychiatric symptoms, and sleep disturbance following a preceding infectious prodrome of mycoplasma pneumonia or group A *Streptococcus* [(GAS), sometimes also groups C and G].[23] BGE frequently affects young children (2–8 years of age), although adolescents have also been described. There is no significant tumor association or sex predilection. Unlike NMDAR encephalitis seizure and cognitive disturbances are less frequent, dominant akinesia, tremor, dystonia, or chorea are more frequent in contrast to the stereotypies and perseverative behavior frequently observed in NMDAR encephalitis, and response to treatment is faster (days to weeks) than anti-NMDAR encephalitis (months). Serum immunoglobulin G (IgG) antibodies to D2R are found in >80% of patients with BGE,[24] by flow cytometry technique, a technique which may not be routinely available. Few patients previously diagnosed as encephalitis lethargica have been reclassified into this group.[25]

Leucine-rich glioma-inactivated 1 encephalitis: These patients present with limbic encephalitis, often with hyponatremia, and about half of the patients have characteristic faciobrachial dystonic seizures (FBDS), a unique identifying feature of this group of disorders.[26] FBDS are very brief (<3 sec) contractions involving unilateral arm, often ipsilateral face (or leg), and occurring up to 100 times a day. Patients usually drop items or may fall down as a result of these.[27,28] FBDS usually predate the onset of cognitive decline and prompt treatment with immunotherapy might prevent progression to limbic encephalitis.[29] Tumor association seems to be low (0–11%) with thymoma and lung cancer probably being most common.

Contactin-associated protein-like 2 related disorder: Caspr2-antibodies cause a more variable syndrome of peripheral or central involvement. CNS symptoms are cognitive decline, seizures, and cerebellar involvement.[30] Peripheral nervous hyperexcitability causes fasciculations and cramps. Morvan's syndrome is a combination of these central and peripheral nervous system symptoms, accompanied by autonomic dysfunction and insomnia. Tumor association is found in 0–32% with thymomas being most common and some of these patients suffer from myasthenia gravis as well.[31-33]

Both LGI1 and CASPR2 have a predilection of affecting elderly males.

Another subset of VGKC-positive patients lacking LGI1 and Caspr2 antibodies, has varied presentation, including epilepsy, pain syndromes, cognitive decline, polyneuropathy, and cramp fasciculation syndromes.[34-36] This clinical heterogeneity has questioned the pathogenicity of these VGKC antibodies.

Stiff person syndrome (SPS): It is a rare autoimmune disorder affecting adults. Clinical suspicion is by new-onset rigidity and spasms involving mostly the trunk, and to a lesser extent the limbs. Classic SPS often presents with lower limb rigidity and episodic spasms spreading to the paraspinal muscles causing debilitating pain, limited mobility, and falls. Impaired breathing and sometimes rhabdomyolysis may result from spasm of back and chest muscles.

Some patients demonstrate prominent stimulus-sensitive myoclonus and follow a progressive course.[37] Progressive encephalomyelitis with rigidity and myoclonus (PERM), also called "SPS plus",[38] is a severe form of SPS with brainstem, autonomic, and long-tract signs. GAD[39-41] antibodies targeted against an intracellular antigen is considered an excellent biomarker of disease but is of uncertain pathogenicity. Similarly, GlyR antibodies, another cell surface antibody, have been identified with diverse involvement including SPS, PERM, isolated brainstem involvement, limbic encephalitis, and sometimes myelitis. DPPX antibodies have also been implicated in this phenotype and gastrointestinal hyper- or hypomobility and marked weight loss are strong indicators of DPPX antibodies.[42]

Autoimmune Movement Disorders (Nonencephalitic)

Sydenham's chorea (SC): SC, considered as a major manifestation of rheumatic fever, is a poststreptococcal autoimmune neuropsychiatric disorder. It is one of the most common cause of new-onset chorea in children occasionally along with some dystonic posturing.[43,44] Although typically generalized it may be asymmetric and in approximately 20% of patients may result in a hemichorea.[44,45] Typical clinical features are hypotonia and motor impersistence and in the most severe cases the patients may be severely hypotonic and appear paralyzed (chorea paralytica).[44,46] They frequently have behavioral changes like personality change, emotional lability, aggression, tearfulness, or an irritable depression,[47] as well as obsessive thoughts which in the untreated chronic form, may become obsessive-compulsive disorder. These patients characteristically lack features of psychosis, severe agitation, or seizures frequently observed in NMDAR encephalitis. An evaluation for carditis is imperative once the condition is diagnosed. However, search for GAS using throat swabs and streptococcal serology although important, may be negative as it is recognized that SC is a latent complication of GAS. IgG binding to the cell surface of live neurone-like cells,[48] and IgG binding to the extracellular domain of D2R (dopamine-2 receptor) are observed in a proportion of SC patients.[49]

Opsoclonus myoclonus ataxia: It is one of the well-described childhood paraneoplastic movement disorder. The diagnosis is made in the presence of three out of the following four features: (1) Opsoclonus, (2) Myoclonus/ataxia, (3) Behavioral change/sleep disturbance, and (4) Neuroblastoma.[50] It commonly presents around 1–3 years, but may occur throughout childhood and adolescence.[51-53] An underlying neuroblastoma is detected in about half of the patients,[51] however, in some patients the syndrome may be postinfectious such as following mycoplasma[52] or hepatitis C virus[54] infection. In many cases, no precipitating cause is identified leading to speculation of a preexisting neuroblastoma which has spontaneously regressed.[55] The clinical course of opsoclonus myoclonus ataxia syndrome (OMAS) usually starts with irritability and ataxia followed by myoclonus of the face, trunk, or extremities[51] followed days to weeks later by opsoclonus. In any child presenting with new-onset ataxia, particularly when there is jerky limb movements, irritability, or sleep disturbance, should be suspected to have OMAS since opsoclonus may be a minor yet important feature. There is some evidence of IgG binding to cell surface antigens in a significant proportion of patients with OMAS,[56] and recently autoantibodies to the extracellular domain of glutamate receptor δ2 (GluD2) in the sera of pediatric patients with OMAS have been identified.

Infection-associated Movement Disorders

Pediatric acute neuropsychiatric syndrome and pediatric autoimmune neuropsychiatric disorders associated with streptococcal infection: A small subgroup of children may develop postinfectious new-onset neuropsychiatric syndromes with acute and often dramatic personality change with dominant emotional symptoms (anxiety, separation anxiety, obsessive-compulsive symptoms, and mood disturbance) and sometimes tics. Since, infections other than streptococcus can induce these episodes, hence, the nomenclature has been changed from PANDAS to PANS. Relapse following subsequent infections can occur. CSF is normal, including CSF neopterin, which is a sensitive marker of inflammation. It is likely that infections trigger a cytokine-induced change in CNS function in patients who are genetically susceptible to neuropsychiatric disease rather than an autoimmune process.

Autoimmune Movement Disorders-associated with Systemic Autoimmune Disorders

Systemic lupus erythematosus (SLE) is associated with neuropsychiatric manifestations including headache, seizures, cognitive disturbance, and movement disorders. Chorea is a well-described complication of lupus[57] and is presumed to be due to autoimmune targeting of the brain. Patients often have antiphospholipid antibodies and may have an overlapping syndrome of SLE and antiphospholipid syndrome.[58] Parkinsonism is also rarely reported in SLE.[59,60] Both lupus chorea and Parkinsonism can be efficiently treated by immune therapy. Although the exact antigenic targets remain to be defined[61] elevated levels of IgG neuronal cell-surface binding antibodies have been demonstrated in patients with antiphospholipid antibodies.

Hashimoto encephalopathy is an immune-responsive (steroid typically) autoimmune encephalopathy[62] in patients with proven autoimmune thyroid disease. A significant proportion of these patients have cell surface antibodies such as NMDAR antibodies.[63] It may be a predisposition for autoimmunity with coexistent autoimmune disorders (and multiple autoantibodies).

Celiac disease, an autoimmune gut disease, has recognized neurological complications and movement disorders associated with it.[64-67] The brain disease is immunological in origin. Antitissue transglutaminase antibodies found in some patients have a questionable pathogenicity for brain disease as the disease is considered to be T cell-mediated.

INVESTIGATIONS

Despite often florid clinical presentation, the findings on standard MRI are surprisingly variable ranging from subtle abnormalities to almost normal. Hyperintensities may be observed in the limbic region as in few cases of NMDAR encephalitis or the basal ganglia and substantia nigra as in BGE.

Cerebrospinal fluid study is frequently undertaken mostly to rule out other differentials and is mostly nonspecific. In about 60–70% of NMDAR encephalitis, there may be pleocytosis with oligoclonal bands whereas in other forms of encephalitis the study may be normal. CSF neopterin is useful but nonspecific marker for inflammation search for disease-specific biomarkers is ongoing with autoantibodies being demonstrated in a few types.

Although autoantibodies are thought to be a key player in the pathogenesis, demonstrating the antibodies, establishing pathogenicity is technically challenging and expensive. Some antibodies are better demonstrated in the CSF and some may be more readily demonstrated in the sera. It is useful to conduct the test in both sera and CSF together. Also, the method applied in detecting antibodies is of utmost importance in picking up the culprit antibody. Screening procedures employ immunohistochemistry or immunoassay or Western blot but they run the risk of detecting nonpathogenic antibodies as they are done by spreading out the denatured proteins. However, cell-based assay is a true reflection of in vivo effects and is the preferred modality whenever available.

Electroencephalogram shows widespread theta-delta activity suggestive of diffuse cerebral dysfunction. In NMDAR encephalitis a very characteristic pattern known as extreme delta brush (slow waves with over-riding fast beta activity) is observed.

Wherever applicable, search for underlying tumors should be undertaken by appropriate modalities.

MANAGEMENT

Successful treatment relies on rapidly recognizing the entity and controlling neuroinflammation which has deleterious effects on the brain. Duration, severity, and relapses are all important predictors of the outcome.

Corticosteroids are used as broad first line agents for controlling inflammation, reducing blood brain barrier permeability, and reducing edema. Methylprednisolone, oral prednisolone, oral dexamethasone, and adrenocorticotropic hormone (ACTH) are used in various combinations, although in selected disorders one agent is preferred over the other, e.g., ACTH in OMAS.[68]

Intravenous immunoglobulin (IVIg) given at a dose of 2 g/kg has a very broad mechanism of action, on autoantibodies, cytokines, T cells, and other cellular functions with broad immune modulatory properties. Similarly, plasma exchange (PLEX) serves to remove antibodies, cytokines, and other immunoactive constituents from the circulation.

In established cases with autoantibodies or reactive lymphocytes, rituximab or cyclophosphamide may be considered for rapid induction. Rituximab targets and depletes CD20 B cells, but its action encompasses effects on T cells and natural killer cells.[69] Cyclophosphamide is a cytotoxic agent effecting proliferating cells such as lymphocytes.

Alternatively mycophenolate mofetil, methotrexate, and azathioprine may be considered for maintenance of immune suppression as steroid sparing agents.

In infection triggered processes, antibiotics are often used with macrolides and tetracyclines having additional anti-inflammatory properties.

In paraneoplastic syndromes, removal of tumor is important but alone insufficient in controlling neuroinflammation.

CONTROVERSIES AND FUTURE

As previously described, there have been demonstrated genetic counterparts of the various encephalitis due to genetic mutations of the target proteins, discovery of neuronal surface antibodies against IgLON5 has opened doors for speculation whether the so called degenerative disease may have an underlying autoimmune basis. Autopsy specimens have revealed presence of hyperphosphorylated three and four repeat tau aggregates in neurons, in the absence of inflammation thus, explaining the poor response to immunotherapy. The IgLON5-antibody-linked tauopathy is characterized by prominent sleep movement disorders, obstructive sleep apnea, dysautonomia, bulbar symptoms, vertical gaze palsy, loss of postural reflexes, and closely mimicking the various degenerative diseases. This may open up avenues for approaching the degenerative disorders in the autoimmune disorder paradigm and new therapeutic opportunities for the diseases.

Although IgG antibodies are considered pathogenic, the role of other categories such as IgA and IgM are yet to be evaluated.

The therapeutic approach is met with variable success depending partially to the type of illness and the location of the antigen. Mostly the treatment is broad spectrum with the same common approach. Whether streamlining, the therapy to particular disease specific approach can improve outcomes needs to be evaluated.

REFERENCES

1. Jain A, Balice-Gordon R. Cellular, synaptic, and circuit effects of antibodies in autoimmune CNS synaptopathies. Handb Clin Neurol. 2016;133:77-93.
2. Standaert DG, Testa CM, Young AB, Penney JB Jr. Organization of N-methyl-D-aspartate glutamate receptor gene expression in the basal ganglia of the rat. J Comp Neurol. 1994;343:1-16.
3. Moscato EH, Peng X, Jain A, Parsons TD, Dalmau J, Balice-GordonRJ. Acute mechanisms underlying antibody effects in anti-N-methyl-D-aspartate receptor encephalitis. Ann Neurol. 2014;76:108-19.
4. Planaguma J, Leypoldt F, Mannara F, Gutierrez-Cuesta J, Martin-Garcia E, Aguilar E, et al. Human N-methyl D-aspartate receptor antibodies alter memory and behaviour in mice. Brain. 2015;138:94-109.
5. Manto M, Dalmau J, Didelot A, Rogemond V, Honnorat J. In vivo effects of antibodies from patients with anti-NMDA receptor encephalitis: further evidence of synaptic glutamatergic dysfunction. Orphanet J Rare Dis. 2010;5:31.
6. Stamelou M, Plazzi G, Lugaresi E, Edwards MJ, Bhatia KP. The distinct movement disorder in anti-NMDA receptor encephalitis maybe related to status dissociatus: a hypothesis. Mov Disord. 2012;27(11):1360-3.
7. Lemke JR, Geider K, Helbig KL, Heyne HO, Schutz H, Hentschel J, et al. Delineating the GRIN1 phenotypic spectrum: a distinct genetic NMDA receptor encephalopathy. Neurology. 2016;86:2171-8.
8. Hutchinson M, Waters P, McHugh J, Gorman G, O'Riordan S, Connolly S, et al. Progressive encephalomyelitis, rigidity, and myoclonus: a novel glycine receptor antibody. Neurology. 2008;71:1291-2.
9. Balint B, Blocker I, Unger M, Stoecker W, Probst C, Komorowski L, et al. Antibody spectrum in stiff person syndrome and related disorders. In: 19th International Congress of Parkinson's Disease and Movement Disorders. USA: Wiley-Blackwell; 2015. p. S263.
10. Piepgras J, Holtje M, Michel K, Li Q, Otto C, Drenckhahn C, et al. Anti-DPPX encephalitis: pathogenic effects of antibodies on gut andbrain neurons. Neurology. 2015;85:890-7.
11. Irani SR, Alexander S, Waters P, Kleopa KA, Pettingill P, Zuliani L, et al. Antibodies to Kv1 potassium channel-complex proteins leucine-rich, glioma inactivated 1 protein and contact in-associated protein-2 in limbic encephalitis, Morvan's syndrome and acquired neuromyotonia. Brain. 2010;133:2734-48.
12. Lai M, Huijbers MG, Lancaster E, Graus F, Bataller L, Balice-Gordon R, et al. Investigation of LGI1 as the antigen in limbic encephalitis previously attributed to potassium channels: a case series. Lancet Neurol. 2010;9:776-85.
13. Ohkawa T, Fukata Y, Yamasaki M, Miyazaki T, Yokoi N, Takashima H, et al. Autoantibodies to epilepsy-related LGI1 in limbic encephalitis neutralize LGI1-ADAM22 interaction and reduce synaptic AMPA receptors. J Neurosci. 2013;33: 18161-74.
14. Horresh I, Poliak S, Grant S, Bredt D, Rasband MN, Peles E. Multiple molecular interactions determine the clustering of Caspr2 and Kv1 channels in myelinated axons. J Neurosci. 2008;28(52):14213-22.
15. Witherick J, Highley JR, Hadjivassiliou M. Pathological findings in a case of stiff person syndrome with anti-GAD antibodies. Mov Disord. 2011;26(11):2138-9.
16. Bien CG, Vincent A, Barnett MH, Becker AJ, Blumcke I, Graus F, et al. Immunopathology of autoantibody-associated encephalitides: clues for pathogenesis. Brain. 2012;135:1622-38.
17. Gresa-Arribas N, Arino H, Martinez-Hernandez E, Petit-Pedrol M, Sabater L, Saiz A, et al. Antibodies to inhibitory synaptic proteins in neurological syndromes associated with glutamic acid decarboxylase autoimmunity. PLoS One. 2015;10:e0121364.
18. Lancaster E, Dalmau J. Neuronal autoantigens-pathogenesis, associated disorders and antibody testing. Nat Rev Neurol. 2012;8:380-90.
19. Khadilkar S, Soni G, Patil S, Huchche A, Faldu H. Autoimmune encephalitis: an update. J Assoc Physicians India. 2017;65:62-9.
20. Dalmau J, Lancaster E, Martinez-Hernandez E, Rosenfeld MR, Balice-Gordon R. Clinical experience and laboratory investigations in patients with anti-NMDAR encephalitis. Lancet Neurol. 2011;10:63-74.
21. Titulaer MJ, McCracken L, Gabilondo I, et al. Treatment and prognostic factors for long-term outcome in patients with anti-NMDA receptor encephalitis: an observational cohort study. Lancet Neurol. 2013;12:157-65.
22. Mohammad SS, Nosadini M, Brilot F, Dale R. Autoimmune Movement Disorders in Children: Clinical Characteristics and Therapeutic Considerations. J Pediatr Neurol. 2015;13(4).
23. Mohammad SS, Ramanathan S, Brilot F, Dale RC. Autoantibody associated movement disorders. Neuropediatrics. 2013;44:336-45.
24. Dale RC, Merheb V, Pillai S, Wang D, Cantrill L, Murphy TK, et al. Antibodies to surface dopamine-2 receptor in autoimmune movement and psychiatric disorders. Brain. 2012;135:3453-68.
25. Dale RC, Church AJ, Surtees RA, Lees AJ, Adcock JE, Harding B, et al. Encephalitis lethargic syndrome: 20 new cases and evidence of basal ganglia autoimmunity. Brain. 2004;127:21-33.
26. Andrade DM, Tai P, Dalmau J, Wennberg R. Tonic seizures: a diagnostic clue of anti-LGI1 encephalitis? Neurology. 2011;76(15):1355-7.
27. Irani SR, Michell AW, Lang B, Pettingill P, Waters P, Johnson MR, et al. Faciobrachial dystonic seizures precede Lgl1 antibody limbic encephalitis. Ann Neurol. 2011;69:892-900.
28. Ismail FS, Popkirov S, Wellmer J, Gronheit W. Faciobrachio-crural dystonic seizures in LGI1 limbic encephalitis: a treatable cause of falls. Neurol Neuroimmunol Neuroinflamm. 2015;2(5): e146.
29. Irani SR, Stagg CJ, Schott JM, Rosenthal CR, Schneider SA, Pettingill P, et al. Faciobrachial dystonic seizures: the influence of immunotherapy on seizure control and prevention of cognitive impairment in a broadening phenotype. Brain. 2013;136:3151-62.
30. Lancaster E, Huijbers MG, Bar V, Boronat A, Wong A, Martinez-Hernandez E, et al. Investigations of caspr2, an autoantigen of encephalitis and neuromyotonia. Ann Neurol. 2011;69(2): 303-11.
31. Becker EB, Zuliani L, Pettingill R, Lang B, Waters P, Dulneva A, et al. Contactin associated protein-2 antibodies in non-paraneoplastic cerebellar ataxia. J Neurol Neurosurg Psychiatry. 2012;83(4):437-40.

32. Klein CJ, Lennon VA, Aston PA, McKeon A, O'Toole O, Quek A, et al. Insights from LGI1 and CASPR2 potassium channel complex autoantibody subtyping. JAMA Neurol. 2013;70(2):229-34.
33. Irani SR, Pettingill P, Kleopa KA, Schiza N, Waters P, Mazia C, et al. Morvan syndrome: clinical and serological observations in 29 cases. Ann Neurol. 2012;72:241-55.
34. Olberg H, Haugen M, Storstein A, Vedeler CA. Neurological manifestations related to level of voltage-gated potassium channel antibodies. J Neurol Neurosurg Psychiatry. 2013;84:941-3.
35. Klein CJ, Lennon VA, Aston PA, McKeon A, Pittock SJ. Chronic pain as a manifestation of potassium channel-complex autoimmunity. Neurology. 2012;79(11):1136-44.
36. Lilleker JB, Jones MS, Mohanraj R. VGKC complex antibodies in epilepsy: diagnostic yield and therapeutic implications. Seizure. 2013;22(9):776-9.
37. Meinck HM, Thompson PD. Stiff man syndrome and related conditions. Mov Disord. 2002;17:853-66.
38. Brown P, Marsden CD. The stiff man and stiff man plus syndromes. J Neurol. 1999;246(8):648-52.
39. Solimena M, Folli F, Denis-Donini S, Comi GC, Pozza G, De Camilli P, et al. Autoantibodies to glutamic acid decarboxylase in a patient with stiff-man syndrome, epilepsy, and type I diabetes mellitus. N Engl J Med. 1988;318(16):1012-20.
40. Solimena M, Folli F. Stiff-man syndrome and type I diabetes mellitus: a common autoimmune pathogenesis? Ann Ist Super Sanita. 1988;24(4):583-6.
41. Blum P, Jankovic J. Stiff-person syndrome: an autoimmune disease. Mov Disord. 1991;6:12-20.
42. Tobin WO, Lennon VA, Komorowski L, Probst C, Clardy SL, Aksamit AJ, et al. DPPX potassium channel antibody: frequency, clinical accompaniments, and outcomes in 20 patients. Neurology. 2014;83:1797-803.
43. Mohammad SS, Fung VS, Grattan-Smith P, Gill D, Pillai S, Ramanathan S, et al. Movement disorders in children with anti-NMDAR encephalitis and other autoimmune encephalopathies. Mov Disord. 2014;29(12):1539-42.
44. Cardoso F, Eduardo C, Silva AP, Mota CC. Chorea in fifty consecutive patients with rheumatic fever. Mov Disord. 1997;12:701-3.
45. Nausieda PA, Grossman BJ, Koller WC, Weiner WJ, Klawans HL. Sydenham chorea: an update. Neurology. 1980;30(3):331-4.
46. El Otmani H, Moutaouakil F, Fadel H, Slassi I. Chorea paralytica: a Videotape case with rapid recovery and good long-term outcome. Acta Neurol Belg. 2013;113(4):515-7.
47. Freeman JM, Aron AM, Collard JE, Mackay MC. The emotional correlates of Sydenham's chorea. Pediatrics. 1965;35:42-9.
48. Brilot F, Merheb V, Ding A, Murphy T, Dale RC. Antibody binding to neuronal surface in Sydenham chorea, but not in PANDAS or Tourette syndrome. Neurology. 2011;76:1508-13.
49. Brimberg L, Benhar I, Mascaro-Blanco A, Alvarez K, Lotan D, Winter C, et al. Behavioral, pharmacological, and immunological abnormalities after streptococcal exposure: a novel rat model of Sydenham chorea and related neuropsychiatric disorders. Neuropsychopharmacology. 2012;37(9):2076-87.
50. Matthay KK, Blaes F, Hero B, Plantaz D, De Alarcon P, Mitchell WG, et al. Opsoclonus myoclonus syndrome in neuroblastoma a report from a workshop on the dancing eyes syndrome at the advances in neuroblastoma meeting in Genoa, Italy, 2004. Cancer Lett. 2005;228:275-82.
51. Tate ED, Allison TJ, Pranzatelli MR, Verhulst SJ. Neuroepidemiologic trends in 105 US cases of pediatric opsoclonus-myoclonus syndrome. J Pediatr Oncol Nurs. 2005;22:8-19.
52. Huber BM, Strozzi S, Steinlin M, Aebi C, Fluri S. Mycoplasma pneumoniae associated opsoclonus-myoclonus syndrome in three cases. Eur J Pediatr. 2010;169(4):441-5.
53. Hero B, Schleiermacher G. Update on pediatric opsoclonus myoclonus syndrome. Neuropediatrics. 2013;44(6):324-9.
54. Ertekin V, Tan H. Opsoclonus-myoclonus syndrome attributable to hepatitis C infection. Pediatr Neurol. 2010;42:441-2.
55. Pike M. Opsoclonus-myoclonus syndrome. Handb Clin Neurol. 2013;112:1209-11.
56. Blaes F, Fühlhuber V, Korfei M, Tschernatsch M, Behnisch W, Rostasy K, et al. Surface-binding autoantibodies to cerebellar neurons in opsoclonus syndrome. Ann Neurol. 2005;58: 313-7.
57. Baizabal-Carvallo JF, Alonso-Juarez M, Koslowski M. Chorea in systemic lupus erythematosus. J Clin Rheumatol. 2011;17(2): 69-72.
58. Plowman EK, Okun MS. Antiphospholipid syndrome and other lupus-related movement disorders. Handb Clin Neurol. 2011;100:237-45.
59. Baizabal-Carvallo JF, Bonnet C, Jankovic J. Movement disorders in systemic lupus erythematosus and the antiphospholipid syndrome. J Neural Transm. 2013;120:1579-89.
60. Kwong KL, Chu R, Wong SN. Parkinsonism as unusual neurological complication in childhood systemic lupus erythematosus. Lupus. 2000;9:474-7.
61. Dale RC, Yin K, Ding A, Merheb V, Varadkhar S, McKay D, et al. Antibody binding neuronal surface in movement disorders associated with lupus and antiphospholipid antibodies. Dev Med Child Neurol. 2011;53(6):522-8.
62. Brain L, Jellinek EH, Ball K. Hashimoto's disease and encephalopathy. Lancet. 1966;2:512-4.
63. Irani SR, Bera K, Waters P, Zuliani L, Maxwell S, Zandi MS, et al. N-methyl-D-aspartate antibody encephalitis: temporal progression of clinical and paraclinical observations in a predominantly non-paraneoplastic disorder of both sexes. Brain. 2010;133:1655-67.
64. Walker RH. Further evidence for celiac disease-associated chorea. Tremor Other Hyperkinet Mov (N Y). 2011;1:93-6.
65. Hall DA, Parsons J, Benke T. Paroxysmal nonkinesigenic dystonia and celiac disease. Mov Disord. 2007;22:708-10.
66. Fung VS, Duggins A, Morris JG, Lorentz IT. Progressive myoclonic ataxia associated with celiac disease presenting as unilateral cortical tremor and dystonia. Mov Disord. 2000;15: 732-4.
67. Deconinck N, Scaillon M, Segers V, Groswasser JJ, Dan B. Opsoclonus-myoclonus associated with celiac disease. Pediatr Neurol. 2006;34:312-4.
68. De Grandis E, Parodi S, Conte M, Angelini P, Battaglia F, Gandolfo C, et al. Long-term follow-up of neuroblastoma-associated opsoclonus-myoclonus-ataxia syndrome. Neuropediatrics. 2009;40(3):103-11.
69. Palanichamy A, Jahn S, Nickles D, Derstine M, Abounasr A, Hauser SL, et al. Rituximab efficiently depletes increased CD20-expressing T cells in multiple sclerosis patients. J Immunol. 2014;193(2):580-6.

CHAPTER 45

Stroke-induced Movement Disorders

Roopa Rajan, Subhash Kaul, Padma MV Srivastava

INTRODUCTION

Strokes are an important cause of secondary movement disorders and nearly 22% of all secondary movement disorders may be of vascular origin. Up to 4% of people suffering from a stroke, ischemic or hemorrhagic, may develop a movement disorder either in the acute setting or later on in the disease course. Stroke-induced movement disorders encompass an entire spectrum of phenotypes and vary from primary movement disorders in their clinical profile, prognosis, and treatment.[1] Substantial heterogeneity and relative rarity of this entity have limited our understanding of the mechanisms of these disorders.

A variety of movement disorders have been described after stroke (**Table 1**).

TABLE 1: Movement disorder phenotypes reported after stroke.

Movement disorder phenotype	*Most common location of vascular insult*
Dystonia	Posterolateral thalamus
Chorea	Caudate
Myoclonus	Frontal lobe
Parkinsonism	Putamen
Tremor	Midbrain
Restless legs syndrome	Pons and putamen
Alien hand syndrome	Parietal lobe
Periodic limb movements	Pons
Stereotypy	Putamen and thalamus
Akathisia	Posterior thalamus
Tics	Caudate

FUNCTIONAL SUBSTRATE FOR MOVEMENT DISORDERS

Although it may seem intuitive that vascular lesions at specific regions of the brain may result in specific movement disorder phenomenologies, it is often not the case. A recent review of 284 cases of poststroke movement disorders revealed poor association between stroke localization and movement disorder phenomenology. This is attributable to the pathophysiology of movement disorders heavily depending on dysfunction of a widely distributed network of neurons. Hence, vascular lesions at remotely different areas may result in similar clinical manifestations. In addition, stroke involving critical areas in the motor network, such as the thalamus, may result in a combination of varying phenomenologies. Not only an acute disruption in neural networks, but also abnormal adaptive responses such as aberrant axonal regeneration, dedifferentiation, and loss of topographic specificity of cortical plasticity, may result in the development of movement disorders after stroke. Regardless of varying phenomenology, all the following regions of the brain have been associated with development of movement disorders after stroke: Caudate, putamen, globus pallidus, thalamus, frontal lobe, corpus callosum, parietal lobe, occipital lobe, temporal lobe, cerebellum, midbrain, pons, and medulla.

EPIDEMIOLOGY

The mean age of onset is typically around 60–70 years, but can range from early childhood to over 90 years. There is no gender predilection. Although there was no correlation with gender, side of lesion, or stroke risk factors, patients who did develop poststroke abnormal movements had significantly more frequent severe motor and sensory deficits during the acute stage of stroke. Age affects the clinical picture with larger proportion of younger patients developing dystonia and older patients developing chorea.

Hemorrhagic strokes appear to be more likely to lead to acute movement disorders than ischemic strokes. About 90% of the acute-onset movement disorders seem to resolve within 6 months. Dystonia and tremor were more common after hemorrhagic strokes, whereas Parkinsonism and restless legs syndrome were more common after ischemic stroke. Movement disorders are usually unilateral and contralateral to the brain lesion (83%) or bilateral. Occasionally, ipsilateral unilateral movement disorders are encountered. This is seen commonly with ipsilateral cerebellar lesions.

The most commonly encountered hyperkinetic movement disorder poststroke is hemichorea with or without hemiballism. This is followed by dystonia as the second most common phenotype. The Lausanne Stroke Registry revealed the following distribution of movement disorder phenotypes: Hemichorea (38%), dystonia (17%), limb shaking (10%), myoclonus-dystonia (10%), stereotypical movements (7%), asterixis (7%), myoclonus (3%), tremor (3%), hemiakathisia (3%), and dysarthria and dyskinetic hand (3%).[2] From the Ecuador Stroke Registry, 4% of the 1,500 stroke patients developed poststroke abnormal movements, 36% developed chorea, 25% developed tremor, and 11% developed Parkinsonism.

PROGNOSIS

Movement disorders may manifest acutely after a stroke or may develop and progress later. Hemiballism and asterixis usually present in the acute setting. Hemiballism can evolve into hemichorea and finally settle as hemidystonia. The latency between the onset of acute stroke and onset of movement disorder can vary from days to even years. Chorea is earliest to manifest and dystonia and Parkinsonism the latest. Delayed progression of dystonia is a well-known phenomenon after static insults of nonvascular origin such as perinatal hypoxia.[3] Younger age at insult is associated with longer delay in the manifestation of movement disorders after a static insult.

In a series of 53 patients reported by Scott and Jankovic, two patients who had strokes in infancy developed dystonia ipsilateral to the hemiparetic limb after a latent period of 42.8 years, whereas adults manifested dystonia after a latency of 1.4 years.[4] Younger age at initial injury was associated with a greater tendency to develop generalized rather than focal or segmental dystonia. Data from the Ecuador Stroke Registry as well as systematic reviews of published cases reveal that older stroke patients tend to develop chorea, whereas the younger patients tend to develop dystonia after stroke.[5]

What is the pathophysiology behind the delayed onset movement disorders after stroke?

Several hypotheses have been proposed:

- Trans-synaptic neuronal degeneration
- Inflammatory changes
- Oxidative stress
- Ephaptic transmission
- Remyelination
- Central synaptic reorganization
- Denervation supersensitivity
- Aberrant neuroplasticity
- Dendritic plasticity and changing patterns of synaptic activity after brain injury
- Deafferentation or loss of proprioceptive input from multiple joints causing impaired synergistic stabilization
- Loss of inhibitory influence of the globus pallidus, pars interna, substantia nigra, and pars reticulata on the thalamus

Changes in neuronal metabolism and plasticity in the aging brain may partly explain the observed relation between age at initial brain insult and the latency and distribution of delayed onset movement disorders.

LOCATION OF THE STROKE AND OUTCOME

Lesions in the striatum or pallidum (44%) followed by the thalamus were the most common cause of poststroke movement disorders in the Lausanne Stroke Registry. The same movement disorder can be caused by lesions in different parts of the brain. Likewise, hemidystonia and hemichorea or hemiathetosis can result from lesions involving areas other than lentiform nucleus or the caudate. One stroke can lead to a combination of different movement disorders such as a combination of chorea, athetosis, and dystonia after a thalamic stroke.

STROKE SUBTYPES

The most common subtype of stroke leading to abnormal movements is small vessel disease with small deep infarcts.[6] However, cardioembolic strokes as well as large vessel atherothrombosis have also been implicated. Chorea and hemiballism have been described in patients with moyamoya disease. Various hypokinetic and hyperkinetic movement disorders have also been described with watershed or border zone infarcts.

Vascular Parkinsonism

Vascular Parkinsonism (VP) is used to describe a heterogeneous group of conditions that manifest clinically with Parkinsonian features, but are presumably of vascular origin as evidenced by historical or imaging evidence of multiple strokes.[7] Pathological data have revealed that a clear history of acute neurological deficits or definite radiological evidence of previous strokes may not be apparent.

In clinic-based series, VP accounts for 3–12% of all cases of Parkinsonism. The age of onset is later than most degenerative Parkinsonian syndromes. Many databases show vascular Parkinsonism to be the second most common cause of Parkinsonism after Parkinson's disease. On the other hand, Parkinsonism is an uncommon manifestation after stroke. In an autopsy study of 220 consecutive patients with ischemic strokes, only five were reported to have Parkinsonian symptoms antemortem.

Vascular Parkinsonism typically presents with lower body Parkinsonism characterized by broad-based shuffling and often freezing of gait and postural instability. Bradykinesia and rigidity are usually bilateral and symmetrical and frequently associated with pyramidal signs, pseudobulbar palsy, incontinence, and cognitive impairment. Rest tremor, a characteristic feature of Parkinson's disease, is uncommon. Patients frequently have vascular risk factors of diabetes and hypertension.

Although the classical picture of VP is as described above, many patients do not fit into the classical phenotype; for instance, 59% of patients with VP had asymmetrical onset. Only 30–48% of patients with VP responded to levodopa; those with symmetric onset of motor symptoms, worse disease severity, no dyskinesias, and increased number of vascular risk factors responded poorly. A unique type of vascular Parkinsonism may have an acute onset temporally associated with basal ganglia infarcts and distinct from the insidious progression of classical VP. About two-thirds of patients with vascular Parkinsonism have a more relentless rather than stepwise progression.

Are there any diagnostic criteria for vascular Parkinsonism?

Two proposed criteria exist to guide the diagnosis of vascular Parkinsonism.[8] The criteria suggested by Zijlmans et al. necessitate the demonstration of Parkinsonism (bradykinesia and one among rigidity, rest tremor, or postural instability) and cerebrovascular disease (on neuroimaging or on clinical history and examination) along with a temporal relationship between the two, i.e., onset of Parkinsonism (acute or insidious) within 1 year of stroke involving the basal ganglia structures or their connections or presence of extensive microangiopathic white matter lesions with lower body Parkinsonism or cognitive impairment. An alternate approach suggested by Winikates and Jankovic includes demonstrating clinical Parkinsonism followed by a vascular score. Points are assigned for diffuse vascular involvement (on pathology or angiography, two points), onset of clinical symptoms (Parkinsonism) within 1 month of stroke (one point), more than one episode of prior strokes (one point), presence of two or more stroke risk factors (one point), and involvement of more than one vascular territory on imaging (one point). A combined score of >2 is required to diagnose VP.

Box 1 Most common imaging findings in vascular Parkinsonism (VP).

- Ischemic changes in multiple vascular territories
- Periventricular white matter ischemia
- Global subcortical ischemic white matter involvement
- Ischemia in the basal ganglia and brainstem
- Cortical atrophy

In patients with VP, the most common site of involvement on imaging is the frontal lobe. The striatum, lentiform nucleus, and pons are other common sites of involvement. Lesions may be unilateral or bilateral. The substantia nigra is typically considered to be spared in VP. However, presynaptic dopaminergic dysfunction on dopamine active transporter-single-photon emission computed tomography (DAT-SPECT) may be seen in up to 70% of patients. Interestingly, the prognosis and treatment response are better in patients with abnormal DAT-SPECT, likely due to the presynaptic component. Hypertension and lesions in the basal ganglia and periventricular regions are associated with poor prognosis (**Box 1**).

Are there any caveats in diagnosing vascular Parkinsonism?

As it is true for other clinically diagnosed disorders, many diseases may mimic VP. To diagnosis VP, it is important to correctly identify true bradykinesia (decremental amplitude on repetitive actions) rather than only slow movement, which may result from spasticity in patients with stroke and corticospinal tract involvement (pseudobradykinesia). Clinically, postural instability gait disorder (PIGD) subtype of Parkinson's disease, corticobasal degeneration, progressive supranuclear palsy (PSP), and normal pressure hydrocephalus are common mimics of VP. Parkinson's disease may be distinguished by the narrow-based rather than wide-based gait, upper body involvement, and robust levodopa response. Presence of typical features of asymmetrical limb dystonia, rigidity and cortical signs (apraxia, cortical sensory loss, and alien limb) in corticobasal syndrome, and vertical (often downgaze) supranuclear palsy point toward alternate diagnoses. Imaging evidence of disproportionate ventricular dilatation is a hallmark of normal pressure hydrocephalus. Pathological changes described in patients with VP were nonspecific. In one series, 12/17 patients with VP had nigral cell loss suggestive of underlying concomitant neurodegenerative Parkinsonism.

Treatment

One-third of patients with VP improve with conventional dopaminergic therapy. Rare cases with abnormal DAT-SPECT imaging are more likely to improve with levodopa.

In one series, four of five patients had early fluctuations and dyskinesias between 1 and 9 months after starting levodopa. Some report spontaneous improvement as well.

All patients with suspected VP merit a trial of levodopa treatment to assess response. Optimal doses and duration of treatment prior to labeling nonresponse are not uniformly described. However, in practice, a minimum dose of 450–600 mg of levodopa for at least 3 months is employed. Higher doses of up to 1,200–2,400 mg or more have been beneficial in occasional patients. Prolonged treatment periods for up to a year may be considered before labeling a patient unresponsive to levodopa. Hallucinations, orthostatic hypotension, and dyskinesias may limit the tolerability of higher doses in individual patients. Improvement in the cardinal motor symptoms and gait merits continuation of therapy. There are no definite predictors of good response to treatment. However, the response is better in patients with asymmetrical disease and rest tremor mimicking Parkinson's disease, those with presynaptic lesions in the substantia nigra, and those with abnormal DAT-SPECT. Apart from levodopa, other medications such as dopamine agonists have limited role in the management of VP. In addition to medications, allied health interventions such as physiotherapy, particularly gait, and posture training are important adjuncts to improve the quality of life in VP.

Unusual Causes of Vascular Parkinsonism

Apart from atherosclerotic vascular disease, Parkinsonism has also been described in genetic vasculopathies such as cerebral autosomal dominant arteriopathy with subcortical infarcts and leukoencephalopathy (CADASIL) and moyamoya disease. Patients with dural arteriovenous fistulae may also rarely present with Parkinsonism along with other clinical features such as cognitive decline, headache, and bladder symptoms. Treatment of the vascular malformation by endovascular or other means may reverse the symptoms in some patients.

Atypical Parkinsonian Syndromes

An atypical Parkinsonian syndrome with clinical features akin to PSP can occur in patients with multiple infarcts. Vascular disease is the second most common cause of this phenotype, next to degenerative PSP. Infarcts in the midbrain, thalamus, basal ganglia regions, or upper brainstem can result in a vascular PSP-like syndrome. Rarely, patients may present with isolated freezing of gait, blepharospasm, or apraxia of eye opening. Even more common than the PSP phenotype is Parkinsonism mimicking corticobasal syndrome with asymmetric rigidity, dystonia, apraxia, cortical sensory loss, and alien limb phenomenon. Contralateral ischemic lesions in the basal ganglia and cortical regions are the second most common cause of this syndrome. Stepwise progression, acute onset, relative stability of symptoms in lieu of relentless progression, and history of strokes help to distinguish vascular etiologies from the typical degenerative atypical Parkinsonism.

Chorea, Ballism, and Athetosis

These are hyperkinetic movement disorder phenomenologies that can occur acutely in the setting of stroke. Hemichorea and hemiballism often appear contralateral to stroke involving the subthalamic region, thalamus, lentiform nucleus, or the caudate. Although classically localized to the subthalamic region, less than one-third of patients with hemiballism have purely subthalamic lesions on imaging. Rarely, ipsilateral hemichorea-hemiballism has been reported following stroke. These movements may appear acutely or during recovery from concurrent hemiparesis. Athetosis is a much debated term clinically and rarely seen in its pure form. Stereotypies and athetoid movements have been reported after stroke in multiple basal ganglia or subcortical regions and often in thalamic stroke.[9] Thalamic lesions causing hemianesthesia may also present with pseudoathetosis.

The clinical course of poststroke hyperkinetic movements is characterized by stabilization and gradual recovery in the majority, though a significant number of patients may be left with persistent deficits. Hemiballism, in particular, can be significantly disabling and injurious to the patient. Dopamine-depleting drugs such as tetrabenazine are the usual first line of management. Anticholinergics, clonazepam, and sodium valproate are other agents that may be helpful. Dopamine receptor blockers, if required, should be used judiciously due to risk of tardive syndromes.[10] Medical management is successful in 45–56% of patients. Functional neurosurgery—stereotactic lesioning or deep brain stimulation has been tried in refractory poststroke hyperkinetic movement disorders. The ventral oralis posterior or intermedius nuclei of thalamus and posteroventral pallidum have been reported to be successful in individual patients, though there is not enough data to recommend its routine use in this population.

Dystonia

Dystonia is unique from other poststroke hyperkinetic movement disorders in that it is a delayed manifestation after stroke. The classical description of poststroke dystonia is a hemidystonia contralateral to the side of stroke. However, poststroke dystonia may be focal (affecting only one limb or cranial region), segmental, or generalized. Poststroke dystonias are typically not task specific, although active movement of the affected body part may worsen the dystonia. In infantile strokes, hemiatrophy may accompany the dystonia resulting in hemidystonia-hemiatrophy syndrome. The mean age of onset of hemidystonia was 14.9 years (range 1–46 years) in a study of 26 patients with hemidystonia-hemiatrophy syndrome. Poststroke dystonia may mimic myoclonus-dystonia with a jerky dystonic unsteady hand and is secondary to lesions in the posterior thalamic nuclei due to posterior choroidal artery infarcts. Dystonic tremor, dystonic athetoid movements, and paroxysmal dystonia have also been described after stroke. Dystonia developing in addition to spasticity has been described as dystonia-spasticity syndrome. Putaminal and thalamic lesions are common culprits for poststroke dystonia, though lesion mapping studies have suggested that involvement of a wide range of locations in the motor network may result in dystonia. Strokes involving the pallidum, thalamic nuclei, brainstem-diencephalic region, or the cerebellum may result in dystonia.

The treatment of poststroke dystonia is symptomatic and does not differ from that for idiopathic dystonia. As for dystonia occurring due to other etiologies, botulinum neurotoxin is useful for focal or segmental dystonias. Particularly, in patients with significant spasticity and disability, botulinum neurotoxin merits consideration. Medications are recommended for patients with more generalized or hemidystonia, sometimes in addition to botulinum neurotoxin. Anticholinergics, baclofen, and benzodiazepines are the commonly used medications. Intrathecal baclofen may be useful in spasticity dystonia. Deep brain stimulation has been attempted in few cases with anecdotal reports suggesting good benefit; however, only modest beneficial effects were noted in the larger case series. Globus pallidus interna and subthalamic nucleus were the commonly used targets.

Tremor

Isolated poststroke tremor that is unaccompanied by other abnormal movements is rare. Although typically a delayed consequence of a stroke, tremor as a part of the acute stroke presentation has been reported anecdotally. Tremor is most often caused by lesions in the posterior thalamus or lesions disrupting the dentatorubrothalamic, cerebellothalamic, or nigrostriatal pathways. Tremor occurring only when writing (task-specific writing tremor) has been described after a small frontal cortical infarct.

Midbrain, rubral, or Holmes tremor has not always been demonstrated to have the classical red nucleus involved, rather lesions anywhere along the dentatorubrothalamic tract or beyond may present with similar tremor. Myorhythmia is a typical slow (1–3 Hz) tremor with rest and postural components that may occur in the setting of pontine or thalamic infarcts. Palatal tremor or myoclonus can result from vascular lesions involving the Guillain–Mollaret triangle.

Medications used for essential tremor such as propranolol, primidone, and topiramate are often tried in poststroke tremor, but the response is often modest. Few patients with Holmes tremor have been reported to benefit from high-dose levodopa. Deep brain stimulation targeting the thalamic nuclei ventralis intermedius, ventralis oralis posterior or both, or the lenticular fasciculus may offer moderate benefits in patients with refractory tremor.

Myoclonus

Poststroke myoclonus is usually focal or segmental with lesions in the midbrain, pons, or thalamus. Secondary palatal myoclonus is mostly due to pontine or bulbar strokes. Myoclonus is most frequently treated with clonazepam and sodium valproate, but levetiracetam, piracetam, primidone, tetrabenazine, acetazolamide, and botulinum toxin injections can be tried.

Asterixis

Asterixis is negative myoclonus manifested as brief lapses of antigravity muscle contractions producing flapping movement of the outstretched limbs. Poststroke asterixis is usually unilateral and affects the upper limb predominantly. Bilateral asterixis has also been described. Asterixis typically develops during the acute phase of the stroke and has been reported after lesions of the basal ganglia, thalamus, frontoparietal cortex, cerebellum, and brainstem strokes. Usually, it is self-limiting.

Transient Paroxysmal Hyperkinesia

Limb shaking transient ischemic attacks (TIAs) occur in patients with severe carotid or vertebrobasilar stenosis. These are characterized by episodic tremors or flapping movements of the upper or lower limbs that resolve spontaneously. Episodes may be precipitated by suddenly assuming upright posture resulting in transient reduction in blood flow. These episodes may be mistaken for seizures or paroxysmal movements.

Stereotypies, Akathisias, and Tics

Rarely, stroke may cause such hyperkinetic movements, particularly thalamic stroke.[11] One interesting phenomenon is punding, which is a form of complex behavioral stereotypy and has been reported in a patient with brainstem stroke in the form of endlessly writing, copying, and organizing recipes as well as purchasing and hoarding food. Akathisia and tics have been managed with clonazepam, clonidine, or dopamine receptor antagonists such as risperidone.

CONCLUSION

In conclusion, both ischemic and hemorrhagic strokes may uncommonly result in the development of movement disorders. Movement disorder phenotypes and the location of vascular insult resulting in a particular phenotype vary. Both hyperkinetic and hypokinetic movement disorders may result from stroke. Management strategies are similar as for symptomatic management of movement disorders of diverse etiologies. Risk factor management for diabetes, hypertension, and lifestyle measures including exercise plays an important role in the prevention of these unusual complications of strokes.

REFERENCES

1. Mehanna R, Jankovic J. Movement disorders in cerebrovascular disease. Lancet Neurol. 2013;12:597-608.
2. Ghika-Schmid F, Ghika J, Regli F, Bogousslavsky J. Hyperkinetic movement disorders during and after acute stroke: the Lausanne stroke registry. J Neurol Sci. 1997;146:109-16.
3. Scott B, Jankovic J. Delayed-onset progressive movement disorders after static brain lesions. Neurology. 1996;46:68-74.
4. Alarcon F, Zijlmans JC, Duenas G, Cevallos N. Post-stroke movement disorders: report of 56 patients. J Neurol Neurosurg Psychiatry. 2004;75:1568-74.
5. Béjot Y, Giroud M, Moreau T, Benatru I. Clinical spectrum of movement disorders after stroke in childhood and adulthood. Eur Neurol. 2012;68:59-64.
6. Suri R, Rodriguez-Porcel F, Donohue K, Jesse E, Lovera L, Dwivedi AK, et al. Post-stroke Movement Disorders: The Clinical, Neuroanatomic, and Demographic Portrait of 284 Published Cases. J Stroke Cerebrovasc Dis. 2018;27:2388-97.
7. Winikates J, Jankovic J. Clinical correlates of vascular parkinsonism. Arch Neurol. 1999;56:98-102.
8. Zijlmans JC, Daniel SE, Hughes AJ, Revesz T, Lees AJ. Clinico-pathological investigation of vascular Parkinsonism, including clinical criteria for diagnosis. Mov Disord. 2004;19:630-40.
9. Gupta N, Pandey S. Post-Thalamic Stroke Movement Disorders: A Systematic Review. Eur Neurol. 2018;79:303-14.
10. Netravathi, M, Pal PK, Devi, IB. A clinical profile of 103 patients with secondary movement disorders: correlation of etiology with phenomenology. Eur Neurol. 2012;19:226-33.
11. Lera G, Scipioni O, Garcia S, Cammarota A, Fischbein G, Gershanik O. A combined pattern of movement disorders resulting from posterolateral thalamic lesions of a vascular nature: a syndrome with clinico-radiologic correlation. Mov Disord. 2000;15:120-6.

CHAPTER 46

Functional Movement Disorders

Meenakshisundaram Umaiorubahan,
Porrselvi Ammaiappan Palanisamy

INTRODUCTION

Functional neurological disorders include seizures, movement disorders, weakness, sensory loss, visual impairment, dizziness, speech disorders, and memory/cognitive problems. Of these, functional movement disorders are nonorganic disorders causing abnormal movements and posturing.[1,2] These disorders occupy a gray zone between the fields of neurology and psychiatry.[3] Patients are often evaluated by numerous specialists and undergo multiple investigations before a diagnosis is even considered[4] and this gets further complicated when the patient has a coexisting organic disorder, as happens in about 10% of the patients.[5] Thus, functional movement disorders cause medical professionals, patients, and caregivers considerable distress, aptly referred to as the "crisis for neurology".[6]

Functional movement disorders have been classified by the Diagnostic and Statistical Manual of Mental Disorders-5 (DSM-5) of the American Psychiatric Association as conversion disorder, or functional neurological symptom disorder, under the general category of somatic symptom and related disorders. It should be noted here that this is an involuntary disorder. When patients make the abnormal movements voluntarily to satisfy a psychological need, it is a factitious disorder. In rare cases, patients may stage the abnormal movements purposely to achieve a specific external goal as in malingering, which is not a psychiatric condition at all.

In the International Classification of Diseases-10 (ICD-10), functional movement disorders are classified as conversion disorder with motor symptom or deficit under dissociative and conversion disorders.

EPIDEMIOLOGY

The accurate prevalence and incidence of functional movement disorders are not known.[7] An incidence of about 5 per 100,000[8] cases has been reported. It has been estimated to comprise between 2% and 20% of the patients attending movement disorder clinics.[3] Functional movement disorders have been reported to account for about 1.5% of all patients seen in neurology clinics and 17% of all functional neurological disorders. Women account for about 70–80% of all patients.[4] The mean age of onset is 37–50 years, although these disorders have been reported in children as well as in the elderly.[1] The most common presentations of functional movement disorders are tremor, myoclonus, gait disorders, and dystonia, with Parkinsonism, tics, and chorea being less common.[1,7,9]

ETIOLOGY AND PATHOPHYSIOLOGY

Although the exact etiopathophysiology of functional movement disorders is unknown, the multifactorial etiology is the basis for the biopsychosocial model. This model includes interactions between biology, psychology, and social factors. Biological factors include age, gender, genetics, physiologic reactions, and tissue health, psychological factors include mental health, emotional health, beliefs, and expectations, while sociological factors include interpersonal relationships, social support dynamics, and socioeconomics.

Imaging studies have shown differences in the patterns of brain activation between patients with weakness and healthy volunteers feigning weakness trying to move their weak leg.[1] Temporal discrimination thresholds and intracortical inhibition have been found to be affected in a similar manner in both organic and functional dystonia. Abnormal cortical plasticity has been found to be exclusively a feature of organic dystonia when compared with functional dystonia on paired associative stimulation (PAS).[10] The brain network system is considered abnormal.

In the previous century, functional movement disorders were largely explained through the concepts of primary gain and secondary gain in the psychodynamic model.[8] From the modern psychiatry point of view, various factors contribute to the generation of somatic complaints that are not of organic origin. They can include traumatic events in childhood or recently, abuse and illness in childhood and adolescence, though how such factors induce the vulnerability to functional neurological disorders are unknown.[2]

In the DSM-5, the need for a psychological stressor to be present for the diagnosis of conversion disorder has been removed as well as the need to exclude malingering or factitious disorder for making a diagnosis[1] because not all cases of functional movement disorders have overt psychopathology.

Functional movement disorders can be voluntary or involuntary in such conversion disorders, though they might seem to be voluntary. In one recent study, it has been found that there was hypoactivity of the temporoparietal junction associated with functional tremor and others including functional myoclonus, gait/balance disturbances, abnormal speech, weakness, and dystonia.[11] This might indicate a lack of appropriate sensorimotor prediction that normally accompanies voluntary movement and integrates the feed-forward system with the feedback system.

During the functional movement, there is low recruitment of the supplementary motor area and high activity in the limbic areas (impaired emotional processing or alexithymia, which causes the misinterpretation of a triggering event to be caused by physical illness rather than as an outcome of the traumatic event).[7] This combined with the lack of appropriate somatosensory processing that may contribute to the misattribution of the movements as being involuntary by the patient.[1]

Teodoro et al.[12] found that when compared to healthy controls, patients with functional movement disorders showed a lack of sensory attenuation at the onset of self-paced movements. Sensory attenuation is the phenomenon by which self-generated stimuli are perceived with lesser intensity. This lack of sensory attenuation in patients may be the reason that patients perceive their movements as involuntary.

DIAGNOSIS

There are three diagnostic criteria that have been reported in literature. The most popular is the *Fahn-Williams diagnostic criteria* proposed in 1988, which categorizes patients into four, based on the levels of diagnostic certainty—documented, clinically established, probable, and possible (**Table 1**). The *Shill-Gerber criteria* (**Table 2**) proposed in 2006 categorizes patients based on historical information such as disproportionate pain or fatigue and presence of an external gain. The *Gupta-Lang criteria* (**Table 3**) proposed in 2009 is based on the electrophysiological findings such as frequency analysis for functional tremor and electromyography-electroencephalography (EMG-EEG) back-averaging for functional myoclonus.[1,4,8,10] Phenotype-specific diagnostic criteria (**Table 4**) for functional movement disorders were proposed in 2015 by Espay and Lang based on the core phenomenological features.[13]

TABLE 1: Fahn-Williams diagnostic criteria.

Documented	Remittance with suggestion, physiotherapy, psychotherapy, and placebos, "while unobserved"
Clinically established	Inconsistent over time/incongruent with clinical condition and other manifestations: Other "false" signs, multiple somatizations, and obvious psychiatric disturbance
Probable	• Inconsistent/incongruent—no other features • Consistent/congruent and "false" neurological signs • Consistent/congruent and multiple somatizations
Possible	Consistent/congruent and obvious emotional disturbance

Source: Adapted from Fahn S, Williams DT. Psychogenic dystonia. Adv Neurol. 1988;50:431-55.

COMMON CLINICAL PRESENTATIONS

Functional Tremor

Functional tremor is the most common type of functional movement disorder and is seen in at least 50% of such patients.[3] Functional tremor, commonly, is a complex type of postural action and resting tremor, which is seen only in organic rubral tremors.[7] Functional tremors are seen in hands, legs, and, sometimes, the whole body. A clinical clue is that there is a sparing of fingers when tremor occurs at the wrist.

Functional Dystonia

Functional dystonia is the second most common type of functional movement disorder. It can be constrained to one part of the body or be generalized,[7] more frequently affecting the lower limbs than the upper limbs. It is seen more often in women than men.[3] It may follow a

TABLE 2: Shill–Gerber criteria.

Clinically proven	Remits with psychotherapy, it is witnessed to remit when the patient feels unobserved or there is premovement Bereitschaftspotential on electroencephalography (EEG) (functional myoclonus only)
Clinically definite	At least three primary criteria and at least one secondary criteria
Clinically probable	Two primary criteria and two secondary criteria
Clinically possible	One primary criterion and two secondary criterion or two primary and one secondary criteria
Primary criteria: Inconsistent with organic disease (false weakness; false sensory signs; inconsistent over time; distractibility; abrupt onset, paroxysmal in nature, or periods of spontaneous remission; astasia–abasia; selective disability; entrainment of tremor to the frequency of repetitive movements; cocontraction sign in tremor; atypical response to a pharmacological agent; and atypical stimulus sensitivity), excessive pain or fatigue, previous exposure to a disease model, and/or potential for secondary gain	Secondary criteria: Multiple somatizations (other than pain and fatigue) and/or obvious psychiatric disturbance

Source: Adapted from Shill H, Gerber P. Evaluation of clinical diagnostic criteria for psychogenic movement disorders. Mov Disord. 2006;21(8):1163-8.

TABLE 3: Gupta–Lang criteria.

1. Documented	Remittance with suggestion, physiotherapy, psychotherapy, and placebos, "while unobserved"
2a. Clinically established plus other features	Inconsistent over time/incongruent with clinical condition and other manifestations: Other "false" signs, multiple somatizations, and obvious psychiatric disturbance
2b. Clinically established minus other features	Unequivocal clinical features incompatible with organic disease with no features suggesting another underlying neurological or psychiatric problem
3. Laboratory-supported definite	Electrophysiological evidence proving a psychogenic movement disorder (primarily in cases of psychogenic tremor and psychogenic myoclonus)
Clinically definite	1 + 2a + 2b

Source: Adapted from Gupta A, Lang AE. Psychogenic movement disorders. Curr Opin Neurol. 2009;22(4):430-6.

minor peripheral injury, dental procedures,[1,3,13] or occur spontaneously[3] and in some cases may be associated with pain and dysautonomic features as seen in complex regional pain syndrome type 1 that develop following immobility.[1,13] Muscle atrophy or joint contractures may be present in chronic functional dystonia. Muscle hypertrophy may rarely be present due to sustained contraction in some patients (organic dystonia when chronic, often leads to muscle hypertrophy).[7] These patients often lack the characteristic clinical features of organic focal dystonia that are task specificity, stereotypy, sensory tricks, morning benefit, and electromyographic findings.

Functional Facial and Cranial Movement Disorders

The most common pattern of functional facial movement disorder was lateral or downward lip protrusion with ipsilateral deviation of the jaw, commonly noted as "lip pulling".[12,14,15] Functional hemifacial spasm, functional blepharospasm, and functional hemilingual spasm can occur and tend to be sustained. In functional hemilingual spasm, the tongue usually deviates toward the side of the facial spasm. Functional palatal tremor (functional palatal myoclonus), in which the tremor is variable in frequency, amplitude, direction, and other characteristics, is entrainable and distractible. Ear clicking is commonly reported. There might be a reported precipitating event such as a sore throat.[14]

Functional Gait

Functional gait disorders often have variability in gait, excessive slowness, and stiffness combined with difficulty to maintain balance, flailing arms, and excessive trunk sway.[7] Patients typically hold energy in efficient postures and tend to hold balance even in very dangerous postures. They seldom report falls.[13] The presence of the "huffing and puffing" sign, while standing and walking, may strongly support the diagnosis of a functional movement disorder when gait is involved.[16] The overall functional gait patterns that have been identified are excessive slowness, astasia-abasia, knee buckling, tightrope walking, trembling walking, and truncal jerking.[17] The "psychogenic toe sign" is characterized by resistance to manipulation of an extended first toe, which can be forcibly flexed only at the expense of associated pain or by extending toes 2–5, which are held in tonic flexion (the organic striatal toe

TABLE 4: Espay and Lang phenotype-specific diagnostic criteria.

Functional phenotype	*Clinically definite, if all present*	*Supportive but neither necessary nor sufficient*	*Laboratory confirmed*
Tremor	• Entrainment or full suppressibility • Distractibility • Tonic coactivation at tremor onset • Pause of tremor during contralateral ballistic movements • Variability in frequency, axis, and/or distribution	• Dual task interference • Increase in tremor amplitude with weight loading	Surface EMG: entrainment (coherence), coactivation, distractibility, variability in tremor frequency and/or axis (e.g., flexion/extension to pronation/supination), and pause during contralateral ballistic movements
Dystonia	• Rapid onset • Fixed dystonia at rest • Variable resistance to manipulation and/or distractibility or absence when unobserved	• Associated pain (except neck) • Complex regional pain syndrome	None established (tentative: Coactivation sign on surface EMG)
Myoclonus	• Variability in duration and/or distribution of jerks or of their latency (if stimulus sensitive) • Entrainment or full suppressibility • Distractibility	Variability in amplitude	• Bereitschaftspotential present on EMG-EEG • EMG bursts >250 ms and of variable duration • Long latency (within voluntary reaction time) in cases of stimulus-sensitive jerks
Tics	• Not fully stereotypical • Interference with speech or voluntary actions	• Lack of premonitory urge • Lack of voluntary control	None established
Parkinsonism	• Marked slowness on examined manual tasks discordant with casual manual tasks (e.g., buttoning, tying shoe laces) • Variable resistance against passive movements without cogwheel rigidity	• "Huffing and puffing" sign • Pincer function preserved • Absence of decrement during finger tapping • Arm held tightly to the side or cradled in front	• Surface EMG for associated tremor • Normal nigrostriatal dopaminergic function on PET or SPECT in cases suspected as having Parkinson's disease (may also be seen in cases of organic dystonic tremor or dopa-responsive dystonia)
Gait impairment	• Knee buckling or astasia–abasia • Bizarre gait plus at least one of the above phenotypes	• Swivel chair test • Excessive slowness or exaggerated effort • Uneconomic postures • Retained balance despite precarious postures	None established

(EEG: electroencephalography; EMG: electromyography; PET: positron emission tomography; SPECT: single-photon emission computed tomography)

Source: Adapted from Espay AJ, Lang AE. Phenotype-specific diagnosis of functional (psychogenic) movement disorders. Curr Neurol Neurosci Rep. 2015;15(6):32.

can be passively manipulated without pain or resistance). Sudden knee buckling without falling is commonly seen in patients with functional gait disorders.[18,19] The clinical clues are inconsistency, "huffing and puffing", and an atypical, chaotic gait.

Functional Myoclonus

Functional myoclonus is reported in about 20% of patients with functional movement disorders.[3] The main features of functional myoclonus are the variability in duration and/or distribution of the jerks or of their latency, especially if they are stimuli sensitive. The clinical clues are variability, suggestibility, and distractibility.

Startle Syndromes

In organic hyperekplexia, patients do not habituate. In functional startle syndromes, patients have an exaggerated initial startle response that habituates with repetitive stimulation or shows inconsistent latencies.[7] The inconsistency is the clinical clue.

LESS COMMON CLINICAL PRESENTATIONS

Functional Parkinsonism

Though Parkinsonism is one of the most common movement disorders encountered, functional Parkinsonism is relatively rare.[20] True bradykinesia is absent. Rigidity may be seen due to the result of voluntary opposition. Gait abnormality and postural instability are present with similarities to functional gait disorders. Reeling backward without falling may also be present.[7] Levodopa-induced motor complications tend not to occur even with prolonged, high-dose therapy.

Functional Tics

The absence of clearly stereotyped movements and increased variability characterize functional tics. They show interference with speech and other voluntary movements unlike in organic tic disorder.[13] Psychogenic myoclonus and psychogenic movements resembling tics (PMRTs) have an older age of onset when compared to organic tics. The lack of premonitory sensation in functional tics is a red flag. Lack of suppressibility is also an important feature.[12]

Functional Chorea

Isolated functional chorea is the rarest of all types of clinical presentations in functional movement disorders. The diagnosis of functional chorea is very difficult to be made with certainty based on clinical evaluation due to the variability that can be seen in organic chorea as well as drug-induced dyskinesias.[13]

Functional Eye Movement Disorders

Functional convergence spasm is the most common type of functional eye movement disorder in which the convergence eye movement reflex persists even when the patient is not looking at a near object. Functional convergence paralysis, functional gaze limitation, and functional and voluntary nystagmus with or without oscillopsia are other types of functional eye movement disorders that have been reported in literature.[14] A convergence spasm is of functional etiology in about 95% of cases.

DIAGNOSTIC CLINICAL CLUES

Common clinical presentations that are associated with functional movement disorders include but are not limited to:[1,7]

- Abrupt onset
- History of a trigger event
- Static course
- Symptoms are reported to begin with or rapidly progress to maximum severity and disability that are inconsistent with examination findings
- Difficult to classify abnormal movements
- Inconsistency over time
- Paroxysmal symptoms
- Whack-a-mole sign—the appearance or worsening of an involuntary movement in a distant body part when the ongoing involuntary movement in an affected body part is suppressed by holding it down[5]
- Weakness (false-give-away weakness), slowness, and false sensory signs
- Increased visual attention toward the affected body part during the movement[10]
- Ability to trigger or relieve the movement with unusual or nonphysiologic intervention such as trigger points on the body and application of a tuning fork
- *Distractibility*: Distracting maneuvers decrease the intensity of the movement in functional movement disorders. (vis-à-vis increase in the intensity of the movement in organic movement disorders). But, distracting maneuvers may not work with chronic functional movement disorders
- Increased movement of the affected body part during observation or examination
- Entrainment—when the patient is asked to perform a voluntary movement at a given frequency in the contralateral limb, the affected limb's movement (especially in functional tremor) will take on the same frequency
- Unresponsiveness to drugs for organic movement disorders
- Response to placebo and suggestion
- Spontaneous remission
- Presence of more than one movement disorder and phenomenological variability between attacks[21]
- History of sexual or physical abuse
- Disease modeling—history of exposure to organic movement disorders of family or friends
- Presence of other unexplained somatic symptoms
- Family history of functional movement disorders[22]
- Comorbid psychopathology
- Presence of secondary gain
- Suggestibility
- Self-inflicted injuries

ELECTROPHYSIOLOGY

Electrophysiological studies have been maximally studied in functional tremor and myoclonus phenotypes. Tremor analysis using surface EMG and accelerometry can help in identifying features associated with functional tremor including entrainment, coactivation of antagonist muscles, variability in tremor frequency, increased tremor amplitude, and frequency with weight loading of the involved limb. Coherence is an important finding. Functional tremor has the same frequency in the affected limb, as the other limb that is performing distracting and entrainment maneuvers.[7,18,23]

In functional myoclonus, surface EMG, EEG, back-averaged EEG, and somatosensory evoked potentials can be helpful. Features associated with functional myoclonus on surface EMG include: (a) Abnormally long and variable latencies between the stimulus and the myoclonic jerk (i.e., a long latency of 100–120 ms from stimulus to jerk), (b) variable patterns of muscle recruitment with each jerk, prolonged myoclonic burst duration, (c) a triphasic pattern of agonist and antagonist muscle activation, and (d) habituation with repeated stimulation. In addition, functional myoclonus is usually but not always preceded by a readiness potential or the Bereitschaftspotential.

IMAGING STUDIES

Neuroimaging methods such as CT and MRI are of little use, except to rule out any structural abnormality. Positron emission tomography (PET) and dopamine transporter-single-photon emission computed tomography (DAT-SPECT) may be useful in functional Parkinsonism.[7,24] Functional MRI during recall of causative life events has revealed an increased activity in the left dorsolateral prefrontal cortex with decreased activity in hippocampal and parahippocampal regions suggesting memory suppression.[25]

FUNCTIONAL MOVEMENT DISORDERS IN CHILDREN

Conversion disorder has been reported in children as young as 4 years, but is more common during adolescence and the peripubertal years.[26] The prevalence of functional or conversion disorders among children has been estimated to have a prevalence of about two to four per 100,000.[27] It is more common in the female sex.[28,29] The symptoms may represent an attention-seeking behavior for secondary gain or may be a mechanism to avoid an aversive experience. In children, the dominant side of the body is more likely to be affected as compared to the nondominant side of the body in adults, probably due to the incomplete lateralization in children. It is usually possible to identify a specific precipitant or trigger event for the conversion symptoms in children.[26,27] Modeling frequently occurs in children and their functional movements closely resemble the phenotype of their model.[27] Typically, the remission occurs in about 3 months since diagnosis and recurrences are rare. When such a conversion disorder recurs in children, a personality disorder, somatization disorder, or any other underlying psychopathology should be looked for and treated appropriately.[26] Functional movement disorders have a better prognosis in children when compared to adults, especially if a trigger is identified.[27]

TREATMENT

Early diagnosis is the key as it obviates unnecessary investigations and medications.

An effective communication of the diagnosis in an empathetic and nonjudgmental manner to the patient and family forms the first line of management following the diagnosis. It is important to remember the key point that the diagnosis should be delivered as like any other diagnosis and that it would be valuable to show the patient how the diagnosis was arrived at.

Acceptance of the diagnosis and a good rapport with the physician and therapists are the strongest predictors for favorable outcome after psychological intervention.[1,3,7] Transcranial magnetic stimulation has been reported to be effective in some patients.[1,3] A combination of physical therapy and psychological intervention such as the symptom-focused cognitive behavioral therapy or psychodynamic psychotherapy has shown promising results.[1-3] Biofeedback techniques using EMG have also shown improvement in some.[2,26] A multidisciplinary approach involving the neurologist, psychiatrist, physiatrist, psychologist, occupational therapist, and social worker is a key to effective management.

PROGNOSIS

The outcome in cases of functional movement disorders is variable and is dependent on various factors including: (a) The nature of the disorder, (b) the presence of an identifiable stressor, (c) chronicity—shorter duration has better prognosis, (d) type of onset—acute onset has better prognosis than an insidious one, (e) the underlying psychopathology—depression or anxiety can be better managed than personality disorders, (f) attitude of the patient and the influence of external factors, (g) quality of support system for the patient, and (h) factors that affect the effectiveness of the treatment such as early diagnosis and perception of efficiency of physician by the patient.[1,2,10]

CONCLUSION

Functional movement disorders are common, real, and disabling. Diagnosis and management of these disorders can be difficult as differentiation from organic movement disorders is sometimes impossible. The term functional is preferred over psychogenic as it is neither judgmental nor assumptive. A keen eye for details is often the decisive diagnostic tool.

REFERENCES

1. Benbadis SR. Psychogenic Movement Disorders. Continuum (Minneap Minn). 2013;19(5):1383-96.
2. Dallocchio C. Psychogenic movement disorders. In: Uehara T (Ed). Psychiatric Disorders: Trends and Developments. Croatia: InTechOpen; 2011.
3. Edwards MJ, Bhatia KP. Functional (psychogenic) movement disorders: merging mind and brain. Lancet Neurol. 2012;11 (3):250-60.
4. Thenganatt MA, Jankovic J. Psychogenic Movement Disorders. Neurol Clin. 2015;33(1):205-24.
5. Hallett M. Functional (psychogenic) movement disorders: clinical presentations. Parkinsonism Relat Disord. 2016;22(1): S149-52.
6. Hallett M. Psychogenic movement disorders: a crisis for neurology. Curr Neurol Neurosci Rep. 2006;6(2):269-71.
7. Miyasaki JM. Functional Movement Disorders. In: Hurtig HI (Ed). UpToDate, Waltham: UpToDate; 2016.
8. Nowak DA, Fink GR. Psychogenic movement disorders: etiology, phenomenology, neuroanatomical correlates and therapeutic approaches. Neuroimage. 2009;47(3):1015-25.
9. Lang AE. General overview of psychogenic movement disorders: epidemiology, diagnosis, and prognosis. In: Lang AE (Ed). Psychogenic Movement Disorders: Neurology and Neuropsychiatry. Philadelphia: Lippincott Williams & Wilkins; 2006.
10. Hallett M. Functional (psychogenic) movement disorders—clinical presentations. Parkinsonism Relat Disord. 2012;22(4): S149-52.
11. Maurer CW, LaFaver K, Ameli R, Epstein SA, Hallett M, Horovitz SG. Impaired self-agency in functional movement disorders: A resting-state fMRI study. Neurology. 2016;87(6):564-70.
12. Teodoro T, Edwards MJ. Functional movement disorders. Curr Opin Neurol. 2016;29(4):519-25.
13. Espay AJ, Lang AE. Phenotype-specific diagnosis of functional (psychogenic) movement disorders. Curr Neurol Neurosci Rep. 2015;15(6):32.
14. Kaski D, Bronstein AM, Edwards MJ, Stone J. Cranial functional (psychogenic) movement disorders. Lancet Neurol. 2015;14(12):1196-205.
15. Fasano A, Valadas A, Bhatia KP, Prashanth LK, Lang AE, Munhoz RP, et al. Psychogenic facial movement disorders: clinical features and associated conditions. Mov Disord. 2012;27(12):1544-51.
16. Laub HN, Dwivedi AK, Revilla FJ, Duker AP, Pecina-Jacob C, Espay AJ. Diagnostic performance of the "huffing and puffing" sign in functional (psychogenic) movement disorders. Mov Disord Clin Pract. 2015;2(1):29-32.
17. Sokol LL, Espay AJ. Clinical signs in functional (psychogenic) gait disorders: a brief survey. J Clin Mov Disord. 2016;3:3.
18. Hallett M. Physiology of psychogenic movement disorders. J Clin Neurosci. 2010;17(8):959-65.
19. Fahn S, Williams DT. Psychogenic dystonia. Adv Neurol. 1988;50:431-55.
20. Jankovic J. Diagnosis and treatment of psychogenic parkinsonism. J Neurol Neurosurg Psychiatry. 2011;82(12): 1300-3.
21. Ganos C, Aguirregomozcorta M, Batla A, Stamelou M, Schwingenschuh P, Münchau A, et al. Psychogenic paroxysmal movement disorders—clinical features and diagnostic clues. Parkinsonism Relat Disord. 2014;20(1):41-6.
22. Stamelou M, Cossu G, Edwards MJ, Murgia D, Pareés I, Melis M, et al. Familial psychogenic movement disorders. Mov Disord. 2013;28(9):1295-8.
23. Kamble NL, Pal PK. Electrophysiological evaluation of psychogenic movement disorders. Parkinsonism Relat Disord. 2016;22 Suppl 1:S153-8.
24. Ellenstein A, Kranick SM, Hallett M. An Update on Psychogenic Movement Disorders. Curr Neurol Neurosci Rep. 2011;11(4):396-403.
25. Pringsheim T, Edwards M. Functional movement disorders: five new things. Neurol Clin Pract. 2017;7(2):141-7.
26. Kirsch DB, Mink JW. Psychogenic movement disorders in children. Pediatr Neurol. 2004;30(1):1-6.
27. Baizabal-Carvallo JF, Fekete R. Recognizing uncommon presentations of psychogenic (functional) movement disorders. Tremor Other Hyperkinet Mov (N Y). 2015;5:279.
28. Shill H, Gerber P. Evaluation of clinical diagnostic criteria for psychogenic movement disorders. Mov Disord. 2006;21(8): 1163-8.
29. Gupta A, Lang AE. Psychogenic movement disorders. Curr Opin Neurol. 2009;22(4):430-6.

SECTION

9

ATAXIAS

CHAPTER 47

Approach to Cerebellar Disorders and Hereditary Ataxia

Achal Kumar Srivastava, Mohammed Faruq, Arpit Agrawal

INTRODUCTION

Incoordination of voluntary motor movements in clinics is commonly described as ataxia (A-taxis; coordination). The commonly identified symptoms of motor incoordination are gait ataxia, intention tremor, dysarthria (slurring of speech), and titubation. Incoordination of movement can arise due to lesions of neuronal axis involving peripheral nerves, spinal cord, and cerebellum. Ataxia may appear due to acquired or genetic etiologies affecting this axis. Ataxias arising due to genetic etiologies are progressive in nature and often involve other regions in the central nervous system in the disease course (see **Box 1** for classification of ataxias). Nearly 200 genetically distinct subtypes are known to cause cerebellar ataxia as a primary abnormality or ataxia as an associated sign with other primary noncerebellar signs of the neurogenetic disorders. Among these, the genes, which are causal for primary ataxia phenotype, nearly 40 loci, are inherited in autosomal dominant and additional 40 loci with autosomal recessive inheritance (see **Box 2** for newly described SCAs). Other than these monogenic form of Mendelian loci, some of the gene defects are transmitted as X-linked and mitochondrial inheritance. Among acquired causes such as stroke, tumor, toxin, infections, drugs, autoimmunity, and vitamin deficiency states are documented.

The critical aspect in diagnosing a patient with ataxia is to carefully evaluate history aimed at determining age of onset of ataxia, progression mode, concurrent risk factor analysis, toxin exposure, family history, and an application of systematic battery of investigations. We have presented in detail the clinical features of ataxias of genetic and nongenetic etiology in their respective subsections.

Box 1 Classification of cerebellar ataxias.

Hereditary group:

- *Autosomal dominant cerebellar ataxias*:
  Spinocerebellar ataxia types 1–31, SCA36, and episodic ataxias
- *Autosomal recessive cerebellar ataxias*:
  Friedreich's ataxia, ataxia telangiectasia, and spastic ataxia
- *Episodic ataxias*
- *Spastic ataxias*
- *Other hereditary forms of ataxias*:
  - X-linked *cerebellar* ataxias
  - Fragile X tremor ataxia syndrome
  - Mitochondrial

Sporadic group:

- *Degenerative progressive*:
  MSA-C and idiopathic late-onset cerebellar ataxia (ILOCA)
- *Toxins-induced cerebellar degeneration*:
  Alcohol, anticonvulsants, anticancer drugs, etc.
- *Autoimmunity-associated cerebellar degeneration*:
  Multiple sclerosis, gluten ataxia, ataxia with anti-GAD antibody
- *Paraneoplastic cerebellar degeneration*
- *Infection-mediated cerebellar degeneration*:
  Postviral infection cerebellitis, enteric fever, adeno/retroviral, malaria, and prions

(GAD: glutamic acid decarboxylase; MSA-C: multiple system atrophy cerebellar type)

Box 2 Clinical features of newly described spinocerebellar ataxia (SCA) subtypes.

- *SCA32*: Gene-unknown, chromosome—7q32-q33, cerebellar ataxia, mental impairment, and azoospermia
- *SCA34*: Young onset, gene—*ELOVL4* (very long-chain fatty acids-like 4 gene), cerebellar ataxia, and papulosquamous erythematous plaques
- *SCA38*: Onset—34–51 years, gene—*ELOVL5* (very long-chain fatty acids-like 5 gene) cerebellar ataxia, and axonal neuropathy
- *SCA40*: Adult onset, gene—*CCDC88C* (coiled-coil domain-containing protein 88C gene), cerebellar ataxia, vertical gaze impairment, and slow progression

(GAD: glutamic acid decarboxylase; MSA-C: multiple system atrophy cerebellar type)

APPROACH TO CEREBELLAR ATAXIA

Major Signs and Symptoms of Cerebellar Ataxia

Ataxia of Lower Limb and Posture

The gait abnormality in cerebellar ataxia resembles to walking impairment in acute alcohol intoxication. At the early stage, patient notices problem such as imbalance, lateral swaying of the body upon walking on narrow path or in a crowded place, or while performing act requiring skilled movements, e.g., cycling, climbing stairs. In advance stage, patient walks with wide base gait even with support with corrections and errors. On examination, patient sways when asked to walk straight on a 10-m walk and associated with wide-based stance of the feet, on natural stance feet are placed wide apart >20 cm. Ataxia can be elicited in patients even earlier on performing tandem gait or one foot stance. Heel-shin test provokes tremor in limb movement; decomposition and lateral movements are seen while sliding the heel on shin. Posture abnormality, truncal tremor, and head tremor may be observed. Various subdivisions and functional anatomy is shown in **Figure 1** which is self explanatory.

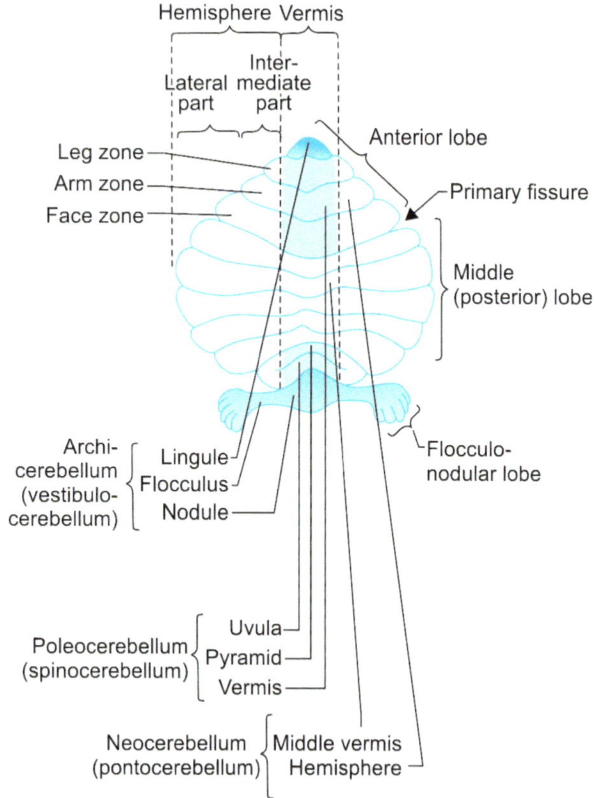

FIG. 1: Functional anatomy of cerebellum.

Kinetic Dysfunction in Upper Limb in Ataxic Disorders

Altered rate, rhythm, and force of contraction of voluntary muscle groups in the upper limb produce cerebellar symptoms, i.e., handshaking on sustaining posture during object holding, e.g., glass of water or a cup of tea. In clinics, upper limb incoordination can be elicited by finger-nose testing, finger-finger testing, examiners finger chasing movements, and dysdiadochokinesia (abnormal rapid alternating hand movements).

Speech Disturbances

The key abnormality in cerebellar speech (dysarthria) is imprecise articulation and phonation, variable loudness, and irregular intervals between syllables. The dysarthric speech in ataxic patients is slurred with uncontrolled volume, pitch, and irregular pause between syllables. There is disarticulation of syllables with distortion of vowels, impaired control over breathing during speech lead to bursting loudness, and equal stress and prolonged pause make speech of the scanning type.

Oculomotor Abnormalities

The observed oculomotor abnormalities include nystagmus, fixation abnormality, impaired saccades, and pursuit movements. Downbeating nystagmus is also observed in some ataxic conditions and is characterized by fast phase of nystagmus toward downgaze in primary position of eyes. Saccadic intrusions and square wave jerks are eye movement fixation abnormalities seen in cerebellar disorders. The saccadic movements are hypermetric or hypometric upon alternating movement toward examiner's finger placed on temporal visual field of the patient.

Other Associated Signs and Symptoms

Apart from ataxia of gait and limbs, other symptoms are also variably experienced by the patients and they include dizziness, headache, cognitive abnormalities, symptoms of autonomic dysfunction, and dysphagia. Among extraneurological manifestations, signs and symptoms with the specific subtype of ataxias may be observed due to muscle involvement, cardiac dysfunction, mental retardation, hypogonadism, and radiosensitivity.

EVALUATION OF CEREBELLAR ATAXIAS

Initial evaluation of an ataxia should comprise of meticulous history taking, determining the family history, age of onset, tempo of the disease progression, and history of concurrent use of drugs, alcohol, and toxin exposure. In addition, history of symptoms apart from ataxia should be obtained. During neurological examination, a detailed survey of distribution of deficits should be undertaken including symmetry of signs (symmetric or asymmetric), type of ataxia (sensory or motor), and presence of ataxia plus signs. Based on history and neurological examination, appropriate investigation can be sought comprising of electrophysiological examinations [nerve conduction studies, electroencephalography (EEG), visual evoked potential (VEP), brainstem auditory evoked response (BAER), and autonomic function tests], radiological investigations [noncontrast computed tomography (NCCT) of the head, MRI, and single-photon emission computed tomography (SPECT)], biochemical tests (drug levels, thyroid function tests, vitamin levels, autoimmune markers, etc.), and genetic testing for hereditary causes. This systematic approach can help in providing insight into the cause of ataxia in the majority of the patients; otherwise, remaining cases can be labeled as idiopathic ataxias. In following section, we describe specific findings expected from ataxia patients.

History

Emphasis should be kept on the disease progression and onset age of the clinical manifestations.

Disease Progression (Tempo) and Onset Age

Generally, acquired causes of ataxias have acute or subacute onset and acute onset cases may be transient or reversible in nature. Infectious etiologies are most common cause for this type of presentation among childhood and young adult cases. In late age, stroke (affecting cerebellum or its connections) and multiple sclerosis (MS) are common causes for acute form of ataxia. Central nervous system (CNS) tumors (posterior fossa), vitamin deficiency (vitamins B1, B12, and E), and autoimmune causes have subacute presentation. In patients with alcohol-induced cerebellar degeneration, symptoms may progress rapidly over months after its onset. Posterior fossa meningioma, glioma, and craniovertebral (CV) junction anomalies develop slowly with features of chronic progression or occasionally static ataxia. Genetic ataxias develop slowly and progress over years and progression of the disease may vary depending upon the type of gene and its mutation. Episodic ataxias have chronic onset, but acute episodes have periodicity and interval between attacks may further diminish with disease progression. Ataxias due to congenital malformations, cerebral palsy, and stroke have static neurological features without any progression.

Distribution of Ataxia Symptoms

Unilateral ataxic features are seen in vascular lesions, cerebellar abscess, neoplastic, demyelinating lesion, acquired immunodeficiency syndrome (AIDS)-related multifocal leukoencephalopathy, and Arnold–Chiari malformation. Drugs, alcohol induced, vitamin deficiency, paraneoplastic cerebellar degeneration (PCD), and genetic causes of ataxia have symmetric distribution of signs and symptoms.

Family History

In the presence of positive family history, genetic causes should be considered and a careful conclusion should be drawn on the particular type of Mendelian inheritance, i.e., autosomal dominant, autosomal recessive, X-linked, or mitochondrial inheritance. A detailed pedigree should be drawn extending up to three generations along with horizontally spread relations of the index cases. Autosomal dominant cerebellar ataxias (ADCAs) are more common than autosomal recessive cerebellar ataxias (ARCAs), mitochondrial, and X-linked ataxias. It is also important to seek information about residence of patient and their family members with regard to their geographical region, since certain genetic mutation is uncommon in certain geographical regions. For example, in India, spinocerebellar ataxia type 12 (SCA12) is a subtype with unique prevalence in Northern India and it is confined to Agrawal ancestry. Similarly, SCA10 is mostly restricted to Brazilian and Mexican population. The identified SCA types in Indian populations are SCA1–3, SCA7, and SCA12. Other genetic ataxias have not been elucidated in India. This may be due to extensiveness of genetic testing of these disorders making it challenging in terms of cost and time or the absence of certain types of genetic ataxias in Indian population. Few genetic factors have also been reported to be associated with multiple system atrophy (MSA), but missing hereditary factors are yet to be elucidated. It is noteworthy that various late-onset genetic ataxic disorders may present with sporadic onset and need appropriate consideration, e.g., late-onset Friedreich ataxia (LOFA), SCA1–3, SCA6–8 with abnormal small expansion mutation and mitochondrial diseases.

Occupational and Substance Abuse History

Due consideration should be given in seeking history pertaining to alcohol abuse [acetaldehyde (ACD)], smoking (vascular causes), and glue sniffing.

Concurrent Drug Intake

Certain drugs, e.g., phenytoin, barbiturates, lithium, immunosuppressants (methotrexate, cyclosporine), chemotherapeutic agents (fluorouracil, cytarabine) have been known to be associated with cerebellar dysfunction manifesting ataxia.

History of Other Systemic Illness

A detailed history should also be obtained for symptoms of other system illness indicating primary disorder (neoplasia) as a cause for paraneoplastic cerebellar disorders. Patients with gluten ataxia may give history pertaining to gastrointestinal upset, chronic diarrhea, loss of weight, etc.

Neurological Examination

Detailed and extensive neurological and neuro-ophthalmological examination is essential to narrow down the final diagnosis. Neurological examination should be focused to ascertain cerebellar or noncerebellar cause of ataxia (sensory, frontal, and vestibular ataxia), symmetry of signs, and cerebellar and ataxia plus features. After having determined the type of ataxia, diagnosis should be further refined based on presence or absence of associated signs (extracerebellar features) such as pyramidal, extrapyramidal, peripheral neuropathy, and oculomotor signs.

Clinical Features and Investigations in Hereditary Ataxias

The clinical presentation of genetic ataxias is complicated and variable. In general, dominant ataxias may have pure cerebellar or cerebellar plus manifestations with widely varying age at onset. Neurological abnormalities over and above the cerebellar features have been observed in various commonly prevalent SCAs (tandem repeat expansion mutation disorders), which help in distinguishing them from each other. Episodic ataxia subtypes differ in their clinical features during episodes, i.e., episodic ataxia type 1 (EA1) (cerebellar ataxia, headache, myokymia, and interictal progression), episodic ataxia type 2 (EA2) (cerebellar ataxia, migraine, and persistent nystagmus), and episodic ataxia type 6 (EA6) (cerebellar ataxia, seizures, and hemiplegic migraine). Among X-linked ataxias, two types have been reported—fragile X-associated tremor/ataxia syndrome (FXTAS) and X-linked adrenoleukodystrophy (X-ALD). The former type is a late-onset disease (>50 years) with predominant manifestation of tremor and ataxia whereas X-ALD has onset at childhood and is characterized by spastic paraplegia, peripheral neuropathy, ataxia, hyperpigmentation, adrenal insufficiency, and hypogonadism. Recessive ataxias appear at early age (<25 years) and have peripheral neuropathy as the most common extracerebellar feature. See **Table 11** which shows diagnostic algorithm to dissect the diagnosis of specific ARCA disorder.

Clinical Manifestations and Investigations in Acquired Causes of Cerebellar Ataxias

The evaluation of sporadic or acquired causes of ataxia requires history taking aimed at identifying potential toxin exposure (drugs, e.g., phenytoin, lithium, alcohol intake, and occupational exposure to agents, e.g., mercury and lead). The history of infectious events in the past or preceding the onset of the disease should be ruled out. The biochemical tests determining vitamins level (vitamins B1, B12, and E) and autoimmune antibodies [antigliadin, antiglutamic acid decarboxylase (GAD)] level should be done. In the late-onset cases, imaging studies are conducted to screen for malignancy along with various antitumor antibodies (anti-Yo, anti-Re, etc.), to rule out PCD. Among late-onset cases, the diagnosis of MSA should be considered based on consensus criteria for MSA. The late-onset chronic cases with negative biochemical testing and genetic screening may be labeled as idiopathic late-onset cerebellar ataxia (ILOCA). The detailed clinical features (cerebellar ± noncerebellar ± extraneuronal) of various acquired causes of ataxia have been described in details below. In brief, following are the key neurological features in predominant acquired causes.

- *Alcoholic cerebellar degeneration*: Central ataxia, lower limb tremor, psychosis, and dementia are predominant neurological features. MRI shows superior cerebellar and cerebral atrophy.[1,2]
- *Drug-induced ataxia*: Mild-to-moderate dose-dependent ataxia, nystagmus, peripheral neuropathy and brisk deep tendon reflexes (DTRs) (phenytoin, carbamazepine, and lithium), generalized cerebellar syndrome, encephalopathy (anticancer drugs), cerebellar ataxia, peripheral neuropathy, myoclonus, encephalopathy, and rest tremor (amiodarone). MRI may show pancerebellar degeneration.[1,2]
- *Autoimmune diseases*: Gait ataxia, peripheral neuropathy and gluten sensitivity (gluten ataxia) and ataxia, nystagmus, and dysarthria (antiglutamate decarboxylase antibody disease).

DETAILED DESCRIPTION OF HEREDITARY AND NONHEREDITARY FORMS OF CEREBELLAR ATAXIA SUBTYPES

Hereditary Ataxias

Genetic Mutations Associated with Hereditary Ataxias

The diagnosis of hereditary ataxias is primarily dependent upon genetic investigations; thus, it is not always possible to have correct diagnostic directions only by clinical means. Diagnostic delineation of the exact etiology should involve battery of investigations comprising biochemical profiling, neuroimaging, and electrophysiological studies along with meticulous history taking, complete family history of illness, geography, and ethnicity along with neurological examination.

There are three distinct categories of mutation mechanisms known till date as the genetic defects for different ataxia causing genes:

1. Tandem nucleotide repeat (TNR) expansion (e.g., SCA1-3, Friedreich ataxia)
2. Point mutations (ataxia telangiectasia, ataxia with oculomotor apraxia, and cerebrotendinous xanthomatosis)
3. DNA structural changes affecting gene dosage (SCA15 caused by *ITPR1* gene deletion)

Of these, TNR expansion mutations are peculiar as ataxia causing factors such that a shared event, their instability by expansion (gain in the length of the repeats), irrespective of their genes predispose a person to develop a common neurodegenerative outcome.[3] There are 12 different genes with TNR expansions known. The other class of mutations are typical genetic changes, i.e., point mutations; single base substitution, deletion, and insertion all affecting protein sequences such that it results in loss of function or gain of function toward toxicity of the respective protein. The last category involves genetic events that affect the normal copy number status of the gene (SCA14) or large deletions (SCA15) in the gene affecting dosages of the respective gene product.

GENETIC SUBCLASSES

There is huge overlap among clinical and genetic features of hereditary ataxias. Following major class of genetic ataxia subtypes allows relevant clinical approach.

Among these classes, (1) SCA—refers to ADCAs, (2) spinocerebellar ataxia recessive (SCAR)—refers to ARCAs, (3) EAs—refer to episodic cerebellar ataxias, and (4) ataxia with spasticity (SPAX)—refers to ataxia with spasticity component.

Spinocerebellar Ataxias

Till date, 46 different SCA subtypes have been identified. Originally, SCAs were classified clinically by Harding[4] into three broad categories of ADCAs—ADCA I-III and later on ADCA-IV was included (**Fig. 2** and **Table 1**). SCAs due to TNR expansion exhibit anticipation, wherein there is an increase in severity and earlier age of onset of disease in successive generations. Once the disease manifests, the rate of progression is variable both among and within same SCAs. Various subclasses of SCAs and their clinical features are described in **Tables 1** to **3**. Among SCAs, TNR expansion-associated SCA has severe symptoms and is rapidly progressive as compared to SCAs caused by conventional point mutation (**Table 4**).

Clinical Features in Spinocerebellar Ataxias

The clinical presentation of genetic ataxia is complicated and variable. In general, dominant ataxia may have pure cerebellar or cerebellar plus manifestations with widely varying age at onset. **Table 2** shows cerebellar plus signs in various commonly prevalent SCAs (tandem repeat expansion mutation disorders), which help in distinguishing them among each other.

Autosomal Dominant Cerebellar Ataxias-I

Following is the description of prevalent ataxia types such as SCA1-3 and SCA12.

Clinical Features

Most prevalent group of SCAs, e.g., SCA1, SCA2, SCA3 belong to this group and have prominent cerebellar ataxias and are associated with one or more features such as peripheral neuropathy in the form of pure sensory (S) in SCA2 or motor (M) and mixed SM neuropathy in SCA1-3; muscle atrophy in SCA2 and facial muscle atrophy in SCA3; pyramidal, i.e., Babinski sign, exaggerated tendon reflexes, and spasticity in SCA1 and SCA3; reduced reflexes in SCA2; extrapyramidal features, i.e., Parkinsonism (SCA2 and SCA3), dystonia, rigidity, dyskinesias prominently in SCA3; and SCA12,[5,6] a unique type, which is confined to Indian population, is characterized by tremor/ataxia syndrome.[7]

Genotype-phenotype Correlation

The genotype-phenotype correlation in some of SCAs shows that the severity of cerebellar and extracerebellar symptoms correlates with the repeat length and disease duration, while oculomotor abnormalities do not correlate with repeat length. In SCA2, repeat lengths in low abnormal range, e.g., 32-38 with interruption are well documented with Parkinsonian phenotype and intermediate repeat of CAG length (27-33 CAG/CAA) has been recently documented with occurrence of amyotrophic lateral sclerosis. In SCA3, four Machado-Joseph disease (MJD)

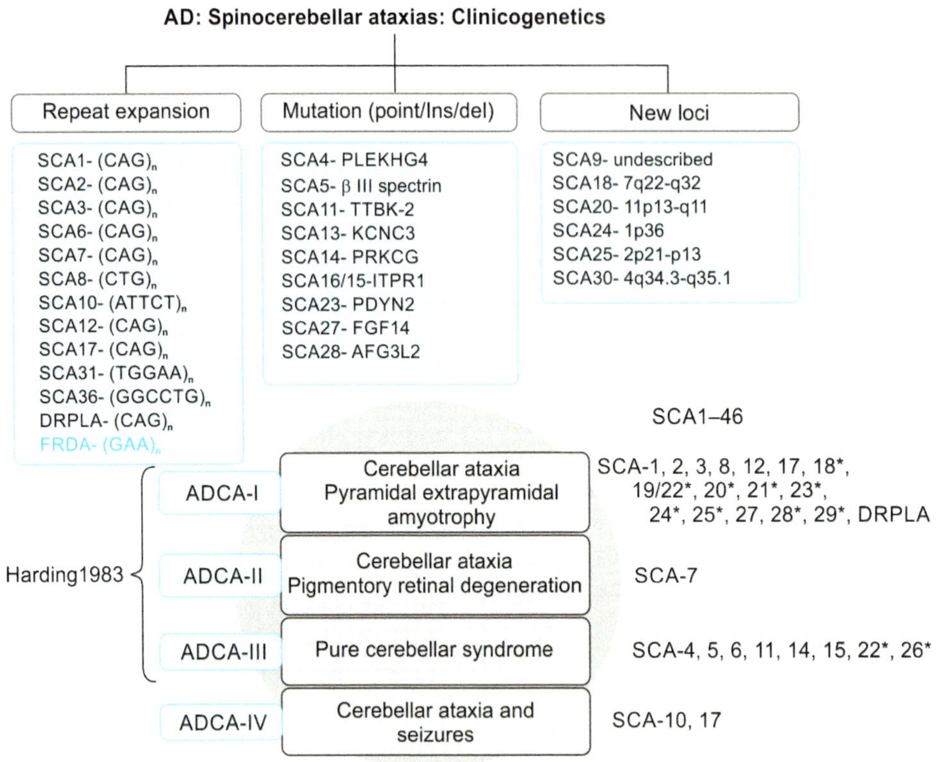

FIG. 2: Various subclasses of autosomal dominantly inherited ataxias.

TABLE 1: Molecular genetics of spinocerebellar ataxias (SCAs) associated with repeat expansion.[5,6,8-11]

SCA types	*Gene*	*Chromosome*	*Mutation*	*Normal allele*	*Reduce penetrance*	*Pathogenic*
Autosomal dominant cerebellar ataxias-I (ADCA-I) (cerebellar ataxia, peripheral neuropathy, ocular movement abnormality, and pyramidal and extrapyramidal involvement)						
SCA1	ATXN1	6p22.3	$(CAG)_n$	29–30	39	40–82
SCA2	ATXN2	12q24.13	$(CAG)_n$	13–29	NR	32–200
SCA3	ATXN3	14q32.12	$(CAG)_n$	13–36	45–51	61–84
SCA8	ATXN8OS	13q21	$(CTG)_n$	15–50	71–80	>80
SCA12	PPP2R2B	5q32	$(CAG)_n$	4–32	40–41	>45
DRPLA	ATN1	12p13.31	$(CAG)_n$	6–35	NR	>48
SCA31	BEAN	16q	$(TGGAA)_n$	NR	NR	2,500–3,800
SCA36	NOP6	20p13	$(GGCCTG)_n$	3–8	NR	1,700–2,300
ADCA-II (cerebellar ataxia, retinal degeneration, and pyramidal and extrapyramidal involvement)						
SCA7	ATXN7	3p14.1	$(CAG)_n$	7–19	34–36	37–306
ADCA-III (pure cerebellar form)						
SCA6	CACNA1A	19p13.13	$(CAG)_n$	<18	19	>20–29
ADCA-IV (cerebellar ataxia + seizures, dementia, and psychomotor disturbances in SCA17)						
SCA10	ATXN10	22q13.31	$(ATTCT)_n$	10–29	280–370	500–4,500
SCA17	TBP	6q27	$(CAG)_n$	25–40	41–48	>49

TABLE 2: Clinically distinguishing signs among spinocerebellar ataxias (SCAs).

Features	*SCA types*
Benign course	SCA6
Pyramidal features	SCA1, 7, 8, and 3
Parkinsonian features	SCA3, 2, 17, 12, and 21
Chorea	SCA2, 1, and 3
Action tremor	SCA12 and 16
Slow saccades	SCA2 and 7 may be in 1, 3
Downbeat nystagmus	SCA6
Peripheral neuropathy	SCA2, 4, 3, 19, and 21
Retinal degeneration	SCA7 and SCA2
Seizure	SCA10
Myoclonus	SCA14 or SCA19
Cognitive impairment	SCA2, 14, 19, 21, and 23

TABLE 3: Clinically distinguishing signs among spinocerebellar ataxias (SCAs).

Features	*SCA types*
Benign course	SCA6
Pyramidal features	SCA1, 7, 8, and 3
Parkinsonian features	SCA3, 2, 17, 12, and 21
Chorea	SCA2, 1, and 3
Action tremor	SCA12 and 16
Slow saccades	SCA2 and 7 may be in 1, 3
Downbeat nystagmus	SCA6
Peripheral neuropathy	SCA2, 4, 3, 19, and 21
Retinal degeneration	SCA7 and SCA2
Seizure	SCA10
Myoclonus	SCA14 or SCA19
Cognitive impairment	SCA2, 14, 19, 21, and 23

TABLE 4: Differentiating features among TNR and non-TNR-associated SCAs.

Conventional mutation SCA	*Repeat expansion SCA*
Variable age at onset (no anticipation)	Variable (intrafamilial); anticipation
Slowly progressive ataxias	Rapid progression
Childhood onset and less severe	Juvenile onset and more severe
Predominant Purkinje cell loss	Diffuse neuronal cell loss

(SCAs: spinocerebellar ataxias; TNR: tandem nucleotide repeat)

variants have been described:[8] MJD type 1: Extrapyramidal (especially dystonic) and pyramidal deficits, early onset (10–30 years), and mean repeat length 80; MJD type 2: Pyramidal and cerebellar deficits, intermediate onset (20–50 years), and mean repeat length 76; MJD type 3: Cerebellar deficits and peripheral neuropathy, late onset (40–75 years), and mean repeat length 73; MJD type 4: Peripheral neuropathy and Parkinsonism, variable onset, and no predilection to a particular pathogenic range; and MJD type 5: Hereditary spastic paraplegic type. Autonomic dysfunction is frequently present in SCA3.

Autosomal Dominant Cerebellar Ataxias-II

Only SCA type 7 is categorized in ADCA-II and cerebellar ataxia and retinal degeneration are hallmark of the disease. Marked pyramidal involvement (hyperreflexia and spasticity) helps to differentiate it from SCA2 and slow saccades can be the earliest finding. In SCA7, highest degree of anticipation is observed and there is significant correlation between repeat length and onset of cerebellar ataxia and retinal degeneration. CAG expansion <49 is associated with gait ataxia preceding retinal degeneration and reverse is observed with >49 repeat expansion. Juvenile cases are reported with repeat expansion beyond 70–80 and CAG >200 or 400 has been described with infantile onset and manifests with multisystemic involvement including failure to thrive, cardiac abnormalities, and respiratory distress.[12-14]

Autosomal Dominant Cerebellar Ataxias-III

Hereditary pure form of cerebellar ataxia is described under this category. SCA6 presents with late onset and slow progression, characterized mainly by pure cerebellar ataxia. Gait ataxia is more pronounced than appendicular ataxia. Oculomotor findings are gaze-evoked nystagmus and impaired pursuit movements in the majority of the patient. Infrequently, downbeat nystagmus, ophthalmoparesis, and hypermetric saccades can be observed.

Prevalence

The relative frequencies of SCAs designated under ADCA category vary geographically and also differ among various ethnicities. In general, among repeat expansion-associated SCAs, SCA1, SCA2, and SCA3 are the most prevalent types worldwide. Among the three, SCA3/MJD seems to be the major subtype worldwide and also represents >70% of the SCA cases in Portugal. On the other hand, dentatorubral-pallidoluysian atrophy (DRPLA) is mostly reported from Japan, SCA10 in Brazil and Mexican population, and SCA12 from India.[5,6] Other TNR-linked subtypes, i.e., SCA6, SCA7, SCA8, SCA17, and SCA31 are relatively less among SCA cohort studied across the world. Except for SCA14 and SCA15, which have been reported in various populations and frequency seems to be higher than anticipated, remaining conventional mutation-associated SCAs are very rare and were observed among only few families.

Penta- and Hexanucleotide Repeat Expansion-associated Spinocerebellar Ataxias[15]

SCA31 and SCA36

The endemic SCA type, SCA31, has been recently genetically characterized from Nagano region of Japan in 2009 by Sato et al. The causative mutation of SCA31 is in *BEAN* gene, which is an expanded pentanucleotide (TGGAA) repeat insertion of 2.5–3.8 kb size in intronic region. Clinically, it is a pure cerebellar variant of SCA (ADCA-III), characterized by ataxia of gait, upper extremities, and dysarthria along with hyperreflexia, hypotonia, and nystagmus. Audiometric evidence of sensorineural loss has been described. Imaging is characterized by isolated cerebellar atrophy without involvement of brainstem. Kobayashi et al. described another unique SCA type with features of cerebellar ataxia and motor neuron disease which they termed SCA36. The reported pathological mutation was a hexanucleotide repeat, GGCCTG expansion (1,700–2,300 repeats, normal repeats 3–8) in intron 1 of *NOP6* on chromosome 20p13. The disease has been found in Japanese population of Chugoku district. The onset of disease was in fourth to fifth decades, with typical features of cerebellar ataxia with tongue fasciculations and atrophy. Some patients may develop atrophy and fasciculations in proximal muscles, but at a later stage. Mild-to-moderate degree of brisk reflexes were noted. Nerve conduction studies were normal; however, neurogenic changes were seen on electromyographic studies in patients with muscle disease. MRI of the brain shows mild cerebellar atrophy.[11]

Nontandem Nucleotide Repeat and Other Genetic Subtypes of Ataxias

Differentiating features among TNR and non-TNR associated ataxias are explained in **Table 3**. Clinical features of other rare and non-TNR- associated SCA subtypes has been provided in tabular form (refer **Table 5**). **Table 6** shows clinical and genetic characteristics of some of the key SCAs associated with conventional mutations (non-TRE SCAs).

Episodic Ataxias

The EAs are characterized by periods (i.e., minutes to hours) of unsteady gait. EAs are often associated with nystagmus or dysarthria. Myokymia, vertigo, or hearing loss may occur in some of the subtypes. Permanent ataxia and even cerebellar atrophy may occur late in the disease course. **Table 7** shows clinical features of various types of EAs and their differentiating features.

Other Genetic Subtypes of Ataxias

Among X-linked ataxias, two types have been reported—FXTAS and X-ALD. The former type is a late-onset disease (>50 years) with predominant manifestation of tremor and ataxia[13,16] whereas X-ALD onsets at childhood age and is characterized by spastic paraplegia, peripheral neuropathy, ataxia, hyperpigmentation, adrenal insufficiency, and hypogonadism. Other rare X-linked ataxias are linked to genes such as *CASK*, *OPHN1*, *SLC9A6*, and Xq25 loci. Clinical and genetic features of X-linked ataxias have been summarized in **Table 8**. **Table 9** shows various differentiating feature of autosomal dominant (AD) or autosomal recessive (AR) ataxia with spasticity (SPAX).

TABLE 5: Clinical features of other rare and non-TNR-associated SCA subtypes.[9]

Early onset <30 years	*late onset >30 years*	*Variable age at onset*
SCA13-with or without mental retardation	SCA11-slow progression	SCA4-sensory neuropathy
SCA13-↓↓DTR	SCA32-azoospermia	SCA5-sensory neuropathy
SCA21-↓↓DTR	SCA23-distal sensory neuropathy	SCA14-extrapymidal, myocionus
SCA27-Orofacial dyskinesia, per cavus	SCA34-papulosquamous erythematous plaques	SCA15-truncal ataxia
SCA29-Cerebellar hypoplasia	SCA35-slow progression	SCA19/22-cogwheel rigidity, amyotrophy
	SCA30-lower limb ↑DTR	SCA20-palatal tremor
	SCA31-SNHL	SCA25-FRDA like
	SCA36-and fasciolingual amyotrophy	SCA26-pure cerebellar
		SCA28-slow progression

(DTR: deep tendon reflex; FRDA: Friedreich's ataxia; SCA: spinocerebellar ataxia; SNHL: sensorineural hearing loss; TNR: tandem nucleotide repeat)

TABLE 6: Clinical and genetic characteristics of some of the key SCAs associated with conventional mutations (non-TRE SCAs).

SCA	*Gene*	*Chromosome*	*Mutation(s)*	*Clinical features*
SCA5	*SPTBN2*	11q13	39-bp Del exon 12, 15-bp del exon 14, and T>C in exon 7	Cerebellar ataxia, sensory impairment, hyporeflexia or hyperreflexia, downbeat or horizontal nystagmus, and impaired smooth pursuit movement
SCA11	*TTBK2*	15q14-q21.3	1 bp (A) insertion and frameshift 2 bp deletion in exon 13	Slow progressive pure cerebellar syndrome, jerky pursuit, and horizontal or vertical nystagmus tendon hyperreflexia without Babinski sign
SCA13	*KCNC3*	19q13	1639C>A and 1554G>A	Early-onset cerebellar ataxia, slow progression, and associated mental retardation (French). Adult late-onset cerebellar ataxia without mental retardation (Filipino) and hyperreflexia without Babinski sign and absence of seizures
SCA14	*PRKCG*	19q13.4-q	Multiple mutations	Cerebellar ataxia, hyperreflexia, cognitive decline, depression, myoclonic jerks, mild extrapyramidal features, and reduction of vibration senses in lower limbs
SCA15	*ITPR1*	3p26.2	Deletion of ITPR1 and SUMF1	Truncal ataxia, head tremor, cognitive impairment, and saccadic eye movements
SCA23	*PDYN2*	20p13	c.414G>T, c.643C>T, c.632T>C, and c.634C>T	Gait impairment, head tremor, gaze fixation instability, very mild dysarthria, action tremor of the hands and a subtle ataxia of the hands and arm, and distal sensory neuropathy
SCA27	*FGF14*	13q34	C.434 T>C in exon 4	Early-onset gait ataxia, dysmetric saccades, nystagmus, emotional outbursts, orofacial dyskinesias, truncal tremor, impairment in memory and executive functioning, depression, and pes cavus
SCA28	*AFG3L2*	18p11.22-q11.2	Multiple mutations in exon 10, exon 15, and exon 16	Slowly progressive early-onset cerebellar ataxia, hyperreflexia, nystagmus, slow saccades, and ophthalmoplegia

(SCAs: spinocerebellar ataxias; TNR: tandem nucleotide repeat)

TABLE 7: Clinical features of episodic ataxia (EA) subtypes.

Disease	*Gene/ Locus*	*Distinguishing clinical features*
EA1	*KCNA1*	• Gait ataxia, attacks lasting seconds to minutes, and startle or exercise induced • Myokymia and no vertigo
EA2	*CACNA1A*	• Gait ataxia, nystagmus, attacks lasting minutes to hours, and posture change induced • Vertigo, later permanent ataxia
EA3	1q42	• Adult onset, vertigo • Tinnitus
EA4	–	Adult onset
EA5	*CACNB4*	Childhood to adolescent onset
EA6	*SLC1A3*	• Seizures and migraine • Childhood onset
EA7	19q13	• Vertigo and Weakness • Seizures • Childhood to adolescent onset

TABLE 8: Clinical and genetic features of X-linked ataxias.[16]

Locus	*Disease*	*Distinguishing clinical features*
FMR1	Fragile X-associated tremor/ataxia syndrome (FXTAS)	Adult onset
ABCB7	X-linked sideroblastic anemia and ataxia (XLSA/A)	• Early childhood onset • Anemia is asymptomatic
CASK	*CASK*-related disorders	• Cognitive deficiency • Microcephaly • Hypotonia • Optic nerve hypoplasia
OPHN1	X-linked mental retardation with cerebellar hypoplasia and distinctive facial appearance	• Infantile onset • Hypotonia • Developmental delay • Seizures
SLC9A6	Syndromic X-linked mental retardation and Christianson type	• Infantile onset • Intellectual disability • Seizures
Xq25-q27.1	X-linked spinocerebellar ataxia 5	• Infantile onset • Cerebellar hypoplasia

TABLE 9: Autosomal dominant (AD) or autosomal recessive (AR) ataxia with spasticity (SPAX).

Disease (MOI)	*Gene*	*Distinguishing clinical features*
SPAX1 (AD)	*VAMP1*	• Initial progressive leg spasticity • Gait ataxia
SPAX2 (AR)	*KIF1C*	Often w/childhood-onset tremor and dysmetria
SPAX3 (AR)	*MARS2*	Periventricular white matter changes
SPAX4 (AR)	*MTPAP*	Optic atrophy
SPAX5 (AR)	*AFG3L2*	Often w/peripheral neuropathy and epilepsy
SPG7 (AR)	*SPG7*	• Vestibular failure • Cerebellar atrophy

Autosomal Recessive Ataxias[17,18]

More than 40 genes are known to cause SCAR. The disease is infantile to juvenile onset (usually <25 years). Clinically, cerebellar ataxias with predominant peripheral neuropathy are observed. Other features are found in different types of SCAR, which help them to distinguish among each other, i.e., cardiac involvement, muscle involvement, immunodeficiency, metabolic derangements, etc., Friedreich's ataxia (FRDA) and ataxia telangiectasia are most prevalent forms of SCAR.[18-20] Four major types of pathological molecular alteration in cellular processes have been illustrated in conjunction with various mutations in respective genes of ARCAs which include: (1) mitochondrial pathology, (2) lipid metabolism alterations, (3) impairment of DNA repair pathway, (4) protein folding, and (5) cerebellar malformation (**Table 10**).

We propose and present clinically diagnostic grouping of these disorders based on neurophysiological and MRI imaging observations, which aims at early diagnosis and investigatory directions of genetically and clinically heterogeneous group of ARCAs (**Table 11**).[12,17]

TABLE 10: Different SCAR types and their underlying molecular defect.[13,14,17,19]

Mitochondrial defect	*Genes*	*Chromosome*
Friedreich's ataxis	FXN	9q13
Infantile onset cerebellar ataxia (IOCA)	C10orf2	10q24
CoQ10 deficinecy adult	UK	UK
Metabolic impairment		
Ataxia with vitamin E deficiency (AVED)	TTPA	8q13.1-13.3
Abetalipoproteinemia (ABL)	MTP	4q22-24
Cerebello tendinous xanthomatosis (CTX)	CYP27	2q33-tex
Late-onset Tay-sachs disease (LOTS)	HEXA	15q23-24
DNA repair defect		
Ataxia Telengiectasia (AT)	ATM	11q22-23
Ataxia Telengiectasia like disorder (ATLD)	MRE11	11q21
Ataxia with occulomotor apraxia 1 (AOA1)	APTX	9p13
Ataxia with occulomotor apraxia 2 (AOA2)	SETX	9q34
Spinocerebellar ataxia with axonal neuropathy (SCAN1)	TDP1	14q31-32
Mitochondrial recessive ataxia syndrome (MIRAS)	POLG	15q22-26
Protein folding defect		
Authosomal recessive ataxia of charlevoix-Saquenay (ARSACS)	SACS	13q11
Marinesco–Sjögren's syndrome (MSS)	SIL1	5q31
Refsum disease	PHYH, PEX7	10pter-11.2, 6q21-22.2

Work Flow for Genetic Investigation Direction in Clinical Setting

Due to larger number of mutations and genetic etiologies, the genetic investigations always remains challenging; however, with help of clinical cues and biochemical features, it is sometimes possible to order a gene-specific investigations (refer **Flowchart 1**). For SCAs, in general, the first-order tests remain the panel testing for trinucleotide repeat expansion ataxia (SCA1-3, SCA6, SCA7, SCA10, SCA12, and SCA17). The second-order tests for SCAs may be adoption of either next generation sequencing (NGS)-based investigations of gene panel sequencing or whole exome sequencing. For recessive ataxia, testing FRDA is straightforward and inconclusive cases can then be subjected to NGS-based testing panel. The work flow we followed at AIIMS-IGIB research collaboration is as following for cost-effective diagnosis (**Flowchart 1**).

Sporadic Cerebellar Ataxias

Sporadic cerebellar ataxias (SpCAs) (without the family history) show late onset or variable age at onset of clinical manifestations of cerebellar ataxia mimicking one or the other hereditary ataxias—recessive (early-onset cases) or dominant (late-onset cases). SpCAs can be caused by acquired events due to drug toxicity, vitamin deficiencies (vitamin B12 and vitamin E), and certain infection-associated cerebellar degeneration. PCD has been associated with certain malignancies and is characterized by presence of serum antibodies (anti-Yo antibody, anti-Hu in lung cell carcinoma, and anti-Tr) (See **Box 3** and **Tables 12** and **13**).[21,22]

TABLE 11: Clinical outline toward approach to cerebellar ataxia with recessive inheritance.

NCV	*MRI*	*Diagnosis*	*Distinguishable features*
Sensory axonal neuropathy	Spinal atrophy	FRDA	Cardiomyopathy
	Spinal/Cerebellar	IOSCA	Seizures
	Normal	AVED	*RP, low vitamin E*, and cardiomyopathy
		ABL	Low lipoproteins *acanthocytes*
Sensory motor axonal neuropathy	Cerebellar atrophy	AT	Telangiectasia, *High AFP*, low Ig, and radiosensitivity
		ATL	Low Ig
		AOA1	Oculomotor apraxia, High cholesterol
		AOA2	Oculomotor apraxia, *high AF**P***, high cholesterol
	Spinal-cerebellar atrophy	ARSACS	Spasticity, *hypermyelinated retinal fibers*
	Cerebellar atrophy + WMH	CTX	*Tendon xanthomas, cataract, High bile alcohol and cholesterol*
Sensory motor demyelinating neuropathy	Cerebellar	MSS	Psychomotor impairment
	Normal	Refsum disease	High phytanic acid

(RP: retinitis pigmentosa; Ig: immunoglobulin)

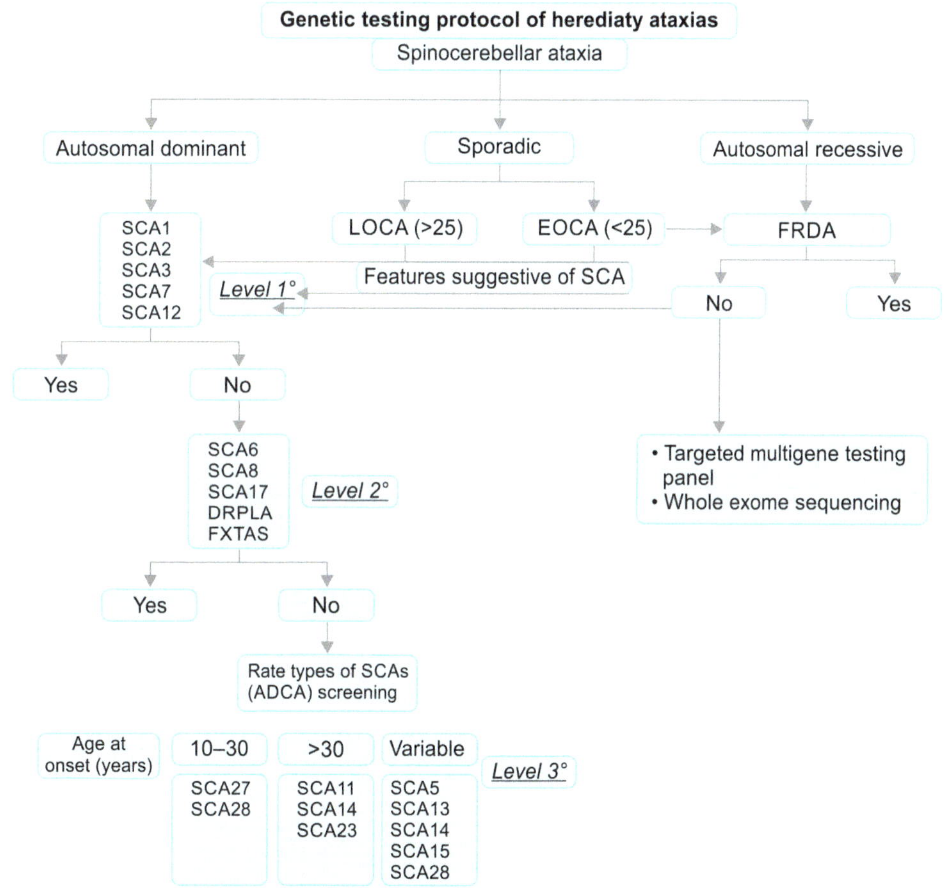

(ADCA: autosomal dominant cerebellar ataxia; EOCA: early-onset cerebellar ataxia; FRDA: Friedreich's ataxia; LOCA: late-onset cerebellar ataxia; SCA: spinocerebellar ataxia)

FLOWCHART 1: Genetic testing workflow for hereditary ataxias.

Box 3 Etiologies of sporadic-onset cerebellar degeneration.

- *Toxins and drugs*: Alcohol, mercury, lead, phenytoin, carbamazepine, amiadarone, anticancer drugs (5-fluorouracil, methotrexate), and cyclosporine[1,23,24]
- *Vitamin deficiency*: Vitamins B1, B12 and E[25,26]
- *Autoimmunity*: Paraneoplastic, antigliadin antibody (Ab), and anti-GAD Ab[27,28]
- *Infection*: Typhoid, malaria, tuberculosis, HIV, and spirochete infection
- *Hereditary SCAs (very late-onset genetic SCAs)*: SCA6, SCA1–3, SCA12, and SCA8
- *Miscellaneous:* Multiple system atrophy-cerebellar (MSA-C) and idiopathic late-onset cerebellar ataxia[29,30]

(GAD: glutamic acid decarboxylase; HIV: human immunodeficiency virus; SCA: spinocerebellar ataxia)

TABLE 12: Clinical features of certain acquired and sporadic causes of ataxias.[25-27,31,32]

Causes	*Agent*	*Clinical features*	*Investigations*
Toxins	Alcohol	Central ataxia, lower limb tremor, psychosis, and dementia	MRI—superior cerebellar and cerebral atrophy
	Mercury and lead	Peripheral neuropathy, gait ataxia, and other nonneural symptoms	History of occupational or accidental chronic exposure and MRI—cerebellar atrophy (Hg—middle and lower cerebellar hemisphere and Pb—pancerebellar atrophy)
Drugs	Anticonvulsant—phenytoin, carbamazepine	Mild-to-moderate dose-dependent ataxia, nystagmus, peripheral neuropathy, and brisk DTR	Serum level of drug, MRI—variable atrophy of cerebellum
	Anticancer drugs—5-fluorouracil and cytosine arabinoside	Generalized cerebellar syndrome and encephalopathy	MRI—pancerebellar atrophy
	Lithium	Cerebellar syndrome, tremors, and hyperreflexia	Serum Li level and history of concomitant treatment—CPZ
	Amiadarone	Cerebellar ataxia, peripheral neuropathy, myoclonus, encephalopathy, and rest tremor	MRI—cerebellar atrophy
Infections	Bacteria—*Salmonella*, *Borrelia*, and *Rickettsia*	Acute/Subacute onset of UL/BL cerebellitis with history of fever and associated signs	Blood study/PCR-based identification of agent and CSF studies
	Viral—EBV, influenza, and HIV	Acute/Subacute onset of UL/BL cerebellitis, eye movement abnormalities, and peripheral neuropathy with preceding or concomitant history of fever and associated signs	PCR-based Ag identification, anti-GQ1b, anti-GM Ab, and CSF studies
Sporadic CJD	Prion protein	Dementia, ataxia, and other neurological abnormality with rapid progression	EEG, CSF-14-3-3 proteins, MRI—cortical, putamen, thalamic and cerebellar atrophy, and PRNP mutations
Cerebellar abscess	Tuberculosis, septic emboli, and cyanotic heart disease	Acute onset unilateral or bilateral cerebellar ataxia, headache, and papilledema	MRI—small diffuse or single hypodense lesion
Autoimmune diseases	Anti-GAD antibodies (Ab)	Mild-to-severe degree of cerebellar ataxia and nystagmus, thyroiditis, and diabetes mellitus	MRI—cerebellar atrophy and serum detection of anti-GAD[33]
Gluten ataxia	IgA/IgG antigliadin Ab, Antiendomyscial Ab, and Ab against tissue transglutaminase	Gait ataxia, peripheral neuropathy, and gluten sensitivity	Serum—IgA, IgG-antigliadin, antiendomyscium, TTG, MRI—cerebellar atrophy and WMH, intestinal biopsy

Continued

Continued

Causes	*Agent*	*Clinical features*	*Investigations*
Vitamin deficiency	Vitamin B1	Acute or subacute onset, psychosis, dementia, confusion, seizures, and peripheral neuropathy	Serum vitamin B1 level and MRI
	Vitamin B12	Sensory ataxia and megaloblastic anemia	Serum vitamin B12 level and peripheral smear
	Vitamin E	Cerebellar syndrome, sensory neuropathy, and reflexia	Vitamin E level
Paraneoplastic disorders	Various antibodies against neuronal molecules	Subacute onset, cerebellar features, and carcinoma detection	Serum/CSF-specific Ab, PET scan—hypometabolism in cerebellar cortex

(CSF: cerebrospinal fluid; DTR: deep tendon reflex; EBV: Epstein-Barr virus; EEG: electroencephalography; GAD: glutamic acid decarboxylase; HIV: human immunodeficiency virus; IgA: immunoglobulin A; PET: positron emission tomography; PCR: polymerase chain reaction; WMH: white matter hyperintensity)

TABLE 13: Paraneoplastic syndrome degeneration (PCD)-associated antibodies and related cancers.[21,22]

Antibodies	*Conditions*
Anti-Yo (Purkinje cell antibody type 1)	Breast and ovarian carcinoma
Anti-Hu (antineuronal nuclear antibody type 1)	Small cell lung carcinoma (SCLC)
Anti-Tr	Hodgkin lymphoma
Anti-mGluR1 (metabotropic glutamate receptor)	Hodgkin lymphoma
Anti-Ri (antineuronal nuclear antibody type 1)	SCLC, breast, ovarian carcinoma
Anti-VGCC (voltage-gated calcium channel)	SCLC
Anti-CRMP5 (collapsin receptor-mediated protein)/Anti-CV2	SCLC
Anti-ZIC4 (zinc finger protein)	SCLC

CONCLUSION

Detailed history and family pedigree along with meticulous clinical examination remains the cornerstone for the diagnosis of ataxias. Even in cases of genetic ataxias, it narrows down the differential diagnosis and helps in focused genetic testing. Recent progress in the elucidation of the genetic and molecular causes of ataxias along with the definition of clinical diagnostic criteria and delineation of characteristic MRI features have greatly facilitated the correct diagnosis of the various forms of sporadic ataxias. Nevertheless, asubstantial number of patients are still tentatively labeled as having SAOA because the disease-causing factors are unknown. Since the delineation of many of the various subcategories of sporadic ataxia was achieved only recently, knowledge of the clinical features, naturalhistory, and epidemiology of these disorders is still very limited. Despite the knowledge of specific causes of ataxia disorders, effective therapies are currently available for only a small proportion of patients. Thus, the greatest challenge for future research is the development of effective therapies for patients with ataxia.

REFERENCES

1. De Marcos FA, Ghizoni E, Kobayashi E, Li LM, Cendes F. Cerebellar volume and long-term use of phenytoin. Seizure. 2003;12(5):312-5.
2. Rittmannsberger H, Leblhuber F. Asterixis induced by carbamazepine therapy. Biol Psychiatry. 1992;32(4):364-8.
3. Cummings CJ, Zoghbi HY. Trinucleotide repeats: mechanisms and pathophysiology. Annu Rev Genomics Hum Genet. 2000;1:281-328.
4. Harding AE. Classification of the hereditary ataxias and paraplegias. Lancet Lond Engl. 1983;1(8334):1151-5.
5. Fujigasaki H, Verma IC, Camuzat A, Margolis RL, Zander C, Lebre AS, et al. SCA12 is a rare locus for autosomal dominant cerebellar ataxia: a study of an Indian family. Ann Neurol. 2001;49(1):117-21.
6. Holmes SE, Hearn EO, Ross CA, Margolis RL. SCA12: an unusual mutation leads to an unusual spinocerebellar ataxia. Brain Res Bull. 2001;56(3–4):397-403.
7. Schöls L, Bauer P, Schmidt T, Schulte T, Riess O. Autosomal dominant cerebellar ataxias: clinical features, genetics, and pathogenesis. Lancet Neurol. 2004;3(5):291-304.

8. Riess O, Rüb U, Pastore A, Bauer P, Schöls L. SCA3: neurological features, pathogenesis and animal models. Cerebellum Lond Engl. 2008;7(2):125-37.
9. Nagaoka U, Takashima M, Ishikawa K, Yoshizawa K, Yoshizawa T, Ishikawa M, et al. A gene on SCA4 locus causes dominantly inherited pure cerebellar ataxia. Neurology. 2000;54(10):1971-5.
10. Stevanin G, Durr A, Benammar N, Brice A. Spinocerebellar ataxia with mental retardation (SCA13). Cerebellum Lond Engl. 2005;4(1):43-6.
11. Kobayashi H, Abe K, Matsuura T, Ikeda Y, Hitomi T, Akechi Y, et al. Expansion of intronic GGCCTG hexanucleotide repeat in NOP56 causes SCA36, a type of spinocerebellar ataxia accompanied by motor neuron involvement. Am J Hum Genet. 2011;89(1):121-30.Fogel BL, Perlman S. Clinical features and molecular genetics of autosomal recessive cerebellar ataxias. Lancet Neurol. 2007;6(3):245-57.
12. Fogel BL, Perlman S. Clinical features and molecular genetics of autosomal recessive cerebellar ataxias. Lancet Neurol. 2007;6(3):245-57.
13. Moghadasian MH. Cerebrotendinous xanthomatosis: clinical course, genotypes and metabolic backgrounds. Clin Investig Med Clin Exp. 2004;27(1):42-50.
14. Verrips A, van Engelen BG, ter Laak H, Gabreëls-Festen A, Janssen A, Zwarts M, et al. Cerebrotendinous xanthomatosis. Controversies about nerve and muscle: observations in ten patients. Neuromuscul Disord NMD. 2000;10(6):407-14.
15. Sato N, Amino T, Kobayashi K, Asakawa S, Ishiguro T, Tsunemi T, et al. Spinocerebellar Ataxia Type 31 Is Associated with "Inserted" Penta-Nucleotide Repeats Containing (TGGAA)n. Am J Hum Genet. 2009;85(5):544-57.
16. Jacquemont S, Hagerman RJ, Leehey M, Grigsby J, Zhang L, Brunberg JA, et al. Fragile X premutation tremor/ataxia syndrome: molecular, clinical, and neuroimaging correlates. Am J Hum Genet. 2003;72(4):869-78.
17. Embiruçu EK, Martyn ML, Schlesinger D, Kok F. Autosomal recessive ataxias: 20 types, and counting. Arq Neuropsiquiatr. 2009;67(4):1143-56.
18. Dürr A, Cossee M, Agid Y, Campuzano V, Mignard C, Penet C, et al. Clinical and genetic abnormalities in patients with Friedreich's ataxia. N Engl J Med. 1996;335(16):1169-75.
19. Pandolfo M. Friedreich ataxia: the clinical picture. J Neurol. 2009;256 Suppl 1:3-8.
20. Schulz JB, Boesch S, Bürk K, Dürr A, Giunti P, Mariotti C, et al. Diagnosis and treatment of Friedreich ataxia: a European perspective. Nat Rev Neurol. 2009;5(4):222-34.
21. Linke R, Schroeder M, Helmberger T, Voltz R. Antibody-positive paraneoplastic neurologic syndromes: value of CT and PET for tumor diagnosis. Neurology. 2004;63(2):282-6.
22. Rojas I, Graus F, Keime-Guibert F, Reñé R, Delattre JY, Ramón JM, et al. Long-term clinical outcome of paraneoplastic cerebellar degeneration and anti-Yo antibodies. Neurology. 2000;55(5):713-5.
23. Mani J, Chaudhary N, Kanjalkar M, Shah PU. Cerebellar ataxia due to lead encephalopathy in an adult. J Neurol Neurosurg Psychiatry. 1998;65(5):797-8.
24. Garretto NS, Rey RD, Kohler G, Cocorullo S, Monteverde DA, Ravera BI, et al. Cerebellar syndrome caused by amiodarone. Arq Neuropsiquiatr. 1994;52(4):575-7.
25. Adachi S, Kawamoto T, Otsuka M, Todoroki T, Fukao K. Enteral vitamin B12 supplements reverse postgastrectomy B12 deficiency. Ann Surg. 2000;232(2):199-201.
26. Harding AE, Muller DP, Thomas PK, Willison HJ. Spinocerebellar degeneration secondary to chronic intestinal malabsorption: a vitamin E deficiency syndrome. Ann Neurol. 1982;12(5):419-24.
27. Hadjivassiliou M, Grünewald RA, Chattopadhyay AK, Davies-Jones GA, Gibson A, Jarratt JA, et al. Clinical, radiological, neurophysiological, and neuropathological characteristics of gluten ataxia. Lancet Lond Engl. 1998;352(9140):1582-5.
28. Marignier R, Chenevier F, Rogemond V, Smitt PS, Renoux C, Cavillon G, et al. Metabotropic glutamate receptor type 1 autoantibody-associated cerebellitis: a primary autoimmune disease? Arch Neurol. 2010;67(5):627-30.
29. Gilman S, Wenning GK, Low PA, Brooks DJ, Mathias CJ, Trojanowski JQ, et al. Second consensus statement on the diagnosis of multiple system atrophy. Neurology. 2008;71(9):670-6.
30. Muzaimi MB, Thomas J, Palmer-Smith S, Rosser L, Harper PS, Wiles CM, et al. Population-based study of late-onset cerebellar ataxia in south east Wales. J Neurol Neurosurg Psychiatry. 2004;75(8):1129-34.
31. Klockgether T. Sporadic ataxia with adult onset: classification and diagnostic criteria. Lancet Neurol. 2010;9(1):94-104.
32. Zerr I, Kallenberg K, Summers DM, Romero C, Taratuto A, Heinemann U, et al. Updated clinical diagnostic criteria for sporadic Creutzfeldt-Jakob disease. Brain J Neurol. 2009;132(Pt 10):2659-68.
33. Lauria G, Pareyson D, Pitzolu MG, Bazzigaluppi E. Excellent response to steroid treatment in anti-GAD cerebellar ataxia. Lancet Neurol. 2003;2(10):634-5.

SECTION

10

OTHER MOVEMENT DISORDERS

CHAPTER 48

Restless Legs Syndrome

Kaushik Sen

INTRODUCTION

Restless legs syndrome (RLS), also known as Willis–Ekbom syndrome, is a neurological sensorimotor disorder that often disturbs sleep.[1] It is characterized by irresistible urge to move the limbs during the period of rest or sleep due to an abnormal unpleasant sensations involving the limbs.[2] The symptoms are transiently relieved by movement but once the patient ceases activity, the symptoms may return. In very severe cases of RLS, prolonged periods of activity may provide minimal to low relief of symptoms.[3] Numerous studies have highlighted primary care physicians' lack of awareness to adequately diagnose the disorder.[4]

HISTORICAL PERSPECTIVE

The symptoms of RLS were first described by Willis in 1685 and then published by Ekbom in 1945.[5] Thomas Willis in 1685 wrote: "*Wherefore to some, when being a bed, they betake themselves to sleep, presently in the arms and legs, leaping and contractions of the tendons, and so great a restlessness and tossing of their members ensure that the diseased are no more able to sleep, than if they were in a place of the greatest torture.*" His descriptions remain so true even today. In 1945, KA Ekbom published his doctoral thesis titled "Restless Legs" and described two important terms: "Asthenia crurum paresthetica" (irritable legs) and "Asthenia crurum dolorosa" (painful legs).[5]

EPIDEMIOLOGY

The prevalence of RLS ranges from 3% to 10% with a higher rate of occurrence in females and in older-aged patients.[6] It is seen most commonly in the third trimester of pregnancy and usually resolves in a month's time following delivery.[2]

The prevalence is probably much lower in Asian population ranging from 0.1% to 1.4%.[7] The first Indian population study on RLS revealed a prevalence of 2.9%.[8] Gupta et al. in 2017 published that RLS was seen in 9.4% of population with higher prevalence among women (13.6% women vs. 4.1% male) and significantly more prevalent at higher altitude (12% at >2,000 m) compared to low altitude (2.5% at 400 m). Most surveys have concluded that the prevalence of RLS increases with age suggesting that the neurodegenerative process may play an important role in RLS. The age varies from childhood to over 90 years of age. Though most patients in clinical practice are middle aged or older, juvenile onset is not rare. About 38–45% of adult patients' complaint about first symptoms before the age of 20 years.[9] It is interesting to note that no gender difference is found in pediatric RLS patients.[10] Sleep, mood, cognition, and quality of life are significantly affected in pediatric RLS patients and attention deficit hyperactivity disorder (ADHD), depressive symptoms, and anxiety are common comorbidities in pediatric RLS patients.[11]

CLASSIFICATION

The RLS includes two groups in general: Primary RLS and secondary RLS (**Table 1**). Primary RLS is considered to be idiopathic when the cause is truly unknown. Among the idiopathic RLS, quite a significant proportion has a family history of RLS, indicating the importance of genetic factors in developing RLS. Secondary RLS should be considered when age of onset is >45 years.[2]

TABLE 1: Causes of secondary restless legs syndrome (RLS).

Common causes	*Uncommon causes*
• Pregnancy	• Cardiovascular disease
• Iron deficiency anemia	• Parkinsonism
• Chronic kidney disease	• Diabetic peripheral neuropathy
	• Obesity
	• Rheumatological disorders
	• Other peripheral neuropathies
	• Multiple sclerosis
	• Spinal cord lesion
	• Radiculopathy
	• Inflammable bowel disease
	• Sjögren's syndrome
	• Migraine
	• Leprosy
	• Drugs such as escitalopram, olanzapine, fluoxetine, tramadol, L-thyroxine, and mirtazapine

CLINICAL PRESENTATIONS

Restless legs syndrome presents as an overwhelming urge to move the body to relieve the unpleasant sensations, primarily when resting, sitting, or sleeping. The uncomfortable feelings are always described by the patients as creeping, crawling, tingling, pooling, or painful, deep inside the limbs, unilaterally or bilaterally occurring with the knees, and the ankles or even the entire lower limbs may be involved.[12] In severe cases, the upper limbs or even the axial parts may be involved. RLS commonly affects sleep, especially in initiating the sleep. It has a significant circadian pattern, which presents as worsening of the symptoms in the evening and temporary remission in the morning after getting up from sleep.[13] Movements such as walking, stretching, or bending the legs relieve the legs at least temporarily and partially.[12] Those with poor nocturnal sleep present with excessive daytime somnolence, poor concentration, and easy fatigability. A significant higher probability of RLS will have associated ADHD, especially in pediatric RLS patients. RLS patients may have cardiovascular diseases and high blood pressure presumably due to higher sympathetic tone. Pain, ADHD, impaired mood and cognition, behavioral changes, and poor scholastic performances are commonly seen in pediatric RLS patients. About 88% of the RLS patients have periodic limb movements during sleep (PLMS). Despite this, PLMS is not an essential criterion for diagnosis of RLS. PLMS is defined as involuntary movements of the patients or their torso during sleep or awake which the patient is not aware of, different from the voluntary limb movements by RLS patients to relieve the discomfort.

DIAGNOSIS

Restless legs syndrome is a purely clinical diagnosis. The diagnostic criterion for RLS has continuously evolved from the broad diagnostic criteria by Ekbom in the 1960 to the first found RLS description established in 1979.[14,15] Present diagnostic criteria are based on revised and updated 2012 version of the National Institutes of Health (NIH) and the International Restless Legs Syndrome Study Group (IRLSSG).[3] This is given below in **Box 1**. To be formally diagnosed with RLS, all five IRLSSG diagnostic criteria must be satisfied.[3]

Supportive Criteria

- A family history of RLS
- A positive response to dopaminergic drugs
- Periodic limb movements during wakefulness or sleep as assessed with polysomnography or leg activity devices

Specifiers for Clinical Course of Restless Legs Syndrome

- *Chronic persistent RLS*: Symptoms occurring at least twice a week on average for the past 1 year when not treated
- *Intermittent RLS*: Symptoms occurring less than twice a week on average for past 1 year when not treated, but at least five lifetime events

Box 1 Essential diagnostic criteria.

- An urge to move the legs, usually accompanied or caused by uncomfortable and unpleasant sensations in the legs. Sometimes, the urge to move is present without the uncomfortable sensations and sometimes the arms or other body parts are involved in addition to legs
- The urge to move or unpleasant sensations begin or worsen during the period of rest or inactivity such as lying or sitting
- The urge to move or unpleasant sensations are partially or totally relieved by movement such as walking or stretching, at least as long as activity continues
- The urge to move or unpleasant sensations are worse in the evening or night than during the day or only occur in the evening or night. When symptoms are severe, the worsening at night may not be noticeable but must have been previously present
- Symptoms are not solely accounted for by another medical or behavioral condition such as leg cramps, myalgia, venous stasis, leg edema, arthritis, positional discomfort, and habitual food habits

Specifiers for Clinical Significance of Restless Legs Syndrome

The symptoms of RLS cause significant distress or impairment in social, occupational, educational, or other important areas of functioning by their impact on sleep, energy or vitality, daily activities, behavior, cognition, or mood.

DIFFERENTIAL DIAGNOSIS

This is given in **Table 2**.

ETIOPATHOGENESIS OF RESTLESS LEGS SYNDROME

Pathogenesis of RLS is complex and poorly understood. However, the following abnormalities are thought to be the pivotal key. These are altered brain iron, dopaminergic dysfunctions, involvement of the central opioid system, adenosinergic system dysfunction, and last, but not least, genetic factors.[16] It is believed that an iron is a cofactor for tyrosine hydroxylase, the rate-limiting enzyme involved in dopamine synthesis, and its abnormal metabolism leads to a decreased production of dopamine, thereby leading to symptoms of RLS. Iron is stored in the endothelial cells at the level of the blood-brain barrier and is required for various other metabolic reactions in the central nervous system (CNS). All dopaminergic cells near the hypothalamus seem to be the major source of dopamine to the spinal cord. These cells possibly have a role to play in generating RLS with the associated circadian rhythm.[16] Functional studies have shown bilateral brainstem and cerebellar activation with contralateral thalamus activation suggesting their involvement in etiopathogenesis of RLS. It was observed that in an iron-deficient state, there was loss of dopaminergic cells in the substantia nigra.

Another proposed mechanism is the involvement of central opioid system, which is thought to be productive for their dopaminergic pathways. It has also been postulated that decreased iron in substantia nigra and thalamus produces CNS hypoadenosinergic state and causes activation of CNS hypoxic pathways leading to altered dopaminergic systems.

A family history of as high as 40–60% has been found in patients of RLS emphasizing the genetic basis of this disease.[17] Various genes have been found using genome-wide association studies within the intronic or intergenic regions of *MEISI* (2p14), *LBXCOR1/MAP2K5* (15q23), *BTBD9* (6p21.2) and *PTPRD* (9p24.1 p23), and neuronal nitric oxide synthase 1 (NOS1) (12q).[17]

INVESTIGATIONS

Though RLS is essentially a clinical diagnosis, certain investigations are needed for giving more support to the diagnosis and to rule out RLS mimics. These are summarized in **Box 2**.

TREATMENT

Before starting the treatment, these aspects should be considered: Lifestyle change, medication effect, and iron deficiency.[18] Lifestyle such as sleep deprivation, alcohol or tobacco use, decreased motility, or medications such as dopamine antagonists, antihistaminics, and antidepressants use can lead to earlier onset or increased severity in RLS symptoms. Treatment of RLS includes pharmacological and nonpharmacological treatment.

TABLE 2: Restless legs syndrome (RLS) mimics.

Common causes	*Uncommon causes*
• Leg cramps (nocturnal)	• Myelopathy
• Positional discomfort	• Myopathy
• Local leg injury	• Vascular or neurogenic claudication
• Arthritis	• Orthostatic tremor
• Leg edema	• Painful legs and moving toes syndrome
• Venous stasis	
• Peripheral neuropathy	
• Radiculopathy	
• Habitual foot tapping or leg rocking	
• Anxiety	
• Myalgia	
• Drug-induced akathisia	

Box 2 Investigations necessary for Restless Legs Syndrome (RLS).

Essential investigations:
- Serum iron and serum ferritin level
- Hemoglobin
- Kidney function test
- Nerve conduction studies
- Blood sugar

Investigations may be needed in selective patients:
- Creatine kinase (CK)
- Calcium and vitamin D levels
- Thyroid function test
- Arterial and venous Doppler of legs
- Neuroimaging studies of brain and spine

Pharmacological Treatment

Dopaminergic agents, especially dopamine agonists such as ropinirole, pramipexole, and rotigotine are commonly used in the treatment of RLS. Pergolide and cabergoline are not recommended due to their association with increased risk of vascular heart disease.[19] Ropinirole has a faster onset with shorter duration, while rotigotine is used usually as a transdermal patch which continuously provides stable plasma drug concentration, resulting in its particular therapeutic effect on patients with symptoms throughout the day.[20] However, rotigotine is not available in India. It is important to note that, though effective, the use of low-dose controlled release of carbidopa/levodopa or plane levodopa-carbidopa should be avoided unless absolutely necessary, as they pose a risk for augmentation and rebound complications.

Alpha-2 delta (α2δ) agonists such as gabapentin, enacarbil, and pregabalin have become increasingly important in treating RLS, for being considered as possible first-line agents for RLS.[20] Hubner et al., in their study in 2013, which was a double-blind study over 12-week period, compared the efficiency of pregabalin, pramipexole, or placebo and demonstrated a better efficiency of pregabalin rather than pramipexole or placebo.[20]

Opioids are effective in treating RLS, but the potential drug abuse and side effects such as respiratory depression and constipation limit its use in routine RLS treatment. Oxycodone-naloxone combination is possibly the most effective opioid. These groups of drugs remain a good option in refractory RLS patients.

Other pharmacological treatment includes iron supplement (both oral and parenteral), some other anticonvulsants such as sodium valproate, and benzodiazepines such as clonazepam. The choice of two major first-line agents should be considered with their side effects. These are summarized in **Boxes 3** and **4**. The recommended doses of the drugs are given in **Table 3**.

Box 3 Selecting agent for initial treatment of RLS.

- *Pregnancy/Risk of pregnancy*: Iron preparation
- *Daytime symptoms*: A long-acting agent or twice daily short-acting agents (dopamine agonist or α2δ ligands)
- *Significant sleep disturbance or comorbid insomnia*: α2δ ligands
- *Increased risk of falls*: Dopamine agonists
- *Painful RLS-associated pain*: α2δ ligands
- *Impulse control disorder*: α2δ ligands
- *Associated Parkinsonism*: Dopamine agonists
- *Very severe RLS symptoms*: Dopamine agonists
- *Excess weight and metabolic syndrome*: Dopamine agonist
- *Comorbid depression*: Dopamine agonist with antidepressant—Bupropion is a good choice
- *Comorbid anxiety*: α2δ ligands
- *Symptomatic PLMS*: Dopamine agonist

(PLMS: periodic limb movements during sleep; RLS: restless legs syndrome)

Box 4 Treatment of RLS during pregnancy and lactation.[21]

Women during pregnancy:
- Nonmedicine treatment
- Iron supplement when serum ferritin <75 μg/L
- Levodopa 100–200 mg in evening or at night
- Clonazepam 0.25–1 mg in evening
- *Refractory cases*: Low-dose oxycodone
- Reassess need for medication periodically and at delivery

Women during lactation:
- Reassess iron status
- Gabapentin 300–900 mg in the evening or at night
- Clonazepam 0.25–1 mg in the evening
- *Refractory cases*: Low-dose tramadol

TABLE 3: Recommended use of dopamine agonists and α2δ ligands.

α2δ ligands	*Initial dose*	*Effective dose range*
Gabapentin enacarbil	600 mg	600–1,200 mg
Pregabalin	75 mg	150–450 mg
Gabapentin	300 mg	900–1,200 mg
Dopamine agonists		
Pramipexole	0.125 mg	0.75 mg
Ropinirole	0.25 mg	4 mg
Rotigotine	1 mg	3 mg

Complications of Long-term Treatment

Augmentation, tolerance, end of dose rebound, and natural progression of the disease are common causes of loss of efficiency of the treatment. Augmentation refers to a worsening of the symptoms that occurs very commonly with RLS patients after long-term treatment with levodopa, dopamine agonists, or even tramadol. Because augmentation worsens over time and RLS is a chronic disease requiring prolong treatment, prescribing α2δ ligands, as a first-line treatment, whenever possible, have slowly gained favor over dopamine agonists.

Whenever dopamine agonists are to be prescribed, they should be prescribed in a lowest possible effective dose.

Augmentation can sometimes be confused for drug tolerance where the therapeutic benefit of the drug diminishes over time. Augmentation shares this quality, but also involves worsening of symptoms beyond the level of severity at the time of initial treatment.[22] This phenomenon can elicit early daytime RLS symptoms and increased intensity of symptoms, distribution of symptoms to other previously unaffected arms with often worsening of symptoms with increased drug dose, and improvement with decreased drug dose. Augmentation is thought to be related to dose and duration of medication and factors such as iron deficiency.

The highest rate of augmentation occurred with levodopa (60–80%).[23] Incidence rate was reported to be higher in the patients who are on short-acting dopamine agonists such as ropinirole or pramipexole than longer-acting dopaminergic agents such as rotigotine. A possible explanation is the masking of earlier symptom onset by longer-acting dopaminergic agents.

Loss of efficiency is the reduction of the drug efficiency over time. In these cases, RLS symptoms are worse than before initiating the treatment; a combination therapy is recommended to decrease the side effects of certain medications as well as to prevent augmentation.

Management of Augmentation

The first step of management will be to rule out iron deficiency state, advice for lifestyle modification, and to take a note of the exacerbating drugs. The next step will be to classify augmentation as mild or severe. Mild augmentation is defined, if the patient satisfies all the following conditions. These are:

- A definite temporal shift of the RLS symptoms
- Dopaminergic dose is maximum recommended dose
- Symptoms cause mild distress
- There has been no prior increase in the dose above what was previously therapeutically effective

Evidence-based guidelines for the management of augmentation were established by the IRLSSG in conjunction with the European Restless Leg Syndrome Study Group (EURLSSG) and Restless Legs Syndrome Foundation (RLSF).[24]

Under mild augmentation, the clinician can keep the original dosage, but splits it between a night-time and daytime dose or starts the dose before symptoms begin. A different approach can be to increase the dopaminergic drug dosage. Alternatively, the clinician can completely change the original dopaminergic medication with α2δ ligands or a long-acting dopamine agonist such as rotigotine.

For severe augmentation symptoms, the guideline suggests three options. One would be to completely switch medication to a long-acting dopamine agonist. The second option involves adding a α2δ ligand and gradually reducing the original dopamine agonist dosage. Although the goal is to abolish the dopaminergic medication while on a α2δ ligand, the patient must be warned that this may cause a temporary worsening of the symptoms. It attempting to eliminate the dopaminergic drug fails, then adding a low dose of dopamine agonist with α2δ ligand can be continued. The third and the last option include a gradual weaning of the dopamine agonist followed by a 10-day washout period. This approach can lead to extreme RLS symptoms that may require a low-dose dopamine agonist to provide some relieve.[24]

Management of Refractory Restless Legs Syndrome

Restless legs syndrome is said to be refractory once the symptoms show minimal improvement with a combination therapy of dopamine agonist and a α2δ ligand or the treatment proves ineffective due to tolerance, augmentation, or adverse drug effect. The clinician should first consider potential factors affecting therapy such as the use of drugs potentiating RLS, a change in sleep habits, or other pathologies disturbing sleep. Opioids are commonly used in treating refractory RLS and if significant iron deficiency exists, which is not correctable by giving oral iron supplements, parenteral iron supplement therapy with ferric carboxymaltose (1,000 mg) is recommended. In addition, nonpharmacological treatment may also be considered.

Nonpharmacological Treatment

Several nonpharmacological treatments are available to RLS patients.

- To maintain proper sleep hygiene
- Exercise
- Pneumatic compression device
- Hemodialysis in end-stage renal disease patients
- Mental alerting activities such as solving crossword puzzles at times of rest or boredom
- Reducing caffeine intake
- For symptomatic relieve—walking, bicycling, and leg massage
- *Novel devices*: A device that promotes vibratory stimulations to the legs (Relaxis pad) was approved by the United States Food and Drug Administration (USFDA) in May, 2014
- Transcranial direct current stimulation
- High-frequency transcranial magnetic stimulation

CONCLUSION

Although major advancements have occurred in etiology, diagnosis, and management of RLS in the last decade, patients are continuously suffering from misdiagnosis and multiple unnecessary referrals. Through advancement in the diagnostic criteria, treatment strategies, and updated guidelines, clinicians now have more resources to diagnose and effectively manage RLS patients. Further advancements in drug therapy guidelines will depend on continued research in investigating long-term pharmacological therapy outcome.

REFERENCES

1. Garcia-Borreguero D, Kohnen R, Silbes MH. The long-term treatment of restless legs syndrome/Willis-Ekbom disease: evidence-based guidelines and clinical consensus best practice guidance: a report from the International Restless Legs Syndrome Study Group. Sleep Med. 2013;14:675-84.
2. Tater P, Pandey S. Restless legs syndrome: a continuing search for better diagnostic criteria. Neurol India. 2018;66:1028-30.
3. Allen RP, Picchietti DL, Garcia-Borreguero D. Restless Legs Syndrome/Willis-Ekbom disease diagnostic criteria: Updated International Restless Leg Syndrome Study Group (IRLSSG) consensus criteria—history, rationale, description and significance. Sleep Med. 2014;15:860-73.
4. Trenkwaldes C. Restless Legs Syndrome: Overdiagnosed or underdiagnosed? Nat Clin Pract Neurol. 2007;3:474-5.
5. Ekbom KA. Restless legs: a clinical study. Acta Med Scand. 1945;158:1-122.
6. Trenkwalder C, Paulus W, Walter AS: The Restless Leg Syndrome. Lancet Neurol. 2005;4:465-75.
7. Shi Y, Yu H, Ding D, Yu P. Prevalence and risk factors of restless legs syndrome among Chinese adults in a rural community of Shanghai in China. PLoS One. 2015;10:e0121215.
8. Panda S, Taly AB, Sinha S, Gururaj G, Girish N, Nagaraja D. Sleep-related disorders among a healthy population in South India. Neurol India. 2012;60:68-74.
9. Walters AS, Hickey K, Maltzman J. A questionnaire study of 138 patients with restless leg syndrome: the Night-Walker Survey. Neurology. 1996;46:92-5.
10. Per H, Gunay N, Ismailogullari S, Oztop DB, Gunay O. Determination of restless leg syndrome prevalence in children aged 13-16 years in the provincial center of Kayseri. Brain Dev. 2017;39:154-60.
11. Pullen SJ, Wall CA, Angstman ER, Munitz GE Kotagal S. Psychiatric comorbidity in children and adolescents with restless leg syndrome: a retrospective study. J Clin Sleep Med. 2011;7:587-96.
12. Trenkwalder C, Paulus W, Walters AS. The restless legs syndrome. Lancet Neurol. 2005;4:465-75.
13. Kushida C, Martin M, Nikam P, Blaisdell B, Wallenstein G, Ferini-Strambi L, et al. Burden of restless legs syndrome on health-related quality of life. Q Life Res. 2007;16:617-24.
14. Ekbom KA. Restless legs syndrome. Neurology. 1960;10:868-73.
15. Sleep Disorders Classification Committee. Association of sleep disorders centres. Sleep. 1979;2:135-7.
16. Guo S, Huang J, Jiang H, Han C, Li J, Xu X, et al. Restless Legs Syndrome: From Pathophysiology to Clinical Diagnosis and Management. Front Aging Neurosci. 2017;9:171.
17. Miyamoto M, Miyamoto T, Iwanami M, Suzuki K, Hirata K. Pathophysiology of restless legs syndrome. Brain Nerve. 2009;61:523-32.
18. Mackie S, Winkelman JW. Long-term treatment of restless legs syndrome (RLS): an approach to management of worsening symptoms, loss of efficiency, and augmentation. CNS Drugs. 2015;29:351-7.
19. Zanettini R, Antonini A, Gatto G, Gentile R, Tesei S, Pezzoli G. Valvular heart disease and the use of dopamine agonists for Parkinson's disease. N Engl J Med. 2007;356:39-46.
20. Hubner A, Krafft A, Gadient S, Werth E, Zimmermann R, Bassetti CL. Characteristics and determinants of restless legs syndrome in pregnancy: a prospective study. Neurology. 2013;80:738-42.
21. Picchietti DL, Hensley JG, Bainbridge JL, Lee KA, Manconi M, Mcgregor JA, et al. Consensus clinical practice guidelines for the restless leg syndrome/Willis-Ekbom disease during pregnancy and lactation. Sleep Med Rev. 2015;22:64-77.
22. Geyer J, Bogan R. Identification and treatment of augmentation in patients with restless leg syndrome: practical recommendation. Postgrad Med. 2017;129:667-75.
23. Garcia-Borreguero D, Silber MH, Winkelman JW, Högl B, Bainbridge J, Buchfuhrer M, et al. Guidelines for the first-line treatment of restless legs syndrome/Willis–Ekbom disease, prevention and treatment of dopaminergic augmentation: a combined task force of the IRLSSG, EURLSSG, and the RLS-foundation. Sleep Med. 2016;21:1-11.
24. Hogl B, Garcia-Borreguero D, Kohnen R, Ferini-Strambi L, Hadjigeorgiou G, Hornyak M, et al. Progressive development of augmentation during long-term treatment with levodopa in restless leg syndrome: results of a prospective multi-center study. J Neurol. 2010;257:230-7.

CHAPTER 49

Movement Disorders in Children

Viraj Sanghi

INTRODUCTION

Evaluating movement disorders is especially challenging in children. Good observational examination skills and phenomenological approaches are essential to reach a diagnosis. Distinguishing normal from abnormal movements in the developing child can be challenging.[1] Movement disorders are categorized into two major groups: (1) Hypokinetic and (2) Hyperkinetic disorders. The hypokinetic disorders are relatively rare in children. The second category, hyperkinetic disorders, is sometimes referred to as dyskinesias. This consists of abnormal, repetitive, and involuntary movements and includes the bulk of pediatric movement disorders. Tics, stereotypies, chorea, dystonia, myoclonus, and tremor all fall into this category. There are a large number of genetic and heredodegenerative diseases, which cause secondary movement disorders in childhood. The management of these disoders must include a detailed history and clinical examination followed by appropriate investigations to determine the underlying etiology (**Flowchart 1**).

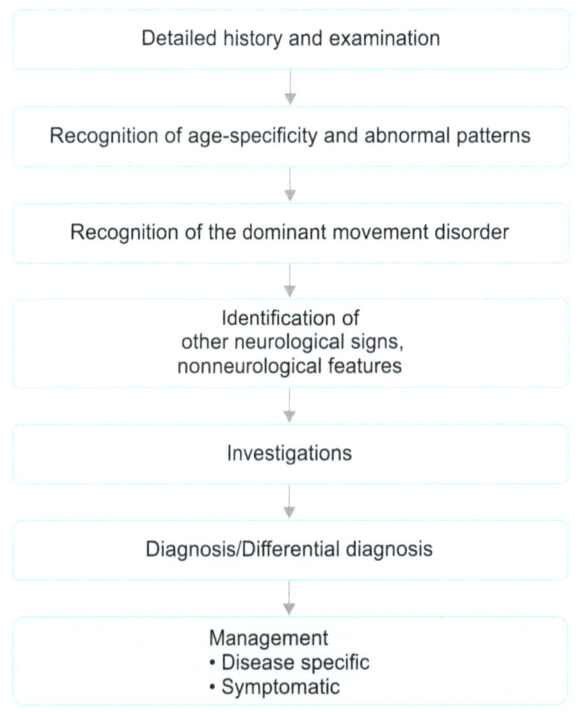

FLOWCHART 1: Stepwise approach to management of pediatric movement disorders.

HYPOKINETIC DISORDERS IN CHILDREN

Hyokinesia is defined as a decrease in the number of movements.[2] Bradykinesia is the decrease in speed of individual movements and rigidity is the increase in the resistance to passive movement uniform throughout direction and speed. These three features form the core features of Parkinsonism. The classic Parkinson's tremor is rare in children. Primary Parkinsonism in children [juvenile Parkinson's disease (PD)] is rare, but must be recognized. Most often, Parkinsonism in children is secondary to a neurologic disorder.

Primary Parkinsonism in Children (Juvenile Parkinson's Disease)

Juvenile Parkinsonism is arbitrarily defined as Parkinsonian symptoms and signs that occur before the age of 21 years. Since the discovery of the first gene for PD 20 years ago, a large number of additional genes have been implicated as monogenic causes for juvenile PD.[3] The most common genes are the *Parkin*, *PINK1*, and *DJ1* genes. Genetic testing of patients with young-onset, hereditary Parkinsonian disorders has become part of clinical practice in many healthcare settings.[3] Currently, there are 27 genes reported in the literature which may be autosomal dominant or recessive (**Table 1**).[4]

Monogenic autosomal dominant Parkinson's disease is seen with mutations of *SNCA*, *LRRK2*, and *VPS35*. Patients with a mutation of *SNCA* may also exhibit cognitive and behavioral dysfunction in addition to autonomic disturbances and myoclonus. Those with a mutation of the *VPS35* may also develop cognitive dysfunction. The newly discovered genes *DNAJC13*, *CHCHD2*, *TMEM230*, and *RIC3* may produce dominant PD. Their roles in pathogenicity are not confirmed as yet.[3]

Autosomal recessive, early-onset PD due to mutations in *PARK2*, *PINK1*, and *DJ1* is well established. These are typically slowly progressive.[4] Newer recessive genes are now described often with more severe and atypical presentations, with intellectual disability, cognitive decline, and neuropsychiatric symptoms being most common. Patients affected by a *SYNJ1* mutation have been described to have early-onset Parkinsonism, typically starting in their early 20s associated with cognitive decline, dystonia, and seizures.[5,6] An Indian family with a different mutation in the *SYNJ1* gene has been described with even earlier onset of tremor and Parkinsonism in their teenage years. The 22q11.2 deletion syndrome has been associated with variable features that may include learning and intellectual disability, autism, schizophrenia, seizures, facial dysmorphism, midline developmental anomalies (palate, larynx, trachea, and/or esophagus), congenital heart disease, and hypocalcemia among other features. Parkinsonism has been described in a few of these patients, typically starting in the fourth or fifth decade of life.[7,8] Additional movement disorders such as tremors, myoclonic jerks, and oculogyric crises may be present either alone or with the Parkinsonism. They may also be more prone to antipsychotic medication-induced movement disorders.[9] Kufor-Rakeb syndrome is a juvenile-onset atypical PD caused by a mutation in the *ATP13A2* gene. Patients with this disease present in adolescence with Parkinsonism, pyramidal signs, supranuclear gaze palsy, dysarthria, dysphagia, and dementia. Brain imaging shows cerebral and cerebellar atrophy.[10]

Mutations in *RAB39B* have been identified in patients and families with X-linked intellectual disability with autism, epilepsy, and/or macrocephaly. The development of tremors, rigidity, and Parkinsonism at variable ages (from early childhood to the fourth decade of life) has been described in some of these individuals and families.[11,12]

TABLE 1: Genes associated with Parkinson's disease or juvenile Parkinsonism.

Autosomal dominant	*Autosomal recessive*	*X-linked*
LRRK2	*PRKN*	*RAB39B*
SNCA	*PINK1*	
VPS35	*DJ1*	
GCH1	*ATP13A2*	
ATXN2	*PLA2G6*	
DNAJC13	*FBXO7*	
TMEM230	*DNAJC6*	
GIGYF2	*SYNJ1*	
HTRA2	*SPG11*	
RIC3	*VPS13C*	
EIF4G1	*PODXL*	
UCHL1	*PTRHD1*	
CHCHD2		
GBA		

Secondary Parkinsonism in Children

The secondary causes of Parkinsonism in children include many disorders (**Table 2**). Hypokinesia and rigidity are usually accompanied by other movement disorders (such as dystonia) and neurological features.

Treatment of Parkinsonism in Children

Juvenile PD responds to treatment with medication in the majority of patients. The mainstay of treatment is Levodopa.[13] Initial responses to treatment are usually good, at least in the early years. Later, escalating dosages may be required. Children may also experience dopa-induced dyskinesias in a manner similar to those seen in adults on long-term therapy. Anticholinergic agents, dopamine agonists (such as pramipexole and ropinirole), and inhibitors of dopamine breakdown (such as entacapone and selegiline) for treating Parkinsonism are also advocated. Amantadine may be used to alleviate mild Parkinsonian symptoms and also dyskinesias associated with the acute or long-term usage of levodopa.[14] Symptomatic therapies such as botulinum toxin for focal dystonias and deep brain stimulation in selected patients can also be tried for improving long-term outcome.[13]

HYPERKINETIC DISORDERS IN CHILDREN

Hyperkinetic movement disorders (dyskinesias) encompass most of the child movement disorders and include tics, chorea/ballismus, dystonia, myoclonus, stereotypies, and tremor. The most frequent movement disorders in children are tics and Tourette syndrome followed by dystonia (**Fig. 1**). Tics may account for more than half of all pediatric movement disorders.[15] It is important to remember that tics and stereotypies do not interfere with voluntary movement unlike the other hyperkinetic movements (**Tables 3** and **4**; **Box 1**).[16]

TABLE 2: Secondary Parkinsonism in children.

Structural	Infectious/ Postinfectious	Toxins/Drugs	Inherited disorders of metabolism	Metals	Autoimmune	Degenerative/ Genetic	Miscellaneous
Mesen-cephalic tumors	Viral encephalitis, e.g., Japanese B encephalitis	Antipsychotics and neuro-leptics, e.g., haloperidol	Neurotransmitter deficiencies, e.g., dopa-responsive dystonias	Wilson's disease	Anti-NMDA receptor	Huntington's disease (HD) (Westphal variant)	Fahr's disease
Hydro-cephalus	Encephalitis lethargica	Antiemetics, e.g., metoclo-pramide	Mitochondrial disorders	NBIA	Anti-VGKC receptor	HD-like diseases	Hypoxic-ischemic encephalopathy
Strokes		Dopamine depletors, e.g., tetrabenazine	Lysosomal storage disorders—Niemann–Pick type C and juvenile NCL	Manganese (acquired/ inherited)	Anti-dopamine 2 receptor	Others, e.g., fragile X, DYT mutations	Trauma

(NBIA: neurodegeneration with brain iron accumulation; NCL: neuronal ceroid lipofuscinosis; NMDA: N-methyl-D-aspartate; VGKC: voltage-gated potassium channel)

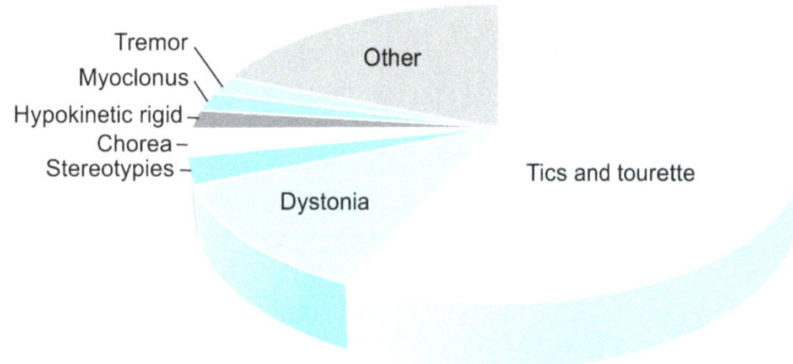

FIG. 1: Relative distribution of pediatric movement disorders by phenomenology.

TABLE 3: Phenomenology of hyperkinetic movement disorders.

Movement disorders	Definition
Chorea/Ballism	Involuntary, chaotic, irregular, random and unpredictable, purposeless movements (or movement fragments) with variable rate and direction. When of very large amplitude, term ballism is used
Dystonia	Sustained or repetitive involuntary muscle contraction that produces abnormal postures and movements. Typically with a twisting quality
Myoclonus	Sudden, brief shock-like movements of one or more muscles
Stereotypy	Patterned, episodic, repetitive, and rhythmic movements
Tremor	Oscillating, rhythmic movements about a fixed point or axis when antagonist muscles contract alternately
Tics	Stereotyped, involuntary, sudden, inopportune, absurd, and irresistible movements or sounds or noises of variable intensity

TABLE 4: Tics versus stereotypies—differentiating clues.

Features	Tics	Stereotypies
Age of onset	6–7 years	<3 years
Common movements	Blink, shrug, grimace, and twist	Hand flap, rocking, and nodding
Vocalizations	Sniffing and throat clearing	Moaning and humming
Duration	Brief and abrupt	More prolonged and continuous
"Urge"	Present	Not present
Distraction	May reduce	Usually stops

These movement disorders will be discussed in further details elsewhere in this book.

SPECIFIC SYNDROMES AND DISEASES

It is important for the practicing clinician to recognize, diagnose, and treat the disorders that commonly produce movement disorders in children. Several of these such as Tourette syndrome, Wilson's disease, neurodegeneration

Box 1 Classification and etiology of stereotypies.

Primary—no specific cause

- Common behaviors—thumb sucking, nail biting, hair twirling, and foot tapping
- Head nodding ("No" movement/"Yes" movement/"Shoulder to shoulder")
- Complex motor stereotypies—hand flapping and rocking

Secondary

- Autism spectrum disorder
- Rett syndrome
- Mental retardation
- Sensory deprivation—congenital blindness/deafness, caging, and constraints
- Lesch–Nyhan disease
- Neuroacanthocytosis
- Drug induced—psychostimulants and tardive dyskinesia
- Bobble-head doll syndrome—third ventricle lesions/tumors, aqueductal stenosis, Dandy–Walker syndrome, and suprasellar cysts
- Psychiatric disorders—obsessive-compulsive disorder (OCD), schizophrenia, and catatonia

with brain iron accumulation (NBIA) group of disorders, paroxysmal dyskinesias, and autoimmune encephalitis are discussed elsewhere in this book. A few other important syndromes and diseases in the pediatric population are discussed here.

Benign Hereditary Chorea

Benign hereditary chorea (BHC) has traditionally been described as an autosomal dominant, nonprogressive disorder characterized by onset of chorea in children with normal intellectual development before 5 years of age. Children with BHC have no regression of skills, no dysmorphic features, and usually have no other neurological abnormalities.[17,18] However, authors have described increasing number of patients with atypical neurologic signs including ataxia, myoclonus, and dystonia in these children.[19] The severity of chorea is variable between and within families. Detailed multigenerational history taking and examination of family members are vital. Neuroimaging is generally normal in BHC. A loss-of-function mutation in the *NKX2-1* gene (also known as *TITF-1* gene) that encodes for thyroid transcription factor 1 on chromosome 14 was first described in 2002.[20] This gene has been implicated in several important molecular pathways essential for brain, thyroid, and lung morphogenesis.[21] Additionally, chromosome 14q13 deletions adjacent to, but not disrupting, *NKX2-1* have been described in patients with BHC. Recently, a mutation in the *MBIP* gene that affects *TITF-1* expression has been described in an Italian family with six subjects of BHC.[22] This mimics haploinsufficiency caused by classical *TITF-1*-related mutations. A broader syndrome consists of the triad of congenital hypothyroidism, neonatal or infantile respiratory distress, and persistent chorea and is known "brain-lung-thyroid syndrome." A large study of BHC in 2014 demonstrated pathogenic mutations in *NKX2-1* in only 26.7% of the cases.[23] In BHC, the chorea tends to improve with age and may respond to Levodopa.

It has been proposed that the term BHC can be abandoned given that: (i) Mutations in the *NKX2-1* may be de novo in 60% of the patients and, thus, not hereditary and (ii) The phenotype has expanded to include many more neurological features. The new term suggested is chorea secondary to *NKX2-1* mutations.[24]

Other early childhood-onset chorea-predominant syndromes have also been described with different genetic mutations. Chorea secondary to *ADCY5* mutation has been described in families with early-onset chorea, myoclonus, dystonia, and facial twitching. This may be de novo or autosomal dominant and is considered to be a nondegenerative disorder.[24] *PDE10A* mutations have also been described in children with early-onset chorea. Dominant mutations in *PDE10A* were associated with symmetric MRI abnormalities in the basal ganglia. Recessive homozygous mutations were associated with an earlier onset and more severe phenotype that included axial hypotonia, cognitive and language delay, and dysarthria. These patients, however, did not have the MRI abnormalities.[24]

Differentiating these early-onset, nondegenerative genetic disorders of chorea from Huntington's disease, ataxia telangiectasia, and dyskinetic cerebral palsy are sometimes challenging and require careful clinical evaluation and genetic testing.

Paroxysmal Kinesigenic Dyskinesia with Infantile Convulsions

Paroxysmal Kinesigenic Dyskinesia-Benign Familial Infantile Epilepsy-Infantile Convulsions and Paroxysmal Choreoathetosis Syndrome Spectrum: PRRT2-related Disorders

The most common form of paroxysmal dyskinesia is paroxysmal kinesigenic dyskinesia (PKD) in which brief, unilateral or bilateral limb dystonia, or choreoathetosis is triggered by sudden movement. Benign familial infantile epilepsy (BFIE) is an autosomal dominant disorder that occurs in infancy and in which seizures usually rebate by 2 years of age.

Attacks of paroxysmal dyskinesia share characteristics with epileptic seizures: The episodes are paroxysmal, they tend to remit, and they usually respond to anticonvulsant medication.[25] They can share a common genetic basis and can be coinherited as a single autosomal dominant trait. The relationship of infantile convulsions and paroxysmal choreoathetosis (ICCA) syndrome and linkage to the pericentromeric region of chromosome 16p12-q12 was first described in four families from northern France in 1997.[25] In these families, benign infantile convulsions were inherited as an autosomal dominant trait along with variably expressed paroxysmal choreoathetosis occurring later in childhood or adolescence. In 2011, a mutation was identified in the *PRRT2* gene (that encodes proline-rich transmembrane protein 2) in eight Chinese families that had PKD.[26] In 2012, mutations in *PRRT2* were described in many more families from different ethnic backgrounds with PKD, BFIE as well as ICCA.[27,28] *PRRT2* is highly expressed in the cerebral cortex, basal ganglia, and cerebellum. The seizures are typically focal motor seizures. Sometimes, generalized tonic-clonic seizures may occur as well as benign myoclonic epilepsy of infancy in rare cases.[29,30] Seizures usually resolve spontaneously by the age of 2 years. They respond well to treatment with valproate or oxcarbazepine, though myoclonic seizures are insensitive to treatment.[29,30] In later years of childhood or adolescence, patients begin having PKD attacks characterized by frequent, brief, and involuntary movements (either dystonia or choreoathetosis or both) that are precipitated by sudden movement or change in velocity of movement (such as sitting to standing, standing to walking, and walking to running). They may experience dozens to hundreds of attacks per day. Usually, these last <5 or 10 seconds but occasionally may be longer. The movement disorder gets significantly better or completely resolves, as the patient grows into middle adult life.[28,31] Avoiding stress, sleep deprivation, and anxiety can help prevent attacks and can lower attack frequency. The movement disorder responds well to treatment with anticonvulsant medications that target voltage-sensitive sodium channels such as carbamazepine, oxcarbazepine, and phenytoin.[31-33] The spectrum of *PRRT2*-related disorders includes hemiplegic migraine.[33,34]

Organic Acidurias

The inherited organic acidurias are a defined group of metabolic diseases that can cause significant movement disorders in children. They can present in the neonatal period with acute crises (either metabolic or encephalopathic) or at a later age with developmental delay, dystonia, and other movement disorders or seizures. The three most common ones such as glutaric aciduria type 1 (GA1), methylmalonic acidemia (MMA), and propionic acidemia (PA) are discussed in further detail here.

Glutaric Aciduria Type 1

Glutaric aciduria type 1 is a rare neurometabolic disorder caused by the deficiency of the enzyme glutaryl-CoA dehydrogenase (GCDH). It is an autosomal recessive disorder caused by mutations in the *GCDH* gene localized on chromosome 19p13.2, which encodes a mitochondrial matrix protein involved in the degradation of L-lysine, L-hydroxylysine, and L-tryptophan. Mutation of the gene results in an excessive accumulation of glutaric acid, 3-hydroxyglutaric acid, glutaconic acid (less frequently), and glutarylcarnitine (C5DC).[35] More than 250 variants in the *GCDH* gene have been reported with a variable frequency among different ethnic groups.[36] There is marked variability in the clinical expression and severity of GA1 even within the same family. Neonates and infants may present with nonspecific neurologic symptoms that include muscular hypotonia and delayed motor development in about half of the cases. Most patients develop an acute encephalopathic crisis during infancy (3–36 months) that is often triggered by an intercurrent infection, immunization, surgical procedure, or other minor illness. The neurologic sequel to this is acute bilateral striatal injury and the development of a complex movement disorder with significant morbidity and mortality.[35-38] This usually consists of generalized dystonia, superimposed on baseline axial hypotonia. With aging, it may evolve to dystonia associated with akinetic-rigid Parkinsonism. Prominent orofacial involvement and speech disorders such as dysarthria and speech apraxia are common in GA1.[39] A hypotonic or choreoathetotic cerebral palsy-like phenotype may be seen in some patients. In a few, neurologic symptoms may develop insidiously without an acute encephalopathy. Patients are at increased risk of epilepsy and seizures may be the initial or sole symptoms in some patients. Some patients may be asymptomatic.[36-38] Macrocephaly is a very frequent finding and may be present at birth or develop in the first few weeks of life.[36-38] MRI findings include brain atrophy, periventricular white matter changes, basal ganglia lesions (volume loss and signal change in bilateral caudate head and lentiform nucleus), and increased fluid collections in bilateral anterior temporal cerebrospinal fluid (CSF) spaces and sylvian fissures.[40-42] Very widely open opercula along with bilateral basal ganglia lesions is almost pathognomonic for GA1 (**Fig. 2**).[40,42] Occasionally, bilateral temporal arachnoid cysts may also be seen. Subdural hemorrhages may also occur in GA1, but these are most common during the age of maximal extent of macrocephaly, i.e., late infancy. It is postulated that disruption of elongated bridging cortical veins by minor head trauma is the underlying pathologic mechanism. In many patients, these are asymptomatic. These infants may be mistakenly diagnosed with shaken baby syndrome and vice versa.[37] Late-onset (beyond the age of 6 years) and adult-onset cases of GA1 have also been reported.[43,44] These may present with nonspecific neurologic features such as headaches, vertigo, transient ataxic gait, reduced fine motor skills, or fainting after exercise, but do not develop striatal injury. In this cohort of patients, periventricular white matter changes are the prominent finding on brain MRI.[37,43,44]

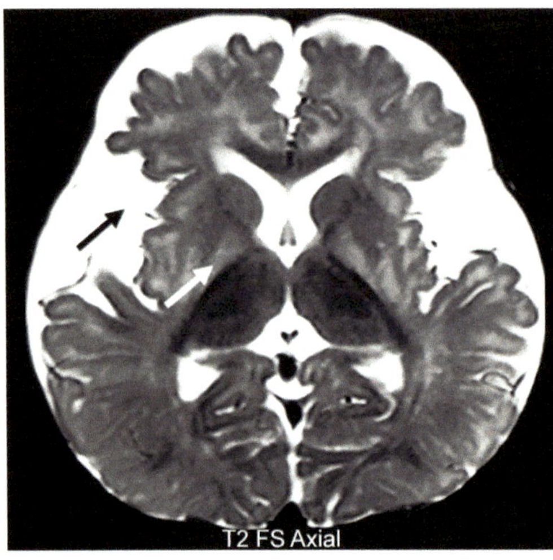

FIG. 2: MRI in glutaric aciduria type 1 [black arrow—widened sylvian fissure; white arrow—basal ganglia (globus pallidus) lesion].

Screening for GA1 by mass spectroscopy is routinely done as part of newborn panels in most countries. The diagnostic metabolite in these screens is elevated C5DC. Further testing must include quantitative analysis of glutaric acid and 3-hydroxyglutaric acid and confirmation of the diagnosis by mutation analysis of the *GCDH* gene and/or *GCDH* enzyme analysis.[37]

Glutaric aciduria type 1 is a treatable neurometabolic disorder. 80–90% of individuals remain asymptomatic, if treatment is initiated in the newborn period before symptom onset. Outcomes are not good when treatment is commenced after symptom onset.[37,38,45-47] Metabolic therapy consists of a low-lysine diet, administration of lysine-free, tryptophan-reduced amino acid mixtures (AAMs), carnitine supplementation, and emergency treatment during episodes. Dystonia can be treated with baclofen, anticholinergic agents such as trihexyphenidyl, benzodiazepines, and botulinum toxin injections.[37] Pallidotomy and deep brain stimulation have been used in patients with severe dystonia with variable outcomes. Valproate and vigabatrin should be avoided when treating seizures due to GA1.

Methylmalonic Acidemia and Propionic Acidemia

The majority of patients with MMA and PA present with an acute metabolic crisis as early as the first day of life or as late as adulthood. Most commonly, this crisis occurs in the neonatal period with severe hyperammonemia and hypoglycemia. After the newborn period, the crises consist more of a metabolic acidosis with ketosis. Periods of intermittent metabolic decompensation are usually precipitated by intercurrent infections and stress. Symptomatic patients without metabolic crises present with a movement disorder, epilepsy, and/or mental retardation.[48]

Isolated methylmalonic acidemia is caused by complete or partial deficiency of the enzyme methylmalonyl-CoA mutase (*mut*^{0} enzymatic subtype or *mut*$^-$ enzymatic subtype, respectively), a defect in the transport or synthesis of its cofactor, adenosylcobalamin (*cblA*, *cblB*, or *cblD*-MMA), or deficiency of the enzyme methylmalonyl-CoA epimerase.

Methylmalonic acidemia may occur in the neonatal period or at any time after that. Apart from the acute metabolic decompensations, patients may present with acute or chronic basal ganglia injury ("metabolic stroke") that causes a disabling movement disorder of dystonia and choreoathetosis. Sometimes, paraparesis or quadriparesis may also occur.[48,49] MRI studies show acute infarcts in bilateral globus pallidus in all patients often along with tiny lacunar infarcts in the substantia nigra (**Fig. 3**).[50] Tubulointerstitial nephritis with renal failure may also occur as a major complication in some patients.

Propionic acidemia is caused by a deficiency of propionyl-CoA carboxylase, a mitochondrial biotin-dependent enzyme, of which the two subunits are encoded by PCCA and PCCB. Clinical presentation and neurological features are similar to MMA.

Treatment of MMA and PA includes lifelong protein-restricted diet (restricted isoleucine, valine, threonine, and methionine) and high calorie intake to reverse catabolism including intravenous (IV) glucose during acute metabolic decompensation. Strategies to reduce ammonia include administration of N-carbamylglutamate, sodium benzoate, and extracorporeal detoxification with venous-venous hemodiafiltration or hemodialysis. Antibiotics (particularly metronidazole) along with laxatives are prescribed to diminish propionyl-CoA carboxylase from gut bacteria through selective bowel decontamination along with carnitine supplementation. Intramuscular hydroxycobalamin injections are administered to selected

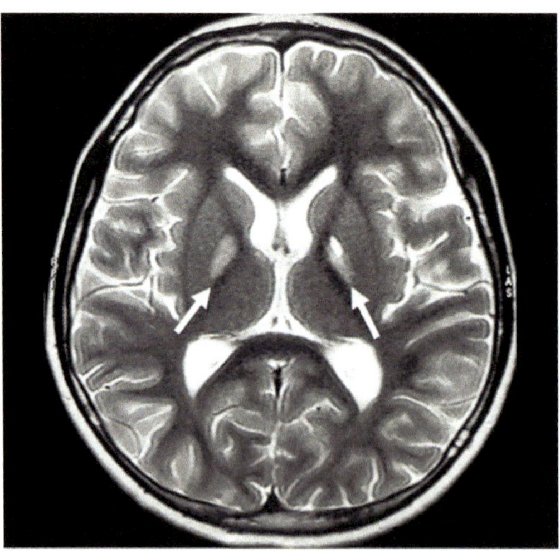

FIG. 3: MRI in methylmalonic acidemia showing bilateral globus pallidus infarcts (white arrows).

cobalamin-responsive MMA patients: *mut*⁻-, cobalamin A-, and cobalamin D-deficient patients.[49,51,52] In very severely affected patients of MMA and PA, liver transplant (or combined liver-kidney transplant in MMA patients) may be considered with some benefits in reducing acute decompensations and basal ganglia strokes but not reversing neurological damage already done.[52-55] New genomic therapies have shown great promise in experimental murine models.[56]

Neurotransmitter Disorders

This is a broad spectrum of relatively uncommon genetic disorders that affect the synthesis and metabolism of neurotransmitters or the cofactors required for their biosynthesis. The chief neurotransmitters involved are the monoamines (serotonin, dopamine, and norepinephrine) and gamma-aminobutyric acid (GABA). Symptoms can start as early as the neonatal period and signs include hypotonia, developmental delay, movement disorders, and/or dysregulated autonomic function or occur later in life presenting as a movement disorder. Neuroimaging studies are usually normal. Quantitative assessment of the neurotransmitter levels in the CSF may be used to make an initial diagnosis of these disorders followed by confirmation with either enzyme activity measurement or mutational analysis of the related genes. Here, the dopa-responsive dystonias (DRDs) are discussed in further detail.

Dopa-responsive Dystonias

The DRDs are a heterogeneous group of inherited disorders of the dopamine synthetic pathway that result in selective nigrostriatal dopamine deficiency without nigral cell loss. They classically manifest in childhood or adolescence as limb-onset, diurnally fluctuating dystonia that exhibits a significant and sustained response to levodopa treatment.[57-60] The clinical spectrum of DRDs has increased to include several distinct disorders (**Table 5**). At the milder end of this spectrum is the most common autosomal dominant GTP cyclohydrolase-1 deficiency (GCH-1-DRD) syndrome and at the more severe end is the much less common autosomal recessive tyrosine hydroxylase deficiency (TH-DRD) syndrome, with intermediate types in between.[61]

Autosomal Dominant GCH-1 Deficiency (Segawa Disease, DYT5a, and DYT/PARK-GCH-1)

This is the "classic" DRD first described by Segawa and colleagues in 1972.[62] An autosomal dominant heterozygous mutation in the gene that encodes for GCH-1 enzyme (located on chromosome 14q22.1-22.2) results in reduced tetrahydrobiopterin (BH4) synthesis, which acts as a cofactor and, thus, in turn, decreases production of tyrosine hydroxylase (TH). This leads to dopamine deficiency. Neopterin level is low and phenlyalanine levels are not elevated.[57,59] GCH-1 deficiency typically manifests in the first decade of life with dystonia that starts in the lower

TABLE 5: Overview of Dopa-responsive disorders.

Group disorders	*Deficiency*	*Inheritance*	*Treatment*
Tetrahydrobiopterin (BH4) disorders	GCH-1	AD	L-DOPA with Carbidopa
	GCH-1	AR	L-DOPA-Carbidopa, 5-HTP, and BH4
	Sepiapterin reductase (SR)	AR	L-DOPA-Carbidopa, 5-HTP, and selegiline
	6-pyruvoyltetrahydropterin synthase (PTPS)	AR	L-DOPA-Carbidopa, 5-HTP, and BH4 (high doses)
	Dihydropteridine reductase (DHPR)	AR	L-DOPA-Carbidopa, 5-HTP, folinic acid, and dietary measures
	Pterin-4a-carbinolamine dehydratase (PCD)	AR	BH4
Monoamine synthesis disorders	Tyrosine hydroxylase (TH)	AR	L-DOPA-Carbidopa and selegiline
	Aromatic L-amino acid decarboxylase (AADC)	AR	Dopamine agonists, selegiline and cofactors (pyridoxine and pyridoxal phosphate)
Monoamine transporter disorders	Dopamine transporter deficiency syndrome (DTDS/SLC6A3)	AR	Dopamine agonists
	Vesicular monoamine transporter 2 (VMAT2/SLC18A2)	AR	Dopamine agonists
Cochaperone defect	DNAJC12	AR	BH4, L-DOPA-Carbidopa, and 5-HTP
Developmental disorder of dopaminergic system	SOX6	De-novo mutation	L-DOPA-Carbidopa

(AD: autosomal dominant; AR: autosomal recessive; GCH-1: GTP cyclohydrolase-1; 5-HTP: 5-hydroxytryptophan)

limbs and then spreads to the upper limbs. Spasticity and brisk reflexes may be seen occasionally leading to a mistaken diagnosis of cerebral palsy. There is a diurnal fluctuation with symptoms worsening, as the day progresses and improving after rest or sleep. Later in the course of the disease, Parkinsonism with tremors and bradykinesia may be seen.[57,59] These patients usually do not suffer from seizures, myoclonus, mental retardation, or autonomic dysfunction.[63] There is a striking and sustained response to treatment with L-DOPA and long-term complications of therapy such as motor fluctuations and dyskinesias are not usually seen.[58-60,63] Flurodopa positron-emission tomography (PET) scans and dopamine transporter imaging show normal uptake patterns in these patients.[59]

Tyrosine Hydroxylase Deficiency (DYT5b/PARK-TH)

TH deficiency is a rare autosomal recessive disorder resulting from cerebral catecholamine deficiency.[57,59,64] Most patients present with a mild-to-moderate phenotype starting in infancy with hypokinesia and rigidity involving all four limbs symmetrically. Ability to walk is not achieved, if treatment is not given. With later onset, within the first few years of life, dystonia is more predominant. Symptoms usually start in one lower limb and then spread to involve the other limbs, trunk, face, and even oropharyngeal musculature. Diurnal fluctuations can occur. Untreated, most children are wheelchair bound in a few years. Oculogyric crises and autonomic disturbances as well as developmental delay may be seen. There is a dramatic response to treatment with L-DOPA in most patients. These patients are exquisitely sensitive to L-DOPA and may experience side effect even at low doses. Those who do not respond may benefit with addition of a monoamine oxidase type B (MAO-B) inhibitor such as selegiline.[57,59,64,65] In rare cases, a severe neonatal-onset encephalopathy with hypokinesia, bradykinesia, and hypotonia is seen. Dystonic crises may occur. Myoclonus, autonomic dysfunction, and tremors may also be seen. Developmental outcomes (motor and cognitive) in this subgroup are much worse with limited response to therapy.[57,64] Rare cases of adult-onset DRD have been reported with either homozygous or heterozygous mutations of the *TH* gene.[66,67]

Autosomal Recessive GCH-1 Deficiency (DYT/PARK-GCH-1)

Compound heterozygous or homozygous mutations in GCH-1 lead to a more severe form of disease presenting in the early neonatal period. The phenotype consists of truncal hypotonia, rigidity, dystonia, Parkinsonism, and even oculogyric crises. Developmental milestones are severely delayed in untreated cases. Hyperphenylalaninemia is present. Treatment is with L-DOPA. Many patients are also treated with 5-hydroxytryptophan (5-HTP) and BH4. The utility of these is not entirely clear.[57,60]

Sepiapterin Reductase Deficiency (DYT/PARK-SPR)

Sepiapterin reductase (SR) deficiency is a very rare autosomal recessive disorder caused by mutations of the *SPR* gene. Onset of the disease is usually in infancy with axial hypotonia, motor developmental delay, and oculogyric crises. Later, dystonia with circadian variation develops. Phenylalanine levels are normal. SR deficiency may be mistaken as cerebral palsy in some patients. Treatment consists of administration of L-DOPA. 5-HTP, MAO-B inhibitors, and selective serotonin reuptake inhibitors (SSRIs) may be tried.[57,60,68]

CONCLUSION

Movement disorders in children thus consist of a very varied and heterogenous group of disorders. The genetic landscape is continually evolving and the list of known genetic disorders is constantly increasing. The field of paediatric movement disorders is thus challenging and exciting.

TABLE 6: Inherited neurometabolic diseases and movement disorders.

Dystonia	*Myoclonus*	*Chorea*	*Parkinsonism*
Wilson's disease	Lafora disease	Mitochondrial cytopathies	Wilson's disease
NBIA	Sialidosis	Lesch–Nyhan disease	Gaucher disease
Glutaric aciduria type 1, MMA, and PA	Mitochondrial cytopathies	Glutaric aciduria type 1, MMA, and PA	Mitochondrial cytopathies
Gaucher disease, Niemann–Pick type C, GM1, and GM2	Niemann–Pick type C, GM1, and GM2		Neurotransmitter disorders
Neurotransmitter disorders	Neuronal ceroid lipofuscinosis		
Mitochondrial cytopathies			
Biotin-thiamine-responsive basal ganglia disease			

(MMA: methylmalonic acidemia; NBIA: neurodegeneration with brain iron accumulation; PA: propionic acidemia)

REFERENCES

1. O'Malley JA, Gilbert DL. Clinical approach to a child with movement disorders. Semin Pediatr Neurol. 2018;25:10-8.
2. García-Cazorla A, Ortez C, Pérez-Dueñas B, Serrano M, Pineda M, Campistol J, et al. Hypokinetic-rigid syndrome in children and inborn errors of metabolism. Eur J Paediatr Neurol. 2011;15(4):295-302.
3. Puschmann A. New Genes Causing Hereditary Parkinson's Disease or Parkinsonism. Curr Neurol Neurosci Rep. 2017;17(9):66.
4. Lunati A, Lesage S, Brice A. The genetic landscape of Parkinson's disease. Rev Neurol (Paris). 2018;174(9):628-43.
5. Krebs C, Karkheiran S, Powell J, Cao M, Makarov V, Darvish H, et al. The Sac1 domain of SYNJ1 identified mutated in a family with early-onset progressive parkinsonism with generalized seizures. Hum Mutat. 2013;34(9):1200-7.
6. Quadri M, Fang M, Picillo M, Olgiati S, Breedveld G, Graafland J, et al. Mutation in the SYNJ1 gene associated with autosomal recessive, early-onset parkinsonism. Hum Mutat. 2013;34(9): 1208-15.
7. Rehman A, Dhamija R, Williams E, Barrett M. 22q11.2 deletion syndrome presenting with early-onset Parkinson's disease. Mov Disord. 2015;30(9):1289-90.
8. Zaleski C, Bassett AS, Tam K, Shugar A, Chow E, McPherson E. The co-occurrence of early onset Parkinson disease and 22q11.2 deletion syndrome. Am J Med Genet A. 2009;149A(3):525-8.
9. Boot E, Butcher N, van Amelsvoort T, Lang A, Marras C, Pondal M, et al. Movement disorders and other motor abnormalities in adults with 22q11.2 deletion syndrome. Am J Med Genet A. 2015;167A(3):639-45.
10. Park J, Blair N, Sue C. The Role of ATP13A2 in Parkinson's Disease: Clinical Phenotypes and Molecular Mechanisms. Mov Disord. 2015;30(6):770-9.
11. Wilson G, Sim J, McLean C, Giannandrea M, Galea CA, Riseley JR, et al. Mutations in RAB39B cause X-linked intellectual disability and early-onset Parkinson disease with alpha-synuclein pathology. Am J Hum Genet. 2014;95(6):729-35.
12. Lesage S, Bras J, Cormier-Dequaire F, Condroyer C, Nicolas A, Darwent L, et al. Loss-of-function mutations in RAB39B are associated with typical early-onset Parkinson disease. Neurol Genet. 2015;1(1):e9.
13. Niemann N, Jankovic J. Juvenile parkinsonism: Differential diagnosis, genetics, and treatment. Parkinsonism Relat Disord. 2019;67:74-89.
14. Paci C, Thomas A, Onofrj M. Amantadine for dyskinesia in patients affected by severe Parkinson's disease. Neurol Sci. 2001;22(1):75-6.
15. Baümer T, Sajin V, Münchau A. Childhood-onset movement disorders: a clinical series of 606 cases. Mov Disord Clin Pract. 2016;4(3):437-40.
16. Fernández-Alvarez E. Movement disorders in children: recent advances in management. Indian J Pediatr. 2009;76:531-6.
17. Kleiner-Fisman G. Benign hereditary chorea. Handb Clin Neurol. 2011;100:199-212.
18. Kleiner-Fisman G, Lang A. Benign hereditary chorea revisited: a journey to understanding. Mov Disord. 2007;22(16): 2297-305.
19. Asmus F, Devlin A, Munz M, Zimprich A, Gasser T, Chinnery P. Clinical differentiation of genetically proven benign hereditary chorea and myoclonus-dystonia. Mov Disord. 2007;22(14):2104-9.
20. Breedveld G, van Dongen J, Danesino C, Guala A, Percy A, Dure L, et al. Mutations in TITF-1 are associated with benign hereditary chorea. Hum Mol Genet. 2002;11(8):971-9.
21. Inzelberg R, Weinberger M, Gak E. Benign hereditary chorea: an update. Parkinsonism Relat Disord. 2011;17(5):301-7.
22. Invernizzi F, Zorzi G, Legati A, Coppola G, D'Adamo P, Nardocci N, et al. Benign hereditary chorea and deletions outside NKX2-1: what's the role of MBIP? Eur J Med Genet. 2018;61(10): 581-4.
23. Thorwarth A, Schnittert-Hübener S, Schrumpf P, Muller I, Jyrch S, Dame C, et al. Comprehensive genotyping and clinical characterisation reveal 27 novel NKX2-1 mutations and expand the phenotypic spectrum. J Med Genet. 2014;51(6):375-87.
24. Mencacci N, Carecchio M. Recent advances in genetics of chorea. Curr Opin Neurol. 2016;29(4):486-95.
25. Szepetowski P, Rochette J, Berquin P, Piussan C, Lathrop GM, Monaco A. Familial infantile convulsions and paroxysmal choreoathetosis: a new neurological syndrome linked to the pericentromeric region of human chromosome 16. Am J Hum Genet. 1997;61(4):889-98.
26. Chen W, Lin Y, Xiong Z, Wei W, Ni W, Tan G, et al. Exome sequencing identifies truncating mutations in PRRT2 that cause paroxysmal kinesigenic dyskinesia. Nat Genet. 2011;43(12):1252-5.
27. Heron S, Grinton B, Kivity S, Afawi Z, Zuberi S, Hughes J, et al. PRRT2 Mutations Cause Benign Familial Infantile Epilepsy and Infantile Convulsions with Choreoathetosis Syndrome. Am J Hum Genet. 2012;90(1):152-60.
28. Lee H, Huang Y, Bruneau N, Roll P, Robertson E, Hermann M, et al. Mutations in PRRT2 responsible for paroxysmal kinesigenic dyskinesias also cause benign familial infantile convulsions. J Hum Genet. 2012;57(5):338-41.
29. Maini I, Iodice A, Spagnoli C, Salerno G, Bertani G, Frattini D, et al. Expanding phenotype of PRRT2 gene mutations: A new case with epilepsy and benign myoclonus of early infancy. Eur J Paediatr Neurol. 2016;20(3):454-6.
30. Yang L, You C, Qiu S, Yang X, Li Y, Liu F, et al. Novel and de novo point and large microdeletion mutation in PRRT2-related epilepsy. Brain Behav. 2020;10(5):e01597.
31. Pan G, Zhang L, Zhou S. Clinical features of patients with paroxysmal kinesigenic dyskinesia, mutation screening of PRRT2 and the effects of morning draughts of oxcarbazepine. BMC Pediatr. 2019;19:439.
32. Mink J. Treatment of paroxysmal dyskinesias in children. Curr Treat Options Neurol. 2015;17(6):350-9.
33. Ebrahimi-Fakhari D, El-Achkar CM, Klein C. PRRT2-associated paroxysmal movement disorders. In: Adam MP, Ardinger H, Pagon R (Eds). Gene Reviews®. Seattle: University of Washington; 1993.
34. Heron SE, Dibbens LM. Role of PRRT2 in common paroxysmal neurological disorders: a gene with remarkable pleiotropy. J Med Genet. 2013;50(3):133-9.

35. Kölker S, Christensen E, Leonard J, Greenberg C, Boneh A, Burlina A, et al. Diagnosis and management of glutaric aciduria type I—revised recommendations. J Inherit Metab Dis. 2011;34(3):677-94.
36. Zayed H, El-Khayat H, Tomoum H, Khalifa O, Siddiq E, Mohammad S, et al. Clinical, biochemical, neuroradiological and molecular characterization of Egyptian patients with glutaric acidemia type 1. Metab Brain Dis. 2019;34(4):1231-41.
37. Boy N, Mühlhausen C, Maier E, Heringer J, Assman B, Burgard P, et al. Proposed Recommendations for Diagnosing and Managing Individuals With Glutaric Aciduria Type I: Second Revision. J Inherit Metab Dis. 2017;40(1):75-101.
38. Kölker S, Garbade S, Greenberg C, Leonard J, Saudubray J, Ribes A, et al. Natural History, Outcome, and Treatment Efficacy in Children and Adults With Glutaryl-CoA Dehydrogenase Deficiency. Pediatr Res. 2006;59(6):840-7.
39. Gitiaux C, Roze E, Kinugawa K, Flamand-Rouvière C, Boddaert N, Apartis E, et al. Spectrum of Movement Disorders Associated With Glutaric Aciduria Type 1: A Study of 16 Patients. Mov Disord. 2008;23(16):2392-7.
40. Brismar J, Ozand P. CT and MR of the brain in glutaric acidemia type I: a review of 59 published cases and a report of 5 new patients. AJNR Am J Neuroradiol. 1995;16(4):675-83.
41. Desai N, Runge V, Crisp D, Crisp M, Naul L. Magnetic resonance imaging of the brain in glutaric acidemia type I: a review of the literature and a report of four new cases with attention to the basal ganglia and imaging technique. Invest Radiol. 2003;38(8):489-96.
42. Twomey EL, Naughten ER, Donoghue VB, Ryan S. Neuro-imaging findings in glutaric aciduria type I. Pediatr Radiol. 2003;33(12):823-30.
43. Boy N, Heringer J, Brackmann R, Bodamer O, Seitz A, Kölker S, et al. Extrastriatal changes in patients with late-onset glutaric aciduria type I highlight the risk of long-term neurotoxicity. Orphanet J Rare Dis. 2017;12(1):77.
44. Gelener P, Severino M, Diker S, Terali K, Tuncel G, Tuzlali H, et al. Adult-onset glutaric aciduria type I: rare presentation of a treatable disorder. Neurogenetics. 2020;21(3):179-86.
45. Couce ML, López-Suárez O, Bóveda MD, Castiñeiras DE, Cocho JA, Garcia-Villoria J, et al. Glutaric aciduria type I: outcome of patients with early- versus late-diagnosis. Eur J Paediatr Neurol. 2013;17(4):383-9.
46. Afroze B, Yunus ZM. Glutaric aciduria type 1—importance of early diagnosis and treatment. J Pak Med Assoc. 2014;64(5):593-5.
47. Larson A, Goodman S. Glutaric acidemia type I. In: Adam MP, Ardinger HH, Pagon RA (Eds). Gene Reviews®. Seattle: University of Washington; 1993.
48. Kölker S, Garcia-Cazorla A, Valayannopoulos V, Lund A, Burlina A, Sykut-Cegielska J, et al. The phenotypic spectrum of organic acidurias and urea cycle disorders. Part 1: the initial presentation. J Inherit Metab Dis. 2015;38(6):1041-57.
49. Manoli I, Sloan JL, Venditti CP. Isolated methylmalonic acidemia. In: Adam MP, Ardinger HH, Pagon RA (Eds). Gene Reviews®. Seattle: University of Washington; 1993.
50. Baker EH, Sloan JL, Hauser NS, Gropman A, Adams D, Toro C, et al. MRI characteristics of globus pallidus infarcts in isolated methylmalonic acidemia. AJNR Am J Neuroradiol. 2015;36(1):194-201.
51. Dimitrov B, Molema F, Williams M, Schmiesing J, Mülhausen C, Baumgartner M, et al. Organic acidurias: major gaps, new challenges, and a yet unfulfilled promise. J Inherit Metab Dis. 2021;44(1):9-21.
52. Haijes HA, van Hasselt PM, Jans JJM, Verhoeven-Duif NM. Pathophysiology of propionic and methylmalonic acidemias. Part 2: Treatment strategies. J Inherit Metab Dis. 2019;42(5):745-61.
53. Yap S, Vara R, Morais A. Post-transplantation Outcomes in Patients with PA or MMA: A Review of the Literature. Adv Ther. 2020;37(5):1866-96.
54. Jiang Y, Sun L. The Value of Liver Transplantation for Methylmalonic Acidemia. Front Pediatr. 2019;7:87.
55. Pillai N, Stroup B, Poliner A, Rossetti L, Rawls B, Shayota B, et al. Liver transplantation in propionic and methylmalonic acidemia: a single center study with literature review. Mol Genet Metab. 2019;128(4):431-43.
56. Chandler RJ, Venditti CP. Gene Therapy for Methylmalonic Acidemia: Past, Present, and Future. Hum Gene Ther. 2019;30(10):1236-44.
57. Brennenstuhl H, Jung-Klawitter S, Assmann B, Opladen T. Inherited Disorders of Neurotransmitters: Classification and Practical Approaches for Diagnosis and Treatment. Neuropediatrics. 2019;50(1):2-14.
58. Wijemanne S, Jankovic J. Dopa-responsive dystonia—clinical and genetic heterogeneity. Nat Rev Neurol. 2015;11(7):414-24.
59. Lee W, Jeon B. Clinical spectrum of dopa-responsive dystonia and related disorders. Curr Neurol Neurosci Rep. 2014;14(7):461.
60. Kim, R, Jeon B, Lee W. A Systematic Review of Treatment Outcome in Patients with Dopa-responsive Dystonia (DRD) and DRD-Plus. Mov Disord Clin Pract. 2016;3(5):435-42.
61. Malek N, Fletcher N, Newman E. Diagnosing dopamine-responsive dystonias. Pract Neurol. 2015;15(5):340-5.
62. Segawa M, Ohmi K, Itoh S, Aoyama M, Hayakawa H. Childhood basal ganglia disease with marked response to L-Dopa: hereditary progressive basal ganglia disease with marked diurnal fluctuation. Shinryo. 1972;24(5):667-72.
63. Lee WW, Jeon B, Kim R. Expanding the Spectrum of Dopa-Responsive Dystonia (DRD) and Proposal for New Definition: DRD, DRD-plus, and DRD Look-alike. J Korean Med Sci. 2018;33(28):e184.
64. Willemsen M, Verbeek M, Kamsteeg E, Rijk-van Andel J, Aeby A Blau N, et al. Tyrosine hydroxylase deficiency: a treatable disorder of brain catecholamine biosynthesis. Brain. 2010;133(Pt 6):1810-22.
65. Dionisi-Vici C, Hoffmann G, Leuzzi V, Hoffken H, Bräutigam C, Rizzo C, et al. Tyrosine hydroxylase deficiency with severe clinical course: clinical and biochemical investigations and optimization of therapy. J Pediatr. 2000;136(4):560-2.
66. Katus LE, Frucht SJ. An unusual presentation of tyrosine hydroxylase deficiency. J Clin Mov Disord. 2017;4:18.
67. Bally JF, Breen DP, Schaake S, Trinh J, Rakovic A, Klein C, et al. Mild dopa-responsive dystonia in heterozygous tyrosine hydroxylase mutation carrier: evidence of symptomatic enzyme deficiency? Parkinsonism Relat Disord. 2020;71:44-5.
68. Friedman J, Roze E, Abdenur J, Chang R, Gasperini S, Saletti V, et al. Sepiapterin reductase deficiency: a treatable mimic of cerebral palsy. Ann Neurol. 2012;71(4):520-30.

CHAPTER **50**

Syndromes of Continuous Muscle Fiber Activity

Satish V Khadilkar, Bhagyadhan Patel, Khushnuma Mansukhani

INTRODUCTION

Syndromes of continuous muscle fiber activity (SCMFA) form an uncommon group of disorders characterized by spontaneous discharges from motor nerve fibers. The initial description of the condition was given by Isaac in 1961. In 1965, Mertens and Zschocke coined the term "neuromyotonia (NMT)" to denote the neural origin of activity in some of the patients who clinically exhibited amyotonia-like stiffness. Morvan used the term "fibrillary chorea" to highlight the involuntary flickering of muscles and also documented central nervous system (CNS) dysfunction (e.g., hallucinations, sleep disturbances, mood changes, encephalopathy) in his patients. Isaacs–Mertens syndrome or SCMFA, Morvan's syndrome, NMT, and cramp fasciculation syndrome (CFS) are grouped under the umbrella of "peripheral nerve hyperexcitability (PNH) syndromes" and the CFS represents a milder form. This group of conditions is presumed to result from antibodies directed against voltage-gated potassium channels (VGKCs) located in the terminal parts of peripheral nerves. Immune-mediated PNH can be secondary to or a part of wider autoimmune disorders and also occur as paraneoplastic syndromes. Rarely, PNH has genetic origins. Some features of PNH can be seen in patients primarily having a peripheral neuropathy or anterior horn cell degeneration and such are termed as "secondary PNH." It is important for clinicians to be aware of PNH, as most of these disorders require long-term supervision, often with immunosuppression and periodic screening for underlying tumors.[1-7]

CLINICAL FEATURES

Overall, PNH syndromes are more common in males with the peak onset in fourth or fifth decade. Uncommonly, these have been reported in younger age groups. SCMFA is characterized by muscle twitching (fasciculations, myokymia), painful cramps, and muscle stiffness (pseudomyotonia, pseudotetany), which lead to muscle hypertrophy in long-standing cases. In severe cases, muscle weakness is present. Overall, the symptoms are more prominent in muscles of lower limb than upper limbs. Sensory disturbances, autonomic dysfunction, and CNS involvement can occur with immune-mediated disorders. Clinical features of PNH are summarized below.

- *Muscle twitching*—this is the most common symptom of SCMFA and represents myokymia and fasciculations. Myokymia is derived from Greek word "kyma," which means a wave. It is characterized by continuous, undulating, and wave-like rippling of muscles, akin to a bag of worms under the skin. It is commonly seen in lower limb muscles, but can be seen in muscles of the upper limbs, trunk, face, and sometimes the tongue. These undulating movements are seen to traverse the breadth of the muscle. The myokymic movements seen in PNH have to be differentiated from fasciculations. Fasciculations are randomly occurring rapid, spontaneous twitches of a single part of a muscle and lack the rhythmic quality of myokymia. Fasciculations occur along the length of muscle fibers as against myokymia. While fasciculations usually denote an anterior horn cell disease, they can also be seen in milder form of illness such as CFS.

- *Painful cramps*—muscle cramps occur very early in the course of illness. These are painful and are associated with muscle spasms, which are worsened on attempting muscle action. Muscle cramps often aggravate on exposure to cold.
- *Muscle stiffness*—patients experience lasting stiffness of muscles, as if the muscle cramps have become long lasting. Due to stiffness, patients can develop difficulty in walking and lose their dexterity. Severe involuntary movements of muscles can lead to persistent contractions of extremities. Spontaneous or evoked "carpopedal spasm-like" posturing of hands can be seen in some patients. Such patients' illness can be mistaken for dystonia and indeed some authors have used the terms such as pseudodystonia or pseudotetany to describe these postures. Clinical features of SCMFA are known to simulate myotonia and patients may exhibit delayed relaxation of muscles after voluntary contraction, e.g., slow release after a handgrip or prolonged eye closure. Importantly, unlike myotonic disorders, there is no percussion myotonia. The absence of percussion myotonia separates them from truly myotonic disorders.
- *Muscle hypertrophy*—continuous muscle activity for sustained periods can result in hypertrophy of skeletal muscles. Most often, calf muscles are hypertrophied but in some patients, muscle enlargement can be seen in forearm and hand muscles as well. The degree of hypertrophy relates to the severity of muscle overactivity.
- *Muscle weakness*—rarely, muscular weakness can occur due to fatigue as a result of continuous muscle fiber activity. Rarely, patients having the Morvan's syndrome have been reported to present with quadriparesis.
- *Sensory complaints*—due to sensory nerve hyperexcitability, a proportion of patients develop paresthesias, dysesthesias, and numbness.
- *Autonomic dysfunction*—hyperhidrosis is the most prevalent and persistent manifestation of autonomic dysfunction. Increased metabolic rate secondary to excessive muscle activity can be a contributory factor to hyperhidrosis. In extreme cases, other dysautonomic features such as tachycardia, hypotension, urinary complaints, constipation, hypersalivation, and lacrimation can be present.
- *Central nervous system involvement*—insomnia and neuropsychiatric features are occasionally seen in patient with SCMFA. Neuropsychiatric features take the forms of hallucinations, confusion, delusions, agitation, and amnesia. A minority of patients are known to develop faciobrachial dystonic seizures or generalized tonic-clonic seizures.[4,5,7-11]

SPECTRUM OF DISORDERS

Medical literature is flooded with terminologies such as idiopathic generalized myokymia, acquired NMT, armadillo syndrome, and syndrome of continuous muscle fiber activity, but PNH is most widely accepted term. Clinical spectrum of PNH is wide. CFS, Issacs' syndrome, and Morvan's syndrome form the three main primary PNH syndromes (**Table 1**). CFS is the milder form, while Isaac's and Morvan's syndrome represent severe form of PNH. A significant proportion of immune-mediated PNH forms parts of systemic autoimmune disorders or occurs in patients having malignancies. In India, contemporary streams of medicine such as Ayurvedic, Homeopathic, and Unani are prevalent and many are known to use metallic oxides having toxic potential. Recently, 32 cases of NMT following the use of Siddha medicine containing mercury compounds have been reported. Secondary PNH can be seen in disorders of peripheral nerves, roots, and anterior horn cells as well as toxin exposure.[1,12-15]

Rarely, PNH syndromes are associated with inherited diseases (**Table 2**).

TABLE 1: Salient features of CFS, Isaacs' and Morvan's syndrome.

Salient features	*CFS*	*Isaacs' syndrome*	*Morvan's syndrome*
Clinical features	Cramps and myalgia, but no weakness	Muscle twitching, cramps, and muscle stiffness	Muscle twitching, cramps, and muscle stiffness
VGKC antibodies	±	++	++
Electrophysiology	Fasciculation at rest; normal MUPs	Myokymia and neuromyotonia	Myokymia and neuromyotonia
Autonomic features	Absent	Present	Present
CNS involvement	Absent	Absent	present
Comorbid illness	Nil; benign syndrome	Thymoma and SCLC	Thymoma, SCLC, and myasthenia gravis

(CFS: cramp fasciculation syndrome; CNS: central nervous system; MUPs: motor unit potentials; SCLC: small cell lung carcinoma; VGKC: voltage-gated potassium channel)

TABLE 2: Disorders associated with myokymia and neuromyotonic discharges.

PNH associated with systemic disorders	• *Associated with other autoimmune disorders*: MG, SLE, CIDP, autoimmune thyroid disease, and rheumatoid arthritis • *Paraneoplastic syndromes*: Thymoma, small cell lung carcinoma, lymphoma, and other hematological malignancies (*Note*: Satoyoshi syndrome is an idiopathic autoimmune disorder that is often included in PNH spectrum)
Secondary PNH	• *Peripheral neuropathy*: CIDP, GBS, entrapment neuropathy such as CTS, radiation plexopathies/neuropathies, and radiculopathy • *Anterior horn cell degeneration*: ALS and SMA • *Toxins*: Heavy metal exposure (gold, lithium, platinum, mercury), penicillamine therapy, alcohol, snake venom, and insecticide • *Miscellaneous*: Thyrotoxicosis
Genetic and hereditary causes	• VGKC (KCNA1) mutations • Familial episodic ataxia type 1 (EA1) • Hereditary neuropathy (HINT1 mutation) • Schwartz–Jampel syndrome (SJS)
Focal myokymia involving face	Multiple sclerosis, brainstem mass lesion (e.g., glioma), cerebellopontine angle mass lesion, basilar invagination, and syringobulbia

(ALS: amyotrophic lateral sclerosis; CIDP: chronic inflammatory demyelinating polyneuropathy; CTS: carpal tunnel syndrome; GBS: Guillain–Barré syndrome; HINT1: histidine triad nucleotide-binding protein 1; MG: myasthenia gravis; PNH: peripheral nerve hyperexcitability; SLE: systemic lupus erythematosus; SMA: spinal muscular atrophy; VGKC: voltage-gated potassium channel)

DIFFERENTIAL DIAGNOSIS

Muscle stiffness and twitching can occur in a number of disorders. **Table 3** highlights salient features of these disorders.

INVESTIGATIONS

The primary step is to confirm electrophysiological changes of PNH, as it can help differentiate it from its mimics (**Table 4** and **Figures 1** to **4**). Further investigations should be directed to detect comorbid autoimmune disorders, neoplasms, and rule out secondary PNH. Following investigations can be of help in PNH (**Table 4**).

MANAGEMENT AND PROGNOSIS

The treatment of PNH is aimed at reducing spontaneous peripheral nerve discharges and management of causative and coexisting illness. Patients having mild illness such as CFS benefit significantly from membrane stabilizing agents alone, while severe forms of PNH require immunosuppressants as well.

Principles of management of PNH syndromes are summarized below.

- *Symptomatic treatment with membrane stabilizing agents*: Antiepileptic medications such as carbamazepine, phenytoin, lamotrigine, pregabalin, gabapentin, and duloxetine help to control pain, cramps, sensory symptoms, muscle twitches, and stiffness. These

TABLE 3: Key clinical features of disorders mimicking SCMFA.[1,16-19]

Disorders mimicking SCMFA	*Key clinical features*
Episodic ataxia type 1	Early onset, positive family history, episodes of cerebellar ataxia, and muscle stiffness lasting for seconds to minutes, which are precipitated by stress and sudden movements and response to acetazolamide
Stiff person syndrome (SPS)	Elderly onset, axial > appendicular board-like rigidity, painful extensor spasms precipitated by external stimuli or sudden movement, hyperlordosis, and continuous firing of normal muscle action potentials simultaneously affecting agonist and antagonist group of muscles favor SPS. There is absence of muscle twitching
McArdle's disease	Early onset, episodic muscle cramps, stiffness, contractures, and weakness aggravated by exercise and relieved by rest. Presence of myoglobinuria and severe elevation of serum creatine kinase (CK) levels favor glycolytic pathway defects
Myotonia congenita	Early onset, familial, muscle stiffness, muscle hypertrophy, presence of action as well as percussion myotonia, and myotonic discharges (lower frequency than neuromyotonic discharges) favor myotonia congenita
Schwartz–Jampel syndrome (SJS)	Early onset, action and percussion myotonia, skeletal deformity, blepharophimosis, absence of myokymia, hyperhidrosis, and presence of myotonic discharges suggest SJS
Amyotrophic lateral sclerosis (ALS) presenting as muscle twitching and spasticity	Elderly onset, fasciculations, muscle cramps, stiffness associated with muscle weakness and wasting, fibrillations, and fasciculations on needle electrode examination (NEE) suggest ALS
Rippling muscle disease	Rippling movements of muscles at rest, on stretching and on percussion, absence of spontaneous activity on needle electrode examination, and presence of muscle weakness favor rippling muscle disease

TABLE 4: Key investigations in PNH syndromes.[1,4,5,8,11,19]	
Nerve conduction studies (NCSs)	• *Sensory*: Normal—except when there is an associated peripheral neuropathy as in Isaacs' syndrome • *Motor*: Normal—except when associated with a peripheral neuropathy as seen in Isaacs' syndrome • *Repetitive CMAPs*: Multiple repetitive discharges are seen, either following the direct muscle response or after the F-wave (depending on the site of the generator). These are called "after discharges" or "repetitive CMAPs." They are the hallmark of peripheral nerve hyperexcitability (PNH) and are essential for the diagnosis of this condition. They may not be seen in all the nerves, are multiple, and do not habituate with repetitive nerve stimulation • *F-waves*: Normal—except—may be difficult to identify, if embedded within the repetitive after discharges (prolonged, if there is an associated peripheral neuropathy)
Needle electrode examination (NEE)	• *Spontaneous activity*: Various types of spontaneous activity can be recorded. The type of activity seen depends on the severity of the PNH. In milder cases, there may be only widespread fasciculation potentials and cramp discharges. As the severity increases, doublets, triplets, and myokymic discharges are within the same muscle at rest. Neuromyotonic discharges seen, persistently mark the most severe part of the spectrum, and are associated with the clinical features of stiffness and persistent contraction of the muscles. Spontaneous activities that can be seen include: • Fasciculation potentials • Myokymic discharges • Doublets, triplets, and multiplets • Neuromyotonic discharges • Neuromyotonic discharges are fast firing motor unit potentials (firing rate: 40–300 Hz) occurring persistently or in bursts, which fire irregularly. Within a burst, the motor unit potential may wane in amplitude and frequency (does not wax). The sound produced depends on the length of the burst and could be defined as "corn-popping sound," "pinging," or "dive bomber." They may occur spontaneously or are induced by tapping or needle movement • Voluntarily evoked motor unit potentials are normal, unless there is denervation associated with the peripheral neuropathy
Routine serum investigations	Presence of hyponatremia suggests VGKC antibodies syndrome. Serum creatine kinase (CK) levels are normal or mildly elevated. In appropriate situations, testing of heavy metal levels in the serum should be ordered, e.g., mercury
Antibody levels	VGKC antibody is found in most patients with Morvan's syndrome, up to 50% in Isaacs' syndrome, and 24% in CFS. CASPR2 antibody is more frequently found than LGI1 antibody in patients with PNH. Patient should undergo testing for antibodies such as AchR, ANA, anti-GAD, RF, and anti-Ro and anti-La
Cerebrospinal fluid (CSF) examination	Usually normal, but CSF examination may show changes of inflammation such as mild elevation in protein levels and lymphocytosis
Electroencephalography (EEG)	EEG may show generalized slowing of the background activity in a small proportion of patients with Morvan's syndrome
Magnetic resonance imaging (MRI)	Except for nonspecific temporal lobe hyperintensities, MRI is usually normal in Morvan's syndrome
Positron emission tomography (PET)	PET scan may show focal or generalized cerebral hypometabolism. Whole-body PET scan can help to detect occult tumors such as thymoma and small cell lung carcinoma

medications can cause side effects such as sedation, dizziness, hyponatremia, sexual dysfunction, and imbalance. Hence, patients need to be monitored closely, as these patients require medications on long-term basis.[1-3,20]

- *Immunotherapy*: Many of the PNH syndromes respond favorably to immunomodulation such as oral or intravenous corticosteroids. In severe cases, patients may need rescue therapies such as intravenous immunoglobulins or plasma exchange to overcome acute stages of illness. Rituximab and cyclophosphamide can be used in severe refractory cases. The information of use of long-term immunosuppressants is less and relapses are known to occur. Patients with severe illness at presentation or relapsing nature of illness may require steroid-sparing agents such as azathioprine, mycophenolate mofetil, or cyclosporine.[1,3,11,20,21]
- *Treatment of underlying illness*: As a significant proportion of these syndromes are paraneoplastic in nature, it is important to fully investigate and address

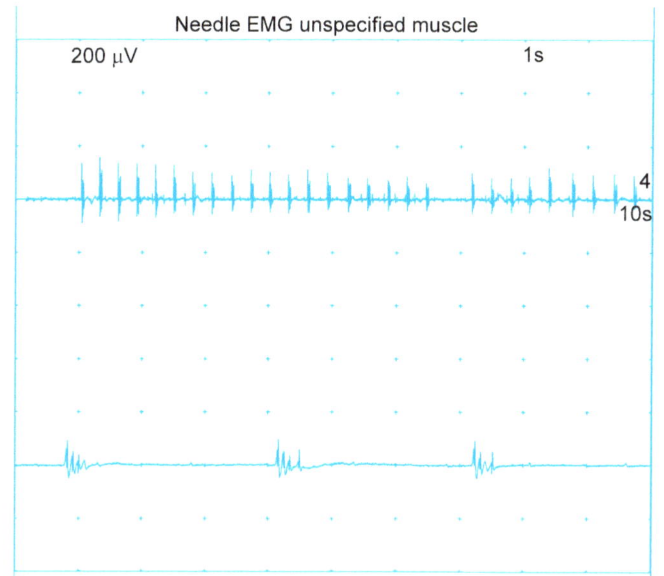

FIG. 1: Myokymic discharges: bursts of few motor units, firing rhythmically.

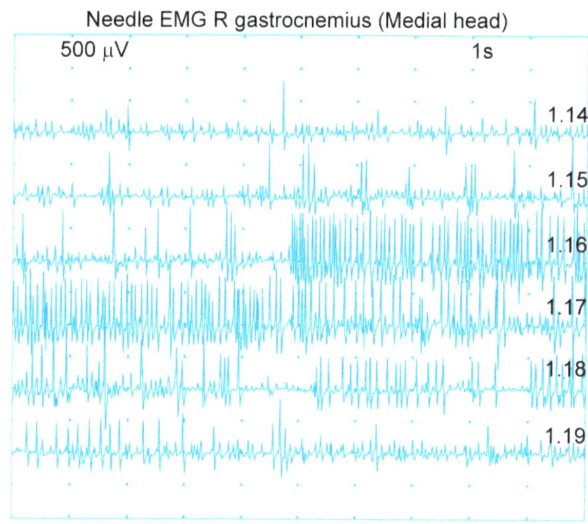

FIG. 3: Continuous motor unit activity seen in a patient with stiff muscle: fast firing rate.

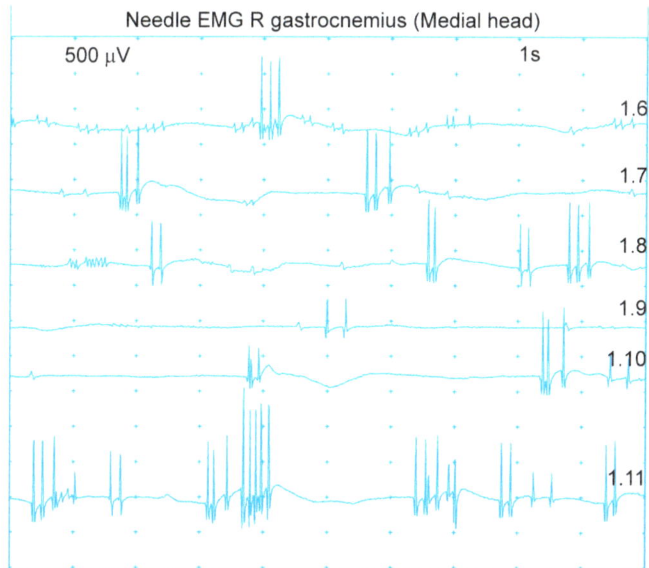

FIG. 2: Multiple discharges seen from the muscle at rest: doublets, triplets, and multiplets.

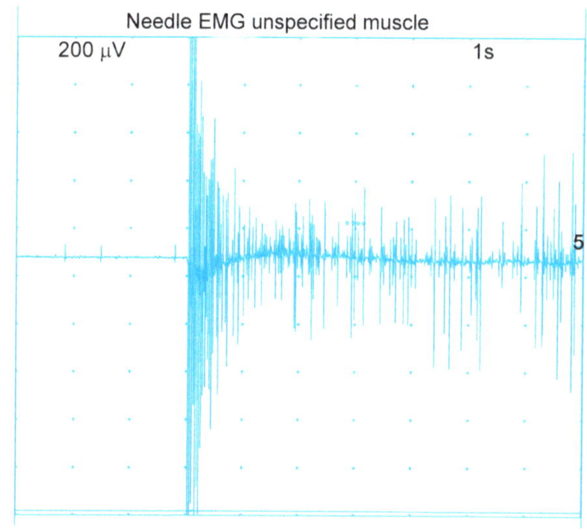

FIG. 4: Waning neuromyotonic discharge.

the underlying illness, as it can positively alter the course of illness.

- *Prognosis*: PNH syndromes such as CFS and Isaacs' syndrome have favorable prognosis, but severe form of PNH with autonomic involvement (arrhythmias and cardiac failure) can be life-threatening. Mortality is higher in patients with underlying tumors. Severe form of PNH may require long-term immunosuppressants and significantly impair the quality of life. While recovery and good outcomes are seen in a proportion of patients, protracted course with fluctuations is not uncommon and counseling to that effect from the early time can prove relevant.[1]

CONCLUSION

The clinical, electrophysiological and laboratory characteristics of this group of disorders are now well characterized. As these immunological diseases respond to immunotherapy and patients can lead a good quality of life, it is important for the clinicians to recognize them early and treat appropriately for optimum results.

REFERENCES

1. Khadilkar SV, Yadav RS, Patel BA. Peripheral nerve hyperexcitability syndromes. In: Khadilkar SV, Yadav RS, Patel BA (Eds). Neuromuscular Disorders: A Comprehensive Review with Illustrative Cases, 1st edition. Singapore: Springer; 2018. pp. 299-309.
2. Sawlani K, Katirji B. Peripheral Nerve Hyperexcitability Syndromes. Continuum (Minneap Minn). 2017;23(5):1437-50.
3. Skeie GO, Apostolski S, Evoli A, Gilhus NE, Illa I, Harms L, et al. Guidelines for treatment of autoimmune neuromuscular transmission disorders. Eur J Neurol. 2010;17(7):893-902.
4. Hart IK, Maddison P, Newsom-Davis J, Vincent A, Mills KR. Phenotypic variants of autoimmune peripheral nerve hyperexcitability. Brain. 2002;125(Pt 8):1887-95.
5. Maddison P. Neuromyotonia. Clin Neurophysiol. 2006;117(10):2118-27.
6. Küçükali CI, Kürtüncü M, Akçay Hİ, Tüzün E, Öge AE. Peripheral nerve hyperexcitability syndromes. Rev Neurosci. 2015;26(2):239-51.
7. Gutmann L, Gutmann L. Myokymia and neuromyotonia 2004. J Neurol. 2004;251(2):138-42.
8. Irani SR, Pettingill P, Kleopa KA, Schiza N, Waters P, Mazia C, et al. Morvan syndrome: clinical and serological observations in 29 cases. Ann Neurol. 2012;72(2):241-55.
9. Lotan I, Djaldetti R, Hellman MA, Benninger F. Atypical case of Morvan's syndrome. J Clin Neurosci. 2016;25(1):132-4.
10. Liewluck T, Klein CJ, Jones LK. Cramp-fasciculation syndrome in patients with and without neural autoantibodies. Muscle Nerve. 2014;49(3):351-6.
11. Abou-Zeid E, Boursoulian LJ, Metzer WS, Gundogdu B. Morvan syndrome: a case report and review of the literature. J Clin Neuromuscul Dis. 2012;13(4):214-27.
12. Gnanashanmugam G, Balakrishnan R, Somasundaram SP, Parimalam N, Rajmohan P, Pranesh MB. Mercury Toxicity Following Unauthorized Siddha Medicine Intake—A Mimicker of Acquired Neuromyotonia—Report of 32 Cases. Ann Indian Acad Neurol. 2018;21(1):49-56.
13. Panagariya A, Kumar H, Mathew V, Sharma B. Neuromyotonia: Clinical profile of twenty cases from northwest India. Neurol India. 2006;54(4):382-6.
14. Chaurasia RN, Abbas A, Shukla R. Toxin-induced continuous muscle fiber activity syndrome. Ann Neurosci. 2008;15:4.
15. Mohanakkannan S, Perumal SR, Velayudham S, Jeyaraj KM, Arunan S. A Case of Morvan's Syndrome Associated with Heavy Metal Poisoning after Ayurvedic Drug Intake. J Neurosci Rural Pract. 2018;9(3):431-3.
16. Pulkes T, Dejthevaporn C, Apiwattanakul M, Papsing C, Hanna MG. Paroxysmal neuromyotonia: a new sporadic channelopathy. Neuromuscul Disord. 2012;22(6):479-82.
17. Jen JC, Graves TD, Hess EJ, Hanna MG, Griggs RC, Baloh RW, et al. Primary episodic ataxias: diagnosis, pathogenesis and treatment. Brain. 2007;130(Pt 10):2484-93.
18. Falace A, Striano P, Manganelli F, Coppola A, Striano S, Minetti C, et al. Inherited neuromyotonia: a clinical and genetic study of a family. Neuromuscul Disord. 2007;17(1):23-7.
19. Ahmed A, Simmons Z. Isaacs syndrome: a review. Muscle Nerve. 2015;52(1):5-12.
20. Hurst RL, Hobson-Webb LD. Therapeutic Implications of Peripheral Nerve Hyperexcitability in Muscle Cramping: A Retrospective Review. J Clin Neurophysiol. 2016;33(6):560-3.
21. Elangovan C, Morawo A, Ahmed A. Current Treatment Options for Peripheral Nerve Hyperexcitability Syndromes. Curr Treat Options Neurol. 2018;20(7):23.

CHAPTER 51

Peripherally Induced Movement Disorders and Other Miscellaneous Movement Disorders

Pankaj A Agarwal, Shruti Agrawal, Sangeeta H Ravat

INTRODUCTION

Movement disorders that originate in the *peripheral* nervous system are a result of lower motor neuronal hyperexcitability. Some specific entities such as restless legs syndrome, neuromyotonia, and stiff-person syndrome have been covered in other chapters in this textbook. This chapter will focus on *hemifacial spasm* (HFS), *hemimasticatory spasm* (HMS), *hereditary geniospasm* (HG), *painful legs and moving toes* (PLMT) syndrome, and *posttraumatic* movement disorders arising after trauma to the peripheral nervous system.

HEMIFACIAL SPASM

Hemifacial spasm is characterized by unilateral irregular clonic or tonic movements of the muscles innervated by the 7th cranial (facial) nerve.[1] The prevalence of HFS has been estimated to be 14.5 per 100,000 women and 7.4 per 100,000 men.[2]

Pathophysiology

Primary HFS is thought to be due to neurovascular in origin, i.e., due to compression of the facial nerve at its root exit zone from the brainstem by an ectatic arterial loop arising from the vertebrobasilar system.[3] Such a loop is often not detected on standard MRI sequences, requiring special MRI sequences for visualization [e.g., constructive interference in steady state/fast imaging employing steady-state acquisition (*CISS/FIESTA*) images] or may even be absent in a small minority of patients, in which case the condition is considered idiopathic. *Secondary HFS* is less common than primary HFS and can occur due to involvement of the facial motor nucleus in the pons by a variety of lesions, or due to injury to the nerve itself, anywhere along its peripheral course, due to nerve trauma, inflammation, demyelination, nerve sheath tumor, or a vascular insult to the nerve.[4]

Clinical Features

Symptom onset is commonly in the fifth decade and females are affected more than males[1,5,6] Most commonly, in a unilateral condition, the left face is more commonly involved due to a higher prevalence of vascular anomalies on the left.[5-7] Bilateral affection is rare but can occur.[8] In primary HFS, the upper eyelid is usually involved before lower hemiface muscles, due to a relatively more dorsal placement of facial nerve fibers that supply the upper face at the root entry zone, and a vascular loop compressing the nerve dorsally. Factors precipitating spasms include speaking, mental stress, chewing, exposure to sunlight, watching television, and hypertension, while sleep commonly relieves spasms. Ipsilateral auditory clicks may be present in HFS and occur due to clonic contractions of the stapedius muscle leading to compression and rarefaction of air in the middle ear. Patients with secondary HFS may have a milder intensity of disease. The *other Babinski sign (OBS)* is classically seen in organic HFS and consists of *concurrent* ipsilateral frontal and orbicularis oculi (O.oc) contraction, thus raising the eyebrow at the same time as ipsilateral eye closure[9] (**Fig. 1A**). Of note, functional (psychogenic) unilateral facial contraction can phenomenologically resemble organic HFS. The two can be differentiated clinically by a lack of the *OBS* in psychogenic facial contraction, wherein the eyebrow may instead be *depressed* due to ipsilateral eye closure and indeed the *contralateral* eyebrow might be elevated[10] (**Fig. 1B**).

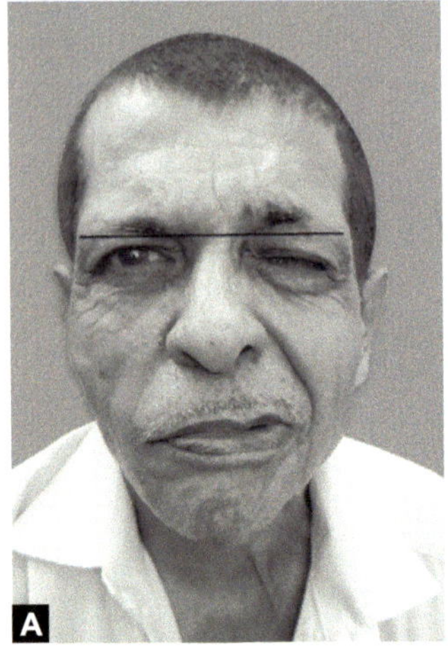

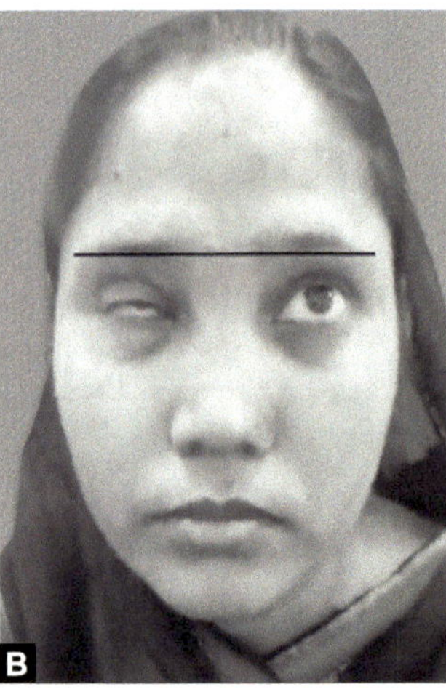

FIGS. 1A AND B: (A) Organic left hemifacial spasm (HFS)—the "other Babinski" sign. Elevation of left eyebrow at the same time as left eye closure due to concurrent contraction of frontalis and orbicularis oculi muscles in HFS; and (B) Functional (psychogenic) right eye closure. The right eyebrow is *relatively* depressed compared to the unaffected left eyebrow. The "other Babinski" sign is, therefore, absent. ***(For color version, see plate 3)***

Other clues for a functional origin include tonic sustained contraction (rather than the fast irregular myoclonus of HFS), higher likelihood of bilateral (or alternating) lower face involvement, suggestibility, distraction, abrupt onset, maximal severity at onset, ipsilateral tongue and/or jaw deviation, and variability in phenomenology.[11]

Treatment

Benefit obtained by oral medication including carbamazepine or clonazepam is modest at best and the most effective treatment is botulinum toxin (BTX) injection. Muscles injected include the O.oc—pretarsal injections are preferred over preseptal O.oc due to higher effectiveness and other muscles such as zygomaticus major and minor, levators of the lip, and risorius; doses range typically from 1.25 to 3.75 units (onabotulinumtoxin A doses) per site. Excessive weakness of facial muscles producing undesirable asymmetry of the lower face, e.g., a crooked smile is the major adverse effect and can be avoided by conservative dosing of toxin, especially for the lower facial muscles. This is also more likely to occur in secondary HFS and, therefore, these patients require lower dosages of toxin than those with primary HFS. Benefit may become apparent after 2–5 days, but is most often within 2 weeks after injection and the typical duration of benefit is 3–6 months, after which injections may need to be repeated. In severe or refractory HFS, surgical treatment, i.e., microvascular decompression (MVD) of the facial nerve can be offered and is generally effective with acceptable overall safety and efficacy and improved quality of life. Adverse effects include postoperative facial weakness and numbness that are usually temporary. Symptom recurrence has been reported in 5–15% of cases.[12,13]

HEMIMASTICATORY SPASM

Hemimasticatory spasm is a rare movement disorder with unilateral paroxysmal and painful involuntary contractions of the muscles of mastication.[14] It was first described by Gowers in 1897 as "masticatory spasms of Romberg".[15] It is twice more common in females and commonly presents in the third or fourth decade of life.[16] An Indian series of seven cases seen over 4 years has recently been reported from Delhi.[17] The masseter and temporalis are the most commonly involved muscles with occasional involvement of medial pterygoid as well[14] and, occasionally, the lateral pterygoid.[18] Triggers for sudden spasms can include speaking, chewing, laughing, yawning, or indeed any jaw movement and attack duration and intensity can vary from brief intermittent painless spasms for several seconds or few minutes to frequent prolonged painful attacks lasting several hours. Prolonged painless spasms can occur. Ipsilateral hemifacial atrophy is seen commonly in up to two-thirds of cases of HMS and localized scleroderma ("morphea") in a third.[17,19] Hypertrophy of the involved masseter and/or temporalis is common. Attacks of HMS can lead to tongue or inner cheek injury by forcefully clenched teeth and in severe cases, tooth dislocation/breakage or temporomandibular joint dislocation.[20]

Pathophysiology

Hemimasticatory spasm is thought to be caused by vascular compression followed by focal demyelination of the motor branch of the trigeminal nerve due to involvement of nerve fibers by structural skin and soft tissue changes causing ipsilateral facial hemiatrophy.[21] Compression of the motor trigeminal branch is found in the infratemporal fossa between the lateral pterygoid muscle and skull surface.[17] Absent or impaired inhibition of the masseter reflex is seen. Rare causes of *secondary* HMS include pontine infarction causing hyperactivity of trigeminal motor nucleus, biopercular syndrome, and cerebellopontine angle hematoma.[17,19,22]

Electromyography

It shows spontaneous bursts of high frequency (100–200 Hz) motor unit action potentials in involved muscles coinciding with clinical spasms.[17,19] An absent or reduced masseter silent period and an impaired inhibition of masseter reflex during muscle spasm may be related to ectopic excitation that is secondary to focal demyelination of trigeminal motor fibers.[19] Blink reflex is normal.

Diagnosis

Because of the rarity of HMS, it is frequently misdiagnosed as HFS, oromandibular dystonia, temporomandibular joint disorder, facial tic or myoclonus, or even focal seizure.[23] Unilateral involvement points to HMS rather than jaw-closing dystonia, where jaw closure contraction is commonly bilateral. Functional (psychogenic) facial contraction is another important differential for HMS and one should look for clues to the former such as jaw *deviation* (rather than jaw *closure* as in HMS), sustained ipsilateral eye closure, tongue deviation to the same side, ipsilateral lower lip eversion with or without platysmal contraction, and variability including alternating side facial involvement. Awareness of HMS and careful history and clinical examination to rule out other possibilities are all important for diagnosis.

Treatment

Carbamazepine or phenytoin may have some effect in controlling spasms and pain.[17,20] However, BTX injection into the affected unilateral masseter and temporalis muscles is the most effective treatment of this disorder and can provide marked relief.[15,17,18,21] MVD has also shown good results in a few patients, though the exact role of surgery is unclear.[24]

HEREDITARY GENIOSPASM

Hereditary geniospasm or "chin trembling" is an autosomal dominant, unusual movement disorder characterized by involuntary, paroxysmal, and often rhythmic up-and-down movements of only the chin and the lower lip due to involvement of bilateral mentalis muscles.[25] Involvement of orbicularis oris and mylohyoid muscles is also described, with partial involvement of the levator labii superioris muscle.[25] Episodes may last for a variable duration ranging from seconds to hours. Triggering factors may be emotion, anxiety, concentration, anger, and stress, but chin tremor can appear without an apparent precipitant. The condition typically manifests in infancy or early life, with episodes tending to reduce in frequency with advancing age.[26,27] Severe chin tremor can lead to bruxism with audible teeth clattering, social embarrassment, and even sleep deprivation.[27-29] People may think that the affected person is going to cry.

The condition was first described in 1894 by Domenico Massaro, who reported 26 cases in the same family in Italy over five generations.[30] In 1922, Percy Stocks reported geniospasm for the first time in a British family.[31] The first report from India was in a child with frequent tongue bite in sleep as a result of parasomnia, which was treated with clonazepam with no effect on chin trembling.[32] Few other Indian reports exist, mostly in children. A family from Maharashtra state has been observed by an author of this chapter (PA) with classic chin trembling of onset in the second (to fourth) decade of life in at least five affected members from three generations, suggestive of autosomal dominant transmission; however, genetic studies have not been performed. HG has been described in the literature using many different terms, including *HG*,[28] *hereditary quivering of the chin*,[29] and *familial trembling of the chin*. Recently, it has been suggested that a better term would be *hereditary chin myoclonus*[28] because the abnormal involuntary movement is related to quick jerks of the mentalis muscle, burst duration is brief (10–25 ms), and there are pauses between individual jerks.[33] Electromyography (EMG) testing of the mentalis and other affected muscles showed rhythmic bursts of involuntary activity and motor units of normal morphology firing at 6–10 Hz for 50–300 ms.[25]

Jarman and colleagues in 1997 identified linkage to markers on the long arm of chromosome 9 in one family and defined an approximately 2.1 cM interval on chromosome 9q13-21.[28] The exclusion of the chromosome 9q13-q21 locus in other families demonstrated that genetic heterogeneity exists with this condition and further linkage studies will be required to identify other chromosomal regions that can cause similar phenotypes.[28]

Diagnosis

Differential diagnoses of HG include tics, facial myokymia, and jaw tremor. Tics do not occur during sleep and each paroxysm is usually preceded by an urge and followed by a feeling of satisfaction.[33] Facial myokymia may occur in association with other neurological conditions such as brainstem tumors and multiple sclerosis, usually affects more than one muscle, and is confined to one side of the face.[26] Jaw tremor, as part of orolingual tremor, can occur in essential tremor (ET) or Parkinson's disease (PD); however, involvement of other body parts will reveal features of ET or PD.[27]

Treatment

Botulinum toxin to the mentalis muscle is the simplest and most effective treatment[34] with low doses (1.25–5 units of onabotulinumtoxinA) employed on both sides and additional doses in other affected muscles, if any. Injections can be repeated every 3–6 months depending on the response. The effect remains overall stable over several years with requirement of similar doses over time.[35]

PAINFUL LEGS AND MOVING TOES SYNDROME

Painful legs and moving toes was first described by Spillane et al. in 1971.[36] Later, variants described include *painful arms and moving fingers*[37] and *painful mouth and moving tongue*.[38] PLMT is a syndrome characterized by pain in both distal lower limbs associated with repetitive toe movements. Pain usually precedes movements, but may appear together or follow each other. It is more common in middle-aged females, though it affects a wide age range (cases reported aged 11-86 years).[39,40] Awareness regarding existence of this entity is important, as patients may be mislabeled as having psychogenic symptomatology.

Pain: It can involve one or both lower limbs. Pain can be described as tearing, throbbing, cramp like, shocking, sharp shooting, tingling, numbness, dull aching, pulling, or bursting. Severity may range from constant discomfort to unbearable pain. About 58% of patients in a study reported various aggravating factors such as various positions (sitting, standing, walking, weight bearing, or bending), diurnal variations, cold temperature, external pressure, Valsalva, or full bladder.[40] Occasional painless variants have been reported.[36,41]

Movements: It commonly involves toes of one lower limb at first before involving both sides. Upper limbs can be affected in 13% of cases.[39] Movements are irregular, nonrhythmic movements, most commonly involving toes with flexion, extension, adduction, abduction, dystonia, myoclonus, or piano-like movements of toes that can be transiently suppressed by distraction or standing. More proximal joints may be involved causing movements in feet or legs. Movements are stereotypical in an individual and can be differentiated from chorea by a lack of flowing character. Hassan et al. have described a patient with involvement of one lower limb followed by shift to the other lower limb with complete resolution of movements in the original limb.[39] Patients with a history of trauma to one limb followed by movements on the contralateral side are also reported.[39]

Pathophysiology

Painful legs and moving toes can be secondary to peripheral neuropathy, radiculopathy, spinal cord or cauda equina injury, injuries to bony and soft tissues of feet, or trauma ranging from a trivial fall to compartment syndromes to limb/pelvic fractures.[42] Other etiologies include Wilson's disease, herpes zoster myelitis, human immunodeficiency virus (HIV), neuroleptics, and chemotherapeutic agents. In about 42% of cases, etiology can be unknown (cryptogenic).[39] The exact pathophysiology is not known, but potential origin in the peripheral nervous system is believed.[43] However, the evolution of the disorder suggests central nervous system integration to perpetuate pain and mediate movements of the digits.

Diagnosis

Clinical examination can be normal or may show reduced or absent reflexes (typically ankle jerks), mild distal limb weakness, hyperreflexia, and impaired rapid alternating movements. PLMT syndrome must be differentiated from restless leg syndrome and periodic leg movement disorder both of which have other specific features. Nerve conduction study results may be normal in the majority or show mild abnormalities of chronic radiculopathy (usually L5), peripheral neuropathy, cramps and fasciculations, isolated fasciculations/fibrillations, mononeuropathy, or evidence of prior poliomyelitis. Enhanced H-reflex is reported.[44] EMG during movements may show irregular phasic bursts of normal motor unit potential firing at a variable rate of 2-200 Hz that lasts for 50 ms to 1 s.

Treatment

Treatment is difficult with the majority of cases proving refractory to medication. Pain is more disabling than the movements. There is evidence of a role of gabapentin[44] with or without levodopa and lorazepam in combination.[39] Movements may show partial response to clonazepam, pramipexole, and ropinirole. Few patients are benefited with localized therapy with epidural corticosteroids or local tibial nerve blockade or with physical therapy including transcutaneous electrical nerve stimulation,[40] massage, cold soaks, chiropraxis, and acupuncture. BTX injection is rarely helpful. Immunosuppressants have not been tried.

PERIPHERAL TRAUMA-INDUCED MOVEMENT DISORDERS

History

Peripheral trauma-induced movement disorders (PTMDs) are rare and unusual movement disorders that are often considered controversial with regard to their origin. PTMD was first described in a naval officer by Gowers in 1888 as "writing spasm"[45] and this was followed by various case reports and series. The role of peripheral trauma as a possible cause of the movement disorder was first highlighted by Jankovic and van der Linden,[46] while the various phenotypes of movements associated with causalgia were described by Schwartzman and Kerrigan.[47] The possibility of a functional or psychogenic component in addition to organicity of these MDs, though pointed out in earlier case series, was highlighted by Bhatia[48,49] in patients with the clinical syndrome of fixed dystonia and causalgia.

Criteria

The following criteria for diagnosis of PTMD were described by Cardoso and Jankovic: (1) Trauma severe enough to cause local symptoms for >2 weeks or needing medical evaluation within the first 2 weeks, (2) trauma location and the movement disorder are colocalized, and

(3) the movement disorder appears within 1 year after the trauma.[50,51] Shortcomings in these criteria have been pointed out[48] including lack of specification of the exact nature of trauma, possibility of a purely coincidental occurrence of the trauma, and an arbitrarily defined time interval criterion between trauma and onset of the MD.

Description

Peripheral trauma-induced movement disorder can occur after soft-tissue injury, fracture, surgery, prolonged immobilization, and constraint-induced therapy.[52] The median age at presentation is 38 years and the majority involve women.[53] The most frequently reported PTMD phenomenology is *dystonia*. In addition, tremor, Parkinsonism, chorea, tics, myoclonus, and PLMT may all be seen. Other PTMDs include a "jumping" postamputation stump and other postamputation dyskinesia, synkinesis secondary to aberrant regeneration, fasciculations, myokymia, contractures including congenital torticollis, and Dupuytren's contractures. Interestingly, PTMDs are often associated with pain and other sensory phenomena including complex regional pain syndrome (CRPS). More than one-third of patients with PTMDs were also diagnosed with CRPS. In such patients, CRPS type I (without nerve injury) is more commonly seen than CRPS type II (with nerve injury).[53] When fixed dystonia is associated with CRPS, it generally has a poor prognosis.[54] The most common site of onset of movement disorder is a limb, followed by the neck and shoulder region, subsequently followed by the trunk and oromandibular region. In 2% of subjects, the MD can start simultaneously in multiple regions. Spread from the original site to other body parts is also described.

Dystonia

Common sites of dystonia in PTMD are the limbs and neck. Interestingly, in PTMD, "fixed" dystonia with tonic-sustained posturing is more common than "mobile" dystonia with typical phasic dystonic movements, contrary to what is observed in typical idiopathic dystonia.[53] Dystonia in PTMD is often associated with pain. Sensory tricks are much more effective in mobile dystonia than in fixed dystonia.

Cervical Dystonia

Two types of posttraumatic cervical dystonia (CD) are described following whiplash-like injury to neck. Acute onset: occurring immediately after or within days following neck trauma and delayed onset: Beginning several months to years later.[55] Other types of dystonia seen are *writer's cramp* after hand injury[56] and *runner's dystonia*[57] starting after trauma to the ipsilateral limb. It may spread to the other leg, but is fairly localized to lower limbs.[53] *Blepharospasm*[58] can follow anterior eye segment disease or local trauma to eye. A "double hit hypothesis" in rat model of blepharospasm is described wherein a preexisting vulnerability of brain (depleted dopamine) is superimposed with environmental stressors to cause blepharospasm.[59] *Oromandibular dystonia* is seen after facial or oral injury.[50,60] Edentulous dyskinesia, particularly in elderly, is a form of peripheral injury-induced oromandibular dystonia.

Laryngeal Dystonia

It is often seen in patients with a long-standing history of occupational voice usage or recurrent upper respiratory tract infection.

Tremor

Tremor is the second most common PTMD. A local injury or a whiplash-like neck injury can lead to arm tremor.[61] Tremor can also spread to other body parts. Distractibility of tremor in PTMD was described in 1990.[47] Tremor may be coexistent with dystonia in the same body part (dystonic tremor) and also be associated with bradykinesia, rigidity, and Parkinsonism. PTMD tremor is generally refractory to treatment. BTX can provide temporary symptomatic relief.

Parkinsonism

The notion of peripheral trauma-induced Parkinsonism was first brought to light in the late 19th century[62] and took nearly one century to gain more recognition.[63] Positron emission tomography in such patients has shown reduced (^{18}F)-fluorodopa uptake in striatum leading to a hypothesis of postsynaptic damage due to possible central reorganization following altered peripheral input.

Tics

Peripheral trauma-induced tics are phenotypically similar to tics seen in Tourette syndrome (TS), but lack other comorbidities associated with TS and are localized to the body part where initial trauma occurred.[64]

Segmental Myoclonus

Postamputation "jumpy" stump and cases with jerking of muscle/muscle groups following thoracic, abdominal, or spine surgery are also described, along with scapular myoclonus after long thoracic nerve injury and shoulder myoclonus after neuralgic amyotrophy.

Pathophysiology

In all these examples of PTMDs, it is postulated that the initial insult to peripheral soft tissue or nerve interferes with normal sensory processing, which eventually leads to spinal or supraspinal reorganization, in turn, leading to chronification of pain, sensory impairments, and abnormal centrally-mediated motor responses.[65] It has also been postulated that PTMDs occur in genetically or otherwise susceptible subjects with a preexistent or subclinical MD.[66] However, over the last few decades, there is an increasing belief that PTMDs may represent a functional (psychogenic) disorder, at least in a large proportion of cases, given several commonalities observed with functional movement disorders in patients without antecedent trauma.[47,48,67]

Treatment

Most cases are refractory to treatment. Chronic fixed dystonia can lead to joint contractures. Only 20% of cases respond to BTX, which can lead to meaningful functional recovery and pain relief.[53] Intrathecal baclofen and spinal cord stimulation can be helpful.[68,69] Surgical therapies tried include peripheral denervation and central ablative and stimulating procedures.[70] Given the likely functional origin in a large group of these patients with PTMD, treatment is along principles of treating functional MDs and includes carefully identifying preceding stressors, if any, and addressing associated psychiatric comorbidity[71] providing comprehensive cognitive and behavioral therapy, arranging specialist physiotherapy as outlined elsewhere for functional MDs.[72]

CONCLUSION

Peripherally induced movement disorders are a heterogeneous group of movement disorders. In this chapter, we have highlighted some of the major syndromes that fall in this broad category. Familiarity with each of these specific clinical syndromes, their differential diagnoses, and approach to their treatment will allow easier recognition of these entities in the clinic, and guide further appropriate management.

REFERENCES

1. Pandey S, Jain S. Clinical features and response to botulinum toxin in primary and secondary hemifacial spasm. Neurol India. 2018;66:1-36.
2. Auger RG, Whisnant JP. Hemifacial spasm in Rochester and Olmstead Country, Minnesota, 1960 to 1984. Arch Neurol. 1990;47:1233-4.
3. Janetta PJ, Abbasy M, Maroon JC, Ramos FM, Albin MS. Etiology and definitive microsurgical treatment of hemifacial spasm. J Neurosurg. 1977;47:321-8.
4. Yaltho TC, Jankovic J. The many faces of hemifacial spasm: differential diagnosis of unilateral facial spasms. Mov Disord. 2011;26:1582-92.
5. Colosimo C, Bologna M, Lamberti S, Avanzino L, Marinelli L, Fabbrini G, et al. A comparative study of primary and secondary hemifacial spasm. Arch Neurol. 2006;63:441-4.
6. Felicio AC, Godeiro-Junior CDO, Borges V, Silva SM, Ferraz HB. Clinical assessment of patients with primary and postparalytic hemifacial spasm: a retrospective study. Arq Neuropsiquiatr. 2007;65:783-6.
7. Batla A, Goyal C, Shukla G, Goyal V, Srivastava A, Behari M. Hemifacial spasm: clinical characteristics of 321 Indian patients. J Neurol. 2012;259:1561-5.
8. Wang A, Jankovic J. Hemifacial spasm: clinical findings and treatment. Muscle Nerve. 1998;21:1740-7.
9. William S, Joseph J. The other Babinski sign in hemifacial spasm. Neurology. 2007;69:402-4.
10. Fasano A, Valadas A, Bhatia KP, Prashanth LK, Lang AE, Munhoz RP, et al. Psychogenic facial movement disorders: clinical features and associated conditions. Mov Disord. 2012;27:1544-51.
11. Baizabal-Carvallo JF, Jankovic J. Distinguishing features of psychogenic (functional) versus organic hemifacial spasm. J Neurol. 2017;264:359-63.
12. Miller LE, Miller VM. Safety and effectiveness of microvascular decompression for treatment of hemifacial spasm: a systematic review. Br J Neurosurg. 2012;26:438-44.
13. Sharma R, Garg K, Agarwal S, Agarwal D, Chandra PS, Kale SS, et al. Microvascular decompression for hemifacial spasm: a systematic review of vascular pathology, long term treatment efficacy and safety. Neurol India. 2017;65:493-505.
14. Christie C, Rodrıguez-Quiroga SA, Arakaki T, Rey RD, Garretto NS. Hemimasticatory spasm: report of a case and review of the literature. Tremor Other Hyperkinet Mov (N Y). 2014;4:210.
15. Gowers WR. A Manual of Diseases of the Central Nervous System, 2nd edition. Philadelphia: Blakiston; 1897. pp. 221-4.
16. Cruccu G, Inghilleri M, Berardelli A, Pauletti G, Casali C, Coratti P, et al. Pathophysiology of hemimasticatory spasm. J Neurol Neurosurg Psychiatry. 1994;57:43-50.
17. Radhakrishnan D, Goyal V, Shukla G, Singh MB, Ramam M. Hemimasticatory spasm: series of 7 cases and review of literature. Mov Disord Clin Pract. 2019;6:316-9.
18. Kumar N, Krueger BR, Ahlskog JE. Hemimasticatory spasm with lateral jaw deviations. Mov Disord. 2008;23:2265-6.
19. Auger RG, Litchy WJ, Cascino TL, Ahlskog E. Hemimasticatory spasm: clinical and electrophysiologic observations. Neurology. 1992;42:2263-6.
20. Thompson PD, Obeso JA, Delgado G, Gallego J, Marsden CD. Focal dystonia of the jaw and the differential diagnosis of unilateral jaw and masticatory spasm. J Neurol Neurosurg Psychiatry. 1986;49:651-6.
21. Gunduz A, Karaali-Savrun F, Uluduz D. Hemimasticatory spasm following pontine infarction. Mov Disord. 2007;22:1674-5.
22. Jin KH, Beom SJ, Kwang-Woo L. Hemimasticatory spasm associated with localized scleroderma and facial hemiatrophy. Arch Neurol. 2000;57:576-80.

23. Hong-Hua Y, Woong-Woo L, Seok JB. Hemimasticatory spasm misdiagnosed as other mimickers: report of two cases. Neurology Asia. 2015;20:73-7.
24. Wang YN, Dou NN, Zhou QM, Jiao W, Zhu J, Zhong J, et al. Treatment of hemimasticatory spasm with microvascular decompression. J Craniofac Surg. 2013;24:1753-5.
25. Carvalho LB, Rampim DB, Chung TM. First Report of Geniospasm in a Five-Generation Brazilian Family: Clinical Features, Electromyography Findings and Botulinum Toxin Treatment. Clin Med Rev Case Rep. 2017;4:191.
26. Soland VL, Bhatia KP, Sheean GL, Marsden CD. Hereditary geniospasm: two new families. Mov Disord. 1996;11:744-6.
27. Jain P, Sharma S, Aneja S. Hereditary chin-trembling. Indian Pediatr. 2015;52:720.
28. Jarman PR, Wood NW, Davis MT, Davis PV, Bhatia KP, Marsden CD, et al. Hereditary geniospasm: linkage to chromosome 9q13-q21 and evidence for genetic heterogeneity. Am J Hum Genet. 1997;61:928-33.
29. Laurance BM, Matthews WB, Diggle JH. Hereditary Quivering of the Chin. Arch Dis Child. 1968;43:249-51.
30. Massaro D. Ventiseicasi de genoispasmoattraverso cinque generazioni: contributoclinicoallo studio dell"ereditáfisiopatologica. I Pissani (Palermo). 1894;1:47-56.
31. Stocks P. Facial spasm inherited through four generations. Biometrika. 1923;14:311-5.
32. Goraya JS, Virdi V, Parmar V. Recurrent Nocturnal Tongue Biting in a Child With Hereditary Chin Trembling. J Child Neurol. 2006;21:985-7.
33. Destee A, Cassim F, Defebvre L, Guieu J. Hereditary chin trembling or hereditary chin myoclonus? J Neurol Neurosurg Psychiatry. 1997;63:804-7.
34. Chalaupka FD, Bartholini F, Mandich G, Mandich G, Turro M. Two new families with hereditary essential chin myoclonus: clinical features, neurophysiological findings and treatment. Neurol Sci. 2006;27:97-103.
35. Grimes DA, Han F, Bulman D, Nicolson ML, Suchowersky O. Hereditary chin trembling: a new family with exclusion of the chromosome 9q13-q21 Locus. Mov Disord. 2002;17:1390-2.
36. Spillane JD, Nathan PW, Kelly RE, Marsden CD. Painful legs and moving toes. Brain. 1971;94:541-6.
37. Verhagen WI, Horstink MW, Notermans SL. Painful arm and moving fingers. J Neurol Neurosurg Psychiatry. 1985;48:384-5.
38. Schwingenschuh P, Bhatia KP. Painful moving tongue in a patient with the painful legs moving toes syndrome. Mov Disord. 2008;23:1324-5.
39. Hassan A, Mateen FJ, Coon EA, Ahlskog JE. Painful legs and moving toes syndrome: a 76-patient case series. Arch Neurol. 2012;69:1032-8.
40. Fan YY, Xu Y, Gao XG. Spontaneous aching pain and peculiar involuntary movements: a case report of painful legs and moving toes and review of the literature. Case Rep Med. 2014;2014:581402.
41. Walters AS, Hening WA, Shah SK, Chokroverty S. Painless legs and moving toes: a syndrome related to painful legs and moving toes? Mov Disord. 1993;8:377-9.
42. Dressler D, Thompson PD, Gledhill RF, Marsden CD. The syndrome of painful legs and moving toes. Mov Disord. 1994;9:13-21.
43. Nathan PW. Painful legs and moving toes: evidence on the site of the lesion. J Neurol Neurosurg Psychiatry. 1978;41:934-9.
44. Tocco P, Tamburin S, Turatti M, Lauriola MF, Zanette G. Painful Legs and Moving Toes Syndrome: Putative Underlying Pathophysiology as a Hint for Combined Pharmacological Treatment? Mov Disord Clin Pract. 2014;1:377-8.
45. Gowers W. A Manual of Diseases of the Nervous System. London: Churchill Livingstone; 1888.
46. Jankovic J, Van der Linden C. Dystonia and tremor induced by peripheral trauma: predisposing factors. J Neurol Neurosurg Psychiatry. 1988;51:1512-9.
47. Schwartzman RJ, Kerrigan J. The movement disorder of reflex sympathetic dystrophy. Neurology. 1990;40:57-61.
48. Bhatia KP, Bhatt MH, Marsden CD. The causalgia dystonia syndrome. Brain. 1993;116:843-51.
49. Ganos C, Edwards MJ, Bhatia KP. Posttraumatic functional movement disorders. Handb Clin Neurol. 2016;139:499-507.
50. Cardoso F, Jankovic J. Peripherally-induced tremor and Parkinsonism. Arch Neurol. 1995;52:263-70.
51. Jankovic J. Peripherally-induced movement disorders. Neurol Clin. 2009;27:821-32.
52. Okun MS, Nadeau SE, Rossi F, Triggs WJ. Immobilization dystonia. J Neurol Sci. 2002;201:79-83.
53. van Rooijen DE, Geraedts EJ, Marinus J, Jankovic J, van Hilten JJ. Peripheral trauma and movement disorders: a systematic review of reported cases. J Neurol Neurosurg Psychiatry. 2011;82:892-8.
54. Ibrahim NM, Martino D, van de Warrenburg BPC, Quinn NP, Bhatia KP, Brown RJ, et al. The prognosis of fixed dystonia: a follow-up study. Parkinsonism Relat Disord. 2009;15:592-7.
55. Tarsy D. Comparison of acute- and delayed-onset posttraumatic cervical dystonia. Mov Disord. 1998;13:481-5.
56. Rosenbaum F, Jankovic J. Focal task-specific tremor and dystonia: categorization of occupational movement disorders. Neurology. 1988;38:522-7.
57. Wu LJ, Jankovic J. Runner's dystonia. J Neurol Sci. 2006;251: 73-6.
58. Martino D, Defazio G, Alessio G, Abbruzzese G, Girlanda P, Tinazzi M, et al. Relationship between eye symptoms and blepharospasm: a multicenter case-control study. Mov Disord. 2005;20:1564-70.
59. Defazio G, Berardelli A, Abbruzzese G, Lepore V, Coviello V, Acquistapace D, et al. Possible risk factors for primary adult onset dystonia: a case-control investigation by the Italian Movement Disorders Study Group. J Neurol Neurosurg Psychiatry. 1998;64:25-32.
60. Schrag A, Bhatia KP, Quinn NP, Marsden CD. Atypical and typical cranial dystonia following dental procedures. Mov Disord. 1999;14:492-6.
61. Ellis RJ. Tremor and other movement disorders after whiplash type injuries. J Neurol Neurosurg Psychiatry. 1997;63:110-2.
62. Factor SA, Sanchez-Ramos J, Weiner WJ. Trauma as an etiology of Parkinsonism: a historical review of the concept. Mov Disord. 1988;3:30-6.
63. Schrag A, Trimble M, Quinn N, Bhatia K. The syndrome of fixed dystonia: an evaluation of 103 patients. Brain. 2004; 127:2360-72.

64. Erer S, Jankovic J. Adult onset tics after peripheral injury. Parkinsonism Relat Disord. 2008;14:75-6.
65. Bohlhalter S, Leon-Sarmiento FE, Hallett M. Abnormality of motor cortex excitability in peripherally-induced dystonia. Mov Disord. 2007;22:1186-9.
66. Fletcher NA, Harding AE, Marsden CD. The relationship between trauma and idiopathic torsion dystonia. J Neurol Neurosurg Psychiatry. 1991;54:713-7.
67. Lang AE, Fahn S. Movement disorder of RSD. Neurology. 1990;40:1476-7.
68. Goldstein DS. Spinal cord stimulation for chronic reflex sympathetic dystrophy. Ann Neurol. 2004;55:5-6.
69. Kemler MA, De Vet HCW, Barendse GAM, Van Den Wildenberg FAJM, Kleef MV. The effect of spinal cord stimulation in patients with chronic reflex sympathetic dystrophy: two years' follow-up of the randomized controlled trial. Ann Neurol. 2004;55:13-8.
70. Jankovic J. Re-emergence of surgery for dystonia. J Neurol Neurosurg Psychiatry. 1998;65:434.
71. Voon V, Lang AE. Antidepressant treatment outcomes of psychogenic movement disorders. J Clin Psychiatry. 2005;66: 1529-34.
72. Espay AJ, Aybek S, Carson A, Edwards MJ, Goldstein LH, Hallett M, et al. Current Concepts in Diagnosis and Treatment of Functional Neurological Disorders. JAMA Neurol. 2018;75:1132-41.

CHAPTER 52

Prion Diseases

Sarosh M Katrak, Azad M Irani

INTRODUCTION

The word "Prion" was coined by Prusiner in 1982 from the amalgam of two words *pro*teinaceous *in*fective particle, which he thought was the agent causing scrapie.[1] The range of prion disorders shares three common properties:

1. Common pathological features of neuronal loss, glial cell proliferation, absence of an inflammatory response, and the presence of spongiform appearance of the neuropil giving rise to the classical spongiform encephalopathy
2. Transmissibility by inoculation into same or different species
3. Abnormal form of prion protein (PrP) as a constituent of the amyloid plaques found in the brain

The range of prion diseases is enumerated in **Box 1**. Scrapie and bovine spongiform encephalopathy are beyond the scope of this chapter. Kuru is now only of historical interest.

Box 1 Range of prion diseases.

- *Scrapie*: Disease of sheep
- Kuru
- Bovine spongiform encephalopathy
- *Creutzfeldt–Jakob disease (CJD)*:
  - Sporadic CJD—(sCJD)
  - Iatrogenic CJD—(iCJD)
- *Familial prion diseases*:
  - Familial Creutzfeldt–Jakob (fCJD) disease
  - Gerstmann–Sträussler–Scheinker (GSS) disease
  - Fatal familial insomnia
- *Variant CJD*: vCJD

BIOLOGY OF PRIONS

Prions are small infectious particles containing protein, but lack nucleic acid. Prion protein is a normal protein found in most cell types in the brain designated as PrP^{c}. It is a glycol protein with unknown function. Prion diseases result from the neuronal accumulation of an abnormally folded isoform of PrP^{c} designated as PrP^{Sc} after scrapie diseases of sheep. Once PrP^{Sc} is present in the brain, it replicates by binding to endogenous PrP^{c} and converting it to PrP^{Sc}.

The coding gene for PrP is located on the short arm of chromosome 20 and one of its two longer exons contains the entire 253 codon region of the gene. A strong link has been established between mutation in the *PrP* gene and forms familial prion diseases with >60 different mutations described.[2] In addition, polymorphism for methionine and valine at codon 129 of the *PrP* gene plays a significant role in determining the host susceptibility and clinical phenotype of familial Creutzfeldt–Jakob disease (fCJD), sporadic CJD (sCJD), and variant CJD (vCJD).[3] Thus, e.g, when the mutant allele of the *PrP* gene coding for asparagine at codon 178, also codes for valine at codon 129, the clinical phenotype is that of fCJD. In contrast, when the mutant allele coding for asparagine at codon 178, also codes for methionine at codon 129, the clinical phenotype is consistent with fatal familial insomnia (FFI). Homozygosity at codon 129 for either valine or methionine is also likely to affect the age at onset, severity, and duration of the illness.[3] Approximately, 90% of sCJD are homozygous for either methionine or valine at codon 129 compared to only 50% of nonaffected individuals. Interestingly, 100% of individuals, with vCJD, are homozygous for methionine at this position.[4,5]

A characteristic biological feature of prions is their resistance to a number of normal decontaminating procedures.

These pathogens are resistant to processes affecting nucleic acids—hydrolysis or shearing—as they do not have any. However, agents digesting or denaturing protein do have activity against prions. The special precautions for decontamination of any material, which has come in contact with prions, have been specified by the Society for Healthcare Epidemiology of America guidelines.[6]

SPORADIC CREUTZFELDT–JAKOB DISEASE

This is the most common form of prion disease accounting for 85–90% of all cases. It has a worldwide distribution and affects approximately 1 individual per million per year. It is a neurodegenerative illness arising from either a spontaneous mutation in the *PrP* gene or a structural protein change in the PrP molecule. The mean age at onset is 57–62 years with a peak incidence in the late sixth to early seventh decade. Rarely, young adults or those above the age of 80 years have been affected.[7]

The cardinal features of sCJD are a rapid mental deterioration and myoclonus. In the initial phases, mental deterioration may be manifest as behavioral abnormalities, mood changes—apathy and depression, and sleep disturbances—hypersomnia or insomnia. With disease progression, there is a rapid deterioration of cognitive abilities and dementia becomes a dominant feature in most patients.

Myoclonus, usually provoked by startle, is present in over 90% of patients and is present at some point of the illness. It may be conspicuous by its absence in the initial phases of the disease. *Sporadic CJD should always be considered in any patient with a rapidly progressive dementia and myoclonus.*

At some phase of the illness, patients may have a variable mixture of extrapyramidal and cerebellar manifestations. Hypokinesia, nystagmus, and ataxia occur in up to two-thirds of patients and are the presenting features in approximately 20–40% of patients. Corticospinal tract involvement including hyperreflexia, spasticity, and a positive Babinski sign develops in about 40–60% of patients. In patients with a younger age at onset (<50 years), prominent psychiatric symptoms are evident at onset and the duration of the disease is more prolonged. Sensory abnormalities, involvement of the cranial nerves, or peripheral nervous system should alert a clinician against a diagnosis of sCJD.

A number of variants/subtypes of sCJD have been defined based on focal neurological deficit reflecting predominant involvement of specific brain regions. These include patients presenting with visual symptoms (Heidenhain variant) and cerebellar ataxia (Oppenheimer-Brownell variant).

Differential Diagnosis

Occasionally, Alzheimer's disease (AD) and frontotemporal dementia (FTD) are associated with myoclonus and a more rapid course. Prominent ataxia or Parkinsonism may suggest diffuse Lewy body disease (DLD), progressive supranuclear palsy (PSP), or multisystem atrophy-parkinsonian/cerebellar (MSA-P/MSA-C) variety. However, none of these neurodegenerative dementias have as rapid a course as sCJD. Other differential diagnosis may be autoimmune limbic encephalitis, paraneoplastic syndromes (PNSs), central nervous system (CNS) vasculitis, and Hashimoto's encephalopathy (HE). These should be excluded because of the potential for therapy in these cases.

Investigations

An electroencephalography (EEG) can provide supportive but not definitive evidence of sCJD. The EEG exhibits changes depending on the stage of the disease. In the early stages, the EEG may show nonspecific diffuse slowing or frontal intermittent rhythmic delta activity (FIRDA). The characteristic EEG pattern is that of periodic slow wave complexes (PSWCs) occurring synchronously at a rate of 1/s (**Fig. 1**). These are observed in 67–95% of patients at sometime during the course of the illness. Hence, multiple EEGs are essential. PSWCs have a specificity and sensitivity of 64% and 91%, respectively, for the diagnosis of sCJD.[8] When seen, PSWCs are relatively specific for sCJD but may also be seen in AD, DLD, toxic metabolic encephalopathy, progressive multifocal leukoencephalopathy (PML), and hypoxic encephalopathy.

Cerebrospinal fluid (CSF) is generally normal in CJD. A mild protein elevation may be seen occasionally but is <100 mg/dL. It is done to rule out other infective etiologies. Multiple biomarkers have been studied, but only a few are of interest. Detection of 14-3-3 protein is the most studied CSF biomarker. It should be considered as an adjunctive rather than an absolute test for the diagnosis of sCJD. A systemic review in 2012 reported a sensitivity of 92% but a specificity of only 80%.[9] False-positive results are reported in AD, vascular dementia, viral encephalitis, and PNS. A variety of other biomarkers—S100 protein, neuronal-specific enolase (NSE), thymosin ß4, and tau protein have been studied. An elevated ratio of total tau to phosphorylated tau had a very high specificity for CJD.[10]

Prion protein diagnostic assays from blood samples are in development. Real-time quaking-induced conversion (RT-QuIC) initiates transition in recombinant PrP into amyloid plaques, which can be monitored in real time. This method is not only useful using blood but also nasal brushing and more recently, eye tissue (retina) from pathologically confirmed cases of sCJD.[11-14]

MRI has proven to be highly sensitive (91%) and specific (96%) for the diagnosis of sCJD. Although hyperintensities

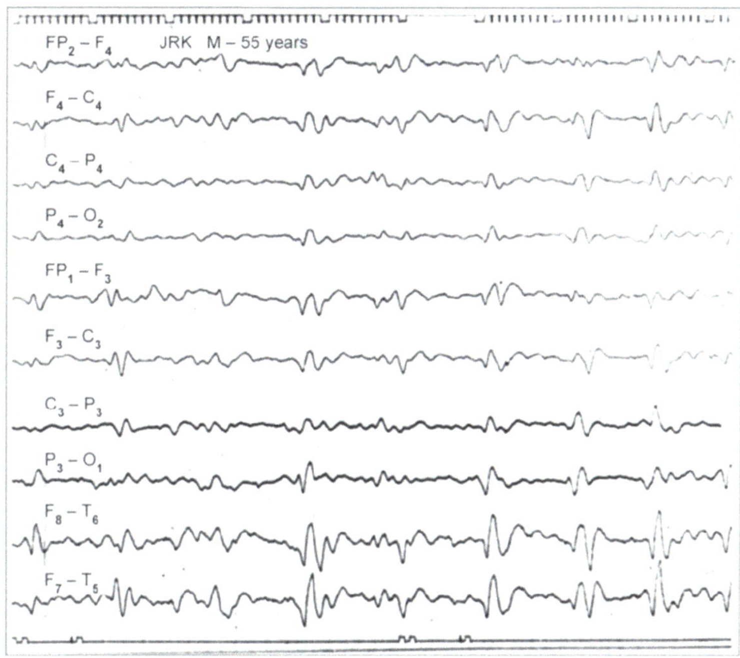

(EEG: electroencephalography; sCJD: sporadic Creutzfeldt–Jakob disease)

FIG. 1: Characteristic EEG in sCJD showing bisynchronous 1/s periodic sharp wave complexes (PSWCs).

(HIs) in the putamen and head of the caudate nucleus were initially described on T2-weighted images, recent small studies have shown that diffusion-weighted imaging (DWI) and fluid attenuation inversion ratio [fluid-attenuated inversion recovery (FLAIR)] sequences are more sensitive for the detection of cortical changes.[15-17] DWI shows "cortical ribboning pattern"—gyral HI in the insular, temporal, and frontal cortices, in addition to HI, in the basal ganglia (**Figs. 2A** to **C**).

These abnormalities are seen even before the onset of characteristic clinical findings of myoclonus or PSWCs in the EEG. In the Heidenhain variant, the cortical ribboning pattern may be seen in the occipital lobes.

For research purposes, diagnostic criteria have been established for sporadic CJD.[18]

Definite diagnosis requires histopathologic confirmation of PrP^{Sc} on brain biopsy or autopsy.

Probable diagnosis requires: (a) Rapidly progressive dementia with two out of the four clinical features: Myoclonus, visual/cerebellar disturbances, pyramidal/extrapyramidal features, or akinetic mutism and (b) A characteristic EEG or 14-3-3 positivity in the CSF or characteristic features on MRI.

Possible diagnosis requires: (a) The clinical features mentioned above and (b) Investigations are either unavailable or negative.

FAMILIAL PRION DISEASES

Three phenotypes of familial prion diseases are well-recognized clinically and neuropathologically:

1. Familial CJD
2. Gerstmann-Sträussler-Scheinker (GSS) disease
3. Fatal familial insomnia

These phenotypes are due to mutation in the *PrP* gene. Over 60 different mutations in the gene have been described in fCJD, of which four point mutations at codons 102, 178, 200, and 210 account for 95% of the familial cases.[2,3] The role of codon 129 in determining host susceptibility and clinical phenotype is already discussed in "Biology of Prion Diseases."

Although GSS is considered a variant of fCJD, it is primarily associated with mutation at codon 102 and rarely at codons 105, 117, and 198. The different mutations in the *PrP* gene are associated with wide variability in age at onset, clinical presentation, and duration of the illness.

Genetics of FFI: It is already discussed in "Biology of Prion Diseases."

Familial Creutzfeldt–Jakob Disease

Familial CJD forms approximately 5–15% of all cases of CJD. Because of an autosomal dominant transmission, a family history is generally positive in these patients. Interestingly, geographical clusters of fCJD have been reported in Libyan Jews in Israel, Spanish families in rural Chile, and in central Slovakia with codon 200 mutations.[19,20] Isolated familial cases have been reported from Canada, France, Japan, UK, USA, Finland, Hungary, and the Netherlands. A large Indian family with D178N mutation has been recently documented.[2] This family of fCJD had a mutant allele coding for asparagine at codon 178 and also coding for valine at codon 129.

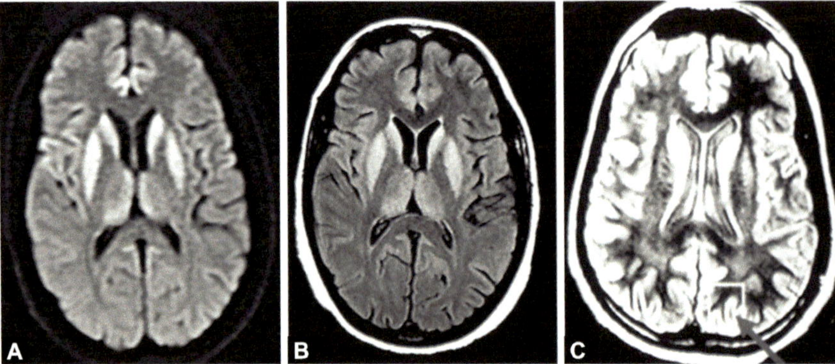

(FLAIR: fluid-attenuated inversion recovery; sCJD: sporadic Creutzfeldt–Jakob disease)

FIGS. 2A TO C: (A) DW image and (B and C) FLAIR images. Figures A and B show hyperintensities of the caudate nucleus, thalamus, and putamen. Also, note early cortical ribboning in the parafalcine frontal cortex, the right frontotemporal cortex, and operculum. Figure C shows extensive cortical ribboning in an advanced stage of sCJD.

Patients with fCJD have an earlier age of onset (mean 46 years) and a more protracted course of illness (mean 23 months). The presenting symptoms may be a behavioral disorder, but dementia is an inevitable feature, although appearing late in the clinical course.

The EEG is nondiagnostic as is the CSF. The 14-3-3 protein may be negative. The DWI on the MRI does show HI of the cortical ribbon in the insular and frontotemporal lobes early in the disease—a feature similar to that of sCJD. The MRI is rather sensitive in cases with characteristic clinical features.

The salient features of the neuropathology are remarkable spongiform degeneration and neuronal loss with gliosis, particularly of the frontal and temporal lobes. Deposition of abnormal PrP is demonstrated by PrP immunostaining. The PrP can be distributed in perivacuolar distribution or a diffuse synaptic pattern.

Gerstmann–Sträussler–Scheinker Disease

This form of prion disease is always familial and is most commonly associated with a point mutation at codon 102. Mutation at other codons 105, 117, 145, 198, 202, and 217 has also been reported.[21]

In the classical form, gait ataxia and dysarthria are the presenting features, followed by a variable degree of pyramidal and extrapyramidal features. Thus, in the initial stages, GSS may mimic spinocerebellar ataxia. These patients may have nystagmus but no myoclonus. Dementia is often a late feature. Variations in the clinical features do occur and are based on the site of mutation. For example, mutation at codon 105 results in clinical features of spastic paraparesis and dementia and has a longer duration of illness, whereas mutations at codons 117 and 198 may have prominent Parkinsonian features together with ataxia and dementia. The duration of the illness is typically 2–7 years, but up to 10 years and more have been described. Because of impaired coordination of swallowing, aspiration pneumonia is a particular risk factor in the terminal stages.

The EEG is unhelpful as GSS lacks periodic discharges and may show nonspecific slow wave abnormalities. The MRI may show nonspecific cerebellar degeneration. The "cortical ribboning pattern" is not seen in GSS. The neuropathological findings of widespread deposits of amyloid plaques and immunoreactivity with anti-PrP antibodies within these plaques are a defining hallmark of GSS pathology. Vacuolation of the neuropils is minimum. The diagnosis is established by genetic testing.

Fatal Familial Insomnia

This is a rare sleep disorder, which is typically familial and lasts for a few months to a few years. Originally, it was reported as a form of familial prion disease, but sporadic cases are known to occur albeit rare.[22]

The main presenting symptom is intractable insomnia, which may be the only symptom for several months. This may lead to panic attacks, hallucinations, confused state, and weight loss. The progression of the disease may be accompanied by several autonomic dysfunctions—pinpoint pupils, sweating, sudden onset of menopause in women or impotence in males, increase in blood pressure and heart rate, and severe constipation. Besides these features, pyramidal and extrapyramidal signs and symptoms are present in the latter half of the disease. Overt dementia is a late feature. The age at onset is between 25 and 60 years with an average of 48 years. The mean survival is 18 months with a range of 7–33 months. Again, the EEG and MRI are unhelpful. The positron emission tomography (PET) scan shows a characteristic hypometabolism or blood flow reduction to the thalamus in the early stages of the disease. Clinical heterogeneity has occurred in a genetically proven Australian family with some members exhibiting intractable insomnia and others none,[23] suggesting that this disease may have a variable presentation.

The diagnosis is achieved by genetic testing. The neuropathological features are those of neuronal loss with gliosis predominantly in the thalamus, inferior olives, and to a lesser degree, the cerebellum. Vacuolation is minimal or absent. Protease-resistant PrP is detectable on immunostaining in specific regions—thalamus and temporal lobes—confirming the diagnosis in a brain biopsy or autopsy.

VARIANT CREUTZFELDT–JAKOB DISEASE

The initial report in 1996 of a new variant of CJD quickly focused attention on human prion diseases, particularly because of its link to bovine spongiform encephalopathy (BSE)—mad cow disease.[24] The bulk of evidence supports the possibility that vCJD represents a bovine-to-human transmission of BSE. As of June 2014, 228 cases of probable or confirmed vCJD have been reported worldwide.[25-28] Fortunately, there is no case report from India.

Variant CJD differs from sCJD by the following features: Considerably younger age at onset, a more protracted clinical course, differences in the presenting symptoms, and differences in the neuropathology.

The mean age at onset, in the original report, was 29 years with a range from 16 to 48 years,[24,29] though cases at age 11 and 74 years have also been reported.[30-32] The presenting symptoms are prominent sensory disturbances and psychiatric disorders. Sensory symptoms include paresthesia or dysesthesia over the face and extremities and at times in a hemibody distribution. Psychiatric disorders may include apathy, depression, anxiety, irritability, and uncommonly frank psychosis with delusions and hallucinations. As the disease progresses, ataxia and dysarthria become obvious. Dementia, involuntary movements, immobility, and mutism are late and practically terminal features.

PrP gene mutations are not reported in vCJD, but almost 100% of the cases are homozygous for methionine at codon 129 of the gene. Another distinguishing feature of vCJD is the prominent involvement of lymphoid tissue—tonsils and appendix. This may facilitate the diagnosis of vCJD by immunostaining of tonsillar tissue for PrP deposits.

Cerebrospinal fluid is rarely helpful for the diagnosis of vCJD, but should be done to rule out other infections. The detection of 14-3-3 protein in the CSF is not a very sensitive marker in these cases. MRI of the brain may show hyperintense signals in the pulvinar of the thalamus (pulvinar sign) and in both the pulvinar and the dorsomedial thalamus (the hockey stick sign) on the FLAIR images. These signs, when present, have a sensitivity and specificity of 78% and 100%, respectively.[33] The EEG is singularly unhelpful. Analysis of the PrP extracted from tonsillar biopsy tissue appears to be a sensitive and specific method for diagnosis of vCJD in the appropriate clinical setting, as is homozygosity for methionine on codon 129.

The initial psychiatric symptoms may be nonspecific. With the onset of neurological symptoms and signs, a long list of differential diagnosis should be considered such as sCJD, PNS, FTD, primary CNS vasculitis, subacute sclerosing panencephalitis (SSPE), multi-infarct dementia, MSA-C, Huntington's disease, HE, and autoimmune limbic encephalitis.

Although vCJD has a more protracted course compared to sCJD, both are progressive and uniformly fatal.

IATROGENIC CREUTZFELDT–JAKOB DISEASE

The diagnosis of this form of prion disease requires a strong association with administration of biological extract or tissue contaminated with prions. Such cases have been reported after injection of human growth hormone (hGH) contaminated with prion,[34] improperly decontaminated depth electrodes[35] or neurosurgical instruments,[36] pituitary-derived gonadotropin,[37] and dura mater grafts.[38]

The length of incubation period and clinical features depend on the portal of entry. With a peripheral route of entry in hGH administration, the mean incubation period can be 12 years or longer. In contrast, with dura mater grafts, where the contaminated material is directly placed in the cranium, the mean incubation period is 6 years. In the peripheral route of infection, the clinical features are often cerebellar ataxia and gait abnormalities. Dementia is a late manifestation and is usually mild. EEG may show only nonspecific diffuse slowing. Patients with dural graft associated iatrogenic CJD (iCJD) tend to be younger than sCJD, but the rest of the features are almost identical.[39]

THERAPY AND MANAGEMENT OF PRION DISEASES

Currently, there is no curative therapy for prion diseases.[40] Several medications have been used to treat prion diseases more out of desperation. These include amantadine, vidarabine, acyclovir, interferons, polyanions, and amphotericin B. Only flupirtine, quinacrine, and doxycycline all given orally have been tested in randomized placebo control clinical trials.[41-43] None was found to be effective in prolonging survival, though flupirtine-treated patients showed some improvement in cognitive function.[41]

Intraventricular pentosan polysulfate has been tried in sCJD without success. It has been used on compassionate grounds on patients with vCJD in UK and Japan. Although it prolongs survival, observational data from UK showed that it did not improve the dementia.[44,45]

As there is no curative therapy, patients can be managed with symptomatic treatment. Selective serotonin reuptake inhibitors are used to treat depression and agitation, atypical antipsychotics, particularly quetiapine, for agitation and psychosis, and clonazepam, levetiracetam, and valproic acid are useful to control myoclonus.

CONCLUSION

Prion diseases may be sporadic, familial or iatrogenic. They share common pathological features and are due to abnormally folded PrP. Sporadic CJD is the most common form of Prion disease and accounts for 85–90% of all cases. It should be one of the prime considerations in cases of rapidly progressive dementia. The other forms are rare and have protean presentations with dementia appearing at varying stages of the illnesses. EEG, CSF, and blood tests help but are not conclusive. The MRI, particularly DWI and FLAIR sequences have a high degree of sensitivity and specificity. RT-QuIC is a promising blood test. Currently there is no curative therapy for prion diseases and they tend to be universally fatal.

REFERENCES

1. Prusiner SB. Novel proteinaceous particles cause scrapie. Science. 1982;216:136-44.
2. Katrak SM, Pauranik A, Desai SB, Mead S, Beck J, Brandner S, et al. Familial Creutzfeldt-Jakob Disease in an Indian Kindred. Ann Indian Acad Neurol. 2019;22:458-61.
3. Brown K, Mastriam JA. The prion diseases. J Geriatr Psychiatry Neurol. 2010;23:277-98.
4. Mead S, Poulter M, Beck J, Webb TE, Campbell TA, Linehan JM, et al. Inherited prion disease with six octapeptide repeat insertional mutation—molecular analysis of phenotypic heterogeneity. Brain. 2006;129:2297-317.
5. Saitoh Y, Ogawa M, Naito Y, Komatsuzaki Y, Tagaya H, Arima K, et al. Discordant clinicopathologic phenotypes in a Japanese kindred of fatal familial insomnia. Neurology. 2010;74:86-9.
6. Rutala WA, Weber DJ, Society for Healthcare Epidemiology of America. Guideline for disinfection and sterilization of prion-contaminated medical instruments. Infect Control Hosp Epidemiol. 2010;31:107-17.
7. Parchi P, Giese A, Capellari S, Brown P, Schulz-Schaeffer W, Windl O, et al. Classification of Creutzfeldt-Jakob disease based on molecular and phenotypic analysis of 300 subjects. Ann Neurol. 1999;46(2):224-33.
8. Steinhoff BJ, Zerr I, Glatting M, Schulz-Schaeffer W, Poser S, Kretzschmar HA. Diagnostic value of periodic complexes in Creutzfeldt-Jakob disease. Ann Neurol. 2004;56:702-8.
9. Muayqil T, Gronseth G, Camicioli R. Evidence-based guideline: diagnostic accuracy of CSF 14-3-3 protein in sporadic Creutzfeldt-Jakob disease: report of the guideline development subcommittee of the American Academy of Neurology. Neurology. 2012;79:1499-506.
10. Skillbäck T, Rosén C, Asztely F, Mattsson N, Blennow K, Zetterberg H, et al. Diagnostic performance of cerebrospinal fluid total tau and phosphorylated tau in Creutzfeldt-Jakob disease: results from the Swedish Mortality Registry. JAMA Neurol. 2014;71:476-83.
11. McGuire LI, Peden AH, Orrú CD, Wilham JM, Appleford NE, Mallinson G, et al. Real time quaking-induced conversion analysis of cerebrospinal fluid in sporadic Creutzfeldt-Jakob disease. Ann Neurol. 2012;72:278-85.
12. Atarashi R, Sano K, Satoh K, Nishida N. Real-time quaking-induced conversion: a highly sensitive assay for prion detection. Prion. 2011;5:150-3.
13. Orrú CD, Bongianni M, Tonoli G, Ferrari S, Hughson AG, Groveman BR, et al. A test for Creutzfeldt-Jakob disease using nasal brushings. N Engl J Med. 2014;371:519-29.
14. Orrù CD, Soldau K, Cordano C, Llibre-Guerra J, Green AJ, Sanchez H, et al. Prion seeds distribute throughout the eyes of sporadic Creutzfeldt-Jakob disease patients. mBio. 2018;9:e02095-18.
15. Yi SH, Park KC, Yoon SS, Kim EJ, Shin WC. Relationship between clinical course and diffusion-weighted MRI findings in sporadic Creutzfeldt-Jakob disease. Neurol Sci. 2008;29:251-5.
16. Shiga Y, Miyazawa K, Sato S, Fukushima R, Shibuya S, Sato Y, et al. Diffusion-weighted MRI abnormalities as an early diagnostic marker for Creutzfeldt-Jakob disease. Neurology. 2004;63: 443-9.
17. Young GS, Geschwind MD, Fischbein NJ, Martindale JL, Henry RG, Liu S, et al. Diffusion-weighted and fluid-attenuated inversion recovery imaging in Creutzfeldt-Jakob disease: high sensitivity and specificity for diagnosis. Am J Neuroradiol. 2005;26:1551-62.
18. Brandel JP, Delasnerie-Lauprêtre N, Laplanche JL, Hauw JJ, Alpérovitch A. Diagnosis of Creutzfeldt-Jakob disease: effect of clinical criteria on incidence estimates. Neurology. 2000;54:1095-9.
19. Goldfarb LG, Korczyn A, Brown P, Chapman J, Gajdusek DC. Mutation in codon 200 of scrapie amyloid precursor gene linked to Creutzfeldt-Jakob disease in Sephardic Jews of Libyan capital and non-Libyan origin. Lancet. 1990;336:637-8.
20. Goldfarb LG, Brown P, Mitrovà E, Cervenáková L, Goldin L, Korczyn AD, et al. Creutzfeldt-Jakob disease associated with the PRNP codon 200Lys mutation: an analysis of 45 families. Eur J Epidemiol. 1991;7:477-86.
21. Webb TE, Poulter M, Beck J, Uphill J, Adamson G, Campbell T, et al. Phenotypic heterogeneity and genetic modification of P102L inherited prion disease in an international series. Brain. 2008;131:2632-46.
22. Mastrianni JA, Nixon R, Layzer R, Telling GC, Han D, DeArmond SJ, et al. Prion protein conformation in a patient with sporadic fatal insomnia. N Engl J Med. 1999;340:1630-8.
23. Mclean CA, Storey E, Gardner RJM, Tannenberg MB, Cervenakova L, Brown P. The D178N (cis-129M) "fatal familial insomnia" mutation associated with diverse clinic-pathologic phenotypes in an Australian kindred. Neurology. 1997;49:552-8.
24. Will RG, Ironside JW, Zeidler M, Cousens SN, Estibeiro K, Alperovitch A, et al. A new variant of Creutzfeldt-Jakob disease in the UK. Lancet. 1996;347:921-5.
25. University of Edinburgh. (2013). National Creutzfeldt-Jakob Disease Surveillance Unit. [online] Available from http://www.cjd.ed.ac.uk/documents/worldfigs.pdf. [Last accessed June, 2021].

26. La Bella V, Collinge J, Pocchiari M, Piccoli F. Variant Creutzfeldt-Jakob disease in an Italian woman. Lancet. 2002;360:997-8.
27. Turner ML, Ludlam CA. An update on the assessment and management of the risk of transmission of variant Creutzfeldt-Jakob disease by blood and plasma products. Br J Haematol. 2009;144:14-23.
28. Gill ON, Spencer Y, Richard-Loendt A, Kelly C, Dabaghian R, Boyes L, et al. Prevalent abnormal prion protein in human appendixes after bovine spongiform encephalopathy epizootic: large scale survey. BMJ. 2013;347:f5675.
29. Collinge J, Rossor M. A new variant of prion disease. Lancet. 1996;347:916-7.
30. Lorains JW, Henry C, Agbamu DA, Rossi M, Bishop M, Will RG, et al. Variant Creutzfeldt-Jakob disease in an elderly patient. Lancet. 2001;357:1339-40.
31. Barbot C, Castro L, Oliveira C, Carpenter S. Variant Creutzfeldt-Jakob disease: the first confirmed case from Portugal shows early onset, long duration and unusual pathology. J Neurol Neurosurg Psychiatry. 2010;81:112-4.
32. Heath CA, Cooper SA, Murray K, Lowman A, Henry C, MacLeod MA, et al. Diagnosing variant Creutzfeldt-Jakob disease: a retrospective analysis of the first 150 cases in the UK. J Neurol Neurosurg Psychiatry. 2011;82:646-51.
33. Knight R, Will R. Prion diseses. J Neurol Neurosurg Psychiatry. 2004;75:i36-42.
34. de Villemeur TB, Gelot A, Deslys JP, Dormont D, Duyckaerts C, Jardin L, et al. Iatrogenic Creutzfeldt-Jakob disease in three growth hormone recipients: a neuropathological study. Neuropathol Appl Neurobiol. 1994;20:111-7.
35. Bernoulli C, Siegfried J, Baumgartner G, Regli F, Rabinowicz T, Gajdusek DC, et al. Danger of accidental person-to-person transmission of Creutzfeldt-Jakob disease by surgery. Lancet. 1977;1:478-9.
36. Will RG, Matthews WB. Evidence for case-to-case transmission of Creutzfeldt-Jakob disease. J Neurol Neurosurg Psychiatry. 1982;45:235-8.
37. Cochius JI, Mack K, Burns RJ, Alderman CP, Blumbergs PC. Creutzfeldt-Jakob disease in a recipient of pituitary-derived gonadotropin. Aust N Z J Med. 1990;20:592-3.
38. Thadani V, Penar PL, Partington J, Kalb R, Janssen R, Schonberger LB, et al. Creutzfeldt-Jakob disease probably acquired from cadaveric dura mater graft. J Neurosurg. 1988;69: 766-9.
39. Belay ED. Transmissible spongiform encephalopathies in humans. Annu Rev Microbiol. 1999;53:283-314.
40. Stewart LA, Rydzewska LH, Keogh GF, Knight RS. Systematic review of therapeutic interventions in human prion disease. Neurology. 2008;70:1272-81.
41. Otto M, Cepek L, Ratzka P, Doehlinger S, Boekhoff I, Wiltfang J, et al. Efficacy of flupirtine on cognitive function in patients with CJD: a double-blind study. Neurology. 2004;62:714-8.
42. Geschwind MD, Kuo AL, Wong KS, Haman A, Devereux G, Raudabaugh BJ, et al. Quinacrine treatment trial for sporadic Creutzfeldt-Jakob disease. Neurology. 2013;81:2015-23.
43. Haïk S, Marcon G, Mallet A, Tettamanti M, Welaratne A, Giaccone G, et al. Doxycycline in Creutzfeldt-Jakob disease: a phase 2, randomised, double-blind, placebo-controlled trial. Lancet Neurol. 2014;13:150-8.
44. Parry A, Baker I, Stacey R, Wimalaratna S. Long-term survival in a patient with variant Creutzfeldt-Jakob disease treated with intraventricular pentosan polysulphate. J Neurol Neurosurg Psychiatry. 2007;78:733-4.
45. Newman PK, Todd NV, Scoones D, Mead S, Knight RS, Will RG, et al. Postmortem findings in a case of variant Creutzfeldt-Jakob disease treated with intraventricular pentosan polysulfate. J Neurol Neurosurg Psychiatry. 2014;85:921-4.

CHAPTER 53

Emergencies in Movement Disorders

Kalyan B Bhattacharyya

INTRODUCTION

Movement disorders are, in general, such as all degenerative disorders in the body, progressive in nature. Acute onset of movement disorders usually indicates a vascular, infective, toxic, immune-mediated, or psychogenic etiology. Some acute movement disorders may present as a medical emergency where immediate care, including admission to intensive care unit, is necessary, since some of them may even turn out to be fatal. The conditions include acute parkinsonism, parkinsonism-hyperpyrexia syndrome, malignant catatonia (MC), dystonic storm, hemiballismus-hemichorea syndrome, tic emergencies, hyperekplexia, serotonin syndrome (SS), and neuroleptic malignant syndrome (NMS), to name a few. The present chapter shall include within its ambit, some of the important conditions, listed above.

ACUTE PARKINSONISM

The usual causes of acute development of a parkinsonian syndrome include infections, autoimmune disorders, toxins, some structural lesions, use of dopamine D2 receptor blocking agents, and psychogenic parkinsonism.

Infections

Constantin von Economo from Rumania gave a classic account of postencephalitic parkinsonism in 1917. He analyzed thousands of such cases, classified the condition into three subgroups namely, *somnolent-ophthalmoplegic, hyperkinetic, and amyostatic* forms, and about the first condition, he wrote:

"...prodromal phenomena consisting of general discomfort, shivering, headache, and slight pharyngitis... Within the next few days, somnolence begins to predominate. The patients, when left to themselves, fall asleep in the act of sitting and standing, and even while walking, or during meals with food in the mouth. If aroused, they wake up quickly and completely, are oriented, and fully conscious, but soon drop back to sleep... Generally, during the first days of illness, cranial nerve palsies appear. Ptosis is one of the first and most frequent symptoms. Rarely observed are supranuclear paralysis, paresis of convergence, nystagmus, optic neuritis, papilledema, pupillary disturbances, and even Argyll Robertson's sign."

Regarding the hyperkinetic form, he wrote:

"...chorea and hemichorea as well as myoclonic twitches were observed... On the other hand, it may find its mental expression in a general, curious restlessness of an anxious or hypomanic type. In most of these cases, there is a very distinct sleep disturbance and generally the condition is one of troublesome sleepiness."

And finally, the amyostatic-akinetic variety is described as:

"...a rigidity, without a real palsy and without symptoms arising from the pyramidal tract. This form of encephalitis lethargica is particularly common in the chronic cases, dominating the clinical picture of parkinsonism... To look at these patients, one would suppose them to be in a state of profound secondary dementia. Emotions are scarcely noticeable in the face, but they are mentally intact".[1]

The cause of this condition has been the subject of much debate. A viral etiology has been considered and some linked it to the pandemic of influenza that occurred around 1919.[2] However, von Economo described it in 1917 and unlike influenza, von Economo's disease was not contagious. The pathological changes were also different and the midbrain being typically affected in von Economo's disease, whereas there is diffuse cerebral congestion in postinfluenza encephalitis.[3]

Recent immunohistochemistry and immunofluorescence studies have failed to detect influenza antigen in the cerebrospinal fluid (CSF) samples of pathologically confirmed cases of von Economo's disease.[4-6] One study showed significant increase in the frequency of HLA-B14 antigen in these cases.[7]

Sometimes, parkinsonism may be the sequel of other viral encephalitis such as Coxsackie B virus, Epstein–Barr virus, Japanese encephalitis virus, polio virus, measles, and finally human immunodeficiency virus (HIV).[8-15] Nonviral agents such as spirochetes, mycoplasma, European tick-borne encephalitis, and other opportunistic infections, complicating HIV infection, may lead to this condition as well.[16-18]

Management

It depends on the identification of the etiology and symptomatic treatment. Usually, it is a difficult condition to treat.

NEUROLEPTIC MALIGNANT SYNDROME

This serious condition was first identified by Delay et al. in the days when haloperidol was frequently used,[19] though subsequent studies confirmed the issue.[20,21] The incidence has gone down substantially after the initiation of the newly developed atypical antipsychotic agents.[22,23] NMS develops in diverse psychiatric ailments as well as in patients with pre-existing catatonia or basal ganglia disorders.[24,25] Exhaustion, agitation, and dehydration predispose to the condition.[26,27] It is important to note that NMS is not a complication of neuroleptic overdose; on the contrary, it may take place with therapeutic dosage.[21]

Pathophysiology

The basic pathophysiological alteration for the development of NMS is the acute reduction of dopamine in the brain and the risk depends on the dose, potency, and the route of administration of the dopamine antagonists.[26-28] Studies of CSF metabolites of the neurotransmitters have confirmed central dopaminergic hypoactivity and it is also observed that these patients have some abnormality in the dopamine D2 receptor gene.[29-32] Changes in the dopamine pathway in response to stress as an additional cofactor can be the cause of NMS as well.[28] Some studies have shown that there is a genetic predisposition for this condition.[33]

Apart from the incontrovertible role of dopamine in the pathogenesis of NMS, there is some evidence that relative excess of glutaminergic transmission, low serum iron, effecting the role of dopamine receptors, and hypoactivity of gamma-aminobutyric acid (GABA) may have important role to play as well and Guerra et al. suggested dysregulation of sympathetic nervous system.[21,28,30,34]

Clinical Features

Classically, NMS presents acutely with rigidity and altered mentation along with autonomic changes and hyperthermia. Younger people and women in the postpartum period are at a greater risk.[35] Obtundation, catatonia, tachycardia, lability in blood pressure, dysarthria, dysphagia, sweating, myoclonic jerks, and fever are other manifestations. Serum creatine phosphokinase is invariably raised, often indicating rhabdomyolysis, leukocytosis, decreased serum iron level, and metabolic acidosis.[21] Generalized slowing in the electroencephalogram is seen in general, while imaging studies are usually noncontributory.[21] It has been shown by some workers that NMS can be triggered within 24 hours of administration of neuroleptics and discontinuation of these drugs resolves the problem, usually within 10 days.[36] Some untreated subjects may develop a persistent catatonic state, even after NMS has subsided.[37] In a large measure, NMS mimics toxic encephalopathy, status epilepticus, heat stroke, malignant hyperthermia, and SS.[37,38]

Management Issues

Management consists of stopping the culprit drugs, cooling and symptomatic management, and starting other medications. Two agents used most frequently include dantrolene sodium and bromocriptine.[39,40] Diuresis for myoglobulinuria and acute renal shutdown is done, since this complication can prove fatal and treatment should need to be reinstituted by low dose of atypical antipsychotics that can be administered with caution. The risk of death is in the range of about 10%.[41]

SEROTONIN SYNDROME

Like NMS, SS is an iatrogenic condition caused by agents which increase synthesis and transmission of serotonin in the brain. It is typically a complication of use of two or more serotonergic drugs such as selective serotonin reuptake inhibitors (SSRIs), selective serotonin-norepinephrine reuptake inhibitors, monoamine oxidase (MAO) inhibitors, tricyclic antidepressants, abuse drugs such as 3,4-methylenedioxymethamphetamine, antimigraine serotonin-augmenting agents such as triptans, and HIV-positive subjects. Clinically, it largely resembles NMS. The condition was first described by Oates et al. in 1960 in patients who were suffering from depression and had been taking concurrently MAO inhibitors and L-tryptophan.[42]

Pathophysiology

Typically, SS occurs in persons who have consumed combination of drugs which synergistically increase serotonin concentration in the synapses. One acute risk is the combination of MAO inhibitors along with 5-hydroxytryptophan (5-HT) or tryptamine agonists, commonly known as the *cheese effect*, with irreversible inhibition of MAO.[43-45] It has been seen that combination of SSRIs and triptans or sibutramine can lead to fatal SS.[46] It was originally believed that an excess of serotonin in the brain and agonism of 5-HT1A receptors in central gray nuclei and medulla were the putative cause, but subsequent studies have shown that overstimulation of 5-HT2A is responsible for this syndrome.[47] The role of norepinephrine has also been questioned, as is that of N-methyl-D-aspartate (NMDA) receptor antagonists and GABA.[48] Finally, an idea, known as *spectrum concept* has been advanced, which states that the side effects are due to increasing serotonin level in the brain and, finally, it turns into toxicity. Thus, it is a dose-dependent phenomenon and some authorities prefer to call the condition serotonin toxicity or serotonin toxidrome, indicating that it is a kind of poisoning with the agent.[49,50]

Symptomatology

They may appear with minutes of elevation of the serotonin level in the brain and there are protean manifestations. There is tachycardia, sweating, mydriasis, myoclonic jerks, brisk tendon reflexes, and shivering. If the condition is more severe, increased bowel movement, hypertension, and hyperthermia may complicate the clinical picture. In severe cases, mental obtundation or hypervigilance, metabolic acidosis, seizures, rhabdomyolysis with renal failure, and disseminated intravascular coagulation may turn out to be the fatal outcome.[43,48] Sometimes, based on the symptom complexes, the clinical features are described as a triad of cognitive features such as agitation, hypomania, confusion, hallucinations, and coma; autonomic features such as shivering, sweating, hyperthermia, tachycardia, nausea, and diarrhea; and somatic symptoms such as myoclonus, hyperreflexia, and tremor.[48] The Hunter Serotonin Toxicity Criteria decision rules have been proposed for diagnosis of SS and it includes spontaneous clonus or inducible clonus plus agitation or diaphoresis or ocular clonus plus agitation or diaphoresis or tremor plus hyperpyrexia or hypertonicity plus temperature above 38°C plus ocular clonus or inducible clonus.[43]

Apart from other closely resembling condition, SS is most frequently confused with NMS, since they share many common features in spite of the fact that pathophysiologically they are vastly different. However, SS has a rapid onset and there is antecedent history of intake of serotonergic drugs, whereas NMS develops over days following administration of dopamine blocking agents.[51] Additionally, lead-pipe rigidity is a feature of NMS, whereas in SS, hyperkinesias and clonus dominate the clinical picture.[52,53] Serum creatine phosphokinase and leukocyte rise are not as high as in NMS.

Management Issues

Firstly, SS is to be managed as an emergency condition, preferably in an intensive care setting. Hyperthermia is treated with cool blankets and antipyretics are of little use, since it is due to severe muscular contraction and not due to problems in hypothalamic heat regulation center. Agitation is controlled with sedatives. In very severe cases, intubation and ventilatory support may be required. The mainstay of therapy includes use of serotonin antagonists such as cyproheptadine.[54,55] Atypical antipsychotics such as olanzapine can be used in severe cases.[48] Most cases recover with 24 hours of recognition and discontinuation of the offending drugs. Myalgia and weakness may persist for some months due to extreme exhaustion.[48]

MALIGNANT CATATONIA

First described by Karl Ludwig Kahlbaum of Germany in 1874, catatonia refers to a state of psychomotor immobility and behavioral abnormality manifested by stupor, while MC was described by Calmeil in 1832.[56] This happens in various neurological disorders, mostly drug induced, and often with psychiatric illnesses. However, diverse conditions such as cerebrovascular accident, seizure disorders, glioma of corpus callosum, infections, head injury, and metabolic conditions are also implicated.[56] The milder form is known as simple and those with hyperthermia and autonomic symptoms are termed as malignant.[56,57] Early clinical descriptions showed a remarkable uniformity.[58,59] There was a prodromal phase lasting for about 2 weeks, which consisted of insomnia, anorexia, mood swings, and uncontrolled and violent motor excitement.[60] The subjects refuse food and there is clouding of consciousness, tachycardia, tachypnea, cyanosis, labile blood pressure, and diaphoresis. Often, there is cutaneous hematoma, catatonic stupor, echolalia, and echopraxia. Later, delusions and hallucinations are common and body temperature rises to the level of 44°C, along with waxy flexibility. This phase lasts for about a week.[56] In one series, all the cases had muscle stiffness, which resembled NMS.[56]

Pathophysiology

A number of authors has assigned the role of a hypodopaminergic state, such as in NMS, as the causative factor for MC.[59,61,62] It has been suggested that the onset of MC is accompanied by an acute reduction of dopaminergic state in the frontal subcortical circuits.[61,62] These circuits possibly represent brain's principal network subserving behavioral patterns of man. There are five such circuits and dopamine is the chief neurotransmitter and additionally, it modulates each circuit through its projections to the striatum.[63-65] Hypodopaminergic state in the motor circuit accounts for muscular rigidity and that in the anterior cingulate circuit possibly predisposes the subject to diminished responsiveness, akinetic state, mutism, hyperthermia, and autonomic disturbances. The same state in the lateral orbitofrontal subcortical circuit may mediate the catatonic features.[65] Finally, some studies indicate that enhanced responsiveness of the dopaminergic system to stress may be a factor for predisposition to MC.[66,67]

Management Issues

The diagnostic workup includes personal and family psychiatric history, medical history, history of drug abuse, and thorough laboratory investigation for relevant precipitating conditions. Benzodiazepines are found highly effective for simple- or antipsychotic-induced catatonia[57,61,68] and it has been suggested by the works of Fricchione et al. and Mann et al. that if benzodiazepines fail to offer any improvement after 5 days, electroconvulsive therapy must be undertaken.[61,68,69] A number of works has indicated that this sort of therapy is most effective, if started early before the progression of the disease to a severe state. Onset of coma or hyperthermia predicts a poor outcome.[56,60] Corticosteroids and adrenocorticotropic hormones have also been used with some success and can be considered, if electroconvulsive therapy turns out to be ineffective.[56,58] Dantrolene and bromocriptine, with or without electroconvulsive therapy, have also been a success in some works.[56] Recently, glutamate antagonists such as amantadine and memantine have been shown to be effective in management.[70]

PROGRESSIVE ENCEPHALOMYELITIS WITH RIGIDITY AND MYOCLONUS SYNDROME

After discussing almost related conditions such as NMS, SS, and MC, a newly described entity, progressive encephalomyelitis with rigidity and myoclonus (PERM) syndrome, merits some consideration.

Moersch et al. described progressive, fluctuating muscular rigidity and spasm in a cohort of 14 cases and named it as *stiff-man syndrome*.[71] Other features include hyperekplexia and brainstem signs.[72] The rigidity and myoclonus are often induced by startle, along with opisthotonus and trismus, consciousness is preserved, and episodes occur in day as well as night, along with moaning and tachypnea.[73] It is a part of the spectrum of stiff-person syndrome with presence of antiglutamic acid decarboxylase (GAD) antibodies in up to 80% of cases. Cases are on record that some of these cases are paraneoplastic in nature with antiamphiphysin, GlyR, and DPPX antibodies as well.[74,75] In hereditary hyperekplexia, mutations in the $\alpha1$ subunit of glycine receptor gene, *GLRA1*, have been observed.[75] These receptors are found in the caudal pontine brainstem and spinal cord and the hyperekplexia is possibly due to interference with the normal inhibitory glycinergic transmission in the nucleus reticularis pontis caudalis.[76] Additional findings include continuous muscle fiber activity in trunk and proximal limb muscles, despite a relaxed state, and brisk deep tendon reflexes.[77]

DYSTONIC STORM

Dystonia, by definition, is an involuntary sustained muscle contraction causing twisting of the body and bizarre posture in a part or throughout the body.[77] However, sometimes, dystonia warrants admission into the intensive care unit. The spasm can last for several hours to days and constitutes a grave emergency. The first such case was reported by Jankovic et al. in 1982 when they described a young boy with severe generalized dystonia along with myoglobinuria and hyperpyrexia and 2 years later, Marsden and his colleagues reported two such cases which they termed as *desperate dystonia*.[78,79] Later, such cases were defined, in general, as *status dystonicus* or *dystonic storm*.[80-82] The risk of this condition correlates with the severity of dystonia and in those where the primary illness is not controlled well.[78] It occurs in primary dystonia with or without DYT1 mutation as well as in secondary dystonia following trauma, encephalitis, cerebral palsy, or the use of neuroleptics.[80,82-85] Neurodegenerative disorders such as Wilson's disease, choreoacanthocytosis, and pantothenate kinase-associated neurodegeneration are also associated with dystonic storm.[80,81,86] Abrupt tapering of drugs such as tetrabenazine, lithium, or anticholinergics can also precipitate the condition.[80,78] Complications include tongue bite, dehydration, cardiac dysfunction, hypotension, aspiration pneumonia, secondary infections, and acute renal failure due to rhabdomyolysis.[80,84,87]

The differential diagnosis of dystonic storm includes NMS, SS, MC, and acute withdrawal from intrathecal baclofen.[80,83,88] Management includes supportive care in the intensive care unit, care of airway, endotracheal intubation and, sometimes, mechanical ventilation. Hyperpyrexia is controlled with cool blankets and antipyretics, while pain is treated with morphine or fentanyl and acute renal failure due to myoglobinuria with dialysis.[80,82,85,78,89]

Hypnotics, midazolam drip, or general anesthetic agents such as propofol is of some use to alleviate the dystonic spasms.[80,81,85] Marsden et al. suggested antidystonic drugs, often known as the *triple cocktail,* which include tetrabenazine, anticholinergics, and a dopamine-blocking drug,[79] while Manji et al. suggested trial of levodopa first followed by the use of triple cocktail.[5] More intensive therapy such as intrathecal baclofen is recommended when oral therapy is not effective.[90,91] Side effects include CSF leak, meningitis, seizures, bradycardia, hypotension, and coma.[92-95]

Surgical procedures such as pallidotomy, thalamotomy, and deep brain stimulation of the globus pallidus have been tried to ameliorate dystonic storm, though their efficacy is not fully clear yet.[96-99] Complications of these procedures include stroke, infections, cognitive impairment, visual field defects, dysarthria, and hypophonia.[100-102] Additionally, the benefit accrued from these procedures takes a long time.[102]

HEMIBALLISMUS-HEMICHOREA SYNDROME

Ballism was defined by Meyers in 1968 as *"repetitive, but constantly varying, large amplitude involuntary movements of the proximal parts of the limbs. This activity is almost ceaseless and movements are often complex and combined"*.[103] This is one of the most dramatic acute movement disorders where the patient presents with sudden flinging movements in one side of the body, usually affecting the proximal muscles. In hemichorea, the movements are only of lesser intensity, affect both the proximal and the distal parts of the limbs of one side, and can coexist with hemiballismus. Usually, this is a disorder of the elderly, affecting both the sexes equally, and the movements can be violent and the patient may hit the limbs against the wall and injure himself. It is nonsuppressible, increases with stress and activity, and disappears during sleep. Monoballism and biballism are also encountered in clinical practice, where in the latter condition, both the sides of the brain are affected.

Hemiballismus-hemichorea syndrome is a comparatively uncommon condition and Dewey et al. in a study of 3,084 patients observed this condition in only 21 subjects, while in another study only 11 cases were recorded in a cohort of 2,000 strokes in the basal ganglia.[104,105]

Etiopathogenesis

Hemiballismus-hemichorea syndrome is an entity where the anatomical substrate is eminently localizable, i.e., the subthalamic nucleus of Luys. However, in more recent times, it has been shown that this condition may be caused by lesions in other areas as well, even outside the basal ganglia.[104-106] Cerebrovascular accident is the most common cause and lacunar infarcts, associated with hypertension and diabetes mellitus, are frequently observed. However, vasculitis and hypercoagulable states are also often implicated. Recently, nonketotic hyperosmolar coma is found to be a common cause of this condition. Classically, the victim is an elderly female and the condition improves with correction of hyperglycemia. Neuroimaging shows high signal intensities in the putamen and globus pallidus, contralateral to the side of the movement, and this too clears up with improvement in the diabetic state. Tumors in the basal ganglia are a rare cause as well.

Hemiballismus-hemichorea syndrome can be induced in experimental animals by ablation of only 20% of the subthalamic nucleus. Lesions in the globus pallidus too can lead to this condition and it has been postulated that this is due to the disruption of the connections between this structure and the subthalamic nucleus. However, a lesion in the globus pallidus internus is shown to ameliorate the movement. Injection of GABA antagonists into various parts of the basal ganglia, affecting the neurons, but not the axons, showed that its administration into the subthalamic nucleus alone led to the development of the abnormal movements and injection into the lateral globus pallidus led to slower movements, akin to what is seen in hyperosmolar nonketotic states.[106] These experiments suggest that lesions in the subthalamic nucleus lead to interruption of the excitatory connections to the globus pallidus internus, which, in turn, results in hypoactivity of this region. This inhibits the thalamus and, consequently, the motor cortex is excited, leading to the involuntary movements.[107] These experiments, however, fail to explain the rather rare occurrence of such movements following lesioning of the subthalamic nucleus for the management of advanced Parkinson's disease.[108] Recent electrophysiological studies have shown that these patients have an abnormal neuronal firing pattern of intermittent bursts followed by pauses and the ballistic movements coincide with increased firing.[109-111]

Prognosis

In spite of the fact that apparently the disease looks rather bizarre, it usually carries a good prognosis. In most cases, the disease is self-limiting within a few months to a year. Hyland et al. reported that in 12 of their 14 patients, the resolution of the symptoms and signs was complete, whereas Johnson et al. observed that stopping treatment after 27 days, only two out of their six patients had recurrence.[112,113] Another group reported that only three of their 11 subjects required long-term therapy.[114] As it has been already said, hemiballismus-hemichorea syndrome, as a complication of hyperosmolar nonketotic coma, resolves with control of hyperglycemia.

Management

Firstly, one must look for reversible causes such as hyperosmolar nonketotic coma or a space-occupying lesion in the subthalamic nucleus. Cerebrovascular accident is managed by antiplatelets, statins, and management of concomitant hypertension or diabetes. Since the violent flinging movements can lead to exhaustion and rhabdomyolysis, attention to such complications is necessary.

Dopamine antagonists are the mainstay for the management of hemiballismus-hemichorea syndrome. Neuroleptics such as haloperidol, perphenazine, pimozide, chlorpromazine, and, in more recent times, tetrabenazine, the most commonly used agent, constitute the mainstay of management for the involuntary movements.[115] However, one of the major problems with these agents, particularly in the elderly, is the development of tardive dyskinesia in the nonaffected limbs, which necessitates reduction of the dopamine antagonists. In general, the improvement rate with these drugs tends to be in the range of about 90%.[116] Atypical neuroleptics such as risperidone, clozapine, and olanzapine are also useful agents, as are sodium valproate, trihexyphenidyl, and amitriptyline. In drug-refractory cases, surgical therapy is recommended and the most frequently performed operation is ventrolateral thalamotomy. In a series of 13 patients, Krauss et al. reported significant improvement in 11 subjects.[117] Globus pallidus internus lesion is another option.[116,117] Deep brain stimulation is the most recent and novel treatment modality, which is employed with some success in a number of cases.[117]

REFERENCES

1. Bhattacharya KB. Eminent Neuroscientists: Their Lives and Works. Kolkata: Academic Publishers; 2011.
2. Ravenholt RT, Foege WH. 1918 Influenza, encephalitis lethargica, and parkinsonism. Lancet. 1982;2:860-2.
3. Caligiuri MP, Ellwanger J. Motor and cognitive aspects of motor retardation in depression. J Affect Disord. 2000;47:83-93.
4. Casals J, Elizan TS, Yahr MD, Harter DH, Duffy PE, Barden H, et al. Postencephalitic parkinsonism: a review. J Neural Transm. 1998;105:645-76.
5. Gamboa ET, Wolf A, Yahr MD. Influenza virus antigen in post-encephalitic parkinsonism brain. Arch Neurol. 1974;31:228-32.
6. Martilla RJ, Hallomen P, Rinne UK. Influenza virus antibodies in parkinsonism: comparison of postencephalitic and idiopathic Parkinson patients and matched controls. Arch Neurol. 1977;34:99-100.
7. Elizan TS, Yahr MD. Histocompatibility antigens and postencephalitic parkinsonism. J Neurol Neurosurg Psychiatry. 1983; 46:688-93.
8. Walters JH. Postencephalitic Parkinson syndrome after meningoencephalitis due to Coxsackie virus group. N Engl J Med. 1960;263:744-7.
9. Hsieh JC, Lue KH, Lee YL. Parkinson-like syndrome as the major presenting symptom of Epstein-Barr virus encephalitis. Arch Dis Child. 2002;87:358-9.
10. Shiraki H, Goto A, Narabayashi H. Etat passé et present de l'enecphalite Japonnaise au Japon. Rev Neurol (Paris). 1963;108:633-96.
11. Shoji H, Watanabe M, Itoh S, Kuwahara H, Hattori F. Japanese encephalitis and parkinsonism. J Neurol. 1993;240:59-60.
12. Barrett AM, Gairdner D, McFarlan AM. An outbreak of encephalitis possibly due to poliomyelitis virus. Br Med J. 1952;1:1317-22.
13. Meyer B. Encephalitis after measles with severe parkinsonism rigidity: recovery. Br Med J. 1943;1:508.
14. Mirsattari SM, Power C, Nath A. Parkinsonism with HIV infection. Mov Disord. 1998;13:684-9.
15. Navia BA, Petito CK, Gold JW, Cho ES, Jordan BD, Price RW. Cerebral toxoplasmosis complicating the acquired immunodeficiency syndrome: clinical and neuropathological findings in 27 patients. Ann Neurol. 1986;19:224-8.
16. Maggi P, de Mari M, Moramarco A, Fiofrentino P, Lamberti P, Angarano G. Parkinsonism in a patient with AIDS and cerebral opportunistic granulomatous lesions. Neurol Sci. 2002;21: 173-6.
17. De Mattos JP, Ross AL, Correa RB, Novis S. Involuntary movements and AIDS: report of seven cases and review of the literature. Arq Neuropsiquitr. 1993;51:491-7.
18. Mansfield KL, Johnson N, Phipps LP, Stephenson JR, Fooks AR, Solomon T. Tick-borne encephalitis virus: a review of an emerging zoonosis. J Gen Virol. 2009;90:1781-94.
19. Delay J, Pichot P, Lemperiere T, Elissade B, Peigne F. Un neuroleptiquemajeur non-phenothiazine et non reserpinique, l'haloperidol, dans le traitement des psychoses. Ann Medico-psychologique. 1960;118:145-52.
20. Caroff SN. The neuroleptic malignant syndrome. J Clin Psych. 1980;41:79-83.
21. Caroff SN, Mann SC. Neuroleptic malignant syndrome. Med Clin North Am. 1993;77:185-202.
22. Caroff SN, Mann SC, Campbell EC, Sullivan KA. Movement disorders associated with atypical antipsychotic drugs. J Clin Psychiatry. 2002;63:12-9.
23. Caroff SN, Mann SC, Campbell EC. Atypical antipsychotics and neuroleptic malignant syndrome. Psychiatr Ann. 2000;30: 314-21.
24. White DAC, Robbins AH. Catatonia: harbinger of the neuroleptic malignant syndrome. Br J Psychiatry. 1991;158:419-21.
25. Caroff SN, Mann SC, McCarthy M, Naser J, Rynn M, Morrison M. Acute infectious encephalitis complicated by neuroleptic malignant syndrome. J Clin Psychopharmacol. 1998;18:349-51.
26. Keck PE, Pope HG, Cohen BM, McElroy SL, Nierenberg AA. Risk factors for neuroleptic malignant syndrome. Arch Gen Psychiatry. 1989;46:914-8.

27. Berardi D, Amore M, Keck PE, Troia M, Dell'Atti M. Clinical and pharmacologic risk factors for neuroleptic malignant syndrome: a case control study. Biol Psychiatry. 1998;44: 748-54.
28. Mann SC, Caroff SN, Fricchione G, Campbell EC. Central dopamine hypoactivity and the pathogenesis of the neuroleptic malignant syndrome. Psychiatr Ann. 2000;30:363-74.
29. Ueda M, Hamamoto M, Nagayama H, Okubo S, Amemiya S, Katayama Y. Biochemical alterations during medication withdrawal in Parkinson's disease with and without neuroleptic malignant syndrome-like syndrome. J Neurol Neurosurg Psychiatry. 2001;71:111-3.
30. Nisijima K, Ishiguro T. Cerebrospinal fluid levels of monoamine metabolites and gamma-aminobutyric acid in neuroleptic malignant syndrome. J Psychiatr Res. 1995;27:233-44.
31. Suzuki A, Kondo T, Otani K, Mihara K, Yasui-Furukori N, Sano A, et al. Association of TaqIA polymorphism of the dopamine D2 receptor gene with predisposition to neuroleptic malignant syndrome. Am J Psychiatry. 2001;158:1714-6.
32. Ram O, Cao Q, Kek PE, Pope HG, Otani K, Addonizio G, et al. Structural change in the dopamine D2 receptor gene in a patient with neuroleptic malignant syndrome. Am J Med Genet. 1995;60:228-30.
33. Otani K, Horiuchi M, Kondo T, Kaneko S, Fukushima Y. Is the predisposition to neuroleptic malignant syndrome genetically transmitted? Br J Psychiatr. 1991;158:850-3.
34. Guerra RJ. Is neuroleptic malignant syndrome a neurogenic form of malignant hyperthermia? Clin Neuropharmacol. 2002;25:183-93.
35. Alexander PJ, Thomas RM, Das A. Is risk of neuroleptic malignant syndrome increased in the postpartum period? J Clin Psychiatr. 1998;59:254-5.
36. Caroff SN, Mann SC. Neuroleptic malignant syndrome. Psychopharmacol Bull. 1988;24:25-9.
37. Strawn JR, Keck PE, Caroff SN. Neuroleptic malignant syndrome. Am J Psych. 2007;164:870-6.
38. Sachdev PS. A rating scale for neuroleptic malignant syndrome. Psychiatr Res. 2005;135:249-56.
39. Caroff SN, Mann SC, Keck PE, Francis A. Residual catatonic state following neuroleptic malignant syndrome. J Clin Psychopharmacol. 2000;20:257-9.
40. Rosenberg MR, Green M. Neuroleptic malignant syndrome: a review of response to therapy. Arch Intern Med. 1989;149: 1927-31.
41. Sakkas P, Davis JM, Janicak PG, Wang JY. Drug-induced treatment of neuroleptic malignant syndrome. Psychopharmacol Bull. 1991;27:381-4.
42. Oates JA, Sjoerdsma A. Neurologic effects of tryptophan in patients receiving a monoamine oxidase inhibitor. Neurology. 1960;10:1076-8.
43. Dunkley EJ, Isbister GK, Sibbritt D, Dawson AH, Whyte IM. The Hunter Serotonin Toxicity Criteria: simple and accurate diagnostic decision rules for serotonin toxicity. Quart J Med. 2003;96:635-42.
44. Fraser J, South M. Life-threatening fluvoxamine overdose in a 4-year-old child. Intensive Care Med. 1999;25:548.
45. Sternbach H. The serotonin syndrome. Am J Psychiatry. 1991;148:705-13.
46. Evans RW. The FDA alert on serotonin syndrome with combined use of SSRIs or SNRIs and Triptans: an analysis of the 29 case reports. MedGenMed. 2007;9:48.
47. Whyte IA. Serotonin Toxicity/Syndrome: Medical Toxicology. Philadelphia: Williams & Wilkins; 2004. pp. 103-6.
48. Boyer EW, Shannon M. The serotonin syndrome. N Engl J Med. 2005;352:1112-20.
49. Gillman PK. The spectrum concept of serotonin toxicity. Pain Med. 2004;5:231-2.
50. Gillman PK. A review of serotonin toxicity data: implications for the mechanisms of antidepressant drug action. Biol Psychiatry. 2006;59:1046-51.
51. Nisijima K, Shioda K, Iwamura T. Neuroleptic malignant syndrome and serotonin syndrome. Prog Brain Res. 2007;162: 81-104.
52. Birmes P, Coppin D, Schmitt L, Lauque D. Serotonin syndrome: a brief review. CMAJ. 2003;168:1439-42.
53. Isbister GK, Dawson A, Whyte IM. Citalopram overdose, serotonin toxicity, or neuroleptic malignant syndrome? Can J Psychiatry. 2001;46:657-9.
54. Christopher F. Recognition and treatment of serotonin syndrome. Can Fam Physician. 2008;54:988-92.
55. Graudins A, Steraman A, Chan B. Treatment of the serotonin syndrome with cyproheptadine. J Emerg Med. 1998;16:615-9.
56. Frucht SJ, Fahn S. Movement Disorder Emergencies: Diagnosis and Treatment, 1st edition. New Jersey: Humana Press; 2007. p. 54.
57. Philbrick KL, Rummans TA. Malignant catatonia. J Neuropsychiatr Clin Neurosci. 1994;6:1-13.
58. Mann SC, Caroff SN, Bleier HR, Welz WK, King MA, Hayashida M. Lethal catatonia. Am J Psychiatr. 1986;143:1374-81.
59. Mann SC, Auriacombe M, Macfadden W, Caroff SN, Campbell EC, Tignol J. Lethal catatonia: clinical aspects and therapeutic intervention. A review of the literature. Encephale. 2001;27: 213-6.
60. Shulack NR. Exhaustion syndrome in excited psychotic patients. Am J Psychiatr. 1946;102:466-75.
61. Fricchione G, Bush G, Fozdar M, Francis A, Fink M. Recognition and treatment of the catatonic syndrome. J Intensive Care Med. 1997;12:135-47.
62. Fricchione G, Mann SC, Caroff SN. Catatonia, lethal catatonia, and neuroleptic malignant syndrome. Psychiatr Ann. 2000;3: 347-55.
63. Alexander GE, DeLong MR, Strick PL. Parallel organization of functionally segregated circuits linking basal ganglia and cortex. Ann Rev Neurosci. 1986;9:357-81.
64. Alexander GE, Crutcher MD, DeLong MD. Basal ganglia-thalamocortical circuits: parallel substrates for motor, oculomotor, prefrontal and limbic functions. Prog Brain Res. 1990;85:119-46.
65. Cummings JL. Frontal-subcortical circuits and human behaviour. Arch Neurol. 1993;50:873-80.
66. Thierry AM, Tassin JP, Blanc G, Glowinski J. Selective activation of the mesocortical dopamine system by stress. Nature. 1976;263:242-44.
67. Lavielle S, Tassin JP, Thierry AM, Blanc G, Herve D, Berthelemy C, et al. Blockade by benzodiazepines of the

selective high increase in dopamine turnover induced by stress in mesocortical dopaminergic neurons of the rat. Brain Res. 1979;168:585-94.

68. Mann SC, Caroff SN, Lazarus A. The pathogenesis of neuroleptic malignant syndrome. Psychiatr Ann. 1991;21:175-80.
69. Leroy A, Naudet F, Vaiva G, Francis A, Thomas P, Amad A. Is electroconvulsive therapy an evidence-based treatment for catatonia? A systemic review and meta-analysis. Eur Arch Psychiatr Clin Neurosci. 2018;268:675-87.
70. Carroll BT, Goforth HW, Thomas C, Ahuja N, McDaniel WW, Kraus MF, et al. Review of adjunctive glutamate antagonist therapy in the treatment of catatonic syndromes. J Neuropsychiatr Clin Neurosci. 2007;19:406-12.
71. Moersch FP, Woltman HW. Progressive fluctuating muscular rigidity and spasm (stiff-man syndrome); report of a case and some observations in 13 other cases. Proc Staff Meet Mayo Clin. 1956;31:421-7.
72. Hutchinson M, Waters P, McHugh G, Gorman S, O'Riordan S, Connolly H, et al. Progressive encephalomyelitis, rigidity, and myoclonus: a novel glycine receptor antibody. Neurology. 2008;71:1291-2.
73. Damásio J, Leite IM, Coutinho E, Water P, Woodhall M, Santos MA, et al. Progressive encephalomyelitis with rigidity and myoclonus: the first pediatric case with glycine receptor antibodies. JAMA Neurol. 2013;70:498-501.
74. Antoine JC, Honnorat AL, Boulesteix JM, de Brouker T, Vial C, Butler M, et al. Antiamphiphysin antibodies are associated with various paraneoplastic neurological syndromes and tumours. Arch Neurol. 1999;56:172-7.
75. Borellini L, Lanfranconi S, Bonato S, Trezzi I, Franco G, Torretta L, et al. Progressive encephalomyelitis with rigidity and myoclonus associated with anti-GlyR antibodies and Hodgkin's lymphoma: a case report. Front Neurol. 2017;8:401.
76. Shiang R, Rya SG, Ya-Zhen Z, Hahn AF, O'Connell P, Wasmuth JJ. Mutations in the α1 subunit of the inhibitory glycine receptor cause the dominant neurologic disorder, hyperekplexia. Nature. 1993;5:351-8.
77. Meinck HM, Thomson PD. Stiff man syndrome and related conditions. Mov Disord. 2002;17:853-66.
78. Jankovic J, Penn AS. Severe dystonia and myoglobinuria. Neurology. 1982;2:1195-7.
79. Marsden CD, Marion MH, Quinn N. The treatment of severe dystonia in children and adults. J Neurol Neurosurg Psychiatr. 1984;47:1166-73.
80. Manji H, Howard RS, Miller DH, Hirsch LP, Carr L, Bhatia K, et al. Status dystonicus: the syndrome and its management. Brain. 1998;121:243-52.
81. Vaamonde J, Narbona J, Weiser R, Garcia MA, Brannan T, Obeso JA. Dystonic storms: a practical management problem. Clin Neuropharmacol. 1994;17:344-7.
82. Opal P, Tinter R, Jankovic J, Leung J, Breakfield XO, Friedman J, et al. Intrafamilial phenotypic variability of the DYT1 dystonia: from asymptomatic TOR1A gene carrier status to dystonic storm. Mov Disord. 2002;17:339-45.
83. Dalvi A, Fahn S, Ford B. Intrathecal baclofen in the treatment of dystonic storm. Mov Disord. 1998;13:611-2.
84. Paret G, Tirosh R, Ben-Zeev B, Verdi A, Brandt N, Barzilav Z. Rhabdomyolysis due to hereditary torsion dystonia. Pediatr Neurol. 1995;13:83-4.
85. Narayan RK, Loubser PG, Jankovic J, Donovan WH. Intrathecal baclofen for intractable torsion dystonia. Neurology. 1991;41:1141-2.
86. Svetel M, Sternic N, Pejovic S, Kostic VS. Penicillamine induced lethal status dystonicus in a patient with Wilson's disease. Mov Disord. 2001;16:568-9.
87. Cavanaugh JJ, Finlayson RE. Rhabdomyolysis due to acute dystonic reaction to antipsychotic drugs. J Clin Psychiatr. 1984;45:356-7.
88. Ford B, Greene P, Louis ED, Petzinger G, Bressman SB, Goodman R, et al. Use of intrathecal baclofen in the treatment of patients with dystonic storm. Arch Neurol. 1996;53:1241-6.
89. Ravi SD, Borge GF, Roach FL. Neuroleptics, laryngeal-pharyngeal dystonia and acute renal failure. J Clin Psychiatry. 1982;43:300.
90. Penn RD. Intrathecal baclofen for spasticity of spinal origin: seven years of experience. J Neurosurg. 1992;77:236-40.
91. Kravitz HM, Corcos DM, Hansen G, Penn RD, Cartwright RD, Gianino J. Intrathecal baclofen: effects on nocturnal muscle spasticity. Am J Phys Med Rehabil. 1992;71:48-52.
92. Delhaas EM, Brouwers JR. Intrathecal baclofen overdose: report of 7 events in 5 patients and review of the literature. Int J Clin Pharmacol Ther Toxicol. 1991;29:274-80.
93. Teddy P, Jamous A, Gardner B, Wang D, Silver J. Complications of intrathecal baclofen delivery. Br J Neurosurg. 1992;6:115-8.
94. Penn RD. Intrathecal baclofen for spasticity of spinal origin: seven years of experience. J Neurosurg. 1992;77:236-40.
95. Siegfried RN, Jacobson L, Chabal C. Development of an acute withdrawal syndrome following the cessation of intrathecal baclofen in a patient with spasticity. Anesthesiology. 1992;77:1048-50.
96. Kupsch A, Kuchn A, Klaffke S, Meissner W, Hammack D, Winter C. Deep brain stimulation in dystonia. J Neurosurg. 2003;250:147-52.
97. Yanni J, Bain PG, Gregory RP, Nandi G, Joint C, Scott RB, et al. Postoperative progress of dystonia patients following globus pallidus internus deep brain stimulation. Eur J Neurol. 2003;10:239-47.
98. Krack P, Vercueil L. Review of functional surgical treatment of severe dystonia. J Neurol. 2001;8:389-99.
99. Ondo WG, Desaloms JM, Jankovic J, Grossman RG. Pallidotomy for generalized dystonia. Mov Disord. 1998;13:693-8.
100. Abosch A, Lozano A. Stereotactic neurosurgery for movement disorders. Can J Neurol Sci. 2003;30:72-82.
101. Beric A, Kelly PJ, Rezai A, Sterio D, Mogilner A, Zonnenshavn M, et al. Complications of deep brain stimulation surgery. Stereotact Funct Neurosurg. 2001;77:73-8.
102. Lozano A, Kumar R, Gross RE, Gilani N, Hutchison WD, Dstrovsky JO, et al. Globus pallidus internus pallidotomy for generalized dystonia. Mov Disord. 1997;12:865-70.
103. Meyer R. Ballismus. In: Vinken J, Bruyn G (Eds). Handbook of Clinical Neurology. Amsterdam: North-Holland Publishing Co.; 1968. pp. 476-90.
104. Dewey RB, Jankovic J. Hemiballism-hemichorea. Clinical and pharmacologic findings in 21 patients. Arch Neurol. 1989;46:862-7.
105. Ghika-Schmidt F, Ghika J, Regli F, Bogousslavsky J. Hyperkinetic movement disorders during and after acute stroke: the Lausanne Stroke Registry. J Neurol Sci. 1997;146:109-16.

106. Ristic A, Marinkovic J, Dragasevic N, Stanisavljevic D, Kostic V. Long-term prognosis of vascular hemiballismus. Stroke. 2002; 33:2109-11.
107. Crossman AR, Sambrook MA, Jackson A. Experimental hemichorea/hemiballismus in the monkey. Studies on the intracerebral site of action in a drug-induced dyskinesia. Brain. 1984;107:579-86.
108. Delong MR. Primate models of movement disorders of basal ganglia origin. Trends Neurosci. 1990;13:281-5.
109. Guridi J. Obeso J. The subthalamic nucleus, hemiballismus, and Parkinson's disease: reappraisal of a neurosurgical dogma. Brain. 2001;124:5-19.
110. Lenz FA, Suarez JI, Metman LV, Reich SG, Karp BI, Hallett M, et al. Pallidal activity during dystonia: somatosensory reorganization and changes in severity. J Neurol Neurosurg Psychiatry. 1998;65:767-70.
111. Suarez JI, Metman LV, Reich SG, Dougherty PM, Hallett M, Lenz FA. Pallidotomy for hemiballismus: efficacy and characteristics of neuronal activity. Ann Neurol. 1997;42:807-11.
112. Vitek JL, Chockkan V, Zhang JY. Neuronal activity in the basal ganglia in patients with generalized dystonia and hemiballismus. Ann Neurol. 1999;46:22-35.
113. Hyland H, Foreman D. Prognosis in hemiballismus. Neurology. 1957;7:381-91.
114. Johnson WG, Fahn S. Treatment of vascular hemiballism and hemichorea. Neurology. 1977;27:634-6.
115. Klawans HL, Moses H, Nausieda PA, Bergen D, Weiner WJ. Treatment and prognosis of hemiballismus. N Engl J Med. 1976;295:1348-50.
116. Krauss JK, Mundinger F. Functional stereotactic surgery for hemiballismus. J Neurosurg. 1996;85:278-86.
117. Postuma RB, Lang AE. Hemiballism: revisiting a classic disorder. Lancet Neurol. 2003;2:661-8.

SECTION

11

BOTULINUM TOXIN IN MOVEMENT DISORDERS

CHAPTER 54

Botulinum Toxin in Movement Disorders

Swetha Tandra, Rukmini Kandadai Mridula, Rupam Borgohain

INTRODUCTION

Botulinum toxins (BoNTs) have been in use for medical purposes for a considerable time, especially in movement disorders after their first discovery in cases of food poisoning who presented with neuromuscular paralysis. It was first used by Dr Alan Scott who was an ophthalmologist in a patient with squint.

The natural BoNT is a high-molecular-weight complex with neurotoxin moiety and complexing proteins.[1] The complexing proteins are hemagglutinins and nonhemagglutinins, which protect the neurotoxin from enzymatic degradation and temperature changes.[2]

TYPES OF BOTULINUM TOXIN

There are seven types of BoNT, A to G. A and B are in clinical use and commercially available.[3] **Table 1** shows the commercially available preparations.

Botulinum toxin is a 150-kDa protein, which needs to be nicked before it becomes active. Among the commercially available preparations, type A (BoNT/A) is 95% nicked but type B is nicked to a much lower level.[4]

MECHANISM OF ACTION

Botulinum toxins are endopeptidases, which cleave the SNARE proteins in presynaptic membrane thus, preventing fusion of vesicles containing acetylcholine with presynaptic membrane. This prevents release of the neurotransmitter acetylcholine. BoNT is taken up by the presynaptic membrane by receptor-mediated endocytosis.[5] BoNT acts at neuromuscular junction, sensory neurons and parasympathetic neurons, and postganglionic sympathetic neurons.[6] Both intrafusal and extrafusal fibers of muscle spindle are affected by BoNT. This causes reduction in the afferent feedback to the alpha motor neuron and, thus, the output of motor neuron.[7] Since the inactivation of SNARE proteins

TABLE 1: Commercial preparations of botulinum toxin.

Trade name	*Botox*	*Dysport*	*Xeomin*	*Myobloc*
Generic name	Onabotulinumtoxin A	Abobotulinumtoxin A	Incobotulinumtoxin A	Rimabotulinumtoxin B
Country of manufacture	United States	France	Germany	United States
Specific activity (U/ng)	20	40	167	75–125
Constituents and excipients	Hemagglutinin, human albumin, saccharose, and sodium chloride	Hemagglutinin, human albumin (20% solution), and lactose	Human albumin and saccharose	Hemagglutinin, human albumin (0.05% solution), sodium chloride, and sodium succinate
Complex size (kDa)	900	900	150	700
Storage of packaged product	–5°C or 2–8°C	2–8°C	Room temperature	2–8°C

is irreversible, the recovery from neuromuscular paralysis occurs only by formation of new nerve twigs and new protein synthesis which usually takes 2-3 months.

PRIMARY AND SECONDARY FAILURES

Primary failure is where the patient does not respond to the first injection of BoNT. Secondary failure is reduction in clinical benefit after initial response. Inappropriate muscle selection and wrong dosing may be the causes. Neutralizing and nonneutralizing antibodies form in some patients, but they are less of a cause for response failure.[8] Neutralizing antibodies may block interaction of BoNT with the neuronal receptor, which is the limiting step of BoNT action thus, leading to loss of efficacy.[9] The efficacy in a patient can be tested by injecting three muscles, i.e., frontalis, corrugators supercilii or extensor digitorum brevis unilaterally with assessment of power of the muscles and action potentials before and after botulinum toxin.[9a] The commercially available assessment of antibodies is done using a mouse lethality assa or the more sensitive mouse hemidiaphragmatic paralysis model (mouse protection assay).[9a]

MUSCLE SELECTION

Appropriate targeting of the muscles affected by dystonia is very important for best response. Muscles can be selected by inspection, palpation, electromyography (EMG), and ultrasound guidance. On inspection and palpation, the contracting muscles can be seen and felt for tone and pain. EMG will show activity at rest and muscles can be directly visualized under ultrasound. Injecting the muscles under EMG or USG guidance has improved the outcome in dystonias such as cervical dystonia.[10] BoNT can be injected directly for blepharospasm and hemifacial spasm.

Blepharospasm

Blepharospasm is dystonic contraction of orbicularis oculi with overflow to procerus and corrugator supercilii.

More than 50 open-label studies recruiting 2,500 patients have shown the efficacy of BoNT in blepharospasm. Approximate doses required are 30-40 A/Ona or 2,500 B/Rima.

Different parts of orbicularis oculi can be differentially affected by spasms. Injecting specifically into the pretarsal portion of orbicularis oculi has improved the response in patients where no improvement was seen with orbital part injection.[11,12]

Average duration of effect lasts up to 3 months and the latency being 3-5 days. Long-term data show that the response to treatment remains stable over time.[13,14]

Hemifacial spasm is twitching of perioral and periocular muscles commonly starting at perioral region. Most patients (95%) have unilateral spasms. Muscles involved are orbicularis oculi, zygomaticus major and minor, orbicularis oris, and platysma. Average doses used are 2.5-5 U A/Ona per site.[15] BoNT injection was shown to reduce the associated features of blepharospasm such as tearing, facial paresthesias, and eye irritation. Side effects are reported in 3-5% of patients, which include ptosis, lagophthalmos, diplopia, and keratitis.[16]

Cervical Dystonia

Cervical dystonia is the most common adult-onset focal dystonia. The dystonia can cause torticollis (turning of head to one side), antecollis (forward bending), laterocollis (head tilt to side), and retrocollis (backward bending). A combination of these movements occurs in most patients. A caput (head)-collis (neck) classification was proposed for the ease of injection.[17] BoNT is shown to be efficacious in cervical dystonia favorably modifying its natural history and in reducing the contractures and pain. Both type A and type B BoNTs are approved for injection in cervical dystonia.[18] A beneficial effect of 66-80% was demonstrated in seven randomized controlled trials encompassing 233 patients and the average dose used was 100-300 A/Ona or 400-800 A/Abo.[19] The beneficial effect ranged from 43 to 68% based on the Toronto Western Spasmodic Torticollis Rating Scale (TWSTRS) as shown in a study by Zoons et al. The common adverse events reported were transient muscle weakness and dysphagia. Dysphagia is more commonly seen in patients where bilateral sternocleidomastoid muscles are injected for antecollis.[20] Patients with antecollis and sagittal shifts have less response to therapy.

Pain is a very prominent symptom in patients with cervical dystonia unlike other focal dystonias. The Cervical Dystonia Patient Registry for Observation of Onabotulinum Toxin A Efficacy (CDPROBE), a prospective registry, showed that most patients reported pain that correlated with the severity of dystonia. This can be relieved in 90% of patients with BoNT injection.[21] Muscles injected in cervical dystonia are shown in **Table 2**.

Laryngeal Dystonia

Abnormal activity of laryngeal muscles leads to laryngeal dystonia. The common clinical subtypes include adductor and abductor spasmodic dysphonia. The less common variants are singer's dystonia and laryngeal breathing dystonia where the patient presents with respiratory stridor.[22] The spasmodic dysphonias are task specific and manifest during speaking. In adduction dystonia, the voice is more strained or strangled and in abductor dystonia, it

TABLE 2: Muscles commonly affected in cervical dystonia, their function, and botulinum toxin (BoNT) doses currently used.

Muscle name	*A/Ona or A/Inco (U)*	*A/Abo (U)*	*B/Rima (U)*
Antecollis:			
Longus colli	15–30	20–60	N/A
Longus capitis	5–15	20–60	N/A
Rectus capitis anterior	2.5–10	10–30	N/A
Sternocleidomastoid	20–50	40–120	1,000–3,000
Laterocollis:			
Anterior scalene	5–30	20–100	500–2,000
Middle scalene	5–30	20–100	500–2,000
Rectus capitis lateralis	N/A	N/A	N/A
Posterior scalene	5–30	20–100	500–2,000
Retrocollis:			
Splenius capitis	40–100	100–350	1,000–4,000
Semispinalis capitis	20–100	60–250	1,000–2,000
Trapezius	25–100	60–300	1,000–4,000
Levator scapulae	20–1,000	60–200	1,000–2,000
Obliquus capitis inferior	10–20	50–80	N/A
Rectus capitis posterior	2.5–10	10–30	N/A

has a breathy and whispering quality. However, laryngeal dystonia should be differentiated from muscle tension dysphonia which can be reversed with voice therapy.[23]

Botulinum toxin can be used to treat laryngeal dystonia. Although there are no randomized controlled trials, several open-label studies have shown efficacy of BoNT/A.[24] The average doses used are 0.5 A/Ona or 1.5 A/Abo. Laryngeal muscles can be injected under EMG guidance bilaterally or unilaterally or can be injected by indirect laryngoscopy without EMG. About 75–95% improvement has been reported; however, the response rate is much less in elderly subjects. BoNT doses and treatment intervals remain stable over long term.[25]

Hoarseness of voice, hypophonia, and dysphagia are the most common side effects, which are transient and subside over time.

Oromandibular Dystonia

Oromandibular dystonia can involve muscles of mastication, tongue, and also pharyngeal muscles. If it is combined with blepharospasm, the term Meige's syndrome is used. Jaw opening, jaw closure, or lateral deviation of jaw can be seen. This can cause difficulty in speaking, chewing, and also injuries to cheek and tongue due to biting.

In a long-term follow-up study by Tan EK and Jankovic, 68% of patients with oromandibular dystonia had improvement with adverse events being reported in 31.5% of patients.[26] The masseter and temporalis muscles are injected in jaw closure dystonia and lateral pterygoid and submental muscles can be injected in jaw opening dystonia. Symptoms such as dysarthria, chewing difficulties, and dental problems improve significantly. The doses injected are lateral pterygoid (7.5 U), masseter (25–50 U), temporalis (15–25 U), anterior digastric (5 U), and medial pterygoid (20 U).[27] Genioglossus is injected in tongue protrusion dystonia. Although lingual muscle injections are associated with risk of dysphagia, the advantage is shown to outweigh the risk with experienced injectors.

Task-specific Dystonias

Task-specific dystonias are focal dystonias that occur only during a skilled motor act. Examples include writer's cramp which is the most common task-specific dystonia, others being musicians dystonia, golfer's dystonia, and typists dystonia. Most of the task-specific dystonias are medically refractory needing BoNT injections. Cohen et al. first demonstrated the efficacy of BoNT in writer's cramp.[28] Majority of subsequent open-label trials with BoNT as therapy in focal dystonias were on writer's cramp. Both flexor and extensor group of muscles can be involved in writer's cramp. Patients with forearm pronation and flexion dystonias had more improvement as shown in an open-label prospective study of 47 patients with writer's cramp.[29] Muscles acting at wrist (pronators and flexors) also should be injected along with forearm group of muscles. Mirror dystonia used as guide for muscle selection for BoNT injection may reduce the difference in outcome between flexor and extensor writer's cramp and is better method for muscle selection than compensatory movements as proposed by Borgohain et al.[30] Most patients (75–80%) report onset of benefit at approximately 1–2 weeks following injection and lasting for 3 months. Majority of patients continue to have benefit with successive injections over years. Repeated BoNT injections may affect reorganization in premotor cortex as shown by some physiologic studies.[31]

Weakness is the most common side effect. Doses used range from 2.5 to 10 U A/Ona or 40–60 U A/Abo.

USE OF BOTULINUM TOXIN IN OTHER MOVEMENT DISORDERS

There is level B recommendation for A/Ona and level U for rest of BoNT formulations in essential tremor.[13] BoNT/A injection led to significant reduction in postural tremor (4–16 weeks); however, kinetic tremor was decreased only at 6-week examination. This resulted in limited functional efficacy.[32]

There is level U recommendation for all four formulations of BoNT in tics.[13] BoNT has been tried in patients with Tourette's syndrome with frequent blinking and blepharospasm and those with painful dystonic tics. There was moderate to marked improvement in the intensity and frequency of tics along with decreased premonitory urge; however, benefit lasted for approximately 2 months.[33] Vocal tics improved in 93% of patients after treatment and 50% of patients being tic free. However, 80% of patients had side effect of hypophonia.[34] In simple motor tics, BoNT decreased tic frequency by 39%; however, there is no subjective improvement among study population.[35]

Dose and location of injection of BoNT for palatal myoclonus depend on response and location of subsequent observed maximal muscular contractions.[36] Most common sites of injection include tensor veli palatini for tinnitus and on either side of uvula for palatal movements.

Meta-analysis had shown that BoNT injection decreased the frequency of bruxism events, decreased bruxism-induced pain events, and satisfy patient self-esteem.[37] It is most commonly injected into temporalis and masseter muscles.

CONCLUSION

In the three to four decades since BoNT was first introduced into clinical use, there has been an explosion in the spectrum of indications that it has been used for along with a considerable number of newer BoNT preparations becoming available. Evidence in the form of controlled trials has also been generated to place the therapy on a firmer footing. A number of previously untreatable or poorly treatable disorders have also found to be better treated with BoNT.

REFERENCES

1. Inoue K, Fujinaga Y, Watanabe T, Ohyama T, Takeshi K, Moriishi K, et al. Molecular composition of Clostridium botulinum type A progenitor toxins. Infect Immun. 1996;64(5):1589-94.
2. Gu S, Rumpel S, Zhou J, Strotmeier J, Bigalke H, Perry K, et al. Botulinum neurotoxin is shielded by NTNHA in an interlocked complex. Science. 2012;335(6071):977-81.
3. Montecucco C, Molgó J. Botulinum neurotoxins: revival of an old killer. Curr Opin Pharmacol. 2005;5(3):274-9.
4. Callaway JE. Botulinum toxin type B (Myobloc): pharmacology and biochemistry. Clin Dermatol. 2004;22(1):23-8.
5. Montecucco C, Schiavo G. Structure and function of tetanus and botulinum neurotoxins. Q Rev Biophys. 1995;28(4):423-72.
6. Naumann M, Jost W. Botulinum toxin treatment of secretory disorders. Mov Disord. 2004;19 Suppl 8:S137-41.
7. Currà A, Trompetto C, Abbruzzese G, Berardelli A. Central effects of botulinum toxin type A: evidence and supposition. Mov Disord. 2004;19 Suppl 8:S60-4.
8. Lange O, Bigalke H, Dengler R, Wegner F, Wohlfarth K. Neutralizing antibodies and secondary therapy failure after treatment with botulinum toxin type A: much ado about nothing?. Clin Neuropharmacol. 2009;32(4):213-8.
9. Dolimbek BZ, Aoki KR, Steward LE, Jankovic J, Atassi MZ. Mapping of the regions on the heavy chain of botulinum neurotoxin A (BoNT/A) recognized by antibodies of cervical dystonia patients with immunoresistance to BoNT/A. Mol Immunol. 2007;44(5):1029-41.

9a. Jankovic J. Botulinum toxin in clinical practice. J Neurol Neurosurg Psychiatry. 2004;75:951-7.

10. Cordivari C, Misra VP, Vincent A, Catania S, Bhatia KP, Lees AJ. Secondary nonresponsiveness to botulinum toxin A in cervical dystonia: the role of electromyogram-guided injections, botulinum toxin A antibody assay, and the extensor digitorum brevis test. Mov Disord. 2006;21(10):1737-41.
11. Albanese A, Bentivoglio AR, Colosimo C, Galardi G, Maderna L, Tonali P. Pretarsal injections of botulinum toxin improve blepharospasm in previously unresponsive patients. J Neurol Neurosurg Psychiatry. 1996;60(6):693-4.
12. Jankovic J. Pretarsal injection of botulinum toxin for blepharospasm and apraxia of eyelid opening. J Neurol Neurosurg Psychiatry. 1996;60(6):704.
13. Hallett M, Albanese A, Dressler D, Segal KR, Simpson DM, Truong D, et al. Evidence-based review and assessment of botulinum neurotoxin for the treatment of movement disorders. Toxicon. 2013;67(4):94-114.
14. Bentivoglio AR, Fasano AL, Ialongo T, Soleti F, Fermo SL, Albanese AL. Fifteen-year experience in treating blepharospasm with Botox or Dysport: same toxin, two drugs. Neurotox Res. 2009;15(3):224-31.
15. Karp BI, Alter K. Botulinum toxin treatment of blepharospasm, orofacial/oromandibular dystonia, and hemifacial spasm. Semin Neurol. 2016;36(1):84-91.
16. Rudzińska M, Wójcik M, Szczudlik A. Hemifacial spasm non-motor and motor-related symptoms and their response to botulinum toxin therapy. J Neural Transm (Vienna). 2010;117(6):765-72.
17. Reichel G. Cervical dystonia: a new phenomenological classification for botulinum toxin therapy. Basal Ganglia. 2011;1(1):5-12.
18. Ramirez-Castaneda J, Jankovic J. Long-term efficacy, safety, and side effect profile of botulinum toxin in dystonia: a 20-year follow-up. Toxicon. 2014;90(4):344-8.
19. Jankovic J. Treatment of cervical dystonia with botulinum toxin. Mov Disord. 2004;19 Suppl 8:S109-15.
20. Zoons E, Dijkgraaf MG, Dijk JM, Van Schaik IN, Tijssen MA. Botulinum toxin as treatment for focal dystonia: a systematic review of the pharmaco-therapeutic and pharmaco-economic value. J Neurol. 2012;259(12):2519-26.
21. Charles PD, Adler CH, Stacy M, Comella C, Jankovic J, Adams AM, et al. Cervical dystonia and pain: characteristics and treatment patterns from CDPROBE (Cervical Dystonia Patient Registry for Observation of Onabotulinumtoxin A Efficacy). J Neurol. 2014;261(7):1309-19.
22. Jinnah HA, Berardelli A, Comella C, DeFazio G, DeLong MR, Factor S, et al. The focal dystonias: current views and challenges for future research. Mov Disord. 2013;28(7):926-43.

23. Altman KW, Atkinson C, Lazarus C. Current and emerging concepts in muscle tension dysphonia: a 30-month review. J Voice. 2005;19(2):261-7.
24. Blitzer A, Brin MF, Stewart CF. Botulinum toxin management of spasmodic dysphonia (laryngeal dystonia): a 12-year experience in more than 900 patients. Laryngoscope. 1998;108(10):1435-41.
25. Cannito MP, Kahane JC, Chorna L. Vocal aging and adductor spasmodic dysphonia: response to botulinum toxin injection. Clin Interv Aging. 2008;3(1):131-51.
26. Tan EK, Jankovic J. Botulinum toxin A in patients with oromandibular dystonia: long-term follow-up. Neurology. 1999;53(9):2102-7.
27. Sinclair CF, Gurey LE, Blitzer A. Oromandibular dystonia: long-term management with botulinum toxin. Laryngoscope. 2013;123(12):3078-83.
28. Cohen LG, Hallett M, Geller BD, Hochberg F. Treatment of focal dystonias of the hand with botulinum toxin injections. J Neurol Neurosurg Psychiatry. 1989;52(3):355-63.
29. Djebbari R, Du Montcel ST, Sangla S, Vidal JS, Gallouedec G, Vidailhet M. Factors predicting improvement in motor disability in writer's cramp treated with botulinum toxin. J Neurol Neurosurg Psychiatry. 2004;75(12):1688-91.
30. Borgohain R, Kanikannan MA, Sattaluri S, Mani J, Surath M. Mirror dystonia (mirror movements) in writer's cramps and therapeutic outcome with botulinum toxin: a prospective study. Mov Disord. 2002;17(1):S293.
31. Byrnes ML, Thickbroom GW, Wilson SA, Sacco P, Shipman JM, Stell R, et al. The corticomotor representation of upper limb muscles in writer's cramp and changes following botulinum toxin injection. J Neurol. 1998;121(5):977-88.
32. Brin MF, Lyons KE, Doucette J, Adler CH, Caviness JN, Comella CL, et al. A randomized, double masked, controlled trial of botulinum toxin type A in essential hand tremor. Neurology. 2001;56(11):1523-8.
33. Jankovic J. Botulinum toxin in the treatment of dystonic tics. Mov Disord. 1994;9(3):347-9.
34. Porta M, Maggioni G, Ottaviani F, Schindler A. Treatment of phonic tics in patients with Tourette's syndrome using botulinum toxin type A. Neurol Sci. 2004;24(6):420-3.
35. Marras C, Andrews D, Sime E, Lang AE. Botulinum toxin for simple motor tics: a randomized, double-blind, controlled clinical trial. Neurology. 2001;56(5):605-10.
36. Sinclair CF, Gurey LE, Blitzer A. Palatal myoclonus: algorithm for management with botulinum toxin based on clinical disease characteristics. Laryngoscope. 2014;124(5):1164-9.
37. Long H, Liao Z, Wang Y, Liao L, Lai W. Efficacy of botulinum toxins on bruxism: an evidence-based review. Int Dent J. 2012;62(1):1-5.

CHAPTER 55

Botulinum Toxin in Spasticity

Nirmal Surya

INTRODUCTION

Spasticity (see **Box 1** for definition) is a relatively common finding in patients with stroke, multiple sclerosis, and cerebral palsy and in those with spinal cord injuries and traumatic brain injuries (**Table 1**).

Box 1 Spasticity is an outcome of upper motor neuron syndrome (UMNS) (spasticity + spastic paresis).[1,2]

- Lance defined spasticity as *"a motor disorder characterized by a velocity-dependent increase in tonic stretch reflexes (muscle tone) with exaggerated tendon jerks, resulting from hyper-excitability of the stretch reflex, as one component of the UMNS"*[1]
- A complete picture of UMNS must also include:
  - Positive symptoms or signs such as flexor spasm, clasp knife phenomenon. Babinski sign, exaggerated cutaneous withdrawal (flexor, pain) reflexes, autonomic hyperreflexia, dystonia, and contractures that may limit voluntary movement and cause discomfort
  - Negative features such as paresis, lack of dexterity, and fatigability

TABLE 1: Epidemiology of spasticity and spasticity-related conditions.[3-7]

Conditions	*Prevalence of spasticity within the condition*
Multiple sclerosis	37–78%
Stroke	35%
Cerebral palsy	>90%
Spinal cord injuries	40%
Traumatic brain injuries	50%

Spasticity can be debilitating for a patient and can seriously affect the quality of life. Furthermore, the burden of spasticity can far extend the patient and place a significant stress on caretakers, financial, and other health resources. Measures for early diagnosis and treatment of spasticity should be an important priority.

Botulinum toxin along with its cosmetic applications is an important therapeutic agent in the management of a variety of neurological conditions such as spasticity, chronic migraine, and cervical dystonia.[8] In the specific contexts of spasticity management, botulinum toxin has been approved by the United States Food and Drug Administration (USFDA) for treatment of upper limb and lower limb spasticity. Botulinum toxin significantly improves a patient's quality of life, alleviates caretaker burden, and is also known to have significant pharmacoeconomic benefits. However, it is important to note that treatment and management of spasticity require a comprehensive neurorehabilitation program (**Fig. 1**) through a multidisciplinary effort and measure to ensure a proactive patient compliance to realistic goal setting.

PHARMACOLOGY OF BOTULINUM TOXIN

Following injections to the affected muscle, botulinum toxin binds irreversibly to the synaptic vesicle protein SV2 (isoforms A, B, and C) on the presynaptic side to gain access into the axons, where it impedes the exocytosis of acetylcholine by interacting with the SNARE apparatus.[9,10] These actions at the neuromuscular junction cause diminution of muscle contraction. It is important to note that botulinum toxins reduce the frequency but not the amplitude of miniature endplate potential (MEPP).

While these effects reduce resistance to passive movement, other neurophysiological effects such as reduced retrograde axonal transport, reduced motoneuronal excitability, decreased Renshaw inhibition, and increased presynaptic inhibition may also contribute to the overall effects of botulinum toxin.[11] Clinically, these effects of botulinum toxin injection last for about 3 months. While the efficacy and safety of botulinum toxin in the management of spasticity are relatively well-established, it is important to note that there are seven immunologically distinct serotypes of botulinum toxin.[12] The serotype that is currently in routine clinical use is botulinum toxin type A. Furthermore, several different products of botulinum toxin type A are currently available and are marketed as Botox® (Allergan), Dysport® (Ipsen Pharmaceuticals), Xeomin® (Merz Pharma GmbH & Co.), Neurobloc® (Solstice Neurosciences Inc.), and Myobloc® (Elan). It is important to note that these products cannot be used interchangeably.[13] Differences in manufacturing processes, formulation techniques, and assay methods render a noninterchangeable uniqueness to botulinum toxin type A preparations.

BOTULINUM TOXIN FOR UPPER LIMB SPASTICITY

Upper limb spasticity is a relatively common presentation in patients with spasticity-prone neurological conditions. While a study by Johansson et al. note that 66% of patients with multiple sclerosis have upper limb motor impairments,[14] Makki et al. note that 83% of children with cerebral palsy have upper limb complications.[15] A study by Opheim et al. notes that spasticity is seen in 25% of stroke patients at day 3 and in 46% patients at 1 year.[16] **Figure 2** depicts the common patterns of upper limb spasticity.[17]

It is encouraging to note that spasticity could be predicted with high sensitivity and specificity as early as 10 days after a stroke using the Fugl-Meyer Assessment for Upper

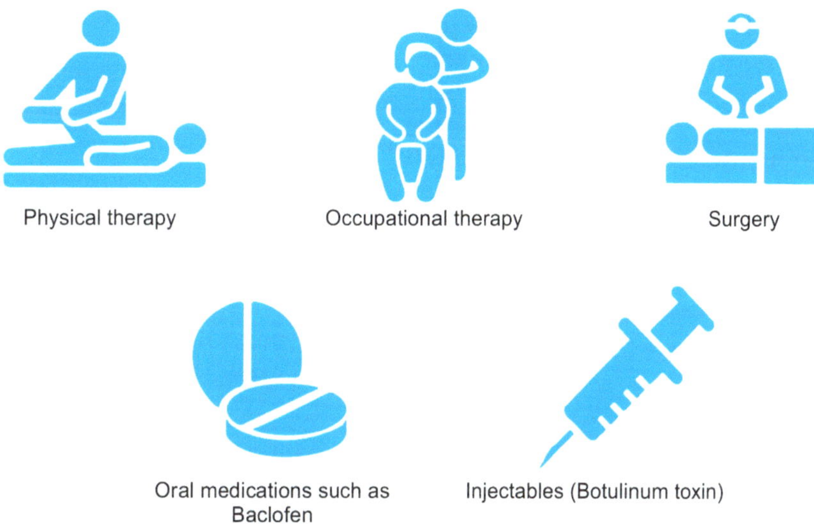

FIG. 1: Components of multidisciplinary spasticity management program.

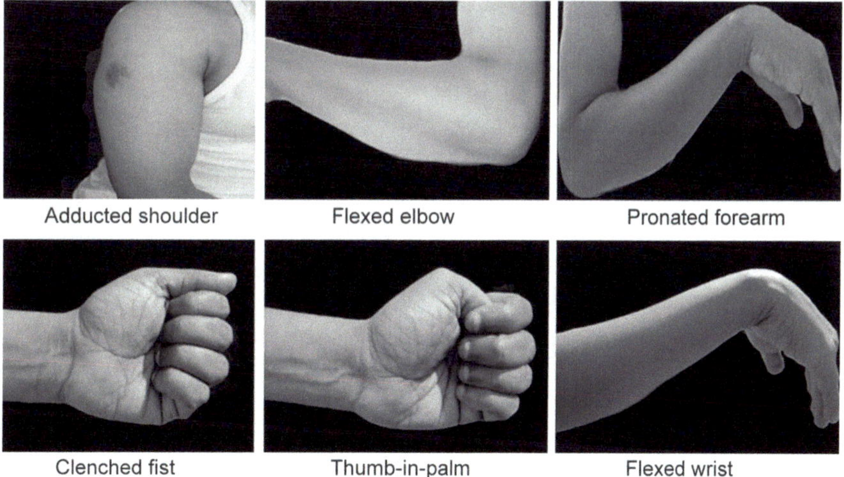

FIG. 2: Common patterns of spasticity in the upper limbs.

Extremity (FMA-UE) scores. Another strand of evidence for early intervention to address poststroke spasticity comes from the BoTULS (Botulinum Toxin for the Upper Limb after Stroke) study, which notes that rehabilitation treatments for spasticity applied within the first 3 months of stroke provide improved results.[18] These data along with highlighting the burden of upper limb spasticity also call for early detection and treatment of spasticity.

EFFICACY AND SAFETY OF BOTULINUM TOXIN IN UPPER LIMB SPASTICITY

With respect to the efficacy of botulinum toxin in the management of upper limb spasticity, a recent meta-analysis of 22 studies (1,804 patients) by Dong et al. suggests that botulinum toxin A produces a statistically significant decrease of muscle tone after each injection as compared to placebo.[19] **Table 2** summarizes the findings of recent clinical studies for the effects of botulinum toxin in upper limb spasticity. Typically, the effects of botulinum toxin wear off in about 3 months time and often warrant repeat injections. While, repeat injections are generally well-tolerated and formation of neutralizing antibodies to botulinum toxin is a rare clinical observation as it is a poor antigen in humans.[20] However, there may be a subset of patients who are persistently resistant to the effects of botulinum toxin. While mutations at the SNARE complex were suggested as a possible cause for this primary resistance, recent studies have failed to identify any such associations.[20] Except for these subsets of patients, repeat administrations of botulinum toxin injections are generally effective in patients with upper limb spasticity. With respect to safety, botulinum toxin is a relatively safe option and is often limited to pain at the injection site. Since botulinum toxin injections provide for a localized effect, systemic side effects are generally not a concern.

Overall, available data indicate that botulinum toxin is an important addition to a comprehensive rehabilitation program and early initiation of such rehabilitation program is important to achieve better outcomes. Furthermore, it is important to ensure proper and pragmatic goal setting along with ensuring a proactive patient participation for successful achievement of treatment targets.

TABLE 2: Summary of placebo-controlled studies demonstrating the effects of botulinum toxin in spasticity.

Authors	*Effects of botulinum toxin*
Brashear et al.[21]	• Improved wrist flexor tone • Improved finger flexor tone • Improvement of at least one point on the Disability Assessment Scale (DAS) in the principal target of treatment
Jahangir et al.[22]	• Improved wrist flexor tone • Improved finger flexor tone • Improvement of at least one point on the DAS in the principal target of treatment
Elovic et al.[23]	• Up to five treatments with botulinum toxin type A every 12 weeks for up to 56 weeks were associated with improved ○ Muscle tone ○ Patients quality of life
Kaňovský et al.[24]	• Improvements in muscle tone (flexors of wrist, elbow, finger and thumb, and forearm pronators) • Repeat treatments well-tolerated for over 89 weeks
Gracies et al.[25]	• Improvements in muscle tone • Improvements in the DAS in the principal target of treatment

SELECTION OF MUSCLES FOR INJECTING BOTULINUM TOXIN

In the United states, botulinum toxin is currently indicated for the treatment of upper limb spasticity in adult patients to reduce the severity of increased muscle tone in elbow flexors (biceps), wrist flexors (flexor carpi radialis and flexor carpi ulnaris), and finger flexors (flexor digitorum profundus and flexor digitorum sublimis).[26] A systematic review of 70 studies with 2,163 adult patients noted that while these on-label muscles were often chosen, clinicians prefer to inject botulinum toxin to a number of off-label muscles (**Table 3**).[26]

BOTULINUM TOXIN FOR LOWER LIMB SPASTICITY

In a recent report, Martin et al. noted that lower limb spasticity was found to occur in one-third of adults after stroke, one-half to two-thirds of patients with multiple sclerosis, and three-fourths of those with cerebral palsy.[27] Lower limb spasticity affects walking and is associated with significant impairments in quality of life and caretaker burden. In a recent internet survey of 281 people with spasticity, 72% reported impact on quality of life, 44% reported loss of independence, and 44% reported depression.[28] While epidemiological data specific to lower limb spasticity is generally scanty, it is a significant healthcare burden that necessitates prompt early diagnosis and treatment with a multidisciplinary approach. The common patterns of spasticity in the lower limb include flexed hip, adducted thighs, extended knee, flexed knee, equinovarus foot, and striatal toe. Several studies have established the efficacy of botulinum toxin in addressing the complications of these patterns.

TABLE 3: List of muscles reported in the literature for botulinum toxin injections in patients with upper limb spasticity.[26]

Shoulder	***Forearm***	***Elbow flexors***
• Infraspinatus • Shoulder adductors • Deltoid • Latissimus dorsi • Levator scapulae • Paraspinous • Pectoralis • Rhomboid • Sternocleidomastoid • Subscapularis • Teres major • Trapezius • Triceps brachii	• Extensor carpi radialis • Extensor carpi ulnaris • Extensor digitorum • Pronator quadrates • Pronator teres • Supinator	• Biceps brachii • Brachialis • Brachioradialis
Wrist flexors	*Finger flexors*	*Thumb*
• Flexor carpi radialis • Flexor carpi ulnaris • Palmaris longus • Wrist flexors	• Finger flexors • Flexor digitorum profundus • Flexor digitorum superficialis • Forearm finger flexor • Interossei volares	• Adductor pollicis • Flexor pollicis brevis • Flexor pollicis longus • Lumbricals • Opponens • Opponens pollicis

EFFICACY AND SAFETY OF BOTULINUM TOXIN IN LOWER LIMB SPASTICITY

A placebo-controlled study by Burbaud et al. in 23 hemiparetic patients noted significant changes with botulinum toxin injections in Ashworth scale scores for ankle extensors and invertors and for active ankle dorsiflexion.[29] This study noted that botulinum toxin injections were less effective in patients with longer duration of spasticity. Thus, early treatment initiation appears extremely important. In another study by Hesse et al. with 12 chronic hemiparetic patients with lower limb spasticity, 400 units of botulinum toxin A were associated with significant improvements from baseline in velocity, stride length, stance symmetry, and the length of the force point of action under the affected foot.[30] These improvements noted on gait analysis are indicative of the usefulness of botulinum toxin injections in improving walking difficulties. Furthermore, this study noted that the effects of botulinum toxin injections lasted for about 8 weeks. Kirazli et al. compared the phenol block and botulinum toxin type A in the treatment of spastic foot after stroke and noted that botulinum toxin type A may be more effective than phenol nerve block in plantar flexor spasticity.[31] In another double-blind, placebo-controlled, and dose-ranging study, botulinum toxin type A significantly reduced muscle tone, limb pain, and dependence on walking aids. However, these effects were greatest in patients receiving 1,500 units of botulinum toxin type A as compared to those receiving 1,000 units or 500 units.[32] In another study by Kaji et al. 300 units of botulinum toxin were associated with significant improvements in spasticity as compared to placebo and the effects with botulinum toxin were better than placebo at weeks 4, 6, and 8.[33] These data demonstrate the usefulness of botulinum toxin in reducing the spasticity of lower limb muscles. Safety data available for botulinum toxin indicates that adverse reactions are generally mild and include myalgias and pain at injection site. Thus, available data indicates that botulinum toxin as part of an early and prompt rehabilitation program would be effective and safe in alleviating the burden and complications of lower limb spasticity.

SELECTION OF MUSCLES FOR INJECTING BOTULINUM TOXIN

Published studies and practice patterns for muscle selection for botulinum toxin injections vary significantly. The choice of "off-label" muscles is usually made on the premise of individualizing treatments for attainment of treatment goals. However, a consensus-based guidance is often required in clinical practice and Esquenazi et al. published a consensus document on the sites of botulinum toxin injections along with the dose.[34] **Table 4** presents a summary of these recommendations.

BOTULINUM TOXIN FOR CEREBRAL PALSY

Cerebral palsy is the most common cause of childhood-onset, lifelong physical disability in most countries, affecting about 1 in 500 neonates with an estimated prevalence of 17 million people worldwide.[35] Cerebral palsy is defined as an "umbrella term covering a group of nonprogressive, but often changing, motor impairment syndromes secondary to lesions or anomalies of the brain arising in the early stages of its development".[36] The motor impairment syndromes seen in children with cerebral palsy can further be categorized into primary and secondary symptoms (**Fig. 3**).[37]

While the management and correction of secondary symptoms often require orthopedic surgery, it is important to delay these procedures until the age of 8–10 years

TABLE 4: Recommendations of Esquenazi et al. for botulinum toxin dosing in lower limb spasticity.[34]

Posture	*Muscles*	*Dose of botulinum toxin (units)*
Adducted thigh	Adductor magnus	75–150
	Adductor longus	75–80
	Adductor brevis	20–25
	Gracilis	25–40
	Iliopsoas	25–150
	Medial hamstrings	50
Flexed knee	Medial hamstrings	125
	Lateral hamstrings	75
	Gastrocnemius	50–200
	Iliopsoas	40–150
	Gracilis	50
Extended knee	Rectus femoris	80–125
	Vastus lateralis	50–70
	Vastus medialis	50
	Vastus intermedius	35–75
	Gluteus maximus	40
Equinovarus foot	Tibialis posterior	100
	Gastrocnemius	125
	Soleus	75–100
	Tibialis anterior	75
	Flexor digitorum longus	20–75
	Flexor digitorum brevis	13–38
	Flexor hallucis longus	25–38
	Extensor hallucis longus	13–50
Plantar flexed foot/ankle	Gastrocnemius	125
	Soleus	75
	Tibialis posterior	25–75
	Long toe flexors	20
Striatal toe	Extensor hallucis longus	50
	Extensor hallucis longus motor point	38
	Flexor digitorum longus	25–30
Flexed toes	Flexor digitorum longus	50–80
	Flexor digitorum brevis	25
	Flexor hallucis longus	40–50
	Flexor hallucis brevis	13

for predictable outcomes. During this presurgical time, a conservative treatment is essential to reduce spasticity. Botulinum toxin has an important place as part of this conservative treatment plan and can complement orthopedic surgery in several individualized clinical paradigms. Details of these aspects are presented in the subsequent sections.

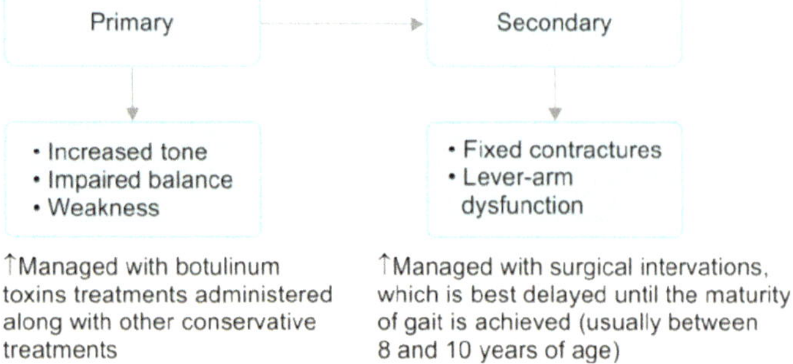

FIG. 3: Motor impairment syndromes seen in children with cerebral palsy.

EFFICACY AND SAFETY OF BOTULINUM TOXIN IN CEREBRAL PALSY

The seminal reports for the use of botulinum toxin in children were published in the early 1990s by Koman et al.[38] and Wall et al.[39] Since then, several studies have established the place of botulinum toxin as a selective option for treating spasticity in children.[40] Spasticity is the main causative factor for development of contractures and bony deformities in children with cerebral palsy.

Thus, the management of cerebral palsy must be focused on reduction of muscle tone to attenuate the development of secondary problems and, thereby, delay or preclude the need for surgical intervention. While botulinum toxin can reduce muscle tone and spasticity in a reversible, selective, and dose-dependent manner, outcomes are better and predictable when it is integrated with other therapies (**Box 2**).[37] Overall, botulinum toxin injections are useful and appropriate for predominantly spastic type of hemiplegia, diplegia, triplegia and quadriplegia, and the Gross Motor Function Classification System (GMFCS) functional levels I-V.Gait improvements are the focus of treatment in functional children (GMFCS level I-III), improving balance, control of sitting, positioning and facilitating hygienic care, and bracing for nonambulatory children (GMFCS level IV and V). **Box 3** lists some of the common treatment goals that can be attained with a comprehensive program that includes botulinum toxin administered to the appropriate muscles.[37]

SELECTION OF MUSCLES FOR INJECTING BOTULINUM TOXIN

Selection of muscles for botulinum toxin injections must be individualized to the specific needs of child assessed after a thorough clinical examination and evaluation of posture, gait, and motion analysis. While the optimal dose of botulinum toxin injections typically depends on the muscle volume and the degree of spasticity, a maximum total dose is 400–600 units for botulinum toxin type A and

Box 2 Integration of botulinum toxin with other treatment modalities for spasticity management.

- Physiotherapy and occupational therapy + botulinum toxin therapy may be more beneficial than occupational and physiotherapy alone[41]
- Botulinum toxin + casting may be better than either treatments alone[42]
- Botulinum toxin can also be effectively combined with selective dorsal rhizotomy[43]
- Botulinum toxin can be helpful in delaying surgeries[44]
- Perioperatively, botulinum toxin helps in reducing spasticity-induced pain[44]

Box 3 A list of common treatment goals in the management of spasticity with botulinum toxin and other conservative treatments.[37]

- Improvements in gait, balance, and posture
- Relief from regional or generalized spasticity
- Facilitation of orthotic management
- Continuation of conservative management until maturity of gait is achieved for orthopedic surgery
- Prevention of hip subluxation by controlling spasticity in hip adductors and flexors
- Treatment of spastic athetoid- and hyperlordosis-related pain
- Relief from perioperative and postoperative pain

TABLE 5: List of upper limb muscles reported in the literature for botulinum toxin injections in patients with cerebral palsy.[45]

Shoulder	*Forearm*	*Elbow flexors*
• Deltoid • Pectoralis • Teres major • Triceps brachii	• Pronator quadratus • Pronator teres	• Biceps brachii • Brachialis • Brachioradialis
Wrist flexors	*Finger flexors*	*Thumb*
• Flexor carpi radialis • Flexor carpi ulnaris	• Flexor digitorum profundus • Flexor digitorum superficialis • Flexor pollicis longus	• Adductor pollicis • Flexor pollicis brevis • Flexor pollicis longus • Opponens pollicis

500–1,000 units for AbobotulinumtoxinA.[37] **Table 5** lists the upper limb muscles commonly injected with botulinum toxin for managing spasticity in children with cerebral palsy.[45] Commonly injected muscles for managing lower limb spasticity are listed include gastrocnemius, soleus, tibialis posterior, and medial and lateral hamstrings. Other lower limb muscles that are commonly injected with botulinum toxin include hip adductors, rectus femoris, and iliopsoas.[37]

A NOTE ON DILUTION AND INJECTION TECHNIQUES

Botulinum toxin type A is commercially available as lyophilized freeze-dried preparations that require refrigeration. It is prepared by dilution with normal saline. Botulinum toxin injections are administered as intramuscular injections into the affected muscles with or without local anesthesia. However, patients experience minimal-to-moderate pain during botulinum toxin injections and local anesthesia can reduce this pain.[46] Conscious sedation or general anesthesia may be used while injecting botulinum toxin in children with cerebral palsy.[47] General anesthesia may be used when multiple levels are involved. With respect to injection techniques, accurate needle placement can be accomplished by palpation with the muscle under stretching and by manual testing.[37] While a few clinicians advocate this technique, others recommend ultrasonography with or without electromyography (EMG) guidance or electrical stimulation as the most appropriate technique to localize and identify the muscles.[48]

COST CONSIDERATIONS

Cost-efficacy of antispasticity treatments is difficult to assess as the costs of botulinum toxin and reimbursement policies differ between countries. Furthermore, the multidisciplinary treatment approaches needed to manage spasticity make it difficult to ascertain the cost-effectiveness of single treatment. While a study by Ward et al. note that botulinum toxin may be a cost-effective option,[49] the results of the BoTULS study indicate that the addition of botulinum toxin type A for management of poststroke upper limb spasticity was not cost-effective at levels of willingness to pay for a quality-adjusted life year (QALY) set by the National Health Service (NHS) decision-makers.[25] In Indian settings, where medical insurance is lean, the cost of treatment with botulinum toxin may be perceived as expensive.[50] However, if affordable, the cost-benefit ratio from botulinum toxin appears to be relatively good.

CONCLUSION

Spasticity, a relatively common presentation in neurology settings, is debilitating for a patient and places a significant stress on caretakers, financial, and other health resources. Spasticity management offers better results upon early diagnosis and prompt initiation of a multidisciplinary treatment approach tailored to pragmatically set treatment targets. Botulinum toxin is an important adjunct in this multipronged approach with over two decades of safety and efficacy data. The anecdotal journey of a potent neurotoxin to a safe and effective drug in neurology is indeed a prominent occurrence in the evidence-based landscape of spasticity management. Used judiciously, this potent neurotoxin can offer significant benefits and relief to patients with spasticity. While patient satisfaction is generally good and cost-benefit ratio favors the use of botulinum toxin in patients who can afford it, measures to reduce cost barriers in economically constrained settings are a much warranted priority.

SUMMARY

- Spasticity is a relatively common presentation in neurology settings
- Steps for early detection and treatment of spasticity are an important health priority
- Rehabilitation programs for spasticity management must set pragmatic treatment targets and motivate a patient for proactive involvement and compliance
- Botulinum toxin injections, as part of these rehabilitation programs, are effective and safe for alleviating the burden of spasticity
- All botulinum toxins are not same; preparations of botulinum toxin injections are unique and not interchangeable
- Used judiciously, this potent neurotoxin can offer significant benefits and relief to patients with spasticity

REFERENCES

1. Lance JW. Pathophysiology of spasticity and clinical experience with baclofen. In: Feldman RG, Young RR, Koella WP (Eds). Spasticity: Disordered Motor Control. Chicago: Year Book Medical Publishers; 1980. pp. 185-204.
2. Trompetto C, Marinelli L, Mori L, Pelosin E, Currà A, Molfetta L, et al. Pathophysiology of spasticity: implications for neurorehabilitation. Biomed Res Int. 2014;2014:354906.
3. Barnes MP, Kent RM, Semlyen JK, McMullen KM. Spasticity in multiple sclerosis. Neurorehabil Neural Repair. 2003;17(1): 66-70.
4. Noreau L, Proulx P, Gagnon L, Drolet M, Laramée MT. Secondary impairments after spinal cord injury: a population-based study. Am J Phys Med Rehabil. 2000;79(6):526-35.
5. Watkins CL, Leathley MJ, Gregson JM, Moore AP, Smith TL, Sharma AK. Prevalence of spasticity post stroke. Clin Rehabil. 2002;16(5):515-22.
6. Wichers MJ, Odding E, Stam HJ, van Nieuwenhuizen O. Clinical presentation, associated disorders and aetiological moments in cerebral palsy: a Dutch population-based study. Disabil Rehabil. 2005;27(10):583-9.
7. Wedekind C, Lippert-Grüner M. Long-term outcome in severe traumatic brain injury is significantly influenced by brainstem involvement. Brain Inj. 2005;19(9):681-4.
8. Bell MS, Vermeulen LC, Sperling KB. Pharmacotherapy with botulinum toxin: harnessing nature's most potent neurotoxin. Pharmacotherapy. 2000;20(9):1079-91.
9. Dong M, Yeh F, Tepp WH, Dean C, Johnson EA, Janz R, et al. SV2 is the protein receptor for botulinum neurotoxin A. Science. 2006;312(5773):592-6.
10. Lu B. The destructive effect of botulinum neurotoxins on the SNARE protein: SNAP-25 and synaptic membrane fusion. Peer J. 2015;3:e1065.
11. Gracies JM. Physiological effects of botulinum toxin in spasticity. Mov Disord. 2004;19 Suppl 8:S120-8.
12. Peng Chen Z, Morris JG, Rodriguez RL, Shukla AW, Tapia-Núñez J, Okun MS. Emerging opportunities for serotypes of botulinum neurotoxins. Toxins (Basel). 2012;4(11):1196-222.
13. Brin MF, James C, Maltman J. Botulinum toxin type A products are not interchangeable: a review of the evidence. Biologics. 2014;8(4):227-41.
14. Johansson S, Ytterberg C, Claesson IM, Lindberg J, Hillert J, Andersson M, et al. High concurrent presence of disability in multiple sclerosis. Associations with perceived health. J Neurol. 2007;254(6):767-73.
15. Makki D, Duodu J, Nixon M. Prevalence and pattern of upper limb involvement in cerebral palsy. J Child Orthop. 2014;8(3):215-9.
16. Opheim A, Danielsson A, Murphy MA, Persson HC, Sunnerhagen KS. Early prediction of long-term upper limb spasticity after stroke: part of the SALGOT study. Neurology. 2015;85(10): 873-80.
17. Simpson DM, Patel AT, Alfaro A, Ayyoub Z, Charles D, Dashtipour K, et al. OnabotulinumtoxinA Injection for Poststroke Upper-Limb Spasticity: Guidance for Early Injectors from a Delphi Panel Process. PM R. 2017;9(2):136-48.
18. Shaw L, Rodgers H, Price C, van Wijck F, Shackley P, Steen N, et al. BoTULS: a multicentre randomised controlled trial to evaluate the clinical effectiveness and cost-effectiveness of treating upper limb spasticity due to stroke with botulinum toxin type A. Health Technol Assess. 2010;14(26):1-113.
19. Dong Y, Wu T, Hu X, Wang T. Efficacy and safety of botulinum toxin type A for upper limb spasticity after stroke or traumatic brain injury: a systematic review with meta-analysis and trial sequential analysis. Eur J Phys Rehabil Med. 2017;53(2): 256-67.
20. Pirazzini M, Carle S, Barth H, Rossetto O, Montecucco C. Primary resistance of human patients to botulinum neurotoxins A and B. Ann Clin Transl Neurol. 2018;5(8):971-5.
21. Brashear A, Gordon MF, Elovic E, et al. Intramuscular injection of botulinum toxin for the treatment of wrist and finger spasticity after a stroke. N Engl J Med. 2002;347(6):395-400.
22. Jahangir AW, Tan HJ, Norlinah MI, Nafisah WY, Ramesh S, Hamidon BB, et al. Intramuscular injection of botulinum toxin for the treatment of wrist and finger spasticity after stroke. Med J Malaysia. 2007;62(4):319-22.
23. Elovic EP, Brashear A, Kaelin D, Liu J, Millis SR, Barron R, et al. Repeated treatments with botulinum toxin type a produce sustained decreases in the limitations associated with focal upper-limb poststroke spasticity for caregivers and patients. Arch Phys Med Rehabil. 2008;89(5):799-806.

24. Kaňovský P, Slawek J, Denes Z, Platz T, Comes G, Grafe S, et al. Efficacy and safety of treatment with incobotulinum toxin A (botulinum neurotoxin type A free from complexing proteins; NT 201) in post-stroke upper limb spasticity. J Rehabil Med. 2011;43(6):486-92.
25. Gracies JM, O'Dell M, Vecchio M, Hedera P, Kocer S, Rudzinska-Bar M, et al. Effects of repeated abobotulinumtoxinA injections in upper limb spasticity. Muscle Nerve. 2018;57(2):245-54.
26. Nalysnyk L, Papapetropoulos S, Rotella P, Simeone JC, Alter KE, Esquenazi A. OnabotulinumtoxinA muscle injection patterns in adult spasticity: a systematic literature review. BMC Neurol. 2013;13:118.
27. Martin A, Abogunrin S, Kurth H, Dinet J. Epidemiological, humanistic, and economic burden of illness of lower limb spasticity in adults: a systematic review. Neuropsychiatr Dis Treat. 2014;10(4):111-22.
28. Barnes M, Kocer S, Fernandez M, Balcaitiene J, Fheodoroff K. An international survey of patients living with spasticity. Disabil Rehabil. 2017;39(14):1428-34.
29. Burbaud P, Wiart L, Dubos JL, Gaujard E, Debelleix X, Joseph PA, et al. A randomised, double-blind, placebo-controlled trial of botulinum toxin in the treatment of spastic foot in hemiparetic patients. J Neurol Neurosurg Psychiatry. 1996;61(3):265-9.
30. Hesse S, Lücke D, Malezic M, Bertelt C, Friedrich H, Gregoric M, et al. Botulinum toxin treatment for lower limb extensor spasticity in chronic hemiparetic patients. J Neurol Neurosurg Psychiatry. 1994;57(11):1321-4.
31. Kirazli Y, On AY, Kismali B, Aksit R. Comparison of phenol block and botulinus toxin type A in the treatment of spastic foot after stroke: a randomized, double-blind trial. Am J Phys Med Rehabil. 1998;77(6):510-5.
32. Pittock SJ, Moore AP, Hardiman O, Ehler E, Kovac M, Bojakowski J, et al. A double-blind randomised placebo-controlled evaluation of three doses of botulinum toxin type A (Dysport) in the treatment of spastic equinovarus deformity after stroke. Cerebrovasc Dis. 2003;15(4):289-300.
33. Kaji R, Osako Y, Suyama K, Maeda T, Uechi Y, Iwasaki M, et al. Botulinum toxin type A in post-stroke lower limb spasticity: a multicenter, double-blind, placebo-controlled trial. J Neurol. 2010;257(8):1330-7.
34. Esquenazi A, Alfaro A, Ayyoub Z, Charles D, Dashtipour K, Graham GD, et al. OnabotulinumtoxinA for Lower Limb Spasticity: Guidance from a Delphi Panel Approach. PM R. 2017;9(10):960-8.
35. Graham HK, Rosenbaum P, Paneth N, Dan B, Lin JP, Damiano DL, et al. Cerebral palsy. Nat Rev Dis Primers. 2016;2:15082.
36. Sankar C, Mundkur N. Cerebral palsy-definition, classification, etiology and early diagnosis. Indian J Pediatr. 2005;72(10):865-8.
37. Molenaers G, Van Campenhout A, Fagard K, De Cat J, Desloovere K. The use of botulinum toxin A in children with cerebral palsy, with a focus on the lower limb. J Child Orthop. 2010;4(3):183-95.
38. Koman LA, Mooney JF, Smith B, Goodman A, Mulvaney T. Management of cerebral palsy with botulinum-A toxin: preliminary investigation. J Pediatr Orthop. 1993;13(4):489-95.
39. Wall SA, Chait LA, Temlett JA, Perkins B, Hillen G, Becker P. Botulinum A chemodenervation: a new modality in cerebral palsied hands. Br J Plast Surg. 1993;46(8):703-6.
40. Hoare BJ, Wallen MA, Imms C, Villanueva E, Rawicki HB, Carey L. Botulinum toxin A as an adjunct to treatment in the management of the upper limb in children with spastic cerebral palsy (UPDATE). Cochrane Database Syst Rev. 2010;1:CD003469.
41. Mathevon L, Bonan I, Barnais JL, Boyer F, Dinomais M. Adjunct therapies to improve outcomes after botulinum toxin injection in children: a systematic review. Ann Phys Rehabil Med. 2019;62(4):283-90.
42. Kanovský P, Bares M, Severa S, Richardson A, Dysport Paediatric Limb Spasticity Study Group. Long-term efficacy and tolerability of 4-monthly versus yearly botulinum toxin type A treatment for lower-limb spasticity in children with cerebral palsy. Dev Med Child Neurol. 2009;51(6):436-45.
43. Park ES, Rha DW, Yoo JK, Kim SM, Chang WH, Song SH. Short-term effects of combined serial casting and botulinum toxin injection for spastic equinus in ambulatory children with cerebral palsy. Yonsei Med J. 2010;51(4):579-84.
44. van Schie PEM, Schothorst M, Dallmeijer AJ, Vermeulen RJ, van Ouwerkerk WJR, Strijers RLM, et al. Short- and long-term effects of selective dorsal rhizotomy on gross motor function in ambulatory children with spastic diplegia. J Neurosurg Pediatr. 2011;7(5):557-62.
45. Park ES, Rha DW. Botulinum toxin type A injection for management of upper limb spasticity in children with cerebral palsy: a literature review. Yonsei Med J. 2006;47(5):589-603.
46. Fung S, Phadke CP, Kam A, Ismail F, Boulias C. Effect of topical anesthetics on needle insertion pain during botulinum toxin type A injections for limb spasticity. Arch Phys Med Rehabil. 2012;93(9):1643-7.
47. Forrester M, Srinivasan J, Mihrshahi S, Waugh M, O'Flaherty S, Rice J, et al. Conscious sedation or general anaesthetic for intramuscular botulinum toxin injections in children—a two centre cross-sectional prospective audit. Eur J Paediatr Neurol. 2012;16(2):215-7.
48. Monnier G, Parratte B, Tatu L, Cosson A, Michel F, Metton G. EMG support in botulinum toxin treatment. Ann Readapt Med Phys. 2003;46(6):380-5.
49. Ward A, Roberts G, Warner J, Gillard S. Cost-effectiveness of botulinum toxin type a in the treatment of post-stroke spasticity. J Rehabil Med. 2005;37(4):252-7.
50. Panicker JN, Muthane UB. Botulinum toxins: pharmacology and its current therapeutic evidence for use. Neurol India. 2003;51(4):455-60.

Index

Page numbers followed by *b* refer to box, *f* refer to figure, *fc* refer to flowchart, and *t* refer to table.

B

C

D

E

I

J

K

L

Q

R

S